中英双语

Essential Obstetrics and Gynaecology

妇 产 科 学

·原书第 6 版·

原 著　[澳] Ian Symonds

　　　　[英] Sabaratnam Arulkumaran

主 译　陈子江　石玉华　杨慧霞

中国科学技术出版社

·北 京·

图书在版编目（CIP）数据

妇产科学：原书第 6 版：中英双语 / (澳) 伊恩·西蒙兹 (Ian Symonds), (英) 萨巴拉特南·阿鲁库马兰 (Sabaratnam Arulkumaran) 原著；陈子江，石玉华，杨慧霞主译 . — 北京：中国科学技术出版社，2023.3

书名原文：Essential Obstetrics and Gynaecology，6E

ISBN 978-7-5046-9892-6

Ⅰ . ①妇⋯ Ⅱ . ①伊⋯ ②萨⋯ ③陈⋯ ④石⋯ ⑤杨⋯ Ⅲ . ①妇产科学—汉、英 Ⅳ . ① R71

中国国家版本馆 CIP 数据核字 (2023) 第 011906 号

著作权合同登记号：01-2023-0387

策划编辑	靳　婷　焦健姿	
责任编辑	靳　婷	
文字编辑	弥子雯	
装帧设计	佳木水轩	
责任印制	徐　飞	

出　　版	中国科学技术出版社
发　　行	中国科学技术出版社有限公司发行部
地　　址	北京市海淀区中关村南大街 16 号
邮　　编	100081
发行电话	010-62173865
传　　真	010-62179148
网　　址	http://www.cspbooks.com.cn

开　　本	889mm×1194mm　1/16
字　　数	1567 千字
印　　张	45
版　　次	2023 年 3 月第 1 版
印　　次	2023 年 3 月第 1 次印刷
印　　刷	北京盛通印刷股份有限公司
书　　号	ISBN 978-7-5046-9892-6 / R·2971
定　　价	458.00 元

Elsevier (Singapore) Pte Ltd.
3 Killiney Road, #08–01 Winsland House Ⅰ, Singapore 239519
Tel: (65) 6349–0200; Fax: (65) 6733–1817

注　意

本译本由中国科学技术出版社完成。相关从业及研究人员必须凭借其自身经验和知识对文中描述的信息数据、方法策略、搭配组合、实验操作进行评估和使用。由于医学科学发展迅速，临床诊断和给药剂量尤其需要经过独立验证。在法律允许的最大范围内，爱思唯尔、译文的原文作者、原文编辑及原文内容提供者均不对译文或因产品责任、疏忽或其他操作造成的人身及（或）财产伤害及（或）损失承担责任，亦不对由于使用文中提到的方法、产品、说明或思想而导致的人身及（或）财产伤害及（或）损失承担责任。

译校者名单

主　　译　陈子江　石玉华　杨慧霞

译 校 者　（以姓氏汉语拼音为序）

陈子江　山东大学附属生殖医院

崔琳琳　山东大学附属生殖医院

高姗姗　山东大学第二医院

管一春　郑州大学第三附属医院

郭　婷　山东大学附属生殖医院

黄　薇　四川大学华西第二医院 / 华西妇产儿童医院

刘见桥　广州医科大学附属第三医院

刘培昊　山东大学附属生殖医院

吕　鸿　山东大学附属生殖医院

孟金来　山东第一医科大学附属省立医院

阮祥燕　首都医科大学附属北京妇产医院

石玉华　广东省人民医院

宋晓翠　山东大学第二医院

谭季春　中国医科大学附属盛京医院

王　珊　山东第一医科大学附属省立医院

颜　磊　山东大学附属生殖医院

杨　欣　北京大学人民医院

杨慧霞　北京大学第一医院

杨一华　广西医科大学第一附属医院

学术秘书　王秋敏　山东大学附属生殖医院

潘　烨　首都医科大学附属北京朝阳医院

内容提要

　　本书引进自 Elsevier 出版社，由澳大利亚产科专家 Ian Symonds 和英国产科专家 Sabaratnam Arulkumaran 共同编写。本书为全新第 6 版，是教科书级别的妇产科著作，包括基础生殖科学、产科学和妇科学三篇，共 21 章，主要阐述了女性骨盆解剖，妊娠期的生理变化，胚胎及胎儿生长发育，围产期孕产妇死亡率，妇科、产科疾病，母体医学，先天性异常与胎儿健康评估，正常妊娠、早孕、产前、产后和新生儿护理，妇科肿瘤，泌尿道脱垂和疾病等主题。为了便于阅读，本书在每章的结尾均总结了要点，既包括了基础知识阐释又涵盖了临床常见问题。本书为中英双语版，临床场景、要点、图表等内容丰富，可作为妇产科专业研究生及住院医师的案头参考书。

原书编著者名单

原著

Ian Symonds

MB BS MMedSci DM FRCOG FRANZCOG

Dean of Medicine-University of Adelaide;

Head of School, Adelaide Medical School;

Visiting Medical Specialist in Obstetrics,

Women's and Children's Hospital,

Adelaide, South Australia

Sir Sabaratnam Arulkumaran

PhD DSc FRCSE FRCOG FRANZCOG(Hon)

Professor Emeritus,

Division of Obstetrics and Gynaecology,

St George's University of London,

London, UK

参编者

Petra Agoston MD
Clinical Fellow in Obstetrics and Gynaecology
St George's University Hospitals NHS Foundation Trust
London, UK

**Sir Sabaratnam Arulkumaran PhD DSc FRCSE FRCOG
   FRANZCOG(Hon)**
Professor Emeritus
Division of Obstetrics and Gynaecology
St George's University of London
London, UK

Shankari Arulkumaran BSc MSc MRCOG MD
Consultant Obstetrician and Gynaecologist
St Mary's Hospital, Imperial College Healthcare NHS Trust
London, UK

Jo Black MB BS MRCPsych
Consultant Perinatal Psychiatrist
Devon Partnership NHS Trust
Exeter, Devon, UK
Associate National Clinical Director for Perinatal Mental
   Health
NHS England

Fiona Broughton Pipkin MA DPhil FRCOG ad *eundem*
Emeritus Professor of Perinatal Physiology
School of Medicine

University of Nottingham
Nottingham, UK

**Karen K.L. Chan MBBChir FRCOG FHKCOG FHKAM
   (O&G) Cert RCOG (Gyn Onc)**
Clinical Associate Professor
Department of Obstetrics and Gynaecology
The University of Hong Kong
Hong Kong, China

**Edwin Chandraharan MBBS MS(Obs & Gyn) DFFP
   DCRM FSLCOG FRCOG**
Lead Consultant, Labour Ward
Consultant Obstetrician and Gynaecologist
St George's University Hospitals NHS Foundation Trust
London, UK

Caroline de Costa AM PhD MPH FRANZCOG FRCOG
Professor of Obstetrics and Gynaecology
James Cook University College of Medicine and Dentistry
Cairns, Queensland, Australia

Stergios K. Doumouchtsis MSc MPH PhD MRCOG
Consultant Obstetrician, Gynaecologist, and Urogynaecologist
Epsom and St Helier University Hospitals NHS Trust
Epsom, Surrey
Honorary Senior Lecturer
St George's University of London

London, UK,

Visiting Professor, University of Athens

Athens, Greece

**Paul Duggan MBChB DipObst MMedSc MD GradCertEd
FRANZCOG**

Associate Professor of Obstetrics and Gynaecology

University of Adelaide

Adelaide, South Australia, Australia

Eloïse Fraison MD

Specialist Registrar in Obstetrics, Gynaecology and
Reproductive Medicine

University of Montpellier

Montpellier, France;

Associate Lecturer

Department of Reproductive Medicine

University of New South Wales

Sydney, New South Wales, Australia

Ian S. Fraser AO DSc MD

Conjoint Professor in Reproductive Medicine

School of Women's and Children's Health,

University of New South Wales

Royal Hospital for Women,

Sydney, New South Wales, Australia

Kevin Hayes MBBS FRCOG

Consultant in Obstetrics and Gynaecology

Reader in Medical Education

St George's University of London

London, UK

**Shaylee Iles BA BSc(Med) MBBS(Hons) UNSW
GradCertClinEd(Flinders) FRANZCOG**

Staff Specialist in Obstetrics and Gynaecology

John Hunter Hospital

Newcastle, New South Wales

Conjoint Lecturer in Obstetrics and Gynaecology

University of Newcastle Australia

Consultant Gynaecologist

Newcastle Gynaecology

Newcastle, New South Wales, Australia

Adonis S. Ioannides MBChB(Hons) PhD FRCSEd

Associate Professor of Clinical Genetics

University of Nicosia Medical School

Nicosia, Cyprus

Jay Iyer MBBS MD DNB MRCOG FRANZCOG

Consultant Obstetrician and Gynaecologist

Townsville and Mater Hospitals

Townsville, Queensland

Adjunct Senior Lecturer, James Cook University

Townsville, Queensland, Australia

David James MA MD FRCOG DCH

Emeritus Professor of Fetomaternal Medicine

University of Nottingham

Nottingham, UK

**Mugdha Kulkarni MBBS DRANZCOG RANZCOG
Trainee**

Urogynaecology Fellow

RANZCOG Trainee

Australia

**William Ledger MA DPhil(Oxon) MB ChB FRCOG
FRANZCOG CREI**

Head and Professor of Obstetrics and Gynaecology

School of Women's and Children's Health

University of New South Wales

Sydney, New South Wales, Australia

Boon H. Lim MBBS FRCOG FRANZCOG

Associate Professor and Senior Staff Specialist

Department of Obstetrics and Gynaecology

Clinical Director

Division of Women, Youth and Children

Canberra Hospital and Health Services

Australian National University

Canberra, Australian Capital Territory, Australia

**Tahir Mahmood CBE MD MBA FRCPE FACOG(Hon)
FEBCOG FRCOG**

Consultant Obstetrician and Gynaecologist

Victoria Hospital

Kirkcaldy, Fife, UK
Senior Lecturer, University of St Andrews
St Andrews, UK

Sambit Mukhopadhyay MD DNB MMedSci FRCOG
Consultant Gynaecologist and Honorary Senior Lecturer
Norwich Medical School
Norfolk and Norwich University Hospitals NHS Foundation
   Trust
Norwich, UK

**Henry G. Murray MB ChB(Hons) DipObstets BMedSci
   DM DDU MRCOG FRANZCOG DDU CMFM**
Clinical Lead and Senior Staff Specialist
Maternity and Gynaecology
John Hunter Hospital
Newcastle, New South Wales, Australia

**Hextan Y.S. Ngan MBBS MD FRCOG FHKCOG
   FHKAM(O&G) CertRCOG(GynOnc)**
Tsao Yin-Kai Professor in Obstetrics and Gynaecology
Chair and Head
Department of Obstetrics and Gynaecology
The University of Hong Kong
Hong Kong, China

**Roger Pepperell MD MGO FRACP FRCOG FRANZCOG
   FACOG(Hon)**
Professor Emeritus in Obstetrics and Gynaecology

University of Melbourne
Melbourne, Victoria, Australia
Retired Professor of Obstetrics and Gynaecology
Penang Medical College
Malaysia

**Ajay Rane OAM MBBS MSc MD PhD FRCS FRCOG
   FRANZCOG CU GAICD**
Professor and Head
Obstetrics and Gynaecology
Consultant Urogynaecologist
James Cook University
Townsville, Queensland, Australia

Ian Symonds MB BS MMedSci DM FRCOG FRANZCOG
Dean of Medicine
University of Adelaide
Head of School
Adelaide Medical School
Visiting Medical Specialist in Obstetrics
Women's and Children's Hospital
Adelaide, South Australia, Australia

Suzanne V.F. Wallace MA BM BCh FRCOG
Consultant Obstetrician
Nottingham University Hospitals NHS Trust
Nottingham, UK

译者前言

由 Ian Symonds 和 Sabaratnam Arulkumaran 联合编写的 *Essential Obstetrics and Gynaecology, 6E* 一书的中英双语版就要与广大同道见面了。本书引进自 Elsevier 出版集团，由国际知名妇产科专家共同编写，是一部国际权威妇产科学经典教科书。该书始于名誉教授 Malcolm Symonds，于 1987 年第一次出版，30 余年来经久不衰，愈增光彩。

本书分为三部分，其中包括生殖医学、产科学和妇科学。新近出版的第 6 版内容更加丰富充实，不仅在各章的内容上进行了更新，涵盖了妇产科学相关研究及最新进展，而且在第 5 版的基础上新增了客观结构化临床技能考核 (OSCE) 站点、自我评估和拓展阅读等内容，更贴近现今医学生的教育模式。本书条理清晰，重点突出，图文并茂，更有学习目标和案例研究，便于读者深入理解和掌握。

作为 *Essential Obstetrics and Gynaecology* 的忠实读者和译者，我们深深体会到全新第 6 版不仅继承了这部经典巨著的精华，而且充分体现了妇产科学及相关学科近几年来的理念更新及技术进步。

本书译者均为具有多年妇产科临床、教学和科研经验的教授、副教授。感谢各位译者在百忙之中按期完成了各自的翻译任务，几经修订才使得本书呈现在读者面前。翻译整理过程中，我们反复推敲斟酌，力求忠于原著，但由于中外术语规范及语言表达习惯有所差异，中文翻译版中可能存在不当之处，恳请广大同行和读者不吝批评指正。

非常感谢原著者编写了如此精彩的著作。衷心感谢出版社对我们的信任和支持。再次感谢所有译者的辛勤付出。希望本书可以为妇产科学相关工作者和医学生提供帮助和启迪，共同促进我国妇产科学的长足发展。

中国科学院院士　陈子江

广东省人民医院　石玉华

北京大学第一医院　杨慧霞

原书前言

本书是 *Essential Obstetrics and Gynaecology* 的第 6 版，距第 1 版出版已有 30 多年。

在过去的 20 年里，对人类生殖的科学理解和临床实践都发生了重大变化。尽管有些方面保持不变，但由于其发展速度之快，我们还是决定邀请妇产科不同领域的专家进行修订再版。除了内容的全面更新，在这一版的自我评估部分还包括了客观结构化临床技能考核（OSCE）站点，它是一种常见的本科生自我评估方式。我们保留了产科和妇科基础生殖科学的普遍整体划分结构，并继续采用第 5 版定义学习成果与 RCOG 国家本科课程一致的格式。拓展阅读部分提供了关键文章和指南的信息，以使读者对主题有更深入的了解。

我们要感谢所有作者的贡献，尤其是 Jo Black 博士，他撰写了有关分娩的精神疾病一章，并从我们的长期撰稿人 Margaret Oates 博士那里更新了这一章。

我们还要感谢 Neville Fields 博士从一名见习医务官的角度对妇科一章所做的评论，感谢 Paul Duggan 副教授对这部分内容的评议。在进行修订的过程中，我们还征询了医学生和初级医务人员的意见，我们要感谢所有参与这次同行评审过程的学生。希望读者就遗漏和争议给我们写信，以便我们可以随时订正。

Ian Symonds
Sabaratnam Arulkumaran

致 谢

编辑们对所有为本教科书的先前版本做出贡献的学者表示感谢；如果没有他们，这个新版本是不可能出现的。我们特别感谢以下为第 5 版做过贡献后不再参加编写的人员。

Kirsten Black

Paddy Moore

Margaret R. Oates

E. Malcolm Symonds

The late Aldo Vacca

我们还要感谢所有在先前的版本中为自我评估问题做出贡献的人。

这是名誉教授 Malcolm Symonds 最初于 1987 年出版的教科书的第 6 版。他的愿景是对女性健康的临床和科学方面进行简要的总结，并且同样适用于医学生、助产士和初级实习生，这确保了这本书的畅销。编辑们想要感谢他 30 多年来对本刊物的核心贡献，以及他作为包括我们在内的许多人的指导者和老师的角色。

献 词

谨以本书献给我们的家庭。

目　录

附录部分

第一篇 生殖科学基础
Essential reproductive science

第1章 女性骨盆解剖
Anatomy of the female pelvis

Caroline de Costa 著 刘培昊 译 石玉华 校

学习目标	LEARNING OUTCOMES
学习本章后你应当能够： **知识标准** • 描述骨性骨盆、外生殖器与内生殖器的解剖结构 • 描述外生殖器与内生殖器的血管、淋巴及神经分布 • 描述盆底与会阴	After studying this chapter you should be able to: **Knowledge criteria** • Describe the anatomy of the bony pelvis, external genitalia and internal genital organs • Describe the blood, lymphatic and nerve supply to the external and internal genital organs • Describe the pelvic floor and the perineum

女性骨盆主要特征的相关知识对于理解生殖与分娩至关重要，对理解各病理过程对盆腔器官及女性健康可能产生的影响也至关重要。

Knowledge of the major features of the female pelvis is essential to the understanding of the processes of reproduction and childbearing and to the effect that various pathological processes may have on the pelvic organs and on the health of the woman.

生殖器官的结构与功能随着个体年龄和激素状态的不同而有很大差异，第 16 章中将会介绍青春期和更年期发生的改变。本章旨在概述女性尤其是性成熟女性的骨盆主要结构。

The structure and function of the genital organs vary considerably with the age of the individual and her hormonal status, as will be apparent in Chapter 16, which covers the changes that take place in puberty and menopause. This chapter aims to outline the major structures comprising the female pelvis, predominantly in the sexually mature female.

一、骨性骨盆 (The bony pelvis)

骨性骨盆包括 1 对髋骨（每块髋骨由髂骨、坐骨和耻骨组成）、骶骨和尾骨（图 1-1）。

The bony pelvis consists of the paired innominate bones (each consisting of an ilium, ischium and pubis) and the sacrum and coccyx (Fig. 1.1).

髋骨前方连接于耻骨联合，后方通过骶髂关节与骶骨相连。这三个关节在未妊娠状态下都是固定的，但孕期出现松动，从而在产程和分娩中有一定的活动性。骶骨向上与第 5 腰椎相连，向下与尾骨相连。

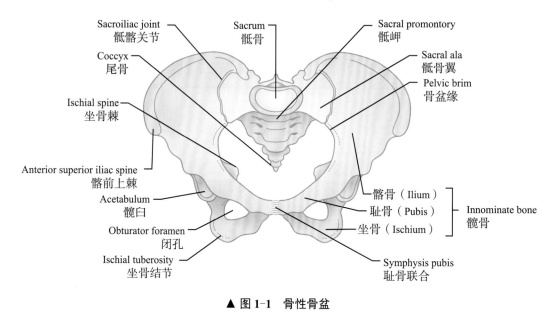

▲ 图 1-1　骨性骨盆

Fig. 1.1　Bony pelvis

The innominate bones are joined anteriorly at the symphysis pubis, and each articulates posteriorly with the sacrum in the sacroiliac joints. All three joints are fixed in the non-pregnant state, but during pregnancy there is a relaxation of the joints to allow some mobility during labour and birth. The sacrum articulates with the fifth lumbar vertebra superiorly and the coccyx inferiorly.

骨性骨盆以骨盆缘为界，分为假骨盆和真骨盆。真骨盆分为三部分：骨盆入口（前方为耻骨上表面，后方为骶骨岬和骶骨翼）、中骨盆（在坐骨棘水平处）和骨盆出口（前方为耻骨联合下缘，侧方为坐骨结节，后方为骶骨尖）。

The bony pelvis is divided into the false pelvis and the true pelvis by the pelvic brim. The true pelvis is divided into three sections: the pelvic inlet (bounded anteriorly by the superior surface of the pubic bones and posteriorly by the promontory and alae of the sacrum); the mid-pelvis (at the level of the ischial spines); and the pelvic outlet (bounded anteriorly by the lower border of the symphysis, laterally by the ischial tuberosities and posteriorly by the tip of the sacrum).

> **！注意**
>
> 坐骨棘在进行阴道检查时易被触及，为产程中评估胎头下降程度提供了参考点。
>
> The ischial spines are easily palpable on vaginal examination during labour and provide the reference point for assessing the descent of the fetal head during labour and birth.

二、外生殖器（The external genitalia）

外阴一词通常指女性外生殖器，包括阴阜、大阴唇、小阴唇、阴蒂、尿道外口、阴道前庭、阴道口和处女膜（图 1–2）。

The term *vulva* is generally used to describe the female external genitalia and includes the mons pubis, the labia majora, the labia minora, the clitoris, the external urinary meatus, the vestibule of the vagina, the vaginal orifice and the hymen (Fig. 1.2).

阴阜由位于耻骨联合上方的纤维脂肪垫组成，在成熟女性中被浓密的阴毛覆盖。阴毛上缘常为直线或向上凸起，这与正常男性分布不同。阴毛通常11—12 岁开始出现。

The mons pubis, sometimes known as the *mons veneris*, is composed of a fibrofatty pad of tissue that lies above the pubic symphysis and, in the mature female, is covered with dense pubic hair. The upper border of this hair is usually straight or convex upwards and differs from the normal male distribution. Pubic hair generally begins to appear between the ages of 11 and 12 years.

大阴唇为 2 条向下、向后延伸的纵向皮肤褶皱，前方起于阴阜，向后延至会阴。阴唇的组成包括被阴毛与汗腺覆盖的外层和含有毛囊皮脂腺的内光滑层。大阴唇包裹尿道口和阴道口所在的外阴裂。

The labia majora consist of two longitudinal cutaneous folds that extend downwards and posteriorly from the mons pubis anteriorly to the perineum posteriorly. The labia are

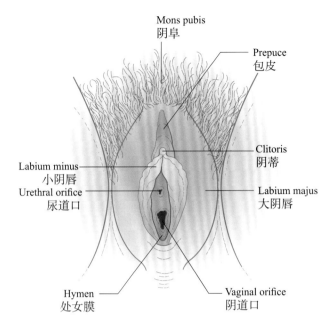

Mons pubis
阴阜

Prepuce
包皮

Clitoris
阴蒂

Labium minus
小阴唇

Urethral orifice
尿道口

Labium majus
大阴唇

Hymen
处女膜

Vaginal orifice
阴道口

▲ 图 1-2　女性外生殖器

Fig. 1.2　**External genital organs of the female**

composed of an outer surface covered by hair and sweat glands and an inner smooth layer containing sebaceous follicles. The labia majora enclose the pudendal cleft into which the urethra and vagina open.

阴唇在阴道口后方合并形成后联合，它与肛门前缘之间的区域构成产科会阴。

Posterior to the vaginal orifice, the labia merge to form the posterior commissure, and the area between this structure and the anterior verge of the anus constitutes the obstetric perineum.

大阴唇与男性阴囊同源。

The labia majora are homologous with the male scrotum.

小阴唇是被大阴唇包绕的皮肤褶皱，前方包裹阴蒂，后方在阴道口后融合形成阴唇系带，即阴道口的后缘。在前方，小阴唇分开包绕阴蒂，前褶皱形成阴蒂包皮，后褶皱形成阴蒂系带。它们富含血管与神经，可勃起。不被毛，但富含皮脂腺。

The labia minora are enclosed by the labia majora and are cutaneous folds that enclose the clitoris anteriorly and fuse posteriorly behind the vaginal orifice to form the posterior fourchette or posterior margin of the vaginal introitus. Anteriorly, the labia minora divide to enclose the clitoris, with the anterior fold forming the prepuce and the posterior fold the frenulum. They are richly vascularized and innervated and are erectile. They do not contain hair but are rich in sebaceous glands.

阴蒂是阴茎的女性同源物，位于小阴唇前缘。阴蒂体含 2 条勃起性组织海绵体，包裹在纤维鞘内。

2 条海绵体在后方分开，附着于耻骨下支。阴蒂的游离端含阴蒂头，阴蒂头由可勃起组织组成，覆盖皮肤，富含感觉神经末梢，因此非常敏感。阴蒂在性刺激和性功能中具有重要作用。

The clitoris is the female homologue of the penis and is situated between the anterior ends of the labia minora. The body of the clitoris consists of two corpora cavernosa of erectile tissue enclosed in a fibrous sheath. Posteriorly, these two corpora divide to lie along the inferior rami of the pubic bones. The free end of the clitoris contains the glans, composed of erectile tissue covered by skin and richly supplied with sensory nerve endings and hence is very sensitive. The clitoris plays an important role in sexual stimulation and function.

阴道前庭是位于小阴唇之间的浅凹。尿道外口位于前庭前方，阴道口位于后方。2 个 Bartholin 腺的腺管开口于阴道前庭，位于阴道口后缘，这些腺体的分泌物在性交中有重要的润滑作用。

The vestibule consists of a shallow depression lying between the labia minora. The external urethral orifice opens into the vestibule anteriorly and the vaginal orifice posteriorly. The ducts from the two Bartholin's glands drain into the vestibule at the posterior margin of the vaginal introitus, and the secretions from these glands have an important lubricating role during sexual intercourse.

Skene 腺管在尿道下 1cm 处与其并行，也开口于阴道前庭。尽管它们有一定的润滑作用，但与 Bartholin 腺相比作用微弱。

Skene's ducts lie alongside the lower 1 cm of the urethra and also drain into the vestibule. Although they have some lubricating function, it is minor compared to the function of Bartholin's glands.

前庭球由 2 个可勃起体组成，位于阴道口两侧，与尿生殖膈表面相接。前庭球由一薄层球海绵体肌覆盖。

The bulb of the vestibule consists of two erectile bodies that lie on either side of the vaginal orifice and are in contact with the surface of the urogenital diaphragm. The bulb of the vestibule is covered by a thin layer of muscle known as the *bulbocavernosus muscle*.

尿道外口位于阴蒂基底部下方 1.5～2cm 处，通常被小阴唇覆盖，也起着引导尿流的作用。除了 Skene 腺管，也常存在一些无腺管的尿道旁腺，有时它们是形成尿道旁囊肿的基础。

The external urethral orifice lies 1.5–2 cm below the base of the clitoris and is often covered by the labia minora, which also function to direct the urinary stream. In addition to Skene's ducts, there are often a number of paraurethral glands without associated ducts, and these sometimes form the basis of paraurethral cysts.

阴道口位于阴道前庭下部，在有性行为前，被处女膜部分覆盖。处女膜是附着在阴道口周围的一层薄膜。处女膜孔和处女膜多种多样。一旦处女膜被穿透，残留物表现为处女膜痕，即阴道口边缘的纤维皮赘结节。

The vaginal orifice opens into the lower part of the vestibule and, prior to the onset of sexual activity, is partly covered by the hymenal membrane. The hymen is a thin fold of skin attached around the circumference of the vaginal orifice. There are various types of openings within the hymen, and the membrane varies in consistency. Once the hymen has been penetrated, the remnants are represented by the *carunculae myrtiformes*, which are nodules of fibrocutaneous material at the edge of the vaginal introitus.

Bartholin 腺是 1 对总状腺体，位于阴道口两侧，直径 0.5～1.0cm。腺管长约 2cm，开口于小阴唇与阴道口间。其功能为在性唤起时分泌黏液。

Bartholin's glands are a pair of racemose glands located at either side of the vaginal introitus and measuring 0.5–1.0 cm in diameter. The ducts are approximately 2 cm in length and open between the labia minora and the vaginal orifice. Their function is to secrete mucus during sexual arousal.

> **！注意** 囊肿形成（Bartholin 囊肿）相对常见，这是腺管阻塞的结果，液体于腺管而非腺体中堆积。
>
> Cyst formation (Bartholin's cysts) is relatively common but is the result of occlusion of the duct, with fluid accumulation in the duct and not in the gland.

严格来说 Bartholin 腺并不在外阴描述的范围内，与产科功能相关的会阴前起阴唇系带，后至肛门，位于会阴体上方，占据肛管和阴道后壁下 1/3 之间的区域。

Although it does not strictly lie within the description of the vulva, the perineum as described in relation to obstetric function is defined as the area that lies between the posterior fourchette anteriorly and the anus posteriorly; it lies over the perineal body, which occupies the area between the anal canal and the lower one-third of the posterior vaginal wall.

三、内生殖器（The internal genital organs）

内生殖器包括阴道、子宫、输卵管和卵巢。这些器官位于盆腔内，向前紧邻尿道、膀胱，向后紧邻直肠、肛管和盆腔结肠（图 1-3）。

The internal genitalia include the vagina, the uterus, the Fallopian tubes and the ovaries. Situated in the pelvic cavity, these structures lie in close proximity to the urethra and urinary bladder anteriorly and the rectum, anal canal and pelvic colon posteriorly (Fig. 1.3).

（一）阴道（The vagina）

阴道是肌性管道，在成熟女性中长 6～7.5cm。它被覆非角化鳞状上皮，穹隆处比阴道口更宽敞。阴道的横断面呈 H 形，延展性极强，尤其是在分娩过程中作为适应容纳胎头的通道时。阴道前方紧邻膀胱三角和尿道。在后方，阴道下段和肛管被会阴体分隔。阴道中 1/3 与直肠壶腹相邻，上段被阴道直肠窝（Douglas 窝）的腹膜覆盖。

The vagina is a muscular tube some 6–7.5 cm long in the mature female. It is lined by non-cornified squamous epithelium and is more capacious at the vault than at the introitus. In cross-section, the vagina is H shaped and is capable of considerable distension, particularly during parturition when it adapts to accommodate the passage of the fetal head. Anteriorly, it is intimately related to the trigone of the urinary bladder and the urethra. Posteriorly, the lower part of the vagina is separated from the anal canal by the perineal body. In the middle third, it lies in apposition to the ampulla of the rectum, and in the upper segment it is covered by the peritoneum of the rectovaginal pouch (pouch of Douglas).

子宫颈凸入阴道穹隆。阴道穹隆分为 4 个区域，

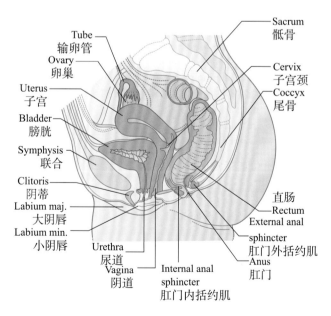

▲ 图 1-3 女性骨盆矢状面示盆腔器官与周围结构关系

Fig. 1.3 **Sagittal section of the female pelvis showing the relationship of the pelvic organs with surrounding structures**

即前穹隆、后穹窿和两个侧穹隆。侧穹隆位于阔韧带基底下，紧邻子宫动脉穿过输尿管的位置。

The uterine cervix protrudes into the vaginal vault. Four zones are described in the vaginal vault: the anterior fornix, the posterior fornix, and the two lateral fornices. The lateral fornices lie under the base of the broad ligament in close proximity to the point where the uterine artery crosses the ureter.

未妊娠的性成熟女性阴道的 pH 在 4.0～5.0，有重要的抗菌作用，可降低盆腔感染发生风险。阴道的功能是性交、分娩和月经血排出。

The pH of the vagina in the sexually mature non-pregnant female is between 4.0 and 5.0. This has an important antibacterial function that reduces the risk of pelvic infection. The functions of the vagina are copulation, parturition and the drainage of menstrual loss.

（二）子宫（The uterus）

子宫是一个中空、肌性、梨形的器官，位于盆腔内，前邻膀胱，后邻直肠和 Douglas 窝。子宫大小取决于女性的激素状态。性成熟女性的子宫长约 7.5cm，最宽处约 5cm。子宫一般处于前倾位，子宫底位置比子宫颈靠前。约 10% 的女性子宫后倾，位于 Douglas 窝内。子宫也可能沿其长轴方向弯曲，向前即前屈，向后即后屈。

The uterus is a hollow, muscular, pear-shaped organ situated in the pelvic cavity between the bladder anteriorly and the rectum and pouch of Douglas posteriorly. The size of the uterus depends on the hormonal status of the female. In the sexually mature female, the uterus is approximately 7.5 cm long and 5 cm across at its widest point. The uterus normally lies in a position of *anteversion* such that the uterine fundus is anterior to the uterine cervix. In about 10% of women, the uterus lies in a position of *retroversion* in the pouch of Douglas. The uterus may also be curved anteriorly in its longitudinal axis, a feature that is described as *anteflexion*, or posteriorly, when it is described as *retroflexion*.

子宫包括子宫体、子宫峡部和子宫颈。

It consists of a body or corpus, an isthmus and a cervi

子宫体由大量平滑肌细胞组成，即肌层，分三层排列。外层平滑肌细胞横穿子宫底进入子宫角，在此处肌纤维合并入输卵管、卵巢和圆韧带的平滑肌外层。中层肌纤维呈环形排列，内层包括纵行、环行和斜行的肌纤维。

The corpus uteri consists of a mass of smooth muscle cells, the *myometrium*, arranged in three layers. The external layers contain smooth muscle cells that pass transversely across

the uterine fundus into the lateral angles of the uterus, where their fibres merge with the outer layers of the smooth muscle of the Fallopian tubes and the ovarian and round ligaments. The muscle fibres in the middle layer are arranged in a circular manner, and the inner layer contains a mixture of longitudinal, circular and oblique muscle fibres.

子宫腔为三角形，前后扁平，因此未妊娠状态下的子宫腔体积约为 2ml。子宫腔被覆子宫内膜，子宫内膜表面为分泌黏液的柱状上皮。子宫内膜的性质取决于月经周期的阶段。月经结束后，增生期内膜仅厚 1～2mm。至月经周期的后半段（分泌期），子宫内膜厚度增长至 1cm。

The cavity of the uterus is triangular in shape and is flattened anteroposteriorly so that the total volume of the cavity in the non-pregnant state is approximately 2 mL. It is lined by endometrium that consists on the surface of mucus-secreting columnar epithelium. The nature of the endometrium depends on the phase of the menstrual cycle. Following menstruation, the endometrium in the proliferative phase is only 1–2 mm thick. By the second half (secretory phase) of the cycle, the endometrium has grown to a thickness of up to 1cm.

子宫内膜腔向下通过子宫颈管与阴道相连，向上通过输卵管与腹膜腔相连。

The endometrial cavity is in contact with the vaginal cavity inferiorly via the cervical canal and superiorly with the peritoneal cavity through the Fallopian tubes.

子宫颈为桶状结构，开口于伸入阴道的宫颈阴道部顶端的子宫颈外口，止于阴道上部的子宫颈内口。子宫颈内口经子宫峡部开口于子宫腔。未经产女性的子宫颈外口为圆形或椭圆形，但是经阴道分娩后变为横向的，这可在临床检查置入窥器时观察到，如取子宫颈样本时。

The cervix is a barrel-shaped structure extending from the external cervical os, which opens into the vagina at the apex of the vaginal portion of the cervix, to the internal cervical os in its supravaginal portion. The internal os opens into the uterine cavity through the isthmus of the uterus. In non-parous women the external os is round or oval, but it becomes transverse following vaginal birth, and this can be noted in clinical examination when a speculum is passed-for example, when taking cervical specimens.

子宫颈管为梭形，被覆分泌黏液的纤毛柱状上皮。柱状上皮和宫颈阴道部的复层鳞状上皮的过渡区形成鳞柱交界。交界的具体部位与女性的激素状态相关。一些子宫颈内衬的腺体分支广泛、分泌黏液。这些腺体的开口阻塞会形成小囊肿，称为 Nabothian 滤泡。

The cervical canal is fusiform in shape and is lined by ciliated columnar epithelium that is mucus secreting. The transition between this epithelium and the stratified squamous epithelium of the vaginal ectocervix forms the squamocolumnar junction. The exact site of this junction is related to the hormonal status of the woman. Some of the cervical glands in the endocervical lining are extensively branched and mucus secreting. If the opening to these glands becomes obstructed, small cysts may form, known as *nabothian follicles*.

子宫颈由平滑肌细胞和纤维组织的环状束组成。外纵行层与阴道肌层融合。

The cervix consists of layers of circular bundles of smooth muscle cells and fibrous tissue. The outer longitudinal layer merges with the muscle layer of the vagina.

子宫峡部连接子宫颈与子宫体，在未妊娠子宫中为长度 2～3mm 的狭长模糊区域。妊娠时，它扩大并参与形成子宫下段，子宫下段是剖宫产术切口的常规部位。分娩时，它成为产道的一部分，但对胎儿娩出无明显助力。

The isthmus of the uterus joins the cervix to the corpus uteri and in the non-pregnant uterus is a narrow, rather poorly defined area some 2–3 mm in length. In pregnancy, it enlarges and contributes to the formation of the lower segment of the uterus, which is the normal site for the incision of caesarean section. In labour it becomes a part of the birth canal but does not contribute significantly to the expulsion of the fetus.

（三）子宫的支持和韧带（Supports and ligaments of the uterus）

子宫和盆腔器官被大量强度不同、重要性不同的韧带与筋膜支撑。盆腔器官同样依赖于盆底的完整性来支撑。人类女性的一个特点是采取直立姿势后，盆底需承担脏器和盆腔器官向下的压力。

The uterus and the pelvic organs are supported by a number of ligaments and fascial thickenings of varying strength and importance. The pelvic organs also depend for support on the integrity of the pelvic floor: a particular feature in the human female is that, an upright posture having been adopted, the pelvic floor has to contain the downward pressure of the viscera and the pelvic organs.

前韧带为筋膜组织，与相邻的腹膜膀胱褶皱一起，起自子宫颈前，经膀胱上表面，延伸至前腹壁的腹腔腹膜。它的支撑作用弱。

The anterior ligament is a fascial condensation that, with the adjacent peritoneal uterovesical fold, extends from the anterior aspect of the cervix across the superior surface of the bladder to the peritoneal peritoneum of the anterior abdominal wall. It has a weak supporting role.

在后侧，宫骶韧带在支撑子宫与阴道穹隆中起主要作用。这些韧带与它们覆盖的腹膜形成子宫直肠窝（Douglas 窝）的侧界。该韧带包括大量纤维组织和非横纹肌，起自子宫颈，延伸至骶骨前侧。

Posteriorly, the uterosacral ligaments play a major role in supporting the uterus and the vaginal vault. These ligaments and their peritoneal covering form the lateral boundaries of the rectouterine pouch (of Douglas). The ligaments contain a considerable amount of fibrous tissue and non-striped muscle and extend from the cervix onto the anterior surface of the sacrum.

在侧方，阔韧带是自子宫侧缘延伸至骨盆侧壁的腹膜皱襞。阔韧带覆盖输卵管、圆韧带和供应子宫、输卵管、卵巢的血管与神经，以及自阔韧带后表面悬挂卵巢的卵巢系膜和卵巢韧带。与前韧带类似，阔韧带的子宫支撑作用弱。

Laterally, the broad ligaments are reflected folds of peritoneum that extend from the lateral margins of the uterus to the lateral pelvic walls. They cover the Fallopian tubes and the round ligaments, the blood vessels and nerves that supply the uterus, tubes and ovaries, and the mesovarium and ovarian ligaments that suspend the ovaries from the posterior surface of the broad ligament. Like the anterior ligaments, the broad ligaments play only a weak supportive role for the uterus.

圆韧带是子宫前面伸出的 2 根纤维肌性韧带。圆韧带在未妊娠状态仅几毫米厚，被阔韧带的腹膜覆盖。它们起自输卵管入口略下方的子宫前侧面，长 10～12cm，沿对角或侧向延伸至骨盆侧壁，在此处进入腹股沟管，止于大阴唇前端。圆韧带对子宫支撑作用弱，但有维持子宫前倾的作用。妊娠时圆韧带增厚增强，在宫缩时刻向前牵拉子宫，调整胎儿长轴以改善胎先露进入盆腔的方向。

The round ligaments are two fibromuscular ligaments that extend from the anterior surface of the uterus. In the non-pregnant state, they are a few millimetres thick and are covered by the peritoneum of the broad ligaments. They arise from the anterolateral surface of the uterus just below the entrance of the tubes and extend diagonally and laterally for 10–12cm to the lateral pelvic walls, where they enter the abdominal inguinal canal and blend into the upper part of the labia majora. These ligaments have a weak supporting role for the uterus but do play a role in maintaining its anteverted position. In pregnancy, they become much thickened and strengthened and during contractions may pull the uterus anteriorly and align the long axis of the fetus in such a way as to improve the direction of entry of the presenting part into the pelvic cavity.

主韧带（宫颈横韧带）是子宫和阴道穹隆的最强支撑，是从子宫颈延伸至骨盆两侧闭孔窝筋膜的密集增厚筋膜组织。一般而言，主韧带合并入覆盖子宫颈和阴道穹隆的大量纤维组织和平滑肌，即子宫旁组织。宫骶韧带也并入子宫旁组织。子宫旁组织邻近子宫颈，其中包括子宫动脉、神经丛和通向膀胱的输尿管。在下方，盆底肌的肌肉活动和会阴体的完整性在预防子宫脱垂中起到至关重要的作用（见第 21 章）。

The cardinal ligaments (transverse cervical ligaments) form the strongest supports for the uterus and vaginal vault and are dense fascial thickenings that extend from the cervix to the fascia over the obturator fossa on each pelvic side wall. Medially, they merge with the mass of fibrous tissue and smooth muscle that encloses the cervix and the vaginal vault and is known as the *parametrium*. The uterosacral ligaments merge with the parametrium. Close to the cervix, the parametrium contains the uterine arteries, nerve plexuses and the ureter passing through the ureteric canal to reach the urinary bladder. Lower down, the muscular activity of the pelvic floor muscles and the integrity of the perineal body play a vital role in preventing the development of uterine prolapse (see Chapter 21).

（四）输卵管（The Fallopian tubes）

输卵管即 Fallopian 管，起自子宫上角，开口于子宫腔的外侧和最上方。输卵管长 10～12cm，位于阔韧带的后表面，向侧方盘绕延伸并最终开口于紧邻卵巢的腹膜腔。

The Fallopian tubes or uterine tubes are the oviducts. They extend from the superior angle of the uterus, where the tubal canal at the tubal ostium opens into the lateral and uppermost part of the uterine cavity. The tubes are approximately 10–12 cm long and lie on the posterior surface of the broad ligament, extending laterally in a convoluted fashion so that, eventually, the tubes open into the peritoneal cavity in close proximity to the ovaries.

输卵管被输卵管系膜覆盖，输卵管系膜是游离于输卵管的阔韧带上缘褶皱，除了输卵管，它还覆盖供应输卵管和卵巢的血管及神经。输卵管系膜中还有各种胚胎期残留物，如卵巢冠、卵巢旁体、Gartner 管和 Morgagni 囊。这些胚胎期残留物的重要性在于如果它们形成卵巢旁囊肿，会与真正的卵巢囊肿难以鉴别。它们常为良性。

The tubes are enclosed in a mesosalpinx, a superior fold of the broad ligament, and this peritoneal fold, apart from the tube, also contains the blood vessels and nerve supply to the tubes and the ovaries. It also houses various embryological remnants such as the epoophoron, the paroophoron, Gartner's duct and the hydatid of Morgagni. These embryological remnants are significant in that they may form para-ovarian cysts, which are difficult to differentiate from true ovarian cysts. They are generally benign.

输卵管被分为以下 4 部分。

The tube is divided into four sections:

- 位于子宫壁内的间质部。

- The *interstitial portion* lies in the uterine wall.

- 峡部是输卵管的缩窄部分，从间质部延伸出，至增宽的下一部分。管腔狭窄，纵行肌层和环状肌层分化良好。

- The *isthmus* is a constricted portion of the tube extending from the emergence of the interstitial portion until it widens into the next section. The lumen of the tube is narrow, and the longitudinal and circular muscle layers are well differentiated.

- 壶腹部是输卵管的宽大部分，肌壁薄。宽大的管腔被覆增厚的黏膜。

- The *ampulla* is a widened section of the tube, and the muscle coat is much thinner. The widened cavity is lined by thickened mucosa.

- 漏斗部是输卵管壶腹的最外侧。它终止于腹部开口，包绕输卵管伞毛，最长者附着于卵巢。

- The *infundibulum* of the tube is the outermost part of the ampulla. It terminates at the abdominal ostium, where it is surrounded by a fringe of fimbriae, the longest of which is attached to the ovary.

输卵管内衬单层纤毛柱状上皮，可协助卵子沿输卵管向下运送。输卵管的神经丰富，且有内在节律性，这种节律性随月经周期阶段不同及是否妊娠而改变。

The tubes are lined by a single layer of ciliated columnar epithelium, which serves to assist the movement of the oocyte down the tube. The tubes are richly innervated and have an inherent rhythmicity that varies according to the stage of the menstrual cycle and whether the woman is pregnant.

（五）卵巢（The ovaries）

卵巢是 1 对杏仁状器官，具有生殖和内分泌功能。

The ovaries are paired, almond-shaped organs that have both reproductive and endocrine functions.

它们长 2.5～5cm，宽 1.5～3.0cm。卵巢位于阔韧带后侧面的一个浅凹，即卵巢窝，卵巢窝紧邻髂外血管和侧骨盆壁的输尿管。每个卵巢均有一个内侧面和一个外侧面，一个前缘和一个游离于腹膜腔的后缘，一个上缘（即输卵管极）和一个下缘（即子宫极）。

They are approximately 2.5–5 cm in length and 1.5–3.0 cm in width. Each ovary lies on the posterior surface of the broad ligaments in a shallow depression known as the *ovarian fossa* in close proximity to the external iliac vessels and the ureter on the lateral pelvic walls. Each has a medial and a lateral surface, an anterior border, a posterior border that lies free in the peritoneal cavity, an upper or tubal pole and a lower or uterine pole.

卵巢的前缘与阔韧带后层通过腹膜皱襞相连，该皱襞叫作卵巢系膜。卵巢系膜内有卵巢的血管和神经。卵巢的输卵管极通过卵巢悬韧带（骨盆漏斗皱襞）与骨盆腔缘相连。下级与子宫外侧通过纤维肌束（即卵巢固有韧带）与子宫外侧相连。

The anterior border of the ovary is attached to the posterior layer of the broad ligament by a fold in the peritoneum known as the *mesovarium*. This fold contains the blood vessels and nerves supplying the ovary. The tubal pole of the ovary is attached to the pelvic brim by the *suspensory ligament* (*infundibulopelvic fold*) of the ovary. The lower pole is attached to the lateral border of the uterus by a musculofibrous condensation known as the *ovarian ligament*.

卵巢表面被立方或低柱状生发上皮覆盖。该表面直接通腹膜腔。

The surface of the ovary is covered by a cuboidal or low columnar type of germinal epithelium. This surface opens directly into the peritoneal cavity.

当卵巢恶性疾病进展时，恶性肿瘤会破坏卵巢表面，肿瘤细胞会直接落入腹膜腔。这种进展是隐匿的且通常无症状，发病晚。鉴于这些特点，卵巢恶性疾病通常预后差，除非诊断时无卵巢外的转移。

The development of malignant disease in the ovary leads to the shedding of malignant cells directly into the peritoneal cavity as soon as the tumour breaches the surface of the ovary. The disease is silent and often asymptomatic and thus presents late. As a result of these characteristics, the prognosis is generally poor unless the disease is diagnosed when it has not extended beyond the substance of the ovary.

生发上皮下是一层致密结缔组织，有效地形成了卵巢囊，即卵巢白膜。卵巢白膜下为卵巢皮质，由基质组织和上皮细胞组成，它们形成成熟或退化阶段的 Graafian 卵泡。这些卵泡也可在卵巢血流丰富的中央部分（即髓质）发现。血管和神经经髓质进入卵巢。

Beneath the germinal epithelium is a layer of dense connective tissue that effectively forms the capsule of the ovary; this is known as the tunica albuginea. Beneath this layer lies the cortex of the ovary, formed by stromal tissue and collections of epithelial cells that form the Graafian follicles at different stages of maturation and degeneration. These follicles can also be found in the highly vascular, central portion of the ovary: the medulla. The blood vessels and nerve supply enter the ovary through the medulla.

四、盆腔器官的血供（The blood supply to the pelvic organs）

（一）髂内动脉（Internal iliac arteries）

骨盆腔器官的血供主要来源于髂内动脉（有时被称为腹下动脉），它起自髂总血管分为髂外动脉和髂内血管的分支点（图 1-4）。

The major part of the blood supply to the pelvic organs is derived from the internal iliac arteries (sometimes known as the *hypogastric arteries*), which originate from the bifurcation of the common iliac vessels into the external iliac arteries and the internal iliac vessels (Fig. 1.4).

髂内动脉起自腰骶关节水平，越过骨盆缘，在腹膜下沿真骨盆腔的后外侧壁持续向下，直到穿过腰大肌和梨状肌。当到达骶神经丛的腰骶干水平，于坐骨大切迹的上缘处分为前干和后干。此后它成为脐动脉，脐动脉在出生后不久闭锁形成侧脐韧带。因此，在胎儿期这是重要的血管网，它通过髂内动脉前干输送血液，后延续为脐动脉连接胎盘。

The internal iliac artery arises at the level of the lumbosacral articulation and passes over the pelvic brim, continuing downward on the posterolateral wall of the cavity of the true pelvis beneath the peritoneum until it crosses the psoas major and the piriformis muscles. It then reaches the lumbosacral trunk of the sacral plexus of nerves and, at the upper margin of the greater sciatic notch, it divides into anterior and posterior divisions. It then continues as the umbilical artery, which, shortly after birth, becomes obliterated to form the lateral umbilical ligament. Thus, in fetal life, this is the major vascular network, which delivers blood via the internal iliac anterior division and its continuation as the umbilical artery to the placenta.

髂内动脉前后干的分支如下。

The branches of the two divisions of the internal iliac artery are as follows.

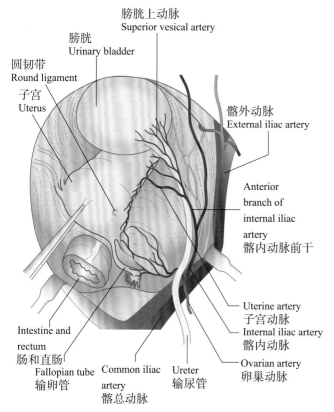

膀胱上动脉
Superior vesical artery

膀胱
Urinary bladder

圆韧带
Round ligament

子宫
Uterus

髂外动脉
External iliac artery

Anterior
branch of
internal iliac
artery
髂内动脉前干

Intestine and
rectum
肠和直肠

Fallopian tube
输卵管

Common iliac
artery
髂总动脉

Ureter
输尿管

Uterine artery
子宫动脉

Internal iliac artery
髂内动脉

Ovarian artery
卵巢动脉

▲ 图 1-4　女性盆腔主要血管

Fig. 1.4　Major blood vessels of the female pelvis

1. 前干分支（Anterior division）

如前所述，髂内动脉前干的结构参与了脐血循环。它分为上、中、下膀胱动脉参与膀胱血供。上、中支居中穿过膀胱的侧面和上面，与对侧分支及子宫、阴道动脉的分支吻合。

The anterior division provides the structure for the umbilical circulation as previously described. It also provides the superior, middle and inferior vesical arteries that provide the blood supply for the bladder. The superior and middle branches, having passed medially to the lateral and superior surfaces of the bladder, anastomose with branches from the contralateral vessels and with the branches of the uterine and vaginal arteries.

它也形成直肠中动脉。

It also forms the middle haemorrhoidal artery.

当妊娠期子宫血流大量增加时，子宫动脉会成为这一支干的主要血管结构。子宫动脉在阔韧带下方腹膜下脂肪内，下行至子宫颈。

The uterine artery becomes the major vascular structure arising from this division during pregnancy, when there is a major increase in uterine blood flow. It initially runs downwards

in the subperitoneal fat under the inferior attachment of the broad ligament towards the cervix.

子宫动脉在输尿管进入膀胱前穿过输尿管，距阴道侧穹隆 1.5～2cm。至与阴道穹隆接触时分出沿着阴道侧壁下行的分支。子宫动脉主干沿子宫外侧壁迁行，众多分支进入子宫，最终侧向分支进入阔韧带，与卵巢动脉吻合，形成卵巢、输卵管和子宫循环供血的循环。

The artery crosses over the ureter shortly before that structure enters the bladder approximately 1.5–2 cm from the lateral fornix of the vagina. At the point of contact with the vaginal fornix, it gives off a vaginal branch that runs downwards along the lateral vaginal wall. The main uterine artery then follows a tortuous course along the lateral wall of the uterus, giving off numerous branches into the substance of the uterus and finally diverging laterally into the broad ligament to anastomose with the ovarian artery, thus forming a continuous loop that provides the blood supply for the ovaries and the tubes as well as the uterine circulation.

还有髂内动脉前区的顶支，其中包括闭孔动脉、阴部内动脉和臀下动脉。

There are also parietal branches of the anterior division of the internal iliac artery, and these include the obturator artery, the internal pudendal artery and the inferior gluteal artery.

2. 后干分支（Posterior division）

髂内动脉后干分为髂腰支、骶外侧支和臀上支，对盆腔器官血供不起主要作用。

The posterior division divides into the iliolumbar branch and the lateral sacral and superior gluteal branches and does not play a major function in the blood supply to the pelvic organs.

（二）卵巢血管（The ovarian vessels）

盆腔器官的其他主要血供来源为卵巢动脉。卵巢动脉起自肾血管和肠系膜下血管之间的主动脉前部。其沿腹膜后的腰大肌表面下降至骨盆缘，在此处穿入骨盆漏斗皱襞，后至卵巢系膜与子宫血管吻合。子宫动脉和卵巢动脉都伴有丰富的静脉丛。

The other important blood supply to the pelvic organs comes from the ovarian arteries. These arise from the front of the aorta between the origins of the renal and inferior mesenteric vessels. They descend behind the peritoneum on the surface of the corresponding psoas muscle until they reach the brim of the pelvis, where they cross into the corresponding infundibulopelvic fold and from there to the base of the mesovarium and on to anastomose with the uterine vessels. Both the uterine and ovarian arteries are accompanied by a rich plexus of veins.

✓ **经验**

子宫和卵巢血管吻合的丰富性意味着需要结扎双侧髂内动脉减少子宫出血，同时通过增加卵巢血管血流量以维持盆腔器官的活力。

The richness of the anastomosis of the uterine and ovarian vessels means that it is possible to ligate both internal iliac arteries and reduce bleeding from the uterus and yet still maintain the viability of the pelvic organs by expanding the blood flow through the ovarian vessels.

五、盆腔淋巴系统（The pelvic lymphatic system）

淋巴管沿血管走行，其特有的淋巴结系统对盆腔恶性疾病非常重要（图 1-5）。

The lymphatic vessels follow the course of the blood vessels but have a specific nodal system that is of particular importance in relation to malignant disease of the pelvis (Fig. 1.5).

来自阴道下部、外阴、会阴和肛门的淋巴引流注入腹股沟浅淋巴结和邻近的股浅淋巴结。

The lymphatic drainage from the lower part of the vagina, the vulva and perineum and anus passes to the superficial inguinal and adjacent superficial femoral nodes.

腹股沟浅淋巴结分为两组，上组与腹股沟韧带平行，下组位于大隐静脉上方。

The superficial inguinal nodes lie in two groups, with an upper group lying parallel with the inguinal ligament and a lower group situated along the upper part of the great saphenous vein.

其中一些淋巴结注入股深淋巴结，股深淋巴结位于股静脉上端的内侧。

Some of these nodes drain into the deep femoral nodes, which lie medial to the upper end of the femoral vein.

其中一个被称为 Cloquet 腺的淋巴结占据股管。

One of these nodes, known as the *gland of Cloquet*, occupies the femoral canal.

在盆腔主要血管旁还有成组的盆壁淋巴结，其中包括髂总淋巴结、髂外淋巴结和髂内淋巴结，它们之后引流至主动脉淋巴结链。

There are also pelvic parietal nodes grouped around the major pelvic vessels. These include the common iliac, external iliac and internal iliac nodes, which subsequently drain to the aortic chain of nodes.

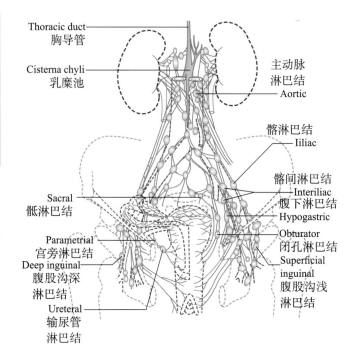

▲ 图 1-5 女性盆腔淋巴引流

Fig. 1.5 Lymphatic drainage of the female pelvis

子宫颈、子宫和阴道上部的淋巴管引流至髂淋巴结，而子宫底、输卵管和卵巢的淋巴管则沿卵巢血管走行，注入主动脉淋巴结。子宫底的部分淋巴管沿圆形韧带走行，注入腹股沟深淋巴结和腹股沟浅淋巴结。

The lymphatics of the cervix, the uterus and the upper portion of the vagina drain into the iliac nodes, whereas the lymphatics of the fundus of the uterus, the Fallopian tubes and the ovaries follow the ovarian vessels to the aortic nodes. Some of the lymphatics from the uterine fundus follow the round ligament into the deep and superficial inguinal nodes.

六、盆腔神经（Nerves of the pelvis）

盆腔和盆腔器官的神经支配既有体神经，也有自主神经。躯体神经有感觉神经和运动神经支配，主要与外生殖器和盆底功能相关，而自主神经则为盆腔器官的交感与副交感神经（图 1-6）。

The nerve supply to the pelvis and the pelvic organs has both a somatic and an autonomic component. While the somatic innervation is both sensory and motor in function and relates predominantly to the external genitalia and the pelvic floor, the autonomic innervation provides the sympathetic and parasympathetic nerve supply to the pelvic organs (Fig. 1.6).

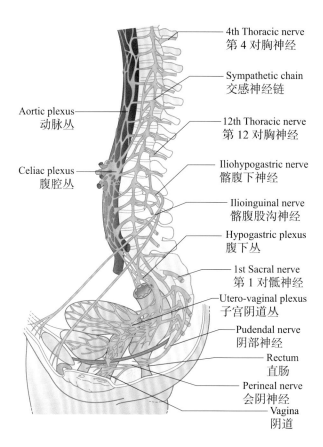

Aortic plexus 动脉丛	4th Thoracic nerve 第 4 对胸神经
Celiac plexus 腹腔丛	Sympathetic chain 交感神经链
	12th Thoracic nerve 第 12 对胸神经
	Iliohypogastric nerve 髂腹下神经
	Ilioinguinal nerve 髂腹股沟神经
	Hypogastric plexus 腹下丛
	1st Sacral nerve 第 1 对骶神经
	Utero-vaginal plexus 子宫阴道丛
	Pudendal nerve 阴部神经
	Rectum 直肠
	Perineal nerve 会阴神经
	Vagina 阴道

▲ 图 1-6　盆腔神经分布

Fig. 1.6　Nerve supply of the pelvis

（一）躯体神经支配（Somatic innervation）

外阴和盆底的躯体神经支配为阴部神经，来自脊髓骶 2、骶 3 和骶 4 节段。这些神经包括传出神经和传入神经。

The somatic innervation to the vulva and pelvic floor is provided by the pudendal nerves that arise from the S2, S3 and S4 segments of the spinal cord. These nerves include both efferent and afferent components.

阴部神经起自腰骶丛，在骶棘韧带下离开骨盆，进入 Alcock 管，穿过坐骨直肠窝进入会阴。运动神经支配肛门外括约肌、会阴浅肌和尿道外括约肌。

The pudendal nerves arise in the lumbosacral plexus and leave the pelvis under the sacrospinous ligament to enter Alcock's canal and pass through the layers of the wall of the ischiorectal fossa to enter the perineum. Motor branches provide innervation of the external anal sphincter muscle, the superficial perineal muscles and the external urethral sphincter.

感觉神经通过阴蒂背神经支配阴蒂。阴唇和会阴皮肤的感觉神经也来自阴部神经分支。另有阴阜和阴唇的皮肤神经支配，来自髂腹股沟神经（腰

1）和生殖股神经（腰 1 和腰 2），以及会阴的皮肤神经支配，来自骶丛的股后皮神经（骶 1、骶 2 和骶 3）。

Sensory innervation is provided to the clitoris through the branch of the dorsal nerve of the clitoris. The sensory innervation of the skin of the labia and of the perineum is also derived from branches of the pudendal nerves. Additional cutaneous innervation of the mons and the labia is derived from the ilioinguinal nerves (L1) and the genitofemoral nerves (L1 and L2) and of the perineum through the posterior femoral cutaneous nerve from the sacral plexus (S1, S2 and S3).

（二）自主神经支配（Autonomic innervation）

交感神经起自胸 10/ 胸 11 水平的节前纤维，通过伴行于卵巢血管的交感神经纤维支配卵巢和输卵管。

Sympathetic innervation arises from preganglionic fibres at the T10/T11 level and supplies the ovaries and tubes through sympathetic fibres that follow the ovarian vessels.

子宫体和子宫颈通过腹下丛接受交感神经支配，腹下丛伴行髂血管，含有发送拉伸信号的神经纤维。

The body of the uterus and the cervix receive sympathetic innervation through the hypogastric plexus, which accompanies the branches of the iliac vessels, and also contain fibres that signal stretching.

支配子宫、膀胱和肛直肠的副交感神经源自骶 1、骶 2 和骶 3，这些神经纤维在控制膀胱和肛门的括约肌系统中起到重要作用。

The parasympathetic innervation to the uterus, bladder and anorectum arises from the S1, S2 and S3 segments; these fibres are important in the control of smooth muscle function of the bladder and the anal sphincter system.

子宫痛觉通过传入胸 11/ 胸 12 和腰 1/ 腰 2 的交感神经介导，感受到的疼痛在下腹部和高位腰椎处。

Uterine pain is mediated through sympathetic afferent nerves passing up to T11/T12 and L1/L2; the pain is felt in the lower abdomen and the high lumbar spine.

子宫颈部疼痛通过传回骶 1、骶 2 和骶 3 的副交感神经介导。会阴疼痛由阴部神经介导，痛感即在会阴部位。

Cervical pain is mediated through the parasympathetic afferent nerves passing backwards to S1, S2 and S3; perineal pain is felt at the site and is mediated through the pudendal nerves.

七、盆底（The pelvic floor）

盆底是跨过真骨盆出口的隔膜，真骨盆内有盆腔器官和一些腹腔器官。盆底开口为阴道、尿道和直肠。盆底在分娩和尿便控制中起到重要作用（图 1-7）。盆底的主要支撑来自肛提肌的组成部分，其中包括以下三个部分。

The pelvic floor provides a diaphragm across the outlet of the true pelvis that contains the pelvic organs and some of the organs of the abdominal cavity. The pelvic floor is naturally breached by the vagina, the urethra and the rectum. It plays an essential role in parturition and in urinary and faecal continence (Fig. 1.7). The principal supports of the pelvic floor are the constituent parts of the levator ani muscles. These are described in three sections:

- 髂尾肌起自盆壁筋膜，由耻骨支后表面延伸至坐骨棘，附着于肛尾韧带和尾骨。

- The iliococcygeus muscle arises from the parietal pelvic fascia, extends from the posterior surface of the pubic rami to the ischial spines and is inserted into the anococcygeal ligament and the coccyx.

- 耻骨直肠肌起自耻骨支的后表面，通向直肠前方的会阴体，与对侧肌纤维交叉。

- The puborectalis muscle arises from the posterior surface of the pubic rami and passes to the centre of the perineal body anterior to the rectum, with some decussation with muscle fibres from the contralateral muscle.

- 耻尾肌起点相似，向后通向直肠侧方和肛尾韧带。

- The pubococcygeus muscle has a similar origin and passes posteriorly to the sides of the rectum and the anococcygeal ligament.

这些肌肉在排便、咳嗽、呕吐和分娩中起着重要作用。

These muscles play an important role in defecation, coughing, vomiting and parturition.

八、会阴（The perineum）

会阴是骨盆下开口的区域，由位于盆底下的所有骨盆结构组成。该区域的前方边界由耻骨联合下缘、耻骨弓和坐骨结节组成，后方边界由骶结节韧带和尾骨组成。

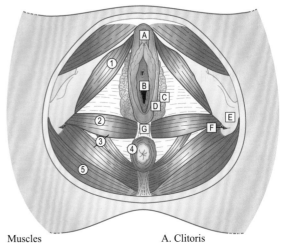

Muscles 肌肉	A. Clitoris 阴蒂
1. Ischiocavernosus 坐骨海绵体肌	B. Vagina 阴道
2. Superficial transverse perineal 会阴浅横肌	C. Bulb of vestibule 前庭球
3. Levator ani pubococcygeus iliococcygeus 肛提耻尾髂尾肌	D. Site of Bartholin's gland Bartholin 腺位置
4. External anal sphincter 肛门外括约肌	E. Ischial tuberosity 坐骨结节
5. Gluteus maximus 臀大肌	F. Pudendal vessels 阴部血管
	G. Perineal body 会阴体

▲ 图 1-7 盆腔肌肉

Fig. 1.7 Muscles of the pelvic floor

The perineum is the region defined as the inferior aperture of the pelvis and consists of all the pelvic structures that lie below the pelvic floor. The area is bounded anteriorly by the inferior margin of the pubic symphysis, the subpubic arch and the ischial tuberosities. Posteriorly, the boundaries are formed by the sacrotuberous ligaments and the coccyx.

会阴被坐骨结节间连线分为前三角和后三角。前部为尿生殖三角，其中包括尿道的一部分；尿生殖膈是盆底肌下方的筋膜，阴道穿过尿生殖膈。后三角或称肛门三角，其中包括肛门、肛门括约肌和会阴体。这两个三角的底部均位于会阴深横肌。

The perineum is divided into anterior and posterior triangles by a line drawn between the two ischial tuberosities. The anterior portion is known as the *urogenital triangle* and includes part of the urethra; the urogenital diaphragm is a condensation of fascia below the level of the pelvic floor muscles and is traversed by the vagina. The posterior or anal triangle includes the anus, the anal sphincter and the perineal body. The two triangles have their bases on the deep transverse perineal muscles.

会阴体是一个纤维肌性的锥形体，位于尿生殖三角与肛门三角交界的中线处。肛提肌、球海绵体肌、会阴浅横肌、会阴深横肌、肛门外括约肌和尿道外括约肌均附着于会阴体。

The perineal body is a pyramidal fibromuscular mass in the midline of the perineum at the junction of the urogenital and anal triangles. The muscles comprising the levator ani, the bulbospongiosus, superficial and deep transverse perineal muscles, external anal sphincter and external urethral sphincter are all attached to the perineal body.

> **！注意**
>
> 在第二产程中，会阴体在支撑阴道后壁和保护肛门外括约肌不被撕裂方面起着重要作用。
>
> During the second stage of labour, the perineal body plays an important role in supporting the posterior vaginal wall and protecting the external anal sphincter from tearing.

坐骨直肠窝是肛管和侧方的坐骨下支围成的腔隙，坐骨下支被闭孔内肌和筋膜覆盖。坐骨直肠窝的后方是臀大肌和骶结节韧带，前方是尿生殖膈的后缘。

The ischiorectal fossa lies between the anal canal and the lateral wall of the fossa formed by the inferior ramus of the ischium covered by the obturator internus muscle and fascia. Posteriorly, the fossa is formed by the gluteus maximus muscle and the sacrotuberous ligament, and anteriorly by the posterior border of the urogenital diaphragm.

阴部神经和阴部内血管穿过被 Alcock 管筋膜层包裹的坐骨直肠窝侧角。

The pudendal nerve and internal pudendal vessels pass through the lateral aspect of the fossa enclosed in the fascial layer of Alcock's canal.

本章概览	Essential information
外生殖器	**The external genitalia**
• 外阴包括以下部分	• The term *vulva* includes:
– 阴阜	– Mons pubis
– 大阴唇	– Labia majora
– 小阴唇	– Labia minora
– 阴蒂	– Clitoris
– 尿道外口	– External urinary meatus
– 阴道前庭	– Vestibule of the vagina
– 阴道口和处女膜	– Vaginal orifice and the hymen
• 外观取决于年龄和激素状态	• Appearance dependent on age and hormonal status
• 大阴唇与男性阴囊同源	• Labia majora homologous with the male scrotum
• 阴蒂为阴茎的女性同源物	• Clitoris female homologue of the penis
– 在性刺激中发挥重要作用	– Important role in sexual stimulation
• 前庭包含以下开口	• The vestibule contains openings of:
– 尿道口	– Urethral meatus
– 阴道口	– Vaginal orifice
– Skene 腺管和 Bartholin 腺管开口	– Skene's and Bartholin's ducts
• 处女膜的薄褶皱皮肤环绕在阴道口边缘	• Hymen thin fold of skin attached around the margins of the vaginal orifice
内生殖器	**The internal genital organs**
• 内生殖器包括以下部分	• The internal genitalia include:
– 阴道	– Vagina
– 子宫	– Uterus
– 输卵管	– Fallopian tubes
– 卵巢	– Ovaries
阴道	**Vagina**
• 内衬鳞状上皮的肌性管道	• Muscular tube lined by squamous epithelium
• 横截面为 H 形	• H shaped in cross-section
• 延展性极强	• Capable of considerable distension
• 相关器官	• Related:
– 前邻尿道和膀胱	– Anteriorly with urethra and bladder
– 后邻肛门、会阴体、直肠、Douglas 窝和盆腔结肠	– Posteriorly with anus, perineal body, rectum, pouch of Douglas and pelvic colon

（续表）

本章概览	Essential information
子宫	**Uterus**
• 子宫颈	• **Cervix**
– 肌纤维圆柱状结构	– Musculofibrous cylindrical structure
– 阴道部和阴道上部	– Vaginal portion and supravaginal portion
– 被覆柱状上皮衬的管道	– Canal lined by columnar epithelium
– 宫颈阴道部被覆复层鳞状上皮	– Ectocervix lined by stratified squamous epithelium
– 外口通向阴道	– · External os opens into vagina
– 内口通向子宫腔	– · Internal os opens into uterine cavity
• 峡部	• Isthmus
– 子宫颈和子宫体之间的交界区	– Junctional zone between cervix and corpus uteri
– 妊娠期间形成子宫下段	– Forms lower segment in pregnancy
• 子宫体	• Corpus uteri
– 有三层平滑肌纤维，具体如下	– Three layers of smooth muscle fibres:
➢ 外层横向纤维	➢ External transverse fibres
➢ 中层圆形纤维	➢ Middle layer circular fibres
➢ 内层纵向纤维	➢ Inner layer longitudinal fibres
– 子宫腔内衬有子宫内膜	– Cavity lined by endometrium
– 高柱状上皮和基质层	– Tall columnar epithelium and stromal layers
– 随月经周期变化	– Change with stage of cycle
子宫支撑	**Supports of the uterus**
• 直接支撑	• Direct supports
– 弱支撑	– Weak
➢ 圆韧带	➢ Round ligaments
➢ 阔韧带	➢ Broad ligaments
➢ 耻骨宫颈韧带	➢ Pubocervical ligaments
– 强支撑	– Strong
➢ 宫骶韧带	➢ Uterosacral ligaments
➢ 主韧带（宫颈横韧带）	➢ Cardinal (transverse cervical) ligaments
– 间接支撑——盆底	– Indirect supports–the pelvic floor
➢ 肛提肌	➢ Levator ani muscles
➢ 会阴体	➢ Perineal body
➢ 尿生殖膈	➢ Urogenital diaphragm
输卵管	**Fallopian tubes (oviducts)**
• 薄肌性管道	• Thin muscular tubes
• 被覆纤毛柱状上皮	• Lined by ciliated columnar epithelium
• 由四个部分组成，具体如下	• Consist of four sections:
– 间质部（子宫壁内）	– Interstitial (intramural)
– 峡部	– Isthmus
– 壶腹部	– Ampulla
– 漏斗部（伞端）	– Infundibulum (fimbriated ends)
卵巢	**The ovaries**
• 成对的杏仁形器官	• Paired almond-shaped organs
• 表面位于腹膜腔	• Surface lies in peritoneal cavity
致密纤维组织囊（白膜）	• Capsule of dense fibrous tissue (tunica albuginea)
• 皮质基质和上皮细胞	• Cortex-stroma and epithelial cells
血供	**Blood supply**
髂内动脉	**Internal iliac arteries**
• 前干	• Anterior division
• 内脏支	• Visceral
– 3 个膀胱分支	– Three vesical branches
– 子宫动脉	– Uterine arteries
• 顶支	• Parietal
– 闭孔动脉	– Obturator artery
– 臀内动脉	– Internal gluteal artery

（续表）

（续表）

本章概览	Essential information
• 后干 　– 髂腰支 　– 骶外动脉 　– 臀下支	• Posterior division 　– Iliolumbar branch 　– Lateral sacral arteries 　– Inferior gluteal branches
卵巢动脉 • 起自肾动脉下方的主动脉 • 与子宫血管吻合丰富	**Ovarian arteries** • From aorta below renal arteries • Rich anastomosis with uterine vessels
盆腔淋巴系统 • 淋巴管与血管伴行 • 腹股沟淋巴结（浅部和深部）接受阴道下部、外阴、会阴和肛门的淋巴引流 • 髂淋巴结和主动脉淋巴结接受子宫颈、子宫下部、阴道上部的淋巴引流 • 子宫底、输卵管和卵巢淋巴注入主动脉淋巴结 • 部分淋巴引流沿圆韧带注入腹股沟淋巴结	**Pelvic lymphatic system** • Lymphatic vessels follow blood vessels • Inguinal nodes (superficial and deep) drain lower vagina, vulva, perineum and anus • Iliac and then aortic nodes drain cervix, lower part uterus, upper vagina • Uterine fundus, tubes and ovaries drain to aortic nodes • Some drainage follows round ligaments to inguinal nodes
神经支配 • 躯体神经支配：来自骶 2、骶 3、骶 4 的阴部神经 • 自主神经支配 • 胸 10、胸 11、胸 12、腰 1、腰 2 的交感神经 • 骶 1、骶 2、骶 3 的副交感神经 • 胸 11、胸 12、腰 1、腰 2、骶 1、骶 2、骶 3 的痛觉神经纤维	**Innervation** • Somatic innervation-pudendal nerves from S2, S3, S4 • Autonomic innervation • Sympathetic outflow T10, T11, T12, L1, L2 • Parasympathetic outflow S1, S2, S3 • Pain fibres through T11, T12, L1, L2, S1, S2, S3
会阴 • 前三角，即泌尿生殖三角，其中包括经行其中的尿道 • 后三角，其中包括肛门、肛门括约肌、会阴体	**Perineum** • Anterior triangle-urogenital triangle includes passage of urethra • Posterior triangle-includes anus, anal sphincters, perineal body

第2章 妊娠与着床
Conception and implantation

Roger Pepperell　著　　刘培昊　宋晓翠　译　　石玉华　校

学习目标	LEARNING OUTCOMES
学习本章后你应当能够：	After studying this chapter you should be able to:
知识标准	**Knowledge criteria**
• 描述配子形成的基本原理	• Describe the basic principles of the formation of the gametes
• 描述正常月经周期的生理	• Describe the physiology of the normal menstrual cycle
• 描述性交、受精和着床的生理	• Describe the physiology of coitus, fertilization and implantation
临床能力	**Clinical competency**
• 为夫妇提供关于受孕时期的建议	• Counsel a couple about the fertile period

一、卵子发生（Oogenesis）

原始生殖细胞最初出现在卵黄囊内，胚胎发育第4周可被识别（图2-1）。胚胎发育44～48天，原始生殖细胞通过发育中的肠的背系肠系膜迁移至生殖嵴。进入含有间充质细胞的生殖结节，间充质细胞出现在中肾的腹侧。生殖细胞形成性索，后发育为卵巢皮质。

Primordial germ cells originally appear in the yolk sac and can be identified by the fourth week of fetal development (Fig. 2.1). These cells migrate through the dorsal mesentery of the developing gut and finally reach the genital ridge between 44 and 48 days post-conception. Migration occurs into a genital tubercle consisting of mesenchymal cells that appear over the ventral part of the mesonephros. The germ cells form sex cords and become the cortex of the ovary.

性索随后分裂为单独的细胞团，至胚胎16周时，这些细胞团发育为初级卵泡，包括中央生殖细胞。

The sex cords subsequently break up into separate clumps of cells and, by 16 weeks, these clumped cells become primary follicles, which incorporate central germ cells.

这些细胞进行快速的有丝分裂，在宫内妊娠20周时数目约700万，被称为卵原细胞。此后，细胞不再进一步分裂，也不再产生。出生时，卵原细胞就已开始减数第一次分裂，成为初级卵母细胞。初级卵母细胞数量逐渐减少，到出生时减少至约100万个，到青春期时减少至约40万个。

These cells undergo rapid mitotic activity, and by 20 weeks of intrauterine life, there are about 7 million cells, known

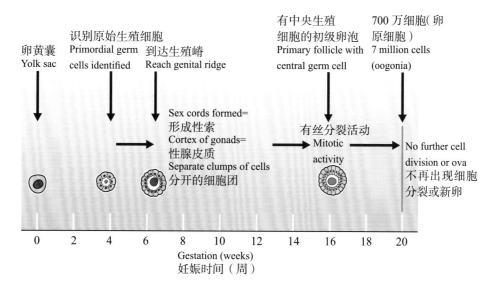

▲ 图 2-1　胚胎和胎儿时期卵原细胞发育

Fig. 2.1　Embryonic and fetal development of oogonia

as *oogonia*. After this time, no further cell division occurs and no further ova are produced. By birth, the oogonia have already begun the first meiotic division and have become primary oocytes. The number of primary oocytes falls progressively and by birth is down to about 1 million and to about 0.4 million by puberty.

1. 减数分裂（Meiosis）

减数分裂过程使每个配子中有 23 条染色体，是正常细胞染色体数目的 1/2。随着卵子被精子受精，染色体数目恢复至正常的 46 条。精卵结合发生在卵母细胞第一次减数分裂完成时；第二次减数分裂于雄配子的 23 条染色体在细胞核内混入雌配子染色体前完成，随后受精卵形成，将发育为胚胎。

The process of meiosis results in 23 chromosomes being found in each of the gametes, half the number of chromosomes found in normal cells. With the fertilization of the egg by a sperm, the chromosome count is returned to the normal count of 46 chromosomes. Fusion of the sperm and the egg occurs when the first of two meiotic divisions of the oocyte has already been completed; with the second meiotic division occurring subsequently and being completed prior to the 23 chromosomes of the male gamete joining those of the female gamete within the nucleus of the cell, the zygote is formed, which will become the embryo.

在减数分裂过程中，连续发生 2 次细胞分裂，每次均分为前期、中期、后期和末期。2 次细胞分裂中的第一次为减数分裂，第二次为改良有丝分裂，通常缺乏前期（图 2-2）。在第一次减数分裂前期末，双染色体联会，产生 1 组 4 个同源染色单体，称为四分体。2 个中心粒运动至相反的两极。中间形成纺锤

体，核膜消失。在减数分裂 I 前期，同源染色体沿整个长度成对进行联会，交叉并进行染色单体交换，这个过程解释了尽管雌配子来源于同一位母亲，两个同性兄弟 / 姐妹间仍存在差异。

In meiosis, two cell divisions occur in succession, each of which consists of prophase, metaphase, anaphase and telophase. The first of the two cell divisions is a reduction division, and the second is a modified mitosis in which the prophase is usually lacking (Fig. 2.2). At the end of the first meiotic prophase, the double chromosomes undergo synapsis, producing a group of four homologous chromatids called a *tetrad*. The two centrioles move to opposite poles. A spindle forms in the middle, and the membrane of the nucleus disappears. During this prophase period of meiosis I, the double chromosomes, which are closely associated in pairs along their entire length, undergo synapsis, crossing over and undergoing chromatid exchange, with these processes accounting for the differences seen between two same-sex siblings despite the fact that the female gametes came from the same mother.

初级卵母细胞保持分裂前期直至性成熟，或更晚至黄体生成素（luteinizing hormone，LH）触发优势卵泡排卵，才自减数分裂 I 开始进展。在减数分裂后期，子染色单体分离并向相反两极移动。减数分裂 II 自精子黏附在卵母细胞表面开始，并在受精的最后阶段前完成。

The primary oocytes remain in suspended prophase until sexual maturity is reached, or even much later, with meiosis I not recommencing until the dominant follicle is triggered by luteinizing hormone (LH) to commence ovulation. In anaphase, the daughter chromatids separate and move towards opposite

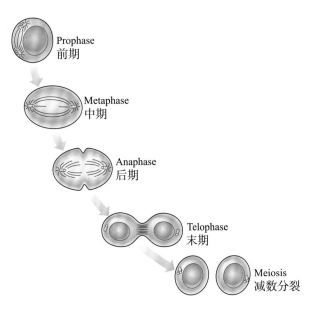

Prophase
前期

Metaphase
中期

Anaphase
后期

Telophase
末期

Meiosis
减数分裂

▲ 图 2-2 初级卵母细胞维持在分裂前期。减数分裂在黄体生成素的刺激下恢复

Fig. 2.2 Primary oocytes remain in suspended prophase. Meiotic division resumes under stimulation by luteinizing hormone

poles. Meiosis II commences around the time the sperm are attached to the surface of the oocyte and is completed prior to the final phase of fertilization.

因此，卵子发生的核内事件与精子发生中的基本相同，但卵子发生中细胞质分裂不均等，只产生 1 个次级卵母细胞。第一次减数分裂后的这个几乎完全由细胞核组成的小细胞，称为第一极体。当卵子进入输卵管时，减数第二次分裂发生，形成次级卵母细胞，同时产生小的第二极体。男性最初细胞内含 46 条染色体，最终形成 4 个精子，大小相同，但每个精子仅含 23 条染色体（见后文精子发生）。

Thus, the nuclear events in oogenesis are virtually the same as in spermatogenesis, but the cytoplasmic division in oogenesis is unequal, resulting in only one secondary oocyte. This small cell consists almost entirely of a nucleus and is known as the *first polar body*. As the ovum enters the Fallopian tube, the second meiotic division occurs and a secondary oocyte forms, with the development of a small second polar body. In the male the original cell containing 46 chromosomes ultimately results in four separate spermatozoa, each being of the same size but containing only 23 chromosomes (see Spermatogenesis, later).

2. 卵巢内卵泡发育（Follicular development in the ovary）

第 1 章介绍了卵巢的大体结构、血供和神经分布。不过，卵巢的显微解剖对于了解卵泡发育和排卵的机制至关重要。

The gross structure and the blood supply and nerve supply of the ovary have been described in Chapter 1. However, the microscopic anatomy of the ovary is important in understanding the mechanism of follicular development and ovulation.

卵巢表面覆盖单层立方上皮。卵巢皮质内含大量卵原细胞，周围环绕以后发育为颗粒细胞的滤泡细胞。卵巢其余部分由间充质核心组成。大部分皮质内的卵细胞不会达到成熟阶段，而是在卵泡发育早期闭锁。在任何时间，均可同时看到成熟和退化的各阶段卵泡（图 2-3）。自青春期后不久至绝经期，每月"丢失"约 800 个初级卵泡，在无超促排卵治疗时，每个月经周期仅 1 个或 2 个卵泡会释放成熟卵子。无论是否妊娠，是否服用口服避孕药，月经规律或闭经，这种进行性的卵泡丢失都会发生，同时，不论妊娠次数或月经周期特征如何，绝经最终都会发生。绝大多数丢失卵泡仅达最低程度的成熟或并未实际成熟。

The surface of the ovary is covered by a single layer of cuboidal epithelium. The cortex of the ovary contains a large number of oogonia surrounded by follicular cells that become *granulosa* cells. The remainder of the ovary consists of a mesenchymal core. Most of the ova in the cortex never reach an advanced stage of maturation and become atretic early in follicular development. At any given time, follicles can be seen in various stages of maturation and degeneration (Fig. 2.3). About 800 primary follicles are 'lost' during each month of life from soon after puberty until menopause, with only one or two of these follicles resulting in release of a mature ovum each menstrual cycle in the absence of ovarian hyperstimulation therapy. This progressive loss occurs irrespective of whether the patient is pregnant, on the oral contraceptive pill, having regular cycles or amenorrhoeic, with menopause occurring at the same time irrespective of the number of pregnancies or cycle characteristics. The vast majority of the follicles lost have undergone minimal or no actual maturation.

卵泡发育的第一阶段以卵子增大同时基质细胞聚集形成卵泡膜细胞为特征。在月经周期第 6 天左右，1 个优势卵泡被选择，最内层颗粒细胞黏附于卵子表面，形成放射冠。颗粒细胞内形成 1 个充满液体的腔，透明的胶质物聚集在卵子周围，形成透明带。卵子位置偏离中心，Graafian 卵泡呈现出典型的成熟形态。卵泡周围的间充质细胞分化为 2 层，形成内膜层和外膜层。

The first stage of follicular development is characterized

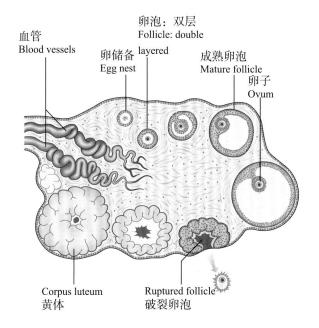

血管
Blood vessels

卵泡：双层
Follicle: double layered

卵储备
Egg nest

成熟卵泡
Mature follicle

卵子
Ovum

Corpus luteum
黄体

Ruptured follicle
破裂卵泡

▲ 图 2-3　Graafian 卵泡的发育和成熟

Fig. 2.3　Development and maturation of the Graafian follicle

by enlargement of the ovum with the aggregation of stromal cells to form the thecal cells. When a dominant follicle is selected at about day 6 of the cycle, the innermost layers of granulosa cells adhere to the ovum and form the *corona radiata*. A fluid-filled space develops in the granulosa cells, and a clear layer of gelatinous material collects around the ovum, forming the *zona pellucida*. The ovum becomes eccentrically placed, and the Graafian follicle assumes its classic mature form. The mesenchymal cells around the follicle become differentiated into two layers, forming the *theca interna and the theca externa*.

随着卵泡增大，它向卵巢表面突出，生发上皮之下的区域变薄。最后，卵子及其周围的颗粒细胞会在排卵时经此区域离开。

As the follicle enlarges, it bulges towards the surface of the ovary and the area under the germinal epithelium thins out. Finally, the ovum, with its surrounding investment of granulosa cells, escapes through this area at the time of ovulation.

卵泡腔内常充满血液，同时颗粒细胞和卵泡膜细胞经历黄素化改变，充满黄色的类胡萝卜素物质。成熟黄体呈现密集血管化和明显空泡化的卵泡膜与颗粒细胞，这是激素存在活性的证据。黄体发育在排卵后约 7 天达顶峰，之后黄体退化，除非胚胎着床，着床后的胚胎产生绒毛膜促性腺激素，维持黄体功能，直至妊娠 10 周左右由胎盘接管这一角色。黄体退变的特征是颗粒细胞空泡化和黄体中心纤维组织增多。最终形成一个白色瘢痕组织，称为白体（图 2-4）。

The cavity of the follicle often fills with blood but, at the same time, the granulosa cells and the theca interna cells undergo the changes of luteinization to become filled with yellow carotenoid material. The corpus luteum in its mature form shows intense vascularization and pronounced vacuolization of the theca and granulosa cells with evidence of hormonal activity. This development reaches its peak approximately 7 days after ovulation, and thereafter the corpus luteum regresses unless implantation occurs, when human chorionic gonadotropin (hCG) production by the implanting embryo prolongs corpus luteum function until the placenta takes over this role at about 10 weeks of gestation. The corpus luteum degeneration is characterized by increasing vacuolization of the granulosa cells and the appearance of increased quantities of fibrous tissue in the centre of the corpus luteum. This finally develops into a white scar known as the *corpus albicans* (Fig. 2.4).

二、排卵相关的激素变化（Hormonal events associated with ovulation）

卵母细胞的成熟、排卵及月经周期中子宫内膜与输卵管的变化都受到一系列相互作用的激素变化的调节（图 2-5）。

The maturation of oocytes, ovulation and the endometrial and tubal changes of the menstrual cycle are all regulated by a series of interactive hormonal changes (Fig. 2.5).

该过程始于促性腺激素释放激素（gonadotrophin-releasing hormone，GnRH）的释放，GnRH 是下丘脑正中隆起产生的一种重要的神经分泌物。该激素是一种十肽，从轴突末端释放到垂体门脉毛细血管，

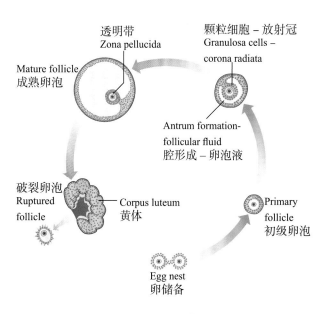

透明带
Zona pellucida

颗粒细胞 – 放射冠
Granulosa cells – corona radiata

Mature follicle
成熟卵泡

Antrum formation-follicular fluid
腔形成 – 卵泡液

破裂卵泡
Ruptured follicle

Corpus luteum
黄体

Primary follicle
初级卵泡

Egg nest
卵储备

▲ 图 2-4　排卵和黄体形成

Fig. 2.4　Ovulation and corpus luteum formation

继而引发垂体释放卵泡刺激素（follide-stimulating hormone，FSH）和黄体生成素（LH）。

The process is initiated by the release of the gonadotrophin-releasing hormone (GnRH), a major neurosecretion produced in the median eminence of the hypothalamus. This hormone is a decapeptide and is released from axon terminals into the pituitary portal capillaries. It results in the release of both follicle-stimulating hormone (FSH) and LH from the pituitary.

GnRH 的释放呈周期性波动，波峰数目的增加与血浆 LH 水平升高有关，血浆 LH 水平升高始于月经周期中期，而雌激素诱导的巨大 LH 峰出现则需要持续的 GnRH 刺激。研究发现月经期血清与尿中肽类激素 kisspeptin 水平可预测排卵。在月经周期前 5 天，kisspeptin 水平低。月经第 11 天左右，优势卵泡直径约 1.2cm 时，出现一个峰值。第二个峰值相对较小，出现在月经第 14 天左右。血清 kisspeptin 水平与 17β- 雌二醇（E$_2$）水平相关性好。kisspeptin 峰可能是排卵前优势卵泡发育的良好标志。

GnRH is released in episodic fluctuations, with an increase in the number of surges being associated with the higher levels of plasma LH commencing just before mid-cycle and continued ongoing GnRH action required to initiate the huge oestrogen-induced LH surge. Kisspeptin levels in the serum and urine have been studied during the menstrual cycle and found to be useful in the prediction of ovulation. During the first 5 days of the cycle, it is low. There is a surge around the eleventh day when the dominant follicle is about 1.2 cm. The second surge, which is smaller, is around the fourteenth day. Serum kisspeptin levels correlate well with 17-β oestradiol (E$_2$) levels. It appears that kisspeptin surge may be a good marker of the dominant follicle development prior to ovulation.

与生殖有关的三种重要激素包括 FSH、LH 和催乳素，由垂体前叶（或称腺垂体）产生。血 FSH 水平在月经期稍高，后水平下降，这是因为优势卵泡生成的雌二醇对 FSH 有负反馈作用。LH 在月经周期的前半阶段保持于相对稳定的水平，而排卵前 35~42h 有一个显著的 LH 峰和一个同步而较小的 FSH 峰（图 2-5）。事实上，LH 峰由 2 个邻近的峰组成，1 个血浆雌二醇峰在 LH 峰前出现。血浆 LH 和 FSH 水平在月经周期后半阶段略低于排卵前，但垂体持续释放 LH 对维持黄体正常功能是必要的。垂体促性腺激素对下丘脑活动的影响是通过促性腺激素与 FSH 和 LH 作用于卵巢而产生的卵巢激素之间的短环路反馈系统实现的。

The three major hormones involved in reproduction are produced by the anterior lobe of the pituitary gland or adenohypophysis and include FSH, LH and prolactin. Blood levels of FSH are slightly higher during menses and subsequently decline due to the negative feedback effect of the oestrogen production by the dominant follicle. LH levels appear to remain at a relatively constant level in the first half of the cycle; however, there is a marked surge of LH 35–42 hours before ovulation and a smaller coincidental FSH peak (see Fig. 2.5). The LH surge is, in fact, made up of two proximate surges, and a peak in plasma oestradiol precedes the LH surge. Plasma LH and FSH levels are slightly lower in the second half of the cycle than in the preovulatory phase, but continued LH release by the pituitary is necessary for normal corpus luteum function. Pituitary gonadotrophins influence the activity of the hypothalamus by a short-loop feedback system between the gonadotrophins themselves and the effect of the ovarian hormones produced due to FSH and LH action on the ovaries.

雌激素的生成在月经周期前半阶段增加，在排卵后下降至卵泡期峰值的 60%，第 2 个高峰出现在黄体期。排卵前孕酮水平低，但在黄体期的大部分时间都是升高的。这些特征如图 2-5 所示。

Oestrogen production increases in the first half of the cycle, then falls to about 60% of its follicular phase peak following ovulation, and a second peak occurs in the luteal phase. Progesterone levels are low prior to ovulation but then become elevated throughout most of the luteal phase. These features are shown in Fig. 2.5.

> ✓ 经验
>
> 特定的反馈机制会调节垂体释放的 FSH 和 LH。这主要是通过卵巢产生的雌激素和孕酮实现的。卵巢功能衰竭时，如绝经期，由于卵巢产生的雌激素和孕酮缺乏，促性腺激素水平显著升高。抑制素 B 水平曾被认为可用于预测不孕女性的卵巢储备，但现已被证实并无太大作用。
>
> Certain feedback mechanisms regulate the release of FSH and LH by the pituitary. This is principally achieved by the oestrogens and progesterone produced by the ovaries. In the presence of ovarian failure, as seen in menopause, the gonadotrophin levels become markedly elevated because of the lack of ovarian oestrogen and progesterone production. Inhibin B levels were thought to predict the ovarian reserve in infertile women but have been shown not to be that useful.

催乳素是由垂体前叶的催乳素细胞分泌的。催乳素水平在月经周期中期略上升，但仍在正常范围内，与黄体期保持相似水平，并趋向于随血浆 17β- 雌二醇水平的改变而变化。催乳素主要通过下丘脑的一个短环路反馈系统控制自身的分泌，该系统可产生催乳素抑制因子多巴胺。在脑中枢作用下，雌激素除了可刺激释放多种神经递质，如 5- 羟色胺、

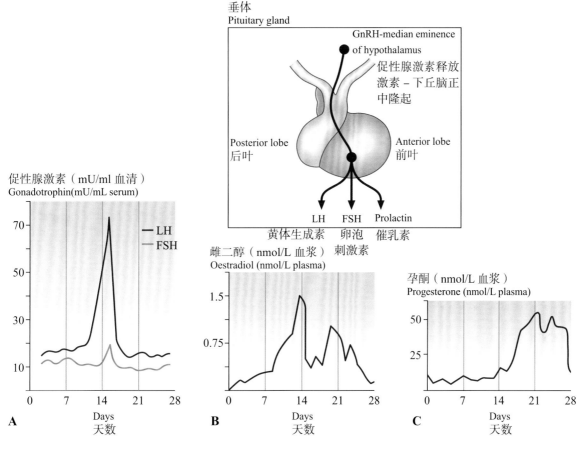

▲ 图 2-5　排卵的激素调节。促性腺激素释放激素（**GnRH**）刺激垂体前叶释放促性腺激素。图示在 28 天的月经周期中，血中黄体生成素（图 **A** 中 **LH**）和卵泡刺激素（**FSH**）、雌二醇（图 **B**）和孕酮（图 **C**）的水平。LSH. 叶黄素刺激素

Fig. 2.5　The hormonal regulation of ovulation. Gonadotrophin-releasing hormone (GnRH) stimulates the release of gonadotrophins from the anterior lobe of the pituitary. Blood levels of (A) luteinizing hormone (LH) and follicle-stimulating hormone (FSH); (B)oestradiol; and (C) progesterone during a 28-day menstrual cycle. LSH, Lutein-stimulating hormone

去甲肾上腺素、吗啡和脑啡肽外，还可刺激催乳素的释放。多巴胺拮抗药（如酚噻嗪、利血平和甲基酪氨酸）也可刺激催乳素释放，而多巴胺激动药（如溴隐亭和卡麦角林）则有相反的作用。

　　Prolactin is secreted by lactotrophs in the anterior lobe of the pituitary gland. Prolactin levels rise slightly at midcycle but are still within the normal range and remain at similar levels during the luteal phase and tend to follow the changes in plasma oestradiol-17 β levels. Prolactin tends to control its own secretion predominantly through a short-loop feedback system on the hypothalamus, which produces the prolactin-inhibiting factor, dopamine. Oestrogen appears to stimulate prolactin release in addition to the release of various neurotransmitters, such as serotonin, noradrenaline (norepinephrine), morphine and enkephalins, by a central action on the brain. Antagonists to dopamine such as phenothiazine, reserpine and methyltyrosine also stimulate the release of prolactin, whereas dopamine agonists such as bromocriptine and cabergoline have the opposite effect.

 经验

高泌乳素血症通过抑制下丘脑 GnRH 的生成和释放而抑制排卵，是继发性闭经和不孕的重要原因。

Hyperprolactinaemia prevents ovulation by an inhibitory effect on hypothalamic GnRH production and release and is an important cause of secondary amenorrhoea and infertility.

促性腺激素的作用（The action of gonadotrophins）

　　FSH 可刺激卵泡生长和发育，且仅与生长卵泡的颗粒细胞结合。在每个月经周期开始成熟的约 30 个卵泡中，有 1 个会变得突出，被称为优势卵泡。颗粒细胞产生雌激素，雌激素反馈抑制垂体的 FSH 释放，仅优势卵泡可获得足以使其继续发育的 FSH。同时，FSH 可刺激 LH 受体。

FSH stimulates follicular growth and development and binds exclusively to granulosa cells in the growing follicle. Of the 30 or so follicles that begin to mature in each menstrual cycle, one becomes pre-eminent and is called the *dominant follicle*. The granulosa cells produce oestrogen, which feeds back on the pituitary to suppress FSH release, with only the dominant follicle then getting enough FSH to continue further development. At the same time, FSH stimulates receptors for LH.

LH 可促进排卵过程，重新激活减数分裂期Ⅰ，维持黄体发育；LH 受体存在于黄体的膜细胞和颗粒细胞。在卵泡生长和成熟过程中，FSH 与 LH 存在密切的相互作用。黄体可生成雌激素和孕酮，直到黄体晚期开始退化（图 2–4）。

LH stimulates the process of ovulation, the reactivation of meiosis I and sustains the development of the corpus luteum; receptors for LH are found in the theca and granulosa cells and in the corpus luteum. There is a close interaction between FSH and LH in follicular growth and maturation. The corpus luteum produces oestrogen and progesterone until it begins to deteriorate in the late luteal phase (see Fig. 2.4).

三、子宫内膜周期（The endometrial cycle）

正常子宫内膜对卵巢甾体激素的波动有周期性反应。子宫内膜分 3 层，月经期间 2 个外层脱落（图 2–6）。

The normal endometrium responds in a cyclical manner to the fluctuations in ovarian steroids. The endometrium consists of three zones, and it is the two outer zones that are shed during menstruation (Fig. 2.6).

基底层是紧密基质薄层，与子宫肌层相互交错，对激素变化的反应不大。在月经期间不会脱落。邻近层（海绵层）含子宫内膜腺体，腺体被疏松基质包围的柱状上皮细胞覆盖。子宫内膜表面覆盖一层致密的上皮细胞（致密层），这层上皮细胞围绕着子宫内膜腺体的开口。子宫内膜周期分为 4 期。

The basal zone (*zona basalis*) is the thin layer of the compact stroma that interdigitates with the myometrium and shows little response to hormonal change. It is not shed at the time of menstruation. The next adjacent zone (*zona spongiosa*) contains the endometrial glands, which are lined by columnar epithelial cells surrounded by loose stroma. The surface of the endometrium is covered by a compact layer of epithelial cells (*zona compacta*) that surrounds the ostia of the endometrial glands. The endometrial cycle is divided into four phases:

1. 月经期。该期为月经周期的前 4 天，在该期子宫内膜最外 2 层脱落。月经来潮前螺旋小动脉出现节段性收缩，使子宫内膜功能层坏死和脱落。血管的变化与雌激素和孕酮水平的下降有关，但这些血管变化的机制由何介导尚不明确。临床上明确的是，

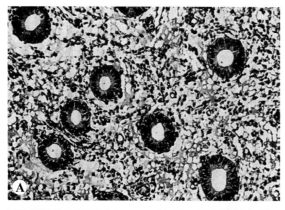
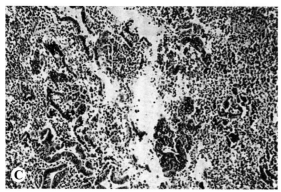
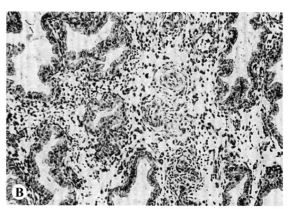

◀ 图 2–6　正常月经的周期性改变。**A.** 增殖期；**B.** 黄体中期；**C.** 月经期

Fig. 2.6　Cyclical changes in the normal menstrual cycle. (A) Proliferative phase. (B) Mid-luteal phase. (C) Menstrual phase

无论是雌激素或是孕酮下降，都会引起子宫内膜外层脱落，从而出现月经，若雌激素和孕酮水平同时下降（如排卵期结束），月经量通常会比较少，若仅雌激素水平下降（如无排卵的月经周期），月经量则通常比较多。

1. Menstrual phase. This occupies the first 4 days of the cycle and results in shedding of the outer two layers of the endometrium. The onset of menstruation is preceded by segmental vasoconstriction of the spiral arterioles. This leads to necrosis and shedding of the functional layers of the endometrium. The vascular changes are associated with a fall in both oestrogen and progesterone levels, but the mechanism by which these vascular changes are mediated is still not understood. What is clear clinically is that the menstruation due to the shedding of the outer layers of the endometrium occurs whether oestrogen or progesterone, or both, fall, with the loss generally being less if both the oestrogen and progesterone levels fall (as at the end of an ovulatory cycle), and heavier when only the oestrogen level falls (as in an anovulatory cycle).

2. 修复期。这个阶段为月经的第 4 天至第 7 天，与盘曲动脉形成新毛细血管床及上皮再生有关。

2. Phase of repair. This phase extends from day 4 to day 7 and is associated with the formation of a new capillary bed arising from the arterial coils and with the regeneration of the epithelial surface.

3. 卵泡期或增殖期。这是子宫内膜生长最旺盛的时期，伴随着腺体的拉长、扩张及基质的发育。该期从月经第 7 天持续至排卵日（通常为月经第 14 天）。

3. Follicular or proliferative phase. This is the period of maximal growth of the endometrium and is associated with elongation and expansion of the glands and with stromal development. This phase extends from day 7 until the day of ovulation (generally day 14 of the cycle).

4. 黄体期或分泌期。该期从排卵后持续至 14 天后下次月经开始。在该期，子宫内膜腺体盘曲，外观呈锯齿状。上皮细胞呈现基底空泡化，到黄体中期（28 天的月经周期中约为第 20 天），这些细胞中可见分泌物。随后分泌物浓缩，当月经来潮时出现基质水肿和假蜕膜反应。月经来潮 2 天内，基质内出现白细胞浸润。

4. Luteal or secretory phase. This follows ovulation and continues until 14 days later when menstruation starts again. During this phase, the endometrial glands become convoluted and 'saw-toothed' in appearance. The epithelial cells exhibit basal vacuolation, and by the mid-luteal phase (about day 20 of a 28-day cycle), there is visible secretion in these cells.

The secretion subsequently becomes inspissated and, as menstruation approaches, there is oedema of the stroma and a pseudodecidual reaction. Within 2 days of menstruation, there is infiltration of the stroma by leukocytes.

已知在无排卵情况下可发生卵泡黄素化，卵母细胞可能会滞留在卵泡中。这被称为滞留排卵或未破卵泡黄素化（luteinized unruptured follice，LUF）综合征，这种情况下孕酮正常生成，月经周期正常。子宫内膜组织学检查一般可精确判断月经周期所处阶段，可为排卵提供重要证据。

It is now clear that luteinization of the follicle can occur in the absence of the release of the oocyte, which may remain entrapped in the follicle. This condition is described as *entrapped ovulation* or luteinized unruptured follicle (LUF) syndrome and is associated with normal progesterone production and an apparently normal ovulatory cycle. Histological examination of the endometrium generally enables precise dating of the menstrual cycle and is particularly important in providing presumptive evidence of ovulation.

四、精子的产生（Production of sperm）

（一）精子发生（Spermatogenesis）

睾丸具有精子发生和雄激素分泌的双重功能。FSH 主要负责刺激精子发生，LH 主要负责刺激睾丸间质细胞和生成睾酮。

The testis combines the dual function of spermatogenesis and androgen secretion. FSH is predominantly responsible for stimulation of spermatogenesis and LH for the stimulation of Leydig cells and the production of testosterone.

精子完全成熟需 64～70 天（图 2-7）。睾丸中可看到精子成熟的所有阶段。自青春期后至老年，经有丝分裂增殖产生大量细胞（称为精原细胞）。这些精原细胞在睾丸内转化为精母细胞，然后开始减数第一次分裂。与女性相同，在这个阶段染色单体发生交换，使所有源于同一细胞的配子都各不相同。精母细胞和精子细胞均来自精原细胞。最终精子生成，被释放入生精小管腔，后进入输精管。最终排精时减数分裂 II 已完成。直到精子通过附睾和精囊，在子宫或输卵管内有合适的内分泌环境，并黏附于卵母细胞，才能实现精子的完全获能，使受精能够发生。

The full maturation of spermatozoa takes about 64–70 days (Fig. 2.7). All phases of maturation can be seen in the testis. Mitotic proliferation produces large numbers of cells

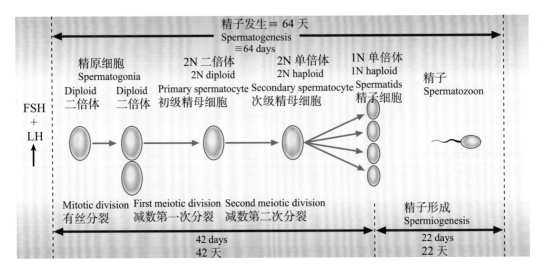

▲ 图 2-7　精子成熟

Fig. 2.7　The maturation cycle of spermatozoa

(called *spermatogonia*) after puberty until late in life. These spermatogonia are converted to spermatocytes within the testis, and then the first meiotic division commences. As in the female, during this phase, chromatid exchange occurs, resulting in all gametes being different despite coming from the same original cell. Spermatocytes and spermatids are produced from the spermatogonia. Spermatozoa are finally produced and released into the lumen of the seminiferous tubules and then into the vas deferens. At the time of this final release, meiosis II has been completed. Full capacitation of the sperm, to enable fertilization to occur, is not achieved until the sperm have passed through the epididymis and seminal vesicles, augmented by a suitable endocrine environment in the uterus or Fallopian tube and finally when the spermatozoon becomes adherent to the oocyte.

（二）精子结构（Structure of the spermatozoon）

精子由头、中段和尾组成（图 2-8）。头部扁平，卵圆形，并覆盖顶体帽，其中包含一些溶素。

The spermatozoon consists of a head, midpiece and tail (Fig. 2.8). The head is flattened and ovoid in shape and is covered by the acrosomal cap, which contains several lysins.

精子核内密集地堆积着精子的遗传物质。中段包含近端和远端 2 个中心粒，构成精子尾的起始部分。远端中心粒在成熟精子中是退化的，但在精子细胞内的是功能性的。精子体部有螺旋结构的线粒体，为精子运动提供"动力源"。

The nucleus is densely packed with the genetic material of the sperm. The midpiece contains two centrioles, proximal and distal, which form the beginning of the tail. The distal centriole is vestigial in mature spermatozoa but is functional in

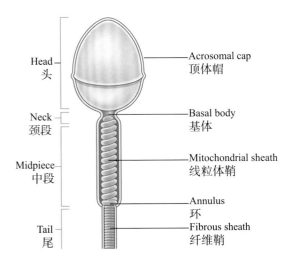

▲ 图 2-8　正常精子结构

Fig. 2.8　Structure of the mature spermatozoon

the spermatid. The body contains a coiled helix of mitochondria that provides the 'powerhouse' for sperm motility.

精子尾由中心 2 条纵向纤维和围绕它们的 9 对纤维组成，这 9 对纤维终止于不同点，直到剩余 1 根卵圆形单纤维。这些有收缩性的纤维可驱动精子。

The tail consists of a central core of two longitudinal fibres surrounded by nine pairs of fibres that terminate at various points until a single ovoid filament remains. These contractile fibres propel the spermatozoa.

（三）精浆（Seminal plasma）

精子的营养储备少，因此需依赖精浆进行营养支持。精浆来源于前列腺、精囊、输精管和尿道球腺。精浆果糖含量高，是精子的主要能量来源。精浆也含高水平氨基酸，尤其是谷氨酸和一些独特的胺，如精胺和亚精胺。

Spermatozoa carry little nutritional reserve and therefore depend on seminal plasma for nutritional support. Seminal plasma originates from the prostate, the seminal vesicles, the vas deferens and the bulbourethral glands. There is a high concentration of fructose, which is the major source of energy for the spermatozoa. The plasma also contains high concentrations of amino acids, particularly glutamic acid, and several unique amines such as spermine and spermidine.

精浆也含高水平的前列腺素，对子宫平滑肌有强刺激作用。正常精液在射精后很快凝结，但在纤溶酶作用下可于 30min 内液化。

Seminal plasma also contains high concentrations of prostaglandins, which have a potent stimulatory effect on uterine musculature. Normal semen clots shortly after ejaculation but liquefies within 30 minutes through the action of fibrinolytic enzymes.

五、受精（Fertilization）

受精过程包括雄配子和雌配子的结合，产生来自配偶双方基因的二倍体。

The process of fertilization involves the fusion of the male and female gametes to produce the diploid genetic complement from the genes of both partners.

（一）精子运输（Sperm transport）

精液在子宫颈附近沉积后，迅速迁移进入子宫颈黏液。这种迁移的速度取决于月经周期中期是否存在可接受精子的黏液。在黄体期，不接受精子进入，因此极少有精子到达子宫腔。在有利的环境下，精子以 6mm/min 的速度移动。这比精子自身的运动速度快得多，因此也必须依赖于子宫腔的支持。只有活动精子才能到达输卵管伞端，发生受精。

Following the deposition of semen near the cervical os, migration occurs rapidly into the cervical mucus. The speed of this migration depends on the presence of receptive mucus in mid-cycle. During the luteal phase, the mucus is not receptive to sperm invasion and, therefore, very few spermatozoa reach the uterine cavity. Under favourable circumstances, sperm migrate at a rate of 6 mm/min. This is much faster than could be explained by the motility of the sperm and must therefore also be dependent on active support within the uterine cavity. Only motile spermatozoa reach the fimbriated end of the tube,

where fertilization occurs

（二）获能（Capacitation）

在精子通过输卵管时，会进入成熟的最后阶段（获能），这使精子能够穿过透明带。这些变化可能是由酶诱导的，如 β- 淀粉酶或 β- 葡糖醛酸糖苷酶可能作用于精子膜，提示存在与精子穿透有关的受体位点。此外，确认了各种其他在精子获能过程中发挥重要作用的因素，如从精子质膜中去除胆固醇，以及精子存在 α 和 β 肾上腺素受体。直到最近，获能仍被认为只能在输卵管内发生。不过，获能也可以在体外相对简单的培养液中被明显非特异的效果诱导。

During their passage through the Fallopian tubes, the sperm undergo the final stage in maturation (capacitation), which enables penetration of the zona pellucida. It seems likely that these changes are enzyme induced, and enzymes such as β-amylase or β-glucuronidase may act on the membranes of the spermatozoa to expose receptor sites involved in sperm penetration. In addition, various other factors that may be important in capacitation have been identified, such as the removal of cholesterol from the plasma membrane and the presence of α- and β-adrenergic receptors on the spermatozoa. Until recently, it was thought that capacitation occurred only in vivo in the Fallopian tubes. However, it can also be induced in vitro by apparently nonspecific effects of relatively simple culture solutions.

附睾尾和精浆中的抑制性物质可阻止获能，这些物质也存在于女性生殖道下游。这些物质似乎可在精卵结合前短暂地保护精子。

Inhibitory substances in the plasma of the cauda epididymis and in seminal plasma can prevent capacitation, and these substances also exist in the lower reaches of the female genital tract. It seems likely that these substances protect the sperm until shortly before fusion with the oocyte.

（三）受精与着床（Fertilization and implantation）

仅少量精子可到达输卵管壶腹部，围绕卵母细胞的透明带。精子黏附于卵母细胞引起顶体反应，该过程中顶体帽失去质膜（图 2-9A）。

Only a small number of spermatozoa reach the oocyte in the ampulla of the tube and surround the zona pellucida. The adherence of the sperm to the oocyte initiates the *acrosome reaction*, which involves the loss of plasma membrane over the acrosomal cap (Fig. 2.9A).

该过程中会释放溶解酶，使卵母细胞膜更易于穿透。一般来说，仅 1 个精子头可与卵母细胞质膜融合，该精子头和中段会通过吞噬作用进入卵母细胞。

The process allows the release of lytic enzymes, which facilitate penetration of the oocyte membrane. Generally, only one sperm head fuses with the oocyte plasma membrane, and by phagocytosis the sperm head and midpiece are engulfed into the oocyte.

精子的头部脱落形成雄原核，最终与卵中的雌原核结合形成合子。原核的核膜分解以促进双方染色体混合。这个过程被称为融合生殖（图 2-9B 和 C），随后几乎立即发生第一次卵裂。

The sperm head decondenses to form the male pronucleus and eventually becomes apposed to the female pronucleus in the female egg to form the *zygote*. The membranes of the pronuclei break down to facilitate the fusion of male and female chromosomes. This process is known as *syngamy* (see Fig. 2.9B, C) and is followed almost immediately by the first cleavage division.

受精后 36h 内，孕体通过输卵管的肌蠕动传输。受精卵经过卵裂，在 16 细胞期变成 1 个实心细胞球，即桑葚胚。桑葚胚内出现充满液体的腔，形成囊胚（图 2-10）。排卵后 6 天，囊胚的胚极附着于子宫内膜，通常靠近子宫腔中部。至排卵后第 7 天，囊胚已经深侵入子宫内膜。

During the 36 hours after fertilization, the conceptus is transported through the tube by muscular peristaltic action. The zygote undergoes cleavage and, at the 16-cell stage, becomes a solid ball of cells known as a *morula*. A fluid-filled cavity develops within the morula to form the *blastocyst* (Fig. 2.10). Six days after ovulation, the embryonic pole of the blastocyst attaches itself to the endometrium, usually near to the mid-portion of the uterine cavity. By the seventh post-ovulatory day, the blastocyst has penetrated deeply into the endometrium.

子宫内膜细胞被细胞滋养层破坏，通过融合与吞噬作用进入滋养层。子宫内膜基质细胞增大、变淡，即为蜕膜反应。

Endometrial cells are destroyed by the cytotrophoblast, and the cells are incorporated by fusion and phagocytosis into the trophoblast. The endometrial stromal cells become large and pale; this is known as the *decidual reaction*.

受精和着床过程就此完成。

The processes of fertilization and implantation are now complete.

六、性交生理学（The physiology of coitus）

正常性唤起在男性与女性中均被分为 4 期，其

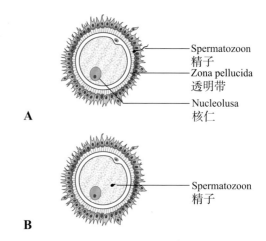

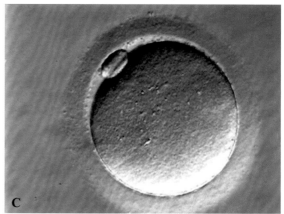

▲ 图 2-9　A. 精子黏附于卵母细胞引起顶体反应；B 和 C. 融合生殖指精子头内的核进入卵母细胞的胞质，形成合子

Fig. 2.9 (A) Adherence of the sperm to the oocyte initiates the acrosome reaction. (B, C) Syngamy involves the passage of the nucleus of the sperm head into the cytoplasm of the oocyte with the formation of the zygote

中包括兴奋期、平台期、高潮期和消退期。男性兴奋期阴茎的静脉收缩，导致勃起。这是通过骶 2 和骶 3 的副交感神经丛介导的。在高潮期，阴茎维持充血状态，睾丸增大，睾丸和阴囊升高。尿道球腺的分泌物使尿道口出现透明液体。这些变化伴随全身特征，其中包括骨骼肌张力增加、通气过度和心动过速。

Normal sexual arousal has been described in four levels in both the male and the female. These levels consist of excitement, plateau, orgasmic and resolution phases. In the male, the *excitement phase* results in compression of the venous channels of the penis, resulting in erection. This is mediated through the parasympathetic plexus through S2 and S3. During the *plateau phase*, the penis remains engorged and the testes increase in size, with elevation of the testes and scrotum. Secretion from the bulbourethral glands results in the appearance of a clear fluid at the urethral meatus. These changes are accompanied by general

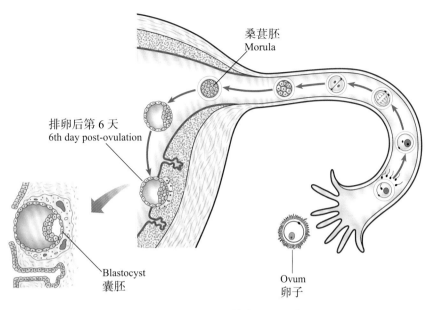

桑葚胚
Morula

排卵后第 6 天
6th day post-ovulation

Blastocyst
囊胚

Ovum
卵子

▲ 图 2-10　从受精至着床的发育阶段
Fig. 2.10　Stages of development from fertilization to implantation

systemic features, including increased skeletal muscle tension, hyperventilation and tachycardia.

! 注意

勃起功能障碍可能是脊髓或大脑神经损伤的结果，也可能是脊柱裂、多发性硬化症和糖尿病神经病变的结果。然而，已知超过 200 种处方药会导致阳痿，占所有病例的 25%。娱乐性药物（如酒精、尼古丁、可卡因、大麻和麦角酰二乙酰胺）也可能导致阳痿；不过，这通常可以通过服用药物枸橼酸西地那非（伟哥）来改善。性刺激可导致局部一氧化氮释放。5- 磷酸二酯酶（PDE₅）抑制药会导致海绵体中环磷酸鸟苷（cGMP）水平升高，可使平滑肌松弛和血液进入海绵体，导致勃起。因此，在无性刺激的情况下，该药物无效。

Erectile dysfunction may result from neurological damage to the spinal cord or the brain and is seen as a result of spina bifida, multiple sclerosis and diabetic neuropathy. However, over 200 prescription drugs are known to cause impotence, and these account for some 25% of all cases. Recreational drugs such as alcohol, nicotine, cocaine, marijuana and LSD may also cause impotence; however, this can usually be improved by the male taking the pharmacological preparation sildenafil citrate (Viagra). Sexual stimulation causes local release of nitric oxide. Inhibition of phosphor diesterase type 5 (PDE5) results in increased levels of cyclic guanosine monophosphate (cGMP) in the corpus cavernosum. This leads to smooth muscle relaxation and inflow of blood to the corpus cavernosum, causing the erection. Hence the drug has no effect in the absence of sexual stimulation.

高潮期是由阴茎头刺激和阴茎体皮肤运动引起的。出现球海绵体肌与坐骨海绵体肌反射性收缩，精液接连射出。出现以阴茎插入为特征的特定肌肉骨骼活动。通气过度和快速呼吸的全身变化持续存在。

The *orgasmic phase* is induced by stimulation of the glans penis and by movement of penile skin on the penile shaft. There are reflex contractions of the bulbocavernosus and ischiocavernosus muscles and ejaculation of semen in a series of spurts. Specific musculoskeletal activity occurs that is characterized by penile thrusting. The systemic changes of hyperventilation and rapid respiration persist.

遗精是交感神经的作用。精液排出是由精囊、射精管和前列腺的平滑肌收缩引起的。

Seminal emission depends on the sympathetic nervous system. Expulsion of semen is brought about by contraction of smooth muscle within the seminal vesicles, ejaculatory ducts and prostate.

在消退期，阴茎勃起迅速平息，过度通气与心动过速也迅速恢复。30%～40% 的人有明显出汗反应。在该阶段，男性对进一步刺激无反应。如果不射精，高潮期可能会延长。

During the *resolution phase*, penile erection rapidly subsides, as do the hyperventilation and tachycardia. There is a marked sweating reaction in some 30–40% of individuals. During this phase, the male becomes refractory to further stimulation. The plateau phase may be prolonged if ejaculation does not occur.

女性兴奋期表现包括乳头和阴蒂勃起、阴道润滑（部分来自阴道渗出液，部分来自 Bartholin 腺分泌物）、大阴唇和小阴唇增厚充血，以及子宫充血。刺激阴蒂和阴唇可进入高潮期，阴道外 1/3 缩窄，阴道穹隆膨起。阴道壁充血并呈紫色，阴道血流量显著增加。高潮时，阴蒂收缩到耻骨联合下，阴道壁和盆底连续收缩，约每秒 1 次，持续几秒钟。同时出现脉率增加、通气过度和特定的骨骼肌收缩。血压升高，意识水平有所下降。高潮时阴道内和子宫内的压力都会增加。

In the female, the *excitement phase* involves nipple and clitoral erection, vaginal lubrication (resulting partly from vaginal transudation and partly from secretions from Bartholin's glands), thickening and congestion of the labia majora and the labia minora and engorgement of the uterus. Stimulation of the clitoris and the labia results in progression to the *orgasmic platform*, with narrowing of the outer third of the vagina and ballooning of the vaginal vault. The vaginal walls become congested and purplish in colour, and there is a marked increase in vaginal blood flow. During orgasm, the clitoris retracts below the pubic symphysis and a succession of contractions occurs in the vaginal walls and pelvic floor approximately every second for several seconds. At the same time, there is an increase in pulse rate, hyperventilation and specific skeletal muscular contractions. Blood pressure rises, and there is some diminution in the level of awareness. Both intravaginal and intrauterine pressures rise during orgasm.

女性高潮期可持续并出现多重高潮。高潮后，盆腔器官的充血迅速消失，心动过速、血压升高和出汗反应可能会持续。

The *plateau phase* may bc sustained in the female and result in multiple orgasms. Following orgasm, resolution of the congestion of the pelvic organs occurs rapidly, although the tachycardia and hypertension, accompanied by a sweating reaction, may persist.

人类性行为的决定因素远复杂于刺激阴蒂或阴茎唤起的简单过程。尽管性交和高潮的频率随年龄增长而下降，但这在一定程度上是因为对伴侣失去兴趣。女性晚年仍可达性高潮，但她的行为实质上是由对男性伴侣的兴趣决定的。男性的性兴趣和性能力也随年龄增长而下降，高龄男性的兴奋和勃起需要更多时间。射精可能变得不那么频繁和有力。

Factors that determine human sexuality are far more complex than the simple process of arousal by clitoral or penile stimulation. Although the frequency of intercourse and orgasm declines with age, this is in part mediated by loss of interest by the partners. The female remains capable of orgasm until late in life, but her behaviour is substantially determined by the interest of the male partner. Sexual interest and performance also decline with age in the male, and the older male requires more time to achieve excitement and erection. Ejaculation may become less frequent and forceful.

常见的性问题会在第 19 章中讨论。

Common sexual problems are discussed in Chapter 19.

本章概览	Essential information
卵子发生 • 原始生殖细胞出现在卵黄囊中 • 至 20 周，卵原细胞达 700 万 • 出生时卵母细胞数量降至 100 万 • 至青春期该数目降至约 40 万 • 配子中染色体数目为正常细胞的一半 • 初级卵母细胞可停滞在减数分裂前期 10～50 年 • 当卵子进入输卵管，减数第二次分裂开始	**Oogenesis** • Primordial germ cells appear in the yolk sac • By 20 weeks, there are 7 million oogonia • Number of oocytes falls to 1 million by birth • Number falls to about 0.4 million by puberty • Chromosome number in gametes is half that of normal cells • Primary oocyte remains in suspended prophase for 10–50 years • The second meiotic division commences as the ovum enters the tube
卵巢内卵泡发育 • 大多数卵子永远不会成熟，每月约有 800 个卵子丢失 • 卵泡周围的基质细胞聚集成卵泡膜细胞 • 最内层的颗粒细胞形成放射冠 • 黄体在排卵后形成	**Follicular development in the ovary** • Most ova never reach advanced maturity, and about 800 are lost each month • Aggregation of stromal cells around follicles become thecal cells • Innermost layers of granulosa cells form the corona radiata • After ovulation, the corpus luteum is formed
激素事件与排卵 • FSH 刺激卵泡生长 • FSH 刺激 LH 受体发育 • LH 刺激排卵，诱导和维持黄体发育 • 卵泡产生雌激素 • 黄体产生雌激素和孕酮	**Hormonal events and ovulation** • FSH stimulates follicular growth • FSH stimulates LH receptor development • LH stimulates ovulation and stimulates and sustains development of the corpus luteum • Follicles produce oestrogen • Corpus luteum produces oestrogen and progesterone

（续表）

本章概览	Essential information

子宫内膜周期
- 月经期：子宫内膜功能层脱落
- 修复期：月经周期第 4～7 天
- 卵泡期：雌激素带来子宫内膜腺体的最大程度生长
- 黄体期：基质中"锯齿状"腺体、假蜕膜反应

精子发生
- 完全成熟需 64～70 天
- 成熟精子源于单倍体精子细胞

精子结构
- 精子头覆盖顶体帽
- 体部含有线粒体螺旋
- 精子尾由 2 根纵向纤维和 9 对纤维组成

精浆
- 源于前列腺、精囊和尿道球腺
- 高浓度果糖为精子运动供能
- 含高水平前列腺素

精子运输
- 快速移动进入接受性宫颈黏液
- 精子以 6mm/min 的速度移动
- 仅活动精子可到达输卵管伞端

获能
- 精子最终在通过输卵管时成熟
- 在附睾尾和精浆中产生抑制性物质

受精
- 少量精子到达卵母细胞
- 精子黏附启动顶体反应
- 精子头与卵母细胞质膜融合
- 精子头和中段被吞入卵母细胞
- 男性和女性染色体混合被称为融合生殖
- 受精 36h 后桑葚胚形成
- 受精 6 天后发生着床

性交生理学
- 阴茎勃起是静脉收缩的结果
- 球海绵体和坐骨海绵体肌收缩引起射精
- 女性性兴奋导致乳头和阴蒂勃起
- 润滑来自阴道渗出物和 Bartholin 腺分泌物
- 性高潮导致阴蒂收缩和盆底肌收缩

The endometrial cycle
- Menstrual phase-shedding of functional layer of endometrium
- Phase of repair-day 4–7 of cycle
- Follicular phase-maximum period of growth of endometrial glands due to oestrogen
- Luteal phase-'saw-toothed' glands, pseudodecidual reaction in stroma

Spermatogenesis
- Full maturation takes 64–70 days
- Mature sperm arise from haploid spermatids

Structure of spermatozoon
- Head is covered by acrosomal cap
- Body contains helix of mitochondria
- Tail consists of two longitudinal fibres and nine pairs of fibres

Seminal plasma
- Originates from the prostate, seminal vesicles and bulbourethral glands
- High concentration of fructose provides energy for sperm motility
- High concentration of prostaglandins

Sperm transport
- Rapid migration into receptive cervical mucus
- Sperm migrate at 6 mm/min
- Only motile sperm reach the fimbriated ends of the tubes

Capacitation
- Final sperm maturation occurs during passage through the oviduct
- Inhibitory substances produced in caudoepididymis and in seminal plasma

Fertilization
- Small number of sperm reaches oocyte
- Adherence of sperm initiates the acrosome reaction
- Sperm head fuses with oocyte plasma membrane
- Sperm head and midpiece engulfed into oocyte
- Fusion of male and female chromosomes is known as syngamy
- Thirty-six hours after fertilization, the morula is formed
- Six days after fertilization, implantation occurs

Physiology of coitus
- Penile erection results from compression of venous channels
- Ejaculation mediated by contractions of bulbocavernosus and ischiocavernosus
- Female excitation results in nipple and clitoral erection
- Lubrication comes from vaginal transudation, Bartholin's glands secretions
- Orgasm results in clitoral retraction and contractions of pelvic floor muscles

第3章　妊娠生理变化
Physiological changes in pregnancy

Fiona Broughton Pipkin　著　　高姗姗　译　　崔琳琳　陈子江　校

学习目标	LEARNING OUTCOMES
学习本章后你应当能够：	After studying this chapter you should be able to:
知识标准	**Knowledge criteria**
• 理解妊娠免疫学	• Understand the immunology of pregnancy
• 描述妊娠期间子宫、阴道和乳房的变化	• Describe the changes in the uterus, vagina and breasts that take place in pregnancy
• 描述心血管、内分泌、呼吸、肾脏和胃肠系统对妊娠的适应性变化	• Describe the adaptations of the cardiovascular, endocrine, respiratory, renal and gastrointestinal systems to pregnancy
临床技能	**Clinical competencies**
• 解释与妊娠期心血管、呼吸、胃肠道和肾脏相关指标有关的各种检验的临床和研究发现	• Interpret the clinical findings and investigatory findings of various tests related to cardiovascular, respiratory, gastrointestinal and renal parameters in pregnancy
专业技能和意见	**Professional skills and attitudes**
• 描述妊娠期的生理性适应对母体健康的影响	• Describe the impact of the physiological adaptation to pregnancy on the wellbeing of the mother

女性在每个排卵周期的黄体期都会出现许多对妊娠的适应性变化，如心率增加和肾血流量增加，因此这些反应是主动性的而不是反应性的，只是在妊娠初期被放大了。这非常有力地表明这些变化是由孕激素驱动的。所有的生理系统都会受到一定程度的影响，并且还会因年龄、胎次、多胎妊娠、社会经济地位和种族等因素而在生理范围内有所不同。

Many maternal adaptations to pregnancy, such as an increased heart rate and renal blood flow, are initiated in the luteal phase of every ovulatory cycle and are thus proactive rather than reactive, simply being amplified during the first trimester should conception occur. This suggests very strongly that they are driven by progesterone. All physiological systems are affected to some degree and will also vary within a physiological range because of factors such as age, parity, multiple pregnancy, socioeconomic status and race.

从目的论的角度来看，这些变化有 2 个主要原因。

From a teleological point of view, there are two main reasons for these changes:

- 为胎儿的营养、生长发育提供合适的环境。

- To provide a suitable environment for the nutrition, growth and development of the fetus.

- 为母亲的分娩过程及随后新生儿营养支持和养育做好保护和准备工作。

- To protect and prepare the mother for the process of parturition and subsequent support and nurture of the newborn infant.

一、妊娠免疫学（Immunology of pregnancy）

妊娠违背了移植免疫学的规则。胎儿是同种异体移植物，根据保护"自我"免受"非自我"侵害的原则，"理应"被母亲排斥。而母亲在应答并破坏其他外来抗原的同时，却不排斥胎儿并赋予了新生儿被动免疫力。子宫不是一个免疫豁免部位，因为植入子宫的其他组织会被排斥。

Pregnancy defies the laws of transplant immunology. The fetus is an allograft that, according to the laws that protect 'self' from 'non-self', 'should' be rejected by the mother. Furthermore, the mother continues to respond to and destroy other foreign antigens and confers passive immunity to the newborn while not rejecting the fetus. The uterus is not an immunologically privileged site, because other tissues implanted in the uterus are rejected.

保护必须自子宫蜕膜化后植入时开始。蜕膜包含所有常见的免疫细胞类型，如淋巴细胞和巨噬细胞，但也包含其他细胞类型，如大颗粒淋巴细胞。巨噬细胞可以引发和引导几乎所有的免疫反应，其中包括 T 细胞和 B 细胞的免疫反应，从而诱导适应性免疫。简单地说，它们能够通过促进或抑制增殖来"杀死或修复"组织，这取决于它们是否将精氨酸代谢为一氧化氮或鸟氨酸。处于"杀死"状态的巨噬细胞被称为 M_1 巨噬细胞，处于"修复"状态的巨噬细胞被称为 M_2 巨噬细胞。M_1 状态在植入时占主导地位，一旦胎盘到胎儿的血液供应充足，便切换为 M_2 状态。

Protection must occur from the time of implantation when the endometrium decidualizes. The decidua contains all the common immunological cell types, e.g. lymphocytes and macrophages, but it also contains additional cell types, e.g. large granular lymphocytes. Macrophages appear to initiate and direct almost all immune responses, including those of T and B cells, inducing adaptive immunity. Crudely speaking, they are able to 'kill or repair' tissues by promoting or inhibiting proliferation, depending on whether they metabolize arginine to nitric oxide or to ornithine. Macrophages in the 'kill' state are known as M_1 *macrophages* and those in the 'repair' state are known as M_2 *macrophages*. The M_1 state predominates around the time of implantation, switching to a predominantly M_2 state once there is an adequate placento-fetal blood supply.

仅有 2 种类型的胎儿胎盘组织与母体组织直接接触，即绒毛和绒毛外滋养层细胞（EVT），并且人类对滋养层细胞实际上没有系统性的母体 T 细胞或 B 细胞反应。浸于母体血液中的绒毛滋养细胞似乎具有免疫学惰性，并且从不表达人类白细胞抗原（human leucocyte antigen，HLA） I 类或 II 类分子。直接与子宫内膜 / 蜕膜组织接触的 EVT 不表达主要的 T 细胞配体、HLA-A 或 HLA-B，但表达 HLA I 类滋养细胞特异性 HLA-G、HLA-C 和 HLA-E，HLA-G 具有很强的免疫抑制性。

Only two types of fetoplacental tissue come into direct contact with maternal tissues: the villous and extravillous trophoblast (EVT), and there are effectively no systemic maternal T- or B-cell responses to trophoblast cells in humans. The villous trophoblast, which is bathed by maternal blood, seems to be immunologically inert and never expresses human leucocyte antigen (HLA) class I or class II molecules. EVT, which is directly in contact with endometrial/decidual tissues, does not express the major T-cell ligands, HLA-A or HLA-B, but does express the HLA class I trophoblast-specific HLA-G, which is strongly immunosuppressive; HLA-C; and HLA-E.

与体循环不同，蜕膜淋巴细胞的主要类型是子宫自然杀伤（NK）细胞。它们表达表面杀伤性免疫球蛋白样受体（KIR），该受体可与滋养细胞上的 HLA-C 和 HLA-G 结合。KIR 具有高度多态性，主要分为两类，即 KIR-A（非激活）和 KIR-B（多次激活）。HLA-E 和 HLA-G 实际上是单态的，但 HLA-C 是多态的，具有两个主要组，即 HLA-C1 和 HLA-C2。因此，母体组织中的多态性 KIR 和胎儿中的多态性 HLA-C 构成了一个潜在多变的受体 – 配体系统。研究表明如果母体的 KIR 单倍型为 AA 而滋养细胞表达任何 HLA-C2，与浅层侵袭相关的流产或先兆子痫风险显著增加。而 KIR-B 则能起到保护作用。HLA-C2 对滋养细胞的迁移具有高度抑制作用，因此可能需要"激活 KIR"来克服。

The main type of decidual lymphocytes are the uterine natural killer (NK) cells, which differ from those in the systemic circulation. They express surface killer immunoglobulin-like receptors (KIRs), which bind to HLA-C and HLA-G on trophoblasts. The KIRs are highly polymorphic, with two main classes: the KIR-A (non-activating) and KIR-B (multiply activating). HLA-E and HLA-G are effectively monomorphic, but HLA-C is polymorphic, with two main groups: the HLA-C1 and the HLA-C2. Thus, the very polymorphic KIR in maternal tissues and the polymorphic HLA-C in the fetus make up a potentially very variable receptor-ligand system. It has been shown that if the maternal KIR haplotype is AA and the trophoblast expresses any HLA-C2, then the possibility of miscarriage or pre-eclampsia, both associated with shallow invasion, is significantly increased. However, even one KIR-B provides protection. HLA-C2 is highly inhibitory to trophoblast migration and thus appears to need 'activating KIR' to overcome it.

在孕早期的蜕膜中发现了 NK 衍生的 CD56$^+$ 颗粒状淋巴细胞。他们释放转化生长因子 β$_2$，也具有免疫抑制活性。

A population of NK-derived, CD56$^+$ granulated lymphocytes is found in first-trimester decidua. They release transforming growth factor-β$_2$, which also has immunosuppressive activity.

胎儿表达父系抗原可以刺激母体抗体的产生。反之，胎儿中存在母体抗体则证实胎盘不是不可通过的免疫屏障。妊娠也可能诱导阻断性抗体，但这些似乎对妊娠的延续并不重要。低级别炎症标志物，如 C 反应肽和 GlycA 升高，表明母亲的基础免疫力增强。正常妊娠可能将适应性免疫反应转向 Th$_2$ 反应，表现为循环白细胞介素（IL）-18 增加，IL-12p70 降低。

The fetus expresses paternal antigens, and these can stimulate the production of maternal antibodies. Conversely, maternal antibodies are present in the fetus, confirming that the placenta is not an impermeable immunological barrier. Pregnancy may also induce blocking antibodies, but these do not appear to be vital to the continuation of pregnancy. Low-grade inflammatory markers such as C-reactive peptide and GlycA are increased, suggesting enhanced maternal innate immunity. Normal pregnancy seems to shift the adaptive immune response towards the Th$_2$ response, with increased circulating interleukin (IL)-18 and lower IL-12p70.

尽管胎儿需要避免受到攻击，但这要付出一定的代价，因为妊娠中被部分抑制的免疫状态使得新的感染、寄生虫病（如疟疾）和潜伏病毒的重新激活更加危险。约 40% 的早产与感染有关。胎盘和蜕膜细胞表达大多数 Toll 样受体（TLR），并且当存在 TLR– 配体活化时，会表达各种细胞因子和趋化因子，如白介素。

While the fetus needs to avoid attack, this carries a cost, as the partly suppressed immune state in pregnancy makes new

infections, parasitic diseases (e.g. malaria) and reactivation of latent viruses potentially more dangerous. Infections are involved in some 40% of pre-term deliveries. The placental and decidual cells express most toll-like receptors (TLRs), and when there is TLR-ligand activation, various cytokines and chemokines, such as the interleukins, are expressed.

胸腺在妊娠期间显示出一些可逆的退化，显然是由孕激素驱动的淋巴细胞从胸腺皮质外移引起的，Th$_1$ 与 Th$_2$ 细胞因子比例向 Th$_2$ 移动。相反，妊娠期间脾脏增大可能是由于红细胞和免疫球蛋白生成细胞的合成加速导致。引流子宫的主动脉旁淋巴结的体积可能会增加，尽管这些淋巴结的生发中心可能会缩小，但这种缩小在分娩后会恢复。

The thymus shows some reversible involution during pregnancy, apparently caused by the progesterone-driven exodus of lymphocytes from the thymic cortex, and the Th$_1$:Th$_2$ cytokine ratio shifts towards Th2. Conversely, the spleen enlarges during pregnancy possibly due to the accelerated production of erythrocytes and immunoglobulin-producing cells. The lymph nodes in the para-aortic chain draining the uterus may increase in size, although the germinal centres of these nodes may shrink, with the shrinkage reversing after delivery.

二、子宫（The uterus）

未妊娠的子宫重 40～100g，在妊娠期间增加，到 20 周时为 300～400g，足月时为 800～1000g。分娩后最初 2 周内恢复迅速，但此后变慢，到 2 个月仍不会完全恢复。子宫由成束的平滑肌细胞组成，被胶原蛋白、弹性纤维和成纤维细胞组成的结缔组织薄片隔开。妊娠期所有组织都会肥厚。肌肉细胞排列最内层为纵向，中间层肌束向各个方向延伸，最外层为圆形和纵向纤维，并与子宫的韧带部分连续（图 3–1）。子宫肌层的生长几乎完全来自于肌肉的肥大和细胞延长，尽管在妊娠初期可能会出现一些增生，肌肉细胞将从非妊娠状态的 50μm 延长至足月 200～600μm。对子宫肌层生长和发育的刺激是不断生长的胎儿、雌激素和孕酮的作用。

The non-pregnant uterus weighs ≈40–100 g, increasing during pregnancy to 300–400 g at 20 weeks and 800–1000 g at term. Involution is rapid over the first 2 weeks after delivery but slows thereafter and is not complete by 2 months. The uterus consists of bundles of smooth muscle cells separated by thin sheets of connective tissue composed of collagen, elastic fibres and fibroblasts. All hypertrophy during pregnancy. The muscle cells are arranged as an innermost longitudinal layer,

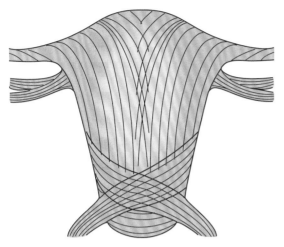

▲ 图 3-1　人体子宫各层肌肉纤维的交叉

Fig. 3.1　Decussation of muscle fibres in the various layers of the human uterus

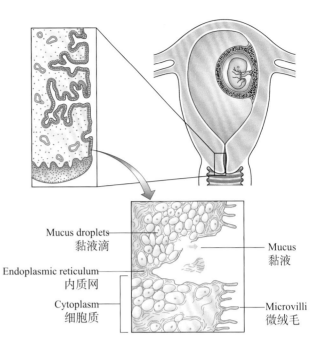

▲ 图 3-2　妊娠期间宫颈的结构与功能

Fig. 3.2　Structure and function of the cervix in pregnancy

a middle layer with bundles running in all directions and an outermost layer of both circular and longitudinal fibres partly continuous with the ligamentous supports of the uterus (Fig. 3.1). Myometrial growth is almost entirely due to muscle hypertrophy and elongation of the cells from 50 μm in the non-pregnant state to 200–600 μm at term, although some hyperplasia may occur during early pregnancy. The stimulus for myometrial growth and development is the effect of the growing conceptus and oestrogens and progesterone.

子宫在功能和形态上分为三个部分，即子宫颈、峡部和子宫体。

The uterus is functionally and morphologically divided into three sections: the cervix, the isthmus and the body of the uterus (corpus uteri).

（一）子宫颈（The cervix）

子宫颈主要是纤维器官，其中子宫肌细胞仅占10%。非妊娠状态的蛋白质总量的 80% 为胶原蛋白，但是到妊娠结束时，胶原蛋白的浓度降低到非妊娠状态的 1/3。子宫颈的主要功能是保留胎儿（图 3-2）。

The cervix is predominantly a fibrous organ with only 10% of uterine muscle cells in the substance of the cervix. Eighty percent of the total protein in the non-pregnant state consists of collagen but, by the end of pregnancy, the concentration of collagen is reduced to one-third of the amount present in the non-pregnant state. The principal function of the cervix is to retain the conceptus (Fig. 3.2).

妊娠期间子宫颈的特征性变化如下。

The characteristic changes in the cervix during pregnancy are:

- 血管增多。

- Increased vascularity.

- 宫颈腺肥大，呈宫颈管柱状上皮增生异位；妊娠期间子宫颈黏液分泌组织增加会导致排出黏厚的宫颈黏液，并在子宫颈中形成黏液抗菌栓。

- Hypertrophy of the cervical glands producing the appearance of a cervical erosion; an increase in mucous secretory tissue in the cervix during pregnancy leads to a thick mucus discharge and the development of an antibacterial plug of mucus in the cervix.

- 妊娠晚期子宫颈的胶原蛋白减少、糖胺聚糖和水累积，导致宫颈成熟的特征性变化。下部随着上部的扩张而缩短，在分娩过程中子宫颈会进一步拉伸和扩张。

- Reduced collagen in the cervix in the third trimester and the accumulation of glycosaminoglycans and water, leading to the characteristic changes of cervical ripening. The lower section shortens as the upper section expands, while during labour there is further stretching and dilatation of the cervix.

（二）峡部（The isthmus）

子宫峡部是子宫颈和子宫体之间的交界区。它在功能上和结构上将宫体的肌纤维连接到子宫颈的致密结缔组织。到妊娠第 28 周时，规律收缩会使峡部逐渐拉伸和变薄，从而初步形成子宫下段。

The isthmus of the uterus is the junctional zone between the cervix and the body of the uterus. It joins the muscle fibres of the corpus to the dense connective tissue of the cervix both functionally and structurally. By the twenty-eighth week of gestation, regular contractions produce some stretching and thinning of the isthmus, resulting in the early formation of the lower uterine segment.

下段在分娩过程中完全形成，是子宫较薄且相对惰性的部分。它对子宫的排挤作用几乎没有贡献，而是实际上成了产道的延伸。由于其在产褥期的相对无血管状态和静止性，它是剖宫产切口的首选部位。

The lower segment is fully formed during labour and is a thin, relatively inert part of the uterus. It contributes little to the expulsive efforts of the uterus and becomes, in effect, an extension of the birth canal. Because of its relative avascularity and quiescence in the puerperium, it is the site of choice for the incision for a caesarean delivery.

（三）子宫体（The corpus uteri）

整个妊娠期间子宫的变化都可以满足胎儿成长的需求，无论是生理大小还是血管适应能力，以提供所需的营养。

The uterus changes throughout pregnancy to meet the needs of the growing fetus both in terms of physical size and in vascular adaptation to supply the nutrients required:

- 排卵月经周期的分泌中期，随着孕酮浓度的升高，子宫内膜上皮和基质细胞停止增殖并开始分化，孕妇白细胞累积，主要是 NK 细胞（见免疫学）。这种蜕膜化对于成功妊娠至关重要。

- As progesterone concentrations rise in the mid-secretory phase of an ovulatory menstrual cycle, endometrial epithelial and stromal cells stop proliferating and begin to differentiate, with an accumulation of maternal leukocytes, mainly NK cells (see Immunology earlier). This decidualization is essential for successful pregnancy.

- 子宫的大小、形状、位置和一致性都会发生变化。在妊娠后期，增大主要发生在子宫底，因此圆韧带往往从子宫的相对尾端出现。子宫从妊娠初期的梨形变为中晚期的球形和卵球形。足月时宫腔从约 4ml 膨胀到 4000ml。子宫肌层在分娩开始之前必须保持相对静止。

- The uterus changes in size, shape, position and consistency. In later pregnancy, the enlargement occurs predominantly in the uterine fundus so that the round ligaments tend to emerge from a relatively caudal

point in the uterus. The uterus changes from a pear shape in early pregnancy to a more globular and ovoid shape in the second and third trimesters. The cavity expands from some 4 mL to 4000 mL at full term. The myometrium must remain relatively quiescent until the onset of labour.

- 所有供应子宫的血管都明显增粗。子宫动脉扩张，其直径是非妊娠状态直径的 1.5 倍。供给胎盘床的弓状动脉增大了 10 倍，而螺旋状小动脉直径达到了妊娠前的 30 倍（见下文）。子宫血流量从妊娠 10 周时的 50ml/min 增加到足月时的 500～600ml/min。

- All the vessels supplying the uterus undergo massive hypertrophy. The uterine arteries dilate so that the diameters are 1.5 times those seen outside pregnancy. The arcuate arteries, supplying the placental bed, become 10 times larger, and the spiral arterioles reach 30 times the pre-pregnancy diameter (see later). Uterine blood flow increases from 50 mL/min at 10 weeks' gestation to 500–600 mL/min at term.

在未妊娠时，子宫血液供应几乎全部来自子宫动脉，但妊娠时，有 20%～30% 血供来自卵巢血管。来自膀胱上动脉的血供很少。子宫和动脉受到自主神经系统的调节，并受到血管扩张药和血管收缩药的直接作用。

In the non-pregnant uterus, blood supply is almost entirely through the uterine arteries, but in pregnancy 20–30% is contributed through the ovarian vessels. A small contribution is made by the superior vesical arteries. The uterine and radial arteries are subject to regulation by the autonomic nervous system and by direct effects from vasodilator and vasoconstrictor humoral agents.

最终向绒毛间隙输送血液的血管（图 3-3）是 100～150 个螺旋状小动脉。每根径向动脉有 2～3 个螺旋状小动脉，每根胎盘子叶有 1～2 个螺旋状小动脉。这些螺旋动脉的重塑对成功妊娠非常重要。滋养细胞分化为绒毛或 EVT。后者可进一步分化为侵袭性 EVT，而侵袭性 EVT 要么是间质性的，迁移到蜕膜，然后分化为子宫肌巨细胞，要么是血管内的，侵犯螺旋动脉管腔。妊娠前 3 个月宫内氧压很低，可刺激 EVT 侵入。

The final vessels delivering blood to the intervillous space (Fig. 3.3) are the 100–150 spiral arterioles. Two or three spiral arterioles arise from each radial artery, and each placental cotyledon is provided with one or two. The remodelling of these spiral arteries is very important for a successful pregnancy. Cytotrophoblast differentiates into villous or EVT.

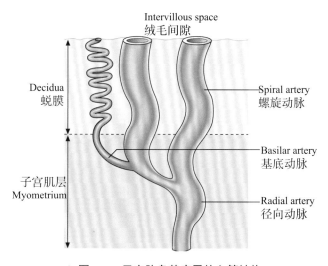

▲ 图 3-3 子宫胎盘基底层的血管结构

Fig. 3.3 Vascular structure in the uteroplacental bed

The latter can differentiate further into invasive EVT, which in turn is either interstitial, migrating into the decidua and later differentiating into myometrial giant cells, or endovascular and invades the lumen of the spiral arteries. The intrauterine oxygen tension is very low in the first trimester, stimulating EVT invasion.

在正常妊娠的最初 10 周，EVT 侵入蜕膜和螺旋小动脉壁，破坏血管壁的平滑肌，使其变为对体液和神经控制无反应的惰性通道（图 3-4）。从 10~16 周，又一波的侵袭发生，延伸至蜕膜部分的血管内腔。从 16~24 周，这种侵袭扩展到螺旋小动脉的肌层部分。这些变化的最终结果是将螺旋小动脉转变为松弛的窦道。

In the first 10 weeks of normal pregnancy, EVT invades the decidua and the walls of the spiral arterioles, destroying the smooth muscle in the wall of the vessels, which then become inert channels unresponsive to humoral and neurological control (Fig. 3.4). From 10 to 16 weeks, a further wave of invasion occurs, extending down the lumen of the decidual portion of the vessel; from 16 to 24 weeks this invasion extends to involve the myometrial portion of the spiral arterioles. The net effect of these changes is to turn the spiral arterioles into flaccid sinusoidal channels.

该过程的失败，特别是在血管的子宫肌层部分中的失败，意味着该部分血管对血管活性刺激保持敏感，并有减少血流的可能。这是先兆子痫和子宫内生长受限的特征，无论后者是否伴发先兆子痫。

Failure of this process, particularly in the myometrial portion of the vessels, means that this portion of the vessels remains sensitive to vasoactive stimuli with the potential for a reduction in blood flow. This is a feature of pre-eclampsia and intrauterine growth restriction, with or without pre-eclampsia.

子宫既有传入神经又有传出神经，尽管它可以在去神经支配的状态下正常工作。宫颈的主要感觉纤维来自 S1 和 S2，而子宫体的主要感觉纤维来自 T11 和 T12 的背侧神经。从子宫颈到下丘脑有 1 条传入通路，因此子宫颈和阴道上部的拉伸刺激了催产素的释放（Ferguson 反射）。子宫颈和子宫血管有丰富的肾上腺能神经供应，而胆碱能神经则局限于子宫颈的血管。

The uterus has both afferent and efferent nerve supplies, although it can function normally in a denervated state. The main sensory fibres from the cervix arise from S1 and S2, whereas those from the body of the uterus arise from the dorsal nerve routes on T11 and T12. There is an afferent pathway from the cervix to the hypothalamus so that stretching of the cervix and upper vagina stimulates the release of oxytocin (*Ferguson's reflex*). The cervical and uterine vessels are well supplied by adrenergic nerves, whereas cholinergic nerves are confined to the blood vessels of the cervix.

（四）子宫收缩（Uterine contractility）

成功妊娠的维持取决于子宫肌层保持静止直到胎儿成熟并能够维持子宫外生命。妊娠期的子宫肌层对扩张的耐受性比非妊娠期的子宫肌层大得多。因此，尽管胎儿的成长使子宫增大，但子宫内压力并没有增加，即使子宫仍有能力产生最大的主动张力。孕酮通过增加肌层细胞的静息膜电位来维持其静息状态，同时减弱电活动的传导并将肌肉活动限制在一小群细胞中。孕激素受体功能似乎在足月时下降。孕酮拮抗药（如米非司酮）可在妊娠早期诱导引产，而前列腺素 $F_{2\alpha}$ 则具有黄体溶解作用。其他机制还包括局部产生的一氧化氮可能通过环鸟苷单磷酸（cGMP）或电压门控钾通道起作用，而一些通过 Gs 受体起作用的松弛激素，如前列环素（PGI_2）、前列腺素（PGE_2）和降钙素基因相关肽则在妊娠期间升高。

The continuation of a successful pregnancy depends on the fact that the myometrium remains quiescent until the fetus is mature and capable of sustaining extrauterine life. Pregnant myometrium has a much greater compliance than non-pregnant myometrium in response to distension. Thus, although the uterus becomes distended by the growing conceptus, intrauterine pressure does not increase, even though the uterus does maintain the capacity to develop maximal active tension. Progesterone maintains quiescence by increasing the resting membrane potential of the myometrial cells while at the same time impairing the conduction of electrical activity and limiting muscle activity to small clumps of cells. Progesterone receptor function appears to decrease towards term. Progesterone antagonists such as mifepristone can induce labour from the

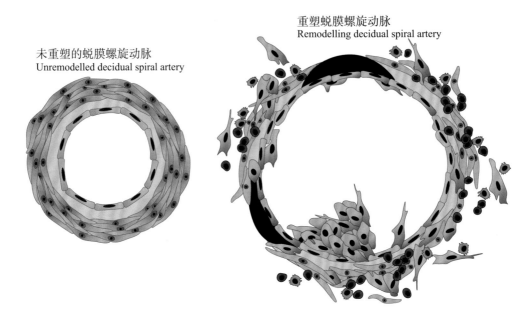

重塑蜕膜螺旋动脉
Remodelling decidual spiral artery

未重塑的蜕膜螺旋动脉
Unremodelled decidual spiral artery

Decidual natural killer (NK) cell
蜕膜自然杀伤细胞
- Regulate EVT invasion
- 调节 EVT 入侵
- Prime vesssl for remodelling
- 启动脉管重塑
- Induce VSMC disorganization/loss
- 诱导 VSMC 瓦解 / 丢失

Decidual macrophage
蜕膜巨噬细胞
- Regulate EVT invasion
- 调节 EVT 入侵
- Accumulate around spiral arteries
- 聚集在螺旋动脉周围
- Phagocytose dead cells
- 吞噬死亡细胞

Extravillous trophoblast (EVT)
绒毛外滋养层细胞
- Invade interstitially/endovascularly
- 侵入间质 / 血管内
- Plug spiral arteries
- 栓塞螺旋动脉
- Remodel extracellular matrix
- 重塑细胞外基质
- Induce EC and VSMC apoptosis
- 诱导 EC 和 VSMC 凋亡

Fibrinoid
类纤维蛋白
- Deposited by EVT
- 由 EVT 存积

Ectracellular matrix
细胞外基质

Endothelial cell (EC)
内皮细胞
- Interact with EVT
- 与 EVT 相互作用
- Temporarily lost from vessel
- 暂时从脉管中丢失

Vascular smooth muscle cell (VSMC)
血平滑肌细胞管
- Lost from vessel
- 从脉管中丢失
- De-differentiate/migrate
- 去分化 / 迁移
- Undergo apoptosis
- 凋亡
- Loss of vessel contractility
- 脉管收缩力的丧失

▲ 图 3-4　在螺旋动脉重塑过程中，血管细胞丢失，动脉增粗，形成了高流量低阻力的血管。这些变化是由母体免疫细胞（蜕膜 NK 细胞和巨噬细胞）及间质性和血管内 EVT 引起的

经许可转载，改编自 Cartwright JE et al. (2010) Reproduction 140:803-813.© Society for Reproduction and Fertility. 版权所有

Fig. 3.4　During spiral artery remodelling, vascular cells are lost, increasing the size of the arteries and creating a high-flow, lowresistance vessel. These changes are brought about by both maternal immune cells (decidual NK cells and macrophages) and by invading interstitial and endovascular EVT.

Adapted from Cartwright JE et al. (2010) Reproduction 140:803-813. © Society for Reproduction and Fertility. Reproduced by permission.

first trimester, as can prostaglandin F2$_\alpha$, which is luteolytic. Other mechanisms include locally generated nitric oxide, probably acting through cyclic guanosine monophosphate (cGMP) or voltage-gated potassium channels, while several relaxatory hormones such as prostacyclin (PGI$_2$), prostaglandin (PGE$_2$) and calcitonin gene-related peptide, which act through the G$_s$ receptors, increase in pregnancy.

（五）子宫肌层活动的发展（The development of myometrial activity）

子宫肌层起合胞体的作用，因此收缩可以通过连接细胞的缝隙产生协调的收缩波。子宫活动在整个妊娠期间都会发生，早在妊娠 7 周就可测量到频繁的低强度宫缩。到中期妊娠，收缩的强度增加，但频率相对较低。在孕晚期，它们的频率和强度都会增加，直到产程第一阶段。妊娠期间的收缩通常是无痛的"紧绷"感（Braxton Hicks 收缩），但有时可能足以产生不适感。它们不会诱发分娩时出现的宫颈扩张。

The myometrium functions as a syncytium so that contractions can pass through the gap junctions linking the cells and produce coordinated waves of contractions. Uterine activity occurs throughout pregnancy and is measurable as early as 7 weeks' gestation, with frequent, low-intensity contractions. As the second trimester proceeds, contractions increase in intensity but remain of relatively low frequency. In the third trimester, they increase in both frequency and intensity, leading up to the first stage of labour. Contractions during pregnancy are usually painless and are felt as 'tightenings' (*Braxton Hicks contractions*) but may sometimes be sufficiently powerful to produce discomfort. They do not produce cervical dilatation, which occurs with the onset of labour.

在妊娠后期，胎儿继续生长，但是子宫停止生长，因此整个子宫壁的张力增加。这会刺激各种基因产物的表达，如催产素和前列腺素 $F_{2\alpha}$ 受体、钠通道和缝隙连接蛋白。促炎细胞因子表达也增加。一旦分娩发动，第一产程后期的宫缩压力可能会达到 100mmHg，并且每 2～3 分钟就会发生 1 次（图 3-5），见第 11 章关于分娩的讨论。

In late gestation, the fetus continues to grow, but the uterus stops growing, so tension across the uterine wall increases. This stimulates expression of a variety of gene products such as oxytocin and prostaglandin F2α receptors, sodium channels and the gap junction protein. Pro-inflammatory cytokine expression also increases. Once labour has begun, the contractions in the late first stage may reach pressures up to 100 mmHg and occur every 2–3 minutes (Fig. 3.5). See Chapter 11 for a discussion of labour and delivery.

三、阴道（The vagina）

阴道内衬的分层鳞状上皮在妊娠期间会发生肥大。表面、中间和基底三层细胞相对比例会发生变化，使中间细胞占主导并且在正常阴道分泌物的细胞群中可见。阴道壁的肌肉组织也变得肥大。与子宫颈一样，结缔组织胶原蛋白减少，而水和糖胺聚糖增加。丰富的静脉血管网络布满阴道壁，呈现微浅蓝色外观。

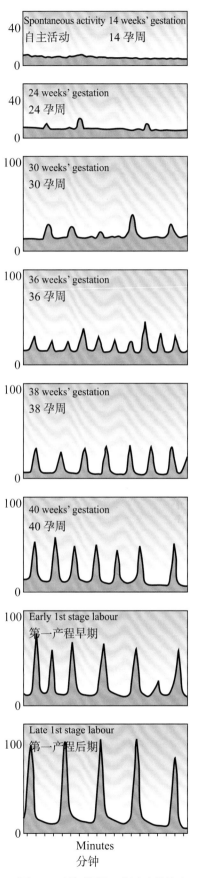

▲ 图 3-5　妊娠期间子宫活动的演变

Fig. 3.5　The evolution of uterine activity during pregnancy

The vagina is lined by stratified squamous epithelium, which hypertrophies during pregnancy. The three layers of superficial, intermediate and basal cells change their relative proportions so that the intermediate cells predominate and can be seen in the cell population of normal vaginal secretions. The musculature in the vaginal wall also becomes hypertrophic. As in the cervix, the connective tissue collagen decreases, while water and glycosaminoglycans increase. The rich venous vascular network in the vaginal walls becomes engorged and gives rise to a slightly bluish appearance.

上皮细胞通常会繁殖并增大，它充满富含糖原的液泡。高雌激素水平会刺激糖原合成和沉积，并且当这些上皮细胞脱落到阴道中时，被称为 Döderlein 菌的乳杆菌会分解糖原以产生乳酸。妊娠期间阴道的 pH 降至 3.5～4.0，这种酸性环境有助于保持阴道免除细菌感染。然而酵母菌感染则可能会在这种环境下盛行，假丝酵母菌感染在孕妇中很常见。

Epithelial cells generally multiply and enlarge and become filled with vacuoles rich in glycogen. High oestrogen levels stimulate glycogen synthesis and deposition, and as these epithelial cells are shed into the vagina, lactobacilli known as *Döderlein's bacilli* break down the glycogen to produce lactic acid. The vaginal pH falls in pregnancy to 3.5–4.0, and this acid environment serves to keep the vagina clear of bacterial infection. Unfortunately, yeast infections may thrive in this environment, and *Candida* infections are common in pregnancy.

四、心血管系统（The cardiovascular system）

心血管系统是在每个排卵月经周期的黄体期都显示出主动适应潜在妊娠的系统之一，远远早于任何生理"需要"之前。许多这些变化在妊娠 12～16 周时几乎已经完成了（图 3-6 和表 3-1）。

The cardiovascular system is one of those that shows proactive adaptations for a potential pregnancy during the luteal phase of every ovulatory menstrual cycle, long before there is any physiological 'need' for them. Many of these changes are almost complete by 12–16 weeks' gestation (Fig. 3.6 and Table 3.1).

（一）心脏的位置和大小（Cardiac position and size）

随着子宫的增长，横膈被向上推动，心脏相应

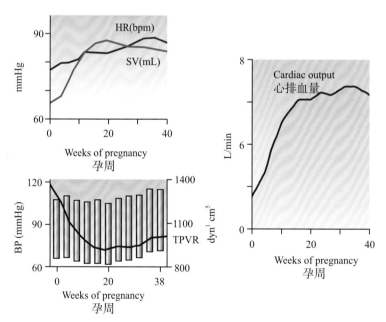

▲ 图 3-6 与正常人妊娠相关的主要血流动力学变化。心排血量明显增加是心率 (HR) 和心搏量 (SV) 不同步升高所致。尽管心排血量增加，血压 (BP) 在妊娠的前半段下降，这意味着整个外周阻力 (TPR) 显著降低

改编自 Broughton Pipkin F (2007) Maternal physiology. In: Edmonds DK (ed) Dewhurst's Textbook of Obstetrics and Gynaecology, 8th edn. Blackwell, Oxford.

Fig. 3.6 Major haemodynamic changes associated with normal human pregnancy. The marked increase in cardiac output results from asynchronous rises in heart rate (HR) and stroke volume (SV). Despite the rise in cardiac output, blood pressure (BP) falls in the first half of pregnancy, implying a very substantial reduction in total peripheral resistance (TPR)

Adapted from Broughton Pipkin F (2007) Maternal physiology. In: Edmonds DK (ed) Dewhurst's Textbook of Obstetrics and Gynaecology, 8th edn. Blackwell, Oxford.)

表 3-1 妊娠期间某些心血管变量的百分比变动

Table 3.1 Percentage change in some cardiovascular variables during pregnancy

	早期妊娠 First trimester	中期妊娠 Second trimester	晚期妊娠 Third trimester
心率 Heart rate	+11	+13	+16
心搏量（ml） Stroke volume (mL)	+31	+29	+27
心排血量（L/min） Cardiac output (L/min)	+45	+47	+48
收缩压（mmHg） Systolic BP (mmHg)	−1	+1	+6
舒张压（mmHg） Diastolic BP (mmHg)	−6	−3	+7
MPAP (mmHg)	+5	+5	+5
总外围电阻（电阻单位） Total peripheral resistance (resistance units)	−27	−27	−29

BP. 血压；MPAP. 平均肺动脉压

数据来自有确定妊娠前数值的研究。显示的平均值是每 3 个月末的平均值，因此不一定是最大值。请注意，在早期妊娠的末尾，变化接近最大

引自 Robson S, Robson SC, Hunter S, et al. (1989) Serial study of factors influencing changes in cardiac output during human pregnancy. Am J Physiol 1989; 256:H1060. Table reproduced from Broughton Pipkin F (2001) Maternal physiology. In: Chamberlain GV, Steer P (eds) Turnbull's Obstetrics, 3rd edn. Churchill Livingstone, London; with permission from Elsevier.

BP, Blood pressure; MPAP, mean pulmonary artery pressure.

Data are derived from studies in which pre-conception values were determined. The mean values shown are those at the end of each trimester and are thus not necessarily the maximal. Note that the changes are near maximal by the end of the first trimester.

Data from Robson S, Robson SC, Hunter S, et al. (1989) Serial study of factors influencing changes in cardiac output during human pregnancy. Am J Physiol 1989; 256:H1060. Table reproduced from Broughton Pipkin F (2001) Maternal physiology. In: Chamberlain GV, Steer P (eds) Turnbull's Obstetrics, 3rd edn. Churchill Livingstone, London; with permission from Elsevier.

地移位，心脏的顶点向上并向左侧移动，偏差约为 15%。放射学上，左上心脏边界变直伴有肺锥突出增加。这些变化导致Ⅲ导联出现倒 T 波，Ⅲ导联和 aVF 出现 Q 波。

As the uterus grows, the diaphragm is pushed upwards and the heart is correspondingly displaced: the apex of the heart is displaced upwards and left laterally, with a deviation of ≈15%. Radiologically, the upper left cardiac border is straightened with increased prominence of the pulmonary conus. These changes result in an inverted T wave in lead Ⅲ and a Q wave in leads III and aVF.

心脏在妊娠早期到晚期之间会增大 70～80ml，约 12%，部分原因是壁厚略有增加，但主要是由于静脉充盈增加。心室容积的增加导致瓣膜环扩张，因此反流流速增加。妊娠期心肌收缩力增加，表现为射血前期缩短，这与心肌纤维延长有关。

The heart enlarges by 70–80 mL, some 12%, between early and late pregnancy, due in part to a small increase in wall thickness but predominantly to increased venous filling. The increase in ventricular volume results in dilatation of the valve rings and hence an increase in regurgitant flow velocities. Myocardial contractility is increased during pregnancy, as indicated by a shortening of the pre-ejection period, and this is associated with lengthening of the myocardial muscle fibres.

（二）心排血量（Cardiac output）

现在可以使用非侵入性方法，如多普勒测速、超声心动图和阻抗心动图，从而可以对整个妊娠期间的心排血量进行标准化的顺序研究。

Non-invasive methods, such as Doppler velocimetry, echocardiography and impedance cardiography, are now available, allowing standardized sequential studies of cardiac output throughout pregnancy.

黄体期心率有小幅上升，到中期妊娠时每分钟心率增加 10～15 次。这可能与孕激素驱动的过度换

气有关（请参阅下文）。因为妊娠进展及心率变异性降低，压力反射敏感性可能下降。最初 3 个月心排血量的增加比心率稍晚一些，在妊娠期间从约 64ml 增加到 71ml。装有人工起搏器并因此具有固定心率的女性，仅凭增加的心排血量就可以很好地补偿妊娠。

There is a small rise in heart rate during the luteal phase, increasing to 10–15 beats/min by mid-pregnancy; this may be related to the progesterone-driven hyperventilation (see later). There is probably a fall in baro-reflex sensitivity as pregnancy progresses and heart rate variability falls. Stroke volume rises a little later in the first trimester than heart rate, increasing from about 64 to 71 mL during pregnancy. Women who have an artificial pacemaker and thus a fixed heart rate compensate well in pregnancy based on increased stroke volume alone.

这两个因素会增加心排血量和心脏指数（与体表面积相关的心排血量）。心排血量的增加大部分发生在妊娠的前 14 周，从 4.5L/min 至 6L/min 增加了 1.5L。第一次妊娠时心排血量较非分娩期变化 35%～40%，而在以后的妊娠中约为 50%。双胎妊娠在整个妊娠期间增加 15%。在健康的妊娠中，出生体重与心排血量的增加、总外周阻力（total peripheral resistonce, TPR）和增强指数的下降有关。相反，妊娠期间患有任何类型高血压的女性，若在分娩时生育婴儿体重低于第十百分位数，其与妊娠相关的血流动力学变化会小得多。

These two factors push up the cardiac output and cardiac index (cardiac output related to body surface area). Most of the rise in cardiac output occurs in the first 14 weeks of pregnancy, with an increase of 1.5 L from 4.5 to 6.0 L/min. The non-labouring change in cardiac output is 35–40% in a first pregnancy and ≈50% in later pregnancies. Twin pregnancies are associated with a 15% greater increase throughout pregnancy. In a healthy pregnancy, the birth weight is associated with the increase in cardiac output and fall in total peripheral resistance (TPR) and augmentation index. Conversely, women with any type of hypertension in pregnancy who deliver babies with birth weights below the tenth centile show much smaller pregnancy-related changes in haemodynamics.

分娩时心排血量可以再增加 1/3（约 2L/min）。产后约 24h 内心排血量保持高水平，然后分娩后约 2 周内后逐渐下降至非妊娠水平。

Cardiac output can rise by another third (≈2 L/min) in labour. The cardiac output remains high for ≈24 hours postpartum and then gradually declines to non-pregnant levels by ≈2 weeks after delivery.

表 3–1 总结了妊娠期间某些心血管变量的百分比变化。

Table 3.1 summarizes the percentage changes in some cardiovascular variables during pregnancy.

> **！注意**
>
> 妊娠会使心排血量显著增加，并可能在患有心脏病的女性中引发心力衰竭。
>
> Pregnancy imposes a significant increase in cardiac output and is likely to precipitate heart failure in women with heart disease.

（三）总外周阻力（Total peripheral resistance）

TPR 不是直接测量的，而是根据平均动脉压除以心排血量计算得出的。增强指数是动脉僵硬度的替代指标，也可以通过脉搏波分析间接测量。测得的 TPR 和增长指数在妊娠 6 周时均下降，故认为后负荷下降。这被"感知"为循环充盈不足，被认为是孕妇循环适应的主要刺激之一。它会激活肾素 - 血管紧张素 - 醛固酮系统，允许必要的血浆容量扩增张（PV，见下文肾功能）。在正常血压的非孕妇中，TPR 约为 1700dyn/(s·cm)；到妊娠中期时降至最低点 40%～50%，此后至足月缓慢上升，妊娠后期达到 1200～1300dyn/(s·cm)。全身性 TPR 下降部分与子宫胎盘床和肾血管系统的血管空间扩张有关。由于血管扩张，在妊娠期间皮肤的血流量也会大大增加。

TPR is not measured directly but is calculated from the mean arterial pressure divided by cardiac output. The augmentation index, a surrogate measure of arterial stiffness, is also measured indirectly from pulse wave analysis. Measured TPR and augmentation index both fall by 6 weeks' gestation, so afterload is assumed to have fallen. This is 'perceived' as circulatory under-filling, which is thought to be one of the primary stimuli to the mother's circulatory adaptations. It activates the renin-angiotensin-aldosterone system and allows the necessary expansion of the plasma volume (PV; see Renal function later). In a normotensive non-pregnant woman, the TPR is around 1700 dyn/s/cm; this falls to a nadir of 40–50% by mid-gestation, rising slowly thereafter towards term, reaching 1200–1300 dyn/s/cm in late pregnancy. The fall in systemic TPR is partly associated with the expansion of the vascular space in the utero-placental bed and the renal vasculature; blood flow to the skin is also greatly increased in pregnancy as a result of vasodilatation.

引起 TPR 下降的血管扩张不是由于交感神经张力的减弱，而是由于从血管收缩激素到血管扩张激素平衡的重大转变所驱动的。参与早期妊娠的血管扩张药包括循环中 PGI_2 和局部合成的一氧化氮，以及后来的心房利钠肽。血管紧张素 II（Ang II）浓度明显升高，但对其升压反应丧失（见内分泌学）。妊娠期血管舒张和血管收缩之间的平衡是血压的关键决定因素，并且是先兆子痫发病机制的核心。

The vasodilatation that causes the fall in TPR is not due to a withdrawal of sympathetic tone but is hormonally driven by a major shift in the balance from vasoconstrictor to vasodilator hormones. The vasodilators involved in early gestation include circulating PGI_2 and locally synthesized nitric oxide and, later, atrial natriuretic peptide. There is also a loss of pressor responsiveness to angiotensin II (AngII), concentrations of which rise markedly (see Endocrinology). The balance between vasodilatation and vasoconstriction in pregnancy is a critical determinant of blood pressure and lies at the heart of the pathogenesis of pre-eclampsia.

（四）动脉血压（Arterial blood pressure）

在月经周期中血压会发生变化。黄体期收缩压升高，在月经开始时达到峰值，而在黄体期的舒张压比卵泡期的舒张压低 5%。

Blood pressure changes occur during the menstrual cycle. Systolic blood pressure increases during the luteal phase of the cycle and reaches its peak at the onset of menstruation, whereas diastolic pressure is 5% lower during the luteal phase than in the follicular phase of the cycle.

妊娠前半期 TPR 下降导致平均动脉压下降约 10 mmHg。其中 80% 发生在妊娠的最初 8 周。此后，还会出现少量的下降，直到妊娠 16～24 周动脉压力达到最低点。此后会再次升高，并可能恢复到孕早期水平。而在发展为先兆子痫的女性中，上升率则更大。

The fall in TPR during the first half of pregnancy causes a fall of some 10 mmHg in mean arterial pressure; 80% of this fall occurs in the first 8 weeks of pregnancy. Thereafter, a small additional fall occurs until arterial pressure reaches its nadir by 16–24 weeks' gestation. It rises again after this and may return to early pregnancy levels. The rate of rise is amplified in women who go on to develop pre-eclampsia.

姿势对孕妇的血压有显著影响，左侧仰卧时血压最低。无论是坐位，仰卧还是左侧卧位，都可以以类似的方式降低妊娠期的血压，但是水平明显不同（图 3-7）。这意味着，如果进行血压比较，进行产前检查的孕妇必须在每次检查时在相同位置记录血压。必须特别注意使用合适尺寸的袖带来测量肱动脉压力。随着年轻女性肥胖发生率的增加，这一点尤为重要。妊娠期间第四和第五 Korotkoff 音之间的间隙变大，并且第五 Korotkoff 音可能很难确定。这两个因素都可能导致妊娠期舒张压测量的差

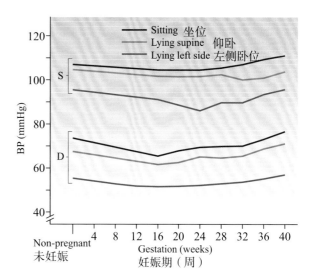

▲ 图 3-7 妊娠期间姿势对血压（BP）的影响

Fig. 3.7　The effect of posture on blood pressure (BP) during pregnancy

异。尽管大多数已发表的血压研究都是基于第四 Korotkoff 音的使用，但是现在建议在消失点清晰时使用第五 Korotkoff 音，而在消失点不清楚的地方使用第四 Korotkoff 音。血压升高时，如先兆子痫时，自动血压计不适合在孕妇中使用。

Posture has a significant effect on blood pressure in pregnancy; pressure is lowest with the woman lying supine on her left side. The pressure falls during gestation in a similar way whether the pressure is recorded sitting, lying supine or in the left lateral supine position, but the levels are significantly different (Fig. 3.7). This means that mothers attending for antenatal visits must have their blood pressure recorded in the same position at each visit if the pressures are to be comparable. Special care must be taken to use an appropriate cuff size for the measurement of brachial pressures. This is especially important with the increasing incidence of obesity among young women. The gap between the fourth and fifth Korotkoff sounds widens in pregnancy, and the fifth Korotkoff sound may be difficult to define. Both these factors may cause discrepancies in the measurement of diastolic pressure in pregnancy. Although most published studies of blood pressure are based on the use of the Korotkoff fourth sound, it is now recommended to use the fifth sound where it is clear and the fourth sound only where the point of disappearance is unclear. Automated sphygmomanometers are unsuitable for use in pregnancy when the blood pressure is raised, as in pre-eclampsia.

当妊娠后期孕妇仰卧时，血压可能会急剧下降。这种现象被称为仰卧低血压综合征。这是由于下腔静脉受压导致下肢静脉回流受限而致心排血量下降。必须注意主动脉压迫也会发生血压下降，并导致妊

娠期肱动脉和股动脉血压之间出现明显差异。当孕妇在妊娠后期从仰卧位转为侧卧位时，血压可能会下降 15%，不过其中有些下降是由于右臂抬高至心脏水平上方而引起的测量假象。

Profound falls in blood pressure may occur in late pregnancy when the mother lies on her back. This phenomenon is described as the *supine hypotension syndrome*. It results from the restriction of venous return from the lower limbs due to compression of the inferior vena cava and hence a fall in stroke volume. It must be remembered that aortic compression also occurs and that this will result in conspicuous differences between brachial and femoral blood pressures in pregnancy. When a woman turns from a supine to a lateral position in late pregnancy, the blood pressure may fall by 15%, although some of this fall is a measurement artefact caused by the raising of the right arm above the level of the heart.

在整个正常妊娠期间，静脉逐渐扩张，并且静脉扩张性和容量增加。妊娠期中心静脉压和上臂静脉压保持不变，但由于妊娠后期子宫和胎先露的压力，下循环静脉压在站立、坐或仰卧时逐渐升高。肺循环可以在不增加压力的情况下吸收高流量血流，因此右心室、肺动脉和毛细血管的压力不会改变。肺阻力在妊娠早期下降，此后没有变化。

There is progressive venodilatation and rises in venous distensibility and capacitance throughout a normal pregnancy. Central venous pressure and pressure in the upper arms remain constant in pregnancy, but the venous pressure in the lower circulation rises progressively on standing, sitting or lying supine because of pressure from the uterus and the fetal presenting part in late pregnancy. The pulmonary circulation can absorb high rates of flow without an increase in pressure, so pressure in the right ventricle and the pulmonary arteries and capillaries does not change. Pulmonary resistance falls in early pregnancy and does not change thereafter.

五、血液（The blood）

血容量测量的是 PV 和红细胞总量。这些指标受到不同的机制调控。PV 的变化在后面讨论（见肾功能）。

Blood volume is a measurement of PV and red cell mass. The indices are under separate control mechanisms. PV changes are considered later (see Renal function).

（一）红细胞（Erythrocytes）

妊娠期间红细胞总量稳定增加，并且在整个妊娠期间这种增加呈线性。细胞数和细胞大小都会增加。循环红细胞的数量从非妊娠女性的约 1400ml 增

加到妊娠期女性的 1700ml，并且是未服用铁剂的女性。多胎妊娠或补充铁剂的女性增加的更多（约 29% vs. 18%）。孕妇中的促红细胞生成素增加，如果不补充铁剂则更多（55% vs. 25%），但是红细胞总量的变化早于此。人胎盘催乳素可能起到刺激造血的作用。

There is a steady increase in red cell mass in pregnancy, and the increase appears to be linear throughout pregnancy. Both cell number and cell size increase. The circulating red cell mass rises from around 1400 mL in non-pregnant women to ≈1700 mL during pregnancy in women who do not take iron supplements. It rises more in women with multiple pregnancies, and substantially more with iron supplementation (≈29% compared with 18%). Erythropoietin rises in pregnancy, more if iron supplementation is not taken (55% compared with 25%), but the changes in red cell mass antedate this; human placental lactogen may stimulate haematopoiesis.

妊娠期间血红蛋白浓度、血细胞容积和红细胞计数下降，因为 PV 的上升比例高于红细胞总量（"生理贫血"，表 9–1）。但是在正常妊娠中，平均血红蛋白浓度保持恒定。血清中铁的浓度下降，但是正常妊娠时，肠道吸收的铁会增加，β_1– 球蛋白转铁蛋白的合成增加也会增强铁结合能力。孕妇膳食中铁的需求量要增加一倍以上。尽管红细胞叶酸浓度下降幅度较小，但血浆叶酸浓度至足月时下降了 1/2，因为肾脏清除率更高。在 20 世纪 90 年代后期，英国 16—64 岁的女性人口中，有 20% 的人血清铁蛋白水平低于 15μg/L，这表明铁储藏量较低。自那时以来似乎没有进行过类似的调查。青少年妊娠可能存在缺铁的风险。即使轻度的母亲贫血也与胎盘 / 出生体重比增加和出生体重下降有关。

Haemoglobin concentration, haematocrit and red cell count fall during pregnancy because the PV rises proportionately more than the red cell mass ('physiological anaemia'; see Table 9.1). However, in normal pregnancy, the mean corpuscular haemoglobin concentration remains constant. Serum iron concentration falls, but the absorption of iron from the gut rises and iron-binding capacity rises in a normal pregnancy, since there is increased synthesis of the β_1-globulin, transferrin. Maternal dietary iron requirements more than double. Plasma folate concentration halves by term because of greater renal clearance, although red cell folate concentrations fall less. In the late 1990s, 20% of the female population aged 16–64 years in the UK was estimated to have serum ferritin levels below 15 μg/L, indicating low iron stores; no similar survey appears to have been undertaken since then. Pregnant adolescents seem to be at risk of iron deficiency. Even relatively mild maternal anaemia is associated with increased placental:birth weight ratios and decreased birth weight.

（二）白细胞（The white cells）

妊娠期间白细胞总数增加。这种增加主要是由于中性粒细胞多形核白细胞增加，并在妊娠 30 周时达到峰值（图 3-8）。分娩期间和分娩后中性粒细胞会进一步大量增多，多形核白细胞数量增加 4 倍。

The total white cell count rises during pregnancy. This increase is mainly due to an increase in neutrophil polymorphonuclear leukocytes that peaks at 30 weeks' gestation (Fig. 3.8). A further massive neutrophilia normally occurs during labour and immediately after delivery, with a fourfold increase in the number of polymorphs.

> **！注意**
> 分娩和产褥期明显的中性粒细胞增多症是正常的，不能认为是由于感染引起的。
> A massive neutrophilia is normal during labour and the immediate puerperium and cannot be assumed to be due to infection.

在妊娠期间，粒细胞的代谢活性也会增加，这可能是由于雌激素作用所致。在正常的月经周期中会有这种改变，中性粒细胞计数也随着月经中期雌激素峰值而增加。妊娠期间嗜酸性粒细胞、嗜碱性

粒细胞和单核细胞保持相对恒定，但在分娩过程中嗜酸性粒细胞显著下降，至分娩时消失。淋巴细胞计数保持恒定，并且 T 细胞和 B 细胞的数量没有改变，但是淋巴细胞功能和细胞介导的免疫力被抑制，这可能是由于覆盖在淋巴细胞表面的糖蛋白浓度增加，从而降低了对刺激物的反应。没有证据表明体液免疫或免疫球蛋白生成被抑制。

There is also an increase in the metabolic activity of granulocytes during pregnancy, which may result from the action of oestrogens. This can be seen in the normal menstrual cycle, where the neutrophil count rises with the oestrogen peak in mid-cycle. Eosinophils, basophils and monocytes remain relatively constant during pregnancy, but there is a profound fall in eosinophils during labour, and they are virtually absent at delivery. The lymphocyte count remains constant, and the numbers of T and B cells do not alter, but lymphocyte function and cell-mediated immunity in particular are depressed, possibly by the increase in concentrations of glycoproteins coating the surface of the lymphocytes, reducing the response to stimuli. There is, however, no evidence of suppression of humoral immunity or the production of immunoglobulins.

（三）血小板（Platelets）

纵向研究表明妊娠期间血小板计数显著下降。血小板数量的减少可能是一种稀释作用，但从约 28 周的血小板体积大幅增加表明妊娠时血小板的破坏增加，因为血液循环中较大和较幼稚的血小板数量

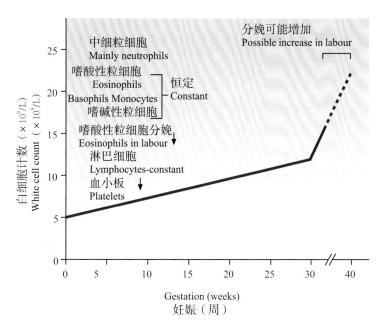

▲ 图 3-8　妊娠与白细胞计数增加有关；这种增加主要发生在多形核白细胞中

Fig. 3.8　**Pregnancy is associated with an increased white cell count; the increase occurs predominantly in polymorphonuclear leukocytes**

增加。妊娠后期原本正常的女性中约有 10% 血小板计数低于 150 000×10⁹/L。在妊娠中晚期，血小板反应性增加，直到分娩后约 12 周才恢复正常。

Longitudinal studies show a significant fall in platelet count during pregnancy. The fall in platelet numbers may be a dilutional effect, but the substantial increase in platelet volume from ≈28 weeks suggests that there is increased destruction of platelets in pregnancy with an increase in the number of larger and younger platelets in the circulation. The platelet count falls below 150,000 ×10⁹/L in ≈10% of otherwise normal women in late gestation. Platelet reactivity is increased in the second and third trimesters and does not return to normal until ≈12 weeks after delivery.

（四）凝血因子（Clotting factors）

妊娠期间的凝血系统发生了重大变化，并有血凝增加的趋势（框 3-1）。在子宫血管床突然、大量出血并危及生命的情况下，凝血能力的提高可能起到挽救生命的作用。不过另一方面，它也增加了血栓形成性疾病的风险。

There are major changes in the coagulation system in pregnancy, with an increased tendency towards clotting (Box 3.1). In a situation where haemorrhage from the uterine vascular bed may be sudden, profuse and life threatening, the increase in coagulability may play a lifesaving role. On the other hand, it increases the risk of thrombotic disease.

妊娠期间许多凝血因子保持不变，但有一些例外情况值得注意（图 3-9）。妊娠期间因子Ⅶ、Ⅷ、Ⅷ：C、Ⅹ 和 Ⅸ（克里斯马斯因子）都会增加，而因子Ⅱ和Ⅴ倾向于保持恒定。因子 Ⅺ 降至非妊娠值的 60%～70%，因子 ⅩⅢ 的浓度降低 50%。可以使因子Ⅴ和Ⅷ失活的蛋白 C 在妊娠期间很可能没有变化，但在孕早期和孕中期，作为辅助因子之一的蛋白质 S 的浓度下降。

Many clotting factors remain constant in pregnancy, but there are notable and important exceptions (Fig. 3.9). Factors VII, VIII, VIII:C, X and IX (Christmas factor) all increase during pregnancy, whereas factors II and V tend to remain constant. Factor XI falls to 60–70% of the nonpregnant values, and concentrations of factor XIII fall by 50%. Protein C, which inactivates factors V and VIII, is probably unchanged in pregnancy, but concentrations of protein S, one of its co-factors, fall during the first two trimesters.

血浆纤维蛋白原水平从非孕期的 2.5～4.0g/L 增加到妊娠晚期的 6.0g/L，并且正常妊娠期间高分子量纤维蛋白 / 纤维蛋白原复合物的浓度增加。妊娠初期红细胞沉降率增加，主要是由于纤维蛋白原的增加。据估计，在胎盘分离过程中消耗了总循环纤维蛋白原的 5%～10%，血栓栓塞是英国孕产妇死亡的主要原因之一。另一方面，在妊娠期间血浆纤溶活性降低。在分娩后 1h 内，活性迅速恢复至非孕水平表明该抑制作用是通过胎盘介导的。

Plasma fibrinogen levels rise from the nonpregnant value of 2.5–4.0 g/L to 6.0 g/L in late pregnancy, and there is an increase in the concentration of high molecular weight fibrin/fibrinogen complex in normal pregnancy. The erythrocyte sedimentation rate is increased in early pregnancy largely because of the increase in fibrinogen. It is estimated that 5%–10% of the total circulating fibrinogen is consumed during the process of placental separation, and thromboembolism is one of the major causes of maternal death in the UK. On the other hand, plasma fibrinolytic activity is decreased during pregnancy. The rapid return of activity to nonpregnant levels within 1 hour of delivery suggests that this inhibition is mediated through the placenta.

框 3-1　凝血系统的常规筛查测试	Box 3.1　Common screening tests for the coagulation system
• 出血时间是皮肤伤口持续出血时间的测量值，是体内血小板与血管相互作用的测试。正常范围是 7～10min	• **Bleeding time is a measure of the length of time** a skin wound continues to bleed and is an in vivo test of platelet-vascular interaction. The normal range is 7–10 minutes.
• 血小板计数是评估急性产科止血失败，尤其是诸如弥散性血管内凝血之类疾病的有价值的筛选测试。低于 100 000/μl 称为血小板减少症	• The **platelet count** is a valuable screening test for assessing acute obstetric haemostatic failure, particularly disorders such as disseminated intravascular coagulation. Values below 100,000 cells/μL are known as thrombocytopaenia.
• 激活部分凝血酶时间是用来监测治疗性肝素水平的测试，通常在 35～45s，但必须与正常对照进行评估	• The **activated partial thromboplastin time** is the test used to monitor therapeutic heparin levels and normally lies between 35 and 45 seconds, but must always be assessed against a normal control.
• 凝血酶原时间用来衡量凝血酶原添加后的凝血时间。这是用来监测华法林的剂量的检验，通常在 10～14s	• **Prothrombin time** measures the clotting time after the addition of thromboplastin. It is the test used to monitor the dosage of warfarin and usually lies between 10 and 14 seconds.
• 在存在严重的消耗性凝血病的情况下，纤维蛋白原的估计很重要，严重的消耗性凝血病可能在严重的胎盘早剥或严重子痫前期的情况下发生。妊娠晚期的正常值在 4.0～6.0g/L	• **Fibrinogen estimation** is important in the presence of severe consumptive coagulopathy, which may occur following severe placental abruption or in cases of severe pre–eclampsia. The normal value in late pregnancy lies between 4.0 and 6.0 g/L.
• 在健康受试者中，纤维蛋白原 / 纤维蛋白降解产物（FDP）较低，但是在存在严重弥散性血管内凝血的情况下，可以检测到高水平的纤维蛋白原 / 纤维蛋白降解产物。该疾病情况下数值可能超过 40μg/L	• **Fibrinogen/fibrin degradation products (FDP)** are low in healthy subjects, but high levels can be detected in the presence of severe disseminated intravascular coagulation. Values in the presence of this disorder may exceed 40 μg/L.

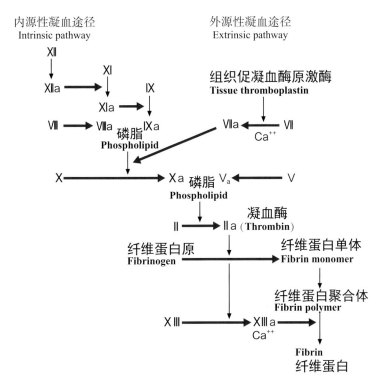

▲ 图 3-9 与人类妊娠相关的凝血途径改变（正常妊娠期间增加的因子以粗体显示）

改编自 Broughton Pipkin F (2007) Maternal physiology. In: Edmonds DK (ed) Dewhurst's Textbook of Obstetrics and Gynaecology, 8th edn. Blackwell, Oxford.

Fig. 3.9 Alterations in the coagulation pathways associated with human pregnancy. Factors that increase during normal pregnancy are shown in bold type.

Adapted from Broughton Pipkin F (2007) Maternal physiology. In: Edmonds DK (ed) Dewhurst's Textbook of Obstetrics and Gynaecology, 8th edn. Blackwell, Oxford.

Plasma fibrinogen levels increase from non-pregnant values of 2.5–4.0 g/L to levels as high as 6.0 g/L in late pregnancy, and there is an increase in the concentration of high-molecular-weight fibrin/fibrinogen complexes during normal pregnancy. The erythrocyte sedimentation rate rises early in pregnancy, mainly due to the increase in fibrinogen. An estimated 5–10% of the total circulating fibrinogen is consumed during placental separation, and thromboembolism is one of the main causes of maternal death in the UK. On the other hand, there is a reduction in plasma fibrinolytic activity during pregnancy; the rapid return to non-pregnant levels of activity within 1 hour of delivery suggests that this inhibition is mediated through the placenta.

> **！注意**
> 妊娠和产褥期凝血趋势增加。
> There is an increased tendency to clotting in pregnancy and the puerperium.

六、呼吸功能（Respiratory function）

横膈水平上升，肋间角从妊娠早期的 68° 增加到妊娠晚期的 103°。虽然在妊娠后期膈肌有向上的压力，但肋部的变化早在子宫增大的压力之前就已经发生了。然而，妊娠期呼吸更多是横膈呼吸而不是肋式呼吸。

The level of the diaphragm rises and the intercostal angle increases from 68 degrees in early pregnancy to 103 degrees in late pregnancy. Although there is upward pressure on the diaphragm in late pregnancy, the costal changes occur well before they could be attributed to pressure from the enlarging uterus. Nevertheless, breathing in pregnancy is more diaphragmatic than costal.

肺活量是指最大吸气后可呼出的最大气体量。由于残气量在妊娠期间略有减少（图 3-10），肺活量略有增加。肺活量与体重有关，并且会因肥胖而减少。吸气量测量潮气量加上吸气储备量。它在妊娠期间逐渐增加约 300ml，而残留量减少约 300ml。这改善了气体混合。妊娠期间 1s 的强制呼气量（FEV_1）和呼气峰值流量保持恒定，患有哮喘的女性似乎不受妊娠的影响。

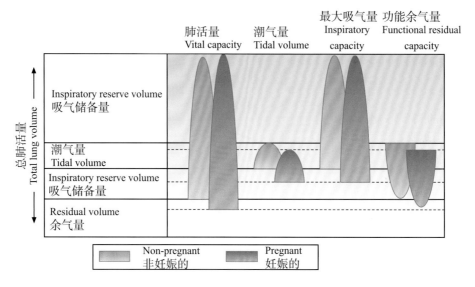

▲ 图 3-10　与人类妊娠相关的肺活量变化。总体而言，吸气储备和潮气量增加，但是以呼气储备和剩余气量减少为代价

改编自 Broughton Pipkin F (2007) Maternal physiology. In: Edmonds DK (ed) Dewhurst's Textbook of Obstetrics and Gynaecology, 8th edn. Blackwell, Oxford

Fig. 3.10　Alterations in lung volumes associated with human pregnancy. Overall, inspiratory reserve and tidal volumes increase at the expense of expiratory reserve and residual volumes

Adapted from Broughton Pipkin F (2007) Maternal physiology. In: Edmonds DK (ed) Dewhurst's Textbook of Obstetrics and Gynaecology, 8th edn. Blackwell, Oxford

Vital capacity describes the maximum amount of gas that can be expired after maximum inspiration. Since residual volume decreases slightly in pregnancy (Fig. 3.10), vital capacity increases slightly. Vital capacity is related to body weight and is reduced by obesity. Inspiratory capacity measures tidal volume plus inspiratory reserve volume. It increases progressively during pregnancy by ≈300 mL, while residual volume decreases by about 300 mL. This improves gas mixing. Forced expiratory volume in 1 second (FEV_1) and peak expiratory flow remain constant in pregnancy, and women with asthma do not appear to be affected by pregnancy.

孕酮使延髓对 $PaCO_2$ 敏感，因此在黄体期和妊娠期会刺激一些过度呼吸。妊娠期间呼吸频率保持恒定，呼吸频率为每分钟 14～15 次，而潮气量则从非孕状态的约 500ml 增加到妊娠后期的约 700ml。妊娠期间增加了约 40%，因此分钟通气量（潮气量和呼吸频率的乘积）也增加了 40%，从约 7.5L/min 增加到 10.5L/min

Progesterone sensitizes the medulla oblongata to P_aCO_2, and so stimulates some over-breathing in the luteal phase and in pregnancy. Respiratory rate remains constant during pregnancy at 14–15 breaths/min, whereas tidal volume increases from about 500 mL in the non-pregnant state to about 700 mL in late pregnancy. Thus, there is ≈40% increase during pregnancy, so the minute ventilation (the product of tidal volume and respiratory rate) also increases by 40%, from about 7.5 to 10.5 L/min.

由于分钟通气量的增加及黄体酮增加红细胞中碳酸酐酶 B 水平，妊娠期动脉 PCO_2 下降。同时，血浆碳酸氢盐浓度下降，因此动脉 pH 保持恒定。随着胎儿新陈代谢的增加，二氧化碳的产量在妊娠中期急剧增加。较低的孕妇 $PaCO_2$ 可使胎盘更有效地将 CO_2 从胎儿转出。

Because of the increase in minute ventilation and the effect of progesterone increasing the level of carbonic anhydrase B in red cells, arterial PCO_2 falls in pregnancy. At the same time, there is a fall in plasma bicarbonate concentration, and the arterial pH therefore remains constant. Carbon dioxide production rises sharply during the third trimester as fetal metabolism increases. The low maternal P_aCO_2 allows more efficient placental transfer of carbon dioxide from the fetus.

肺泡通气的增加导致孕妇的 PO_2 有小幅度的升高（约 5%）。这种增加被红细胞中 2,3- 二磷酸甘油酸（2,3–DPG）增加引起的母体氧解离曲线右移所抵消。这有助于将氧卸给胎儿，胎儿 PO_2 低得多，而且由于胎儿血红蛋白对 2,3–DPG 的敏感性较低，氧解离曲线明显向左偏移。

The increased alveolar ventilation results in a small (≈5%) rise in maternal PO_2. This increase is offset by the rightward shift of the maternal oxyhaemoglobin dissociation curve caused by an increase in 2,3-diphosphoglycerate (2,3-DPG) in the erythrocytes. This facilitates oxygen unloading to the fetus, which has both a much lower PO_2 and a marked leftwards shift of the oxyhaemoglobin dissociation curve due to the lower sensitivity of fetal haemoglobin to 2,3-DPG.

由于母婴需求的增加，耗氧量增加了约 16%。由于血液中携氧能力提高约 18%（见上文），因此动静脉内的氧气差异实际上有所降低。

There is an increase of ≈16% in oxygen consumption by term due to increasing maternal and fetal demands. Since the increase in oxygen-carrying capacity of the blood (see earlier) is ≈18%, there is actually a fall in arteriovenous oxygen difference.

总而言之，呼吸系统疾病，尤其是阻塞性气道疾病对母亲健康的影响远小于心脏疾病，但严重的脊柱后凸畸形等严重限制肺部空间的疾病除外。

Overall, respiratory diseases and especially obstructive airway diseases have far fewer implications for the mother's health than cardiac disorders, with the exception of conditions such as severe kyphoscoliosis, where the lung space is severely restricted.

妊娠通常不会对患有呼吸道疾病的女性造成任何额外的风险。

Pregnancy does not generally impose any increased risk on women with respiratory disease.

七、肾功能（Renal function）

（一）解剖学（Anatomy）

到孕晚期，肾实质体积增加 70%，并且大多数女性的肾盏、肾盂和输尿管明显扩张。这与血容量的扩大一起导致肾脏体积的增加。孕早期发生这种变化是由于受到孕酮的影响而不是反压的影响。这是生理性的。但是，输尿管扩张在骨盆边缘结束，提示在妊娠后期可能有一些反压的影响。右侧这些变化总是更明显，表明有解剖上的影响。输尿管并没有低张或是运动能力低下，相反输尿管会出现平滑肌肥大和结缔组织增生。偶尔会发生膀胱输尿管反流，而反流与输尿管扩张的同时存在与尿潴留和尿路感染的高发生率相关。

Renal parenchymal volume increases by 70% by the third trimester, and there is marked dilatation of the calyces, renal pelvis and ureters in most women. This, together with the expansion of vascular volume, results in increased renal size. The changes occur in the first trimester under the influence

of progesterone rather than the effect of back pressure. This is physiological. However, the ureteric dilatation ends at the pelvic brim, suggesting that there may be some effect from back pressure in later pregnancy. These changes are invariably more pronounced on the right side, suggesting an anatomical contribution. The ureters are not hypotonic or hypomotile, and there is hypertrophy of the ureteral smooth muscle and hyperplasia of the connective tissue. Vesicoureteric reflux occurs sporadically, and the combination of reflux and ureteric dilatation is associated with a high incidence of urinary stasis and urinary tract infection.

（二）生理（Physiology）

在排卵月经周期中，肾血流量（renal blood flow，RBF）和肾小球滤过率（glomerular filtration rate，GFR）都会增加，并且如果受孕，则可以保持这种增加。妊娠最初 3 个月的 RBF 增加 50%～80%，孕中期保持在这个水平，此后下降约 15%（图 3-11）。肌酐清除率是一个有效的 GFR 指标，但其值明显低于通过菊糖清除率获得的值（金标准）。最后一次月经后 4 周，24h 肌酐清除率增加了 25%，第 9 周增加了 45%。在孕晚期，较非孕期值有一些下降，但小于 RBF 的下降。因此滤过率在孕早期下降，孕中期稳定，至足月上升到非孕期数值。

Both renal blood flow (RBF) and glomerular filtration rate (GFR) increase during an ovulatory menstrual cycle, and this increase is maintained should conception occur. RBF increases by 50%–80% in the first trimester, is maintained at these levels during the second trimester and falls by ≈15% thereafter (Fig. 3.11). Creatinine clearance is a useful indicator of GFR but gives values that are significantly less than those obtained by inulin clearance (gold standard). The 24-hour creatinine clearance has increased by 25% 4 weeks after the last menstrual period and by 45% at 9 weeks. In the third trimester, there is some decrease towards non-pregnant values, but less than the fall in RBF. The filtration fraction thus falls in the first trimester, is stable in the second and rises towards non-pregnant values towards term.

妊娠期必须保持水分以增加血浆容量。饮水的渗透压阈值在第 4 周到第 6 周之间下降，这会刺激饮水，从而稀释了体液。血浆渗透压（约 10mOsm/kg）显著下降。然而精氨酸加压素（arginine vasopressin，AVP）仍保持一定循环浓度，使水在肾髓质集合管被重新吸收，直到 Posm 低于新的渗透性口渴阈值时，建立起一个新的稳定状态。妊娠期钠潴留会促进水分潴留（见下文）。站立的抗利尿效果较非妊娠者更明显。

Water retention must occur to allow the increase in

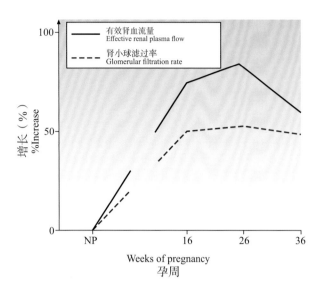

▲ 图 3-11　妊娠期肾功能的变化在孕早期结束时已基本完成

改编自 Broughton Pipkin F (2007) Maternal physiology. In: Edmonds DK (ed) Dewhurst's Textbook of Obstetrics and Gynaecology, 8th edn. Blackwell, Oxford

Fig. 3.11　The changes in renal function during pregnancy are largely complete by the end of the first trimester

Adapted from Broughton Pipkin F (2007) Maternal physiology. In: Edmonds DK (ed) Dewhurst's Textbook of Obstetrics and Gynaecology, 8th edn. Blackwell, Oxford

plasma volume. The osmotic threshold for drinking falls between weeks 4 and 6, which stimulates water intake and thus dilution of body fluids. There is a marked fall in plasma osmolality (≈10 mOsm/kg). However, arginine vasopressin (AVP) continues to circulate at concentrations that allow water to be reabsorbed in the renal medullary collecting ducts until the P_{osm} falls below the new osmotic thirst threshold, when a new steady state is established. Water retention is facilitated by the sodium retention of pregnancy (see later). Standing upright is significantly more antidiuretic than in non-pregnant subjects.

　　PV 未孕时为 2600ml，至孕 32～34 周增加到峰值，并在分娩后 4 周恢复到未孕水平。第一次妊娠的总增加量约为 50%，而第二次或以后的妊娠总增加量为 60%。膨胀越大，婴儿的平均出生体重就越大。总的来说，细胞外液总量增加了约 16%，因此 PV 的增加是不成比例的。多胎妊娠与血浆容量显著增加有关。患有妊娠高血压或先兆子痫的女性血浆容量较低，胎儿生长受限时也是如此，但何时出现下降尚不清楚。

　　PV increases in pregnancy to a peak between 32 and 34 weeks, from a non-pregnant level of 2600 mL, and returns to non-pregnant levels by 4 weeks after delivery. The total increase is ≈50% in a first pregnancy and 60% in a second or subsequent pregnancy. The bigger the expansion is, the bigger,

on average, the birth weight of the baby. The total extracellular fluid volume rises by about 16% by term, so the percentage rise in PV is disproportionately large. Multiple pregnancies are associated with a significantly higher increase in plasma volume. Women with established gestational hypertension or pre-eclampsia have lower plasma volumes, as do pregnancies exhibiting impaired fetal growth, but it is not yet established when the decrease occurs.

> **！注意**
>
> GFR 明显升高，PV 增大，说明正常妊娠血浆中肌酐、尿素等多种溶质浓度下降。在解释实验室报告时应记住这一点。
>
> The marked increase in GFR and the expansion of the PV mean that plasma concentrations of a variety of solutes, such as creatinine and urea, fall in normal pregnancy. This should be remembered when interpreting laboratory reports.

　　由于 GFR 的增加，钠的过滤负荷增加了 5000～10 000mmol/d。肾小管的重吸收与 GFR 增加一致（见下文肾素 - 血管紧张素系统），每天保留 3～5mmol 的钠进入胎儿和母体存储。钠的总净增量为 950mmol，主要存储在母体中。但是，由于血浆容量明显增加，钠的血浆浓度在妊娠期间会略有下降。钾离子也发生类似的变化，净增量约 350mmol。

　　The filtered load of sodium increases by 5000–10,000 mmol/day because of the increase in the GFR. Tubular reabsorption increases in parallel with the GFR (see Renin-angiotensin system later), with the retention of 3–5 mmol of sodium per day into the fetal and maternal stores. The total net sodium gain amounts to 950 mmol, mainly stored in the maternal compartment. However, the plasma concentration of sodium falls slightly in pregnancy because of the marked rise in plasma volume. A similar change occurs with potassium ions, with a net gain of approximately 350 mmol.

　　妊娠期间肾小管功能也发生显著变化。尿酸通过肾小球自由过滤，但大部分随后被重吸收。但是，在孕妇中，GFR 后尿酸滤过会增加一倍，并且肾小管重吸收减少，因此到妊娠中期，血清尿酸浓度下降 25%。妊娠期间的正常值范围为 148～298µmol/L，上限约为 330µmol/L。在妊娠后期，肾脏排出的过滤尿酸比例逐渐变小，因此妊娠后半期血清尿酸浓度升高是正常的。尿素也有类似的情况，部分尿素在肾单位中被重新吸收。

　　Renal tubular function also changes significantly during pregnancy. Uric acid is freely filtered through the glomerulus, but most is later reabsorbed. However, in pregnancy, uric acid filtration doubles, following the GFR, and there is a decrease in net tubular reabsorption, so serum uric acid concentrations fall by 25% to mid-pregnancy. The normal values in pregnancy range from 148–298 μmol/L, with an upper limit of ≈330 μmol/L. In later gestation, the kidney excretes a progressively smaller proportion of the filtered uric acid, so some rise in serum uric acid concentration during the second half of pregnancy is normal. A similar pattern is seen in relation to urea, which is also partly reabsorbed in the nephron.

妊娠期葡萄糖排泄增加，间歇性糖尿在正常妊娠中常见，与血糖水平无关。在妊娠期间肾小管的重吸收可能不完全。其他糖类，如乳糖和果糖的排泄量也会增加。

Glucose excretion increases during pregnancy, and intermittent glycosuria is common in normal pregnancy, unrelated to blood glucose levels. Tubular reabsorption is probably less complete during pregnancy. The excretion of other sugars, such as lactose and fructose, is also increased.

✓ 经验　糖尿可能是正常妊娠的特征。
Glycosuria may be a feature of normal pregnancy.

大概在 1,25- 二羟基维生素 D 浓度增加的影响下，钙的肾小管重吸收得到了增强。即使这样，正常妊娠的尿钙排泄量比未妊娠女性高 2～3 倍。肾碳酸氢盐的重吸收和氢离子排泄在妊娠期间似乎没有改变。尽管孕妇可以使尿液酸化，但尿液通常呈弱碱性。

The tubular reabsorption of calcium is enhanced, presumably under the influence of the increased concentrations of 1,25-dihydroxyvitamin D. Even so, urinary calcium excretion is twofold to threefold higher in normal pregnancy than in the non-pregnant woman. Renal bicarbonate reabsorption and hydrogen ion excretion appear to be unaltered during pregnancy. Although pregnant women can acidify their urine, it is usually mildly alkaline.

总蛋白和白蛋白排泄从孕早期至 36 周均增加。因此，在妊娠晚期，总蛋白排泄可接受的上限为 200mg/24h。总的来说，至少有 1/8 的女性表现出明显的蛋白尿，但不是临床上定义的高血压（"妊娠期蛋白尿"），尽管她们的血压还是显著高于那些没有蛋白尿的女性。这可能反映了肾小球通透性增加或肾小管功能的改变。用试纸评估妊娠期蛋白尿的变异性较大。

Both total protein and albumin excretion rise from the first trimester to at least 36 weeks. Thus in late pregnancy, an upper limit of normal of 200 mg total protein excretion/24 hour collection is accepted. Overall, at least one woman in eight will show significant proteinuria without clinically defined hypertension by term ('gestational proteinuria'), although their blood pressure increases more than that of women who do not show clinically significant rises in proteinuria. This may reflect increased glomerular permeability or altered tubular handling. Using dipsticks to assess proteinuria in pregnancy gives highly variable data.

八、消化系统（The alimentary system）

妊娠期间胃分泌减少，胃动力低下，因此胃排空被延迟。小肠和大肠也会出现运动能力下降，结肠对水和钠的吸收增加，导致便秘的可能性增大。胃灼热常见，可能与下食管括约肌穿过横膈的移位和它随着腹内压升高而降低的反应有关。孕妇在全身麻醉诱导期间更容易误吸胃内容物。

Gastric secretion is reduced in pregnancy and gastric motility is low, so gastric emptying is delayed. Decreased motility also occurs in both the small and large bowel, and the colonic absorption of water and sodium is increased, leading to a greater likelihood of constipation. Heartburn is common and may be related to the displacement of the lower oesophageal sphincter through the diaphragm and its decreased response as the intra-abdominal pressure rises. Pregnant women are more prone to aspiration of the gastric contents during the induction of general anaesthesia.

在雌激素刺激下，白蛋白、血浆球蛋白和纤维蛋白原的肝合成增加，尽管血浆体积增加，但后两者的增加也足以提升血浆浓度。球蛋白含量存在明显的个体差异。肝对循环氨基酸的提取减少。妊娠期间，胆囊体积增大，排空较慢，但胆汁分泌没有变化。

Hepatic synthesis of albumin, plasma globulin and fibrinogen increases under oestrogen stimulation-the latter two increase sufficiently to give increased plasma concentrations despite the increase in plasma volume. There are marked individual differences in the globulin fractions.

九、血液中的营养（Nutrients in blood）

（一）孕妇的糖代谢（Maternal carbohydrate metabolism）

葡萄糖是胎儿生长和营养的主要基质，因此妊娠期间的糖代谢对胎儿的发育非常重要。肠道对葡萄糖的吸收和胰岛素的半衰期似乎都没有改变。然而，到孕 6～12 周时，空腹血糖浓度较未妊娠时下降 0.5～1mmol/L；胎儿血糖浓度比这低约 20%。母亲的血浆胰岛素浓度升高，有利于脂肪堆积。在妊娠最初 3 个月结束时，摄入糖类后血糖的增加低于未妊娠状态（图 3-12）。孕妇在妊娠后期会产生胰岛素抵抗，任何葡萄糖刺激都会产生额外的胰岛素，但不会像非妊娠女性那样迅速降低血糖水平。这导致了一种分解代谢状态，孕妇血糖和游离脂肪酸（free fatty acid，FFA）浓度升高，这都是胎儿生长所必需的。胰岛素抵抗是激素驱动的，可能是通过人胎盘催乳素或皮质醇引起的。第 9 章将讨论孕妇糖尿病的管理。

Glucose is the major substrate for fetal growth and nutrition, so carbohydrate metabolism in pregnancy is very important for fetal development. Neither the absorption of glucose from the gut nor the half-life of insulin seem to change. However, by 6–12 weeks' gestation, fasting plasma glucose concentrations have fallen to about 0.5–1 mmol/L lower than non-pregnant values; fetal concentrations run ≈20% lower than this. The mother's plasma insulin concentrations rise, favouring fat accumulation. By the end of the first trimester, the increase in blood glucose following a carbohydrate load is less than outside pregnancy (Fig. 3.12). Pregnant women develop insulin resistance later in pregnancy, so any given glucose challenge will produce extra insulin, which does not reduce the blood glucose levels as quickly as the response in non-pregnant women. This results in a catabolic state, with raised maternal blood glucose and free fatty acid (FFA) concentrations, both of which are needed for fetal growth. The insulin resistance is hormonally driven, possibly via human placental lactogen or cortisol. The management of the pregnant woman with diabetes is discussed in Chapter 9.

除了将葡萄糖移入细胞外，胰岛素还降低了氨基酸和 FFA 的循环水平（请参阅后文的内分泌学）。

As well as moving glucose into the cells, insulin reduces the circulating level of amino acids and FFAs (see Endocrinology later).

（二）血浆蛋白的变化（Changes in plasma proteins）

妊娠前 3 个月的总蛋白浓度从 7～6g/dl 下降了约 1g/dl，尽管氮潴留有所增加。这是由于胰岛素浓度的增加，但也因为胎盘摄取和转移氨基酸给胎儿糖异生和蛋白质合成。这种下降很大程度上与白蛋白浓度的下降成正比，并与相应的胶体渗透压的下降有关。但下降并不足以影响载药能力。

The total protein concentration falls by about 1 g/dL during the first trimester from 7 to 6 g/dL, even though there is

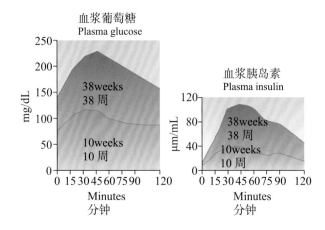

▲ 图 3-12　正常孕妇在妊娠早期和晚期对 50 克口服葡萄糖负荷的反应

在妊娠早期，血浆胰岛素反应正常，与非妊娠状态相比，血浆葡萄糖浓度相对降低。然而在妊娠晚期，尽管血浆胰岛素反应显著增强，但血浆葡萄糖浓度在延迟后仍达到较高水平，这种模式可以解释为相对胰岛素抵抗 [改编自 Broughton Pipkin F (2007) Maternal physiology. In: Edmonds DK (ed) Dewhurst's Textbook of Obstetrics and Gynaecology, 8th edn. Blackwell, Oxford.]

Fig. 3.12　Responses in normal pregnant women to a 50-g oral glucose load during early and late gestation

During early pregnancy there is a normal plasma insulin response, with a relative reduction in plasma glucose concentrations compared with the non-pregnant state. However, during late pregnancy, plasma glucose concentrations reach higher levels after a delay, despite a considerably enhanced plasma insulin response, a pattern that could be explained by relative resistance to insulin. (Adapted from Broughton Pipkin F (2007) Maternal physiology. In: Edmonds DK (ed) Dewhurst's Textbook of Obstetrics and Gynaecology, 8th edn. Blackwell, Oxford.)

increased nitrogen retention. This is partly due to the increased insulin concentrations, but also because of placental uptake and transfer of amino acids to the fetus for gluconeogenesis and protein synthesis. This fall is largely proportional to the fall in albumin concentration and is associated with a corresponding fall in colloid osmotic pressure. The fall is insufficient to affect drug-carrying capacity.

（三）氨基酸（Amino acids）

除丙氨酸和谷氨酸外，孕妇血浆中的氨基酸水平低于非妊娠水平。氨基酸向胎儿的主动转运是蛋白质合成和糖异生的基础。

With the exception of alanine and glutamic acid, amino acid levels in maternal plasma decrease below non-pregnant values. There is active transport of amino acids to the fetus as building blocks for protein synthesis and gluconeogenesis.

（四）脂类（Lipids）

血清总脂质浓度从大约 600mg/dl 上升到 1000mg/dl。最大的变化是 36 周时极低密度脂蛋白（VLDL）甘油三酯增加了约 3 倍，VLDL 胆固醇增加了 50%。足月出生体重和胎盘体重与孕妇 VLDL 甘油三酯水平直接相关。在整个孕期，总脂肪酸（FA）浓度升高，饱和脂肪酸和单不饱和脂肪酸的比例也升高，但 ω-6 脂肪酸的比例会下降。FFA 的水平在孕妇中尤其不稳定，可能会受到禁食、劳累、情绪紧张和吸烟的影响。与体重指数（BMI）正常的女性相比，超重女性的整个妊娠过程中的脂质氧化更高。

The total serum lipid concentration rises from about 600 to 1000 mg per 100 mL. The greatest changes are the approximate threefold increases in very-low-density lipoprotein (VLDL) triglycerides and a 50% increase in VLDL cholesterol by 36 weeks. Birth weight and placental weight are directly related to maternal VLDL triglyceride levels at term. Total fatty acid (FA) concentration rises throughout pregnancy, as does the proportion of saturated and monounsaturated FAs, but the proportion of omega-6 FAs falls. Levels of FFAs are particularly unstable in pregnancy and may be affected by fasting, exertion, emotional stress and smoking. Lipid oxidation is higher throughout pregnancy in women who are overweight than in those with normal body mass index (BMI).

正常妊娠的高脂血症不会引起动脉粥样硬化，尽管妊娠可以诱发病理性高脂血症。母体通常可以通过增加内源性抗氧化物质免受孕期脂质过氧化增加的潜在有害影响，尽管这在子痫前期中可能是不够的。此外，还需要从膳食中摄取足够的抗氧化物质，如维生素 A、类胡萝卜素和维生素 A 原类胡萝卜素。妊娠期间，脂溶性维生素水平上升，而水溶性维生素水平则趋于下降。

The hyperlipidaemia of normal pregnancy is not atherogenic, although pregnancy can unmask pathological hyperlipidaemia. Mothers are usually protected from the potentially harmful effects of increasing lipid peroxidation in pregnancy by an increase in endogenous antioxidants, although this may be inadequate in pre-eclampsia. An adequate dietary intake of antioxidants such as vitamin A, the carotenoids and provitamin A carotenoids is also needed. Levels of fat-soluble vitamins rise in pregnancy, whereas levels of water-soluble vitamins tend to fall.

胆汁盐有助于膳食脂肪和脂溶性维生素的吸收。血清胆汁酸随着妊娠的进展而增加，其中初级胆汁酸的增加最多。核法尼醇 X 受体（FXR）主要负责胆汁酸稳态。在妊娠期间其活性降低。

Bile salts facilitate the absorption of dietary fats and fat-soluble vitamins. Serum bile acids rise as pregnancy progresses, with the primary bile acids showing the greatest increase. The nuclear Farnesoid X receptor (FXR) is mainly responsible for bile acid homeostasis; its activity is reduced during pregnancy.

脂肪在妊娠初期沉积。它也被当作一种能量来源，主要由母体在妊娠中晚期用于高代谢需求和在哺乳期使用，以便为生长中的胎儿提供葡萄糖。储备脂肪的总量为 2～6kg，主要在孕中期沉积，并受瘦素的调节。它主要沉积在背部、大腿上部、臀部和腹壁。

Fat is deposited early in pregnancy. It is also used as a source of energy, mainly by the mother from mid to late pregnancy for the high metabolic demands and during lactation so that glucose is available for the growing fetus. Total fat accretion is ≈2–6 kg, mainly laid down in the second trimester, and is regulated by the hormone leptin. It is deposited mainly over the back, the upper thighs, the buttocks and the abdominal wall.

（五）钙（Calcium）

孕妇血浆总钙下降是因为白蛋白浓度下降，但未结合的离子钙未改变。1,25- 二羟基胆钙化固醇的合成增加，促进胃肠道钙的吸收增强，在孕 24 周增加一倍，然后稳定下来。

Maternal total plasma calcium falls because albumin concentration falls, but unbound ionized calcium is unchanged. Synthesis of 1,25-dihydroxycholecalciferol increases, promoting enhanced gastrointestinal calcium absorption, which doubles by 24 weeks, after which it stabilizes.

十、孕妇体重增加（Maternal weight gain）

妊娠是一种合成代谢状态。体重指数正常的女性在妊娠期间平均体重约增加 12.5kg。许多女性在孕早期体重没有增加，与食欲不振和孕吐导致的食物摄入减少相关。而正常妊娠 18 周内平均增重为每周 0.3kg，18～28 周平均增重为每周 0.5kg，之后体重轻微减重约为每周 0.4kg，直到足月（图 3-13）。由于多种因素的影响，正常妊娠中孕妇体重增加的范围可能从接近 0 到平均增加体重的 2 倍。呼吸比 [RQ，即二氧化碳的产生 / 氧气的消耗；用于计算基础代谢率（basal metabolic rete，BMR）] 给出了在妊娠期间糖类与脂肪氧化比例变化的概念。体重正常的女性到妊娠结束时，BMR 升高约 5%。图 3-14 总结了足月孕产妇和胎儿对体重增加的相对贡献。

Pregnancy is an anabolic state. The average weight gain over pregnancy in a woman of normal BMI is ≈12.5 kg. Many women during the first trimester do not gain any weight because of reduced food intake associated with loss of appetite and morning sickness. However, in normal pregnancy, the

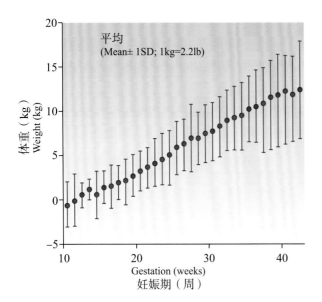

▲ 图 3-13　正常妊娠中孕妇体重增加 [平均值 ±1 SD (标准差)]

经 许 可 转 载， 引 自 James D, Steer P, Weiner C, et al (2010) High Risk Pregnancy: Management Options. Elsevier Saunders, St Louis . Elsevier.

Fig. 3.13　Maternal weight gain (mean ± 1 SD [standard deviation]) in normal pregnancy.

From James D, Steer P, Weiner C, et al (2010) High Risk Pregnancy: Management Options. Elsevier Saunders, St Louis © Elsevier. Reproduced by permission.

average weight gain is 0.3 kg/week up to 18 weeks, 0.5 kg/week from 18 to 28 weeks and thereafter a slight reduction with a rate of ≈0.4 kg/week until term (Fig. 3.13). The range of maternal weight gain in normal pregnancy may vary from near zero to twice the mean weight gain because of variation in the multiple contributory factors. The respiratory quotient (RQ: carbon dioxide production/oxygen consumption; used to calculate basal metabolic rate (BMR)) gives an idea of changes in the proportion of carbohydrate vs. fat oxidized during pregnancy. The BMR rises by ≈5% by the end of pregnancy in a woman of normal weight. Figure 3.14 summarizes the relative maternal and fetal contributions to weight gain at term.

在所有系统中，重量增加的很大一部分是由于水潴留。平均总增加量约为 8.5L，初产妇和经产妇相同。结缔组织水化增加导致关节松弛，尤其是骨盆韧带和耻骨联合。子宫和乳房等组织的大小会增加。

Much of this weight increase in all systems arises from the retention of water; the mean total increase is ≈8.5 L and is the same in primigravid and multiparous women. The increased hydration of connective tissue results in laxity of the joints, particularly in the pelvic ligaments and the pubic symphysis. Tissues such as the uterus and breasts increase in size.

大量体重增加通常与水肿和液体潴留有关。然而，总体体重增加与出生体重呈正相关，尽管这可能与潜在的血浆容量增加有关系。尽管急性体重过

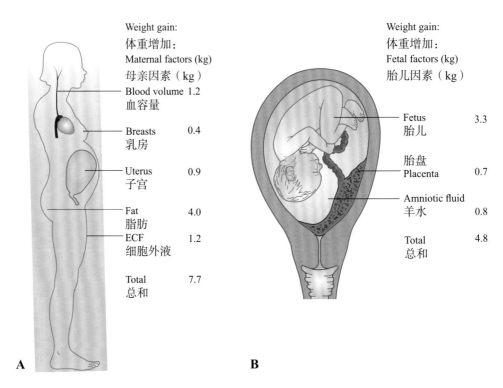

▲ 图 3-14　孕妇（A）和胎儿（B）对足月体重增加的贡献。ECF. 细胞外液

Fig. 3.14　(A) Maternal and (B) fetal contributions to weight gain at term. ECF, Extracellular fluid

度增加可能与先兆子痫的发展有关，但轻度水肿与良好的胎儿结局有关。

High weight gain is commonly associated with oedema and fluid retention. However, overall weight gain has a positive association with birth weight, although this may relate to the underlying rise in plasma volume. Although acute excessive weight gain may be associated with the development of pre-eclampsia, mild oedema is associated with a good fetal outcome.

体重未增加更为危险，这可能与羊水体积减小、胎盘小、胎儿生长受损和不良结局有关。

Far more sinister is failure to gain weight, which may be associated with reduced amniotic fluid volume, small placental size, impaired fetal growth and an adverse outcome.

> **！注意**　急性体重增加表明体液潴留。体重增加不足与胎儿生长受限有关。
>
> Acute excess weight gain indicates fluid retention. Poor weight gain is associated with fetal growth restriction.

蛋白质和蛋白质的沉积量不能超过胎儿和胎盘的生长，以及特定靶器官（如子宫和乳房）大小的增加所需。

No more protein is laid down than can be accounted for by fetal and placental growth and by the increase in size in specific target organs such as the uterus and the breasts.

在欧洲，有 20%～40% 的孕妇体重增加超过建议值。令人惊讶的是，能量摄入和母亲体重增加之间的相关性很差，一般不建议试图在妊娠期间减肥，因为这可能导致必需营养素的限制，进而可能对胎儿的生长发育产生不良影响。

Between 20% and 40% of pregnant women in Europe are gaining more weight than recommended. Surprisingly, the correlation between energy intake and maternal weight gain is poor, and it is generally not advisable to attempt to promote weight loss in pregnancy, as it may result in a parallel restriction of essential nutrients, which in turn may have undesirable effects on fetal growth and development.

产后体重（Postpartum weight）

分娩后体重立即减轻约 6kg，这是由于水和液体的流失及减去受孕产物造成的。利尿发生在产褥初期，去除了妊娠期间残留的水分。从大约第 3 天起，体重每天下降约 0.3kg/d 直到第 10 天，至第 10 周稳定在约比孕前体重高约 2.3kg，继续哺乳的女性每天下降约 0.7kg。利尿发生在产褥期早期，排出妊娠期

间残留的水分。到分娩后 6～18 个月，妊娠导致的体重增加仍会保留 1～2kg，但是约 20% 的女性可以保留 5kg 或更多。肥胖女性通常在妊娠期间体重增重较少，但产后保留更多。

Immediately following delivery, there is a weight loss of ≈6 kg, which is accounted for by water and fluid loss and by the loss of the products of conception. Diuresis occurs during the early puerperium, removing the water retained during pregnancy. From approximately day 3, body weight falls by ≈0.3 kg/day until day 10, stabilizing by week 10 at ≈2.3 kg above pre-pregnancy weight, or 0.7 kg in women who are continuing to lactate. By 6–18 months after delivery, 1–2 kg of pregnancy-related weight gain will still be retained, but in about one-fifth of women, 5 kg or more can be retained. Obese women usually put on less weight during pregnancy but retain more postpartum.

经产妇体重增加比初产妇约少 0.9kg。但是，对近 3000 名女性进行了 5 年的随访发现，在这段时间内，经产妇比未产妇增加了 23kg。

Weight gain is about 0.9 kg less in multigravidae than in primigravidae. However, a 5-year follow-up of nearly 3000 women found that parous women gained 23 kg more than nulliparae during this time.

十一、乳房（The breasts）

妊娠最初的一些体征和症状发生在乳房，其中包括乳房压痛、体积增大、乳头增大、乳晕血管增多和色素沉着。

Some of the first signs and symptoms of pregnancy occur in the breasts, including breast tenderness, an increase in size, enlargement of the nipples and increased vascularity and pigmentation of the areola.

乳晕中有妊娠期间肥大的皮脂腺（Montgomery 结节）。乳晕富含感觉神经，确保在哺乳时向下丘脑发送脉冲，从而刺激垂体后叶释放催产素从和乳汁的排出。

The areola contains sebaceous glands that hypertrophy during pregnancy (Montgomery's tubercles). The areola is richly supplied with sensory nerves, which ensures that suckling sends impulses to the hypothalamus and thus stimulates the release of oxytocin from the posterior lobe of the pituitary gland and the expulsion of milk.

（一）妊娠期间乳房发育(Breast development during pregnancy)

高浓度的雌激素及生长激素和糖皮质激素会刺激妊娠期的导管增生（图 3-15）。在雌激素主导的乳房中，黄体酮和催乳素刺激腺泡的生长。分泌活动

是在妊娠期间开始的，并由催乳素和胎盘催乳素促进，因此从 3～4 个月及分娩后的最初 30h，乳房可排出浓稠、有光泽的富含蛋白质的液体，称为初乳。但是，在妊娠期间，高水平的雌激素和孕酮会阻止 α- 乳清蛋白在乳腺中的转录，抑制全乳分泌。

High oestrogen concentrations, with growth hormone and glucocorticoids, stimulate ductal proliferation during pregnancy (Fig. 3.15). Alveolar growth is stimulated in the oestrogen-primed breast by progesterone and prolactin. Secretory activity is initiated during pregnancy and is promoted by prolactin and placental lactogen so that from 3 to 4 months onwards and for the first 30 hours after delivery, a thick, glossy, protein-rich fluid known as *colostrum* can be expressed from the breast. However, full lactation is inhibited during pregnancy by the high levels of oestrogen and progesterone that block the alveolar transcription of α-lactalbumin.

（二）哺乳期的开始（The initiation of lactation）

催乳素直接作用于乳腺细胞以刺激所有乳成分的合成，包括酪蛋白、乳白蛋白和脂肪酸。分娩后孕激素和雌激素水平的突然降低使催乳素以不受抑制的方式发挥作用，它的释放是通过哺乳来促进的，到第 5 天乳汁流量充分，在接下来的 3 周内进一步增加。每天生产 500～1000ml 乳汁，母亲每天需要约 500kcal 的额外热量来维持这一水平；另外 250kcal/d 来自母亲的脂肪储存。母乳喂养的母亲，妊娠后期所堆积的内脏脂肪和增加的胰岛素抵抗、脂质和甘油三酸酯逆转得更快、更彻底。

Prolactin acts directly on alveolar cells to stimulate the synthesis of all milk components, including casein, lactalbumin and fatty acids. The sudden reduction of progesterone and oestrogen levels following parturition allows prolactin to act in an uninhibited manner, and its release is promoted by suckling, with the development of the full flow of milk by day 5 and a further gradual increase over the next 3 weeks. Some 500–1000 mL of milk is produced daily, and the mother needs about 500 kcal extra per day to maintain this; a further 250 kcal/day are derived from the maternal fat stores. The visceral fat accumulation and increased insulin resistance, lipid and triglyceride levels of later pregnancy reverse more quickly, and more completely, in breast-feeding mothers.

哺乳还促进下丘脑视上核和室旁核的特定神经元释放催产素，催产素刺激肌上皮细胞收缩继而导致排乳反射。母亲看到婴儿或听到婴儿的哭声，或者只是想着喂奶，也会刺激排乳反射。它也可能被儿茶酚胺释放或不良的情绪和环境因素所抑制。使

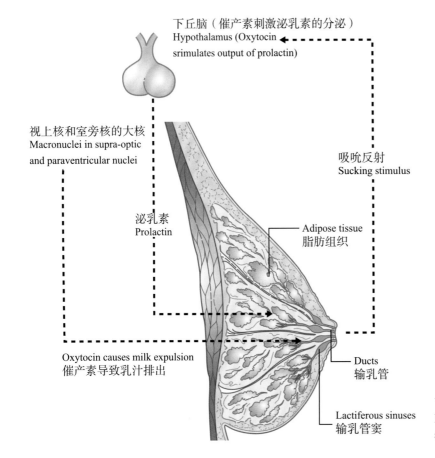

下丘脑（催产素刺激泌乳素的分泌）
Hypothalamus (Oxytocin srimulates output of prolactin)

视上核和室旁核的大核
Macronuclei in supra-optic and paraventricular nuclei

吸吮反射
Sucking stimulus

泌乳素
Prolactin

Adipose tissue
脂肪组织

Oxytocin causes milk expulsion
催产素导致乳汁排出

Ducts
输乳管

Lactiferous sinuses
输乳管窦

◀ 图 3-15 调节乳汁产生和排出的因素
Fig. 3.15 Factors regulating milk production and expulsion

用多巴胺激动药，如溴隐亭，可抑制泌乳素的释放，并使产奶停止。

Suckling also promotes the release of oxytocin from specialized neurons in the supraoptic and paraventricular nuclei of the hypothalamus, and this in turn results in the milk-ejection reflex as the oxytocin stimulates the myoepithelial cells to contract. The milk-ejection reflex can also be stimulated by the mother seeing the infant or hearing its cry or just thinking about feeding! It may also be inhibited by catecholamine release or by adverse emotional and environmental factors. The administration of a dopamine agonist such as bromocriptine inhibits the release of prolactin and abolishes milk production.

十二、皮肤（The skin）

妊娠期皮肤变化的特征是在脸上出现黑素细胞刺激激素（melanocyte-stimulating hormone，MSH）刺激的色素沉着（称为黄褐斑），乳头乳晕和前腹壁的白线，出现黑中线。妊娠纹主要出现在腹壁的应力线上，也出现在大腿和乳房的侧面。妊娠纹是由下角质层胶原纤维破坏造成的，与妊娠期间肾上腺皮质激素的分泌增加有关，而与腹腔扩张引起的皮肤皱褶的压力和张力无关。

The characteristic feature of skin changes in pregnancy are the appearance of melanocyte-stimulating hormone (MSH)-stimulated pigmentation on the face, known as *chloasma*, the areola of the nipples and the linea alba of the anterior abdominal wall, giving rise to the *linea nigra*. Stretch marks (*striae gravidarum*) predominantly occur in the lines of stress of the abdominal wall but also occur on the lateral aspects of the thighs and breasts. Striae gravidarum result from the disruption of collagen fibres in the subcuticular zone and are related more to the increased production of adrenocortical hormones in pregnancy than to the stress and tension in the skin folds associated with the expansion of the abdominal cavity.

皮肤血流量显著增加，并且血流介导的扩张增加。这些变化可以使热量更有效地流失，尤其是在妊娠晚期，处于发育中的胎儿，其核心温度比母亲的温度高约1℃，增加了热量的产生。

Skin blood flow increases markedly, and flow-mediated dilatation is increased. These changes allow more efficient heat loss, especially in late pregnancy, when the developing fetus, whose core temperature is ≈1°C higher than the mother's, contributes to increasing heat production.

十三、内分泌变化（Endocrine changes）

胎盘大量生产性类固醇激素以主导内分泌谱，

但是在妊娠期间母亲所有的内分泌器官也发生了显著变化。认识到这些变化是很重要的，这样这些变化就不会被解释为功能异常。

Massive production of sex steroids by the placenta tends to dominate the endocrine picture, but there are also significant changes in all the maternal endocrine organs during pregnancy. It is important to be aware of these changes so that they are not interpreted as indicating abnormal function.

（一）胎盘激素（Placental hormones）

人绒毛膜促性腺激素是妊娠的信号。胎儿胎盘单位合成了大量的雌激素和孕酮，都是子宫生长、静止和乳房发育所需要的。但是，雌激素也刺激甲状腺激素和糖皮质激素结合球蛋白的合成。皮质醇结合球蛋白（cortisolbinding globulin，CBG）在整个孕期都会增加，达到非孕期水平的2倍，而甲状腺结合球蛋白（thyroid-binding globulin，TBG）在孕早期结束时增加一倍，并在整个孕期保持升高状态。雌激素还刺激血管内皮生长因子（vascular endothelial growth factor，VEGF）及其受体和血管生成。反过来，在胎盘绒毛毛细血管床的发育过程中，VEGF似乎与其他胎盘产生的激素和血管生成素-2相互作用。胎盘特异性抗血管生成的可溶性fms样酪氨酸激酶-1（sFLT-1）e15a可拮抗VEGF和胎盘生长因子的活性。过多的话，就会导致内皮功能障碍。过氧化物酶体增殖物激活受体-γ（PPARγ）在人绒毛和胞外细胞滋养层中表达，并与天然配体（如花生酸类、FA和氧化低密度脂蛋白）结合并被激活。

Human chorionic gonadotrophin is the signal for pregnancy. The fetoplacental unit synthesizes very large amounts of oestrogen and progesterone, both being needed for uterine growth and quiescence and for breast development. However, oestrogen also stimulates the synthesis of binding globulins for thyroxine and corticosteroids; cortisolbinding globulin (CBG) increases throughout pregnancy to reach twice non-pregnant levels, while thyroid-binding globulin (TBG) is doubled by the end of the first trimester and remains elevated throughout pregnancy. Oestrogens also stimulate vascular endothelial growth factor (VEGF) and its receptors and angiogenesis. In turn, VEGF appears to interact with other placentally produced hormones and angiopoietin-2 in the development of the placental villous capillary bed. The placentally specific form of the anti-angiogenic soluble fms-like tyrosine kinase-1 (sFLT-1) e15a antagonizes the activity of VEGF and placental growth factor. In excess, this can lead to endothelial dysfunction. The peroxisome proliferator-activated receptor-γ (PPARγ) is expressed in human villous and extravillous cytotrophoblast and binds to, and is activated by, natural ligands such as eicosanoids, FAs and oxidized low-density lipoproteins.

（二）垂体（The pituitary gland）

1. 解剖学（Anatomy）

垂体前叶和后叶具有不同的胚胎学起源，垂体前叶起源于发育中的口腔中的 Rathke 囊，而垂体后叶则来自形成第三脑室底部的神经组织的向下生长。专门的血管门静脉系统将两个部分连接起来。初产妇妊娠期间垂体腺增大了约 30%，而经产女性的垂体则增大了 50%。重量的增加主要是由于垂体前叶的变化。

The anterior and posterior pituitary glands have different embryological origins, with the anterior pituitary arising from Rathke's pouch in the developing oral cavity, while the posterior pituitary is derived from a down-growth of neural tissue that forms the floor of the third ventricle. A specialized vascular portal system connects the two parts. The pituitary gland enlarges during pregnancy by ≈30% in primigravid women and 50% in multiparous women. The weight increase is largely due to changes in the anterior lobe.

2. 垂体前叶（Anterior pituitary）

垂体前叶可产生 3 种糖蛋白（促黄体激素、促卵泡激素和促甲状腺激素）和 3 种多肽和肽类激素 [生长激素、催乳激素和肾上腺皮质营养激素（adrenocorticotrophic hormone，ACTH）]。雌激素水平的增加刺激了催乳素细胞的数量和分泌活性。催乳素的释放受催乳素抑制因子（如多巴胺）的控制。妊娠期催乳素的合成和血浆浓度稳定增长，在分娩时激增，随后随着胎盘雌激素消失而下降。继续母乳喂养的女性的催乳素水平仍高于基础水平。

The anterior pituitary produces three glycoproteins (luteinizing hormone, follicular-stimulating hormone and thyroid-stimulating hormone) and three polypeptide and peptide hormones (growth hormone, prolactin and adrenocorticotrophic hormone (ACTH). The increased oestrogen levels stimulate the number and secretory activity of the lactotrophs. Prolactin release is controlled by prolactin inhibitory factors such as dopamine. There is a steady rise in prolactin synthesis and plasma concentration, with a surge at the time of delivery, and a subsequent fall with the disappearance of placental oestrogens. Levels of prolactin remain raised above basal in women who continue to breast-feed.

妊娠期间血浆 ACTH 水平升高，但仍处于非妊娠期的正常范围内。部分增加可能是由于胎盘的合成。黑素细胞刺激激素（melanocyte-stimulation hormone，MSH）在垂体中间叶合成，与 ACTH 共享一个前体（促阿片黑素皮质激素），并在妊娠期间增加。

Plasma levels of ACTH rise in pregnancy but remain within the normal non-pregnant range. Some of the increase may be the result of placental production. Melanocyte-stimulating hormone (MSH), synthesized in the pituitary intermediate lobe, shares a precursor (pro-opiomelanocortin) with ACTH and rises in pregnancy.

绒毛膜促性腺激素的上升抑制了促性腺激素的分泌，生长激素的分泌也受到了抑制。妊娠期甲状腺素水平保持恒定。

Gonadotrophin secretion is inhibited by the rising chorionic gonadotrophin, as is the secretion of growth hormone. Thyrotrophin levels remain constant in pregnancy.

3. 垂体后叶（Posterior pituitary）

垂体后叶释放 AVP 和催产素。妊娠早期血浆渗透压下降，胎盘产生的亮氨酸氨基肽酶（produced leucine aminopeptidase，PLAP）使 AVP 清除率增加 4 倍。但是，一旦达到新的基线渗透压浓度，AVP 就会对水合过度和水合不足做出适当的反应（见血浆容量）。

The posterior pituitary releases AVP and oxytocin. Plasma osmolality falls in early pregnancy and clearance of AVP increases fourfold because of a placentally produced leucine aminopeptidase (PLAP). However, AVP responds appropriately to over- and under-hydration once the new baseline osmolality is reached (see Plasma volume earlier).

催产素刺激子宫收缩。其孕期的低水平也是由于 PLAP 的高浓度。分娩中的催产素水平不会升高，但是子宫催产素受体的表达上调，因此对催产素的敏感性增强。这似乎与雌激素与孕激素的比例有关，因为雌激素结合位点上调而孕酮使其下调。另外，子宫颈的扩张刺激催产素的释放，从而增强子宫活动。催产素在哺乳过程中也起着重要作用，因为它是在刺激乳头后释放出来的。作用于乳腺泡周围的肌上皮细胞，使这些细胞收缩并排出乳汁。

Oxytocin stimulates uterine contractions. Concentrations are low during gestation, again because of the high concentrations of PLAP. Oxytocin levels are not raised in labour, but there is an upregulation of uterine oxytocin receptors, so there is enhanced sensitivity to oxytocin. This appears to be related to the oestrogen:progesterone ratio, as oestrogen upregulates binding sites and progesterone downregulates them. In addition, dilatation of the cervix stimulates the release of oxytocin, thus reinforcing uterine activity. Oxytocin also plays an important role in lactation, as it is released following stimulation of the nipples. It then acts on the myoepithelial cells surrounding the breast alveoli, causing these cells to contract and eject milk.

（三）下丘脑（Hypothalamus）

下丘脑合成各种"释放激素"，如促甲状腺激素释放激素（thyrotropin-releasing hormone，TRH）和促性腺激素释放激素。妊娠期血清催乳素和促甲状腺激素（TSH）对 TRH 的平均反应略小于非妊娠期的反应，并且在整个妊娠期较平稳。促肾上腺皮质激素释放激素（corticotrophin-releasing hormone，CRH）刺激 ACTH 的释放。下丘脑和胎盘都会合成 CRH。血浆 CRH 水平在妊娠晚期大幅升高，这可能是分娩开始的诱因之一。

The hypothalamus synthesizes a variety of 'releasing hormones' such as thyrotropin-releasing hormone (TRH) and gonadotropin-releasing hormone. The mean serum prolactin and thyroid-stimulating hormone (TSH) responses to TRH in pregnancy are somewhat smaller than the non-pregnant response and are similar across pregnancy. Corticotrophin-releasing hormone (CRH) stimulates the release of ACTH. Both hypothalamus and placenta synthesize CRH. Plasma levels of CRH increase greatly in the third trimester and may be one of the triggers for the onset of labour.

（四）甲状腺（The thyroid）

孕妇甲状腺肿大的比例高达 70%，具体比例视碘摄入量而定。正常妊娠时，尿碘排泄增加，碘甲状腺原氨酸转移到胎儿。这反过来导致了母亲体内血浆无机碘水平的下降。与此同时，甲状腺从血液中吸收的碘增加了 2 倍，造成了碘的相对缺乏，这可能是导致腺体代偿性滤泡增大的原因（图 3-16）。

The thyroid gland enlarges in up to 70% of pregnant women, the percentage varying depending on iodine intake. In normal pregnancy, there is increased urinary excretion of iodine and transfer of iodothyronines to the fetus. This in turn results in a fall of plasma inorganic iodide levels in the mother. At the same time, the thyroid gland triples its uptake of iodide from the blood, creating a relative iodine deficiency, which is probably responsible for the compensatory follicular enlargement of the gland (Fig. 3.16).

由于 TBG 升高，妊娠期的总三碘甲状原氨酸（T_3）和甲状腺素（T_4）升高，而游离 T_3 和 T_4 是只有妊娠初期升高，随后降至非孕水平。TSH 可能会略有增加，但倾向于保持在正常范围内。T_3、T_4 和 TSH 不能穿过胎盘屏障，因此，孕妇和胎儿的甲状腺功能之间没有直接关系。但是，碘和抗甲状腺药物确实可以穿过胎盘，而长效甲状腺刺激剂（LATS）也可以。因此，胎儿受碘摄入水平和母亲自身免疫性疾病的影响。

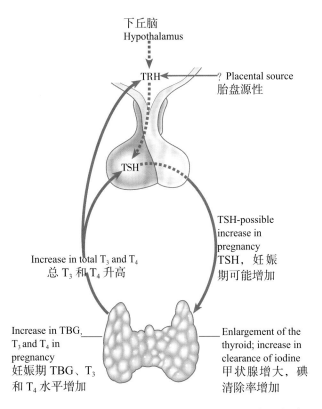

▲ 图 3-16　妊娠期间的甲状腺功能。T_3. 三碘甲状原氨酸；T_4. 甲状腺素；TBG. 甲状腺结合球蛋白；TRH. 促甲状腺激素释放激素；TSH. 促甲状腺激素

Fig. 3.16　Thyroid function in pregnancy. T3, Tri-iodothyronine; T4, thyroxine; TBG, thyroid-binding globulin; TRH, thyrotropinreleasing hormone; TSH, thyroid-stimulating hormone

As a result of the increase in TBG, total tri-iodothyronine (T_3) and thyroxine (T_4) levels increase in pregnancy, although free T_3 and T_4 rise in early pregnancy and then fall to remain in the non-pregnant range. TSH may increase slightly but tends to remain within the normal range. T_3, T_4 and TSH do not cross the placental barrier, and there is therefore no direct relationship between maternal and fetal thyroid function. However, iodine and anti-thyroid drugs do cross the placenta, as does the long-acting thyroid stimulator (LATS). Hence, the fetus may be affected by the level of iodine intake and by the presence of autoimmune disease in the mother.

降钙素是另一种甲状腺激素。在孕早期上升，在孕中期达到高峰然后下降，但变化幅度不大。它可能有助于调节 1,25- 二羟基维生素 D。

Calcitonin is another thyroid hormone. It rises during the first trimester, peaks in the second and falls thereafter, although the changes are not large. It may contribute to the regulation of 1,25-di-hydroxy vitamin D.

（五）甲状旁腺（The parathyroids）

甲状旁腺激素（parathyroid hormone，PTH）调

节近曲小管 1,25- 二羟基维生素 D 的合成。妊娠期间 PTH 下降，但是 1,25- 二羟基维生素 D 增加了 1 倍。胎盘来源的 PTH 相关蛋白（PTHrP）也存在于母体循环中，并通过 PTH 受体起作用，进而影响钙稳态。

Parathyroid hormone (PTH) regulates the synthesis of 1,25-dihydroxy vitamin D in the proximal convoluted tubule. There is a fall in intact PTH during pregnancy but a doubling of 1,25-dihydroxy vitamin D. Placentally derived PTH-related protein (PTHrP) is also present in the maternal circulation and affects calcium homeostasis by acting through the PTH receptor.

（六）肾素 – 血管紧张素系统（RAS）(The renin-angiotensin system (RAS))

RAS 在黄体期被激活，是最早"识别"妊娠的激素之一。GFR 的增加和高孕激素导致致密斑钠负荷增加，刺激肾素的释放。同时，雌激素刺激血管紧张素原的合成。Ang Ⅱ 的增加会刺激醛固酮合成并从肾上腺皮质释放，这抵消了孕激素在远端小管的利尿钠作用，并导致钠潴留和 PV 扩张。Ang Ⅱ 升高对血压的潜在影响被血管对 Ang Ⅱ 敏感性的平行降低所抵消。而正常妊娠中对 Ang Ⅱ 敏感性的下降在子痫前期患者中消失了，这类患者的敏感性甚至在高血压发生前就增加了。

The RAS is activated in the luteal phase and is one of the first hormones to 'recognize' pregnancy. The increased GFR and high progesterone cause an increased sodium load at the macula densa, which stimulates renin release. At the same time, oestrogens stimulate angiotensinogen synthesis. The resultant increase in AngII stimulates aldosterone synthesis and release from the adrenal cortex, which counters the natriuretic effect of progesterone at the distal tubule and results in sodium retention and PV expansion. The potential effect of the raised AngII on blood pressure is offset by a parallel, specific reduction in vascular sensitivity to AngII. The decreased sensitivity to AngII in normal pregnancy is lost in pre-eclampsia, where sensitivity increases even before the onset of hypertension.

Ang Ⅱ 直接通过 2 个对应的受体 AT_1 和 AT_2 亚型起作用。AT_1 受体促进血管生成、肥大和血管收缩，AT_2 受体促进细胞凋亡。AT_2 的表达在早期的胎盘中占主导地位，该系统可能参与了植入和血管重塑。

AngII acts through two directly opposing receptors, the AT1 and AT2 subtypes. AT1 receptors promote angiogenesis, hypertrophy and vasoconstriction, and AT2 receptors promote apoptosis. AT2 expression dominates in the early placenta, where the system may be involved in implantation and vascular re-modelling.

（七）肾上腺（The adrenal gland）

肾上腺的大小保持不变，但功能发生变化。像垂体一样，肾上腺有 2 个不同的胚胎起源。间叶皮质和肾上腺髓质，后者起源于迁移的神经嵴细胞。皮质激素会影响髓质激素（如糖皮质激素刺激肾上腺素的合成）；相反，肾上腺素可能在"压力"下增加 ACTH 释放。

The adrenal glands remain constant in size but exhibit changes in function. Like the pituitary gland, the adrenal gland has two distinct embryological origins: the mesenchymal cortex and the adrenal medulla, which originates from migratory neural crest cells. Cortical hormones can influence medullary ones (e.g. glucocorticoids stimulate adrenaline synthesis); conversely, adrenaline may increase ACTH release under 'stress'.

ACTH 的上升刺激了皮质醇的合成，血浆总皮质醇浓度从 3 个月上升至足月。大部分皮质醇与 CBG 或白蛋白结合；即使如此，平均游离（活化）皮质醇浓度在妊娠期间也会增加，昼夜变化消失。正常的胎盘合成一种妊娠特异性的 11β- 羟类固醇脱氢酶，该酶抑制母体皮质醇向胎儿的转移。过度转移可能会抑制胎儿的生长。

The rising ACTH stimulates cortisol synthesis, and plasma total cortisol concentrations rise from 3 months to term. Much of this cortisol is bound to CBG or to albumin; even so, mean free (active) cortisol concentrations do also increase during pregnancy, with the loss of diurnal variation. The normal placenta synthesizes a pregnancy-specific 11 β-hydroxysteroid dehydrogenase, which inhibits transfer of maternal cortisol to the fetus; excess transfer is thought to inhibit fetal growth.

血浆中肾小球源性的醛固酮会在整个妊娠过程中逐渐升高（见"肾素 – 血管紧张素系统"）。在妊娠 8 周时，胎儿胎盘单位源性的弱盐皮质激素类脱氧皮质酮也明显增加。

Plasma aldosterone from the zona glomerulosa rises progressively throughout pregnancy (see The renin-angiotensin system earlier); there is also a substantial increase in the weak mineralocorticoid deoxycorticosterone that is apparent by 8 weeks' gestation and may reflect production by the fetoplacental unit.

雌激素引起的性激素结合球蛋白（SHBG）产量增加，导致总睾酮水平增加。

The oestrogen-induced increase in the production of sex hormone-binding globulin (SHBG) results in an increase in total testosterone levels.

改进的测量技术表明，从孕早期到孕晚期血浆儿茶酚胺浓度逐渐下降。妊娠期站立和等长运动时去甲肾上腺素（主要反映交感神经活动）的升高有一定程度的减弱，但肾上腺素反应（主要是肾上腺素）没有改变。然而，在分娩过程中，由于压力和肌肉活动，肾上腺素和去甲肾上腺素的浓度往往大幅增加。

Improved measurement techniques have shown that plasma catecholamine concentrations fall from the first to the third trimester. There is some blunting of the rise in noradrenaline (reflecting mainly sympathetic nerve activity) seen on standing and isometric exercise in pregnancy, but the adrenaline response (predominantly adrenal) is unaltered.

However, there are often massive increases in both adrenaline and noradrenaline concentrations during labour as the result of stress and muscle activity.

十四、结论（Conclusion）

有时许多相互依赖的、较大的综合性改变在妊娠之前就已经开始了。要理解不正常的变化，就必须了解正常的变化。

Many of the sometimes very large, inter-dependent and integrated changes in maternal physiology begin even before conception. One needs a good understanding of the normal changes to understand the abnormal.

本章概览	Essential information
总论 • 许多对妊娠的适应性变化在黄体期就开始了，即主动适应	**General** • Many pregnancy adaptations are initiated in the luteal phase, i.e. are proactive
免疫反应 • 子宫不是免疫豁免部位 • 滋养细胞不会引起同种异体反应 • 胎儿与母体循环间具有非免疫原性界面 • 产妇的免疫反应是局部调控的 • 胸腺在妊娠期退化 • 引流子宫的淋巴结增大	**Immunological responses** • The uterus is not an immunologically privileged site • Trophoblast does not elicit allogeneic responses • Fetus has a non-immunogenic interface with maternal circulation • Maternal immune response is locally manipulated • Thymus involutes in pregnancy • Lymph nodes draining the uterus enlarge
子宫颈的变化 • 血管增加 • 胶原蛋白减少 • 糖胺聚糖和水的积累 • 宫颈腺肥大 • 黏液分泌增加	**Changes in the cervix** • Increased vascularity • Reduction in collagen • Accumulation of glycosaminoglycans and water • Hypertrophy of cervical glands • Increased mucus secretions
妊娠子宫的血管变化 • 子宫血管过度增大 • 从妊娠 10 周至足月，子宫血流量从 50ml/min 增至 500ml/min • 滋养层侵袭螺旋小动脉直至妊娠 24 周 • 100～150 个螺旋状小动脉向绒毛间隙输送血液 • 每个胎盘子叶有 1 个螺旋小动脉	**Vascular changes in the pregnant uterus** • Hypertrophy of the uterine vessels • Uterine blood flow from 50 to 500 mL/min 10 weeks to term • Trophoblast invasion of spiral arterioles up to 24 weeks • 100–150 spiral arterioles supply intervillous space • One spiral arteriole per placental cotyledon
子宫收缩 • 被孕激素抑制 • 静息膜电位增加 • 传导受损 • 7 周开始宫缩，频繁、低强度 • 妊娠晚期，更强、更频繁 • 分娩时，宫缩会导致宫颈扩张	**Uterine contractility** • Suppressed by progesterone • Increased resting membrane potential • Impaired conduction • Contractions by 7 weeks-frequent low intensity • Late pregnancy-stronger and more frequent • In labour, contractions produce cervical dilatation
心排血量 • 最初 3 个月增加 40% • 分娩时进一步可达 2L/min • 双胎妊娠增加 15% • 心率每分钟提高 15 次 • 心排血量从 64ml 增加到 71ml	**Cardiac output** • 40% increase in the first trimester • Further increase of up to 2 L/min in labour • 15% increment with twin pregnancy • Heart rate increased by 15 beats/min • Stroke volume increases from 64 to 71 mL

（续表）

本章概览	Essential information
总外周阻力 • 在前 4～6 周下降，在妊娠中期减半 • 允许血容量扩增 • 激素驱动	**Total peripheral resistance** • Falls in first 4-6 weeks, halving by mid–pregnancy • Allows expansion of blood volume • Hormonally driven
动脉血压 • 第五 Korotkoff 音现在是舒张压测量的首选 • 妊娠中期前平均血压持续下降 • 仰卧低血压在妊娠后半段很常见	**Arterial blood pressure** • Korotkoff sound 5 is now preferred for diastolic pressure measurement • Mean blood pressure falls to mid–pregnancy • Supine hypotension is common in the second half of pregnancy
血液 • 红细胞的数量根据铁的摄入量增加 20%～30% • 浓度指标下降，如血细胞比容 • 白细胞计数缓慢增加，但是在分娩和分娩过程中通常会发生大量中性粒细胞增多 • 妊娠和产褥期凝血倾向增加	**The blood** • Red cell mass rises by ≈20-30% depending on iron intake • Concentration measures fall, e.g. haematocrit • White cell count rises slowly, but massive neutrophilia is usual around labour and delivery • There is an increased tendency to clotting in pregnancy and the puerperium
呼吸功能 • 每分钟通气量增加 40% • 母体 $PaCO_2$ 下降，使胎儿能更好地交换气体 • 对于患呼吸系统疾病的女性来说妊娠通常不是问题	**Respiratory function** • Minute ventilation rises by 40% • Maternal P_aCO_2 falls, allowing better gas exchange from the fetus • Pregnancy is not usually a problem for women with respiratory disease
肾功能 • 在妊娠早期，GFR 上升约 50%，RPF 上升 50% • 血浆中许多溶质的浓度下降，可反应在实验室结果上 • 少量糖尿和轻度蛋白尿（≤200mg/ml）在妊娠期很常见	**Renal function** • GFR rises by ≈50% and RPF by 50% in the first trimester • Plasma concentration of many solutes falls-effect on interpretation of lab results • Some glycosuria and mild proteinuria (≤200 mg/mL) are common in pregnancy
血液中的营养 • 葡萄糖是主要的胎儿能量底物 • 白蛋白在整个妊娠过程中都会下降；球蛋白升高约 10% • 除丙氨酸和谷氨酸外，其他氨基酸减少 • 妊娠是高脂血症状态 • 游离脂肪酸升高 • 脂溶性维生素的浓度增加，水溶性维生素的含量下降	**Nutrients in blood** • Glucose is the major fetal energy substrate • Albumin falls throughout pregnancy; globulin rises by ≈10% • Amino acids decrease, except alanine and glutamic acid • Pregnancy is a hyperlipidaemic state • Free fatty acids are raised • Concentration of fat-soluble vitamins rises; that of water-soluble vitamins falls
内分泌变化 • 胎盘是内分泌的动力源，可合成类固醇，多肽和前列腺素 • 胎盘产生促肾上腺皮质激素释放激素和促肾上腺皮质激素 • 胎盘亮氨酸氨基肽酶在妊娠期间降低催产素 • 胎盘促性腺激素可抑制生长激素、LH 和 FSH 水平 • 垂体增大 • 催乳素分泌增加 • 甲状腺功能增强 • 醛固酮和脱氧皮质酮水平升高	**Endocrine changes** • Placenta is an endocrine powerhouse, synthesizing steroids, polypeptides and prostanoids • Placenta produces CRH and ACTH • Placental leucine aminopeptidase lowers oxytocin during pregnancy • Growth hormone, LH and FSH levels are suppressed by placental gonadotrophins • Pituitary gland enlarges • Increased secretion of prolactin • Thyroid function increases • Aldosterone and deoxycorticosterone levels rise

第 4 章　胎盘和胎儿的生长发育
Placental and fetal growth and development

Adonis S. Ioannides　著　　刘见桥　译　　崔琳琳　陈子江　校

学习目标	LEARNING OUTCOMES
学习本章后你应当能够：	After studying this chapter you should be able to:
知识标准	**Knowledge criteria**
• 描述正常胎盘的形成过程	• Describe normal placental development
• 描述脐带结构和子宫胎盘血流	• Describe the structure of the umbilical cord and uteroplacental blood flow
• 列出胎盘转运的机制和功能	• List the placental transfer mechanisms and functions
• 描述胎儿正常发育顺序	• Describe the sequence of normal fetal development
• 了解羊水的形成及临床意义	• Understand the formation and clinical significance of amniotic fluid

一、早期胎盘发育（Early placental development）

卵子受精、卵裂后形成桑葚胚，桑葚胚的卵裂球之间积聚液体形成囊腔，形成囊胚。

After fertilization and egg cleavage, the *morula* is transformed into a *blastocyst* by the formation of a fluid-filled cavity within the ball of cells.

囊胚的表面为原始细胞滋养层。胚胎发育的第7天，随着滋养层细胞侵入子宫内膜，囊胚植入到子宫内膜（图 4-1）。滋养细胞的外层形成合体滋养细胞层。与合体滋养细胞层接触后，子宫内膜间质细胞体积变大，颜色变浅，这个过程称为蜕膜反应。

在这个过程中，一些子宫内膜细胞被滋养细胞吞噬。

The outer layer of the blastocyst consists of primitive cytotrophoblast, and by day 7, the blastocyst penetrates the endometrium as a result of trophoblastic invasion (Fig. 4.1). The outer layer of the trophoblast becomes a syncytium. In response to contact with the syncytiotrophoblast, the endometrial stromal cells become large and pale, a process known as the *decidual reaction*. Some endometrial cells are phagocytosed by the trophoblastic cells.

蜕膜反应的性质和功能尚不完全清楚，但蜕膜细胞可能限制了滋养层细胞的侵袭，最早为发育中的胎盘提供营养物质。

The nature and function of the decidual reaction remain uncertain, but it seems likely that the decidual cells both limit the invasion of trophoblastic cells and serve an initial

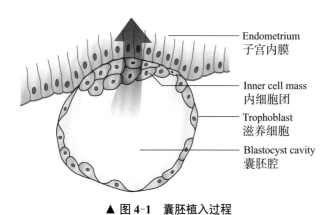

▲ 图 4-1　囊胚植入过程

Fig. 4.1　Implantation of the blastocyst

nutritional function for the developing placenta.

在胎盘的发育过程中，细胞滋养层细胞（Langhans 细胞）中心索向蜕膜的基底层生长，穿透子宫内膜微静脉和毛细血管，形成腔隙。当腔隙充满母体血液时，提示绒毛间隙开始形成。

During development of the placenta, cords of cytotrophoblast, or *Langhans cells*, grow down to the basal layers of decidua and penetrate some of the endometrial venules and capillaries. The formation of lacunae filled with maternal blood presages the development of the intervillous space.

向下侵袭的滋养细胞中心索形成初级绒毛，随后分支形成次级绒毛，最后形成三级绒毛，悬浮在绒毛间隙中。

The invading cords of trophoblast form the primary villi, which later branch to form secondary villi and, subsequently, free-floating tertiary villi.

胚外中胚层细胞长入绒毛的中心索，形成绒毛内毛细血管网。将发育中的胎儿与胎盘连接起来的体蒂形成脐血管。脐血管长入绒毛，与绒毛毛细血管相连接，建立胎盘循环。

The central core of these villi is penetrated by a column of mesoblastic cells that become the capillary network of the villi. The body stalk attaching the developing fetus to the placenta forms the umbilical vessels, which advance into the villi to join the villous capillaries and establish the placental circulation.

滋养细胞包绕着囊胚。发育成胎盘的滋养细胞局部增厚并广泛分支，形成"叶状绒毛膜"。然而，最终扩张形成胎膜外层的滋养细胞，叫作"平滑绒毛膜"。此处绒毛萎缩，表面变光滑（图 4-2）。胎盘下面的蜕膜叫作底蜕膜，胎膜与子宫肌层之间的蜕膜被称为包蜕膜。

Although trophoblastic cells surround the original blastocyst, the area that develops into the placenta becomes thickened and extensively branched and is known as the *chorion frondosum*. However, in the area that subsequently expands to form the outer layer of the fetal membranes, or *chorion laeve*, the villi become atrophic and the surface becomes smooth (Fig. 4.2). The decidua underlying the placenta is known as the *decidua basalis* and the decidua between the membranes and the myometrium is known as as the *decidua capsularis*.

二、胎盘进一步发育（Further placental development）

到了排卵后第 6 周，滋养层细胞已经侵入 40~60 个螺旋小动脉内。来自母体的血液促使悬浮的次级毛细血管和三级毛细血管进入帐篷形的母体胎盘小叶。通过固定绒毛将这些"帐篷"固定在蜕膜板上。母体小动脉的血液喷射到绒毛膜板，然后回流至基板上的母体静脉。最终形成约 12 个大型母体胎盘小叶和 40~50 个较小的胎盘小叶（图 4-3）。

By 6 weeks after ovulation, the trophoblast has invaded some 40–60 spiral arterioles. Blood from the maternal vasculature pushes the free-floating secondary and tertiary capillaries into a tent-shaped *maternal cotyledon*. The tents are held down to the basal plate of the decidua by anchoring villi, and the blood from arterioles spurts towards the chorionic plate and then returns to drain through maternal veins in the basal plate. There are eventually about 12 large maternal cotyledons and 40–50 smaller ones (Fig. 4.3).

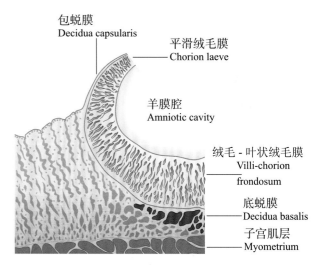

▲ 图 4-2　早期胎盘的发育。叶状绒毛膜形成胎盘的绒毛，平滑绒毛膜形成胎膜的绒毛膜部分

Fig. 4.2　Development of early placentation. The chorion frondosum forms the placental villi. The chorion laeve forms the chorionic portion of the fetal membranes

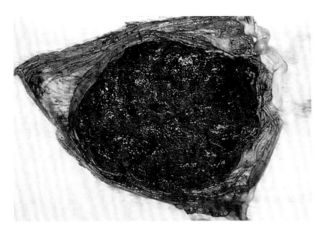

▲ 图 4-3　足月胎盘的母体面及胎盘小叶

Fig. 4.3　Maternal surface of the full-term placenta showing cotyledons

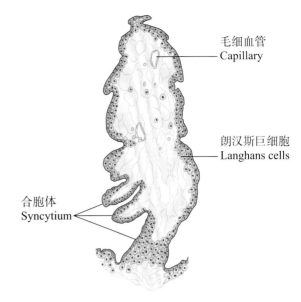

毛细血管
Capillary

朗汉斯巨细胞
Langhans cells

合胞体
Syncytium

▲ 图 4-4　绒毛膜绒毛是胎盘的功能单位

Fig. 4.4　The chorionic villus is the functional unit of the placenta

（一）绒毛（The villus）

虽然绒毛排列成母体胎盘小叶，但胎盘的功能单位仍然是绒毛干或胎儿胎盘小叶。图 4-4 所示为绒毛干的末端（也称末端绒毛或绒毛膜绒毛）。最初约有 200 个绒毛干从叶状绒毛膜发出，其中约有 150 个在母体胎盘小叶的挤压下功能逐渐丧失，留下约 12 个大的胎盘小叶和 40～50 个小的胎盘小叶，成为胎盘的功能单位。

Despite the arrangement of villi into maternal cotyledons, the functional unit of the placenta remains the *stem villus* or *fetal cotyledon*. The end unit of the stem villus, sometimes known as the terminal or chorionic villus, is shown in Fig. 4.4. There are initially about 200 stem villi arising from the chorion frondosum. About 150 of these structures are compressed at the periphery of the maternal cotyledons and become relatively functionless, leaving a dozen or so large cotyledons and 40–50 smaller ones as the active units of placental function.

成熟胎盘的绒毛膜绒毛总表面积约为 $11m^2$。因大量微绒毛的存在，胎盘胎儿面和绒毛的表面积增大。绒毛中心索由紧密排列的梭形成纤维细胞构成的基质和分枝状的毛细血管组成。基质中还含有被称为 Hofbauer 细胞的吞噬细胞。在妊娠早期，绒毛的外层是合体滋养细胞，内层是细胞滋养细胞。随着妊娠的进展，细胞滋养层消失，最后只留下一层薄薄的合体滋养层。合胞体细胞簇（也称合胞体结）的形成，以及妊娠晚期细胞滋养细胞的再次出现，可能是缺氧所致。有证据表明，在近足月时合胞体细胞的凋亡加速，尤其在胎儿生长受限时明显加速。

The estimated total surface area of the chorionic villi in the mature placenta is approximately $11m^2$. The surface area of the fetal side of the placenta and of the villi is enlarged by the presence of numerous microvilli. The core of the villus consists of a stroma of closely packed spindleshaped fibroblasts and branching capillaries. The stroma also contains phagocytic cells known as *Hofbauer cells*. In early pregnancy, the villi are covered by an outer layer of syncytiotrophoblast and an inner layer of cytotrophoblast. As pregnancy advances, the cytotrophoblast disappears until only a thin layer of syncytiotrophoblast remains. The formation of clusters of syncytial cells, known as *syncytial knots*, and the reappearance of cytotrophoblast in late pregnancy are probably the result of hypoxia. There is evidence that the rate of apoptosis of syncytial cells accelerates towards term and is particularly increased where there is evidence of fetal growth impairment.

（二）脐带结构（Structure of the umbilical cord）

脐带由 2 条脐动脉和 1 条脐静脉组成（图 4-5）。两条脐动脉将含氧量低的血液从胎儿运送到胎盘，并将含氧量高的血液经脐静脉运送回胎儿。在分娩的新生儿中，单脐动脉的发生率约为 1/200。单脐动脉的新生儿中，心血管异常的发生率为 10%～15%。脐血管周围包绕着一种亲水的黏多糖——Wharton 胶，脐带的最外层覆盖的是羊膜上皮。脐带长度为 30～90cm。

The umbilical cord contains two arteries and one vein (Fig. 4.5). The two arteries carry deoxygenated blood from the fetus to the placenta and the oxygenated blood returns to the fetus via the umbilical vein. Absence of one artery occurs in about 1 in 200 deliveries and is associated with a 10–15% incidence of cardiovascular anomalies. The vessels are surrounded by a hydrophilic mucopolysaccharide known as *Wharton's jelly*, and the outer layer covering the cord consists of amniotic epithelium. The cord length varies between 30 and 90 cm.

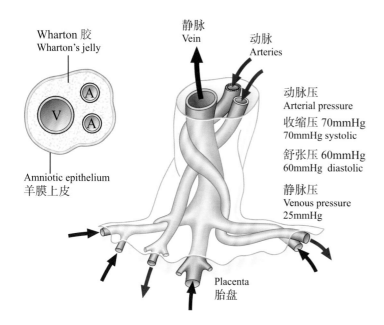

静脉
Vein

动脉
Arteries

Wharton 胶
Wharton's jelly

动脉压
Arterial pressure

收缩压 70mmHg
70mmHg systolic

舒张压 60mmHg
60mmHg diastolic

静脉压
Venous pressure
25mmHg

Amniotic epithelium
羊膜上皮

Placenta
胎盘

◀ 图 4-5　脐带的血管结构。静脉输送含氧血液，两条动脉输送缺氧血液

Fig. 4.5　Vascular structure of the umbilical cord. The vein carries oxygenated blood, and the two arteries carry deoxygenated blood

血管呈螺旋状生长，这种生长方式的功能优势为避免血管缠绕、减少扭曲，从而保护血管的功能。

The vessels grow in a helical shape. This configuration has the functional advantage of protecting the patency of the vessels by absorbing torsion without the risk of kinking or snarling of the vessels.

对脐血管的血压测量显示，孕晚期的动脉收缩压约为 70mmHg，舒张压约为 60mmHg，脉压相对较低。而静脉压异常高，达到 25mmHg 左右。如此高的静脉压保证了静脉血的流动，并保证绒毛毛细血管内压能超过脐静脉压。

The few measurements that have been made in situ of blood pressures in the cord vessels indicate that the arterial pressure in late pregnancy is around 70 mmHg systolic and 60 mmHg diastolic, with a relatively low pulse pressure and a venous pressure that is exceptionally high, at approximately 25 mmHg. This high venous pressure tends to preserve the integrity of the venous flow and indicates that the pressure within the villus capillaries must be in excess of the cord venous pressures.

> **！注意**
>
> 毛细血管压力高说明：在近端，胎儿面的绒毛毛细血管超过了绒毛膜蜕膜腔内压。因此，绒毛表面的任何损伤都会导致胎儿血细胞进入母体循环，但母体细胞很少会进入胎儿血管内。
>
> The high capillary pressures imply that, at the point of proximity, the fetal pressures exceed the pressures in the choriodecidual space so that any disruption of the villus surface means that fetal blood cells enter the maternal circulation and only rarely do maternal cells enter the fetal vascular space.

脐带血管常有假结，假结由动脉折叠而成。偶尔脐带血管形成真结而影响其血流量，但大部分时候不会对胎儿造成任何明显的不良影响。

The cord vessels often contain a false knot consisting of a refolding of the arteries; occasionally, blood flow is threatened by a true knot, although such formations are often seen without any apparent detrimental effects on the fetus.

足月胎儿的脐血流量约为 350 ml/min。

In the full-term fetus, the blood flow in the cord is approximately 350 mL/min.

三、子宫胎盘血流（Uteroplacental blood flow）

在妊娠的前 10 周，滋养层细胞侵入螺旋小动脉，破坏血管壁的一些平滑肌，随后这些血管松弛扩张。母体血液进入绒毛间隙，在母体心室收缩期，血液从动脉喷向胎盘的绒毛膜板，然后返回到胎盘床的静脉开口。绒毛间隙的特点是压力低及血流量大，平均压力约为 10mmHg。足月时子宫血流量为 500~750ml/min（图 4-6）。

Trophoblastic cells invade the spiral arterioles within the first 10 weeks of pregnancy and destroy some of the smooth muscle in the wall of the vessels, which then become flaccid dilated vessels. Maternal blood enters the intervillous space, and during maternal systole, blood spurts from the arteries towards the chorionic plate of the placenta and returns to the venous openings in the placental bed. The intervillous space is characterized by low pressures, with a mean pressure estimated

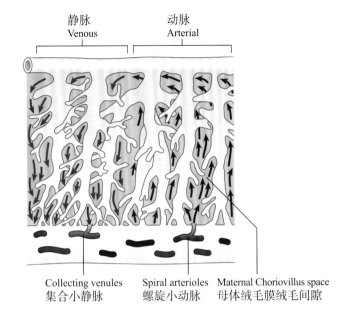

静脉
Venous　　　　动脉
　　　　　　　Arterial

Collecting venules　Spiral arterioles　Maternal Choriovillus space
集合小静脉　　　　螺旋小动脉　　　　母体绒毛膜绒毛间隙

▲ 图 4-6　血流从螺旋小动脉喷出至绒毛模板，然后回流至集合小静脉

Fig. 4.6　Blood from the spiral arterioles spurts towards the chorionic plate and returns to the collecting venules

at 10 mmHg and high flow. Assessments of uterine blood flow at term indicate values of 500–750 mL/min (Fig. 4.6).

调节胎儿胎盘和子宫血流的因素（Factors that regulate fetoplacental and uterine blood flow）

胎儿胎盘循环受胎儿心脏及主动脉、脐血管和绒毛血管的影响，因此影响这些解剖结构的因素都可能影响胎儿循环。如脐带水肿、胎儿大血管内血栓形成和钙化，或者急性脐带受压或脐带阻塞等急性事件，都可能会直接对胎儿产生致命的影响。然而，影响胎儿健康更常见的因素来源于子宫胎盘循环。利用多普勒超声对这些因素进行评估，极大增加了我们对子宫血流调节机制的理解。

The fetoplacental circulation is affected by the fetal heart and aorta, the umbilical vessels and the vessels of the chorionic villi, so factors that affect these structures may affect the fetal circulation. Such factors as oedema of the cord, intramural thrombosis and calcification within the large fetal vessels or acute events such as acute cord compression or obstruction of the umbilical cord may have immediate and lethal consequences for the fetus. However, the more common factors that influence the welfare of the fetus arise in the uteroplacental circulation. Access to these factors by the use of Doppler ultrasound has greatly improved our understanding of the control mechanisms of uterine blood flow.

子宫血流量的调节对胎儿的健康至关重要。子

宫胎盘循环包括子宫动脉及其分支至螺旋小动脉、绒毛间隙血流及其静脉回流。

The regulation of uterine blood flow is of critical importance to the welfare of the fetus. The uteroplacental blood flow includes the uterine arteries and their branches down to the spiral arterioles, the intervillous blood flow and the related venous return.

子宫血流受阻会导致胎儿生长发育障碍，严重时会导致胎儿死亡。影响子宫胎盘血流量的急性因素包括母体出血、子宫强直收缩（异常强而持久的收缩），以及去甲肾上腺素和肾上腺素等物质的作用。血管紧张素 II 在生理水平下会增加子宫血流量，因为它直接促进胎盘释放促血管扩张物质前列腺素，但在高浓度下会导致血管收缩。

Impairment of uterine blood flow leads to fetal growth impairment and, under severe circumstances, to fetal death. Factors that influence uteroplacental blood flow acutely include maternal haemorrhage, tonic or abnormally powerful and prolonged uterine contractions and substances such as noradrenaline (norepinephrine) and adrenaline (epinephrine). Angiotensin II increases uterine blood flow at physiological levels, as it has a direct effect on the placental release of vasodilator prostaglandins, but in high concentrations it produces vasoconstriction.

最常见的情况是，孕晚期母体仰卧位时会压迫下腔静脉，使子宫胎盘血管床的血流量突然下降，从而导致胎儿急性窒息。

At the simplest level, acute fetal asphyxia can be produced by the effect of the mother lying in the supine position in late pregnancy, causing compression of the maternal inferior vena cava and hence a sudden reduction in blood flow through the uteroplacental bed.

慢性病理学方面，子宫胎盘循环受损的主要原因是滋养层细胞侵入不充分，急性动脉粥样硬化影响螺旋小动脉，从而导致胎盘缺血、胎盘过熟和胎盘梗死。

In terms of chronic pathology, the main causes of impaired uteroplacental circulation are inadequate trophoblast invasion and acute atherosis affecting the spiral arterioles, resulting in placental ischaemia, advanced maturation and placental infarction.

四、胎盘转运（Placental transfer）

胎盘在胎儿的生长发育及调节母体对妊娠的适应中起着至关重要的作用。胎盘是胎儿营养、排泄、

呼吸和激素合成的器官。

The placenta plays an essential role in the growth and development of the fetus and in regulating maternal adaptation to pregnancy. The placenta is an organ of fetal nutrition, excretion, respiration and hormone synthesis.

通过胎盘膜的物质转移受物质分子量、溶解度和离子电荷控制。实际的转运通过以下方式来实现，即简单扩散、易化扩散、主动转运和胞饮作用（图 4-7）。

Transfer of materials across the placental membrane is governed by molecular mass, solubility and the ionic charge of the substrate involved. Actual transfer is achieved by simple diffusion, facilitated diffusion, active transport and pinocytosis (Fig. 4.7).

（一）简单扩散（Simple diffusion）

母体和胎儿血液之间的交换是由滋养层细胞调节的。必须记住的是，在绒毛膜绒毛中将胎儿和母体血液分隔开的不是简单的半透膜，而是代谢活跃的细胞层。然而，对于一些物质来说，它确实像半透膜，因为这些物质通过简单扩散进行交换。

Transfer between maternal and fetal blood is regulated by the trophoblast, and it must be remembered that the layer separating fetal from maternal blood in the chorionic villus is not a simple semipermeable membrane but a metabolically active cellular layer. However, with regard to some substances, it does behave like a semipermeable membrane, and substances pass by simple diffusion.

尽管存在一些例外情况，但小分子物质通常以这种方式穿过胎盘，其运动是由化学或电化学梯度决定的。溶质的转运量可用 Fick 扩散方程来描述。

$$\frac{Q}{t} = \frac{KA \; (C^1 - C^2)}{L}$$

Although there are some exceptions, small molecules generally cross the placenta in this way, and movement is determined by chemical or electrochemical gradients. The quantity of solute transferred is described by the Fick diffusion equation:

其中 Q/t 是单位时间内转运的量，K 是特定物质的扩散常数，A 是可用的总表面积，C^1 和 C^2 表示溶质浓度的差异，L 表示膜的厚度。

where Q/t is the quantity transferred per unit of time, K is a diffusion constant for the particular substance, A is the total surface area available, C^1 and C^2 indicate the difference in concentrations of solute and L represents the thickness of the membrane.

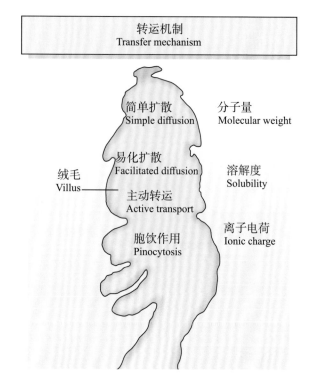

▲ 图 4-7 决定通过胎盘运送物质和气体的因素

Fig. 4.7 **Factors that determine transfer of materials and gases across the placenta**

这种计算方法特别适用于气体的转运，尽管氧气的浓度梯度会因绒毛滋养细胞摄取氧气被扩大。

This method is applicable particularly to transfer of gases, although the gradient of oxygen, for example, is exaggerated by the fact that oxygen is extracted by the villous trophoblast.

（二）易化扩散（Facilitated diffusion）

有些化合物在胎盘中的转运速度比简单扩散的预期速度快得多。转运总是顺着浓度梯度的方向进行，但速度加快了。葡萄糖的转运与这一机制有关，只能通过酶催化过程和特定转运系统的积极作用来解释。

Some compounds are transported across the placenta at rates that are considerably enhanced above the rate that would be anticipated by simple diffusion. Transport always occurs in favour of the gradient, but at an accelerated rate. This mechanism pertains to glucose transport and can only be explained by the active involvement of enzyme processes and specific transport systems.

（三）主动转运（Active transport）

一些化合物逆化学梯度进行转运，这过程一定涉及一个能量依赖性的主动转运系统。氨基酸和水溶性维生素是用这个机制进行转运的。胎儿血液中这些物质的化合物浓度高于母体血液中的浓度证明了这一点。这种转运机制可被细胞毒素抑制且具有构象特异性。

Transfer against a chemical gradient occurs with some compounds and must involve an active transport system that is energy dependent. This process occurs with amino acids and water-soluble vitamins and can be demonstrated by the presence of higher concentrations of the compound in the fetal blood as compared with maternal blood. Such transfer mechanisms can be inhibited by cell poisons and are stereo-specific.

（四）胞饮作用（Pinocytosis）

人们观察到，大分子化合物分子量大，看似不可能通过绒毛膜，但它们也能完成跨膜转运。在这种情况下，微滴被吞入滋养层细胞的细胞质中，然后被挤压到胎儿循环中。球蛋白、磷脂和脂蛋白都是通过这一过程转运的。胞饮作用在免疫活性物质的转运中也起着特别重要的作用。蛋白质（占能量供应的 10%）合成的主要原料氨基酸，也是通过主动运输转运的。

Transfer of high-molecular-mass compounds is known to occur even where such transfer would be impossible through the villus membrane because of the molecular size. Under these circumstances, microdroplets are engulfed into the cytoplasm of the trophoblast and then extruded into the fetal circulation. This process applies to the transfer of globulins, phospholipids and lipoproteins and is of particular importance in the transfer of immunologically active material. The major source of materials for protein synthesis, which also accounts for some 10% of energy supplies, is amino acids transferred by active transport.

（五）完整细胞的转运（Transport of intact cells）

在母体循环中常见到胎儿红细胞，尤其是在分娩后。这种转运发生在滋养细胞膜破裂之后，因此也可能在流产时或胎盘早剥后发生。尽管在胎儿循环中可以发现一些母体细胞，但这种情况比较少见。如前所述，胎儿毛细血管压力较大，绒毛间隙压力较低，这种浓度差决定了物质比较容易从胎儿毛细血管向绒毛间隙转运。

Fetal red cells are commonly seen in the maternal circulation, particularly following delivery. This transfer occurs through fractures in the integrity of the trophoblastic membrane and may also therefore occur at the time of abortion or following placental abruption. Although some maternal cells can be found in the fetal circulation, this is much less common. As previously mentioned, the pressure gradient favours movement from the relatively high pressure of the fetal capillaries to the low-pressure environment of the intervillous space.

（六）水和电解质的转运（Water and electrolyte transfer）

水很容易通过胎盘，一次就可以达到平衡。水通过胎盘的驱动力包括静水压、胶体渗透压和溶质渗透压。

Water passes easily across the placenta, and a single pass allows equilibrium. The driving forces for movement of water across the placenta include hydrostatic pressure, colloid osmotic pressure and solute osmotic pressure.

1. 钠（Sodium）

胎儿静脉血浆中的钠浓度高于母体静脉血浆中的浓度。因此，胎盘可能通过绒毛滋养细胞胎儿面 Na/K-ATP 酶的作用，主动调节钠的转运。

The concentration of sodium is higher in the venous plasma of the fetus than in the maternal venous plasma. It therefore seems that the placenta actively regulates sodium transfer, probably through the action of Na/K ATPase on the fetal surface of the villus trophoblast.

2. 钾（Potassium）

钾的转运也是细胞膜调控的，但其机制尚不清楚。胎儿血钾水平显著高于母体血钾水平，尤其是在胎儿缺氧和酸中毒的情况下。为使酸碱保持平衡，胎儿血钾水平会显著升高，浓度梯度增加。有证据表明在胎盘母体面存在载体介导的转运，胎盘钾的转运可能受到细胞内 Ca^{2+} 的调节。

The transfer of potassium is also controlled at the cell membrane level, but the mechanism remains obscure. Fetal plasma potassium levels are significantly higher than maternal plasma levels. In particular, fetal plasma levels become significantly raised in the presence of fetal hypoxia and fetal acidosis with an exaggerated gradient if the acid-base balance remains normal. There is evidence for a carrier-mediated transfer at the maternal surface of the placenta, and the transfer of placental potassium may also be modulated by intracellular Ca^{2+}.

3. 钙（Calcium）

钙主动转运通过胎盘，胎儿血钙水平显著高于母体血钙。

Calcium is actively transported across the placenta, and there are higher concentrations in fetal plasma than in maternal plasma.

五、胎盘的功能（Placental function）

胎盘有 3 种主要功能。

* 气体交换。
* 胎儿营养供应及代谢产物的清除。
* 内分泌功能。

The placenta has three major functions:

* gaseous exchange
* fetal nutrition and removal of waste products
* endocrine function

（一）气体交换（Gaseous exchange）

气体通过简单扩散方式进行交换，气体交换的主要决定因素是胎儿和母体血流量、可用于气体交换的胎盘表面积，以及胎盘膜的厚度。

As the transfer of gases occurs by simple diffusion, the major determinants of gaseous exchange are the efficiency and flow of the fetal and maternal circulation, the surface area of the placenta that is available for transfer and the thickness of the placental membrane.

1. 氧气转运（Oxygen transfer）

当 氧 分 压（oxygen partial pressure，PO_2）为 90～100mmHg 时，进入绒毛间隙的母体血液平均氧饱和度为 90%～100%。如此高的氧浓度有助于把氧气转运到胎儿循环。胎盘本身消耗了一部分氧气后，剩余的氧气供胎儿循环使用。胎儿血红蛋白与成人血红蛋白相比，对氧气有更高的亲和力，同时胎儿的血红蛋白浓度更高。以上这些因素都有助于胎儿在 30～40mmHg 的低氧分压下迅速摄取氧气。

The average oxygen saturation of maternal blood entering the intervillous space is 90–100% at a Po_2 of 90–100 mmHg, and these high levels of oxygen favour transfer to the fetal circulation. After the placenta itself has utilized some of this oxygen, the remainder is available to the fetal circulation. Fetal haemoglobin has a higher affinity for oxygen than does adult haemoglobin, and haemoglobin concentration is higher in the fetus. All of these factors favour the rapid uptake of oxygen by the fetus at Po_2 levels as low as 30–40 mmHg.

氢离子浓度会影响血红蛋白的氧饱和度。脱氧的血液从胎儿体内进入胎盘循环时，氢离子浓度增加，导致母体来源的氧气在胎儿胎盘床的释放增加。随着 H^+ 浓度、PCO_2 和温度的增加，氧解离曲线右移，称为 Bohr 效应（图 4-8）。氧主要以氧合血红蛋白的形式运输，因为溶液中几乎没有游离氧。

The extent to which haemoglobin can be saturated by oxygen is affected by hydrogen ion concentration. The increase that occurs in deoxygenated blood arriving in the placental circulation from the fetus favours the release of maternal oxygen in the fetoplacental bed. The oxygen dissociation curve is shifted to the right by the increase in H+ concentration, Pco_2 and temperature, and this is known as the *Bohr effect* (Fig. 4.8). Oxygen is predominantly transported in the form of oxyhaemoglobin, as there is little free oxygen in solution.

2. 二氧化碳传递（Carbon dioxide transfer）

二氧化碳（carbon dioxide，CO_2）易溶于血液，能通过胎盘迅速转运。PCO_2 差约为 5mmHg。CO_2 在溶液中以碳酸氢盐、碳酸，或者氨基甲酰血红蛋白的形式进行运输。影响氧释放的因素亦会影响 CO_2 与血红蛋白的结合。因此，氨基甲酰血红蛋白含量升高会导致氧的释放。这种现象被称为 Haldane 效应。

Carbon dioxide is readily soluble in blood and transfers rapidly across the placenta. The partial pressure difference is about 5 mmHg. Transport of carbon dioxide may occur in solution as either bicarbonate or carbonic acid. It is also transported as carbamino-haemoglobin. The binding of CO_2 to haemoglobin is affected by factors that influence oxygen release. Thus, an increase in carbamino-haemoglobin results in the release of oxygen. This is known as the *Haldane effect*.

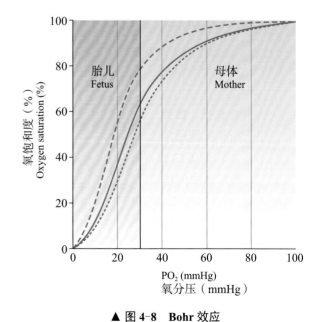

▲ 图 4-8 Bohr 效应

Fig. 4.8 The Bohr effect

3. 酸 – 碱平衡（Acid-base balance）

H⁺、乳酸和碳酸氢根离子等酸碱平衡调节因子也能通过胎盘。因此，母体在饥饿和脱水状态下发生的酸中毒可能也会引起胎儿酸中毒。然而，在母体酸碱平衡处于正常状态时，胎儿也可能因缺氧发生酸中毒。

Factors involved in the regulation of acid-base balance such as H⁻, lactic acid and bicarbonate ions also move across the placenta. As a consequence, acidosis associated with starvation and dehydration in the mother may also result in acidosis in the fetus. However, the fetus may become acidotic as the result of oxygen deprivation in the presence of normal maternal acid-base balance.

（二）胎儿营养及代谢产物的清除（Fetal nutrition and removal of waste products）

1. 糖代谢（Carbohydrate metabolism）

源于母体循环的葡萄糖是胎儿和胎盘氧化代谢的主要底物，供应胎儿 90% 的能量需求。易化扩散确保葡萄糖快速地穿过胎盘。在妊娠晚期，胎儿每千克体重中约有 10g 用于储存能量。多余的葡萄糖都以糖原或脂肪的形式储存在体内。糖原储存于肝脏、肌肉、胎盘及心脏中，而脂肪沉积在心脏周围及肩胛骨后方。

Glucose transferred from the maternal circulation provides the major substrate for oxidative metabolism in the fetus and placenta and provides 90% of the energy requirements of the fetus. Facilitated diffusion ensures that there is rapid transfer of glucose across the placenta. In late pregnancy, the fetus retains some 10 g/kg body weight, and any excess glucose is stored as glycogen or fat. Glycogen is stored in the liver, muscle, placenta and heart, whereas fat is deposited around the heart and behind the scapulae.

动物实验表明，糖类的转运具有选择性。总的来说，葡萄糖和单糖通常能够快速穿过胎盘，而蔗糖、麦芽糖和乳糖等二糖不能通过胎盘。山梨醇、甘露醇、去糖醇和中间肌醇等糖醇类物质也不能通过胎盘。

Animal studies have shown that the transfer of sugars is selective. Generally, glucose and the monosaccharides cross the placenta readily, whereas it is virtually impermeable to disaccharides such as sucrose, maltose and lactose. The placenta is also impermeable to sugar alcohols such as sorbitol, mannitol, deleitol and meso-inositol.

正常妊娠期女性禁食时，母体静脉血葡萄糖浓度约为 4.0mmol/L，此时胎儿脐静脉血葡萄糖浓度约为 3.3mmol/L。向母体注射葡萄糖会使母体及胎儿血糖浓度均升高，直至胎儿血糖浓度达到 10.6mmol/L，之后便不会随母体血糖浓度升高而继续升高了。

In the fasting normal pregnant woman, blood glucose achieves a concentration of approximately 4.0 mmol/L in the maternal venous circulation and 3.3 mmol/L in the fetal cord venous blood. Infusion of glucose into the maternal circulation results in a parallel increase in both maternal and fetal blood until the fetal levels reach 10.6 mmol/L, when no further increase occurs, regardless of the values in the maternal circulation.

调节葡萄糖稳态的重要激素包括胰岛素、胰高血糖素、人胎盘催乳素和生长激素，这些激素均不能通过胎盘。因此，母体血糖水平似乎是胎儿葡萄糖代谢的主要调节因素。胎盘本身消耗葡萄糖，并可能消耗多达 50% 的转移到胎儿胎盘单位的葡萄糖。

The hormones that are important in glucose homeostasis-insulin, glucagon, human placental lactogen and growth hormone-do not cross the placenta, and maternal glucose levels appear to be the major regulatory factor in fetal glucose metabolism. The placenta itself utilizes glucose and may retain as much as half of the glucose transferred to the fetoplacental unit.

妊娠中期，胎盘消耗的约 70% 的葡萄糖通过糖酵解代谢，10% 通过磷酸戊糖途径代谢；其余葡萄糖通过合成糖原和脂肪储存起来。足月时，胎盘的葡萄糖消耗下降 30%。

In mid-pregnancy, approximately 70% of this glucose is metabolized by glycolysis and 10% via the pentose phosphate pathway; the remainder is stored by glycogen and lipid synthesis. By full term, the rate of placental glucose utilization has fallen by 30%.

胎儿肝脏储存的糖原在整个妊娠期稳定地增加。至足月时，胎儿肝糖原储存量为母体储存量的 2 倍。但在胎儿出生后的最初数小时，其含量迅速降低至成人水平。

Glycogen storage in the fetal liver increases steadily throughout pregnancy and by full term is twice as high as the storage in the maternal liver. A rapid fall to adult levels occurs within the first few hours of life.

胎儿窒息时，无氧糖酵解通路被激活，此时胎儿的糖原储备便成为极其重要的能量来源。

Fetal glycogen reserves are particularly important in providing an energy source in the asphyxiated fetus when anaerobic glycolysis is activated.

2. 脂肪代谢（Fat metabolism）

脂肪不溶于水，因此在血液中以与白蛋白结合的游离脂肪酸，或者脂蛋白的形式进行运输。脂蛋白包含甘油三酯，甘油三酯附着在其他脂质或蛋白质上，并包装成乳糜微粒。

Fats are insoluble in water and are therefore transported in blood either as free fatty acids bound to albumin or as lipoproteins consisting of triglycerides attached to other lipids or proteins and packaged in chylomicrons.

胎儿需要利用脂肪酸来构建细胞膜，以及沉积脂肪组织。作为新生儿期的能量来源，这一点尤为重要。

The fetus needs fatty acids for cell membrane construction and for deposition in adipose tissue. This is particularly important as a source of energy in the immediate neonatal period.

研究表明，游离脂肪酸以非选择性的方式通过胎盘。胎儿的必需脂肪酸来源于母体循环。胎盘能将亚麻酸转化为花生四烯酸。母体饥饿时，胎儿体内甘油三酯动员增加。

There is evidence that free fatty acids cross the placenta and that this transfer is not selective. Essential fatty acids are also transferred from the maternal circulation, and there is evidence to suggest that the placenta has the ability to convert linoleic acid to arachidonic acid. Starvation of the mother increases mobilization of triglycerides in the fetus.

3. 蛋白质代谢（Protein metabolism）

胎儿能够利用游离氨基酸合成蛋白质。这些氨基酸来源于胎盘的逆浓度梯度转运。因此，胎儿血液中游离脂肪酸的浓度较母体血液高。

Fetal proteins are synthesized by the fetus from free amino acids transported across the placenta against a concentration gradient. The concentration of free amino acids in fetal blood is higher than in the maternal circulation.

胎盘不参与胎儿蛋白质的合成，尽管它确实合成一些转移到母体循环中的蛋白质激素，如绒毛膜促性腺激素和人胎盘催乳素。到足月时，人类胎儿已积累了约 500g 蛋白质。

The placenta takes no part in the synthesis of fetal proteins, although it does synthesize some protein hormones that are transferred into the maternal circulation: chorionic gonadotrophin and human placental lactogen. By full term, the human fetus has accumulated some 500 g of protein.

免疫球蛋白（immunoglobulins，Ig）由胎儿的淋巴组织合成。妊娠 20 周，胎儿血循环中首次出现 IgM，随后 IgA、IgG 依次出现。

Immunoglobulins (Ig) are synthesized by fetal lymphoid tissue, and IgM first appears in the fetal circulation by 20 weeks' gestation, followed by IgA and finally IgG.

IgG 是唯一能通过胎盘的 γ- 球蛋白，这种现象可能与胎盘对 IgG 的选择性有关。目前没有证据表明促生长激素能够通过胎盘。

IgG is the only gamma-globulin to be transferred across the placenta, and this appears to be selective for IgG. There is no evidence of placental transfer of growth-promoting hormones.

4. 尿素和氨（Urea and ammonia）

胎儿血液中尿素浓度比母体中高约 0.5mmol/L。足月时，通过胎盘的尿素清除率约为 0.54mg/(min·kg)（译者注：原著表述似有误，已修改）。

Urea concentration is higher in the fetus than in the mother by a margin of about 0.5 mmol/L, and the rate of clearance across the placenta is approximately 0.54 mg^{-1} min^{-1} kg fetal weight at term.

氨易通过胎盘，同时有证据证明母体内氨是胎儿氮的来源之一。

Ammonia transfers readily across the placenta, and there is evidence that maternal ammonia provides a source of fetal nitrogen.

（三）胎盘的激素合成（Placental hormone production）

胎盘作为一个内分泌器官具有重要功能，它负责合成蛋白质类激素和类固醇类激素。胎儿也参与了多种激素的合成过程。在这个过程中，胎儿作为一个单位参与胎儿和胎盘的功能。

The placenta plays a major role as an endocrine organ and is responsible for the production of both protein and steroid hormones. The fetus is also involved in many of the processes of hormone production, and in this capacity the conceptus functions as a unit involving both fetus and placenta.

1. 蛋白质激素（Protein hormones）

(1) 绒毛膜促性腺激素（Chorionic gonadotrophin）：人绒毛膜促性腺激素（human chorionic gonadotrophin，hCG）是由滋养细胞产生的，其化学结构与促黄体生成素非常相似。它是一种糖蛋白，含有 α 和 β 2 个不同的亚基。妊娠 10～12 周，孕妇尿液和血液中 hCG

达到峰值；32～36 周时，hCG 出现一个小的亚高峰。孕 7 天时，母体血浆中即可检测到 hCG 的 β 亚单位。

Human chorionic gonadotrophin (hCG) is produced by trophoblast and has a structure that is chemically very similar to that of luteinizing hormone. It is a glycoprotein with two non-identical α and β subunits and reaches a peak in maternal urine and blood between 10 and 12 weeks' gestation. A small sub-peak occurs between 32 and 36 weeks. The β subunit of hCG can be detected in maternal plasma within 7 days of conception.

该激素唯一已知的功能似乎是维持孕期的黄体功能。黄体负责合成孕酮，直到这种分泌功能被胎盘取代。

The only known function of the hormone appears to be the maintenance of the corpus luteum of pregnancy, which is responsible for the production of progesterone until such time as this production is taken over by the placenta.

该激素可通过使用包被红细胞或乳胶颗粒的凝集抑制技术进行测量。这构成了现代标准化妊娠试验的基础（见第 18 章）。97% 的孕妇月经消失 2 周后，尿 hCG 检测阳性。居家妊娠检测试剂盒最低能够检测到 25～50U/L 的 β-hCG。

The hormone is measured by agglutination inhibition techniques using coated red cells or latex particles, and this forms the basis for the standard modern pregnancy test (see Chapter 18). This will be positive in urine by 2 weeks after the period is missed in 97% of pregnant women. Home pregnancy test kits are able to detect 25–50 IU/L of β hCG.

(2) 人胎盘催乳素（Human placental lactogen）：人胎盘催乳素（human placental lactogen，hPL），又名绒毛膜生长激素，是一种分子量为 22 000 的肽类激素，其化学性质与生长激素相似。它由合体滋养细胞产生，血浆 hPL 水平在整个妊娠期间稳步上升。目前，这种激素的功能还不确定。它能增加游离脂肪酸和胰岛素的水平。在妊娠晚期 hPL 水平的急剧升高与血糖升高及糖耐量异常有关。这也解释了迟发性糖尿病的病因。

Human placental lactogen (hPL), or chorionic somatomammotrophin, is a peptide hormone with a molecular weight of 22,000 that is chemically similar to growth hormone. It is produced by syncytiotrophoblast, and plasma hPL levels rise steadily throughout pregnancy. The function of the hormone remains uncertain. It increases levels of free fatty acids and insulin. The level tends to rise steeply in the third trimester and is linked to higher blood sugars and abnormal glucose tolerance tests, i.e. helping to unmask late-onset diabetes.

血浆 hPL 水平已被广泛用于胎盘功能的评估，因为胎盘功能衰竭时 hPL 水平较低。妊娠期最后 2 周，正常妊娠中血清 hPL 水平会下降。然而，由于这些指标鉴别胎盘功能较差，目前较少用于胎盘功能的检测。现阶段，hPL 常用免疫分析法进行测定。

Plasma hPL levels have been extensively used in the assessment of placental function, as the levels are low in the presence of placental failure. In the last 2 weeks of gestation, the levels in the serum fall in normal pregnancy. However, the use of these measurements as placental function tests has largely fallen into disfavour because of their low discriminant function. The hormone is measured by immunoassay.

2. 类固醇激素（Steroid hormones）

(1) 孕酮（Progesterone）：至妊娠 17 周，胎盘成为孕酮的主要来源。孕酮的生物合成主要依赖于母体胆固醇的供应。在母体血浆中，90% 的孕酮与蛋白质结合，在肝脏和肾脏代谢。10%～15% 的孕酮以孕二醇形式在尿液中排出。足月时，胎盘每天能合成约 350mg 孕酮。血浆孕酮水平在整个妊娠期间增加，到足月时达到 150mg/ml 左右。尿中孕二醇或血浆孕酮的测定曾被用作评估胎盘功能的一种方法。但由于在正常妊娠中孕酮正常水平范围较大，尚未证明其有效性。

The placenta becomes the major source of progesterone by the seventeenth week of gestation, and the biosynthesis of progesterone is mainly dependent on the supply of maternal cholesterol. In maternal plasma, 90% of progesterone is bound to protein and is metabolized in the liver and the kidneys. Some 10–15% of progesterone is excreted in the urine as pregnanediol. The placenta produces about 350 mg of progesterone per day by full term, and plasma progesterone levels increase throughout pregnancy to achieve values around 150 mg/mL by full term. The measurement of urinary pregnanediol or plasma progesterone has been used in the past as a method of assessing placental function but has not proved to be particularly useful because of the wide scatter of values in normal pregnancies.

(2) 雌激素（Oestrogens）：在孕妇尿液中发现了 20 多种不同的雌激素，但主要的雌激素是雌酮、17β- 雌二醇和雌三醇。尿液中分泌的雌激素比例升高最多的是雌三醇。而尿液中雌酮的排泄量增加了 100 倍，雌三醇排泄量增加了 1000 倍。

Over 20 different oestrogens have been identified in the urine of pregnant women, but the major oestrogens are oestrone, oestradiol-17β and oestriol. The largest increase in urinary oestrogen excretion occurs in the oestriol fraction.

Whereas oestrone excretion increases 100-fold, urinary oestriol increases 1000-fold.

尿液雌激素的增加很少来源于卵巢，因为胎盘是孕期雌激素的主要来源。雌三醇的底物来自胎儿肾上腺。脱氢表雄酮（dehydroepiandrosterone，DHEA）先在胎儿肾上腺皮质中合成，随后进入胎儿肝脏并发生 16- 羟基化。这些前体物质与磷酸腺苷磷酸硫酸盐结合有助于溶解，胎盘中活化的硫酸酯酶引起游离雌三醇的释放。

The ovary makes only a minimal contribution to this increase, as the placenta is the major source of oestrogens in pregnancy. The substrate for oestriol production comes from the fetal adrenal gland. Dehydroepiandrosterone (DHEA) synthesized in the fetal adrenal cortex passes to the fetal liver, where it is 16-hydoxylated. Conjugation of these precursors with phosphoadenosyl phosphosulphate aids solubility, and active sulphatase activity in the placenta results in the release of free oestriol.

雌二醇和雌酮由合体滋养细胞直接合成。尿和血浆中雌三醇水平在整个妊娠期间逐渐升高，直到妊娠 38 周开始下降。

Oestradiol and oestrone are directly synthesized by the syncytiotrophoblast. Urinary and plasma oestriol levels increase progressively throughout pregnancy until 38 weeks' gestation, when some decrease occurs.

目前，多样化的超声评估已基本取代了雌三醇，成为评估胎盘功能的主要方法。

The use of oestriol measurements has now largely been replaced by the use of various forms of ultrasound assessment.

(3) 皮质类固醇（Corticosteroids）：目前，少有证据表明胎盘能分泌皮质类固醇。患 Addison 病或肾上腺切除术后，母体尿液中 17- 羟皮质类固醇和醛固酮消失。在正常妊娠期，皮质醇的生成量显著增加。这至少在一定程度上是由于血液中皮质类固醇结合球蛋白水平升高，导致了皮质醇的结合能力显著增加。

There is little evidence that the placenta produces corticosteroids. In the presence of Addison's disease or following adrenalectomy, 17-hydoxycorticosteroids and aldosterone disappear from the maternal urine. In normal pregnancy, there is a substantial increase in cortisol production, and this is at least in part due to the raised levels of transcortin in the blood so that the capacity for binding cortisol increases substantially.

(4) 促肾上腺皮质激素释放激素（Corticotrophin-releasing hormone）：在妊娠中期和妊娠晚期，母体血浆中促肾上腺皮质激素释放激素（corticotrophin-releasing hormone，CRH）水平逐渐升高。母体血浆中，高亲和力 CRH 结合蛋白（CRH-binding protein，CRH-BP）的存在降低了 CRH 的所有生物学效应。CRH-BP 的浓度在妊娠的最后 4～5 周下降，因此游离 CRH 的水平有所升高。

A progressive increase in the levels of corticotrophin-releasing hormone (CRH) in maternal plasma has been noted in the final two trimesters of pregnancy. Any biological effects of CRH are diminished by the presence of a high-affinity CRH-binding protein (CRH-BP) in maternal plasma, although the concentrations of CRH-BP fall in the last 4–5 weeks of pregnancy, and as a consequence, free levels of CRH appear to rise.

六、胎儿生长发育（Fetal development）

（一）生长（Growth）

妊娠 10 周，发育中胚胎的细胞数量大量增加，但实际增加的体重很小。此后体重迅速增加直到足月，足月胎儿的最终体重约为 3.5kg。

Up to 10 weeks' gestation, a massive increase in cell numbers occurs in the developing embryo, but the actual gain in weight is small. Thereafter a rapid increase in weight occurs until the full-term fetus reaches a final weight of around 3.5 kg.

母体妊娠期间，胎儿的蛋白质不断积累。然而，就胎儿脂肪组织而言，情况却大不相同。游离脂肪酸储存在颈部、肩胛骨和胸骨后方以胎儿及肾脏周围的棕色脂肪中。白色脂肪形成了覆盖足月胎儿身体的皮下脂肪。在妊娠 24～28 周，胎儿体内脂肪储存仅占体重的 1%；然而，到妊娠 35 周时，脂肪组织质量占胎儿体重的 15%。

Protein accumulation occurs in the fetus throughout pregnancy. However, the situation is very different as far as fetal adipose tissue is concerned. Free fatty acids are stored in brown fat around the neck, behind the scapulae and the sternum and around the kidneys. White fat forms the subcutaneous fat covering the body of the full-term fetus. Fat stores in the fetus between 24 and 28 weeks' gestation make up only 1% of the body weight, whereas by 35 weeks, it makes up 15% of body weight.

胎儿的生长速度在近足月时逐渐减慢。胎儿的实际大小是由多种因素决定的，其中包括胎盘的功能、子宫胎盘血流的充足性，以及胎儿内在的遗传和种族因素。

The rate of fetal growth diminishes towards term. Actual

fetal size is determined by a variety of factors, including the efficiency of the placenta, the adequacy of the uteroplacental blood flow and inherent genetic and racial factors in the fetus.

正常的胎儿生长和出生体重取决于胎龄及体质变量，如母亲的身高、体重、胎次和种族出身。胎儿的预计出生体重取决于以上因素的组合，每一次妊娠都有所不同。计算机生成的"个性化"增长曲线概述了如何达到这一预测体重及其上、下限。图 4-9 基于左上角所示的特征，分别展示了"Mrs Small"和"Mrs Average"的胎儿相关指标的增长曲线图。图中显示中位数及第九十位、第七十位的百分位线，概述了每次妊娠的宫高及体重测量的正常范围。在每张图表上绘制了同一胎儿连续的体重测量值。"Mrs Small"生长轨迹尚可，而"Mrs Average"的胎儿生长缓慢，应当对后者的胎儿发育进行关注，并行进一步检查和（或）干预。

Normal fetal growth and birth weight are determined by gestational age as well as constitutional variables such as maternal height, weight, parity and ethnic origin. The projected birth weight depends on a combination of these factors and is different for each pregnancy. The computergenerated 'customized' growth curve outlines how this weight is to be reached, together with upper and lower limits. Fig. 4.9 shows two growth charts, for 'Mrs Small' and 'Mrs Average', respectively, based on the sets of characteristics displayed in the top-left corner. The median as well as the 90th and 70th centile lines are shown, outlining different normal ranges for fundal height and fetal weight measurements for each pregnancy. The same series of fetal weight measurements is plotted on each chart and shows an acceptable growth trajectory for 'Mrs Small' but slow growth for 'Mrs Average', which should raise concern for the fetus and prompt further investigation and/or intervention.

妊娠 12 周，胎儿的特征性外观如图 4-10 所示。皮肤半透明状，几乎没有皮下脂肪，因此皮肤血管清晰可见。此时，胎儿已经能对刺激作出反应。上肢已达到最终的相对长度，外生殖器外部清晰可见，但仍未分化。

The characteristic appearance of the fetus at 12 weeks' gestation is shown in Fig. 4.10. The skin is translucent, and there is virtually no subcutaneous fat so that the blood vessels in the skin are easily seen, but even at this stage, the fetus reacts

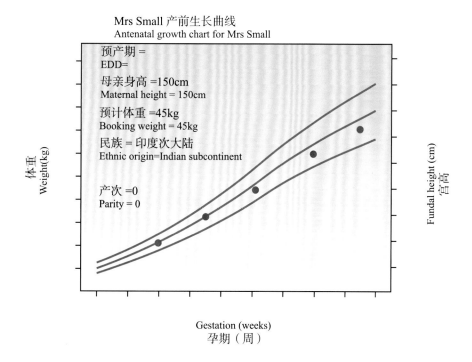

▲ 图 4-9A　根据胎次、母亲身高、体重和种族绘制的胎儿体重和胎龄图。EDD. 预产期

图片由 Jason Gardosi 提供，引自 Gardosi, J, Chang A, Kalyan B, et al (1992) Customised antenatal growth charts. The Lancet, 339 (8788): 283-287.

Fig. 4.9A　Fetal weight and gestational age plotted on the basis of parity, maternal height and weight and ethnic group. EDD; Estimated date of delivery.

Courtesy Jason Gardosi. Adapted from Gardosi, J., Chang A., Kalyan B., et al (1992) Customised antenatal growth charts. The Lancet, 339 (8788):283-287

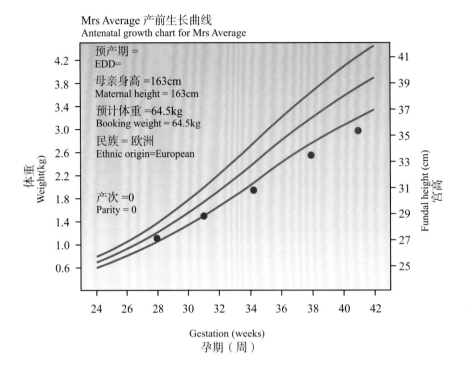

Mrs Average 产前生长曲线
Antenatal growth chart for Mrs Average

▲ 图 4-9B　根据胎次、母亲身高、体重和种族绘制的胎儿体重和胎龄图。EDD. 预产期

图片由 Jason Gardosi 提供，引自 Gardosi, J, Chang A, Kalyan B, et al (1992) Customised antenatal growth charts. The Lancet, 339 (8788): 283-287

Fig. 4.9B　Fetal weight and gestational age plotted on the basis of parity, maternal height and weight and ethnic group. EDD; Estimated date of delivery

Courtesy Jason Gardosi. Adapted from Gardosi, J., Chang A., Kalyan B., et al (1992) Customised antenatal growth charts. The Lancet, 339 (8788):283-287

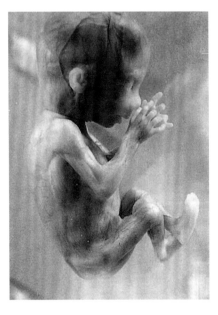

▲ 图 4-10　妊娠 12 周，胎儿对刺激有反应。上肢达到最终的相对长度，胎儿外生殖器可辨别

Fig. 4.10　At 12 weeks' gestation, the fetus reacts to stimuli. The upper limbs reach their final relative length, and the sex of the fetus is distinguishable externally

to stimuli. The upper limbs have already reached their final relative length, and the external genitals are distinguishable externally but remain undifferentiated.

妊娠 16 周（图 4-11），顶臀径长为 122mm，下肢已达最终相对长度。此时，外生殖器可辨别。

By 16 weeks' gestation (Fig. 4.11), the crown-rump length is 122 mm and the lower limbs have achieved their final relative length. The external genitalia can now be differentiated.

妊娠 24 周（图 4-12），顶臀径长 210mm。胎儿眼睑分开，皮肤不透明，由于缺乏皮下脂肪而起皱纹，身体覆盖着细毛。妊娠 28 周，眼睛睁开，头皮长出毛发。

By 24 weeks' gestation (Fig. 4.12), the crown-rump length is 210 mm. The eyelids are separated, the skin is opaque but wrinkled because of the lack of subcutaneous fat and there is fine hair covering the body. By 28 weeks, the eyes are open and the scalp is growing hair.

（二）心血管系统（The cardiovascular system）

在妊娠 3 周末，在中胚层发育的成对心内膜管。

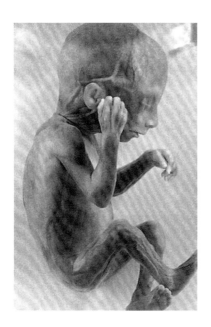

▲ 图 4-11　妊娠 16 周，胎儿顶臀径长 122mm。下肢达到最终的相对长度，眼睛面向前方

Fig. 4.11　At 16 weeks' gestation, the crown-rump length is 122 mm. The lower limbs achieve their final relative length, and the eyes face anteriorly

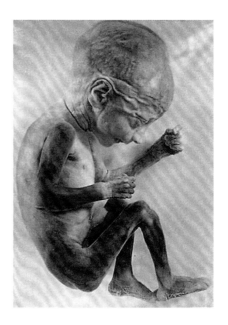

▲ 图 4-12　妊娠 24 周，胎儿肺部开始分泌表面活性物质。眼睑分开，身体由细毛覆盖

Fig. 4.12　At 24 weeks' gestation, the fetal lungs start to secrete surfactant. The eyelids are separated, and fine hair covers the body

由于胚胎折叠而靠得更近，并在第 4 周融合形成单个心管。妊娠 4～5 周，心率为每分钟 65 次。单一心管中形成许多沟槽（沟）和膨大，成为心腔和流出道的前体；这些前体通过折叠和成环的过程重新排列，形成成人心脏的空间关系。分隔和瓣膜发育最终把心脏的各个腔室分开。

The paired endocardial tubes that develop in the mesoderm towards the end of the third week of gestation are brought closer together as a result of embryonic folding and fuse to form a single cardiac tube during week 4. By 4–5 weeks' gestation, a heartbeat is present at a rate of 65 beats/min. A number of grooves (sulci) and expansions form in this single tube, marking the precursors of the cardiac chambers and outflow tract, which are rearranged by a process of folding and looping resulting in the spatial relationships of the adult heart. Septation and valvular development complete the definition of the chambers.

妊娠 11 周，形成较完整的血液循环系统，心率增加至每分钟 140 次左右。在成熟胎儿循环中，进入右心房的静脉回流约有 40% 通过卵圆孔直接流入左心房（图 4-13）。血液从右心房泵入右心室，随后被排出到肺动脉中。在此，肺动脉血通过动脉导管进入主动脉或直接进入肺血管。这两种血管联系允许含氧血液通过脐静脉进入心脏，从而在很大程度上绕过收缩的肺循环，转而泵入体循环。

The definitive circulation has developed by 11 weeks' gestation, and the heart rate increases to around 140 beats/min. In the mature fetal circulation, about 40% of the venous return entering the right atrium flows directly into the left atrium through the foramen ovale (Fig. 4.13). Blood pumped from the right atrium into the right ventricle is expelled into the pulmonary artery, where it passes either into the aorta via the ductus arteriosus or into the pulmonary vessels. These two connections allow oxygenated blood entering the heart via the umbilical vein to largely bypass the constricted pulmonary circulation and be pumped into the systemic circulation instead.

成熟胎儿的心排血量约为 200mg/(min·kg)。胎儿与成人血液循环不同，其心排血量完全取决于心率而不是每搏输出量。胎心率的自主控制在妊娠晚期成熟，副交感神经倾向于降低基础胎心率。

In the mature fetus, the fetal cardiac output is estimated to be 200 mg^{-1} min^{-1} kg body weight. Unlike the adult circulation, fetal cardiac output is entirely dependent on heart rate and not on stroke volume. Autonomic control of the fetal heart rate matures during the third trimester, and parasympathetic vagal tonus tends to reduce the basal fetal heart rate.

（三）呼吸系统（The respiratory system）

妊娠第 4 周开始，原始的前肠管向腹侧外翻，形成喉气管沟，开始发育为呼吸系统。妊娠第 4 周末，未来支气管和肺的原基在喉气管沟的尾端出现

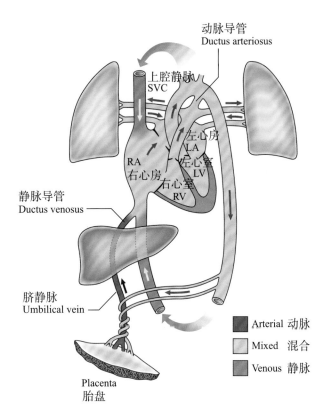

▲ 图 4-13　动脉血、静脉血和混合血的分布

LA. 左心房；LV. 左心室；RA. 右心房；RV. 右心室；SVC. 上腔静脉

Fig. 4.13　Fetal circulation showing the distribution of arterial, venous and mixed blood.

LA, Left atrium; LV, left ventricle; RA, right atrium; RV, right ventricle; SVC, superior vena cava.

分叉。呼吸道发生是指腹侧气管与背侧的食管从头端分离到分叉处，之后继续分支发育形成支气管肺芽，进而形成呼吸道的各分支和肺泡。分支形态发生的时期包括胚胎期、假腺期、小管期和囊状期、肺泡成熟期。肺泡成熟期从妊娠 36 周开始，持续到胎儿出生后。

The respiratory system develops from the primitive foregut tube as a ventral evagination, the laryngotracheal groove, at the start of the fourth week of gestation. By the end of the fourth week, the primordia of the future bronchi and lungs appear as a bifurcation at the caudal end of the laryngotracheal groove. Respiratory morphogenesis involves the separation of the ventral trachea from the dorsal oesophagus cranial to the bifurcation and successive branching of the bronchopulmonary buds to form the respiratory tree and alveoli. Branching morphogenesis comprises the embryonic, pseudoglandular, canalicular and saccular phases, followed by a period of alveolar maturation that starts at about the thirty-sixth week of gestation and continues into the postnatal period.

胎儿呼吸运动最早可在妊娠 12 周时检测到。至妊娠中期，已形成规律的呼吸模式。妊娠 34 周，呼吸运动以每分钟 40～60 次的速度发生，中间存在呼吸暂停期。这些呼吸运动很浅，此时羊水只进入细支气管。偶尔会有较大的液体流入支气管树，但由于肺泡液的分泌使得发育中的肺泡内维持高压，液体不会流入肺泡。但也有例外，缺氧情况下，喘气可能导致羊水进入肺泡更深的位置。在这种情况下，液体中通常有胎粪。

Fetal respiratory movements can be detected from as early as 12 weeks' gestation, and by mid-trimester, a regular respiratory pattern is established. By 34 weeks' gestation, respiration occurs at a rate of 40–60 movements/min with intervening periods of apnoea. These respiratory movements are shallow, with movement of amniotic fluid only into the bronchioles. There are occasional larger flows of fluid into the bronchial tree, but this does not extend into the alveoli because of the high pressure maintained in the developing alveoli from the secretion of alveolar fluid. An exception to this situation may result from episodes of hypoxia, when gasping may lead to the inhalation of amniotic fluid deeper into the alveoli. This fluid may often, under these circumstances, be meconium stained.

高碳酸血症和母体血糖水平升高会刺激胎儿呼吸，如母体处于饭后状态；而缺氧会减少呼吸运动的次数，比如母亲吸烟时。

Fetal breathing is stimulated by hypercapnia and by raised maternal glucose levels, as in the post-prandial state, whereas hypoxia reduces the number of respiratory movements, as does maternal smoking.

胎儿呼吸暂停的发生频率在近足月过程中有所增加。此时，正常胎儿呼吸运动可能暂停长达 120min。

The occurrence of fetal apnoea increases towards term, when breathing movements may be absent for as long as 120 minutes in a normal fetus.

胎儿肺泡由 2 种主要的肺泡上皮细胞覆盖。气体交换发生在 Ⅰ 型细胞，而 Ⅱ 型细胞分泌一种磷脂表面活性物质，这种表面活性物质对维持肺泡的功能至关重要。表面活性剂主要的成分是鞘磷脂和卵磷脂。妊娠 32 周时，卵磷脂的合成达到功能水平，尽管卵磷脂最早可能在妊娠 24 周时开始合成。在某些情况下，如妊娠期糖尿病，胎儿肺泡表面活性物质的产生可能会延迟；母体服用皮质类固醇可以加速这一过程。

The fetal pulmonary alveoli are lined by two main types of alveolar epithelial cell. Gaseous exchange occurs across the type I cells, and the type II cells secrete a surface-active phospholipid surfactant that is essential in maintaining the functional patency of the alveoli. The principal surfactants are sphingomyelin and lecithin; production of lecithin reaches functional levels by 32 weeks' gestation, although it may begin as early as 24 weeks. In some circumstances, such as in the diabetic pregnancy, the production of surfactant may be delayed, and the process can be accelerated by the administration of corticosteroids to the mother.

羊水中卵磷脂浓度的测定可用于评价胎儿肺功能成熟程度，且这是一种有用的方法。

The measurement of lecithin concentration in the amniotic fluid provides a useful method of assessing functional fetal lung maturity.

（四）胃肠道（The gastrointestinal tract）

在妊娠第 4 周，胚胎折叠将扁平的内胚层转化为原始消化管。原始消化管最初通过卵黄管与卵黄囊相连。头部通过口咽膜关闭，尾部通过泄殖腔膜关闭。口腔是由口咽膜破裂形成的。在后肠中，发育中的尿直肠隔将泄殖腔分为腹侧的尿生殖窦和背侧的原始直肠。前肠、中肠和后肠的区域划分是由它们对应的血液供应来定义的。在妊娠第 6～10 周或 11 周，中肠的快速生长导致部分肠管进入脐带底部形成生理性疝。在这期间肠道旋转的结果将决定肠道在腹腔的最终解剖位置。十二指肠内胚层的增厚和随后的出芽促使胰腺、肝脏和胆囊发育。

Embryonic folding converts the flat endodermal layer into the primitive gastrointestinal tube during the fourth week of gestation. The tube is initially connected to the yolk sac by the vitellointestinal duct and is closed at both its cranial and caudal ends by the oropharyngeal and cloacal membranes, respectively. The mouth is formed by the breakdown of the oropharyngeal membrane, and in the hindgut, the developing urorectal septum divides the cloaca into a ventral urogenital sinus and a dorsal rectum. The foregut, midgut and hindgut regions are defined by the boundaries of their corresponding blood supply. Rapid growth of the midgut leads to a physiological herniation of part of the intestine into the base of the umbilical cord during the period between the sixth and the tenth to eleventh weeks of gestation. The final anatomical position of the bowel in the abdominal cavity is the result of intestinal rotation during this period. Thickening of the duodenal endoderm and subsequent budding lead to the development of the pancreas, liver and gallbladder.

胎儿肠道和肠道功能的发育贯穿整个孕期，妊娠 16～20 周时出现黏膜腺体，预示着肠道功能最初的发育开始。妊娠 26 周时大部分消化酶已经存在，但直至新生儿期胃肠道才显现淀粉酶的活性。妊娠

中期胎儿吞下羊水，肠道蠕动建立。羊水中的细胞和蛋白质消化形成胎儿粪便，称为胎粪。

The development of the fetal gut and gut function proceeds throughout pregnancy, and by 16–20 weeks' gestation, mucosal glands appear, heralding the earliest onset of gut function. By 26 weeks' gestation most of the digestive enzymes are present, although amylase activity does not appear until the neonatal period. The fetus swallows amniotic fluid, and peristaltic gut movement is established by mid-pregnancy. The digestion of cells and protein in amniotic fluid results in the formation of fetal faeces known as *meconium*.

正常情况下，胎粪停留在肠道内。随着胎儿成熟度的增加，胎粪也出现在羊水中。当羊水量减少，胎儿出现应激或窒息时，胎粪也会出现在羊水中。

Meconium normally remains in the gut and appears in the amniotic fluid with increasing maturity and also under conditions of fetal stress and asphyxia when the quantity of amniotic fluid may be less.

（五）肾脏（The kidney）

在妊娠第 4 周初，肾脏从中胚层开始发育。肾脏发育分 3 个阶段，分别为前肾、中肾和后肾（永久肾）。这三个阶段按照从头到尾的方向依次发育。前肾无功能且会退化。中肾由多个中肾小管组成，这些中肾小管发育为功能单元，并引流至成对的中肾管（Wolffian 管）中，其尾端连接原始泌尿生殖窦。与男性不同，女性的中肾管会退化，男性中肾管尾部则大部分发育为睾丸输出小管、附睾、输精管和精囊。后肾的发育始于妊娠第 5 周，从中肾管输尿管芽出芽开始。输尿管芽将形成肾脏的集合系统，并与泌尿生殖窦形成的未来膀胱部分相连。输尿管芽向侧面生长，通过一系列上皮 – 间充质相互作用诱导肾实质发育，中间中胚层的大量细胞称为后肾胚芽。

The kidneys start developing in the intermediate mesoderm at the beginning of the fourth week of gestation. Three distinct phases of nephrogenesis have been described with the sequential development of the pronephros, mesonephros and metanephros (the definitive kidney) in a craniocaudal direction. The pronephros is not functional and regresses. The mesonephros consists of multiple mesonephric tubules that develop into functional units and drain into paired mesonephric (Wolffian) ducts, which themselves caudally connect to the primitive urogenital sinus. In the female, the mesonephric duct all but degenerates in contrast to the male, where its caudal-most part develops into the efferent ducts, epididymis, vas deferens and seminal vesicle. Development of the metanephros begins at the start of the fifth week of gestation with the budding of ureteric buds from the mesonephric duct.

The ureteric buds will form the collecting system of the kidneys and connect to the part of the urogenital sinus that will form the future urinary bladder. The ureteric buds grow laterally and induce development of the renal parenchyma through a series of reciprocal epithelial-mesenchymal interactions with a mass of cells in the intermediate mesoderm known as the *metanephric blastema.*

妊娠 22 周，肾皮质肾小球旁区首次出现功能性肾小体，并出现滤过功能。直至妊娠 36 周，肾脏形成完成。随着肾小球数目的增加和胎儿血压的升高，肾小球的滤过增加。

Functional renal corpuscles first appear in the juxtaglomerular zone of the renal cortex at 22 weeks' gestation, and filtration begins at this time. The formation of the kidney is completed by 36 weeks' gestation. Glomerular filtration increases towards term as the number of glomeruli increases and fetal blood pressure rises

在胎儿时期，只有 2% 的心排血量流向肾脏，因为大部分由肾脏完成的排泄功能通常是通过胎盘完成的。

In the fetus, only 2% of the cardiac output perfuses the kidney, as most of the excretory functions normally served by the kidney are met by the placenta.

在接受肾小球滤过前，胎儿肾小管具有主动转运的功能。因此，肾小球滤过前，一些尿液可能在肾小管中产生。肾小管重吸收的效率很低，胎儿循环中低至 4.2mmol/L 的葡萄糖浓度即可溢入胎儿尿液中。

The fetal renal tubules are capable of active transport before any glomerular filtrate is received, and thus some urine may be produced within the tubules before glomerular filtration starts. The efficiency of tubular reabsorption is low, and glucose in the fetal circulation spills into fetal urine at levels as low as 4.2 mmol/L.

胎儿尿液是羊水的重要组成部分。

Fetal urine makes a significant contribution to amniotic fluid.

（六）特殊感觉（The special senses）

耳的胚胎学是复杂的，外耳和中耳发育自第一和第二鳃弓及其相关的裂和袋，内耳则源自称为耳板的外胚层结构。从第 10 周开始，外耳可通过超声观察到。中耳和 3 个听小骨在 18 周时完全形成，此时它们均已骨化。内耳的组成部分，包括耳蜗、膜迷路及骨迷路，都在妊娠 24 周时发育完成。胎儿对声音的感知必须通过行为反应来衡量。通常认为，

胎儿在妊娠 24 周首次对声音刺激发生反应。尽管一些观察研究表明早在第 16 周时胎儿就可能有感知。但从内耳的发育时间表来看，这似乎是不太可能的。

The embryology of the ear is complex with the external and middle ear deriving from the first and second pharyngeal arches and the associated cleft and pouch and the internal ear from an ectodermal structure known as the *otic placode.* The external ear can be visualized using ultrasound from 10 weeks onwards. The middle ear and the three ossicles are fully formed by 18 weeks, when they also become ossified; the contents of the inner ear, including the cochlear and the membranous and bony labyrinth, are all fully developed by 24 weeks' gestation. The perception of sound by the fetus has to be gauged by behavioural responses, and it is generally agreed that the first responses to acoustic stimuli occur at 24 weeks' gestation, although some observations have suggested that there may be perception as early as 16 weeks. In view of the developmental timetable of the inner ear, this seems unlikely.

> **！注意**
>
> 有充分的证据表明胎儿可以听到母亲的声音。母体腹壁内传播的声音确实比从腹壁外传来的声音响亮得多。利用回声平面功能磁共振成像的研究表明，母亲在孕晚期诵读童谣会引起胎儿颞叶血管变化。在孕晚期，母亲们可能要注意她们对胎儿所说的话！
>
> There is good evidence that the fetus can hear the mother's voice, and indeed sounds delivered internally are much louder than sounds delivered from outside the maternal abdominal wall. Studies with echoplanar functional magnetic resonance imaging have demonstrated temporal lobe vascular changes in the fetus in response to the mother reciting nursery rhymes in late pregnancy. Perhaps mothers should beware what they say to the fetus in late pregnancy!

眼由外胚层（神经外胚层、神经嵴和表面外胚层）和中胚层发育而来。视觉感知更难评估，但似乎在孕晚期，胎儿确实会对穿透母体腹壁的光线产生一些感知。妊娠期间确实可以观察到胎儿的眼部运动。这是观察到的胎儿各种行为状态的重要组成部分，这个问题会在第 10 章讨论。

The eye develops both from ectoderm (neuroectoderm, neural crest and surface ectoderm) and mesoderm. Visual perception is much more difficult to assess, but it seems likely that some perception to light through the maternal abdominal wall does develop in late pregnancy. Certainly, fetal eye movements can be observed during pregnancy and form an important part of the observations made concerning various fetal behavioural states, a subject that is discussed in Chapter 10.

七、羊水（Amniotic fluid）

（一）形成（Formation）

羊膜腔在妊娠早期发育。早在妊娠第 7 天就可在人类胚胎中发现羊膜腔。羊膜腔发育的第一个征象可在囊胚的内细胞团中看到。

The amniotic sac develops in early pregnancy and has been identified in the human embryo as early as 7 days. The first signs of the development of the amniotic cavity can be seen in the inner cell mass of the blastocyst.

妊娠早期，羊水可能是胎儿和母体细胞外间隙的透析液，因此 99% 是水。它也含有细胞和蛋白质成分。有证据表明，妊娠 24 周胎儿皮肤开始角化时，水分可能通过胎儿皮肤渗透发生明显转移。妊娠后半期胎儿肾脏开始出现功能时，胎儿尿液成为羊水的重要组成部分。因此，当胎儿肾脏缺失，如肾发育不全时，总会出现羊水量过少的情况，即羊水过少。

Early in pregnancy, amniotic fluid is probably a dialysate of the fetal and maternal extracellular compartments and therefore is 99% water. It does have a cellular and protein content as well. There is evidence that up to 24 weeks' gestation, when keratinization of fetal skin begins, significant transfer of water may occur by transudation across the fetal skin. In the second half of pregnancy after the onset of kidney function, fetal urine provides a significant contribution to amniotic fluid volume. Certainly, when the kidneys are missing, as in renal agenesis, the condition is invariably associated with minimal amniotic fluid volume, a condition known as *oligohydramnios*.

人们对正常妊娠中胎儿对羊水量的调节作用知之甚少。目前已知胎儿能吞食羊水并在肠道吸收，妊娠晚期胎儿会将尿液排泄到羊膜腔中（图 4-14）。

The role of the fetus in the regulation of amniotic fluid volume in normal pregnancy is poorly understood, but the fetus swallows amniotic fluid, absorbs it in the gut and, in later pregnancy, excretes urine into the amniotic sac (Fig. 4.14).

必须注意的是，这是一种高度变化的状态。因为羊膜腔中的羊水每 2～3 小时就会更新 1 次。因此，任何干扰羊水形成或排出的因素都可能导致羊水容量的急剧变化。

It must be noted that this is a highly dynamic state, as the total volume of water in the amniotic sac is turned over every 2–3 hours. Any factor that interferes with either formation or removal of amniotic fluid may therefore result in a rapid change in amniotic fluid volume.

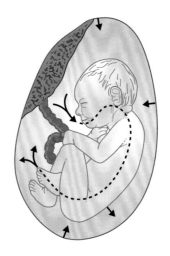

▲ 图 4-14　分泌到羊膜腔中的羊水被胎儿吞下，通过肠道吸收，并通过胎儿尿液排出

Fig. 4.14　Amniotic fluid secreted into the amniotic sac is swallowed by the fetus, absorbed through the gut and excreted through fetal urine.

与羊水摄入能力受损相关的先天畸形，通常与羊水量过多有关，这种情况被称为羊水过多。

Congenital abnormalities that are associated with impaired ability to ingest amniotic fluid are commonly associated with excessive amniotic fluid volume, a condition known as *polyhydramnios*.

综上所述，羊水是通过羊膜和胎儿皮肤分泌及渗出、胎儿尿液排入羊膜腔中形成的。羊水循环是通过胎儿肠道、皮肤和羊膜对羊水的重吸收实现的。

In summary, amniotic fluid is formed by the secretion and transudation of fluid through the amnion and fetal skin and from the passage of fetal urine into the amnioticsac. Circulation of amniotic fluid occurs by reabsorption of fluid through the fetal gut, skin and amnion.

（二）容量（Volume）

到妊娠第 8 周时，羊水已积累了 5～10ml。此后，随着胎儿生长和胎龄的增加，容量迅速增加，在妊娠 38 周时达到最大容量 1000ml。随后，羊水容量逐渐减少。到 42 周时，可能会降到 300ml 以下。评估羊水容量是超声评估胎儿健康的标准构成部分。

By 8 weeks' gestation, 5–10 mL of amniotic fluid has accumulated. Thereafter, the volume increases rapidly in parallel with fetal growth and gestational age up to a maximum volume of 1000 mL at 38 weeks. Subsequently, the volume diminishes so that by 42 weeks, it may fall below 300 mL. The estimation of amniotic fluid volume forms a standard part of the ultrasound assessment of fetal wellbeing.

（三）羊水容量检测的临床价值（Clinical significance of amniotic fluid volume）

1. 羊水过少（Oligohydramnios）

羊水量的减少通常与羊水分泌障碍有关。因此，羊水过少是胎盘功能受损的标志，除外胎儿过熟，也可能与胎膜早破伴慢性羊水丢失有关。

The diminution of amniotic fluid volume is most commonly associated with impaired secretion of fluid and therefore is a sign of the impairment of placental function, with the exception of the effect of post-maturity. It may be associated with the pre-term rupture of the membranes with chronic loss of amniotic fluid.

羊水过少通常与宫内胎儿生长受限有关，因此是胎儿危险的重要标志。

Oligohydramnios is commonly associated with intrauterine fetal growth restriction and is therefore an important sign of fetal jeopardy.

羊水过少也与先天性畸形有关，如肾脏发育不全，胎儿无法生成尿液。

It is also associated with congenital abnormalities such as renal agenesis, where there is no production of fetal urine.

羊水过少与胎儿的各种结构和功能问题有关。出生时肺发育不全和呼吸困难也与羊水过少有关。还可能导致身体畸形，如马蹄内翻足、颅骨畸形和歪颈。分娩时，羊水过少导致宫缩时脐带异常受压，导致胎儿缺氧。一些医疗机构尝试用羊水输注来避免这些问题的出现，但这些技术的有效性仍需进一步验证。

Oligohydramnios is associated with various structural and functional problems in the fetus. It may be associated with pulmonary hypoplasia and respiratory difficulties at birth. It may also cause physical deformities such as club foot, skull deformities and wry neck. In labour it has been associated with abnormal cord compression during contractions and hence with fetal hypoxia. Amniotic fluid infusions are used in some units to try and avoid these problems, but the efficacy of these techniques remains in doubt.

2. 羊水过多（Polyhydramnios）

羊水过多通常是慢性起病，但有时也可能是急性的。

The presence of excessive fluid commonly arises as a chronic condition but may on occasions be acute.

急性羊水过多较为罕见，往往出现在妊娠中期或妊娠晚期的初期，通常导致早产。这种情况对于母亲来说是痛苦的，可能导致呼吸困难和呕吐。子宫剧烈膨胀，可能需要通过羊膜腔穿刺术来缓解压力。然而，这只能提供短暂的缓解，需要进行重复操作。其通常伴有潜在的先天异常，其中一种罕见的病因是先天性尿崩症。也可以使用吲哚美辛对母亲进行药物治疗，剂量为每天 1～3mg/kg。但长期使用吲哚美辛可能导致肾动脉和肺动脉血管收缩，因此只能使用数天。

Acute polyhydramnios is a rare condition that tends to arise in the second trimester or the early part of the third trimester and commonly results in the onset of pre-term labour. The condition is painful for the mother and may cause dyspnoea and vomiting. The uterus becomes acutely distended, and it may be necessary to relieve the pressure by amniocentesis. However, this only gives short-term relief and nearly always requires repeated procedures. There is often an underlying congenital abnormality. A rare cause is congenital diabetes insipidus. It could also be managed medically with indomethacin to the mother at a dose of 1–3 mg/kg body weight per day. Indomethacin over a prolonged period may cause renal and pulmonary arterial vasoconstriction and hence should be used only for a few days.

慢性羊水过多可能发生在有大胎盘的妊娠中，如多胎妊娠、胎盘绒毛膜血管瘤或母亲患有糖尿病。也可能是特发性的，没有明显的潜在原因，胎儿也可能是完全正常的。然而，在约 30% 的病例中，伴有明显的先天性异常。慢性羊水过多可见于以下胎儿或胎盘异常，按发生率递减顺序排列。

- 无脑儿。
- 食管闭锁。
- 十二指肠闭锁。
- 枕骨裂脑露畸形。
- 脑积水。
- 膈疝。
- 胎盘绒毛膜血管瘤。

Chronic hydramnios may arise in those pregnancies where there is a large placenta, such as occurs in multiple pregnancy, chorioangioma of the placenta or a mother with diabetes. It may also be idiopathic, with no obvious underlying cause, and the fetus may be entirely normal. However, in approximately 30% of all cases, there is a significant congenital anomaly. Chronic hydramnios is seen with the following fetal or placental anomalies, in decreasing order of frequency:

- anencephaly
- oesophageal atresia
- duodenal atresia

- iniencephaly
- hydrocephaly
- diaphragmatic hernia
- chorioangioma of the placenta

羊水过多本身与某些并发症有关，这些并发症包括以下情况。

- 胎位不稳定。
- 脐带脱垂或肢体脱垂。
- 胎盘早剥时羊水突然释放。
- 子宫过度扩张相关的产后出血。
- 母体不适和呼吸困难。

Hydramnios itself is associated with certain complications, and these include the following:

- unstable lie
- cord prolapse or limb prolapse
- placental abruption if there is sudden release of amniotic fluid
- postpartum haemorrhage associated with over-distension of the uterus
- maternal discomfort and dyspnoea

（四）羊水检测的临床价值（Clinical value of tests on amnioticfluid）

羊水的生化和细胞学成分都可以用于各种临床检测。然而，许多以前使用的检测已被超声检查、脐带穿刺术和绒毛活检等操作所取代。

Both the biochemical and cytological components of amniotic fluid can be used for a variety of clinical tests. However, many of the tests previously used have been replaced by ultrasonography and procedures such as cordocentesis and `chorionic villus biopsy.

羊水中含有 2 种不同类型的细胞。第一种来自胎儿，第二种来自羊膜。胎源性细胞较大，很可能是无核的。而羊膜源性细胞较小，囊状核中有明显的核仁。在妊娠 32 周之前，这些细胞所占比例较大。

Amniotic fluid contains two distinct types of cells. The first group is derived from the fetus and the second from the amnion. Cells of fetal origin are larger and more likely to be anucleate, whereas those derived from the amnion are smaller, with a prominent nucleolus contained within the vesicular nucleus, and are found in proportionately greater numbers prior to the thirty-second week of gestation.

伊红染色的细胞来源于羊膜，在妊娠早期最多。妊娠 38 周后，这些细胞的数量下降至不到细胞总数

的 30%。

Cells that stain with eosin are most prominent in early gestation and are derived from the amnion. After 38 weeks' gestation, numbers of these cells fall to less than 30% of the total cell population.

嗜碱性细胞的数量随着孕周增加而增加，但在妊娠 38 周后也趋于减少。这些细胞的大量存在与女性胎儿有关，可能来源于胎儿阴道。

Basophilic cells increase in number as pregnancy progresses but also tend to decrease after 38 weeks. The presence of large numbers of these cells has been related to the presence of a female fetus; the fetal vagina is thought to be the possible source.

妊娠 38 周后，羊水中出现大量嗜酸性无核细胞。这些细胞被 Nile 蓝硫酸盐染成橙色，可能来自成熟的皮脂细胞。

After 38 weeks, a large number of eosinophilic anucleate cells appear. These cells stain orange with Nile blue sulphate and are thought to be derived from maturing sebaceous cells.

这些细胞过去曾被用于评估胎龄，但现在已被超声成像和胎儿生长评估所取代。

These cells have been used in the past as a method of assessing gestational age, but this has now been replaced as a method by ultrasound imaging and the assessment of fetal growth.

八、羊膜腔穿刺术（Amniocentesis）

羊水是通过羊膜腔穿刺获得的。这项操作是在无菌条件下，通过局部麻醉，用一根细针穿过母体前腹壁进入宫腔抽取羊水。羊膜腔穿刺可用于诊断染色体异常，通常在妊娠第 14～16 周进行。这项操作必须在超声引导下进行，以确定最佳和最易获得羊水的位置，并尽可能避免接触胎盘和胎儿。操作需抽出多达 10ml 的羊水，在手术前后均需检查胎儿心搏的情况（图 4-15）。

Amniotic fluid is obtained by the procedure of amniocentesis. This procedure involves inserting a fine-gauge needle under aseptic conditions through the anterior abdominal wall of the mother under local anaesthesia. The procedure, when used for diagnostic testing for chromosomal abnormalities, is commonly performed at 14–16 weeks' gestation. The procedure must be performed under ultrasound guidance in order to identify the best and most accessible pool of amniotic fluid and, where possible, to avoid the placenta and the fetus. Up to 10 mL of fluid is withdrawn, and the

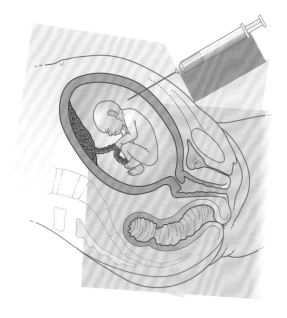

▲ 图 4-15 超声引导下，将针插入羊膜腔抽取羊水，操作过程需尽可能避免接触胎盘

Fig. 4.15 Amniotic fluid is obtained by the procedure of amniocentesis by inserting a needle into the amniotic sac under ultrasound guidance, avoiding the placenta where possible

presence of a fetal heartbeat is checked both before and after the procedure (Fig. 4.15).

羊膜腔穿刺适应证（Indications for amniocentesis）

1. 染色体异常和性连锁疾病（Chromosomal abnormalities and sex-linked diseases）

对从羊水中提取的胎儿细胞进行培养可确定胎儿核型。这可以检查染色体异常，如 Down 综合征、Turner 综合征及各种嵌合体。以前这种方法被用于鉴定胎儿性别，以辅助诊断性连锁疾病，如血友病和 Duchenne 肌营养不良，但在目前的实践中并不常用。早在妊娠 10 周前，胎儿性别就可以通过无创方法获取游离胎儿 DNA 来确定。在孕早期的最后阶段，通过评估生殖结节的角度可证实。

The fetal karyotype can be determined by the culture of fetal cells obtained from amniotic fluid. This can reveal chromosome abnormalities such as those found in Down syndrome, Turner syndrome and various mosaics. In the past, it was used for the determination of fetal sex to assist in the management of sex-linked disorders such as, haemophilia and Duchenne muscular dystrophy, but this is not common in current practice. Fetal sex can be determined non-invasively using free fetal DNA, even before 10 weeks, and this is supported towards the end of the first trimester by assessing the angle of the genital tubercle.

2. 代谢异常（Metabolic disorders）

有许多罕见的代谢异常，如 Tay-Sachs 病和半乳糖血症，可以通过从羊水中提取胎儿细胞来诊断。

There are a number of rare metabolic disorders, such as Tay-Sachs disease and galactosaemia, that can be diagnosed using fetal cells obtained from amniotic fluid.

3. 胎儿肺成熟度评估（Estimation of fetal lung maturity）

在妊娠 28 周后及早产前，新生儿发生呼吸窘迫综合征的风险较高，羊水中的卵磷脂或卵磷脂 / 鞘磷脂比值可被用于评估胎儿肺功能成熟度。然而，这种情况下目前的常规做法是给母亲使用糖皮质激素。由于糖皮质激素能有效促进胎肺成熟，目前很少用这个方法来检测胎肺的成熟度。其他用羊水来检测胎儿成熟度的方法已被超声所取代。

The estimation of lecithin or the lecithin/sphingomyelin ratio in amniotic fluid has been used to measure functional lung maturity in the fetus after 28 weeks' gestation and prior to premature delivery and where there is a significant risk of the child developing respiratory distress syndrome. However, it is now routine practice to give the mother corticosteroids under these circumstances. Such is the efficacy of this procedure that it has reduced the need to use the test. Other tests for fetal maturity based on amniotic fluid have now been abandoned in favour of ultrasound techniques.

本章概览	Essential information
胎盘的早期发育 • 囊胚在第 7 天植入 • 胎盘绒毛由 Langhans 细胞形成	**Early placental development** • Implantation of the blastocyst occurs by day 7 • Formation of placental villi takes place from Langhans cells
胎盘的进一步发育 • 母体胎盘小叶在排卵后 6 周形成 • 绒毛干仍然是胎盘的功能单位	**Further placental development** • Maternal cotyledons form by 6 weeks after ovulation • Stem villi remain the functional unit of the placenta
脐带结构 • 包含 2 条动脉和 1 条静脉，被 Wharton 胶所包绕，被覆上皮细胞	**Umbilical cord structure** • Contains two arteries and a vein surrounded by Wharton's jelly and covered in epithelium
子宫胎盘血流 • 平均压力为 10mmHg，足月时血流量为 500~750ml/min • 可因出血、子宫收缩和肾上腺素 / 去甲肾上腺素受损 • 损伤可导致胎儿生长受限和潜在的窒息	**Uteroplacental blood flow** • Mean pressure 10 mmHg and flow at term 500-750 mL/min • Can be impaired by haemorrhage, uterine contractions and adrenaline/noradrenaline • Impairment leads to fetal growth restriction and possible asphyxia
胎盘交换与功能 • 气体交换是通过简单扩散来实现的 • 即使血压很低，胎儿循环也能迅速吸收氧气 • 胎儿营养 / 排泄	**Placental transfer and function** • Gaseous exchange comes about by simple diffusion • Oxygen rapidly taken up by the fetal circulation even at low pressure • Fetal nutrition/excretion
内分泌功能 • hCG，在妊娠 10~12 周达到峰值 • hPL • 孕酮，足月时胎盘分泌约 350mg/d • 雌激素，胎盘为其主要来源，20 种不同的激素	**Endocrine function** • hCG-reaches peak between 10 and 12 weeks' gestation • hPL • Progesterone-placenta produces about 350 mg/day at term • Oestrogens-placenta major source, 20 different hormones
胎儿发育 • 胎儿生长速度在 10 周后增加，近足月时再次变慢 • 胎心在妊娠 4~5 周出现 • 足月时心排血量为 200ml/(min·kg)（译者注：原著表述似有误，已修改），完全取决于心率 • 妊娠中期出现规律呼吸模式 • 34 周时，呼吸频率为每分钟 40~60 次 • 肺的主要表面活物质为鞘磷脂和卵磷脂 • 卵磷脂的产生在妊娠 32 周时达到功能水平 • 母体糖尿病可能会延迟肺表面活性物质的产生 • 大多数消化酶在妊娠 26 周时出现 • 胎儿肾在妊娠 36 周时完全形成，但大部分排泄功能由胎盘完成 • 对声音的感知始于妊娠 16~24 周	**Fetal development** • Rate of fetal growth increases after 10 weeks and diminishes again towards term • Heartbeat present at 4-5 weeks • Cardiac output at term 200 mL^{-1} min^{-1} kg, entirely dependent on heart rate • Regular respiratory pattern by mid-trimester • 40-60 movements/min at 34 weeks • Principal surfactants sphingomyelin and lecithin • Production of lecithin reaches functional levels by 32 weeks • Surfactant production may be delayed by maternal diabetes • Most digestive enzymes present by 26 weeks • Fetal kidney completely formed by 36 weeks, but most excretory functions performed by the placenta • Perception of sound begins between 16 and 24 weeks
羊水 • 胎儿尿液是主要成分 • 羊水每 2~3 小时更新 1 次 • 羊水过少 • 与宫内生长受限和先天性畸形有关，如肾发育不全 • 可能引起分娩时肺发育不全、足畸形、颅骨畸形、斜颈和胎儿缺氧 • 羊水过多 • 可能与多胎妊娠，糖尿病或先天异常有关 • 可能导致胎位不固定、脐带脱垂、胎盘早剥或产后出血	**Amniotic fluid** • Fetal urine major contributor • Total volume turned over every 2-3 hours • Oligohydramnios • Associated with intrauterine growth restriction and congenital abnormalities, e.g. renal agenesis • May cause pulmonary hypoplasia, club foot, skull deformity, wry neck and fetal hypoxia in labour • Polyhydramnios • May be associated with multiple pregnancy, diabetes or congenital abnormality • May cause unstable lie, cord prolapse, placental abruption or postpartum haemorrhage
临床检测 • 羊膜腔穿刺术有助于检测染色体异常 • 羊膜腔穿刺术也可以检测胎儿性别 • 当可能出现先兆早产时，可用于评估胎肺成熟度	**Clinical tests** • Amniocentesis may help to detect chromosome abnormalities • Amniocentesis also detects fetal sex • Can be used to estimate fetal lung maturity where premature delivery is likely

第 5 章　围产期和产妇死亡

Perinatal and maternal mortality

Boon H. Lim　著　　　刘见桥　译　　　崔琳琳　陈子江　校

学习目标	LEARNING OUTCOMES
学习本章后，您应该能够掌握：	After studying this chapter you should be able to:
知识标准 • 了解孕产妇死亡率和围产期死亡率的定义 • 列出孕产妇和围产期死亡的主要原因 • 描述影响围产期和孕产妇死亡的社会经济因素	**Knowledge criteria** • Understand the definitions of maternal and perinatal mortality • List the main causes of maternal and perinatal mortality • Describe the socioeconomic factors that affect perinatal and maternal mortality
临床能力 • 解释孕产妇、围产期数据及其对各种卫生服务的影响	**Clinical competencies** • Interpret maternal and perinatal data and the implications on the various health services
专业技能和态度 • 反思在不同的国家和文化中，影响这些的直接原因、间接原因及社会人口因素的差异	**Professional skills and attitudes** • Reflect on the differences in the direct and indirect causes and the sociodemographic factors that influence these in different countries and cultures

一、围产期死亡（Perinatal mortality）

（一）概述（Introduction）

围产期死亡率是孕产妇保健、健康和营养的一个重要指标；它还反映了产科、新生儿和儿科护理的质量。了解围产期死亡率统计数据至关重要，有助于制订高质量的死因监测方法，使卫生保健系统能够制订预防战略，帮助临床医生和父母了解新生儿的死亡原因，以便为未来妊娠规划有效的监测战略。

Perinatal mortality is an important indicator of maternal care, health and nutrition; it also reflects the quality of obstetric, neonatal and paediatric care. The understanding of perinatal mortality statistics is vital in enabling the development of a high-quality approach to the surveillance of the causes of deaths, allowing health care systems to develop prevention strategies and to help clinicians and parents to understand the cause of death of their newborn in order to plan effective monitoring strategies for future pregnancies.

（二）定义（Definitions）

世界卫生组织（WHO）意识到围产期与新生儿死亡在国家间对比的重要性。他们协调卫生统计数据的汇编，并鼓励成员国在比较统计数据时采用相同的定义。然而，一些国家对围产期死亡的定义仍然存在差异，这反映了各个国家对生存能力和资源定义的差异。

The World Health Organization (WHO), in recognizing the importance of international comparison of perinatal and neonatal mortality, coordinates the compilation of health statistics and encourages member countries to rely on the same definitions when comparing the statistics. However, there remain differences in the definitions of perinatal mortality between some countries, reflecting the definition of viability and resources in the individual countries.

这些定义来自《国际疾病分类（第 10 版）》（ICD-10）。主要的定义如下。

The definitions are drawn from the tenth revision of the *International Classification of Diseases* (ICD-10). The key definitions are:

(1) 活产：不论妊娠时长，妊娠物从母体中完全排出或取出时有呼吸或有任何其他生命迹象，如心搏、脐带搏动或随意肌确切的运动，无论脐带是否被切断或胎盘是否附着，均视为活产。

Live birth: Complete expulsion or extraction from its mother of a product of conception, irrespective of the duration of the pregnancy, which, after such separation, breathes or shows any other evidence of life, such as beating of the heart, pulsation of the umbilical cord or definite movement of voluntary muscles, whether or not the umbilical cord has been cut or the placenta is attached; each product of such a birth is considered liveborn.

(2) 死胎 / 胎儿死亡：不论妊娠时长，妊娠物从母体中完全排出或取出前死亡。死亡的定义为胎儿没有呼吸或其他任何其他生命迹象，如心搏、脐带搏动或随意肌的确切运动。

Stillbirth or fetal death: Death prior to the complete expulsion or extraction from its mother of a product of conception, irrespective of the duration of pregnancy; the death is indicated by the fact that after such separation the fetus does not breathe or show any other evidence of life, such as beating of the heart, pulsation of the umbilical cord or definite movement of voluntary muscles.

世卫组织推荐的国际定义是：在妊娠≥28 周后出生，或者出生体重 1000g 的婴儿没有生命迹象。

ICD-10 提供的进一步定义将出生体重优先于孕周，具体如下。

The definition recommended by the WHO for international comparison is a baby born with no signs of life at or after 28 weeks' gestation (or birth weight of 1000 g). Further definition provided by ICD-10 gave priority of birth weight over gestation as follows:

- 晚期死胎：1000g 或以上、28 周或以上、体长 35cm 或以上的胎儿死亡。
- Late fetal death-1000 g or more, 28 weeks or more or 35 cm or more
- 早期死胎：500g 或以上、22 周或以上、体长 25cm 或以上的胎儿死亡。
- Early fetal death-500 g or more or 22 weeks or more or 25 cm or more
- 流产：孕 22 周之前的妊娠丢失。
- Miscarriage as a pregnancy loss before 22 completed weeks of gestational age

(3) 围产期：从妊娠 22 周（154 天）开始，到出生后 7 天。

Perinatal period: Commences at 22 completed weeks (154 days) of gestation and ends 7 completed days after birth.

(4) 新生儿期：从出生开始到出生后 28 天。新生儿死亡可分为早期新生儿死亡和晚期新生儿死亡，前者发生在出生后第 7 天（0～6 天）；后者发生在出生后第 7 天之后，第 28 天之前（7～27 天）。

Neonatal period: Begins with birth and ends 28 complete days after birth. Neonatal deaths may be subdivided into early neonatal deaths, occurring during the first 7 days of life (0–6 days), and late neonatal deaths, occurring after the seventh day but before the twenty-eighth day of life (7–27 days).

在英国，相关的定义有所不同，反映在存活率和生存能力概念的区别。目前适用于英格兰和威尔士的定义如下。

In the UK, the definitions are different, reflecting the survival rates and concept of viability. The present legal definitions that apply to England and Wales are as follows:

(5) 死胎：在妊娠 24+0 周或之后分娩的婴儿没有生命迹象，无论何时死亡。

Stillbirth: A baby delivered at or after 24+0 weeks gestational age showing no signs of life, irrespective of when the death occurred.

- 产前死胎：在妊娠 24+0 周或之后分娩的婴儿，

没有生命迹象，已知在分娩护理开始前死亡。

- *Antepartum stillbirth:* A baby delivered at or after 24+0 weeks gestational age showing no signs of life and known to have died before the onset of care in labour.

- **产时死胎：** 在妊娠 24+0 周或之后分娩的婴儿，没有生命迹象，已知在分娩护理开始时还未死亡。

- *Intrapartum stillbirth:* A baby delivered at or after 24+0 weeks gestational age showing no signs of life and known to have been alive at the onset of care in labour.

(6) 新生儿死亡：活产婴儿（出生时胎龄≥20+0 周，无法准确估计孕周时出生体重≥400g），出生后 28 天内死亡。

Neonatal death: A liveborn baby (born at 20+0 weeks gestational age or later, or with a birth weight of 400 g or more where an accurate estimate of gestation is not available) who died before 28 completed days after birth.

- **新生儿早期死亡：** 活产婴儿（出生时胎龄≥20+0 周，无法准确估计孕周时出生体重≥400g），出生后 7 天内死亡。

- *Early neonatal death:* A liveborn baby (born at 20+0 weeks gestational age or later, or with a birth weight of 400 g or more where an accurate estimate of gestation is not available) who died before 7 completed days after birth.

- **新生儿晚期死亡：** 活产婴儿（出生时胎龄≥20+0 周，无法准确估计孕周时出生体重≥400g），出生后第 7 天至第 28 天前死亡。

- Late neonatal death: A liveborn baby (born at 20+0 weeks gestational age or later, or with a birth weight of 40 g or more where an accurate estimate of gestation is not available) who died after 7 completed days but before 28 completed days after birth.

(7) 围产期死亡：胎儿或新生儿在妊娠 24 周开始至出生后 7 天内死亡。

Perinatal death: Death of a fetus or a newborn in the perinatal period that commences at 24 completed weeks' gestation and ends before 7 completed days after birth.

在澳大利亚和新西兰，死胎被定义为"出生时胎龄≥20+0 周，无法准确估计孕周时出生体重≥400g，妊娠产物从母亲体内完全排出或取出前死亡"。即在胎儿从母体分离后，没有呼吸或任何其他生命迹象，如心脏搏动、脐带搏动或随意肌确切的运动，提示胎儿死亡。

In Australia and New Zealand, stillbirth is defined as 'Death prior to the complete expulsion or extraction from its mother of a product of conception of 20 or more completed weeks of gestation or of 400 g or more birth weight where gestation is not known. The death is indicated by the fact that after such separation the fetus does not breathe or show any other evidence of life, such as beating of the heart, pulsation of the umbilical cord, or definite movement of voluntary muscles'.

在澳大利亚，围产期始于妊娠 20 周（140 天），结束于出生后满 28 天。

In Australia, the perinatal period commences at 20 completed weeks (140 days) of gestation and ends 28 completed days after birth.

（三）死亡率（Mortality rates）

目前的定义如下。

The current definitions are as follows:

死胎率（SBR）：每 1000 名新生儿中的死胎数。

Stillbirth rate (SBR): The number of stillbirths per 1000 total births

新生儿死亡率（NMR）：每 1000 名活产中出生后 28 天内发生的新生儿死亡数。

Neonatal mortality rate (NMR): The number of neonatal deaths occurring within the first 28 days of life per 1000 live births

围产期死亡率（PNMR）：每 1000 名新生儿（包括活产和死胎）中的死胎和早期新生儿死亡数（出生后第 1 周发生的死亡数）。

Perinatal mortality rate (PNMR): The number of stillbirths and early neonatal deaths (those occurring in the first week of life) per 1000 total births (live births and stillbirths)

（四）全球情况（The global picture）

2000 年，联合国成员国承诺努力实现一系列千年发展目标（MDG），其中包括在 2015 年将 1990 年的孕产妇死亡率（MMR；每 10 万活产中孕产妇死亡人数）降低 3/4。这一目标（千年发展目标 5A）和实现普遍获得生殖健康（千年发展目标 5B）共同构成了千年发展目标 5（MDG5）的两个目标：改善产妇健康。令人失望的是，在千年发展目标结束时，自 2000 年以来死胎率的下降速度一直慢于孕产妇死亡率及 5 岁以下儿童死亡率。2000—2015 年，全球死胎数量下降了 19.4%，年降幅（ARR）为 2%，低于同期孕产妇死亡率（ARR=3.0%）和 5 岁以下儿童死亡率（ARR=3.9%）。

In 2000, the United Nations (UN) member states pledged to work towards a series of Millennium Development Goals (MDGs), including the target of a three-quarters reduction in the 1990 maternal mortality ratio (MMR; maternal deaths per 100,000 live births), to be achieved by 2015. This target (MDG 5A) and that of achieving universal access to reproductive health (MDG 5B) together formed the two targets for MDG 5: Improve maternal health. Disappointingly, at the end of the MDG era, stillbirth rates declined more slowly since 2000 than either maternal mortality or mortality in children younger than 5 years. Worldwide, the number of stillbirths declined by 19.4% between 2000 and 2015, representing an annual reduction rate (ARR) of 2%. This rate of reduction was lower when compared with that for MMR (ARR = 3.0%) and under-5 mortality rate (ARR = 3.9%) for the same period.

为了改进孕产妇死亡的分类，世卫组织对 ICD-10 的定义进行了一些修改。这就是 ICD 孕产妇死亡率。

In an attempt to improve the classification of maternal deaths, the WHO applied some modifications to the definitions of ICD-10. This is known as *ICD-Maternal Mortality (MM)*.

这一定义将发生在妊娠、分娩和产褥期的死亡定义为女性在妊娠期间或终止妊娠后 42 天内的死亡，而不区分死亡原因（产科和非产科）。

This defined death occurring during pregnancy, childbirth and the puerperium as the death of a woman while pregnant or within 42 days of termination of pregnancy, irrespective of the cause of death (obstetric and non-obstetric).

2015 年，全球有 260 万死胎，每天超过 7178 例死亡，死胎率（SBR）为 18.4‰。98% 的死胎发生在中低收入国家。死胎率最高的是冲突地区和紧急地区。约 60% 的死胎发生在农村地区。撒哈拉以南非洲的死胎率约为发达国家的 10 倍（29‰ vs. 3‰）。

In 2015, there were 2.6 million stillbirths globally, with more than 7178 deaths a day, representing a stillbirth rate (SBR) of 18.4 per 1000 births. Ninety-eight percent occurred in low- and middle-income countries. The highest stillbirth rates are in conflict and emergency areas. About 60% of stillbirths are in rural areas. The SBR in sub-Saharan Africa is approximately 10 times that of developed countries (29 versus 3 per 1000 births).

在每年出生的 1.33 亿活产婴儿中，有 280 万在出生后第 1 周死亡。这些死亡的模式类似于产妇死亡的模式；这与保健专业人员接生技术低有关。主要位于非洲和南亚的 10 个国家，2015 年死胎率占全球的 2/3；新生儿死亡率占 68%，孕产妇死亡率占 58%。

Among the 133 million babies born alive each year, 2.8 million die in the first week of life. The patterns of these deaths are similar to the patterns for maternal deaths; this correlates with areas of low-skilled health professional attendants at birth. Ten countries, many of these in Africa and South Asia, account for two-thirds of stillbirths and most neonatal (62%) and maternal (58%) deaths estimated in 2015.

为了继续降低全球围产期死亡率，2014 年年中的世界卫生大会启动了"每一个新生儿行动计划"（ENAP），该计划得到了所有国家的认可。ENAP 的目标是到 2030 年将所有国家的新生儿死亡率降低到每 1000 名活产 12 例或更少，死胎率降低到每 1000 名活产 12 例或更少。减少新生儿和死胎的目标都作为核心指标纳入了《2015—2030 年全球女性、儿童和青少年健康战略》（图 5–1）。

In an effort to continue to improve the perinatal mortality rates worldwide, the Every Newborn Action Plan (ENAP) was launched in mid-2014 with a World Health Assembly resolution, endorsed by all countries. ENAP targets the reduction of the NMR to 12 or fewer per 1000 live births and stillbirths to 12 or fewer per 1000 births in all countries by 2030. Both the neonatal and stillbirth reduction targets are included as core indictors in the Every Woman, Every Child Global Strategy for Women's, Children's and Adolescents' Health (2015–2030) (Fig. 5.1).

在过去 30 年里，发达国家的围产期死亡率（PNMR）一直在稳步下降。在英国，MBRRACEUK（"通过英国各地的审计和保密调查降低母婴风险"的缩写）发布了 2015 年第三次全国围产期死亡统计报告。该报告显示，围产期死亡率为 5.61‰，其中死胎率为 3.87‰，孕产妇死亡率为 1.74‰。死胎率自 2013 年以来一直呈下降趋势，产妇死亡率下降很少。

Developed countries have seen a steady fall in the PNMR over the last 30 years. In the United Kingdom, MBRRACEUK (Mothers and Babies: Reducing Risks through Audits and Confidential Enquiries across the UK) published the third annual report of the national perinatal mortality statistics for 2015. This showed a PNMR of 5.61 per 1000 births, comprising an SBR of 3.87 and an NMR of 1.74 per 1000 births. Whilst the SBR has shown a downward trend since 2013, the NMR has only marginally reduced.

据报道，2015 年新西兰围产期死亡率为 9.7‰。虽然这一数据为自 2007 年以来"围产期和孕产妇死亡率审查委员会"收集数据以来的最低水平，但在统计上没有显示出明显的改善趋势。

The perinatal-related mortality rate in 2015 in New Zealand was reported as 9.7/1000 births. Whilst this rate

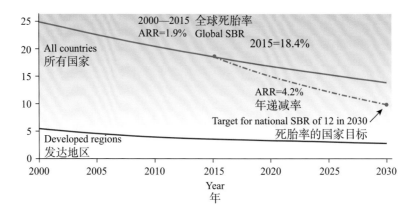

▲ 图 5-1　至 2030 年 "每一个新生儿行动计划" 中终结可预防性死胎目标的全球进程

ARR. 年递减率；SBR. 死胎率 [经许可转载，引自 www.thelancet.com/pb/assets/raw/Lancet/stories/series/stillbirths2016-exec-summ. pdf (Accessed 10 October 2018)]

Fig. 5.1　Global progress towards Every Newborn Action Plan target to end preventable stillbirths by 2030

ARR, Annual reduction rate; SBR, stillbirth rate. [Reproduced with permission. From www.thelancet.com/pb/assets/raw/Lancet/stories/series/stillbirths2016-exec-summ.pdf (Accessed 10 October 2018)]

was the lowest since data were collected by the Perinatal and Maternal Mortality Review Committee in 2007, it did not show a statistically significant trend in improvement.

澳大利亚卫生和福利研究所（AIHW，2017 年）报告说，在 1993—2012 年的 20 年期间，围产期死亡率的稳定在每 1000 名活产中约 10 例死亡。2015 年，每 1000 例分娩中有 9 例围产期死亡，共计 2849 例围产期死亡。这包括 2160 例胎儿死亡（死胎）和 689 例新生儿死亡，即每 1000 例分娩中有 7 例胎儿死亡，每 1000 例活产中有 2 例新生儿死亡。

The Australian Institute of Health and Welfare (AIHW, 2017) reported that in the 20-year period from 1993 to 2012, the overall PNMR remained stable at around 10 deaths per 1000 live births. In 2015, there were 9 perinatal deaths for every 1000 births, a total of 2849 perinatal deaths. This included 2160 fetal deaths (stillbirths), or 7 fetal deaths per 1000 births, and 689 neonatal deaths, a rate of 2 neonatal deaths per 1000 live births.

（五）影响围产期死亡率的因素（Factors that influence perinatal mortality rates）

影响围产期死亡率的因素主要是孕产妇保健、健康和营养。这些因素包括社会人口特征、产妇年龄、贫困和偏远、种族和肥胖。吸烟对出生体重和围产期死亡率也有显著的不利影响。

PNMRs are influenced by maternal care, health and nutrition. Factors include socio-demographic characteristics, maternal age, deprivation and remoteness, ethnicity and obesity. Smoking also has a significant adverse effect on birth weight and perinatal mortality.

（六）社会人口特征（Sociodemographic characteristics）

与北美和新西兰等许多发达国家一样，澳大利亚土著人口的围产期死亡率仍然很高。土著和托雷斯海峡岛民（Torres Strait Islander）的疾病负担平均是非土著民的 2.3 倍。虽然 1993—2012 年，土著母亲所生婴儿的围产期死亡率下降了 20%，但土著或托雷斯海峡岛民母亲所生婴儿的死亡率儿乎是非原住民母亲所生婴儿的 2 倍（每 1000 名新生儿中有 17.1 人死亡 vs. 9.6 人死亡）。

Like many developed nations, such as those in North America and New Zealand, the PNMRs of the indigenous populations in Australia remain high. The Aboriginal and Torres Strait Islander populations have, on average, 2.3 times the disease burden of non-indigenous people. Whilst there was a 20% decrease in the perinatal death rate of babies born to indigenous mothers between 1993 and 2012, the PNMR of babies born to mothers who identified as Aboriginal or Torres Strait Islander was almost double that of babies of non-indigenous mothers (17.1 versus 9.6 deaths per 1000 births).

1. 孕产妇年龄（Maternal age）

孕产妇年龄的两个极端都与围产期死亡率的增加有关。在澳大利亚，低龄母亲和 45 岁以上母亲的死胎率是 30—34 岁母亲死胎率的 2 倍多（分别为 13.9‰ 和 17.1‰ vs. 6.4‰）。在英国，人们注意到了一个略有不同的趋势。虽然在 2013—2015 年期间，年轻母亲（＜ 20 岁）的死胎率有所下降（从每 1000 名新生儿中的 5.28 例下降到 4.65 例）。但同期新生儿死亡率略有增长（每 1000 名新生儿中 2.35～2.95 例死胎）。高龄母亲（>40 岁）中，婴儿死亡率在此期间保持不变，而孕产妇死亡率略有下降（从每 1000 例活产中的 2.66 例降至 2.52 例）。要关注这种影响，因为在发达国家，越来越多的女性在推迟生育。

Maternal age at both extremes is associated with an increase in perinatal mortality. In Australia, the stillbirth rates for babies of teenage mothers and mothers older than 45 was more than double that for mothers aged 30–34 (13.9 and 17.1 versus 6.4 deaths per 1000 births, respectively). In the UK, a slightly different trend was noted. Whilst there has been a reduction in the rate of stillbirth for the youngest mothers (<20 years of age) over the period 2013–2015 (from 5.28 to 4.65 stillbirths per 1000 total births), a similar-sized increase in the NMR occurred over the same period (2.35–2.95 per 1000 live births). For older mothers (>40 years age), the SBR has remained static over this period, whereas the NMR has shown a small reduction (from 2.66 to 2.52 per 1000 live births). It is important to note this effect as more women are delaying childbearing in developed countries.

2. 贫困（Deprivation）

在英国，母亲的社会经济地位对围产期死亡率也有显著的影响。最贫困地区的死胎率为非贫困地区 1.7 倍（5.05‰ vs. 3.0‰），新生儿死亡率为 1.6 倍（2.28‰ vs. 1.41‰）（表 5-1）。

The socioeconomic status of the mothers also has a

表 5-1　按母亲年龄和社会经济程度分层的死胎和新生儿死亡率之比：英国及皇家属地（2015 年）

Table 5.1　Ratios of mortality rates for stillbirth and neonatal death by mother's age and socioeconomic deprivation quintile of residence: United Kingdom & Crown Dependencies, for births in 2015

母亲特点 Mother's characteristics	2015 年死亡率风险值 [§] Ratio of mortality rates (RR) [§] 2015	
母亲年龄 Mother's age (in years)	死胎 Stillbirths	新生儿死亡 Neonatal deaths
<20	1.28（1.06～1.55）	1.85（1.44～2.36）
20—24	1.17（1.04～1.30）	1.27（1.08～1.49）
25—29	1.03（0.94～1.13）	1.05（0.91～1.21）
30—34	—	—
35—39	1.20（1.08～1.34）	1.16（0.99～1.36）
≥40	1.55（1.32～1.82）	1.58（1.24～2.01）
五等分的社会经济程度 * Socioeconomic deprivation quintile*		
1（最富有） 1-Least deprived	参照 Reference	参照 Reference
2	1.08（0.96～1.23）	1.07（0.89～1.28）
3	1.23（1.09～1.39）	1.13（0.94～1.36）
4	1.48（1.31～1.66）	1.42（1.19～1.68）
5（最贫困） 5-Most deprived	1.68（1.50～1.89）	1.61（1.36～1.91）

§. 排除妊娠终止和小于 24+0 周的分娩；*. 根据母亲分娩时的邮政编码，按属地对低收入家庭的孩子进行评估（引自 MBRRACE-UK Perinatal Mortality Surveillance Report, UK Perinatal Deaths for Births from January to December 2015. Leicester: The Infant Mortality and Morbidity Studies, Department of Health Sciences, University of Leicester. 2017.）

§. Excluding teminations of pregnancy and births <24+0 weeks gestational age. *. Based on mothers' postcodes at time of delivery, using the Children in Low-Income Families Local Measure. From MBRRACE-UK Perinatal Mortality Surveillance Report, UK Perinatal Deaths for Births from January to December 2015. Leicester: The Infant Mortality and Morbidity Studies, Department of Health Sciences, University of Leicester. 2017.

statistically significant effect on the perinatal mortality rates in the UK. Mothers in the most deprived areas were 1.7 times (5.05 versus 3.0 per 1000 births) more likely to have a stillbirth and 1.6 times (2.28 versus 1.41 per 1000 births) more likely to have a neonatal death compared with mothers in the least deprived areas (Table 5.1).

3. 种族（Ethnicity）

在英国的报告中指出，种族因素在死胎率和新生儿死亡率方面具有显著性差异。其中黑种人和亚裔母亲的风险最高。种族差异可能与就业和贫困状况有关。虽然在 2013—2015 年，死胎率和新生儿死亡率总体有小幅下降，英国黑种人群体的死胎率却从每 1000 例分娩中的 7.02 例增加到 8.17 例。

A statistically significant ethnic distribution compared with the general maternity population in the rates of stillbirths and neonatal mortality, with mothers of black and Asian ethnic origins being at highest risks, was noted in the UK report. Ethnic differences may be linked to employment and deprivation status. Whilst a small reduction in mortality rates over time can be seen for most of the characteristics for both stillbirth and NMR, an increase was noted in the rate of stillbirth for the black British ethnic group from 7.02 to 8.17 per 1000 total births in the period of 2013–2015.

4. 母亲其他特征（Other maternal characteristics）

吸烟是一个重要的独立危险因素。在澳大利亚，母亲吸烟的婴儿中，围产期死亡率比母亲不吸烟的婴儿高出近 50%（每 1000 名新生儿中的死亡人数为 13.3 人 vs. 8.9 人）。2015 年，英国总死胎和新生儿死亡中约 20% 的母亲在妊娠期间确定有吸烟。美国国家健康和保健卓越研究所（NICE，2010）建议对所有孕妇常规进行一氧化碳监测。这是美国国家医疗服务体系"死胎护理"的一部分，用于确定女性在预约服务时的吸烟状况，并鼓励她们戒烟。这对死胎率的影响仍在监测之中。

Smoking is an important independent risk factor. In Australia, the PNMR was almost 50% higher among babies whose mothers smoked compared with those who did not (13.3 versus 8.9 deaths per 1000 births). In the UK, around one-fifth of the mothers of both stillbirths and neonatal deaths were identified as smoking throughout pregnancy in 2015. The National Institute for Health and Care Excellence (NICE, 2010) recommends the use of routine carbon monoxide (CO) monitoring in all pregnant women. This forms part of the Stillbirth Care Bundle in the National Health Service to determine the smoking status of women at booking and to help encourage them to quit. The effect of this on the stillbirth rates is still being monitored.

体重指数（BMI）可能是导致围产期死亡率的一个因素，但并不是所有的出生数据都被收集。2015 年，英国 25% 的死胎母亲和 19% 的新生儿死亡母亲属于肥胖人群。产次、早产、出生时的胎位和分娩方式各方面没有统计学差异。既往的产科病史，如早产、中期妊娠丢失、复发性流产和先兆子痫是影响围产期死亡率的重要因素。

Body mass index (BMI) may be a factor in contributing to the PNMR, but the data are not universally collected for all births. In the UK, in 2015, 25% of mothers who had stillbirths and 19% of mothers who had neonatal deaths fell into the obese group. There was no statistical difference in outcomes when parity, early booking, presentation at birth or mode of delivery was compared. Past obstetric history such as pre-term birth, mid-trimester loss, recurrent miscarriage and pre-eclampsia were important factors.

（七）死胎的原因（Causes of stillbirths）

死胎在围产期死亡中所占比例最大。为了帮助理解死胎的影响因素，对死胎的原因进行分类至关重要。如果按照传统的分类系统，如 Wigglesworth 和 Aberdeen（产科）分类系统，高达 2/3 的死胎可被归类为不明原因死胎。随着现在很多新分类系统的开发，被归类为不明原因死胎的数量明显减少。

Stillbirths are the largest contributor to perinatal mortality. It is important to classify the causes of stillbirths in order to help with the understanding of the antecedents. The traditionally used systems such as the Wigglesworth and the Aberdeen (Obstetric) classifications consistently reported up to two-thirds of stillbirths as being from unexplained causes. Many newer classifications have been developed that have resulted in a significant reduction of the numbers of stillbirths being classified as unexplained.

在澳大利亚和新西兰，由澳大利亚和新西兰围产期协会（Perinatal Society of Australia and New Zealand, PSANZ）制定的围产期死亡分类（perinatal death classification, PDC）和新生儿死亡分类（neonatal death classification, NDC）被用来对所有的死胎和新生儿死亡进行分类。根据这一分类系统，先天畸形是 2011—2012 年澳大利亚居民死胎的主要原因（占死胎的 26.3%），而自发性早产是当地土著和托雷斯海峡岛民围产期死亡的主要原因（占死胎的 26.8% 和新生儿死亡的 48.0%）。MBRRACE-UK 使用死因及相关因素（cause of death & associated conditions, CODAC）分类系统对死胎和新生儿死亡进行分类。CODAC 系统有一个编码死因的三级层级树。与 2014 年 MBRRACE-UK 围产期死亡监测报告相比，2015 年采用这个系统对先天畸形死因分类进行修订后，先天畸形导致死胎和新生儿死亡的比例上升，分别由 6.4% 上升至 8.8%，以及由 27.9% 上升至 33.1%。2015 年的数据还显示，胎盘原因在死胎中占比 27.1%，但仍有 39.5% 被归入不明原因死胎（图 5-2）。对数据的进一步分析显示，在不明原因的死胎中，几乎 1/3 的死胎存在潜在的生长受限（1190 人中有 360 例，30.2%），这凸显了在孕期密切监测胎儿生长发育的重要性。

In Australia and New Zealand, the Perinatal Society of Australia and New Zealand Perinatal Death Classification (PSANZ-PDC) and the Perinatal Society of Australia and New Zealand Neonatal Death Classification (PSANZ-NDC) are used to classify all stillbirths and neonatal deaths. Using this classification, the leading cause of stillbirths in Australia was noted to be congenital abnormalities (26.3% of stillbirths) during the period 2011–2012. The leading cause of perinatal deaths among babies of Aboriginal and Torres Strait Islander mothers was spontaneous pre-term birth (26.8% of stillbirths and 48.0% of neonatal deaths). MBRRACE-UK uses the Cause of Death & Associated Conditions (CODAC) classification system to classify both stillbirths and neonatal deaths. The CODAC system has a threelevel hierarchical tree of coded causes of death. Using this system, a revision of the cause of death classification for congenital anomalies in 2015 has resulted in an increase in the percentage for stillbirths and neonatal deaths from congenital abnormalities when compared with the MBRRACE-UK perinatal mortality surveillance report for births in 2014: 8.8% of stillbirths and 33.1% of neonatal deaths compared with 6.4% and 27.9%, respectively, in 2014. Placental causes account for 27.1% of all stillbirths in 2015, but 39.5% still fall into the 'Unknown' group (Fig. 5.2). Further analysis of the data showed that almost one-third of stillbirths with an unknown primary cause of death were potentially growth restricted (360 out of 1190, 30.2%), highlighting the importance of close monitoring of growth during pregnancy.

世卫组织报告（2015）指出，在全球范围内，死胎的主要原因如下。

- 分娩并发症。

- 过期妊娠。

- 孕期孕产妇感染（疟疾、梅毒和艾滋）。

- 孕产妇疾病（尤其是高血压、肥胖症和糖尿病）。

- 胎儿生长受限。

- 先天畸形。

On a global scale, the WHO report (2015) states that the major causes of stillbirth include:

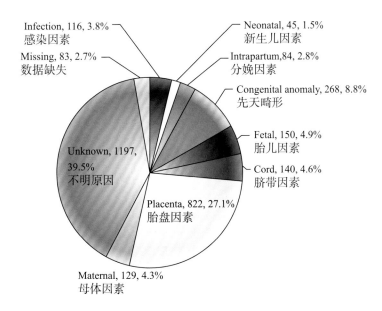

▲ 图 5-2　按 CODAC 一级死因分类的死胎：英国及皇家属地，2015 年出生人数

引自 MBRRACE-UK Perinatal Mortality Surveillance Report, UK Perinatal Deaths for Births from January to December 2015. Leicester: The Infant Mortality and Morbidity Studies, Department of Health Sciences, University of Leicester. 2017.

Fig 5.2　Stillbirths by CODAC Level 1 cause of death: United Kingdom & Crown Dependencies, for births in 2015.

From MBRRACE-UK Perinatal Mortality Surveillance Report, UK Perinatal Deaths for Births from January to December 2015. Leicester: The Infant Mortality and Morbidity Studies, Department of Health Sciences, University of Leicester. 2017.

- childbirth complications
- post-term pregnancy
- maternal infections in pregnancy (malaria, syphilis and HIV)
- maternal disorders (especially hypertension, obesity and diabetes)
- fetal growth restriction
- congenital abnormalities

在死胎之前，母亲通常会感觉到胎动减少（decreased fetal movement，DFM）。DFM 也与不良围产期结局密切相关。虽然这一领域的证据仍在不断涌现，但一些研究表明，通过提高产妇、临床医生和社区对 DFM 重要性的认识，可以降低死胎率。

Stillbirths are often preceded by maternal perception of decreased fetal movement (DFM). DFM is also strongly linked to adverse perinatal outcomes. While evidence is still emerging in this area, some studies indicate that a reduction in stillbirth rates may be achieved by increasing maternal, clinician and community awareness about the importance of DFM.

产时死胎（Intrapartum stillbirth）

根据世卫组织的估计，产时死胎占全世界死胎总数的 50%。据估计，不同地区产时死胎的比例各不相同，发达地区为 10%（英国为 5.3%），而南亚可达 59%。大多数产时死胎是可以预防的，因此改善产时的护理对于防止再出现 130 万产时死胎至关重要。

The WHO estimations have shown that intrapartum stillbirths account for half of all stillbirths worldwide. Estimated proportions of intrapartum stillbirths vary from 10% (5.3% in the UK) in developed regions to 59% in South Asia. Improved care at birth is essential to prevent 1.3 million intrapartum stillbirths, most of which are preventable.

分娩并发症是绝大部分产时死胎的原因，通过提供经过适当培训的助产士和设施，这些在很大程度上是可以避免的。发达国家的大多数分娩都是在有资质的机构和合格卫生人员在场的情况下进行的。在全球范围内，熟练助产士的覆盖率从 2000 年的 61% 上升至 2016 年的 78%。然而，尽管全球和区域内的情况稳步改善，仍有数百万的分娩没有得到助产士、医生或训练有素的护士的帮助。在非洲撒哈拉以南地区，2016 年只有接近 50% 的活产是在熟练助产士的帮助下分娩的。

Complications of childbirth are the cause of almost all the intrapartum deaths; these are largely avoidable through the provision of appropriately trained birth attendants and facilities. Most deliveries in developed countries take place in institutions

and in the presence of qualified health personnel. Globally, coverage of skilled attendants during childbirth increased from 61% in 2000 to 78% in 2016. However, despite steady improvement globally and within regions, millions of births were not assisted by a midwife, a doctor or a trained nurse. In sub-Saharan Africa, approximately only half of all live births were delivered with the assistance of a skilled birth attendant in 2016.

（八）新生儿死亡的原因（Causes of neonatal deaths）

新生儿死亡人数从 1990 年的 460 万人下降到 2009 年的 330 万人，但在过去 10 年中仅略有下降。自 2000 年联合国千年发展计划（UNMDG）制定以来，对女性和儿童的保健投资更多，其中对存活母亲（每年增长 2.1%）和 5 岁以下儿童（每年增长 2.3%）的投资多于对新生儿的投资（每年增长 1.7%）。每年的 5 岁以下儿童死亡中，近 41% 发生在新生儿期（出生后的 28 天内），其中又有 3/4 发生在出生后的第 1 周。在发展中国家，近 50% 的母亲和新生儿在产时和产后即刻无法得到专业的护理。几乎所有的新生儿死亡（99%）都发生在低收入和中等收入国家，特别是非洲和南亚，这些国家在减少新生儿死亡方面取得的进展最小。在全球范围内，新生儿死亡的 3 个主要原因是感染（36%，其中包括败血症 / 肺炎、破伤风和腹泻）、早产（28%）和产时窒息（23%）。不同的国家之间存在一些差异，这取决于各国的护理配置。

Newborn deaths dropped from 4.6 million in 1990 to 3.3 million in 2009, but fell only slightly during the last decade. More investment into health care for women and children since 2000, when the UN MDGs were set, resulted in more rapid progress for the survival of mothers (2.3% per year) and children under 5 years (2.1% per year) than for newborns (1.7% per year). Every year nearly 41% of all under-5 child deaths are among newborn infants, babies in their first 28 days of life or infants in the neonatal period. Three-quarters of all newborn deaths occur in the first week of life. In developing countries, nearly half of all mothers and newborns do not receive skilled care during and immediately after birth. Virtually all (99%) newborn deaths occur in low- and middle-income countries, especially in Africa and South Asia, where the least progress in reducing neonatal deaths has been made. Globally, the three major causes of neonatal deaths are infections (36%, which includes sepsis/pneumonia, tetanus and diarrhoea), pre-term (28%) and birth asphyxia (23%). There is some variation between countries depending on their care configurations.

在英国，2015 年约 44% 的新生儿死亡归因于新生儿原因。在新生儿死亡原因分类中，新生儿死亡人数最多的分别是极早产、神经和心肺疾病（图

5-3）。在澳大利亚，新生儿死亡（2011—2012 年）的主要原因是先天畸形（33.1%）。而在 PSANZ-NDC 分类系统中极早产是导致新生儿死亡的主要因素（33.5%）。低出生体重虽然不是新生儿死亡的直接原因，但却是重要的相关因素。有 15%～20% 的新生儿体重低于 2500g，其发生率从发达国家的 6% 到欠发达国家的 30% 以上不等。

In the UK, approximately 44% of the neonatal deaths in 2015 were attributed to a neonatal cause. The classifications for causes of death with the largest numbers of neonatal deaths were extreme prematurity, neurological and cardio-respiratory conditions (Fig. 5.3). In Australia, the leading cause of neonatal deaths (2011–2012) was congenital abnormality (33.1%). An additional PSANZ-NDC of extreme prematurity was the leading condition contributing to deaths in the neonatal period (33.5%). Low birth weight, although not a direct cause of neonatal death, is an important association. Around 15–20% of newborn infants weigh less than 2500 g, ranging from 6% in developed countries to more than 30% in the poorly developed countries.

世界各地为了改善围生期死亡率已实施了许多战略，然而结果上的差距仍然存在。各项千年计划（MDG）已经取得了不同程度的成功。改善结局的关键仍然是提供高分娩期高质量护理的覆盖率。通过预防孕产妇和新生儿死亡、预防死胎和残疾的发生，以及改善儿童发育，能够获得 4 倍的回报。通过提高产前护理和计划生育的质量，能够最大限度地提高母婴健康和儿童长期健康。

Many strategies have been implemented in an attempt to improve the PNMRs across the world. Yet disparities in outcomes still persist. The objectives of the various MDGs have been realized with varying degrees of success. The key to improving outcomes remains in the provision of high coverage of high-quality care during labour and birth. This gives a quadruple return on investment by preventing maternal and neonatal deaths, and also stillbirths and disability, with improvements in child development. Improved quality of antenatal care and family planning are also important to maximize maternal and fetal wellbeing and the long-term wellbeing of the child.

二、孕产妇死亡（Maternal mortality）

ICD-10 将孕产妇死亡定义为女性在妊娠期或妊娠终止后 42 天内死亡，无论妊娠期长短和妊娠部位，

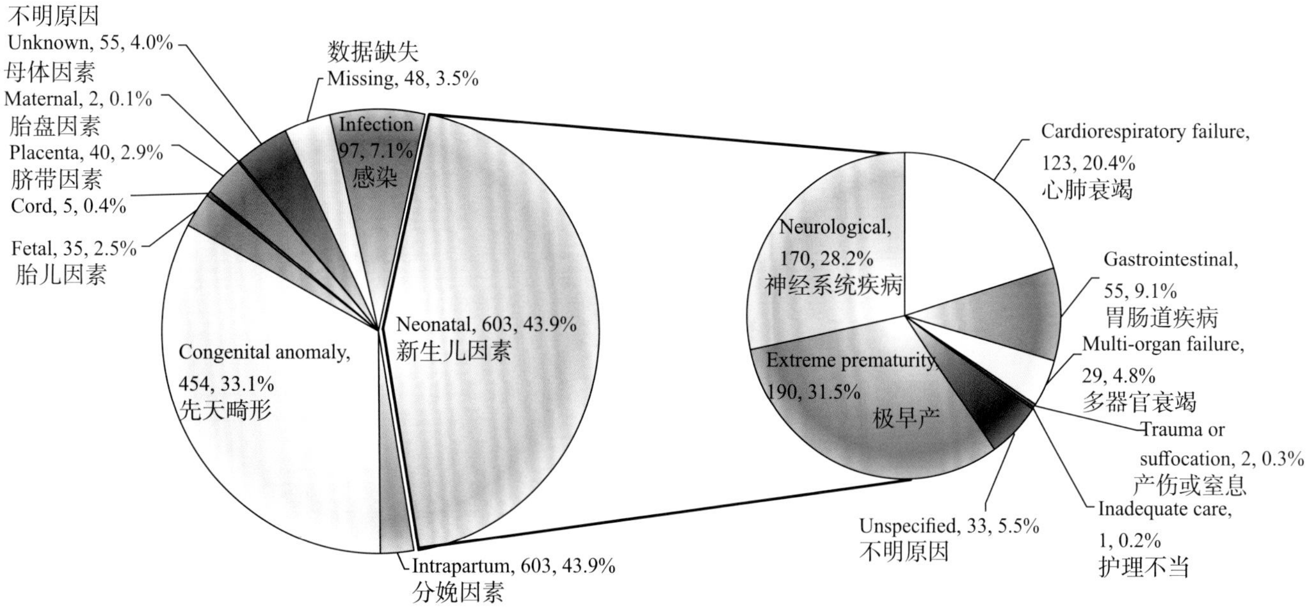

▲ 图 5-3　按 CODAC 一级和二级死因分类的新生儿死亡：英国及皇家属地，2015 年出生人数

（引自 MBRRACE-UK Perinatal Mortality Surveillance Report, UK Perinatal Deaths for Births from January to December 2015. Leicester: The Infant Mortality and Morbidity Studies, Department of Health Sciences, University of Leicester. 2017.）

Fig. 5.3　Neonatal deaths by CODAC Level 1 and Level 2 cause of death: United Kingdom & Crown Dependencies, for births in 2015.

(From MBRRACE-UK Perinatal Mortality Surveillance Report, UK Perinatal Deaths for Births from January to December 2015. Leicester: The Infant Mortality and Morbidity Studies, Department of Health Sciences, University of Leicester. 2017.)

且死因与妊娠及其治疗有关或原有疾病因此加重，但不包括由于意外或偶然因素导致的死亡。

The Tenth Revision of the ICD defines a maternal death as the death of a woman while pregnant or within 42 days of termination of pregnancy, irrespective of the duration and the site of the pregnancy, from any cause related to or aggravated by the pregnancy or its management but not from accidental or incidental causes.

孕产妇死亡可分为以下两类。

- 直接产科死亡：由于妊娠状态（妊娠、分娩和产褥期）的产科并发症、医疗干预、疏忽、处理不当或由上述的任何一项引起的一系列事件导致的死亡。

- 间接产科死亡：由于以前已存在的疾病或在妊娠期间新发生的疾病导致的死亡，这些疾病虽非直接由产科原因引起，却由于妊娠的生理影响而加重。

Maternal deaths are subdivided into two groups:

- *Direct obstetric deaths:* Those resulting from obstetric complications of the pregnancy state (pregnancy, labour and the puerperium); from interventions, omissions or incorrect treatment; or from a chain of events resulting from any of the above.

- *Indirect obstetric deaths:* Those resulting from pre-existing disease or a disease that developed during pregnancy and which was not due to direct obstetric causes but which was aggravated by the physiological effects of pregnancy.

晚期孕产妇死亡：指女性在终止妊娠后超过 42 天但不到 1 年，由直接或间接原因造成的死亡。

Late maternal death is the death of a woman from direct or indirect causes more than 42 days but less than 1 year after termination of pregnancy.

意外死亡：发生在妊娠或产褥期间非疾病和妊娠相关的意外死亡（引自 ICD-10）。

Coincidental (fortuitous): Deaths from unrelated causes that occur in pregnancy or the puerperium (from ICD-10).

为了改善对孕产妇死亡的分类，世界卫生组织对 ICD-10 的定义进行了一些修改，并称为 ICD- 产妇死亡率（ICD-Maternal Mortality，ICD-MM）。

In an attempt to improve the classification of maternal deaths, the WHO applied some modifications to the definitions of ICD-10. This is known as *ICD-Maternal Mortality (ICD-MM).*

它将发生在妊娠、分娩和产褥期的死亡定义为

女性在妊娠期间或终止妊娠后 42 天内死亡，不论死亡原因（产科和非产科）。

This defined death occurring during pregnancy, childbirth and the puerperium as the death of a woman while pregnant or within 42 days of termination of pregnancy, irrespective of the cause of death (obstetric and non-obstetric).

这些新的编码建议很可能被纳入第 11 版 ICD（ICD-11）。

The proposals for the new codes are likely to be incorporated into the 11th Revision of the ICD (ICD-11).

（一）孕产妇死亡率（Maternal mortality rates）

MMR 的国际定义是每 10 万名活产中直接和间接死亡的人数。

The international definition of the MMR is the number of direct and indirect deaths per 100,000 live births.

由于缺乏关于孕产妇死亡的准确报告，获取准确的 MMR 数据仍然是一项全球性的挑战。为了改善孕产妇健康而进行的规划和病因分析，要求建立一套准确且国际可比的孕产妇死亡率评价标准。过去 10 年，许多国家通过民事登记系统、调查、人口普查和专业的研究文献等渠道在收集数据方面取得了显著进展。这些为了登记孕产妇死亡数据而付出的努力是值得称赞的，这提供了有价值的新数据。然而，在缺乏民事登记系统的情况下，用于评估孕产妇死亡率的方法不同，导致通过各个渠道产生的各项指标无法直接进行比较。迄今为止，各国在这方面的进展仍然不足，这是由于许多国家依旧缺乏民事登记系统，而有这种系统的地方，持续存在的漏报也对数据的准确性造成重大挑战。

Obtaining accurate MMR data remains a global challenge due to a lack of accurate reporting of maternal deaths. Planning and accountability for improving maternal health require accurate and internationally comparable measures of maternal mortality. Many countries have made notable progress in collecting data through civil registration systems, surveys, censuses and specialized studies over the past decade. This laudable increase in efforts to document maternal deaths provides valuable new data, but the diversity of methods used to assess maternal mortality in the absence of civil registration systems prevents direct comparisons among indicators generated. To date, insufficient progress has been made, as many countries still lack civil registration systems, and where such systems do exist, underreporting continues to pose a major challenge to data accuracy.

建立准确且标准化的直接评价方法来评估孕产

妇死亡率仍存在挑战。鉴于此，WHO 联合世界各地许多非政府组织和大学成立了机构间孕产妇死亡率估算小组（maternal mortality estimation inter-agency group，MMEIG），目的是为了更好地估算 1990—2015 年孕产妇死亡数，以审查全球、区域和国家的孕产妇死亡情况及相关进展。为了提供更准确的 MMR 估计数，MMEIG 对以前的估计方法进行了改进，以最大限度地利用国家层面的数据。

Given the challenges of obtaining accurate and standardized direct measures of maternal mortality, the Maternal Mortality Estimation Inter-Agency Group (MMEIG), comprising WHO and many non-governmental organizations and universities across the world, was established to provide better estimates for 1990–2015 to examine the global, regional and country progress of MM. To provide increasingly accurate estimates of MMR, previous estimation methods have been refined to optimize use of country-level data.

英国等发达国家的优势在于拥有准确的人口数据，其中包括活产和死产数，并将其 MMR 定义为每 10 万名孕产妇中直接或间接死亡的人数，将孕产妇数量作为更准确的分母来表明处于危险之中的女性的数量。

Developed countries such as the UK have the advantage of accurate denominator data, including both live births and stillbirths, and have defined their MMRs as the number of direct and indirect deaths per 100,000 maternities as a more accurate denominator to indicate the number of women at risk.

此处孕产妇的定义是指在任何孕周的活产和孕 24 周及以后死胎的孕产妇数量，要求依法上报。这使得人们能够获得关于 MMR 的详细情况，且能比较其在一段时间内的变化趋势。

Maternities are defined as the number of pregnancies that result in a live birth at any gestation or stillbirths occurring at or after 24 completed weeks of gestation and are required to be notified by law. This enables a more detailed picture of MMRs to be established and is used for the comparison of trends over time.

改善孕产妇健康是 WHO 2000 年峰会通过的 8 项 MDG 之一。评估改善孕产妇健康进展情况的两个目标（MDG 5）分别是在 1990—2015 年将 MMR 降低 75%，以及在 2015 年实现生殖健康的普及。

Improving maternal health is one of the eight MDGs adopted at the WHO 2000 Millennium Summit. The two targets for assessing progress in improving maternal health (MDG 5) are reducing MMR by 75% between 1990 and 2015 and achieving universal access to reproductive health by 2015.

由 WHO、联合国儿童基金会（United Nations Children's Fund，UNICEF）、联合国人口基金（United Nations Population Fund, UNFPA）、世界银行集团和联合国人口司（United Nations Population Division, UNPD）在 2015 年发布的题为"产妇死亡率趋势（1990—2015）"的年报中报道，1990 年以来，全球孕产妇死亡率下降了 44%，从每 10 万活产 385 例死亡下降到 216 例死亡（从估计的 532 000 例下降到 303 000 例），年均下降 2.3%（表 5-2），这是非常令人鼓舞的。虽然这数据令人印象深刻，但 MDG 5 的目标是 2015 年 MM 下降 3/4，也就是年均下降率达 5.5%。而目前的数据还未达到 MDG 5 中 MM 目标（年下降率 5.5%）的 1/2。每个地区的 MMR 都有所改善。几乎所有的孕产妇死亡都是可以预防的。然而，在极端富裕和贫穷的国家之间，差距仍然存在。2015 年，非洲撒哈拉以南地区的 MM 水平仍然高得令人无法接受。在全球孕产妇死亡人数中，这一地区约占 66%（20.1 万人次），南亚约占 22%（6.6 万人次）。在高收入国家，孕产妇死亡的终生风险为 1/3300，而在低收入国家，这一比例为 1/41。

In the 2015 report issued by the WHO, the United Nations Children's Fund (UNICEF), the United Nations Population Fund (UNFPA), the World Bank Group and the United Nations Population Division (UNPD) entitled *Trends in Maternal Mortality: 1990–2015*, it is encouraging to note that from 1990, the global MMR declined by 44%-from 385 deaths to 216 deaths per 100,000 live births (from an estimated 532,000 to an estimated 303,000), representing an average annual rate of reduction of 2.3% (Table 5.2). While impressive, this is less than half of the 5.5% annual rate needed to achieve the three-quarters reduction in MM targeted for 2015 in MDG 5. Improvements in MMR have been achieved in every region. Almost all maternal deaths are preventable. However, disparities still occur between the richest and poorest countries, with levels of MM remaining unacceptably high in sub-Saharan Africa, which accounts for approximately 66% (201,000), and southern Asia (22% (66,000)), of the global maternal deaths in 2015. The lifetime risk of maternal death in highincome countries is 1 in 3300, compared with 1 in 41 in low-income countries.

在全球范围内，孕产妇死亡的主要原因如图 5-4 所示。

- 出血，是死因的首位，占所有死亡人数的 27%。
- 高血压疾病。
- 脓毒血症。
- 不安全的流产。
- 栓塞。

表 5–2　联合国千年发展计划按区域分层的孕产妇死亡率（MMR，每 10 万活产中孕产妇死亡人数）和
孕产妇死亡人数比较（1990 年和 2015 年）

Table 5.2　Comparison of maternal mortality ratio (MMR, maternal deaths per 100,000 live births) and number of maternal deaths,
by United Nations Millennium Development Goal region, 1990 and 2015

联合国千年发展目标区域 United Nations Millennium Development Goal region	1990		2015		1990 年至 2015 年百分比变化 Percentage change between 1990 and 2015
	孕产妇死亡率 MMR	孕产妇死亡数 Maternal deaths	孕产妇死亡率 MMR	孕产妇死亡数 Maternal deaths	
世界 World	385	532 000	216	303 000	44
发达地区 Developed regions	23	3500	12	1700	48
发展中地区 Developing regions	430	529 000	239	302 000	44

引自 Trends in Maternal Mortality 1990 to 2015: Estimates by WHO, UNICEF, UNFPA, World Bank Group and the United Nations Population Division (WHO 2015).

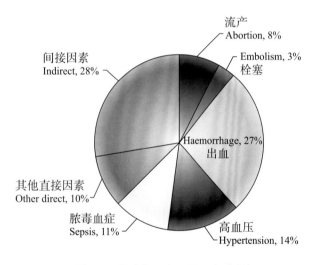

▲ 图 5-4　孕产妇死亡原因：全球通报

（经许可转载，引自 Trends in maternal mortality: 1990 to 2015: estimates by WHO, UNICEF, UNFPA, World Bank Group and the United Nations Population Division, 2015.）

Fig 5.4　Causes of maternal mortality-the global picture.

(Reproduced with permission. From Trends in maternal mortality: 1990 to 2015: estimates by WHO, UNICEF, UNFPA, World Bank Group and the United Nations Population Division, 2015.)

Globally, the major causes of maternal death are (Fig. 5.4):

- haemorrhage, the leading cause, accounting for 27% of all deaths
- hypertensive disorders
- sepsis
- unsafe abortion
- embolism

在英国，自 1952 年英格兰和威尔士引入《孕产

妇死亡机密调查》后，每 3 年发布一次报告。60 多年来一直代表着详细调查和改善孕产妇保健的国际黄金标准。自 2012 年以来，MBRRACE-UK 一直在出版来自英国和爱尔兰的《孕产妇死亡率和发病率的机密调查》，标题为"关怀母亲，拯救生命"（Saving Lives，Improving Mothers' Care）。在 2017 年 12 月发布的第四次年度报告中，公布了 2013—2015 年孕产妇死亡的监测数据。在澳大利亚，AIHW 也每 3 年报告一次类似的孕产妇死亡数据。最近一次发布于 2017 年，涵盖了 2012—2014 年的数据。

In the UK, the Confidential Enquiry into Maternal Deaths has been publishing triennial reports since it was introduced in England and Wales in 1952 and has represented a gold standard internationally for detailed investigation and improvement in maternity care for over 60 years. Since 2012, MBRRACE-UK has been publishing the Confidential Enquiries into Maternal Mortality and Morbidity from the UK and Ireland entitled Saving Lives, Improving Mothers' Care. In the fourth annual report released in December 2017, surveillance data on maternal deaths from 2013 to 2015 were published. In Australia, similar data on MM are reported every 3 years by the AIHW. The latest report was published in 2017, covering the period 2012–2014.

在 2013—2015 年，英国 240 名女性在妊娠期或妊娠终止后 42 天内死亡，其中 38 名为意外死亡。因此，在这三年中，2 305 920 名孕产妇中有 202 名女性死于直接和间接产科原因。孕产妇死亡率为每 10 万名孕产妇 8.76 人。这与 2012—2014 年每 10 万名孕产妇 8.54 人的死亡率相当。

In the UK, 240 women died in 2013–2015 during or

within 42 days of the end of pregnancy. The deaths of 38 women were classified as coincidental. Thus, in this triennium, 202 women died from direct and indirect causes among 2,305,920 maternities, a maternal death rate of 8.76 per 100,000 maternities. This is comparable to the rate of 8.54 per 100,000 maternities in 2012–2014.

比较 2003—2005 年和 2013—2015 年两个时间段的数据，孕产妇死亡率总体下降了 37%，其中直接死亡率下降了 44%，间接死亡率下降了 31%。2013—2015 年孕产妇的总死亡率和直接死亡率与 2010—2012 年没有显著差异，而 2013—2015 年孕产妇的间接死亡率明显低于 2010—2012 年（图 5-5）。

There was an overall 37% decrease in maternal death rates between 2003–2005 and 2013–2015. The direct maternal death rate has decreased by 44% since 2003–2005, and there was a 31% decrease in the rate of indirect maternal deaths. The rates of overall mortality and direct maternal death in the 2013–2015 triennium were not significantly different from the rates in 2010–2012. However, the indirect maternal death rate was significantly lower in 2013–2015 than 2010–2012 (Fig. 5.5).

（二）英国孕产妇死亡的主要原因（Major causes of maternal death in the UK）

2013—2015 年，英国孕产妇死亡的 5 个主要直接原因，按发病率排序如下。

- 血栓形成和血栓栓塞。
- 出血。
- 精神因素，如自杀。
- 与妊娠相关的感染，如败血症。
- 羊水栓塞。

The five major direct causes of maternal death in the UK (2013–2015), in order of importance, are as follows:

1. thrombosis and thromboembolism
2. haemorrhage
3. psychiatric causes-suicides
4. pregnancy-related infections-sepsis
5. amniotic fluid embolism

自上一个 3 年期以来，因间接原因死亡的孕产妇人数基本保持不变。孕产妇在分娩后 1 年内死亡的 3 种最常见的间接原因是心脏病、其他间接原因和神经系统疾病。许多心脏病患者有与生活方式相关的危险因素，如肥胖、吸烟和年龄。

The number of indirect maternal deaths has remained largely unchanged since the last triennium. The three commonest indirect causes of maternal death in the year following delivery are cardiac disease, other indirect causes and neurological conditions. Many of the women with cardiac disease had lifestyle-related risk factors such as obesity, smoking and maternal age.

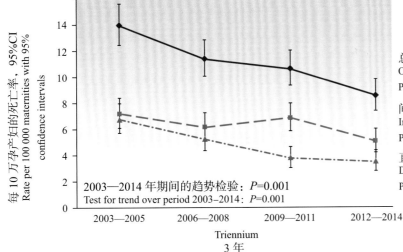

总孕产妇死亡率随时间变化趋势的 *P*=0.018
Overall maternal death rate
P-value for trend over time = 0.018

间接孕产妇死亡率随时间变化趋势的 *P*=0.220
Indirect maternal death rate
P-value for trend over time = 0.220

直接孕产妇死亡率随时间变化趋势的 *P*=0.031
Direct maternal death rate
P-value for trend over time =0.031

▲ 图 5-5　英国 2003—2014 年每 10 万名孕产妇的直接和间接孕产妇死亡率（使用 ICD-MM）

（经许可转载，引自 MBRRACE-UK. Saving Lives, Improving Mothers' Care-Lessons learned to inform maternity care from the UK and Ireland Confidential Enquiries into Maternal Deaths and Morbidity 2013-15. Oxford: National Perinatal Epidemiology Unit, University of Oxford 2017.）

Fig.5.5　**Direct and indirect maternal mortality rates per 100,000 maternities, UK 2003–2014 (using ICD-MM).**

(Reproduced with permission. From MBRRACE-UK. Saving Lives, Improving Mothers' Care - Lessons learned to inform maternity care from the UK and Ireland Confidential Enquiries into Maternal Deaths and Morbidity 2013-15. Oxford: National Perinatal Epidemiology Unit, University of Oxford 2017.)

（三）澳大利亚的孕产妇死亡情况（The situation in Australia）

澳大利亚也有类似的趋势，MMR 从 2003—2005 年的每 10 万名女性 8.4 人下降到 2012—2014 年的 6.8 人。土著女性的 MMR（每 10 万例产妇 18.7 人）是非土著女性（每 10 万例产妇 6.3 人）的 3 倍。

Similar trends have occurred in Australia, with a fall in the MMR from 8.4 per 100,000 women giving birth in 2003–2005 to 6.8 in 2012–2014. The MMR in indigenous women (18.7 per 100,000 women giving birth) remains three times higher than in the non-indigenous population (6.3 per 100,000).

在澳大利亚（2012—2014 年），孕产妇死亡最常见的直接原因是肺栓塞、产科出血和高血压疾病。非产科因素的出血和心血管疾病则是孕产妇死亡最常见的间接原因。自 2000 年以来，土著和托雷斯海峡岛民女性与其他澳大利亚女性相比，孕期死于心血管疾病、自杀、高血压疾病、产科出血、败血症及死于早孕期的可能性更高。

In Australia (2012–2014), direct maternal deaths were most frequently due to pulmonary thromboembolism, obstetric haemorrhage and hypertensive disorders. Nonobstetric haemorrhage and cardiovascular disease were the most common groups of indirect maternal death causes. Since 2000, Aboriginal and Torres Strait Islander women have been significantly more likely than other Australian women to die in relation to pregnancy from cardiovascular causes, suicide, hypertensive disorders, obstetric haemorrhage, sepsis and in early pregnancy.

本章概览	Essential information
围产期死亡率	**Perinatal mortality**
• 全球死胎率：18.4/1000 产次	• Global stillbirth rate: 18.4/1000 births
• 英国死胎率（2015）：3.87/1000 产次	• UK stillbirth rate, 2015: 3.87/1000 births
• 新生儿死亡率：1.74/1000 产次	• Neonatal death rate: 1.74/1000 births
• 围产期死亡率：5.61/1000 产次	• Perinatal mortality rate: 5.61/1000 births
• 澳大利亚围产期死亡率（2015）：7.0/1000 产次	• Australian perinatal mortality rate, 2015: 7.0/1000 births
病因学（MBRRACE–UK 2015）	**Aetiology (MBRRACE-UK 2015)**
• 死产	• Stillbirths
– 不明原因：39.5%	– Unexplained: 39.5%
– 胎盘因素：27.1%	– Placental: 27.1%
– 先天畸形：8.8%	– Congenital anomaly: 8.8%
• 新生儿死亡	• Neonatal deaths
– 新生儿原因，其中包括极早产、神经系统和心肺因素：43.9%	– Neonatal causes, including extreme prematurity, neurological and cardio-respiratory causes: 43.9%
– 先天畸形：33.1%	– Congenital anomaly: 33.1%
– 感染：7.1%	– Infection: 7.1%
孕产妇死亡率	**Maternal mortality**
• 英国机密调查（2013—2015）	• UK Confidential Enquiry 2013–2015
– 直接死亡：每 10 万例孕产妇 3.82 人	– Direct deaths: 3.82 per 100,000 maternities
– 间接死亡：每 10 万例孕产妇 4.94 人	– Indirect deaths: 4.94 per 100,000 maternities
• AIHW（2012—2014）	• AIHW 2012–2014
– 直接死亡：每 10 万例产妇 3.45 人	– Direct deaths: 3.45 per 100,000 women giving birth
– 间接死亡：每 10 万例产妇 3.35 人	– Indirect deaths: 3.35 per 100,000 women giving birth
英国孕产妇死亡常见的直接原因	**Commonest causes of direct deaths in the UK**
• 血栓形成和血栓栓塞	1. Thrombosis and thromboembolism
• 出血	2. Haemorrhage
• 精神因素：自杀	3. Psychiatric causes-suicides
• 妊娠相关感染：败血症	4. Pregnancy-related infections-sepsis
• 羊水栓塞	5. Amniotic fluid embolism
英国孕产妇死亡常见的间接原因	**Commonest indirect causes in the UK**
• 心脏病	• Cardiac disease
• 其他间接原因	• Other indirect causes
• 神经系统疾病	• Neurological conditions

第二篇　产科学基础
Essential obstetrics

第 6 章　产科病史采集与检查
History taking and examination in obstetrics

Petra Agoston　Edwin Chandraharan　著　　郭　婷　译　　杨慧霞　校

学习目标	LEARNING OUTCOMES
学习本章后你应当能够：	After studying this chapter you should be able to:
知识标准	**Knowledge criteria**
• 解释本次妊娠详细病史的相关性	• Explain the relevance of a detailed history of the index pregnancy
• 讨论既往产科、内科、妇科病史及家族史的重要性	• Discuss the importance of previous obstetric, medical, gynaecological and family history
• 解释如何进行详细、全面的产科及骨盆检查	• Explain how to conduct a detailed, general, obstetric and pelvic examination
• 讨论妊娠期症状及体征的病理生理学基础	• Discuss the pathophysiological basis of symptoms and physical signs in pregnancy
临床能力	**Clinical competency**
• 详细记录当前或既往妊娠过程中正常及并发症的产科病史	• Take a detailed obstetric history in a normal pregnancy and a pregnancy with complications in the index or previous pregnancy
• 对正常妊娠和有母胎并发症的患者进行全身检查和产科检查，其中包括：	• Carry out general and obstetric examination in a normal pregnancy and that with maternal or fetal complications, including:
－ 测量血压	－ Measure blood pressure in pregnancy
－ 尿液分析及解释	－ Perform and interpret urinalysis in pregnancy
－ 腹部检查（孕周超过 20 周）	－ Perform an abdominal examination in women during pregnancy (over 20 weeks)
－ 胎儿心脏超声检查	－ Auscultate the fetal heart
• 综合病史、化验及检查结果，制订处理方案	• Summarize and integrate the history, examination and investigation results and formulate a management plan
• 用患者能理解的语言向其解释	• Provide explanations to patients in a language they can understand
专业技能和态度	**Professional skills and attitudes**
• 思考有效的言语和非言语沟通要素	• Reflect on the components of effective verbal and nonverbal communication
• 理解灵活处理的必要性，并愿意根据新信息接受建议	• Understand the need to be flexible and be willing to take advice in the light of new information
• 识别产科中的急性不适患者	• Recognize the acutely unwell patient in obstetrics

在对女性进行妊娠、分娩和产褥期管理时，正确区分妊娠相关的正常解剖、生理变化及病理状态是至关重要的。产科的基本临床技能包括按逻辑顺序进行有效的言语和非言语交流：询问病史、体征检查（全身、系统和产科检查），以及区分正常的妊娠相关变化与异常改变，得出初步诊断。同步、准确、详细和清晰的临床记录是"基本临床技能"的基石。这种系统化的方法有助于提高管理效率，确保在需要时得到多学科的支持。

It is vital to differentiate the normal anatomical and physiological changes associated with pregnancy from pathological conditions whilst managing a woman during pregnancy, childbirth and puerperium. Basic clinical skills in obstetrics include effective verbal and non-verbal communication in a logical sequence: history, eliciting physical signs (general, systemic and obstetric examinations), differentiating normal pregnancy-associated changes from abnormal deviation and arriving at a provisional diagnosis. Contemporaneous, accurate, detailed and legible clinical note-keeping is a cornerstone of 'basic clinical skills'. Such a systematic approach will aid effective management by ensuring a multidisciplinary input when required.

一、相关全面病史采集（Taking a relevant and comprehensive history）

相关和准确的病史记录有助于医生做出诊断，是临床实践的基石。需要注意的是，在妇科和产科的全面病史采集过程中往往会涉及隐私问题。因此，在问诊过程中需要与患者建立良好的关系，并在取得患者信任后，在问诊即将结束时询问隐私或敏感的问题。

Taking a relevant and accurate history forms a cornerstone of good clinical practice, as it helps arrive at a diagnosis. It is essential to appreciate that taking a comprehensive history in obstetrics and gynaecology involves eliciting confidential and often very 'personal' information. Therefore, it is essential to build a good rapport with the woman during the consultation and ask confidential and sensitive information towards the end of this history-taking process, after establishing mutual trust and confidence.

二、产科病史（Obstetric history）

在进行产科病史采集时，最好先询问当前（本次）妊娠的详细情况，然后再询问既往产科病史（包括分娩方式及并发症）和妇科病史。

It is advisable to commence obstetric history taking by eliciting details of the current (or index) pregnancy followed by previous obstetric (including modes of birth and complications) and previous gynaecological history.

（一）当前妊娠史（History of present pregnancy）

末次月经（last menstrual period，LMP）第 1 天的日期为临床医生提供了当前妊娠时间的概念，即妊娠期。然而，这一信息往往不准确，除非这些日期与重大的生活事件有关或该女性在积极备孕，否则很多女性并不会记录她们的月经日期。因此，除了询问末次月经，还应在早孕期或中孕早期进行超声检查，以确定妊娠时间和胎龄。

The date of the first day of the last menstrual period (LMP) provides the clinician with an idea of how advanced the current pregnancy is, i.e. period of gestation. However, this information is often inaccurate, as many women do not record the days on which they menstruate unless the date of the period is associated with a significant life event or the woman has been actively trying to conceive. Hence, in addition to LMP, an ultrasound scan in the first or early second trimester should be used to date the pregnancy and to confirm the gestational age.

月经史还应包括月经周期，因为排卵发生在月经前第 14 天。月经和排卵之间的时间间隔（月经周期的增殖期）可能存在很大差异，而排卵后的阶段（分泌期）则相对恒定（12～14 天）。

Menstrual history should also include the duration of the menstrual cycle, as ovulation occurs on the fourteenth day before menstruation. The time interval between menstruation and ovulation (the proliferative phase of the menstrual cycle) may vary substantially, whereas the post-ovulatory phase (secretory phase) is fairly constant (12–14 days).

月经周期是指本次月经第 1 天至下次月经第 1 天之间的时间间隔。正常女性的月经周期从 21 天到 35 天不等，但大部分女性 28 天自然来潮 1 次。

The length of the menstrual cycle refers to the time interval between the first day of the period and the first day of the subsequent period. This may vary from 21 to 35 days in normal women, but menstruation usually occurs every 28 days.

要注意妊娠前的避孕方式，使用性激素避孕可能引起停药后第 1 个月经周期的排卵延迟。月经开始（初潮）的年龄可能与女性妊娠有关，以决定生育的开始。

It is important to note the method of contraception prior to conception, as hormonal contraception may be associated with a delay in ovulation in the first cycle after discontinuation. The age of onset of menstruation (the *menarche*) may be relevant in teenage pregnancies to determine the onset of fertility.

预产期（estimated date of delivery，EDD）可以从末次月经的第 1 天开始计算，在此基础上加 9 个月零 7 天。但是，应用该算法的基础是末次月经时间是准确的，并且月经周期是 28 天（图 6-1）。从受孕之日起，女性平均妊娠期为 269 天。因此，对于月经周期为 28 天的女性而言，若从末次月经第 1 天开始算起，妊娠期则为 283 天（加上从末次月经到受孕前的 14 天）。预产期也可以根据末次月经第 1 天减去 3 个月再加 7 天来计算。需要注意的是，只有 40% 的女性在预产期前后 5 天内分娩，而近 2/3 的女性在预产期前后 10 天内分娩。因此，根据月经周期计算预产期仅为女性的分娩时间提供了一个大概的范围。

The estimated date of delivery (EDD) can be calculated from the first day of the LMP by adding 9 months and 7 days to this date. However, to apply this Naegele's rule, the first day of the menstrual period should be accurate and the woman should have had regular 28-day menstrual cycles (Fig. 6.1). The average duration of human gestation is 269 days from the date of conception. Therefore, in a woman with a 28-day cycle, this is 283 days from the first day of the LMP (14 days are added for the period between menstruation and conception). In a 28-day cycle, the EDD can be calculated by subtracting 3 months from the first day of the LMP and adding on 7 days (or alternatively, adding 9 months and 7 days). It is important to appreciate that only 40% of women will deliver within 5 days of the EDD and about two-thirds of women deliver within 10 days of the EDD. The calculation of the EDD based on a woman's LMP is therefore, at best, a guide to a woman as to the date around which her delivery is likely to occur.

如果女性的月经周期小于或大于 28 天，预产期应减去或加上适当的天数。例如，月经周期为 35 天，则预产期推迟 7 天。

If a woman's normal menstrual cycle is less than 28 days or is greater than 28 days, an appropriate number of days should be subtracted from or added to the EDD. For example, if the normal cycle is 35 days, 7 days should be added to the EDD.

1. 妊娠症状（Symptoms of pregnancy）

月经周期规律的女性出现继发性闭经，则提示妊娠可能。除此之外，妊娠相关的解剖、生理、生化、内分泌和代谢的变化可能会导致以下症状（表 6-1）。

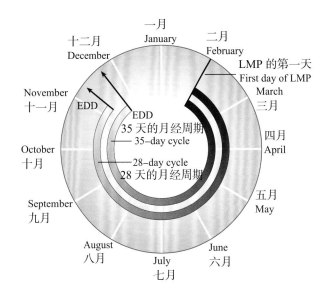

▲ 图 6-1　预产期（EDD）计算

LMP. 末次月经

Fig. 6.1　Calculation of the estimated date of delivery（EDD）

LMP. Last menstrual period

A history of secondary amenorrhoea in a woman who has been having a regular menstrual cycle serves as a self-diagnostic tool for pregnancy. In addition to this, anatomical, physiological, biochemical, endocrine and metabolic changes associated with pregnancy may result in the following symptoms (Table 6.1).

2. 假性妊娠（Pseudocyesis）

假性妊娠是指未孕女性出现妊娠症状及体征，其往往是由于强烈的妊娠欲望或妊娠恐惧引发的下丘脑性闭经所致。在现代产科实践中，随着超声检查在早孕期的广泛应用，极少假性妊娠患者能进入晚孕期，这种情况多因未及时就诊所致。

Pseudocyesis refers to development of symptoms and many of the signs of pregnancy in a woman who is not pregnant. This is often due to an intense desire for or fears of pregnancy that may result in hypothalamic amenorrhoea. In modern obstetric practice, with the widespread use of ultrasound scanning in early pregnancy, it is unlikely to proceed into late pregnancy unless the woman presents late to a booking clinic.

妊娠试验及超声结果阴性均可证实未妊娠。然而要解决引发假性妊娠的潜在焦虑，必须要给予患者共情的态度和支持。被告知真实情况后，患者的月经通常会恢复。

The presence of a negative pregnancy test and ultrasound scan information will provide confirmation that the woman is

表 6-1　妊娠症状

Table 6.1　Symptoms of pregnancy

妊娠的症状 Symptoms of pregnancy	病因 Explanation	鉴别诊断 Deviation from normal
闭经 Amenorrhoea	受精发生后，卵巢黄体增大，孕激素分泌增加。妊娠期孕激素和雌激素水平都将上升，它们会抑制排卵，导致闭经 As the fertilization occurs, the corpus luteum enlarges and will increase the production of progesterone. As both progesterone and oestrogen levels rise in pregnancy, they suppress further ovulation, leading to amenorrhoea.	下丘脑 - 垂体激素变化 Hypothalamo-hypophyseal hormonal changes 卵巢变化 [多囊卵巢综合征（PCOS）、早绝经等] Ovarian changes (polycystic ovarian syndrome (PCOS), premature menopause, etc.) 子宫瘢痕、宫腔内粘连 Uterine scarring, intrauterine adhesions 避孕 Contraception 低 / 高体质量指数 (BMI) Low/high body mass index (BMI) 压力 Stress
恶心和呕吐 Nausea and vomiting	继发于人类绒毛膜促性腺激素 (hCG) 上升后，通常发生在预期月经过后的前 2 周内。虽然通常被描述为晨起恶心，但呕吐可能发生在一天中的任何时间，并且通常因闻到食物气味或看到食物而诱发 It is believed to be secondary to a rise in human chorionic gonadotropin (hCG) and commonly occurs within the first 2 weeks of missing the first period. Although it is commonly described as morning sickness, vomiting may occur at any time of the day and is often precipitated by the smell or sight of food.	妊娠剧吐是严重或持续性的呕吐，导致孕妇脱水、酮尿症和电解质失衡。这种情况需要及时诊断、补充水分和纠正代谢和电解质紊乱 Hyperemesis gravidarum is severe or persistent vomiting leading to maternal dehydration, ketonuria and electrolyte imbalance. This condition needs prompt diagnosis, rehydration and correction of metabolic and electrolyte derangements. 胃肠道感染和食物中毒也可能出现这些症状 Gastrointestinal infections and food poisoning can also present with these symptoms.
尿频 Frequent micturition	一般是由于妊娠子宫对膀胱的压迫所致。妊娠 12 周后，随着子宫升到耻骨联合上方，尿频减轻 It is considered to be due to the pressure on the bladder exerted by the gravid uterus. It tends to diminish after the first 12 weeks of pregnancy as the uterus rises above the symphysis pubis. 受孕后不久血浆渗透压下降，孕早期排泄水的能力下降。孕妇直立坐位时，水负荷加重，孕晚期尿频症状减轻。但在孕早期这可能引发尿频 Plasma osmolality falls soon after conception, and the ability to excrete a water load is altered in early pregnancy. There is an increased diuretic response after water loading when the woman is sitting in the upright position, and this response declines by the third trimester. However, it may be sufficient to cause urinary frequency in early pregnancy.	尿路感染（UTI）可增加排尿频率，并出现相关症状（排尿困难、血尿） Urinary tract infections (UTIs) can present with persistence of increased frequency, as well as associated symptoms (dysuria, haematuria).
过度疲惫 Excessive lassitude or lethargy	一般认为孕酮会导致嗜睡和疲劳。这是妊娠早期的常见症状，甚至可能在月经推迟之前就表现出来。通常在妊娠 12 周后消失 It is thought that progesterone can cause lethargy and fatigue. It is a common symptom in early pregnancy and may become apparent even before the first period is missed. Often, it disappears after 12 weeks of gestation.	甲状腺功能减退也会有类似的影响，感觉过度疲劳的孕妇应行甲状腺功能检测 Hypothyroidism can have similar effects, and expectant mothers with excessive fatigue should be tested for it.

（续表）

妊娠的症状 Symptoms of pregnancy	病因 Explanation	鉴别诊断 Deviation from normal
乳房敏感和增大 Breast tenderness and heaviness	由于血清孕酮和催乳素水平升高所致。这增加了乳房的泌乳及储水能力 It is due to the effect of increasing serum progesterone and prolactin increasing the breast tissues to be ready for lactation, as well as an increased retention of water.	有的女性在月经前期会有类似表现，也可能由于感染、脓肿、损伤或扭伤引起，或者某些药物（避孕药、抗抑郁药）的不良反应 This can be experienced in the premenstrual phase of the cycle. It can also be caused by infections, abscesses or injuries and sprains. It can also be a side effect of some medicines (contraceptives, antidepressants).
胎动 Fetal movements	第一次感觉胎儿活动称为胎动。在第 1 次妊娠期间，通常要到妊娠 20 周才能注意到胎动，第 2 次及其以上的妊娠要到 18 周才能注意到胎动。但是，许多孕妇可能在 18 周之前就出现胎动，还有一些女性可能在妊娠 20 周以后，完全没有意识到胎动 First perception of fetal movements is called *quickening*. It is not usually noticed until 20 weeks' gestation during the first pregnancy and 18 weeks in the second or subsequent pregnancies. However, many women may experience fetal movements earlier than 18 weeks, and others may progress beyond 20 weeks of gestation without being aware of fetal movements at all.	妊娠期间，胎动减少和突然增加都可能是不正常的。胎动减少可能由慢性胎儿窘迫引起，如先兆子痫，而胎动突然增加可能是胎盘早剥的征兆，尽管这种情况没有详细的文献记录 Both the lack of fetal movements and a sudden increase in their activity can be abnormal in pregnancy. A decrease can be caused by chronic fetal distress, as in pre-eclampsia, while a sudden increase may be a sign of placental abruption, although this is not well documented.
异食症 Pica	这是对某种特定食物的异常渴望。在妊娠期间，由于激素水平的变化，这种特殊的渴望被认为是正常的 Pica is an abnormal desire for a particular food. In pregnancy, particular cravings are considered to be normal; they are thought to be due to hormonal changes.	异食的对象可以是非营养物质，如土壤、金属、纸张或墙漆。这可能是缺铁的表现 Its subject can also be a non-nutrient, like soil, metals, paper or wall paint. It can be a sign of iron deficiency.

not pregnant. However, a sympathetic approach and support are essential to resolve the underlying anxieties that led to pseudocyesis. Menstruation usually returns after the woman is informed of her condition.

（二）既往产科病史（Previous obstetric history）

孕次一词是指女性妊娠的次数，与妊娠结局无关，其中包括终止妊娠、流产或异位妊娠等。初孕妇是指第 1 次妊娠的女性，经孕妇是指有 2 次或 2 次以上妊娠史的女性。

The term *gravidity* refers to the number of times a woman has been pregnant, irrespective of the outcome of the pregnancy, i.e. termination, miscarriage or ectopic pregnancy. A *primigravida* is a woman who is pregnant for the first time, and a *multigravida* is a woman who has been pregnant on two or more occasions.

必须将孕次与产次区分开来，产次是指妊娠 24 周以上分娩的或出生体重大于 500g 的活产儿和死产儿的数目。因此，初产妇是指第一次妊娠 24 周后分娩婴儿的女性。

This term *gravidity* must be distinguished from the term *parity*, which describes the number of live-born children and stillbirths a woman has delivered after 24 weeks or with a birth weight of 500 g. Thus, a *primipara* is a woman who has given birth to one infant after 24 weeks.

经产妇是指生育 2 个或 2 个以上婴儿的女性，而未经产妇是指未于妊娠 24 周后分娩婴儿的女性。多产妇被用来描述生育过 5 个或 5 个以上婴儿的女性。

A multiparous woman is one who has given birth to two or more infants, whereas a nulliparous woman has not given birth after 24 weeks. The term *grand multipara* has been used to describe a woman who has given birth to five or more infants.

因此，如果 1 名女性曾经 3 次分娩单胎，并且流产 2 次，那么将被描述为 G5P3，称为经孕经产妇。

Thus, a pregnant woman who has given birth to three viable singleton pregnancies and has also had two miscarriages would be described as gravida 5 para 3: a multigravid multiparous woman.

产妇是指正在经历分娩的女性，产褥期产妇是指既往 42 天内经历过分娩的女性。

A *parturient* is a woman in labour, and a *puerpera* is a woman who has given birth to a child during the preceding 42 days.

病史应记录既往所有妊娠情况，其中包括流产及每次妊娠周数。特别需要记录既往产科并发症、引产、产程、胎方位及分娩方式等细节问题，以及每个婴儿的出生体重和性别。

A record should be made of all previous pregnancies, including previous miscarriages, and the duration of gestation in each pregnancy. In particular, it is important to note any previous antenatal complications, details of induction of labour, the duration of labour, the presentation and the method of delivery, as well as the birth weight and sex of each infant.

应注意每个婴儿在出生时的状况及是否需要进入新生儿监护室观察。同时，应详细询问分娩期及产褥期并发症，如产后出血、泌尿生殖道感染、深静脉血栓（deep vein thrombosis，DVT）和会阴裂伤等。必须认识到这些并发症存在再次发生的风险，并可能影响再次妊娠的处理方式，如有 DVT 史的女性需要在产前和产后进行血栓预防。

The condition of each infant at birth and the need for care in a special care baby unit should be noted. Similarly, details of complications during labour, as well as puerperium, such as postpartum haemorrhage, infections of the genital tract and urinary tract, deep vein thrombosis (DVT) and perineal trauma, should be enquired. It is vital to appreciate that these complications may have a recurrence risk and may influence the management of subsequent pregnancies; e.g. history of DVT requires thromboprophylaxis during the antenatal and postnatal periods.

三、既往内科病史（Previous medical history）

应考虑基础疾病对妊娠的影响，以及妊娠相关的解剖、生化、内分泌、代谢和血液学变化对基础疾病的影响。

The effects of pre-existing medical conditions on pregnancy, as well as the effect of anatomical, biochemical, endocrine, metabolic and haematological changes associated with the physiological state of pregnancy on pre-existing medical conditions, should be considered.

糖尿病、肾病、高血压、心脏病、多种内分泌疾病（如甲状腺毒症和 Addison 病）及传染病（如结核、艾滋病、梅毒、甲型或乙型肝炎）的病程进展可能因妊娠而发生变化。反之，这些疾病也可能对产妇和围产儿造成不利影响（见第 9 章）。

The natural course of diabetes, renal disease, hypertension, cardiac disease, various endocrine disorders (e.g. thyrotoxicosis and Addison's disease) and infectious diseases (e.g. tuberculosis, HIV, syphilis and hepatitis A or B) may be altered by pregnancy. Conversely, they may adversely affect both maternal and perinatal outcome (see Chapter 9).

家族史（Family history）

大多数女性能够意识到常见遗传性疾病的家族携带情况，没有必要向她们详细列举疾病风险，以免引起过度的焦虑情绪。一般性地询问家族中是否存在遗传性疾病就足够了，除非夫妇中一方（或双方）为领养，存在不了解的家族史情况。

Most women will be aware of any significant family history of the common genetically based diseases, and it is not necessary to list all the possibilities to the mother, as it may increase her anxiety. A general enquiry as to whether there are any known inherited conditions in the family will be sufficient, unless one partner (or both) is adopted and not aware of his/her family history.

通过人口统计资料 [如产妇年龄、增加的体重指数（body mass index，BMI）]、产科、内科和外科既往史（如腹腔镜手术、剖宫产术、子宫肌瘤切除术）及家族史收集详细信息，将有助于进行适当的孕期检查并制订相应的管理计划。

Detailed and relevant information obtained with regard to demographics (e.g. maternal age; increased body mass index [BMI]); past obstetric, medical and surgical history (e.g. laparotomy, caesarean section, myomectomy); and family history will help in performing appropriate tests, as well as in making a care plan.

四、检查（Examination）

妊娠期间的检查包括一般检查、系统检查（心血管系统、呼吸系统、一般腹部检查，特殊情况下还包括神经系统检查）和详细的产科检查（子宫及其内部）（表 6-2）。

Examination during pregnancy involves general, systemic (cardiovascular system, respiratory system, general abdominal and, in specific circumstances, a neurological examination) and detailed obstetric (uterus and its contents) examinations (Table 6.2).

（一）一般系统检查（General and systemic examination）

在初次就诊时，如预约就诊，应进行全面的

妊娠期血压的测量 Measuring blood pressure in pregnancy	知识链接 ABC

测量血压时，患者取仰卧位和左侧卧位，以避免子宫压迫下腔静脉（图 6-2）。如果记录坐位血压，则应在每次就诊时以同一姿势、同一手臂记录血压。姿势对血压的影响已在第 3 章中指出。晚孕期静脉压迫可引起晕厥和恶心，这与体位性低血压有关，这种症状被称为仰卧位低血压综合征。如果长时间没有认识到这一点，子宫胎盘循环减少可能会继发胎儿受损。

Blood pressure is recorded with the patient supine and in the left lateral supine position to avoid compression of the inferior vena cava by the gravid uterus (Fig. 6.2). If blood pressure is to be recorded in the sitting position, it should be recorded in the same position for all visits and on the same arm. The effect of posture on blood pressure has been noted in Chapter 3. Vena caval compression in late pregnancy may cause symptoms of syncope and nausea, and this is associated with postural hypotension, the condition being known as the supine hypotensive syndrome. If this is not recognized for a prolonged period, fetal compromise may occur secondary to a reduction in uteroplacental circulation.

虽然过去舒张压一直以 Korotkoff 第四音，即声音开始消失时的压力值来表示，但现在一致认为，如果 korotkoff 第五音，即声音消失的点是清晰的，则应该用它来代表舒张压。如果声音持续减弱而无法确定声音消失的点，则应当使用第四音。

Although in the past the diastolic pressure has always been taken as Korotkoff fourth sound, where the sound begins to fade, it is now agreed that where the fifth sound, i.e. the point at which the sound disappears, is clear, this should be used to represent the diastolic pressure. If the point at which the sound disappears cannot be identified because it continues towards zero, then the fourth sound should be used.

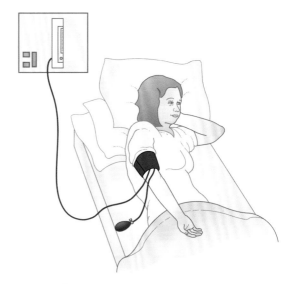

▲ 图 6-2　左侧卧位血压的记录标准

Fig. 6.2　Blood pressure recording standardized in the left lateral position

骨盆检查不再作为常规产检的一部分。

Routine pelvic examination to confirm pregnancy and gestation at booking is not indicated in settings where an ultrasound scan is freely available. If a routine cervical smear is due at the time of booking, this can usually be deferred until after the puerperium, as interpretation of cervical cytology is more difficult in pregnancy. Clinical assessment of the size and shape of the pelvis may be useful in specific circumstances such as a previous fractured pelvis, but not in routine practice. Hence, it is generally no longer carried out as part of the routine antenatal examinations.

早孕期的窥视检查适用于评估出血情况（见第 18 章）。晚孕期的骨盆检查适用于评估宫颈功能（见第 11 章）、诊断分娩及发现胎膜破裂情况（见第 11 章）。晚孕期如果出现产前出血，在排除前置胎盘之前，禁忌进行阴道指检。

A speculum examination in early pregnancy is indicated in the assessment of bleeding (see Chapter 18). Pelvic examination in later pregnancy is indicated for cervical assessment (see Chapter 11) and the diagnosis of labour and to confirm ruptured membranes (see Chapter 11). Digital vaginal examination is contraindicated in later pregnancy in cases of antepartum haemorrhage until placenta praevia can be excluded.

阴道指检在正常分娩中的应用将在第 12 章讨论。

The role of vaginal examination in normal labour is discussed in Chapter 12.

早孕期骨盆检查的方法与未妊娠女性相同，详见第 15 章。

身体检查，以确定是否存在与产前护理有关的躯体问题。

At the initial visit to the clinic, i.e. the booking visit, a complete physical examination should be performed to identify any physical problems that may be relevant to the antenatal care.

应在初次及后续产检时记录身高和体重，这将有助于计算 BMI[BMI= 体重（kg）/ 身高的平方（m^2）]。

Height and weight are recorded at the first and all subsequent visits, and this will help in the calculation of BMI (BMI = weight in kg/height in m^2).

（二）骨盆检查（Pelvic examination）

在可以使用超声的情况下，并不建议通过常规骨盆检查来确定妊娠情况。如果就诊时需进行宫颈涂片检查，通常可以推迟到产褥期后进行，因为妊娠期的宫颈细胞学变化比较难解释。对骨盆的大小和形状的临床评估主要在特殊情况下使用，如既往出现过骨盆骨折，而在常规检查中并不使用。因此，

表 6-2　妊娠期间的检查

Table 6.2　Examination in pregnancy

系统 System	原因 Change and explanation	鉴别诊断 Deviation from normal
	面部：许多妊娠期女性在前额和脸颊上出现一种名为"黄褐斑"的褐色色素沉着，特别是在经常暴露在阳光下的地方（图 6-3）。产后色素沉着逐渐消失 **Face:** Many women develop a brownish pigmentation called *chloasma* over the forehead and cheeks, particularly where there is frequent exposure to sunlight (Fig. 6.3). The pigmentation fades after puerperium.	黄褐斑也可能是艾迪生病、血色病或狼疮的症状，也可能是光敏感药物的副作用 Chloasma (or melasma) can also be a symptom of Addison's disease, haemochromatosis or lupus and a side effect of light-sensitive drugs.
皮肤 Skin	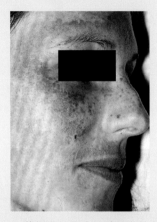 ▲ 图 6-3　黄褐斑，额头和脸颊上的色素沉着 Fig. 6.3　Chloasma: facial pigmentation over the forehead and cheeks. 腹部：腹部检查通常能看到妊娠纹（图 6-4）。瘢痕最初出现在皮肤的压力线上，略呈紫色。妊娠纹也可延伸至大腿和臀部，并延伸至乳房。在妊娠后期，这些瘢痕呈银白色 **Abdomen:** Examination of the abdomen commonly shows the presence of stretch marks, or *striae gravidarum* (Fig. 6.4). The scars are initially purplish in colour and appear in the lines of stress in the skin. These scars may also extend on to the thighs and buttocks and on to the breasts. In subsequent pregnancies, the scars adopt a silvery-white appearance. 白线常有着色，称为黑线。这种色素沉着往往在第一次妊娠后持续存在 The linea alba often becomes pigmented and is then known as the *linea nigra*. This pigmentation often persists after the first pregnancy.	妊娠纹也可发生在快速减肥或体重增加时，也可出现在身体的其他部位 Stretch marks can also occur during rapid weight loss or weight gain and can also be found on other parts of the body. 皮质醇会使结缔组织松弛，因此，若皮质醇分泌增加，如 Cushing 综合征或摄入较多皮质类固醇激素类药物，也会出现妊娠纹 The hormone cortisone weakens the connective tissue; therefore increased production, e.g. Cushing's syndrome or higher intake of corticosteroid medications, can also present with stretch marks.
	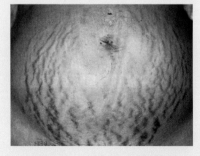 ▲ 图 6-4　前腹壁上的妊娠纹 Fig. 6.4　Striae gravidarum on the anterior abdominal wall	

（续表）

系统 System	原因 Change and explanation	鉴别诊断 Deviation from normal
心脏和肺 Heart and lungs	心脏：正常妊娠的高血流动力学状态引起的良性"血流杂音"是很常见的，没有临床意义。通常能够在心尖区听到柔和的收缩期杂音，偶尔也会在第二肋间听到乳房内血管发出的杂音，该杂音随听诊器的压力增加而消失（图 6-5） **Heart:** Benign 'flow murmurs' due to the hyperdynamic circulation associated with normal pregnancy are common and are of no significance. These are generally soft systolic bruits heard over the apex of the heart, and occasionally a mammary souffle is heard, arising from the internal mammary vessels and audible in the second intercostal spaces. This will disappear with pressure from the stethoscope (Fig. 6.5). **▲ 图 6-5　正常妊娠时有血流杂音** **Fig. 6.5　Flow murmurs in normal pregnancy** 肺部：呼吸系统的检查包括评估呼吸频率和呼吸肌运动情况 **Lungs:** Examination of the respiratory system involves assessment of the rate of respiration and the use of any accessory muscles of respiration.	其他心脏杂音可能是严重心脏病的表现。如果在收缩期听到杂音，可能存在主动脉 / 肺动脉狭窄或二尖瓣 / 三尖瓣反流，而舒张期杂音可能是由二尖瓣 / 三尖瓣狭窄或主动脉 / 肺动脉反流引起的。由于妊娠期心血管疾病恶化可能引发心力衰竭，因此在出现这些杂音时需行心脏病学检查 Other cardiac murmurs can be signs of severe cardiac disease. If a murmur is heard in systole, it can indicate aortic or pulmonary stenosis or mitral or tricuspid regurgitation, whereas a murmur in diastole can be caused by mitral or tricuspid stenosis or aortic or pulmonary regurgitation. In these cases, cardiology review is necessary, as worsening of these conditions due to the cardiovascular changes in pregnancy can lead to heart failure. 肺部病变可能对母体和胎儿造成不利影响，因此应在孕期尽早发现 Gross lung pathology may adversely affect maternal and fetal outcome and should therefore be identified as early in the pregnancy as possible.
头颈部 Head and neck	黏膜：由于贫血是妊娠常见并发症，应检查黏膜表面和结膜是否苍白 **Mucosa:** The colour of the mucosal surfaces and the conjunctivae should be examined for pallor, as anaemia is a common complication of pregnancy. 牙齿：应注意牙齿的一般状况，因为妊娠常伴随牙龈炎，必要时需转诊。尽管仍存在争议，但牙周炎和牙龈炎也与感染和早产风险增加有关 **Teeth:** The general state of dental hygiene should also be noted, as pregnancy is often associated with hypertrophic gingivitis and dental referral may be needed. Periodontitis and gingivitis can be associated with increased risk of infection and pre-term birth, although this is still debated in the literature. 颈部：妊娠期常出现一定程度的甲状腺肿大，这种轻微的甲状腺肿大一般不伴随其他甲状腺疾病的相关症状 **Neck:** Some degree of thyroid enlargement commonly occurs in pregnancy, but unless it is associated with other signs of thyroid disease, mild thyroid enlargement can generally be observed.	贫血的原因也可能是长期消化道出血、痔疮和月经出血过多（闭经或痛经），也可能是血液病的表现 Anaemia can also occur due to prolonged gastrointestinal bleeding, haemorrhoids and excessive menstrual bleeding (menorrhagia or dysmenorrhoea). It can be a sign of various haematological conditions as well. 卫生和饮食不当也可导致牙龈肿大。感染引起的炎症变化也有类似表现 Gingival hypertrophy can occur due to poor hygiene and inadequate diet. Inflammatory changes due to infections can have similar presentation. 也可能是某些药物的不良反应，如抗惊厥药、抗高血压药或免疫抑制药等 It can develop as a side effect of some medications, such as anticonvulsants, antihypertensives or immunosuppressants. 若出现甲状腺功能亢进症（腹泻、精神紧张、多动、出汗、体重减轻等）或甲状腺功能减退症（疲倦、体重增加、对寒冷敏感度增加）的症状，需要进一步检查 If signs of hyperthyroidism (diarrhoea, nervousness, hyperactivity, sweating, weight loss etc.) or hypothyroidism (tiredness, weight gain, increased cold sensitivity) appear, further investigations are needed.

（续表）

系统 System	原因 Change and explanation	鉴别诊断 Deviation from normal
乳房 Breasts	妊娠期乳房会出现特征性的表现，其中包括体积增大、血管增多、Montgomery 小管发育、乳头乳晕色素沉着（图 6-6）。 The breasts show characteristic signs during pregnancy, which include enlargement in size with increased vascularity, the development of Montgomery's tubercles and increased pigmentation of the areolae of the nipples (Fig. 6.6). ▲ 图 6-6　早孕期乳房的生理变化，如乳晕出现色素沉着、Montgomery 小管发育 Fig. 6.6　Physiological changes in the breast in early pregnancy. The areola becomes pigmented and Montgomery's tubercles develop	虽然没有必要进行常规乳房检查，但需要询问乳头内翻的情况，因为可能会引起后续的哺乳困难。此外，若孕妇出现其他乳房症状则需要关注其病理意义，如乳房囊肿或实性结节。据报道，妊娠期乳腺癌进展快，预后差。因此，应对存在乳房"肿块"的患者进行详细的乳房检查 Although routine breast examination is not indicated, it is important to ask about inversion of nipples, as this may give rise to difficulties during suckling, and to look for any pathology such as breast cysts or solid nodules in women who complain of any breast symptoms. Breast cancer during pregnancy is reportedly associated with rapid progression and poor prognosis. Hence, any complaint of a 'lump' in the breast should prompt a detailed breast examination.
腹部 Abdomen	应排除肝大、脾大及肾肿大 Hepatosplenomegaly should be excluded, as well as any evidence of renal enlargement. 子宫在妊娠 12 周后才能作为腹部器官被触摸到 The uterus does not become palpable as an abdominal organ until 12 weeks' gestation.	其他任何异常结果都需要进一步检查 Any other abnormal examination findings require further investigations. 由于不断增大的子宫会改变腹部解剖结构，使妊娠期阑尾炎的诊断更为困难，因此在对腹痛患者进行检查时需要格外注意 The diagnosis of appendicitis in pregnancy is difficult, as the growing uterus alters the anatomy; therefore extra caution is needed when examining a patient with abdominal pain.
四肢和骨骼改变 Limbs, skeletal changes	四肢：应检查腿部是否出现水肿和静脉曲张，还应该检查是否有下肢缩短的迹象，因为随着腹部隆起可能会导致步态异常 Limbs: The legs should be examined for oedema and for varicose veins. They should also be examined for any evidence of shortening of the lower limbs, as this may give problems with gait as the abdomen expands. 脊柱：孕妇的站姿会随着胎儿的生长和腹部的膨隆而改变，出现驼背，特别是为了应对发育中胎儿的重量，出现上半身向后倾斜而腰椎前凸的姿势（图 6-7）。其往往导致腰背疼痛，有时还会引起坐骨神经痛 Spine: Posture also changes in pregnancy as the fetus grows and the maternal abdomen expands, with a tendency to develop some kyphosis and, in particular, to develop an increased lumbar lordosis as the upper part of the trunk is thrown backwards to compensate for the weight of the developing fetus (Fig. 6.7). This often results in the development of backache and sometimes gives rise to sciatic pain.	引起水肿的其他原因还包括肝脏、心脏和肾脏疾病。避孕药、皮质类固醇药物、营养不良和长期固定体位也可导致水肿 Other causes of oedema are liver, heart and kidney disease. Contraceptive pills, corticosteroids, malnutrition and prolonged immobility or standing can present with oedema. 其他脊柱畸形可能是先天性、退行性、特发性或疾病（肿瘤、感染）引起。这些异常可能会改变骨盆径线，影响分娩。此时，应充分告知患者可选择的分娩方式 Other spinal deformities can be congenital, degenerative, idiopathic or caused by a disease (tumours, infections). They can interfere with labour as the pelvic diameters change in these conditions. The patient should be informed about her options for delivery.

（续表）

系统 System	原因 Change and explanation	鉴别诊断 Deviation from normal
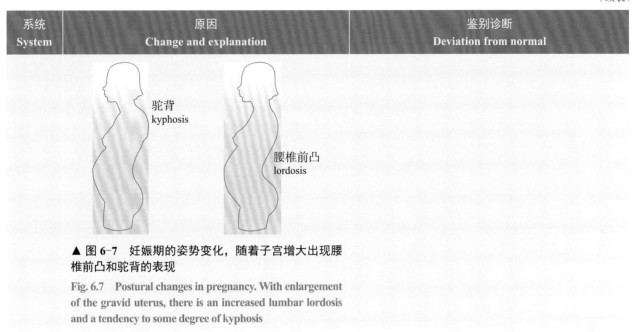		

▲ 图 6-7　妊娠期的姿势变化，随着子宫增大出现腰椎前凸和驼背的表现

Fig. 6.7　Postural changes in pregnancy. With enlargement of the gravid uterus, there is an increased lumbar lordosis and a tendency to some degree of kyphosis

The technique of pelvic examination in early pregnancy is the same as that for the non-pregnant woman and is described in Chapter 15.

通过检查外阴排除其他异常病变，并评估既往妊娠相关的会阴损伤。静脉曲张是比较常见的外阴变化，这在妊娠过程中可能会进一步加重。

The vulva should be examined to exclude any abnormal lesions and to assess the perineum in relation to any damage sustained in previous pregnancies. Varicosities of the vulva are common and may become worse during pregnancy.

妊娠期间，随着阴道壁复层鳞状上皮增厚，上皮细胞中糖原含量进一步增加，阴道壁会变得更加粗糙。

The vaginal walls become more rugose in pregnancy as the stratified squamous epithelium thickens with an increase in the glycogen content of the epithelial cells.

阴道旁的血管分布也明显增加，使阴道壁外观呈现紫红色。随着阴道渗出增加、上皮细胞脱落及宫颈黏液分泌增多，阴道分泌物也明显增多。

There is also a marked increase in the vascularity of the paravaginal tissues so that the appearance of the vaginal walls becomes purplish-red. There is an increase in vaginal secretions, with increased vaginal transudation, increased shedding of epithelial cells and some contribution from enhanced production of cervical mucus.

宫颈逐渐变软，同时出现血管分布增加的征象。宫颈的增大与血管分布增多、结缔组织水肿、细胞增生和肥大有关。宫颈内的腺体含量增加，占宫颈实质的 50%，并且产生黏稠的宫颈黏液栓堵塞宫颈口（图 6-8）。

The cervix becomes softened and shows signs of increased vascularity. Enlargement of the cervix is associated with an increase in vascularity, as well as oedema of the connective tissues and cellular hyperplasia and hypertrophy. The glandular content of the endocervix increases to occupy half the substance of the cervix and produces a thick plug of viscid cervical mucus that occludes the cervical os (Fig. 6.8).

1. 骨盆的评估（Assessment of the bony pelvis）

常规的产前临床检查或通过放射性手段检测骨盆对分娩结局的预测价值不大。但对产程进展缓慢的病例，通过骨盆检查评估是否存在胎儿头盆不称的情况是有必要的。对于既往存在骨盆外伤或骨盆

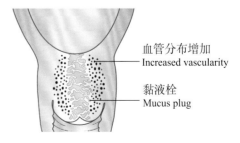

血管分布增加
Increased vascularity

黏液栓
Mucus plug

▲ 图 6-8　孕期宫颈的变化，腺体含量增加及黏稠的宫颈黏液栓

Fig. 6.8　Cervical changes in pregnancy include increased glandular content and a thick mucus plug

发育异常的女性，临床骨盆检测对分娩结局依然具有预测价值。各骨盆径线可以通过影像学检查获得较为准确的数字。

Routine antenatal clinical or radiological pelvimetry has not been shown to be of value in predicting the outcome of labour. However, it is important to assess the pelvis and fetus for possible disproportion when managing cases of delayed progress in labour. Clinical pelvimetry may be of value where there has been previous trauma or abnormal development of the bony pelvis. Precise information about the various dimensions could be obtained by imaging.

骨盆由骶骨、尾骨和两侧髋骨组成。髂耻线以上的骨盆区域称为假骨盆，以下的区域为真骨盆，后者对妊娠和分娩非常重要。真骨盆的盆壁由后方的骶骨，侧方的坐骨、坐骨切迹及韧带，前方的耻骨、闭孔窝及坐骨的升支和耻骨支构成（图 6-9）。

The bony pelvis consists of the sacrum, the coccyx and two innominate bones. The pelvic area above the iliopectineal line is known as the *false pelvis*, and the area below the pelvic brim is the true *pelvis*. The latter is the important section in relation to childbearing and parturition. Thus, the wall of the true pelvis is formed by the sacrum posteriorly, the ischial bones and the sacrosciatic notches and ligaments laterally, and anteriorly by the pubic rami, the obturator fossae and membranes, the ascending rami of the ischial bones and the pubic rami (Fig. 6.9).

临床的骨盆测量包括骨盆入口（骶骨岬）、中骨盆（骨盆侧壁包括坐骨棘、坐骨棘间径和骶骨曲度）及骨盆出口（耻骨弓角度和坐骨结节间径）。

Clinical pelvimetry involves assessment of the pelvic inlet (sacral promontory), mid-cavity (pelvic side walls including the ischial spines, the interspinous diameter and the hollow of the sacrum) and the pelvic outlet (subpubic angle and the intertuberous diameter).

在正常女型骨盆中，由于骶骨是均匀弯曲的，所以中骨盆为胎头提供了最大空间。骶骨触摸起来曲度应当是均匀的。

In a normal female or gynaecoid pelvis, because the sacrum is evenly curved, maximum space for the fetal head is provided in the pelvic mid-cavity. The sacrum should feel

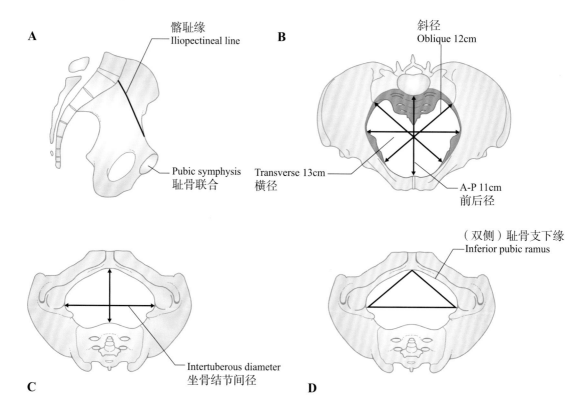

▲ 图 6-9　A. 真骨盆入口以骶骨岬、髂耻线、坐骨的耻骨支和耻骨联合为界。B. 真骨盆入口径线尺寸。C. 骨盆出口以耻骨支下缘、坐骨结节及骶结节韧带为界。D. 双侧耻骨支下缘应成 **90°** 夹角

Fig. 6.9　(A) Inlet of the true pelvis is bounded by the sacral promontory, iliopectineal lines, pubic rami and pubic symphysis. (B) Dimensions of the inlet of the true pelvis. (C) Pelvic outlet bounded by the inferior pubic rami and the ischial tuberosities and the sacrosciatic ligaments. (D) The inferior pubic rami should form an angle of 90 degrees

evenly curved.

如果骶骨触之平坦，那么骨盆出口可能会缩窄，如男型骨盆，可能会导致胎头下降时发生嵌顿。

If the sacrum feels flat, then the pelvis may contract towards the pelvic outlet, as in the android or male-like pelvis, and may lead to impaction of the fetal head as it descends through the pelvis.

2. 骨盆平面（The planes of the pelvis）

真骨盆的形状和大小，最好通过骨盆的 4 个平面来评估。

The shape and the dimensions of the true pelvis are best understood by consideration of the four planes of the pelvis.

（1）骨盆入口平面：后方以骶骨岬为界，侧方以髂耻线为界线，前方系耻骨支及耻骨联合的上缘。该平面在正常女型骨盆中几乎为圆形，但横径略大于前后径。

Plane of the pelvic inlet. The plane of the pelvic inlet, or pelvic brim, is bounded posteriorly by the sacral promontory, laterally by the iliopectineal lines and anteriorly by the superior pubic rami and upper margin of the pubic symphysis. The plane is almost circular in the normal gynaecoid pelvis but is slightly larger transversely than anteroposteriorly.

骨盆入口的真结合径或前后径是指骶岬前缘中点与前方耻骨联合上缘中点之间的距离（图 6-10）。直径约为 11cm。产科结合径是最短也是最具临床意义的径线，即骶骨岬中点与耻骨联合后表面最近点之间的距离。

The true conjugate or anteroposterior diameter of the pelvic inlet is the distance between the midpoint of the sacral promontory and the superior border of the pubic symphysis anteriorly (Fig. 6.10). The diameter measures approximately 11 cm. The shortest distance, and the one of greatest clinical significance, is the obstetric conjugate diameter. This is the distance between the midpoint of the sacral promontory and the nearest point on the posterior surface of the pubic symphysis.

通过临床检查无法测量这些径线；唯一可以进行临床评估的骨盆入口处径线是耻骨联合下缘到骶岬中点的距离。这被称为对角径，约比产科结合径长 1.5cm。在实际操作中，临床检查一般无法触及骶岬，能摸到的最高点是骶骨的第二节或第三节。如果很容易摸到骶岬，则说明骨盆入口缩窄（图 6-11A）。

It is not possible to measure either of these diameters by clinical examination; the only diameter at the pelvic inlet that is amenable to clinical assessment is the distance from the inferior margin of the pubic symphysis to the midpoint of the sacral

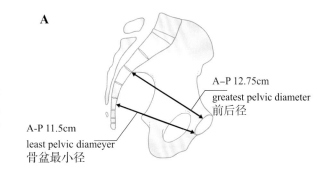

A

A–P 12.75cm
greatest pelvic diameter
前后径

A-P 11.5cm
least pelvic diameyer
骨盆最小径

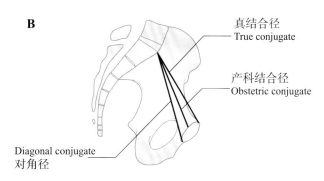

B

真结合径
True conjugate

产科结合径
Obstetric conjugate

Diagonal conjugate
对角径

▲ 图 6-10　A. 中骨盆及骨盆出口前后径（A-P）；B. 骨盆入口结合径

Fig. 6.10　(A) Anteroposterior (A-P) diameters of the mid-cavity and pelvic outlet. (B) Conjugate diameters of the pelvic inlet

promontory. This is known as the *diagonal conjugate diameter* and is approximately 1.5 cm greater than the obstetric diameter. In practical terms, it is not usually possible to reach the sacral promontory on clinical examination, and the highest point that can be palpated is the second or third piece of the sacrum. If the sacral promontory is easily palpable, the pelvic inlet is contracted (Fig. 6.11A).

（2）骨盆最大平面：骨盆最大平面的临床意义不大，前后径和横径约为 12.7cm。前后径从耻骨联合后方中点延伸至骶骨第二节和第三节的交界处。横径从侧方穿过髋臼中央。

Plane of greatest pelvic dimensions. The plane of greatest pelvic dimensions has little clinical significance and has an anteroposterior and transverse diameter of approximately 12.7 cm. The anteroposterior diameter extends from the midpoint of the posterior aspect of the pubic symphysis to the junction of the second and third pieces of the sacrum. The transverse diameter passes laterally through the middle of the acetabuli.

这一平面对骨盆形状的唯一提示是骶骨的曲度和骶坐骨切迹的形状，应成 90° 夹角。这通常允许两根手指沿着骶棘韧带进入，此韧带从坐骨棘延伸至骶骨第二节和第三节的侧方。

The only indication of the shape of the pelvis at this level is the curvature of the sacrum and the shape of the sacrosciatic notch, which should subtend at an angle of 90 degrees. This normally allows the admission of two fingers along the sacrospinous ligaments, which extend from the ischial spines to the lateral aspects of the second and third pieces of the sacrum.

（3）骨盆最小平面：是胎儿头部最可能发生嵌顿的平面。其前后径从耻骨联合下缘开始延伸，横跨坐骨棘间径。前后径和坐骨棘间径在临床上均可评估，其中坐骨棘间径是骨盆最狭窄的径线（10cm）。应触诊坐骨棘感知其是否突出，并对坐骨棘间径进行评估（图 6-11B）。

Plane of least pelvic dimensions. The plane of least pelvic dimensions represents the level at which impaction of the fetal head is most likely to occur. The anteroposterior diameter extends from the inferior margin of the pubic symphysis and transects the line drawn between the ischial spines. Both the transverse (interspinous) and the anteroposterior diameters can be assessed clinically, and the interspinous diameter is the narrowest space in the pelvis (10 cm). The ischial spines should be palpated to see if they are prominent and to make an estimate of the interspinous diameter (Fig. 6.11B).

3. 骨盆出口（Outlet of the pelvis）

骨盆出口由 2 个三角形平面构成。前方三角以耻骨弓下缘为界，一般成 90° 夹角。出口横径是指两侧坐骨结节之间的距离，即坐骨结节间径，一般不小于 11cm。后方三角的底边为坐骨结节间径，两边由骶骨尖及骶结节韧带构成。

The outlet of the pelvis consists of two triangular planes. Anteriorly, the triangle is bounded by the area under the pubic arch, and this should normally subtend at an angle of 90 degrees. The transverse diameter is the distance between the ischial tuberosities i.e. the intertuberous diameter, which is normally not less than 11 cm. The posterior triangle is formed anteriorly by the intertuberous diameter and posterolaterally by the tip of the sacrum and the sacrosciatic ligaments.

临床上，可通过握拳并将拳置于坐骨结节间，评估坐骨结节间径。耻骨弓角度可通过将双手大拇指沿耻骨下缘放置，或者将检查手的两指置于耻骨弓下方进行评估。

Clinically, the intertuberous diameter can be assessed by placing the knuckles of the clenched fist between the ischial tuberosities. The subpubic angle can be assessed by placing the index fingers of both hands along the inferior pubic rami or by inserting two fingers of the examining hand under the pubic arch.

（三）常规随访中的产检（Obstetric examination at subsequent routine visits）

在随后的产检中，应记录血压，并检测尿液中的蛋白质和葡萄糖水平。记录孕妇体重是评估胎儿生长状况的方法之一，尤其是在超声检查没有普及的地方。妊娠 18 周后，孕妇体重平均增速应为每周 0.5kg 左右。

At all subsequent antenatal visits, the blood pressure should be recorded and the urine tested for protein and glucose. It is good practice to record maternal weight at each visit, especially in clinical settings where recourse to ultrasound scan for assessment of fetal growth is not freely available. Maternal weight should increase by an average of approximately 0.5 kg/week after the eighteenth week of gestation.

体重的快速和过度增长几乎都与液体潴留有关，体重不变或体重下降可能提示胎儿生长异常。体重增长过快往往与水肿有关，且水肿在面部、手部（戒

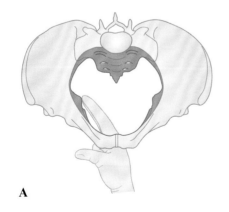
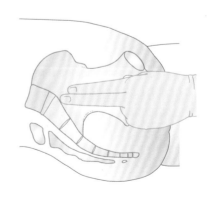

A   **B**

▲ 图 6-11　**A.** 骨盆最小平面处的坐骨棘临床检查；**B.** 骨盆入口评估

Fig. 6.11 **(A)** Clinical assessment of the ischial spines at the plane of least pelvic dimensions. **(B)** Assessment of the pelvic inlet

指摘除变得困难）、前腹壁、小腿和脚踝处尤为明显。骶骨垫上的"非依赖性"水肿在妊娠期很少见，如果出现，应排除先兆子痫等原因。

Rapid and excessive weight gain is nearly always associated with excessive fluid retention, and static weight or weight loss may indicate the failure of normal fetal growth. Excessive weight gain is often associated with signs of oedema, and this is most readily apparent in the face, the hands (where it may become difficult to remove rings), on the anterior abdominal wall and over the lower legs and ankles. 'Non-dependent' oedema over the sacral pad is rare in pregnancy and, if present, causes such as pre-eclampsia should be excluded.

五、腹部触诊（Abdominal palpation）

（一）宫底触诊（Palpation of the uterine fundus）

评估胎龄是孕妇腹部检查的第一步。评估胎儿大小的方法有多种。

The estimation of gestational age is the first step in examination of the abdomen in the pregnant woman. Several methods are employed to assess the size of the fetus.

妊娠 12 周时，子宫在耻骨联合上方首次可触及，妊娠 24 周时宫底到达脐水平线。妊娠 36 周时，宫底在胸骨剑突平面处可触及，然后保持在这一位置直到临产，或者随着胎先露部分入盆而略微下降。

The uterus first becomes palpable above the symphysis pubis at 12 weeks' gestation, and by 24 weeks' gestation it reaches the level of the umbilicus. At 36 weeks' gestation, the uterine fundus is palpable at the level of the xiphisternum and then tends to remain at this level until term or to fall slightly as the presenting part enters the pelvic brim.

所有临床评估胎龄的方法都存在不准确性，特别是与孕妇脐部相关的早期评估，且宫底高度受到多种因素的影响，如多胎妊娠、羊水过多、胎儿过小或羊水过少等。

All methods of clinical assessment of gestational age are subject to considerable inaccuracies, particularly in the early assessment related to the position of the umbilicus, and the fundal height will be affected by the presence of multiple fetuses, excessive amniotic fluid or, at the other extreme, the presence of a small fetus or oligohydramnios.

（二）耻骨联合 – 宫底高度测量（Measurement of symphysial-fundal height）

直接测量腹围或耻骨联合 – 宫底高度，为评估胎儿生长状况和胎龄提供了更为可靠的方法。

Direct measurement of the girth, or the symphysial-fundal height, provides a more reliable method of assessing fetal growth and gestational age.

运用平均值 ± 标准差，可以描述百分位数 10%～90% 的胎儿。在不同研究中，该方法检测小于孕龄儿的敏感度为 20%～70%。将同一个人的连续测量值绘制在胎儿生长表上，可以更容易地发现生长受限的胎儿。妊娠 36 周后，若将此方法用于随机观察，准确率将大大降低。对于大于胎龄儿，该方法的预测价值也较低。但是，该方法简单易行，且在没有其他更为精确的检测技术时尤为适用。

Using two standard deviations from the mean, it is possible to describe the tenth and ninetieth centile values. The sensitivity of this method for the detection of small for gestational age babies varies from 20% to 70% in different studies. Serial measurements by the same person plotted on customized growth charts are more likely to detect growth-restricted babies. The accuracy is considerably reduced as a random observation after 36 weeks' gestation. The predictive value is also lower for large-for-dates infants. However, the technique is simple and easily applicable and is particularly useful where other, more precise techniques are not available.

耻骨联合 – 宫底高度测量 Measurement of symphysial-fundal height	知识链接 ABC

左手尺侧缘置于子宫底。子宫底与耻骨联合上缘之间的距离以厘米为单位进行测量。为了减小观察者偏差，测量宫底至耻骨联合上缘的距离时，卷尺的厘米刻度侧朝下。然后将卷尺倒转过来，以厘米为单位读取距离。妊娠 20 周时，平均宫高约为 20cm，且每周增加 1cm，因此 36 周时，胎底高度将为 36cm（图 6-12）。

The ulnar border of the left hand is placed on the uterine fundus. The distance between the uterine fundus and the top of the pubic symphysis is measured in centimetres. To minimize observer bias, the distance is measured from the fundus to the superior edge of the symphysis pubis with the side of the tape measure with the centimetre measures facing downwards. The tape measure is then turned over to show the distance in centimetres. The mean fundal height measures approximately 20 cm at 20 weeks and increases by 1 cm/week so that at 36 weeks the fundal height will be 36 cm (Fig 6.12).

（三）腹围测量（Measurement of abdominal girth）

腹围测量是另一种评估方法，需围绕孕妇的脐水平进行测量。若未孕时的平均腹围长度是 60cm，妊娠 24 周之前不会出现明显的增长。此后，腹围每周增加 2.5cm，至足月时腹围将达 100cm。

Measurement of girth provides another method of

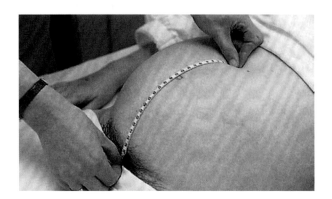

▲ 图 6-12　耻骨联合 - 宫底高度测量

Fig. 6.12　Measurement of symphysial-fundal height

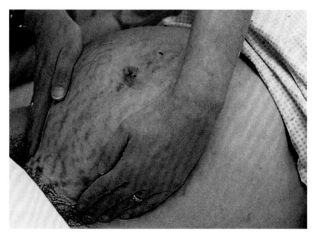

▲ 图 6-13　先露部位和胎背触诊

Fig. 6.13　Palpation of the presenting part and the fetal back

assessment. The measurement of girth is made at the level of the maternal umbilicus. Assuming that the average nonpregnant girth is 60 cm, no significant increase will occur until 24 weeks' gestation. Thereafter the girth should increase by 2.5 cm weekly so that at full term the girth will be 100 cm.

若未孕时的腹围大于或小于 60cm，则必须做出适当的调整。因此，一名腹围为 65cm 的女性在妊娠36 周后，腹围的测量值应为 95cm。

If the non-pregnant girth is greater or smaller than 60 cm, then an appropriate allowance must be made. Thus, a woman with a 65-cm girth would have a measurement of 95 cm at 36 weeks' gestation.

六、胎儿部位触诊（Palpation of fetal parts）

妊娠 24 周前通常无法触及胎儿部位。当行胎儿触诊时，必须注意，由于羊水的存在，需在掌指关节处手指屈曲做"下压"动作。触诊的目的是描述胎儿与母体躯干及骨盆的关系（图 6-13）。

Fetal parts are not usually palpable before 24 weeks' gestation. When palpating the fetus, it must be remembered that the presence of amniotic fluid necessitates the use of 'dipping' movements with flexion of the fingers at the metacarpophalangeal joints. The purpose of palpation is to describe the relationship of the fetus to the maternal trunk and pelvis (Fig. 6.13).

（一）胎产式（Lie）

胎产式指的是胎儿身体长轴与子宫长轴的关系（图 6-14）。面向孕妇双脚，检查者左手沿母体腹部左侧放置，右手放在子宫右外侧。先用左手再用右手向中线方向进行系统性的触诊，可以感受到来自胎儿背部的抵抗或胎儿不规则的肢体特征。

The term *lie* describes the relationship of the long axis of the fetus to the long axis of the uterus (Fig. 6.14). Facing the feet of the mother, the examiner's left hand is placed along the left side of the maternal abdomen and the right hand on the right lateral aspect of the uterus. Systematic palpation towards the midline with the left and then the right hand will reveal either the firm resistance of the fetal back or the irregular features of the fetal limbs.

如果胎产式是纵向的，胎头或胎臀在骨盆入口上方或骨盆入口处可触及。如果是倾斜位，胎儿身体长轴与子宫长轴成 45° 夹角，在孕妇髂窝处可以摸到胎儿先露部位。横位时，胎儿与母体成直角，胎儿的头和足在母体侧面可触摸到。

If the lie is *longitudinal*, the head or breech will be palpable over or in the pelvic inlet. If the lie is *oblique*, the long axis of the fetus lies at an angle of 45 degrees to the long axis of the uterus and the presenting part will be palpable in the iliac fossa. In a *transverse* lie, the fetus lies at right angles to the mother and the poles of the fetus are palpable in the flanks.

在确定了胎产式和胎背的位置后，接下来重要的是双手交替用力，以感知胎头和胎臀。胎头坚硬、圆润、不连续。它可以在检查者手间"跳跃"，在早期妊娠中被描述为"触诊抵抗"。臀部则较软，略散，并且不存在触诊抵抗。胎头应当在孕妇下腹部或宫底处寻找。检查者面向孕妇的脚，在先露处用力。如果先露部位是胎头，需注意其是否容易触摸，是否需要深压。

Having ascertained the lie and the location of the fetal back, it is now important to feel for the head and breech by firm pressure with alternate hands. The head is hard, round and discrete. It can be 'bounced' between the examining hands

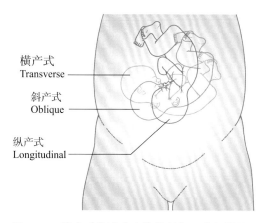

▲ 图 6-14　胎产式指胎儿身体长轴与子宫长轴的关系

Fig. 6.14　Fetal lie describes the relationship of the long axis of the fetus to the long axis of the uterus

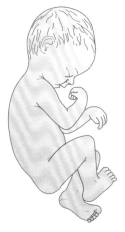

▲ 图 6-15　胎儿的正常姿势是屈曲

Fig. 6.15　The normal attitude of the fetus is one of flexion

and is described as being 'ballotable' in earlier gestations. The buttocks are softer and more diffuse, and the breech is not ballotable. The head should be sought in the lower abdomen or in the uterine fundus. Facing the mother's feet, firm pressure is applied over the presenting part. If the head is presenting, note is made as to whether it is easily palpable or whether it is necessary to apply deep pressure.

胎儿的正常姿态是屈曲的（图 6-15），但在某些情况下，如"横产式"，它可能表现为伸展的姿态。

The normal attitude of the fetus is one of flexion (Fig. 6.15), but on occasions, as with the 'flying fetus', it may exhibit an attitude of extension.

（二）胎先露（Presentation）

纵产式的胎儿先露部位是头部或臀部。横产式的胎儿先露部位是肩部。

In a longitudinal lie, the presenting part may be the head (*cephalic*) or the breech (*podalic*). In a transverse lie, the presenting part is the shoulder.

根据俯曲或仰伸的程度，胎头的不同部位会显露在骨盆入口处。当胎头充分俯曲时，先露部是枕部，即位于前后囟门之间的区域，侧面是双顶骨顶点。如果胎头完全仰伸，则面部显露于骨盆入口处（面先露），如果胎头位于两个姿势之间，则为额部显露（额先露）。额部是指鼻基底与前囟门之间的区域。枕先露时，骨盆入口处的胎头径线为枕下前囟径（表 6-3，图 6-16）。如果胎头倾斜，径线为枕额径。如果额先露，径线为枕额径。只有宫颈扩张至可以触及颅缝和前囟门时，才能通过阴道检查准确地判定胎先露和胎姿势。因此，这种检查仅适用于

孕妇即将分娩时。

Depending on the degree of flexion or deflexion, various parts of the head will present to the pelvic inlet. Where the head is well flexed, the presentation is the vertex, i.e. the area that lies between the anterior and posterior fontanelles anteroposteriorly and biparietal eminences laterally. If the head is completely extended, the face presents to the pelvic inlet (*face presentation*), and if it lies between these two attitudes, the brow presents (*brow presentation*). The brow is the area between the base of the nose and the anterior fontanelle. The diameter of presentation for the vertex is the suboccipitobregmatic diameter (Table 6.3, Fig. 6.16). If the head is deflexed, the occipitofrontal diameter presents. With a brow presentation, the verticomental diameter presents to the pelvic inlet. Presentation and position can be accurately determined only by vaginal examination when the cervix has dilated and the suture lines and fontanelles can be palpated. This situation only really pertains when the mother is well established in labour.

表 6-3　不同先露的径线

Table 6.3　Diameters of presentation

先露部位 Presenting part	径线 Diameter	长度（cm） Size (cm)
枕先露 Vertex	枕下前囟径 Suboccipitobregmatic	9.5
额先露 Brow	枕颏径 Verticomental	13.5
面先露 Face	颏下前囟径 Submentobregmatic	9.5
颅顶倾斜 Deflexed vertex	枕额径 Occipitofrontal	11.7

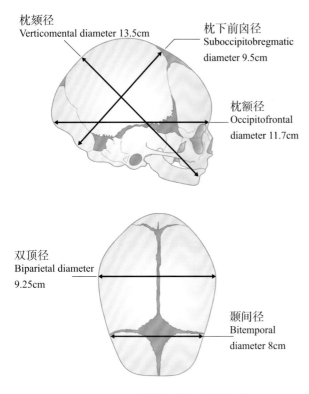

▲ 图 6-16 成熟胎头先露部的径线

Fig. 6.16 Diameters of presentation of the mature fetal skull

（三）胎方位（Position）

胎方位是指先露部位指示点与母体骨盆入口的位置关系。它不能与胎先露相混淆。它进一步描述了先露部位与母体骨盆的关系，在产程中尤为重要。各先露部位的指示点如下。

先露部位	指示点
枕部	枕骨
面部	颏部
臀部	骶骨
肩部	肩胛骨

由此，在枕先露中，描述了 6 个不同的胎方位（图 6-17）。

The position of the fetus is a description of the relationship of the denominator of the presenting part to the inlet of the maternal pelvis. It must not be confused with the presentation. It provides a further description of the relationship of the presenting part to the maternal pelvis and is of particular importance during parturition. The denominators for the various presentations are as follows:

Presentation	Denominator
Vertex	Occiput
Face	Chin (mentum)
Breech	Sacrum
Shoulder	Acromion

Thus, in a vertex presentation, six different positions are described (Fig. 6.17).

自骨盆下方观察，多观察到左右枕横位、左右枕前位及左右枕后位。很少能直接观察到正枕前或正枕后位，除非是在第二产程晚期。

Viewed from below the pelvis, these include the right and left occipitotransverse positions as well as left and right anterior and posterior positions. Except in the advanced second stage, it is very rare for the head to be identified in a direct anterior or posterior position.

面先露以颏骨标记胎方位，臀先露以前骶骨标记胎方位。额先露时没有合适的胎方位描述，因为缺乏典型的骨性标志。当额先露纠正为其他的胎方位后，沿用其他胎方位的阴道分娩机制。

With a face presentation, the prefix *mento-* is included, and with a breech presentation the prefix is sacro-. No such description is given to a brow presentation, as there is no defined peripheral prominence to define as denominator. There is no mechanism of vaginal delivery in a brow presentation unless it is corrected.

通过腹部触诊可以确定胎儿前肩的位置。如果胎肩靠近中线且容易触及，则为前位。如果不易触及，且胎儿四肢感比较明显，则可能是后位。

The position can be determined from abdominal palpation by palpating the anterior shoulder of the fetus. If this is near the midline and easily palpable, the position is anterior. If it is not easily palpable and the limbs are prominent, the position is probably posterior.

但是，分娩发动后通过扩张的宫颈触诊颅缝、前囟门或胎臀，大部分可以准确地确定先露部所处的位置。

However, the position of the presenting part can be most accurately determined by palpating the suture lines and fontanelles, or the breech presentation through the dilated cervix once labour has started.

此时，胎头的俯曲程度也可以确定。腹部触诊时，仰伸或伸展的胎头往往感觉很大，且枕部与胎背之间的颈沟也较容易识别。

The degree of flexion of the head can also be determined. On abdominal palpation, a deflexed or extended head tends to feel large, and the nuchal groove between the occiput and the

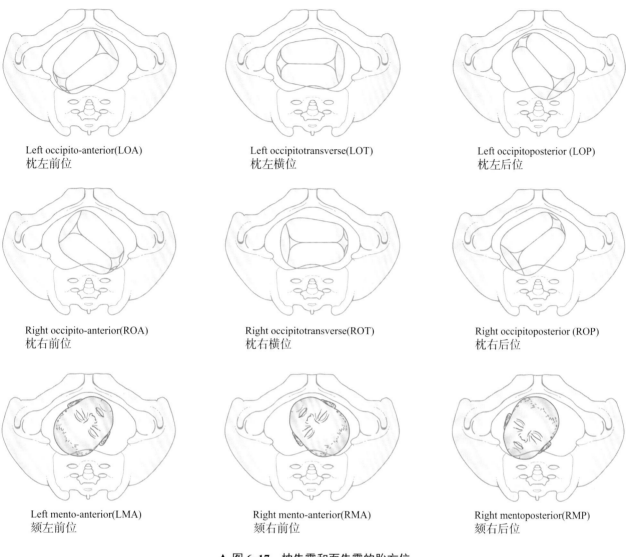

Left occipito-anterior(LOA)
枕左前位

Left occipitotransverse(LOT)
枕左横位

Left occipitoposterior (LOP)
枕左后位

Right occipito-anterior(ROA)
枕右前位

Right occipitotransverse(ROT)
枕右横位

Right occipitoposterior (ROP)
枕右后位

Left mento-anterior(LMA)
颏左前位

Right mento-anterior(RMA)
颏右前位

Right mentoposterior(RMP)
颏右后位

▲ 图 6-17　枕先露和面先露的胎方位

Fig. 6.17　Positions of the head in vertex and face presentations viewed from below.

fetal back is easily identified.

（四）胎头位置与衔接（Station and engag-ement）

头部所处位置在骨盆缘上方被分成 5 阶描述（图 6-18）。当胎头最大横径（双顶径）通过真骨盆的入口时，胎头即已衔接。衔接的胎头通常是固定的，只有 2/5 的部分可以触摸到。在孕妇腹部通常难以摸到。

The station of the head is described in fifths above the pelvic brim (Fig. 6.18). The head is *engaged* when the greatest transverse diameter (the biparietal diameter) has passed through the inlet of the true pelvis. The head that is engaged is usually fixed and only two-fifths palpable. It is usually difficult to feel abdominally.

（五）胎心听诊（Auscultation）

胎心听诊是产科检查的一项常规内容。现在的标准做法是使用手持式多普勒超声检查设备，该设备会发出电信号，以便识别和计数胎心。如果使用电子胎心监护转换器，需配合使用 Pinard 胎儿听诊器证实胎心音（图 6-19）。孕晚期胎心音听诊最好在孕妇脐部以下与胎儿前肩上方区域（约位于孕妇脐与髂前上棘距离的中部）或胎后位时的中线区域。如果是臀部先露，在孕妇脐水平听诊胎心音最好。听诊后需记录胎心率及节律。

Auscultation of the fetal heart rate is a routine part of the obstetric examination. It is now standard practice to use a hand-held Doppler ultrasound device that will produce an electronic signal to enable the heartbeat to be recognized

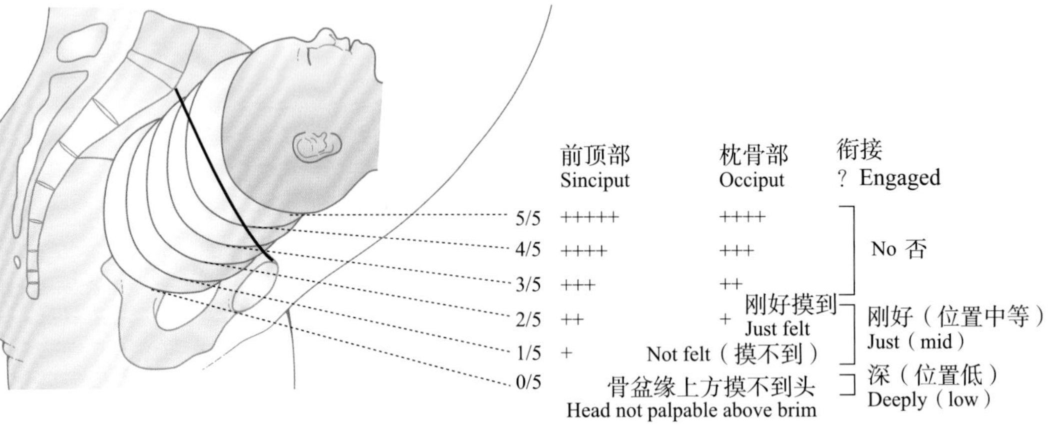

	前顶部 Sinciput	枕骨部 Occiput	衔接 ? Engaged
5/5	+++++	++++	No 否
4/5	++++	+++	No 否
3/5	+++	++	
2/5	++	+ 刚好摸到 Just felt	刚好（位置中等） Just（mid）
1/5	+	Not felt（摸不到）	
0/5		骨盆缘上方摸不到头 Head not palpable above brim	深（位置低） Deeply（low）

▲ 图 6-18　胎头衔接时的位置

Fig. 6.18　Stations of the fetal head

！注意

小的胎头即便已衔接，也可是活动的。胎头较大可能会被卡在骨盆入口边缘而不能衔接。一般来说，未衔接的胎头在腹部比较容易摸到，而在头先露且已充分衔接的情况下，很难摸到胎头。

有些情况下胎头位置难以确定，这可能由于胎头在母体肋下，如臀先露；或胎头已充分衔接；或罕见的无脑儿。

在上述情况下，由于已衔接胎头的前部可在坐骨棘水平触及，因此应行阴道检查。

A small head may still be mobile even though it is engaged. A large head may be fixed in the pelvic brim and yet not be engaged. As a general rule, a head that is easily palpable abdominally is not engaged, whereas a head that is presenting and is deeply engaged is difficult to palpate.

Where it is difficult to locate the head, this may either be because the head is under the maternal rib cage, as with a breech presentation, or because it is deeply engaged with 0/5'th of the head palpable or a rare case of anencephaly.

Under these circumstances, a vaginal examination should be performed, as the leading part of the engaged head will be palpable at the level of the ischial spines.

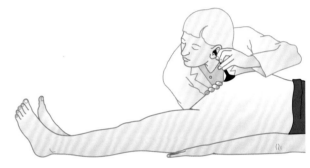

▲ 图 6-19　胎心听诊

Fig. 6.19　Auscultation of the fetal heart

and counted. If the transducer of an electronic fetal monitor is used, the fetal heart sounds should be confirmed with a Pinard fetal stethoscope (Fig. 6.19). The fetal heart sounds are best heard in late pregnancy below the level of the umbilicus over the anterior fetal shoulder (approximately halfway between the umbilicus and the anterosuperior iliac spine) or in the midline where there is a posterior position. With a breech presentation, the sound is best heard at the level of the umbilicus. The rate and rhythm of the heartbeat should be recorded.

本章概览	Essential information
孕妇人口统计资料 • 年龄、身高和体重（身体质量指数） • 社会经济地位、家庭支持 • 吸烟、滥用药物、酗酒或家庭暴力史 • 抑郁症或自杀未遂的病史 • 参与社会关爱服务的情况	**Maternal demographics** • Age, height and weight (BMI) • Socioeconomic status, support at home • History of smoking, substance misuse and alcohol–related or domestic violence • Previous history of depression or attempted suicides • Involvement with social care services
产科病史：当前妊娠 • 月经史（末次月经的日期、月经周期、受孕前使用药物避孕的情况） • 根据 Naegele 规则确定预产期（EDD）。（EDD= 末次月经的第 1 天减 3 个月加 7 天，或加 9 个月和 7 天） • 从末次月经计算闭经时间，以计算胎龄	**Obstetric history: present pregnancy** • Menstrual history (date of LMP, length and regularity of menstrual cycle, use of hormonal contraception prior to conception) • Establish EDD using Naegele's rule (EDD = subtract 3 months/add 7 days to LMP or add 9 months and 7 days to LMP) • Calculate the period of amenorrhoea from LMP to calculate the gestational age
妊娠相关症状的问诊 • 恶心、呕吐、尿频、过度疲倦、乳房胀痛 • 胎动感及胎动频率	**Enquire about common symptoms associated with pregnancy** • Nausea and vomiting, frequency of micturition, excessive lassitude, breast tenderness • Onset (quickening) and frequency of fetal movements
异常妊娠相关症状的问诊 • 脚部肿痛或泛红（深静脉血栓） • 头痛、视觉障碍、上腹痛或尿量减少（子痫前期） • 阴道流血（产前出血） • 漏液（胎膜早破）	**Enquire about symptoms that may be associated with abnormal pregnancy** • Painful swelling of feet or redness (DVT) • Headaches, visual disturbances, epigastric pain or reduced urine output (pre-eclampsia) • Vaginal bleeding (antepartum haemorrhage) • Leakage of fluid (pre-labour rupture of membranes)
既往产科病史 • 既往妊娠丢失（流产、异位妊娠及终止妊娠） • 既往活产数，即产次 • 死胎 / 死产或新生儿死亡 • 分娩方式 (经阴顺产、经阴人工助产、人工助产失败和剖腹产术) • 胎龄、出生体重和婴儿性别 • 既往产前或产后并发症	**Previous obstetric history** • Previous pregnancy losses (miscarriages, ectopic pregnancies and terminations) • Previous viable pregnancies, i.e. parity • Stillbirths or neonatal deaths • Method of delivery (spontaneous vaginal, assisted vaginal, failed assisted vaginal and abdominal) • Gestational age, birth weight and sex of infants • Previous antenatal or postnatal complications
既往内科病史 • 糖尿病（妊娠期、胰岛素依赖性、非胰岛素依赖性）、心脏病、高血压、肾病、传染病，如艾滋病、乙型或丙型肝炎 • 深静脉血栓或肺栓塞 • 精神疾病	**Previous medical history** • Diabetes mellitus (gestational, insulin dependent, noninsulin dependent), cardiac disease, hypertension, renal disease, infectious disease such as HIV or hepatitis B or C • DVT or pulmonary embolism • Psychiatric illness
检查 • 一般检查（苍白、发绀、黄疸、牙齿和甲床）和系统检查（心血管系统、呼吸系统、腹部检查） • 收缩期杂音是常见的，其他的则需要全面的心脏检查 • 乳房和乳头检查（如果有临床指征）	**Examination** • General examination (pallor, cyanosis, icterus, teeth and nail beds) and systemic examination (cardiovascular system (CVS), respiratory system (RS), abdominal) • Systolic flow murmurs are common; others would need full cardiological examination and investigations • Examine breasts and nipples if clinically indicated
窥器下检查 • 排除产前出血的局部原因（宫颈息肉、增生）和胎膜早破（根据病史）	**Speculum examination** • To exclude local causes of antepartum bleeding (cervical polyps, growths) and pre-labour rupture of membranes (based on the history)

119

（续表）

本章概览	Essential information
阴道检查 • 骨盆测量，评估宫颈扩张和胎先露下降情况（评估产程进展） **产科触诊** • 大体观（腹部形状、黑线、妊娠纹、手术瘢痕和胎动） • 触诊（耻骨联合–宫底高度测量，感知胎先露部位，确定胎产式、胎方位和衔接情况，预估羊水量及预计胎儿体重） • 胎心听诊	**Vaginal examination** • Clinical pelvimetry and to assess cervical dilatation and descent of the presenting part (to assess progress of labour) **Obstetric palpation** • Inspection (shape of the abdomen, linea nigra, striae gravidarum, surgical scars and fetal movements) • Palpation (measure symphysial-fundal height, feel for presenting part, determine lie, position and engagement of the presenting part, amniotic fluid volume and estimated fetal weight) • Auscultation of fetal heart

（续表）

第 7 章　正常妊娠与产前保健
Normal pregnancy and antenatal care

Shaylee Iles　著　　谭季春　译　　杨慧霞　校

学习目标	LEARNING OUTCOMES

学习本章后你应当能够：

知识标准
- 描述常规孕前保健的目的和模式
- 列出孕前保健的关键要素
- 比较妊娠人群结构的变化
- 讨论既往产科史对产前保健的重要性
- 列出产前保健的常规检查，其中包括胎儿发育异常的筛查
- 讨论妊娠期滥用药物的风险
- 讨论抗 D 免疫预防的作用

临床能力
- 实施常规预约的产前检查
- 提供有关孕期生活方式的产前教育

专业技能与态度
- 思考社会和文化因素与妊娠之间相互作用的重要性
- 思考孕期安全用药的原则

After studying this chapter you should be able to:

Knowledge criteria
- Describe the aims and patterns of routine antenatal care
- List the key elements of pre-conceptual care
- Contrast the changing demographics of pregnancy
- Discuss the significance of previous obstetric history on planning antenatal care
- List the routine investigations used in antenatal care, including screening for fetal abnormality
- Discuss the risks of substance misuse in pregnancy
- Discuss the role of anti-D immunoprophylaxis

Clinical competencies
- Carry out a routine antenatal booking visit
- Provide antenatal education on general lifestyle advice in pregnancy

Professional skills and attitudes
- Consider the importance of the interaction between social and cultural factors and pregnancy
- Consider principles of safe prescribing in pregnancy

一、常规产前检查的目的和模式（Aims and patterns of routine antenatal care）

通过产前管理可以改善女性的生育结局这一概念始于 1911 年的爱丁堡，却在最近才被关注。许多群体尤其是生活在偏远和资源贫乏的地区的人，要么缺乏产前保健，要么由于社会或宗教的原因无法实施产前保健。不幸的是，产前保健往往在那些最需要的群体中不能够得到应用，尤其在处于营养不良或营养过剩的群体中。

The concept that the reproductive outcomes of a woman might be improved by antenatal supervision is surprisingly recent and was first introduced in Edinburgh in 1911. In many societies, particularly in isolated and low-resource settings, antenatal care either is not available or, for social or religious reasons, is not used when it is available. Unfortunately, it is often least available in those communities where the need is greatest and where antenatal disorders, particularly those linked to malnutrition or over-nutrition, are most common.

妊娠和分娩是正常的生理事件，在它们的任何阶段都可能出现并发症。产前保健旨在发现、预防或治疗这些不良结局，确保在整个妊娠期间和产褥期母儿健康，同时在帮助父母做好抚养和照顾婴儿的准备。

The basic assumption is that pregnancy and birth are normal physiological events in which complications may, and do, arise at any stage. Antenatal care aims to detect, prevent or treat these adverse outcomes in order to ensure optimal health of the mother and fetus throughout pregnancy and in the puerperium. It also aims to prepare parents for the transition to parenting and care of the infant.

实现这些目标的方式将根据母体的初始健康状况和病史而有所不同，其方法是将筛查、教育和情感支持，以及在整个妊娠期间监测胎儿生长和母体健康相结合。

The ways by which these objectives are achieved will vary according to the initial health and history of the mother and are a combination of screening tests, educational and emotional support and monitoring of fetal growth and maternal health throughout the pregnancy.

在现代产前保健中，访视时间，特别是在妊娠的前 28 周，访视的时间与产前需要筛查的项目密切相关。在无并发症的妊娠女性中，初始产检建议每 4 周检查 1 次，直至 28 周；此后每 2 周检查一次直至 36 周；36 周后每周 1 次。与访视时间表相比，访视次数减少未对母体或围产期结局产生不利影响，尽管母体满意度可能有所降低。

In modern antenatal care, the timing of visits, particularly in the first 28 weeks of pregnancy, is closely geared to attendance for screening tests. In uncomplicated pregnancy, a reduction in the number of visits compared to the original suggested schedule of 4 weekly until 28 weeks, 2 weekly until 36 weeks and weekly thereafter has not been shown to adversely affect maternal or perinatal outcome, although maternal satisfaction may be reduced.

产前保健通过各种不同的机构提供，可能由全科医生、助产士和产科医生提供，通常是共同管理

的模式。产科医生或母胎医学专家对高危妊娠应给予更多关注。在首次产前访视时评估孕妇的危险分级，并制订相应的保健计划。咨询和转诊指南，如由澳大利亚助产士学院或英国国家卫生与临床优化研究所（NICE）制订的指南，可以成为评估风险和确定最优护理模式的有效工具。在妊娠过程中，妊娠风险和最优的医疗保健提供者可能会发生变化。

Antenatal care is provided through a variety of different mechanisms and may be provided by general practitioners, midwives and obstetricians, often in a pattern of shared care. Pregnancies that are considered to be high risk should receive a high proportion of their care by obstetricians or specialists in fetomaternal medicine. Risk stratification should be assessed at the earliest antenatal visits and care planned accordingly. Guidelines for consultation and referral, such as those produced by the Australian College of Midwives or the National Institute for Health and Clinical Excellence (NICE), can be a useful tool to assess risk and determine the most suitable model of care. Pregnancy risk and the most suitable care provider may alter during the course of pregnancy.

二、孕前保健和维生素补充（Pre-conceptual care and vitamin supplementation）

理想情况下，应在孕前由专业保健人员为所有女性提供孕前保健和咨询。这一角色通常由全科医生担任。这提供了进行筛查试验的机会及备孕和早孕期保健的建议。不幸的是，尽管避孕措施已广泛使用，但仍有约 50% 的妊娠是计划外的。

Ideally, all women would present prior to conception to allow their health care professional to provide them with pre-pregnancy care and counselling. This role is often best provided by the woman's usual general practitioner. This appointment allows for an opportunity to undertake screening tests and provide advice regarding conception and early pregnancy care. Unfortunately, despite widely available contraception, approximately half of all conceptions are not planned.

产前保健的重要组成部分包括评估风疹、水痘和百日咳免疫接种的必要性。如果既往接种过疫苗或无法确定是否感染的女性，可能需要进行血清学检查。如果血清学为阴性或需进行疫苗接种的女性，可以接种疫苗。由于这些疫苗是减毒活病毒疫苗，建议女性在接种后 28 天内采取充分的避孕措施以推迟妊娠。由于与妊娠期流感感染相关的严重疾病发病率逐渐增加，建议对计划妊娠或已妊娠的女性按季节接种流感疫苗。如果需要的话，此次就诊也是

常规宫颈癌筛查的理想时机。

Essential components of pre-conceptual care include the assessment of the need for immunization for rubella, varicella and pertussis. If the history of past vaccination or infection is uncertain, serology may be required. If serology is negative or immunization is due, this can then be provided. As these vaccines are live attenuated viral vaccines, it is recommended that the woman use adequate contraception to defer conception for 28 days following administration. Administration of the influenza vaccine on a seasonal basis to women who are intending to be or who are pregnant is also recommended due to the increased incidence of serious morbidity associated with influenza infection in pregnancy. This visit is also an ideal opportunity to undertake routine cervical cancer screening if due.

此时还应给予有关饮食和维生素补充的建议。建议所有女性在孕前至少 1 个月开始补充叶酸（每日 400～500μg），补充至妊娠后 3 个月，以作为降低神经管缺陷发生率的有效手段。某些高风险人群，如服用抗癫痫药的女性、肥胖女性、糖尿病女性或既往孕育过神经管缺陷胎儿的女性，可能建议服用更高剂量的叶酸（每日 5mg）。在膳食碘缺乏的国家或地区，也建议每天补充碘 150μg，以帮助胎儿脑发育。可考虑在高危人群（包括肤色较深或在长期室外遮阳的人群）中筛查维生素 D 缺乏症，必要时给予补充。

Dietary and vitamin supplementation advice should also be given at this time. It is recommended that all women take a folic acid supplement (400–500 μg daily) for at least 1 month prior to conception and the first 3 months of pregnancy as an effective means of reducing the incidence of neural tube defects. Certain risk groups may be recommended to take a higher dose (5 mg daily), such as those on anti-epileptic agents, obese women, diabetic women or women with a past history of neural tube defects. Iodine supplementation of 150 μg per day is also recommended in countries or regions where there is a dietary deficiency of iodine to aid in the development of the fetal brain. Consideration of screening for vitamin D deficiency in at-risk populations (including those with darker skin tones or who are always covered while outside) can be considered, with supplementation given if required.

此时可以对孕产妇的医疗状况（包括药物使用情况）进行审查并优化。这为探讨妊娠与医疗条件之间的互相影响提供了机会。所用药物可能需要更换或适当减量。转诊至专科医生处进行治疗优化是较恰当的。

Maternal medical conditions, including medications, can be reviewed and optimized at this time. This provides an opportunity to discuss the impact of pregnancy on the medical condition, as well as the impact of the medical condition on pregnancy. Medication may need to be altered or doses reduced where appropriate. Referral to specialist physician colleagues for treatment optimization may be appropriate.

此时也应提供关于合理饮食和规律运动的建议以优化孕前健康状况。还应开展关于合法和非法药物使用的探索和讨论。

Optimization of pre-conceptional health with advice on a nutritious diet and regular moderate exercise should also be provided at this time. Exploration and discussion around the use of licit and illicit substances should also be explored.

三、妊娠人口结构的变化（Changing demographics of pregnancy）

孕产妇年龄是产科保健结局的重要决定因素，年龄过大或过小均会使风险增加。发达国家女性分娩的中位年龄持续上升，目前刚超过 30 岁。自 1990 年以来，40 岁以上女性的生育率增加了 2 倍，现已超过了 20 岁以下女性的生育率。25 岁以下女性（包括青春期女性）的生育率目前处于英国自 1938 年有记录以来的最低水平。在发达国家，女性推迟生育是大势所趋。其原因是复杂的，其中包括一些社会、经济和教育因素。30—34 岁年龄组生育率最高。

Maternal age is an important determinant of outcome in obstetric services, with increased risk being associated with both extremes of maternal age. The median age of women giving birth in developed countries has continued to rise and currently sits at just over 30 years. Fertility rates for women over 40 have trebled since 1990 and now exceed the fertility rate for women under 20 years. Fertility in women under 25 (including amongst adolescent women) is now at the lowest rate since recording began in the UK in 1938. The tendency for women to delay childbearing until later in life is seen consistently across developed countries. The reasons for this are complex and due to a number of social, economic and educational factors. Fertility rates are highest in the 30–34 years age group.

随着平均生育年龄的增长，辅助生殖技术（assisted reproductive technology，ART）的应用逐渐增加。在澳大利亚和英国，大约 3.6% 的出生婴儿是通过 APT 辅助诞生的试管婴儿。此外，多胎妊娠率已趋于平稳，目前约占所有产妇的 1.6%。以前多胎妊娠率快速上升主要是由于辅助生殖技术使用的增加和孕妇年龄的增加。然而，由于单胚胎移植应用的增加，辅助生殖技术受孕的孕妇中多胎妊娠率有所下降。大多数多胎妊娠仍然源于自然受孕。

Use of assisted reproductive technologies (ARTs)

has increased along with the rise in median birthing age. Approximately 3.6% of babies born are conceptions assisted by ART in Australia and the UK. In addition, rates of multiple pregnancies have plateaued, currently around 1.6% of all mothers. The previous rapidly rising rates were largely due to the increases in ART and increasing maternal age. However, rates of multiples in ART pregnancy are declining due to the increased use of single-embryo transfer. The majority of multiple pregnancies remain due to spontaneous conceptions.

每个女性所生婴儿的数量仍然很低，75% 的母亲只生育 1 个或 2 个婴儿。初产妇的中位年龄也在持续上升，目前在 28 岁左右。

The absolute number of babies born to each woman continues to be low, with 75% of mothers giving birth to their first or second baby. The median age of first-time mothers also continues to rise and is currently around 28 years.

女性是产前保健的积极参与者，超过 98% 的女性至少接受一次产前访视，92% 的女性接受 5 次或 5 次以上访视。约 8.7% 的妊娠会发生早产，其中 80% 以上的早产发生在 32～36 周。

Women are active participants in antenatal care, with over 98% having at least one antenatal visit and 92% having five or more visits. Pre-term birth occurs in around 8.7% of all pregnancies, with more than 80% occurring between 32 and 36 weeks.

随着孕妇年龄的增加和体重指数（BMI）的增加，剖宫产率有逐年上升的趋势。

Rates of caesarean section as a proportion of births increase with increasing maternal age and with increasing body mass index (BMI).

四、预约访视（The booking visit）

详细的产前病史和常规临床检查已在前一章已做过讨论。然而，在首次访视时，最好在妊娠前 10 周内进行母体身高、体重等的测量，这对预测妊娠结局很有价值。低 BMI[<20，其中 BMI 为体重（kg）除以身高的平方（m²）] 的女性发生胎儿生长受限和围产期死亡的风险增加。高 BMI（BMI>30）的女性产前、产时和产后风险增加，BMI 达到 30 后风险递增。

The details of antenatal history and routine clinical examination are discussed in the preceding chapter. However, certain observations should be obtained at the first visit and it is preferable that these observations be made within the first 10 weeks of pregnancy. The measurement of maternal height and weight is important and has value in prediction of pregnancy outcomes. Women with a low BMI (less than 20, where BMI is estimated as weight (kg) divided by height (m²)) are at an increased risk of fetal growth restriction and perinatal mortality. Women with a high BMI are recognized as being at increased antenatal, intrapartum and postnatal risk, with the risks beginning to rise from a BMI of 30.

应尽早进行初始血压测量，以确定既往是否存在高血压，或作为妊娠后期高血压监测的参照值。

The initial measurement of blood pressure should be taken as early as possible to determine the presence of preexisting hypertension or as a reference point for hypertension detected at later gestations.

五、既往产科史，包括分娩方式（Consideration of past obstetric history, including mode of delivery）

应记录所有妊娠史，其中包括流产和终止妊娠，以及每次妊娠的持续时间。尤其重要的是要注意既往的所有产前并发症、分娩阵痛发作的细节、分娩过程持续时间、每个婴儿的出生时间、分娩方式、出生体重和性别。分娩方式（自然分娩、助产或剖宫产）对此次分娩存在影响，所以必须明确。查阅既往手术记录有助于此次妊娠的咨询。

A record should be made of all previous pregnancies, including previous miscarriages and terminations, and the duration of gestation in each pregnancy. In particular, it is important to note any previous antenatal complications, details of onset of labour, the duration of labour, the presentation and the method of delivery and the birth weight and gender of each infant. The mode of delivery (spontaneous, assisted or caesarean section) has implications for the current birth and must be explored. Previous operation records should be sought if relevant to aid in appropriate counselling for this pregnancy.

应注意每个婴儿出生时的状况和在婴儿特殊护理病房的护理需求。

The condition of each infant at birth and the need for care in a special care baby unit should be noted.

产褥期并发症，如产后出血、会阴大面积损伤或伤口破裂、生殖道感染、深静脉血栓形成或哺乳困难，均可能与此次妊娠相关。

Complications of the puerperium, such as postpartum haemorrhage, extensive perineal trauma or wound breakdown, infections of the genital tract, deep vein thrombosis or difficulties with breast-feeding, may all be relevant to the current pregnancy.

六、推荐的常规筛查试验 (Recommended routine screening tests)

建议从首次访视开始就进行一些基本筛查，必要时会在妊娠期重复进行。现今省略这些检测通常被认为是不合规的，因此它们具有法医学重要性和临床相关性。国家循证指南可用于指导医疗保健从业者。

Beginning at the first visit, a number of screening tests are recommended. Some will be repeated later in the pregnancy. The omission of offering these tests will generally now be considered to be evidence of substandard practice, so they have medicolegal importance as well as clinical relevance. National evidence-based guidelines are available to guide the health care practitioner.

(一) 血液学检查 (Haematological investigations)

全血细胞计数 (Full blood count)

贫血是妊娠期间的一种常见疾病，在大多数群体中，贫血是由于铁缺乏，或者是因为储存铁耗竭或铁摄入量减少所致。妊娠期病理性贫血大多数是由于铁缺乏所致。叶酸或维生素 B_{12} 缺乏、血红蛋白病（镰状细胞性贫血或地中海贫血）或各种寄生虫感染并不常见。

Anaemia is a common disorder in pregnancy and in most communities will be due to iron deficiency, either because of the depletion of iron stores or because of reduced iron intake. The majority of cases of pathological anaemia in pregnancy are due to iron deficiency. However, it may also less commonly be due to folate or vitamin B_{12} deficiency, haemoglobinopathies (sickle cell or thalassemia) or various parasitic infections.

应在首次访视时进行全血细胞计数检测，并在妊娠 28～36 周时重复进行。储存铁不足的女性应在妊娠早期开始口服补铁。那些不能耐受口服铁剂的女性应考虑静脉输注铁。对那些常见地中海贫血和镰状细胞贫血等疾病的种族应常规提供血红蛋白病的筛查。

A full blood count should be performed at the first visit and repeated at 28 and 34–36 weeks' gestation. Women who have deficient iron stores should be given oral supplements of iron starting early in pregnancy. Those women unable to tolerate oral iron supplements should be considered for iron infusion. Screening for haemoglobinopathies should be routinely offered to those racial groups where conditions such as thalassaemia and sickle cell disease are common.

(二) 血型和抗体 (Blood group and antibodies)

所有孕妇均应测定血型，并在妊娠早期进行红细胞抗体筛查。在 Rh 阴性血女性中，应在首次产前检查时（最好在孕早期）进行 Rh 抗体筛查，随后在妊娠 28 周时重复筛查。ABO 抗体也可能引起胎儿和新生儿的异常，但这一问题目前仍无法解决。

Blood group should be determined in all pregnant women, and screening for red cell antibodies should be undertaken early in pregnancy. In Rhesus (Rh)-negative women, screening for Rh antibodies should be performed at the first visit (preferably in the first trimester) and then repeated at 28 weeks' gestation. ABO antibodies may also cause problems in the fetus and newborn, but no method is available to counter this problem.

抗 D 免疫球蛋白的使用 (The use of anti-D immunoglobulin)

约 15% 的高加索女性为 Rh 阴性血，并且有在妊娠期或妊娠后即刻产生抗 D 抗体的风险。抗 D 抗体的形成可能对后来胎儿的健康甚至存活构成风险，这是由于预先形成的抗体穿过胎盘并攻击 Rh 阳性胎儿的红细胞。这对胎儿和新生儿将产生毁灭性的影响，其中包括胎儿贫血、水肿、新生儿贫血、黄疸、核黄疸或胎儿宫内死亡。自 20 世纪 60 年代开始便有强有力的证据表明，产后给予抗 D 免疫球蛋白（抗 D Ig）可显著降低该并发症的发生率。

Around 15% of Caucasian women will be Rh negative and be at risk of developing anti-D antibodies during or immediately following pregnancy. The formation of anti-D antibodies may pose a risk to the wellbeing and even survival of a subsequent fetus due to the pre-formed antibodies crossing the placenta and attacking the red blood cells of an Rh-positive fetus. The effects on the fetus and newborn can be devastating and include fetal anaemia, hydrops, neonatal anaemia, jaundice, kernicterus or fetal death in utero. There is very strong evidence dating from the 1960s that postpartum administration of anti-D immunoglobulin (anti-D Ig) can dramatically reduce the incidence of this complication.

直到最近几年，抗 D 免疫球蛋白仅用于妊娠期发生致敏事件的女性或在产后给予分娩 Rh 阳性婴儿的女性。产后 72h 内给药，可将 Rh 同种免疫的风险降低至约 1.5%。首次给药前，应通过流式细胞术（如果有）或 Kleihauer-Betke 试验对母胎出血的程度和进一步给药剂量进行定量。

Until the past few years, anti-D Ig was given only to women with a sensitizing event in pregnancy or postnatally to women delivered of an Rh-positive infant. Given within 72 hours of birth, this dose reduces the risk of Rh isoimmunization to around 1.5%. Quantitation of the degree of fetomaternal haemorrhage and the need for further doses should be undertaken by flow cytometry (where available) or the Kleihauer-Betke test prior to administration of the first dose.

致敏事件包括正常分娩、流产、终止妊娠、异位妊娠、侵入性产前诊断、腹部创伤、产前出血或外倒转术。致敏作用也可在女性不自觉时发生于妊娠期间。因此现在抗 D 免疫球蛋白已容易获得，在妊娠 28 周和 34 周给予抗 D 免疫球蛋白预防已成为标准操作（图 7-1）。

Sensitizing events include normal delivery, miscarriage, termination of pregnancy, ectopic pregnancy, invasive prenatal diagnosis, abdominal trauma, antepartum haemorrhage or external cephalic version. Sensitization during pregnancy can also occur without the woman being aware of such an event. Hence, now that anti-D Ig is readily available, it has become standard practice to give anti-D Ig prophylaxis at 28 and 34 weeks' gestation (Fig. 7.1).

这将阻止几乎所有 Rh 阳性胎儿的母体免疫，只有 0.2% 的 Rh 阴性女性例外，在这些女性中，胎儿细胞的输入量超过了给予的抗体剂量。这是对前述适应证的补充。

This will prevent maternal immunization by an Rh-positive fetus in all but 0.2% of Rh-negative women, in whom the infusion of cells from the fetus overwhelms the dose of antibody administered. This is in addition to the earlier noted indications.

（三）感染疾病筛查（Infection screening）

1. 风疹（Rubella）

所有 11—14 岁的女孩通常由学校组织进行风疹疫苗接种。有研究表明，约 2.5% 的澳大利亚女性在妊娠期间血清学检查阴性。多数被发现为免疫力低下。约 50% 的无免疫性女性以前接种过疫苗。所有血清阴性和弱阳性女性应在产褥期立即进行免疫接种。使用风疹病毒减毒活疫苗进行单剂量皮下注射。虽然没有证据表明在风疹疫苗接种前后受孕女性的婴儿的异常率显著增加，但通常建议在疫苗接种后 1 个月内避免妊娠。应建议无免疫性的女性避免与感染者接触。所有临床疑似感染都应该采集双份血清进行检测，最好使用初次访视时采集的原始样本。

All girls are offered rubella vaccination between the ages of 11 and 14 years, often through a school-based vaccination programme. In pregnancy, around 2.5% of women in the Australian population are found to be seronegative. A greater proportion are found to have low levels of immunity. Around 50% of non-immune women will have been previously vaccinated. All seronegative and low-level seropositive women should be offered immunization in the immediate puerperium. Vaccination is performed with a live attenuated rubella virus vaccine and involves a single dose injected subcutaneously. Although there is no evidence to suggest any significant increase in abnormality rate in the babies in women who have conceived immediately before or following rubella vaccination, it is generally recommended that pregnancy be avoided for 1 month after vaccination. Non-immune women

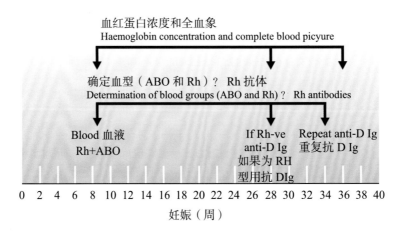

▲ 图 7-1　血红蛋白评估和 Rh 抗体检测和给药的常规检测时间

Ig. 免疫球蛋白；Rh. 恒河猴

Fig. 7.1　Schedules for routine tests of haemoglobin estimation and detection and administration of Rh antibodies

Ig, Immunoglobulin; Rh, Rhesus.

should be advised to avoid contact with infected individuals. Any clinically suspected infection should be investigated with paired sera, preferably with the original sample taken at the time of booking.

2. 梅毒（Syphilis）

建议对梅毒进行常规筛查。虽然其相对罕见，但是可以治疗的，如果未治疗会有严重的新生儿后遗症。在某些地区，发病率的升高意味着在妊娠 28 周和 36 周时应同样推荐进行检测。有许多非特异性和特异性检查梅毒的方法，能否使用应咨询当地病理学实验室。

Routine screening for syphilis is recommended practice. Although relatively rare, the condition is treatable and has major neonatal sequelae if left untreated. Increasing rates in some jurisdictions mean that testing at 28 and 36 weeks' gestation may also be recommended. A number of nonspecific and specific tests exist, and advice should be sought from the local pathology laboratory as to availability.

3. 肝炎（Hepatitis）

建议对妊娠女性进行乙型肝炎和丙型肝炎的全面筛查。所有婴儿均建议进行乙肝疫苗接种，对于高危婴儿，建议进行乙肝疫苗接种及给予乙型肝炎免疫球蛋白（HBIG）。在 90% 的病例中，完成完整的疫苗接种计划可保护高危婴儿免受乙型肝炎感染。可用于治疗丙肝感染的新型药物意味着对丙肝的检测是一项重要的公共卫生措施（见第 9 章）。

Universal screening for hepatitis B and C in pregnancy is recommended. Hepatitis B vaccination, as well as the administration of hepatitis B immunoglobulin (HBIG), is recommended for at-risk infants, and hepatitis B vaccination for all infants. Completion of the full vaccination schedule protects at-risk infants from hepatitis B infection in 90% of cases. Newer agents available to treat hepatitis C infection mean detection of this condition is an important public health measure. (see the chapter 9 on maternal medical conditions).

4. 人类免疫缺陷病毒（Human immunodeficiency virus）

检测 HIV 的试验基础是检测 HIV 抗体。如果检测结果为阳性，应进行 HIV RNA 检测，以确定病毒载量并监测治疗疗效。

The basis of tests for the detection of HIV is the detection of HIV antibodies. A positive test should always be followed up with an HIV RNA test to determine the disease load and monitor treatment efficacy.

由于抗体经胎盘传播，母体血清阳性，婴儿的血清通常也是阳性，但这可能并不意味着婴儿有活动性感染。但是，如果不使用积极的管理方案，高达 45% 的婴儿将感染 HIV。由于治疗可有效将传播率降至 2% 以下，因此对所有女性进行常规筛查对于预防新生儿 HIV 感染作用很大。这些管理方案包括对检测到病毒载量的女性进行剖宫产、避免母乳喂养和在产前产时对孕妇及新生儿进行抗逆转录病毒治疗（见第 9 章）。

Seropositive mothers always have seropositive babies due to transplacental transmission of antibodies, but this may not indicate active infection in the baby. However, up to 45% of babies will have contracted HIV if active management programmes are not used. As treatment is highly effective in reducing transmission rates to less than 2%, there is a strong case for routine screening of all women. These strategies include caesarean section with any detectable viral load, avoidance of breast-feeding and antiretroviral therapy in both the antenatal and intrapartum period as well as for the newborn. (see the chapter 9 on maternal medical conditions).

5. B 组链球菌（Group B *Streptococcus*）

B 组链球菌（GBS）是一种革兰阳性菌，是胃肠道常见的共生菌。高达 25% 的妊娠女性可从阴道培养出 GBS，这也可能导致尿路感染。在阴道分娩过程中，存在传播给新生儿的风险。早产和胎膜破裂时间延长会增加这种风险。新生儿感染的发生率为 1‰～2‰，可导致严重的败血症，并伴有显著的发病率和死亡率。90% 的感染发生在出生后数天内，但在 3 月龄时可能出现迟发症状。

Group B *Streptococcus* (GBS) is a gram-positive bacterium that is a common commensal carried in the gastrointestinal tract. It can be cultured from the vagina in up to 25% of women in pregnancy and may also be a cause of urinary tract infection. During vaginal delivery, there is a risk of transmission to the neonate. This risk is increased in pre-term delivery and prolonged rupture of membranes. Neonatal infection occurs in 1–2 per 1000 births and can result in overwhelming sepsis associated with significant morbidity and mortality. Ninety percent of infections present within the first days of life, but late presentations at up to 3 months of age can occur.

病原体可由阴道和直肠拭子检出，并通过产时静脉应用青霉素治疗降低垂直传播率。许多中心推荐在 34～36 周使用阴道下部和肛周拭子进行 GBS 筛查，但没有得到普及。

The organism can be detected on vaginal and rectal

swabs and the rate of vertical transmission reduced by the use of intrapartum antibiotic treatment with intravenous penicillin. Screening for GBS using a low vaginal and perianal swab taken between 34 and 36 weeks is recommended by many centres but is not universal practice.

6. 尿路感染（Urinary tract infection）

已有证据表明筛查无症状菌尿的是有益的。病原菌每 1000ml 超过 10 000 个表明存在明显的菌尿。妊娠期间包括急性肾盂肾炎在内的上行性尿路感染的发生率增加，这与妊娠丢失和早产增加以及母体发病率增加相关。早期治疗无症状的菌尿可降低此类感染的发生率，从而改善孕产妇的健康。

Screening for asymptomatic bacteriuria is of proven benefit. The presence of pathogenic organisms in excess of 10,000 organisms/mL indicates significant bacteriuria. The incidence of ascending urinary tract infection, including acute pyelonephritis, is increased in pregnancy and is associated with increased pregnancy loss and pre-term birth, as well as maternal morbidity. Early treatment of asymptomatic bacteriuria reduces the incidence of such infections and thus improves maternal health.

7. 妊娠期糖尿病（Gestational diabetes mellitus）

妊娠期糖尿病（GDM）与胎死宫内及分娩期并发症和新生儿并发症的增加有关。筛选程序遵循以下 2 种途径之一。

- 根据病史筛选（澳大利亚妊娠期糖尿病标准：ADIPS），具体如下。
  - 既往妊娠期高血糖。
  - 既往血糖水平升高。
  - 种族，如亚洲人、印度人、澳洲原住民、托雷斯海峡岛民、太平洋岛民、毛利人、中东人、非白种非洲人。
  - 糖尿病 (DM) 家族史（直系亲属患 DM 或姐妹患 GDM）。
  - 巨大儿生产史，既往胎儿的出生体重超过 4.5kg 或 >第 90 百分位数。
  - 肥胖（孕前 BMI>30）。
  - 多囊卵巢综合征 (PCOS)。
  - 母亲年龄 >40 岁。
  - 药物，如皮质类固醇、抗精神病药物。

Gestational diabetes mellitus (GDM) is associated with an increased incidence of intrauterine fetal death, as well as intrapartum and neonatal complications. Screening programmes follow one of two pathways:

- Selection by history (Australasian Diabetes in Pregnancy Criteria: ADIPS):
  - Previous hyperglycaemia in pregnancy
  - Previously elevated blood glucose level
  - Ethnicity: Asian, Indian, Aboriginal, Torres Strait Islander, Pacific Islander, Maori, Middle Eastern, nonwhite African
  - Family history of diabetes mellitus (DM) (first-degree relative with DM or sister with GDM)
  - Previous macrosomic infant with a birth weight in excess of 4.5 kg or >90th centile
  - Obesity (pre-pregnancy BMI >30)
  - Polycystic ovarian syndrome (PCOS)
  - Maternal age >40 years
  - Medications: corticosteroids, anti-psychotics

在这些情况下，应使用 75g 或 100g 负荷剂量的葡萄糖进行葡萄糖耐量试验（GTT）。除非之前已经确诊，否则应在预约访视时进行检测并在妊娠 28 周时再次进行检测。

Under these circumstances, a full glucose tolerance test (GTT) should be performed using either a 75-g or 100-g loading dose of glucose. The test should be performed at the booking visit and again at 28 weeks' gestation unless diagnosed prior.

或者

Or

- 普遍筛查：对所有妊娠 26～28 周女性进行筛查，将比单独通过危险因素筛查发现更多的糖耐量受损或糖尿病女性。按照国际妊娠糖尿病协会 (IADPSG) 规定的诊断标准进行完整的 GTT。

- Universal screening: The screening of all women at 26–28 weeks' gestation will identify more women with impaired glucose tolerance or diabetes than those screened by risk factors alone. The full GTT is done with criteria for diagnosis as outlined by the International Association of Diabetes in Pregnancy Study Groups (IADPSG).

大多数地区只进行高危人群的筛查，是因为筛查整个人群存在实际困难和成本问题，特别是在大型产科医院。

Most jurisdictions who choose to only screen at-risk

populations do so because of the practical difficulties and costs of screening the whole population, particularly in large maternity hospitals.

七、胎儿异常筛查（Screening for fetal anomaly）

结构性异常占所有围产儿死亡的 20%～25%，约占出生后第一年死亡的 15%。因此，有充分的理由在适当情况下尽早发现和终止妊娠。常见结构异常包括心脏、颅脑、脊柱、肾脏和胃肠道系统异常。

Structural fetal anomalies account for some 20–25% of all perinatal deaths and for about 15% of all deaths in the first year of life. There is therefore a strong case to be made for early detection and termination of pregnancy offered where this is appropriate. Common structural anomalies include those of the cardiac, craniospinal, renal and gastrointestinal systems.

这些异常通常可通过超声扫描检测到，这将在"先天性异常"中讨论。最常在 18～22 周时进行胎儿异常超声检查。

These anomalies are generally detectable by ultrasound scanning, and this will be discussed in the chapter on congenital abnormalities. This is most commonly done at the 18–22-week fetal anomaly ultrasound.

非整倍体和早期结构评估（Aneuploidy and early structural assessment）

1. 颈项透明层厚度和生化筛查（Nuchal translucency and biochemical screening）

21 三体综合征（唐氏综合征）筛查已成为大多数产前服务的常规项目。此类筛查合理的重要性是提供侵入性检测，然后在有非整倍体证据情况下终止妊娠。如果不能选择终止妊娠，筛查的价值会降低，但阳性结果可以帮助父母为下一个孩子的出生做好准备。筛查使用生化和超声检查。重要的是，女性要了解这些只是筛查试验，有其局限性。筛查不会检测出所有病例，同样高风险结果也不一定意味着婴儿会受到影响。尽管唐氏综合征在 35 岁以上的妊娠女性的胎儿中发病率增加，但是仅根据年龄进行筛查并不能发现大部分受影响的胎儿，建议对所有女性进行筛查。唐氏综合征筛查的主要方式是使用超声测量颈项透明层，即测量胎儿颈后液体的厚度（图 10-7）。结合孕妇年龄和生化检查结果，为

该胎儿评估 21 三体、13 三体和 18 三体的风险（见第 10 章）。本试验检测 21 三体的敏感性为 95%。

The offer of screening for trisomy 21 (Down's syndrome) has become routine in most antenatal services. The logical consequence of such a programme is to offer invasive testing and then termination of pregnancy where there is evidence of aneuploidy. Although the value of the test is reduced if termination is not an option, a positive result can help parents prepare for the birth of an additionalneeds child. Screening is by the use of biochemical and ultrasound tests. It is important that women understand that these are screening tests and therefore have their limitations. They will not detect every case, and high-risk results do not necessarily mean that the baby is affected. Despite the increased incidence of Down's syndrome in mothers over 35 years, screening on the basis of age alone will not detect most affected fetuses, and it is recommended to offer screening to all women. The major modality for screening for Down's syndrome is the use of ultrasound measurement of nuchal translucency, a measurement of fluid behind the fetal neck (see Chapter 10, Fig. 10.7). This is combined with maternal age and the results of biochemical tests to provide a risk for this fetus of trisomy 21, 13 and 18 (see Chapter 10). The sensitivity of this test for the detection of trisomy 21 is 95%.

2. 无创产前检测（NIPT）[Non-invasive prenatal testing (NIPT)]

自 2011 年以来，非整倍体筛查已经可以在母体血液中检测出胎儿游离 DNA 的存在。从孕 10 周开始，可以在母血中获得足够的胎儿 DNA 片段，21 三体的检测灵敏度超过 99%，而 18 三体和 13 三体的检测率略低。性染色体检测也被报道用于性别鉴定。值得注意的是，这也是一种筛选试验，在做出临床决策之前需要进行有创性检查（如绒毛取样或羊膜穿刺术）。目前在大多数司法管辖区，这是一项自费检查；但预计在未来几年内，成本效益分析导致政府将决定资助这项检测，使它作为一种常规的产前检查。目前，该检测的其他商业应用包括检测其他常见的遗传病，如囊性纤维化（cystic fibrosis，CF）、脊髓性肌萎缩症（spinal muscular atrophy，SMA）和脆性 X 染色体综合征。全部染色体的三体全面筛查也同样有效。这是一个快速变化的领域，预计在短期至中期，许多其他遗传性疾病将能够用这种技术进行检测。

Since 2011, aneuploidy screening has become available on maternal blood, which detects the presence of fetal cell-free DNA. Able to be done from 10 weeks' gestation to allow for an adequate fetal fraction in the sample, the sensitivity for detection of trisomy 21 is over 99%, with marginally lower rates for trisomy 18 and 13. Sex chromosome identification allowing for gender determination is also reported. It is important to note that this is also a screening test, and onfirmatory testing with invasive tests (such as chorionic villus sampling or amniocentesis) is required before clinical decision-making can occur. In most jurisdictions this is currently available as a privately funded test; however, it is anticipated that over the next few years, the cost-benefit analysis will result in governments deciding to fund this test as part of routine antenatal investigation. Other commercial applications of this test currently available include testing for other common genetic concerns such as cystic fibrosis (CF), spinal muscular atrophy (SMA) and fragile X. Full screening for trisomy of all chromosomes is also available. This is an area of rapid change, and it is anticipated that many other genetic conditions will be able to be tested with this technology over the short to medium term.

值得注意的是，NIPT 并不能取代使用超声进行的颈项透明层厚度的结构评估，因此，若选择 NIPT 进行非整倍体的筛查，建议同时进行早期结构超声检查（非颈项透明层厚度检查）。这样就可以发现多胎妊娠和主要的结构畸形。

It is important to note that NIPT does not replace the structural assessment that is done with the ultrasound component of the nuchal translucency assessment, and hence if NIPT is chosen for aneuploidy screening, an early structural ultrasound (without measurement of the nuchal translucency) should also be recommended. This allows for multiple gestations and major structural malformations to be detected.

八、常规产前检查时间表（Schedules of routine antenatal care）

随访（Subsequent visits）

尽管产前保健的模式会因环境和妊娠的正常与否而不同，但常规的访视模式应部分围绕筛查流程的要求以及母亲的孕产史和病史进行。所有访视均应测量血压，并记录耻骨联合到宫底的高度，但这种检查对胎儿发育迟缓监测的能力有限。如果每次就诊时都进行连续的超声测量，检出率会更高，但这对于非高危妊娠的女性来说是不可行的或不必要的。表 7–1 列出了推荐的产前检查流程。

Although the pattern of antenatal care will vary with circumstances and with the normality or otherwise of the pregnancy, a general pattern of visits will partly revolve around the demands of the screening procedures and the obstetric and medical history of the mother. The measurement of blood pressure is performed at all visits, and the measurement of symphysis/

fundal height should be recorded, accepting that this observation has a limited capacity to detect fetal growth restriction. Serial ultrasound measurements would have a greater detection rate if performed at every visit, but this is not practicable or necessary for women who are not considered to be at high risk. A suggested regime for antenatal visits is listed in Table 7.1.

一般来说，如果通过早期超声准确确定妊娠日期，从而确定胎龄，则 41 周后引产可降低胎盘功能不全并发症的发生率，如羊水粪染、产时缺氧和胎儿窘迫，以及胎儿和新生儿死亡的风险。巨大儿和严重会阴裂伤的发生率也降低了。Meta 分析表明，41 周后引产会减少剖宫产分娩，增加器械助产和产时镇痛的使用。

In general, where pregnancies have been accurately dated by early ultrasound so that the gestational age is certain, induction of labour after 41 weeks reduces the incidence of complications of placental insufficiency, such as meconium staining, intrapartum hypoxia and fetal compromise, and the risk of fetal and neonatal death. Rates of macrosomia and major perineal trauma are also reduced. Meta-analysis suggests that there is reduction in caesarean deliveries with induction of labour after 41 weeks; however, instrumental births and intrapartum usage of analgesia are increased.

九、产前教育（Antenatal education）

产前保健的一个重要组成部分是对母亲及其伴侣进行有关妊娠、分娩和婴儿护理的教育。作为教育的一部分，这一过程应在孕前开始，并持续到整个孕期和产褥期。实现这一目标的方法多种多样，但通常可以在孕期定期举办产前培训班来满足这些需求。参与常规产前护理和分娩的工作人员最好也是向女性提供产时护理的人员，以便将护理和教育的过程视为一个整体（表 7–2）。

An important and integral part of antenatal care is the education of the mother and her partner about pregnancy, childbirth and the care of the infant. This process should start before pregnancy as part of school education and should continue throughout pregnancy and the puerperium. There are various ways by which this can be achieved, but commonly, the needs are met by regular antenatal classes during the course of the pregnancy. It is preferable that those staff who are involved in general antenatal care and delivery be part of the team that provides intrapartum care to the woman so that the processes of care and education are seen as one entity (Table 7.2).

（一）饮食建议（Dietary advice）

孕期饮食的重要性是毋庸置疑的。在一个极端

表 7-1　产前保健访视

Table 7.1　Visits for antenatal care

8～12 周 8–12 weeks	初次访视，确认妊娠、在孕产史中寻找风险因素；有指征时进行宫颈筛查、提供一般健康、吸烟和饮食建议；讨论并组织筛选程序；检查孕妇体重，并给出推荐的叶酸和碘补充剂建议；如果不确定，标注扫描日期 Initial visit, confirmation of pregnancy, search for risk factors in maternal history. Cervical screening where indicated, advice on general health, smoking and diet. Discuss and organize screening procedures. Check maternal weight and give advice on recommended folic acid and iodine supplements. Dating scan if uncertainty exists.
11～14 周 11–14 weeks	通过 ± 颈后透明层扫描和血液检查或 NIPT 和结构超声（如要求）筛查三倍体；确认访视安排；如果有任何贫血证据，提供膳食补充剂铁 Screening for trisomies with ± nuchal translucency scan and blood tests or NIPT and structural ultrasound if requested. Confirm booking arrangements. Offer dietary supplements of iron if any evidence of anaemia.
16 周 16 weeks	检查所有血液结果；在妊娠 18～20 周进行常规超声异常扫描 Check all blood results. Offer routine ultrasound anomaly scan to be performed between 18 and 20 weeks' gestation
20 周 20 weeks	检查超声结果、BP、宫底高度 Check ultrasound result, BP, fundal height.
24 周 24 weeks	检查 BP、宫底高度、胎儿活动情况 BP, fundal height, fetal activity.
28 周 28 weeks	检查 BP、宫底高度、胎儿活动、全血细胞计数和抗体筛查；如果 Rh 阴性，给予抗 D 免疫球蛋白；葡萄糖耐量试验 BP, fundal height, fetal activity, full blood count and antibody screen. Administer anti-D if Rh negative. Glucose tolerance test.
32 周 32 weeks	检查 BP、宫底高度、胎儿活动和胎儿生长扫描（如胎儿生长模式可疑异常或胎盘低置） BP, fundal height, fetal activity and fetal growth scan where pattern of fetal growth is in doubt or low-lying placenta on anomaly scan
34 周 34 weeks	检查 BP、宫底高度、胎儿活动、Rh 阴性女性抗 D 免疫球蛋白第二剂、全血细胞计数 BP, fundal height, fetal activity, also second dose of anti-D for Rh-negative women, full blood count
36 周 36 weeks	检查 BP、宫底高度、胎儿活动、B 组链球菌阴道和肛周拭子；确定先露 BP, fundal height, fetal activity, group B Streptococcus vaginal and perianal swab determine presentation
38 周 38 weeks	检查 BP、宫底高度、胎儿活动、产妇健康 BP, fundal height, fetal activity, maternal wellbeing
40 周 40 weeks	检查 BP、宫底高度、胎儿活动、产妇健康 BP, fundal height, fetal activity, maternal wellbeing
41 周 41 weeks	检查 BP、宫底高度、胎儿活动、阴道检查评估宫颈是否良好、心电图、羊水指数；在引产和持续评估方面进行个体化护理 BP, fundal height, fetal activity, assessment by vaginal examination as to cervical favourability, cardiotocograph, amniotic fluid index. Individualize care with regard to induction of labour and ongoing assessment.

BP. 血压；NIPT. 无创产前检测

改编自 Kean L (2001) Routine antenatal management. Curr Obstet Gynaecol 11:63-69.

BP, Blood pressure; NIPT, non-invasive prenatal testing.

Adapted from Kean L (2001) Routine antenatal management. Curr Obstet Gynaecol 11:63-69.

情况下，严重营养不良会导致宫内生长受限、贫血、早产和胎儿畸形。较轻程度的营养不良也可能与胎儿畸形发生率增加有关，尤其是神经管缺陷，因此提供饮食指导并确保在整个妊娠期和产褥期保持适当质量和数量的饮食是很重要的。然而，在发达国家，营养过剩和母亲肥胖的问题更为常见。值得注意的是，尽管热量摄入过多，但由于选择性的摄入，维生素和矿物质缺乏在这些人中也很常见。

表 7–2 孕期一般生活方式建议

Table 7.2 General lifestyle advice in pregnancy

健康行为 Health behaviour	建议 Recommendation
营养 Nutrition	孕期每日食用推荐量的五大类食物和饮用大量的水是很重要的 Eating the recommended number of daily servings of the five food groups and drinking plenty of water are important during pregnancy. 额外摄入五大类食物可能有助于增加过瘦女性的体重，但在超重或肥胖女性中应受到限制 Additional servings of the five food groups may contribute to healthy weight gain in women who are underweight, but these should be limited by women who are overweight or obese. 少量或适量的咖啡因不太可能对胎儿造成伤害 Small to moderate amounts of caffeine are unlikely to harm the fetus.
运动 Exercise	孕期进行低到中等强度的体育活动有很多益处，且对妊娠或胎儿无负面影响 Low-to moderate-intensity physical activity during pregnancy has a range of benefits and is not associated with negative effects on the pregnancy or baby.
吸烟 Smoking	主动和被动吸烟均会对妊娠和胎儿产生负面影响；强烈建议戒烟 Smoking and passive smoking can have negative effects on the pregnancy and the baby. Smoking cessation is strongly recommended.
饮酒 Alcohol	不饮酒是最安全的选择 Not drinking alcohol is the safest option for women who are pregnant.
非法药物 Illicit substances	非法药物和非医疗用药（如阿片类药物）对妊娠和胎儿有负面影响 Illicit substances and non-medical use of medications (e.g. opioids) have negative effects on the pregnancy and the baby.

改编自 Department of Health (2018) *Clinical Practice Guidelines: Pregnancy Care*. Canberra: Australian Government Department of Health, page 84.

Adapted from Department of Health (2018) *Clinical Practice Guidelines: Pregnancy Care*. Canberra: Australian Government Department of Health, page 84.

There can be no doubt about the importance of diet in pregnancy. At one extreme, gross malnutrition is known to result in intrauterine growth restriction, anaemia, prematurity and fetal malformation. Lesser degrees of malnutrition may also be associated with an increased incidence of fetal malformations, particularly neural tube defects, and it is therefore important to provide guidance on diet and to ensure that a diet of appropriate quality and quantity is maintained throughout pregnancy and the puerperium. However, in the developed world, the concerns of overnutrition and maternal obesity are much more frequently encountered. Of note, despite excessive caloric consumption, it is not uncommon for vitamin and mineral deficiencies to also be encountered in this population, largely due to choice of intake.

显然，饮食的性质会因文化因素和实际体型的不同而有很大的差异，但我们可以提供一些一般原则，以满足母亲和发育中的胎儿的需要。

Clearly, there will be substantial variation in the nature of the diet depending on cultural factors and actual physical size, but general principles can be provided as advice to meet the needs of the mother and of the developing fetus.

在孕早期，应提供有关李斯特菌风险的建议，并建议避免高风险食物，如软奶酪、熟食肉类、自助沙拉和冰淇淋。

Advice should be given early in pregnancy regarding *Listeria* risk and advice given to avoid high-risk foods such as soft cheeses, delicatessen meats, salad bars and soft-serve ice cream.

1. 能量摄入（Energy intake）

为满足母体和胎儿新陈代谢的需要，在妊娠中晚期，总能量摄入每日应达到为 2000~2500kcal。哺乳期女性产褥期的每日能量需求可能增加到 3000kcal。

A total energy intake of 2000–2500 kcal/day is necessary during the last two trimesters of pregnancy because of the demands of both maternal and fetal metabolism. This requirement may increase to 3000 kcal in the puerperium in lactating women.

2. 蛋白质（Protein）

除阿根廷和澳大利亚等一些国家外，一级蛋白质在大多数国家价格都很昂贵，因此在欠发达国家很可能缺乏。选择不吃肉和肉制品的人的饮食也可能有缺陷。动物蛋白来自肉、家禽、鱼、蛋和奶酪。植物蛋白存在于坚果、小扁豆、菜豆和豌豆中。平均每天应获取 60～80g。那些只从蔬菜中摄取蛋白质的女性可能需要补充维生素 B_{12}。这些人更易出现缺铁性贫血。

First-class protein is expensive in most countries, with some notable exceptions such as Argentina and Australia, and is therefore likely to be deficient in less developed nations. It is also likely to be deficient in the diet of those who choose to avoid meat and meat products. Animal protein is obtained from meat, poultry, fish, eggs and cheese. Vegetable protein occurs in nuts, lentils, beans and peas. An average of 60–80 g daily is desirable. Those women deriving their protein intake solely from vegetable sources are likely to need vitamin B_{12} supplementation. Iron-deficiency anaemia is also found more commonly in this group.

3. 脂肪（Fats）

脂肪是均衡饮食的重要组成部分。必需脂肪酸可能在细胞生长和预防孕期高血压的发展中发挥重要作用。脂肪也是重要的能量来源和脂溶性维生素的来源，其中包括维生素 A、维生素 D 和维生素 K。

Fats provide an important component of a balanced diet. Essential fatty acids may play an important part in cellular growth and in preventing the development of hypertension during pregnancy. Fats are also an important source of energy and a source of fat-soluble vitamins, including vitamins A, D and K.

动物脂肪存在于肉、蛋和奶制品中，含有高比例的饱和脂肪。另一方面，植物脂肪很重要，因为它们含有亚油酸和亚麻酸等不饱和脂肪。

Animal fats are found in meat, eggs and dairy products and contain a high percentage of saturated fats. Vegetable fats, on the other hand, are important because they contain unsaturated fats such as linoleic and linolenic acids.

4. 碳水化合物（即糖类）（Carbohydrates）

糖类是母体和胎儿的主要能量来源，因此是孕期必不可少的饮食成分。然而，过量摄入糖类会导致体重增加和脂肪堆积，因此饮食中均衡摄入糖类

是至关重要的。尤其要记住的是，母体和胎儿的血糖水平之间有着密切的关联，葡萄糖是胎儿的主要能量来源。

Carbohydrates are the primary source of energy for both mother and fetus and are therefore an essential dietary component during pregnancy. However, excessive carbohydrate consumption can result in excessive weight gain and fat accumulation, so a balanced dietary intake of carbohydrate is an essential. In particular, it should be remembered that there is a close correlation between maternal and fetal blood glucose levels and that glucose is the major source of energy for the fetus.

5. 矿物质和维生素（Minerals and vitamins）

除了叶酸和碘，孕期不需要常规补充铁和其他维生素。但是，如果多胎妊娠或有证据表明饮食缺乏，则应从妊娠的前 3 个月开始补充铁和维生素。

Other than folic acid and iodine, routine supplementation with iron and other vitamins should not be necessary during pregnancy. However, where there is evidence of dietary deficiency or in cases of multiple gestations, iron and vitamin supplements should be given from the first trimester onwards.

所有女性在预约产检时都应得到关于孕期适当体重增长的建议。目标体重增加取决于孕前体重，并考虑到胎儿体重、羊水、胎盘、子宫、血容量和母乳喂养的脂肪储备。

All women should be given advice at the booking visit regarding appropriate weight gain in pregnancy. Target weight gains depend on pre-pregnancy weight and make allowance for the weight of the fetus, amniotic fluid, placenta, uterus, blood volume and fat stores for breast-feeding.

对于理想体重增加的建议，见表 7-3。

Recommendations for ideal weight gain are found in Table 7.3.

（二）孕期运动（Exercise in pregnancy）

应鼓励孕妇在孕期进行合理的活动。随着妊娠的进展，腹部大小的变化和对母亲身体平衡的限制会限制运动，但在妊娠早期，没有必要将体育活动限制在避免过度劳累和疲劳的常识限度之外。但对于有流产史的女性可能例外。游泳是一种有益的运动形式，尤其是在孕晚期，因为水可以支撑孕妇增大的腹部。

Pregnant women should be encouraged to undertake reasonable activity during pregnancy. This will be limited with advancing gestation by the physical restrictions imposed by

表 7-3　美国医学研究所（IOM）2009 年妊娠期
体重增加目标

Table 7.3　U.S. Institute of Medicine (IOM) 2009 gestational
weight gain targets

孕前 BMI（kg/m²） Pre-pregnancy BMI(kg/m²)	推荐的体重增加（kg） Recommended weight gain (kg)
＜18.5	12.5～18.0
18.5～24.9	11.5～16
25.0～29.9	7.0～11.5
≥30.0	5.0～9.0

✓ 经验

如果出现营养不良，通常是因为饮食的选择，而不是经济的压力。这可以通过补充叶酸和孕期多种维生素来解决。在某些城市环境中，叶酸缺乏往往是营养不良的一部分，应在妊娠早期预测，以便补充铁和叶酸。

Where deficiencies do arise, this is generally because of dietary choice rather than from economic pressures. This situation can be overcome by giving folic acid and pregnancy multivitamin supplements. In some urban environs, folate deficiency tends to be part of a pattern of malnutrition and should be anticipated in early pregnancy so that supplements of iron and folic acid can be given.

the changes in abdominal size and by the balance restrictions imposed on the mother, but during early pregnancy there is no need to limit sporting activities beyond the common-sense limits of avoiding excessive exertion and fatigue. There may be exceptions to this situation in women with a history of previous pregnancy losses. Swimming is a useful form of exercise, particularly in late pregnancy, when the water tends to support the enlarged maternal abdomen.

十、孕期药物使用和滥用（Substance use and misuse in pregnancy）

（一）吸烟（Smoking）

吸烟对胎儿的生长发育有不良影响，因此孕期禁止吸烟。影响的机制如下（图 7-2）。

Smoking has an adverse effect on fetal growth and development and is therefore contraindicated in pregnancy. The mechanisms for these effects are as follows (Fig. 7.2):

- 一氧化碳对胎儿的影响：一氧化碳对血红蛋白的亲和力是氧气的 200 倍。新鲜空气中含有

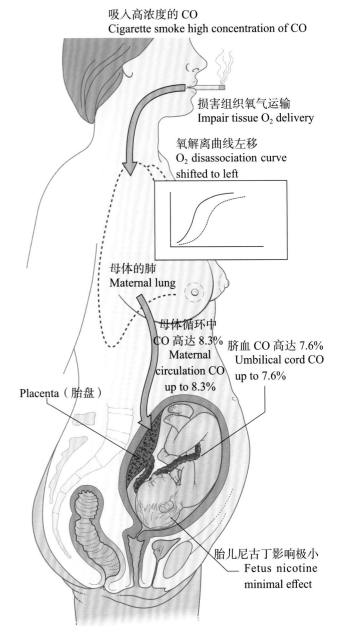

▲ 图 7-2　吸烟对胎儿胎盘单位的影响

Fig. 7.2　The effects of smoking on the fetoplacental unit

0.5ppm 的一氧化碳，但在香烟烟雾中可检测到高达 60 000ppm 的一氧化碳。一氧化碳使胎儿和母体血红蛋白的氧离解曲线左移。母体一氧化碳饱和度在母体中可能上升到 8%，在胎儿中可能上升到 7%，因此对氧转移有特定的干扰。

- *The effect of carbon monoxide on the fetus*. Carbon monoxide has an affinity for haemoglobin 200 times greater than oxygen. Fresh air contains up to 0.5 ppm of carbon monoxide, but in cigarette smoke values as high as 60,000 ppm may be detected. Carbon monoxide shifts the oxygen dissociation curve to the left in both fetal and maternal haemoglobin. Maternal carbon monoxide saturation may rise to 8% in the mother and 7% in the fetus so that there is specific interference with oxygen transfer.

- 尼古丁作为血管收缩物对子宫胎盘血管系统的影响：关于尼古丁输注对心输出量影响的动物研究表明，高剂量的尼古丁输注会导致心输出量和子宫胎盘血流量下降。然而，当尼古丁浓度比吸烟者高出 5 倍时，影响不显著，因此尼古丁不太可能通过减少子宫胎盘血流量而产生任何不良影响。

- *The effect of nicotine on the uteroplacental vasculature as a vasoconstrictor.* Animal studies on the effect of infusions of nicotine on cardiac output have shown that high-dose infusions produce a fall in cardiac output and uteroplacental blood flow. However, at levels up to five times greater than those seen in smokers, there are no measurable effects, and it is therefore unlikely that nicotine exerts any adverse effects by reducing uteroplacental blood flow.

- 吸烟对胎盘结构的影响：主要是胎盘形态的一些改变。滋养层基底膜不规则增厚，部分胎儿毛细血管管径缩小。这些不持续或不明显的变化与胎盘体积的明显缩小无关。被动吸烟女性的形态结构变化尚未得到证实。

- *The effect of smoking on placental structure.* Some changes are seen in the placental morphology. The trophoblastic basement membrane shows irregular thickening, and some of the fetal capillaries show reduced calibre. These changes are not consistent or gross and are not associated with any gross reduction in placental size. The morphological changes have not been demonstrated in those women subjected to passive smoking.

- 对围产儿死亡率的影响：孕期吸烟会减轻婴儿出生体重和缩短身长。吸烟直接增加围产儿的死亡率，那些每天吸烟多达 20 支的女性，这一风险被量化为 20%，而每天吸烟超过 20 支的女性，这一风险达到 35%。

- *The effect on perinatal mortality.* Smoking during pregnancy reduces the birth weight of the infant and reduces the crown-heel length. Perinatal mortality is increased as a direct effect of smoking, and this risk has been quantified at 20% for those women who smoke up to 20 cigarettes per day and 35% in excess of one packet per day.

建议妊娠期戒烟。对于吸烟但戒烟困难的女性，可以考虑使用尼古丁替代疗法（贴片）使伤害最小化。

Women should be advised to stop smoking during pregnancy. The use of nicotine replacement therapy (patches) as a harm-minimization option for women who smoke and feel unable to quit can be considered.

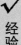

> **经验** 矛盾的是，有大量的证据表明，孕期吸烟的女性患先兆子痫的概率大大降低。然而，如果她们确实患上了先兆子痫，围产期死亡的风险会显著增加。
>
> Paradoxically, there is a considerable volume of evidence to show that women who smoke in pregnancy have a substantially reduced chance of developing pre-eclampsia. However, if they do develop pre-eclampsia, there is a significantly increased risk of perinatal loss.

（二）酒精摄入（Alcohol intake）

每天摄入 8 种或 8 种以上标准含酒精饮料可导致胎儿酒精综合征（fetal alcohol syndrome，FAS）。这种婴儿的特征包括生长受限、各种结构缺陷，特别是面部缺陷、多关节畸形和心脏畸形。长期饮酒的女性，由于饮食摄入不足，通常会伴有维生素和矿物质的缺乏。越来越多的人意识到胎儿酒精谱系障碍（fetal alcohol spectrum disorder，FASD），这可归因于孕期饮酒对神经发育和行为的一系列影响，呈剂量依赖性。所有备孕和妊娠期女性都应被询问饮酒情况，并被告知可能对胎儿产生的不利影响。妊娠期间饮酒安全程度的有关研究尚无明确结论，因此建议不饮酒是最安全的。

Fetal alcohol syndrome (FAS) has been attributed to consumption of eight or more standard drinks per day. Features in the infant include growth restriction, various structural defects and, in particular, facial defects, multiple joint anomalies and cardiac defects. Women who drink alcohol at this rate often have concomitant vitamin and mineral deficiencies due to inadequate diet. Increasingly, there is awareness of fetal alcohol spectrum disorder (FASD), a range of neurodevelopmental and behavioural effects attributable to alcohol consumption in pregnancy in a dose-dependent manner. All women considering pregnancy, and during pregnancy, should be asked about consumption of alcohol and provided education on the potential for adverse effects on the fetus. Research is not clear as to what level of alcohol consumption is safe in pregnancy, so a recommendation to abstain from any consumption is the safest choice.

（三）非法用药（Illicit drug use）

常见的妊娠期滥用的非法药物有苯丙胺、类阿片、可卡因和大麻。这些药物对母体和胎儿都有不良反应，其包括与生活方式和营养不良有关的不良影响。

The common forms of illicit substance misuse that occur during pregnancy are from amphetamines, opioids, cocaine and marijuana. All of these drugs have adverse effects on both the mother and the fetus, including the adverse effects related to lifestyle and malnutrition.

安非他明的使用，特别是冰毒，已成为妊娠期滥用最严重的药物，这与社会广泛使用增加相关。妊娠期使用会增加流产、早产、生长受限、胎盘早剥、胎死宫内和胎儿发育异常的风险。建议转诊到药物依赖性服务机构寻求治疗建议。

Amphetamine use, especially crystal methamphetamine (Ice), has become the most significantly misused drug in pregnancy, paralleling increased use in wider society. Use in pregnancy is associated with an increased risk of miscarriage, pre-term birth, growth restriction, placental abruption, fetal death in utero and developmental anomalies. Referral to a drug dependency service for advice on cessation is recommended.

阿片类药物成瘾与胎儿宫内生长受限、围产期死亡和早产的发生率增加有关。除海洛因外，滥用羟考酮和氢吗啡酮等处方类阿片药物也引起越来越多的关注。此外，许多宫内阿片暴露的婴儿会出现新生儿戒断症状。母亲应被转介到戒毒所戒除海洛因并进行美沙酮或丁丙诺啡替代治疗。

Opioid addiction is associated with an increased incidence of intrauterine growth restriction, perinatal death and pre-term labour. In addition to heroin, misuse of prescription opioids such as oxycodone and hydromorphone is causing increasing concern. Furthermore, many infants with intrauterine opioid exposure will suffer from neonatal withdrawal manifestations. The mother should be referred to a drug dependence service for withdrawal of heroin and replacement with methadone or buprenorphine.

吸食可卡因可引起母亲心律失常、中枢神经系统损害、胎盘早剥、胎儿生长受限和早产。对可卡因上瘾的管理旨在戒除。

Cocaine usage may induce cardiac arrhythmias and central nervous system damage in mothers as well as placental abruption, fetal growth restriction and pre-term labour. Management of cocaine addiction is directed at withdrawing the drug.

大麻对妊娠没有明显的不良影响，尽管 9– 四氢大麻酚的活性成分已被证明对动物有致畸作用。这通常与大量的烟草使用有关，同前所述，这会产生严重的有害影响。

Marijuana has no apparent adverse effect on pregnancy, although the active ingredient of 9-tetrahydrocannabinol has been shown to have teratogenic effects in animal studies. Consumption is usually associated with significant tobacco use, which has major detrimental effects as outlined earlier.

（四）孕期性生活（Coitus in pregnancy）

在正常妊娠的任何阶段都没有性生活的禁忌证，除了腹部大小变化造成的生理困难。然而，在有先兆流产或有反复流产史的情况下，避免性交是明智的。由于性生活有引起感染的危险，若有胎膜早破迹象和孕期流血史的女性，最好避免性生活。患有前置胎盘的女性也应避免性生活。

There are no contraindications to coitus in normal pregnancies at any stage of gestation other than the physical difficulties imposed by changes in abdominal size. It is, however, sensible to avoid coitus where there is evidence of threatened miscarriage or a previous history of recurrent miscarriage. Because of the risk of introducing infection, it is also advisable to avoid coitus where there is evidence of pre-labour rupture of the membranes and where there is a history of antepartum haemorrhage. Women with a known placenta praevia are also advised to avoid intercourse.

十一、乳房护理（Breast care）

除外有可能对胎儿或母亲造成不良后果的特定禁忌证，应鼓励所有女性进行母乳喂养。既往的乳房损伤或破裂或乳头严重内陷可能会使母乳喂养困难。部分药物可通过母乳对婴儿造成损害，这种情况下禁止母乳喂养。一些母体感染，如艾滋病病毒感染，是禁止母乳喂养的。然而，这些情况并不常见，在大多数情况下，母亲应知道母乳喂养对母体及胎儿皆有益处。

Breast-feeding should be encouraged in all women unless there are specific contraindications that would have adverse fetal or maternal consequences. Previous damage or surgery to the breasts or grossly inverted nipples may make breast-feeding difficult. There are also a small number of medications that are concentrated in breast milk and may be hazardous for the infant, in which case breast-feeding is contraindicated. In some maternal infections, such as HIV, breast-feeding is contraindicated. However, these circumstances are uncommon and, in most conditions, the mother should be advised of the benefits to both her child and herself of breast-feeding.

在产前，应鼓励孕妇保持良好的个人卫生，其中包括乳房护理。特别是在妊娠晚期，尤其是在经产女性中，初乳可能从乳头溢出。乳房应该用合适的孕妇胸罩支撑。对于有潜在哺乳困难的高危因素，如困难喂养史或乳房手术史的女性，在产前应提供哺乳咨询。

In the antenatal period, good personal hygiene, including breast care, should be encouraged. Colostrum may leak from the nipples, particularly in the third trimester, especially in multiparous women. The breasts should be supported with an appropriate maternity brassiere. Antenatal referral to a lactation consultant for women who have risk factors for potentially encountering difficulty with breast-feeding, such as previous difficulty or breast surgery, should be offered.

十二、社会文化意识（Social and cultural awareness）

妊娠和分娩是目前接受产前护理的女性生活复杂性的一部分。广泛的支持性讨论将使卫生保健从业人员能够了解女性及其生活的其他方面，其中包括社会和文化因素，这些因素可能对其妊娠结局产生深远影响。不同的文化信仰和期望、社会经济地位和支持、相互竞争的生活优先次序和教育水平都会对妊娠结局产生强烈影响。认可和尊重文化多样性将有助于向所有女性提供适当和及时的产前及围产期护理。

Pregnancy and childbirth form one part of the complexities of life for the women who present for antenatal care. Supportive and extensive discussion will enable health care practitioners to develop an understanding of the woman and the other aspects in her life, including social and cultural factors, which may have a profound impact on her pregnancy outcome. Different cultural beliefs and expectations, socioeconomic status and supports, competing life priorities and levels of education can all impact strongly on pregnancy outcome. Acknowledgement and respect of cultural diversity will assist in providing appropriate and timely antenatal and peripartum care to all women.

十三、孕期安全处方（Safe prescribing in pregnancy）

使用处方药和非处方药，以及补充和替代药物是很常见的。有些女性需要对已有疾病进行持续治疗，如癫痫或哮喘。有些疾病可能在妊娠过程中重新出现并需要治疗，如妊娠期糖尿病和血栓栓塞。简单的镇痛药、解热药、抗组胺药和镇吐药都很常见。这里不讨论有关单个药物的风险和益处。关于妊娠期和哺乳期药物种类的安全性，大多数药物处方中都有大量信息。可靠的网上资源通常很有帮助，如 www.motherisk.org 可随时使用。孕期用药最安全的方法是经常进行检查。很多药物在妊娠或哺乳期使用是没有不良后果的。

The use of prescription and over-the-counter medications, as well as complementary and alternative medications, is common. Some women will require ongoing treatment of pre-existing medical conditions, e.g. epilepsy or asthma. Some conditions may develop de novo in pregnancies that require therapy, e.g. gestational diabetes and thromboembolism. Simple analgesics, antipyretics, antihistamines and antiemetics are all commonly consumed. A discussion of the risks and benefits of individual medications is beyond the scope of this text. Extensive information is available in most drug formularies about the safety of categories of drugs in pregnancy and lactation. Reputable online resources such as www.motherisk.org are available around the clock and are often helpful. The safest course before prescribing in pregnancy is to always check. Many medications have been shown to have no adverse outcomes when used in pregnancy or lactation.

本章概览	Essential information
产前保健的基本目标	**Basic aims of antenatal care**
• 确保母体的最佳健康状态	• To ensure optimal maternal health
• 发现和治疗疾病，确保母儿健康	• To detect and treat disorders to ensure a healthy mother and infant
孕前保健	**Pre-conception care**
• 风疹、水痘、百日咳和流感免疫接种	• Immunization for rubella, varicella, pertussis and influenza as indicated
• 补充叶酸和碘	• Folic acid and iodine supplementation
• 优化母体的健康状态	• Optimization of maternal health

（续表）

本章概览	Essential information
妊娠人口结构的变化 • 产妇年龄持续增加 • 辅助生殖技术使用的增加	**Changing demographics of pregnancy** • Increasing maternal age • Increasing use of ART
常规筛查项目 • 血液学调查，检测易感人群中的贫血和血红蛋白病 • 血型和抗体；预防溶血性疾病	**Routine screening tests** • Haematological investigations to detect anaemia, and haemoglobinopathies in susceptible groups • Blood group and antibodies; prevention of Rhesus disease
传染病筛查 • 风疹、水痘、梅毒、乙型和丙型肝炎、艾滋病病毒、B 族链球菌	**Infection screening** • Rubella, varicella, syphilis, hepatitis B and C, HIV, GBS
筛查母体疾病 • 糖尿病 • 尿路感染	**Screening for maternal disorders** • Diabetes • Urinary tract infection
胎儿异常检查 • 颈项透明层厚度 • NIPT • 孕中期超声检查 • 侵入性诊断性检测	**Testing for fetal anomalies** • Nuchal translucency • NIPT • Second-trimester ultrasound • Invasive diagnostic testing
产前教育 • 饮食建议 • 运动 • 孕期药物使用 　– 吸烟 　– 饮酒 　– 非法药物 • 性生活	**Antenatal education** • Dietary advice • Exercise • Substance use in pregnancy 　– Smoking 　– Alcohol 　– Illicit drugs • Coitus

第 8 章　产科疾病

Obstetric disorders

Henry G. Murray　著　　孟金来　译　　杨慧霞　校

学习目标	LEARNING OBJECTIVES
学习本章后你应当掌握：	After studying this chapter you should be able to:
知识标准	**Knowledge criteria**
• 描述妊娠期主要产科并发症的病理生理学、病因和表现：	• Describe the pathophysiology, aetiology and presentation of the major antenatal complications of pregnancy:
－ 妊娠期高血压疾病	– Hypertension in pregnancy
－ 产前出血和胎盘植入	– Antepartum haemorrhage and placenta accreta
－ 多胎妊娠，臀位	– Multiple pregnancy, breech presentation
－ 胎位异常、不稳定胎位和过期妊娠	– Abnormal and unstable lie and prolonged pregnancy
临床能力	**Clinical competencies**
• 上述产科并发症的初步诊治与处理	• Plan initial investigations and management of these obstetric disorders
• 患产科疾病的孕妇检查、血液和尿液检测的结果	• Interpret the investigation results of scan, blood and urine tests performed in cases of obstetric disorders
• 向孕妇及家属阐明产科疾病的愈后	• Explain to the mother and her partner the consequences of the obstetric disorder
专业技能及态度	**Professional skills and attitudes**
• 当因产科疾病而发生不良事件时，应对孕妇及其家属表示同情	• Empathize with the woman and her family should an adverse event occur as a result of an obstetric disorder

一、妊娠期高血压疾病（Hypertensive disorders of pregnancy）

妊娠期高血压疾病仍然是发达国家最常见的妊娠并发症，也一直是导致孕产妇死亡的主要原因之一。不同国家受到多种因素的影响其发病率差异较大，其中包括产次、种族和食物摄入量。在英国，10%～15% 的孕妇会发生妊娠期高血压，4%～13% 的人会发展为子痫前期，即高血压伴蛋白尿的发生。虽然大多数高血压发生都与妊娠有关，并在终止妊娠后消失，但也有一些患有其他形式高血压的孕妇，如原发性高血压或因肾脏疾病引起的高血压，高血压将会持续存在。高血压疾病可能会影响妊娠过程甚至影响妊娠结局。

Hypertensive disorders remain the commonest complication of pregnancy in the developed world and are consistently one of the main causes of maternal death. The incidence varies substantially in different countries and is influenced by a number of factors, including parity, ethnic group and dietary intake. In the UK, the condition occurs in 10–15% of all pregnancies, and 4–13% of the population will develop pre-eclampsia, i.e. hypertension with proteinuria. While most episodes of hypertension are specifically related to the pregnancy and will resolve when the pregnancy is completed, some women who suffer from other forms of hypertension, e.g. essential hypertension or that due to renal disease, will continue to have raised blood pressure (BP). These diseases may influence the outcome of the pregnancy, and the progress of the disease may be influenced by the pregnancy.

对轻度患者，高血压在妊娠晚期出现，对孕妇和胎儿影响小。

In its mildest form, hypertension alone arising in late pregnancy appears to be of minimal risk to mother or child.

但对重度患者，会并发胎盘早剥、抽搐、蛋白尿、重度水肿甚至危及生命的严重后果，也可能导致脑出血、肝肾衰竭及弥散性血管内凝血（disseminated intravascular coagulopathy，DIC），甚至可能导致胎儿及产妇死亡。

In its most severe form, the condition is associated with placental abruption, convulsions, proteinuria, severe oedema and life-threatening hypertension, which may result in cerebral haemorrhage, renal and hepatic failure, as well as disseminated intravascular coagulopathy (DIC). This may lead to fetal and maternal death.

关于抽搐和妊娠之间的联系在古希腊和埃及的著作中有描述。1897 年，Vasquez 首次对子痫进行了描述，症状为抽搐、高血压和蛋白尿。

The association between convulsions and pregnancy was described in ancient Greek and Egyptian writings. The first description of eclampsia, with the occurrence of convulsions, hypertension and proteinuria, was given by Vasquez in 1897.

（一）定义（Definitions）

妊娠期高血压是指收缩压≥140mmHg 和（或）舒张压≥90mmHg，2 次测量时间至少间隔 4h。舒张压是在 Korotkoff 第五音时测得的，在妊娠的状况下，听不到该音；在这种情况下，有必要使用第四音。

Hypertension in pregnancy is defined as a systolic pressure above 140 mmHg or a diastolic pressure above 90 mmHg on two or more occasions at least 4 hours apart. Diastolic pressure is taken at the fifth Korotkoff sound. At times in pregnancy, there is no fifth sound; in these circumstances, it is necessary to use the fourth sound.

高血压的其他定义还包括收缩压上升至少 30mmHg 和（或）舒张压上升至少 15mmHg。若收缩压低于 140mmHg 或舒张压低于 90mmHg，尚无证据表明这些孕妇会发生不良后果。

Some definitions of hypertension also include reference to a rise in systolic pressure of at least 30 mmHg or a rise in diastolic pressure of at least 15 mmHg. There is no evidence that these women have adverse outcomes if the systolic BP remains less than 140 mmHg or diastolic less than 90 mmHg.

蛋白尿是指 24h 尿蛋白浓度大于 0.3g/L，或间隔至少 6h 的两次或两次以上随机采样尿蛋白浓度大于 1g/L。

Proteinuria is defined as the presence of urinary protein in concentrations greater than 0.3 g/L in a 24-hour collection or in concentrations greater than 1 g/L on a random sample on two or more occasions at least 6 hours apart.

水肿是指出现了凹陷性水肿或在一周内体重增加超过 2.3kg。水肿部位在四肢，特别是脚部、脚踝及手指，或者腹壁和面部（图 8-1）。水肿在无妊娠并发症中也很常见。这不是妊娠高血压疾病的特征性表现。因此，目前它已不作为诊断妊娠期高血压疾病的一部分。

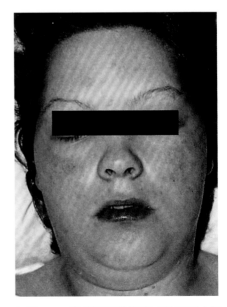

▲ 图 8-1　重度子痫前期患者的面部水肿

Fig. 8.1　Facial oedema in severe pre-eclampsia

Oedema is defined as the development of pitting oedema or a weight gain in excess of 2.3 kg in a week. Oedema occurs in the limbs, particularly in the feet and ankles and in the fingers, or in the abdominal wall and face (Fig. 8.1). Oedema is very common in otherwise uncomplicated pregnancies. This is the least useful sign of hypertensive disease. It has therefore been dropped from many classifications of pregnancy-induced hypertension.

（二）分类（Classification）

高血压的分类如下。

The various types of hypertension are classified as follows:

- 妊娠期高血压其特点是在妊娠 20 周后或产后 24h 内出现高血压，之前无任何高血压诊断；根据定义，血压应该在妊娠结束 12 周后恢复正常，但多数产妇通常在分娩后 10 天内血压就恢复了正常。

- 子痫前期是指妊娠 20 周后出现高血压伴有蛋白尿。首次妊娠的女性更常见。

- 子痫是子痫前期基础上发生不能用其他原因解释的抽搐。

- 慢性高血压并发子痫前期是指可能是由各种病理原因引起的，妊娠前已存在高血压的情况。

- 并发的子痫前期 – 子痫是患有慢性高血压或肾脏疾病的孕妇并发子痫前期。

- 未分类高血压包括那些随机产生的妊娠期高血压病例，这些病例没有足够的分类信息。

- Gestational hypertension is characterized by the new onset of hypertension without any features of pre-eclampsia after 20 weeks of pregnancy or within the first 24 hours postpartum. Although by definition the blood pressure should return to normal by 12 weeks after pregnancy; it usually returns to normal within 10 days after delivery.

- Pre-eclampsia is the development of hypertension with proteinuria after the twentieth week of gestation. It is more commonly a disorder of women in their first pregnancy.

- Eclampsia is defined as the development of convulsions secondary to pre-eclampsia in the mother.

- Chronic hypertensive disease is the condition in which hypertension has been present before pregnancy and may be due to various pathological causes.

- Superimposed pre-eclampsia or eclampsia is the development of pre-eclampsia in a woman with chronic hypertensive disease or renal disease.

- Unclassified hypertension includes those cases of hypertension arising in pregnancy on a random basis where there is insufficient information for classification.

> **！注意**
>
> 蛋白尿的发展是改变母婴预后的关键因素。那些单独患有高血压的女性往往胎儿发育正常，婴儿预后良好；而那些伴有蛋白尿孕妇的胎盘改变与胎儿生长受限的发生有关，胎儿预后较差。从治疗的角度来看，只有在终止妊娠后才能做出最终诊断，所以必须假定所有患有高血压的孕妇都被认为存在风险。
>
> The critical factor that changes the prognosis for the mother and infant is the development of proteinuria. Those women who develop hypertension alone tend to have normal fetal growth with a good prognosis for the infant, whereas those who develop proteinuria have placental changes that are associated with intrauterine growth restriction and a poorer fetal prognosis. From a management point of view, the final diagnosis can only be made after the pregnancy has been completed, so the assumption must be made that any woman who develops hypertension must be considered to be at risk.

（三）子痫前期和子痫的发病机制和病理（Pathogenesis and pathology of pre-eclampsia and eclampsia）

子痫前期病因和发病机制尚未完全阐明。几乎身体的各个主要系统都参与该疾病的发生。因此，每个系统似乎都有变化，但不一定会对此产生重要作用。

The exact nature of the pathogenesis of pre-eclampsia remains uncertain. Nearly every major system in the body is affected by the advanced manifestations of the condition. Therefore, every system that is studied appears to show changes without necessarily doing more than manifesting secondary effects.

如图 8-2 所示，该疾病的病理生理学有如下 2 个特点。

- 全身小动脉痉挛：特别是在子宫、胎盘和肾脏的血管床。

- 弥散性血管内凝血。

The pathophysiology of the condition, as outlined in Figure 8.2, is characterized by the effects of:

- Arteriolar vasoconstriction, particularly in the vascular

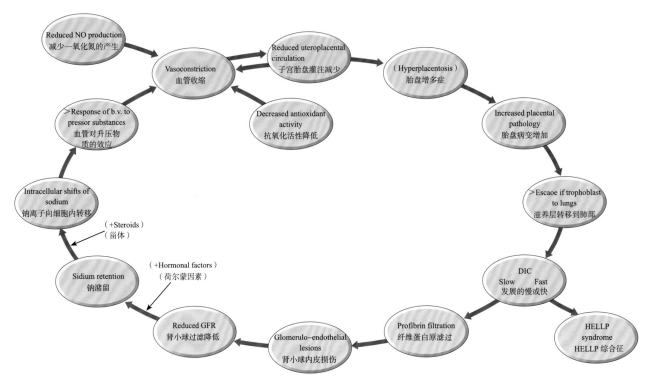

▲ 图 8-2　子痫前期发病机制中的循环

b.v. 血管；DIC. 弥散性血管内凝血；GFR. 肾小球滤过率；HELLP. 溶血 – 肝酶升高 – 血小板减少；NO. 一氧化氮

Fig. 8.2　The cycle of changes involved in the pathogenesis of pre-eclampsia.

b.v., Blood vessels; DIC, disseminated intravascular coagulation; GFR, glomerular filtration rate; HELLP, haemolysis-elevated liver enzymes-low platelets; NO, nitric oxide.

bed of the uterus, placenta and kidneys

• DIC

血压由心输出量（每搏量 × 心率）和外周血管阻力决定。心输出量在正常妊娠时显著增加，但血压通常在妊娠中期下降。因此，最重要的调节因素是妊娠期间外周阻力的降低。如果没有这种效应，所有孕妇将会患上高血压！

Blood pressure is determined by cardiac output (stroke volume × heart rate) and peripheral vascular resistance. Cardiac output increases substantially in normal pregnancy, but blood pressure normally falls in the mid-trimester. Thus, the most important regulatory factor is the loss of peripheral resistance that occurs in pregnancy. Without this effect, all pregnant women would presumably become hypertensive!

交感神经张力保持不变，外周阻力由体液血管扩张物质和血管收缩物质之间的平衡决定。在妊娠时，血管紧张素 II 的敏感性降低，血管紧张素 II 通常对抗局部活性血管扩张物质前列腺素的作用，导致全身血管扩张。然而，任何使肾素 – 血管紧张素系统活性或降低组织前列腺素活性的因素增加都会

导致血压升高，从而阻碍正常的妊娠变化。

As sympathetic tone appears to remain unchanged, peripheral resistance is determined by the balance between humoral vasodilators and vasoconstrictors. In pregnancy, there is a specific loss of sensitivity to angiotensin II, which normally counters the effect of locally active vasodilator prostaglandins, resulting in systemic vasodilatation. However, any factors that increase the activity of the renin-angiotensin system or reduce the activity of tissue prostaglandins will result in raising of the BP, thus countering the normal pregnancy changes.

子痫前期孕妇对血管紧张素 II 具有一定的敏感性，而且有证据表明血小板血管紧张素 II 受体升高，增加了血管收缩和血小板聚集的机会。

Pre-eclamptic women appear to retain some sensitivity to infused angiotensin II, and there is evidence that platelet AII receptors are increased, all of which increases the chance of vasoconstriction and platelet aggregation.

目前证据表明，子痫前期是一种内皮功能障碍的疾病。一氧化氮（NO）或内皮源性舒张因子（EDRF）是一种有效的血管扩张物质。在子痫前期中，NO 合成降低，可能是因为 NO 合成酶活性受到抑制。

Current evidence also suggests that pre-eclampsia is a disease of endothelial dysfunction. Nitric oxide (NO) or endothelial-derived relaxing factor (EDRF) is a potent vasodilator. In pre-eclampsia, NO synthesis is reduced, possibly because of an inhibition of NO synthetase activity.

另一个需要考虑的因素是脂质过氧化物对内皮细胞的损害作用，正常情况下，抗氧化物质会阻碍这些作用，但在子痫前期，抗氧化活性低，全身内皮损伤，导致血管内液体流失。这些变化发生在妊娠中期，通常早于孕妇血压升高之前。

A further area of consideration is the damaging effect of lipid peroxides on the endothelium. Normally, the production of antioxidants limits these effects, but in preeclampsia, antioxidant activity is decreased and endothelial damage occurs throughout the body, resulting in fluid loss from the intravascular space. All these changes occur in the second trimester long before a rise in BP is measurable in the mother.

一旦胎盘床发生血管收缩，就会导致胎盘损伤，并随之释放滋养层因子进入外周循环。滋养层因子富含凝血酶素，可引起不同程度的 DIC。这一过程会导致病理改变，最显著的部位在肾、肝和胎盘床。肾损伤导致钠和水潴留，其中大部分液体由于血管内皮损伤而移动到细胞外间隙，从而导致液体外渗。事实上，重度子痫前期患者的血管内空间会随血浆容量的减少而减少。同时，钠潴留的增加会导致血管对血管收缩物质的敏感性增加，从而发生恶性循环，进一步促进血管收缩和组织损伤，最终可能导致急性肾衰竭合并肾小管或皮质坏死、肝衰竭合并门静脉周围坏死、急性心力衰竭和肺水肿，甚至随着血压失控而发生脑出血。

Once vasoconstriction occurs in the placental bed, it results in placental damage and the consequent release of trophoblastic material into the peripheral circulation. This trophoblastic material is rich in thromboplastins, which precipitate variable degrees of DIC. This process gives rise to the pathological lesions, most notably in the kidney, liver and placental bed. The renal lesion results in sodium and water retention, with most of this fluid moving to the extracellular space due to vascular endothelial damage which permits fluid extravasation. In fact, the intravascular space is reduced in severe pre-eclampsia as plasma volume diminishes. At the same time, increased sodium retention results in increased vascular sensitivity to vasoconstrictor influences, which promotes further vasoconstriction and tissue damage in a vicious circle of events that may ultimately result in acute renal failure with tubular or cortical necrosis, hepatic failure with periportal necrosis, acute cardiac failure and pulmonary oedema, and even cerebral haemorrhage as BP becomes uncontrolled.

随着血管进一步收缩，胎盘梗死进一步加重，胎儿生长受限、胎盘早剥发病率增加，甚至导致胎儿死亡。

As the vasoconstriction progresses, the placenta becomes grossly infarcted, and this results in intrauterine growth restriction, increased risk of abruption and sometimes fetal death.

为什么有些孕妇会患有子痫前期，而有些则不会？在女性身上是否存在遗传易感性？第二个问题的答案几乎是肯定的。在美国、冰岛和苏格兰进行的纵向研究表明，患有子痫前期或子痫女性的女儿有 25% 的概率患上这种疾病，这一风险是其他女性患有该病风险的 2.5 倍。数据表明，母亲单一的隐性基因与子痫前期发生有关。然而，这些数据也支持另一个假设，即该病具有部分外显率的显性遗传。虽然目前已找出各种不同的基因位点，但需较长期的研究对其进一步探索，以确定明确的潜在基因。事实上，单一的子痫前期致病基因不会存在；可能是几个基因之间有相互作用，外部环境因素加强这种可能性。这些因素包括自身免疫性疾病、动静脉血栓栓塞性疾病及潜在的慢性肾脏疾病或原发性高血压。另外，食物热量摄入也可能是一个潜在的危险因素。

Why do some women develop pre-eclampsia and others do not? Is there a genetic predisposition in some women? The answer to this second question is almost certainly yes. Longitudinal studies in the United States, Iceland and Scotland have shown that the daughters of women who have suffered from pre-eclampsia or eclampsia have themselves a one in four chance of developing the disease, a risk that is 2.5 times higher than in the daughters-in-law of such women. The data suggest that a single recessive maternal gene is associated with pre-eclampsia. However, the data could also support a hypothetical model of dominant inheritance with partial penetrance. Although various gene loci have been proposed, further long-term studies are ongoing to try and identify the correct candidate gene. It is in fact unlikely that there is a single pre-eclampsia gene; it is probable that there are interactions between several genes, with external environmental factors enhancing this predisposition. These factors include autoimmune conditions, diseases that increase venous and arterial thromboembolic disease (thrombophilias) and the existence of underlying chronic renal disease or essential hypertension. Dietary intake may also be a factor.

1. 肾损害（The renal lesion）

组织学上的肾脏病变是子痫前期最特异的特征

（图 8-3），具体包括以下 3 点。

- 内皮细胞的肿胀和增生，导致毛细血管阻塞。

- 毛细血管间或系膜细胞的肥大和增生。

- 纤维物质（原纤维蛋白）沉积在基底膜上和内皮细胞之间。

The renal lesion is, histologically, the most specific feature of pre-eclampsia (Fig. 8.3). The features are:

- Swelling and proliferation of endothelial cells to such a point that the capillary vessels are obstructed.
- Hypertrophy and hyperplasia of the intercapillary or mesangial cells.
- Fibrillary material (profibrin) deposition on the basement membrane and between and within the endothelial cells.

因此，特征性的表现是毛细血管细胞增多和血管减少。发生子痫前期的初产妇中只有 71% 发生这种病变，但经产妇中有 29% 会发生该病变。经产妇慢性肾脏疾病的发病率要比初产妇高得多。

The characteristic appearance is therefore one of increased capillary cellularity and reduced vascularity. The lesion is found in 71% of primigravid women who develop pre-eclampsia but in only 29% of multiparous women. There is a much higher incidence of women with chronic renal disease in multiparous women.

肾小球病变通常有蛋白尿发生和肾小球滤过率降低有关，从而导致血清肌酐升高。肾血流量减少和近端肾小管病变导致尿酸排出障碍，从而导致高尿酸血症发生。

The glomerular lesion is always associated with proteinuria and with reduced glomerular filtration resulting in a raised serum creatinine. Decreased renal blood flow and proximal tubular changes result in impaired uric acid secretion, leading to hyperuricaemia.

2. 胎盘病变（Placental pathology）

胎盘梗死可发生在正常妊娠状态下，但在子痫前期中更为常见。胎盘有以下 5 点特征（图 8-4）。

- 合胞节或芽增加。

- 合胞体受损增加。

- 细胞滋养层细胞增多。

- 滋养层基底膜增厚。

- 绒毛坏死。

Placental infarcts occur in normal pregnancy but are considerably more extensive in pre-eclampsia. The characteristic features in the placenta (Fig. 8.4) include:

- increased syncytial knots or sprouts
- increased loss of syncytium
- proliferation of cytotrophoblast
- thickening of the trophoblastic basement membrane
- villous necrosis

在子宫胎盘床中，正常的绒毛外滋养层细胞沿着螺旋小动脉的管腔表面侵袭，但没有超越蜕膜肌层交界，螺旋动脉和蜕膜层的血管明显收缩（图 8-5）。这些变化会使胎盘灌注量减少，导致胎盘缺氧。

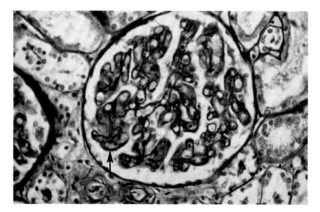

▲ 图 8-3 子痫前期肾脏改变包括内皮细胞肿胀，肾小球无血管化和基底膜下纤维蛋白沉积（箭）

Fig. 8.3 Renal changes in pre-eclampsia include endothelial swelling (E), apparent avascularity of the lomerulus and fibrin deposition (arrow) under the basement membrane.

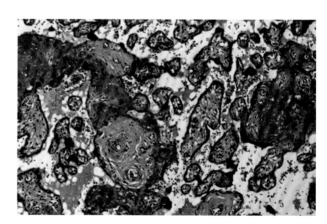

▲ 图 8-4 子痫前期胎盘改变包括合体结节增多、细胞滋养层细胞增殖和滋养细胞基底膜增厚

Fig. 8.4 Placental changes in pre-eclampsia include an increase in syncytial knots, proliferation of cytotrophoblast and thickening of trophoblastic basement membrane.

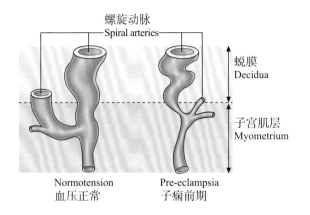

螺旋动脉
Spiral arteries

蜕膜
Decidua

子宫肌层
Myometrium

Normotension
血压正常

Pre-eclampsia
子痫前期

▲ 图 8-5　滋养细胞侵袭螺旋状小动脉导致血管扩张，这一过程参与子痫前期的发病机制

Fig. 8.5　Trophoblast invasion of the spiral arterioles results in dilatation of these vessels. This process is defective in pre-eclampsia.

In the uteroplacental bed, the normal invasion of extravillous cytotrophoblast along the luminal surface of the maternal spiral arterioles does not occur beyond the deciduomyometrial junction, and there is apparent constriction of the vessels between the radial artery and the decidual portion (Fig. 8.5). These changes result in reduced uteroplacental blood flow and in placental hypoxia.

3. 弥散性血管内凝血（Disseminated intravascular coagulation）

在重度子痫前期和子痫病例中，许多器官的毛细血管床上可以看到血栓的形成。大脑可以识别多个血小板和纤维蛋白血栓。在肝脏的门静脉周围区域、脾和肾上腺皮质也可以看到类似的变化。某些情况下可能会出现血小板减少，只有 10% 的子痫孕妇的血小板计数降至 100 000/ml 以下。由于纤维蛋白产量增加和纤溶功能受损，纤维蛋白沉积和循环系统中纤维蛋白降解产物增多。可以明确的是，虽然这些变化不是子痫前期的病因，但它们在疾病的病理过程中起到了重要作用。

In severe pre-eclampsia and eclampsia, thrombosis can be seen in the capillary bed of many organs. Multiple platelet and fibrin thrombi can be identified in the brain. Similar changes are seen in the periportal zones of the liver and in the spleen and the adrenal cortex. Thrombocytopenia may occur in some cases, but in only 10% of eclamptic women does the platelet count fall below 100,000/mL. There is an increase in fibrin deposition and in circulating fibrin degradation products as a result of increased fibrin production and impaired fibrinolysis. There seems to be little doubt that while these changes are not the cause of preeclampsia, they do play an important role in the pathology of the disease.

（四）其他与妊娠期高血压有关的因素（Other associations with pregnancy hypertension）

据推测，子痫前期可能是由于母体对胎盘反应异常。近亲婚配中子痫前期的发生率较低，第二次婚姻中首次妊娠期高血压的发病率较高。子痫前期孕妇的人类白细胞抗原（HLA）–G 水平有所改变。

It has been postulated that pre-eclampsia may be due to an abnormality of the maternal host response to placentation. There is a lower incidence of pre-eclampsia in consanguineous marriages and an increased incidence of hypertension in first pregnancies of second marriages. Levels of human leukocyte antigen (HLA)-G are altered in preeclamptic women.

细胞介导的免疫反应也被证明参与了重度子痫前期发生。然而，还有许多其他因素独立于潜在的免疫因素，如种族、气候条件和遗传或家族因素。其中，在子痫前期中发现游离脂肪酸的增加、糖尿病和肥胖在子痫前期发生中可能有致病作用。

Indices of cell-mediated immune response have also been shown to be altered in severe pre-eclampsia. However, there are many other factors that operate independently from any potential immunological factors, such as race, climatic conditions and genetic or familial factors. One of these includes raised free fatty acids found in pre-eclampsia and their possible causative role in the increased incidence of pre-eclampsia in women with diabetes and obesity.

1. HELLP 综合征（The HELLP syndrome）

子痫前期的严重并发症是一种被称为 HELLP 的综合征。该综合征有 3 种临床表现，溶血、肝酶水平升高和血小板计数降低。这是 DIC 的进一步发展的结果，会导致溶血和血小板减少，肝脏内皮细胞功能障碍 / 缺氧，导致肝脏氨基转移酶释放，特别是丙氨酸氨基转移酶的释放。

A severe manifestation of pre-eclampsia occurs in a variant known as the *HELLP syndrome*. In this syndrome, there is a triad of manifestations that include haemolysis (H), elevated levels of liver enzymes (EL) and a low platelet count (LP). This manifestation is an extension of the DIC causing the haemolysis and low platelets and the endothelial dysfunction/hypoxia in the liver resulting in the release of liver transaminases, especially the alanine aminotransferase (ALT).

血小板减少进展迅速，若任其发展，可能会导致大脑和肝出血。这种并发症需要及时干预，并在高血压控制稳定后立即考虑终止妊娠。

The thrombocytopenia is often rapidly progressive and if left to become severe may result in haemorrhage into the brain and the liver. The syndrome demands intervention and immediate consideration of termination of the pregnancy after any treatable manifestations like hypertension are controlled.

（五）妊娠期高血压和子痫前期的治疗（ Management of gestational hypertension and pre-eclampsia ）

治疗的目的是预防子痫的发生，将孕妇和胎儿可能发生的风险降至最低。达到这些目标有赖于密切关注孕妇及胎儿的情况，若继续妊娠的风险超过干预风险时，及时终止妊娠。

The object of management is to prevent the development of eclampsia and to minimize the risks of the condition to both the mother and the fetus. The achievement of these objectives depends on careful scrutiny of the condition of both the mother and the fetus and timely intervention to terminate the pregnancy when the risks of continuation outweigh the risks of intervention.

1. 测量血压（ Blood pressure measurement ）

在产检时，首先要注意的是血压升高。因体位的变化对血压值有一定影响，所以每次就诊时应以恒定的体位记录血压值。最舒适的体位是坐位，使用与妊娠期血压测量相匹配的血压计，并在右上臂使用合适大小的袖带。自动血压仪在妊娠期测量血压时可能不可靠。

A rise in BP is usually the first sign to be noted at the antenatal visit. BP should be recorded in a constant position at each visit, as it is posture dependent. The most comfortable position is seated, using a sphygmomanometer compatible with BP measurement in pregnancy and a cuff of an appropriate size applied to the right upper arm. Automated BP machines can be unreliable in measuring BP in pregnancy.

如果血压升高，应在短时间休息后重复测量。如果血压仍然升高，则需要继续密切观察。若高度怀疑子痫前期，可以通过住院来确诊，如果有不确定意义的高血压，可以到日间病房就诊，或者由助产师或家庭全科医生仔细检查是否患有高血压。建议这类孕妇休息，卧床休息可以改善肾脏灌注量和子宫胎盘血流量，会使尿量增多和血压有所改善，但没有证据表明卧床休息可改善母体或胎儿的整体预后。

If the pressure is elevated, the measurement should be repeated after a short period of rest. If the BP remains elevated, then continuing close observation is essential. This may be achieved by hospital admission if significant preeclampsia is suspected, a visit to a 'day ward' for hypertension of uncertain significance or careful scrutiny at home by a visiting midwife or the family general practitioner for the possibility of white coat

hypertension. The woman should be advised to rest. However, although bed rest improves renal blood flow and uteroplacental flow and commonly results in a diuresis and mild improvement in the BP, it has not been shown to improve overall outcomes in the mother or the fetus.

蛋白尿超过 1+ 或尿蛋白 / 肌酐比值超过 30mg/mmol 是密切监测孕妇妊娠状况的绝对指征，因为这种变化是孕妇和胎儿发生风险的分界线。

The development of more than 1+ proteinuria or a spot urinary protein/creatinine ratio of more than 30 mg/mmol is an absolute indication for close surveillance of the pregnancy, as this change constitutes the dividing line between minimal risk and significant risk to both mother and baby.

如果高血压持续或恶化，胎儿已足月或即将足月，应当终止妊娠。如果认为孕妇可以继续妊娠，则应考虑使用降压药治疗。切记，子痫前期延长孕周完全是为了胎儿的利益。

If the hypertension persists or worsens and the mother is at or close to term, the fetus should be delivered. If it is considered that the fetus would benefit from further time in utero and there is no maternal contraindication, treatment with antihypertensive drugs should be considered. It must be remembered that prolonging the pregnancy in pre-eclampsia is solely for the benefit of the fetus.

2. 降压药物治疗（ Antihypertensive drug therapy ）

在出现急性高血压危象时，用药控制血压是必不可少的。但发生轻度妊娠期高血压和子痫前期的情况时，药物的疗效是有争议的。有证据表明，在妊娠期间治疗轻度或中度慢性高血压可降低其发展为重度高血压的风险。

In the presence of an acute hypertensive crisis, controlling the BP with medication is essential, but in the case of mild gestational hypertension and moderate pre-eclampsia, their role is more contentious. There is, however, convincing evidence that the treatment of mild or moderate chronic hypertension in pregnancy reduces the risk of developing severe hypertension and the need for hospital admission.

对于患有妊娠期高血压的孕妇，降压药物的治疗应仅限于那些对保守治疗无效的孕妇，若情况允许，可卧床休息。早期降压治疗可能降低发展为肾性高血压的风险。治疗的目的是将产妇及胎儿的发病率和死亡率降至最低。收缩压或舒张压超过 170mmHg 或 110mmHg 的血压必须进行紧急处理，目的是降低脑出血和子痫的风险。最近，人们还认为，如果血压保持在 160/100mmHg 以上，孕妇存在脑出血的风险，降压治疗是必不可少的。根据英国产妇死亡调查 2011 年的数据表明，血压在 150/100mmHg 以上的孕妇需要治疗。

In women with gestational hypertension, treatment with antihypertensive drugs should be confined to those women who fail to respond to conservative management, including stopping work if that is possible. Early antihypertensive treatment possibly reduces the risk of progression to severe proteinuric hypertension. Management is based on the principle of minimizing both maternal and fetal morbidity and mortality. BPs of more than 170 mmHg systolic or 110 mmHg diastolic must be treated as a matter of urgency to lower the risk of intracerebral haemorrhage and eclampsia. Until recently it was believed that if BP stays above 160/100 mmHg, antihypertensive treatment is essential, as there is a risk of maternal cerebral haemorrhage. Data from the UK maternal death enquiry 2011 clearly show that treatment is warranted at levels above 150/100mmHg.

常用的药物包括以下几种。

- 甲基多巴（口服）。

- 肼苯哒嗪（口服和静脉注射）。

- α 受体拮抗药和 β 受体拮抗药联合使用，如拉贝洛尔（口服或静脉注射）。

- α 受体拮抗药，如哌唑嗪（口服）。

- 钙通道阻滞药，如硝苯地平（口服）。

注意：血管紧张素转化酶抑制药（ACEI）在妊娠期间是禁用的。

在需要紧急治疗的情况下，静脉推注 5mg 肼屈嗪或 20mg 拉贝洛尔。口服药物控制血压时可能需要一定时间。

The drugs most commonly used are:
- methyldopa (oral)
- hydralazine (oral and intravenous (IV))
- combined alpha- and beta-blockers such as labetalol (oral or IV)
- alpha-blocker such as prazosin (oral)
- calcium channel blockers such as nifedipine (oral)

Note: Angiotensin-converting enzyme (ACE) inhibitors are contraindicated in pregnancy.

Where acute control is required, an IV bolus of hydralazine 5 mg or labetalol 20 mg should be administered. Oral medications can take a variable time to control BP.

类固醇：若妊娠小于 34 周且伴有严重高血压，需终止妊娠的孕妇，每次给予倍他米松 12mg（译者注：原书剂量似有误，已修改）肌内注射，两次间隔 12～24h，以尽量减少早产儿的并发症，如呼吸窘迫综合征（RDS）、脑室出血和坏死性小肠结肠炎的发生。

Steroids: Where a woman is less than 34 weeks' gestation and her hypertensive disease is severe enough that early delivery is contemplated, betamethasone 11.4 mg intramuscularly (IM), two doses 12–24 hours apart. Should be given to minimize neonatal consequences of prematurity like respiratory distress syndrome (RDS), intraventricular haemorrhage and necrotizing enterocolitis.

3. 孕产妇研究（Maternal investigations）

对于孕妇监测最重要几点如下。

- 每 4h 测量 1 次血压，直到血压恢复正常。

- 定期检测尿液中是否含有尿蛋白。最初筛查方法根据用试纸或尿蛋白 / 肌酐比值，一旦确定尿液中含有尿蛋白，则应当收集 24h 尿样，24h 内尿蛋白超过 0.3g/L 为异常。

- 孕妇血清学筛查子痫前期。

The most important investigations for monitoring the mother are:
- The 4-hourly measurement of BP until such time that the BP has returned to normal.
- Regular urine checks for proteinuria. Initially, screening is done with dipsticks or spot urinary protein/creatinine ratio, but once proteinuria is established, 24-hour urine samples should be collected. Values in excess of 0.3 g/ L over 24 hours are abnormal.
- Maternal serum screening for pre-eclampsia.

（六）实验室研究（Laboratory investigations）

- 全血计数，特别是血小板计数和溶血。

- 肾功能和肝功能的监测。

- 尿酸测量：疾病进展的有效指标。

- 重度子痫前期和（或）血小板减少的凝血研究。

- 存在重度高血压的情况，特别是在没有蛋白尿的情况下应进行儿茶酚胺测定，排除嗜铬细胞瘤。

- Full blood count with particular reference to platelet count and haemolysis.
- Tests for renal and liver function.
- Uric acid measurements: a useful indicator of progression

in the disease.

- Clotting studies where there is severe pre-eclampsia
- and/or thrombocytopaenia.
- Catecholamine measurements in the presence of severe hypertension, particularly where there is no proteinuria, to rule out phaeochromocytoma.

（七）胎盘研究（Fetoplacental investigations）

子痫前期是胎儿生长受限和围产儿死亡的重要原因，因此使用以下方法监测胎儿健康至关重要。

- 超声检测

  - 每 2 周测量 1 次胎儿的发育状况。测量的胎儿双顶径、头围、腹围和股骨长度等参数。

  - 每周 2 次测量羊水量和胎儿多普勒检查。

  - 在临近分娩时进行胎心监测（CTG）检查。

Pre-eclampsia is an important cause of fetal growth restriction and perinatal death, and it is therefore essential to monitor fetal wellbeing using the following methods:

- Serial ultrasounds for:
  - Measurements of fetal growth every 2 weeks. Parameters measured are fetal biparietal diameter, head circumference, abdominal circumference and femur length.
  - Measurements of liquor volume and fetal Doppler studies up to twice weekly.
  - Daily cardiotocography (CTG) in advanced cases close to requiring delivery.

（八）胎儿多普勒（Doppler flow studies）

- 每次对胎儿进行评估时常使用多普勒波形测量、评估胎儿健康 / 氧合状态。脐动脉血流阻力是衡量胎盘血管完整性的一种指标，阻力增大是衡量小血管疾病的一种指标。胎儿大脑中动脉血流通常有高阻力模式，阻力下降与血管扩张和胎儿缺氧有关。当脐血管阻力超过中脑血管阻力时 [脑 / 胎盘比例（CPR）＜ 1]，胎儿将面临缺氧相关的并发症风险，因此这些参数对评估是否继续妊娠观察还是终止妊娠具有非常重要的参考价值。因子痫前期而出现生长受限的胎儿比正常生长的胎儿更有可能发生心肺异常。在任何情况下，胎儿脐动脉舒张期断流或反流提示有严重血管疾病，可能严重危及胎儿。若 CTG 出现异常，必须考虑终止妊娠。

- The use of serial Doppler waveform measurements in the fetus with every assessment of liquor is an essential part of assessment of the fetal wellbeing/oxygenation status. The resistance to flow in the umbilical artery is a measure of placental blood vessel integrity, with raised resistance being a measure of small-vessel disease. The fetal middle cerebral artery normally has a high resistance pattern, and a fall in resistance relates to vasodilatation and fetal hypoxia. Where the resistance in the umbilical vessels exceeds that in the middle cerebral vessels (cerebral/placental ratio (CPR) is less than 1), the fetus is at significant risk of morbidity associated with hypoxia. Consideration

病例分析	Case study
F 夫人长期患有不孕症，之后怀上了她的第一个孩子。她在妊娠前曾在医院行腹腔镜输卵管检查，但在妊娠过程中，没有任何迹象表明她患有高血压。妊娠 32 周时，她因急性头痛和严重高血压于晚上 10 时入院，血压值为 220/140mmHg。无蛋白尿，无反射亢进。没有胎儿生长受限迹象。一开始试图用静脉注射肼屈嗪和拉贝洛尔控制血压。终止妊娠后，她的血压值仍然很高且无法控制，随后出现心力衰竭，并于第二天早上 7 时死亡。尸检发现右侧肾上腺有一个巨大的嗜铬细胞瘤。	Mrs F was pregnant with her first child after a long history of subfertility. She had been admitted to hospital before her pregnancy for tubal evaluation by dye laparoscopy, but at no time then or subsequently during her pregnancy had she shown any evidence of hypertension. At 32 weeks' gestation, she was admitted to hospital at 10 PM with acute headache and severe hypertension, with a BP reading of 220/140 mmHg. There was no proteinuria and no hyper–reflexia. There was no evidence of fetal growth restriction. Despite initial attempts to control her BP with intravenous hydralazine and labetalol, and despite delivery of the fetus, her hypertension remained severe and uncontrollable and she went into high–output cardiac failure and died at 7 AM the following morning. Autopsy revealed a large phaeochromocytoma in the right adrenal gland.
这是一种非常罕见的妊娠期高血压。除非能及早发现并切除肿瘤，否则预后很差。这次，她发现得太晚了。所有产前血压记录均正常。虽然在这种情况中，血压值是正常的情况下是有参考价值的，重度高血压出现在妊娠早期，应当检测尿儿茶酚胺	This is an extremely rare form of hypertension in pregnancy. It has an appalling prognosis unless it is detected early and the tumour removed. In this case, it presented late. All other antenatal recordings of BP had been normal. Although it would not have helped in this case as the BP readings were always normal, where hypertension is severe and presents early in pregnancy, it is always worth checking urinary catecholamines.

must be given to very close observation or delivery of these pregnancies, regardless of the fetal growth parameters, albeit that fetuses that are growth restricted from maternal pre-eclampsia are more likely to have an abnormal CPR than an appropriately grown fetus. At any time, absent or reverse flow in diastole in the umbilical artery of the fetus indicates severe vessel disease, with probable severe fetal compromise, and delivery of the fetus must be considered if the CTG is abnormal.

- 作为一项单因素研究，14 周后对母体进行多普勒超声检测并未显示能有效纠正子痫前期的发生。

- As a single investigation, doppler ultrasound of maternal vessels after 14 weeks has not been shown to add to the ability to effectively treat maternal pre-eclampsia.

- 每日对子痫前期患者进行胎心监测：胎心监测结果与多普勒一起评估。胎心监测是检测胎儿健康的有效工具。正常的反应性示踪是确保胎儿无缺氧的表现。反复减速和基线变异性丧失是提示胎儿缺氧的强烈指征。较轻微的胎心监测结果异常可能被过度解释，导致过度诊断胎儿损害。因此，解读胎心监测时应当谨慎。

- Antenatal CTG measured daily in admitted cases of pre-eclampsia: CTG recordings are used in conjunction with Doppler assessment. The measurement of the antenatal CTG (fetal heart rate in relation to uterine activity) provides a useful tool in the detection of fetal wellbeing. A normal reactive trace is an assurance of a non-hypoxic fetus. A trace with recurrent decelerations and a loss of baseline variability is a strong indication of fetal metabolic acidaemia. Lesser anomalies on CTG trace can be over-interpreted, leading to an over-diagnosed fetal compromise. The CTG recording must therefore be interpreted with care.

妊娠高血压综合征的各种治疗流程如图 8-6 所示。该流程图显示了各种进展途径及其治疗方案。轻度高血压的最初表现可以通过保守治疗得到改善，但也可能迅速发展为重度子痫前期，最终发展为子痫。

A summary of the various management strategies for pregnancy-related hypertension is shown in Figure 8.6. This flow diagram shows the various pathways of progression and their management. An initial presentation of mild hypertension may improve with conservative management, or it may progress rapidly to the severe forms of preeclampsia and ultimately eclampsia.

（九）子痫前期的预防（Prevention of pre-eclampsia）

毫无疑问，谨慎的评估和监测可以在很大程度上预防子痫发生，但对子痫前期的预防应该是治疗上的"金标准"。

There is no doubt that careful management and anticipation can largely prevent the occurrence of eclampsia, but preventing pre-eclampsia should be the gold standard of care.

预防子痫前期的首要时机是在 12 周产检时。研究发现，孕 12 周时母体子宫动脉阻力增加，同时母体高血压和低妊娠相关血浆蛋白 –A（PAPP-A）和胎盘生长因子（PlGF）水平与不良妊娠结局有关，尤其是早发性子痫前期（32 周前子痫前期）。阿司匹林 100～150mg 的治疗已被证明可以改善妊娠结局，甚至可以延迟胎儿分娩至足月。

The first opportunity to prevent pre-eclampsia is at the 12-week scan. In the mother, the finding of increased resistance in the uterine arteries at 12 weeks, along with a finding of maternal hypertension and low pregnancy-associated plasma protein-A (PAPP-A) and Placental Growth Factor (PlGF) levels, has been associated with poor pregnancy outcome, in particular early-onset pre-eclampsia (significant pre-eclampsia before 32 weeks). Treatment with aspirin 100–150 mg has been shown to improve the pregnancy outcome by delaying the need for fetal delivery to close to term.

一些证据表明，钙补充可以降低普通人群中子痫前期的发病率，但仅限于营养不良的女性。

There is some evidence that calcium supplements may reduce the risk of pre-eclampsia in the general population, but only in women who have dietary deficiency.

在患有原发性高血压的孕妇和既往患有子痫前期的孕妇中，阿司匹林被证明可降低后续妊娠中子痫前期的发病率。

In women with essential hypertension and those with pre-eclampsia in previous pregnancies, aspirin has been shown to reduce the incidence of pre-eclampsia in subsequent pregnancies.

对于在上一次妊娠中患有重度子痫前期的女性，应在产后进行血栓形成的筛查，因为有潜在血栓形成倾向的发生率，在之后的妊娠中除阿司匹林外使用低分子肝素治疗可能获益。

In women who have had severe pre-eclampsia in the previous pregnancy, a thrombophilia screen should be undertaken postnatally, as there is an incidence of underlying thrombotic tendencies that may also benefit from the use of

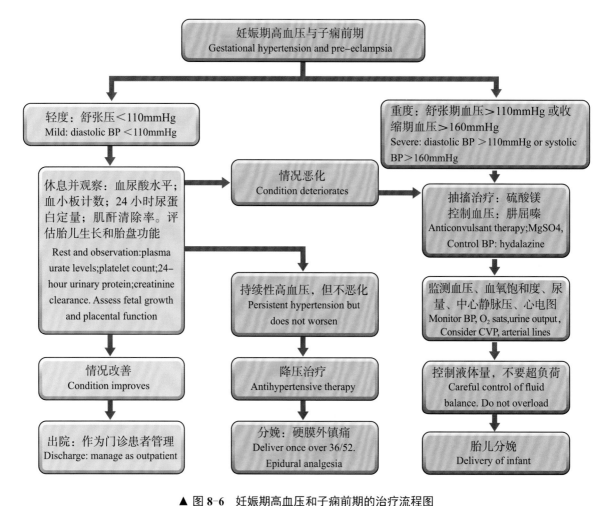

▲ 图 8-6　妊娠期高血压和子痫前期的治疗流程图

Fig. 8.6　Flow diagram of the management of gestational hypertension and pre-eclampsia. BP, Blood pressure; CVP, central venous pressure.

low-molecular-weight heparin therapy in addition to aspirin in a subsequent pregnancy.

（十）子痫前期和子痫症状（Symptoms of preeclampsia and eclampsia）

子痫前期通常是一种无症状的状态。然而，有些症状不容忽视，其中包括头痛、视物模糊、呕吐和右上腹疼痛。在这些症状中，最重要的是上腹疼痛，无论是在妊娠期间还是在产褥期（图 8-7）。

Pre-eclampsia is commonly an asymptomatic condition. However, there are symptoms that must not be overlooked, and these include frontal headache, blurring of vision, sudden onset of vomiting and right epigastric pain. Of these symptoms, the most important is the development of epigastric pain-either during pregnancy or in the immediate puerperium (Fig. 8.7).

若孕妇表现出头痛、血压明显升高和反射亢进，且血象证实实患有重度子痫前期，就必须考虑终止妊

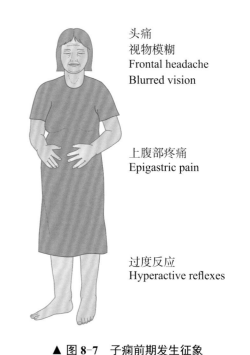

▲ 图 8-7　子痫前期发生征象

Fig. 8.7　Presenting signs of impending eclampsia.

娠。最初的治疗是静脉给药控制血压，并以 1g/h 的剂量静脉滴注硫酸镁 4g，持续静滴 20min，直到分娩 24h 后抽搐的风险消除为止，以预防子痫抽搐的发生。

Where a woman presents with headache, markedly raised BP and hyperreflexia, and has blood testing confirming severe pre-eclampsia, delivery of the fetus must be considered. The initial treatment is to control the BP with IV medication and prevention of seizures with an infusion of magnesium sulphate 4 g IV over 20 minutes with 1 g/h until the risk of seizures has ceased 24 hours after delivery (see also Eclampsia later).

> **！注意**
> 上腹痛的发生通常被误诊或忽视，但这是重度子痫前期和子痫的一个重要特征。通常发生在妊娠晚期，有时会误诊为消化不良、胃灼热或胆结石。除非记录血压并检测尿液中的蛋白质含量，否则疼痛的重要性就会被忽视，直到女性出现抽搐发作。
>
> The occurrence of epigastric pain is commonly misdiagnosed or overlooked as a feature of severe pre-eclampsia and impending eclampsia. Occurring often in the late second or the early third trimester, an erroneous diagnosis of indigestion, heartburn or gallstones is sometimes made, and unless the BP is recorded and the urine checked for protein, the significance of the pain can be overlooked until the woman presents with seizures.

（十一）终止妊娠（Induction of labour）

在妊娠合并高血压疾病的情况下，考虑母体和（或）胎儿 / 胎盘状况的原因，应考虑终止妊娠。

- 母体
  - 妊娠＞37 周。
  - 血压不可控。
  - HELLP 综合征。
  - 持续肝功能损害。
  - 血小板降低。
  - 溶血导致血红蛋白下降。
  - 肾功能恶化（肌酐＞90mmol/L）。
  - 子痫。
  - 急性肺水肿。

- 胎儿 / 胎盘
  - 胎心监测异常。
  - 脐动脉舒张末血流消失或反流。
  - 胎儿血管多普勒示大脑 / 胎盘比值异常。
  - 超声检查 2 周以上胎儿无生长。
  - 胎盘早剥或胎儿窘迫。

In a pregnancy complicated by hypertensive disease, delivery of the fetus should be considered for the following maternal and/or fetal/placental reasons:

- maternal
  - gestation >37 weeks
  - uncontrollable BP
  - HELLP syndrome
  - rising liver dysfunction
  - falling platelets
  - falling haemoglobin due to haemolysis
  - deteriorating renal function (creatinine >90 mmol/L)
  - eclampsia
  - acute pulmonary oedema
- fetal/placental
  - fetal compromise on CTG tracing
  - absent or reversal of end diastolic flow in the umbilical artery
  - abnormal cerebro/placental ratio on Doppler scanning of the fetal vessels
  - no fetal growth over more than 2 weeks on ultrasound
  - placental abruption with fetal compromise

若决定终止妊娠，选择是经阴道分娩还是剖宫产。这一决定将取决于临床情况的严重性。若时间允许，妊娠＜34 周的孕妇应使用产前类固醇激素，以最大限度地减少新生儿发病率。在特殊情况下，如子痫或严重的胎儿宫内窘迫，不应为了使用类固醇激素而推迟分娩。同样，若胎儿＜30 周妊娠分娩的，在子宫下段剖宫产（LUSCS）或顺产过程中，应考虑在分娩前 1h 内负荷量并静滴硫酸镁，硫酸镁可以保护新生儿大脑神经。当硫酸镁用于预防母体抽搐（子痫）时，硫酸镁起到保护新生儿大脑的作用，则不需要加量。

If the decision has been made to proceed to delivery, the choice will rest with either the induction of labour or delivery by caesarean section. This decision will be determined by the seriousness of the clinical situation. If there is time, antenatal steroids should be given for gestations of less than 34 weeks to minimize neonatal morbidity. In an extreme situation like eclampsia or severe fetal compromise, delivery should not be delayed in order to administer steroids. Similarly, where a fetus is to be delivered at a gestation of less than 30 weeks, a loading dose and infusion of magnesium sulphate should be considered in the hour before delivery by lower uterine segment caesarean section (LUSCS) or during an induced labour, as it provides neuroprotection for the neonatal brain. Where an infusion of magnesium sulphate is being used as prophylaxis against maternal seizures (eclampsia), this infusion acts to protect the neonatal brain and no further dosing is required.

若宫颈成熟度不适合引产时（Bishop 评分低于 7 分），通常可以通过将前列腺素 E 制剂放入阴道后穹隆或通过宫颈使用机械气囊导管（Foley 导管）来使其成熟。

If the cervix is unsuitable for surgical induction (Bishop score of less than 7), it can often be ripened by the introduction of a prostaglandin E preparation into the posterior fornix of the vagina or the use of a mechanical balloon catheter (Foley catheter) through the cervix.

如果宫颈 Bishop 评分大于 7，则可以通过人工破膜和使用催产素引产（见第 11 章）。

If the cervix has a Bishop score of greater than 7, labour is induced by artificial rupture of membranes and oxytocin infusion (see Chapter 11).

（十二）并发症（Complications）

并发症分类如下。

- 胎儿

    - 生长受限、缺氧、死亡。

- 母体

    - 重度子痫前期与流向各个重要器官的血流减少有关。若孕妇治疗不当和（或）胎儿未能及时分娩，并发症包括肾功能衰竭 (肌酐升高 / 少尿 / 无尿)、肝功能衰竭、肝内出血、癫痫发作、DIC、成人急性呼吸窘迫综合征 (ARDS)、脑出血 / 梗死和心力衰竭。

- 胎盘

    - 梗死、早剥。

Complications can be grouped as follows:
- fetal
    - growth restriction, hypoxia, death
- maternal
    - severe pre-eclampsia is associated with a fall in

blood flow to various vital organs. If the mother is inadequately treated and/or the fetus is not delivered in a timely manner, complications include renal failure (raised creatinine/oliguria/anuria), hepatic failure, intrahepatic haemorrhage, seizures, DIC, adult RDS (ARDS), cerebral haemorrhage/ infarction and heart failure

- placental
    - infarction, abruption

（十三）子痫（Eclampsia）

妊娠期子痫前期的抽搐发作即子痫。子痫是一种可以预防的疾病，它的发生通常意味着未能认识到子痫前期的早期恶化迹象。虽然这在初次孕女性中更为常见，但它可能发生在产前、产中或产后的任何妊娠期间，并且有发生胎儿宫内死亡和孕妇死于脑出血或肝肾衰竭的严重风险。

The onset of convulsions in a pregnancy complicated by pre-eclampsia denotes the onset of eclampsia. Eclampsia is a preventable condition, and its occurrence often denotes a failure to recognize the early worsening signs of preeclampsia. Although it is more common in primigravid women, it can occur in any pregnancy during the antepartum, intrapartum or postpartum period. It carries serious risks of intrauterine death for the fetus and of maternal death from cerebral haemorrhage and/or renal and hepatic failure.

所有患者都必须在医院进行治疗，最好是在有重症监护设施的医院进行治疗。除非可以证明由其他原因引发，任何在妊娠期间因抽搐入院的孕妇或因高血压而昏迷入院的孕妇都应被认为患有子痫。

All cases must be managed in hospital and preferably in hospitals with appropriate intensive care facilities. Any woman admitted to hospital with convulsions during the course of pregnancy or who is admitted in a coma associated with hypertension should be considered to be suffering from eclampsia until proved otherwise.

（十四）子痫前期的治疗（Management of eclampsia）

子痫的三个基本指导原则如下。

- 控制抽搐。

- 控制血压。

- 终止妊娠。

The three basic guidelines for management of eclampsia are:
- Control the fits.
- Control the BP.
- Deliver the infant.

病例分析	Case study
并非所有妊娠期间发生抽搐的孕妇都诊断为子痫。Marilyn D 是一位单身母亲，她被两个朋友送进急诊室，并在同一家医院生产，她的产前记录显示，到目前为止，她妊娠过程顺利。妊娠 34 周，入院时血压为 140/90mmhg。尿液中有微量的蛋白质。星期六晚上，她被送进了医院，她的朋友说他们在去医院的路上把车停了下来，由于她的抽搐发作的很严重，所以把 Marilyn 放在了路边的人行道上。	Not all women admitted with seizures in pregnancy are eclamptic. Marilyn D was a single mother who was brought into an accident and emergency department by two friends with a statement that she had fitted on two occasions. She was booked for confinement at the same hospital, and her antenatal records showed that her pregnancy had so far been uncomplicated. She was 34 weeks pregnant, and on admission her BP was 140/90 mmHg. There was a trace of protein in the urine. She was brought into hospital on a Saturday night, and her friends stated that they had stopped the car on the way into hospital and laid Marilyn down on the pavement by the roadside because of the violence of her seizure.
经密切监测 Marilyn 的血压稳定在 110/75mmHg，生化指标检验正常后，决定继续观察，24h 内无进一步发展。对该病例进一步讨论，发现她服用了包括安非他命在内的多种违禁药物，这是一个医学生提出的诊断！	After careful assessment of the BP that settled to 110/75 mmHg and normal biochemical testing, it was decided to proceed with observation, and within 24 hours, there were no further fits. Further discussion with Marilyn revealed that she had taken a mixture of illicit drugs, including amphetamines: a diagnosis that was suggested by one of the medical students!

1. 控制抽搐发作（Control of fits）

过去，人们使用各种药物控制抽搐的发生。

- 子痫发作通常是自限性的。急诊处理是为了确保患者安全，保护气道。

- 硫酸镁是解痉的首选药物。这种药能有效地抑制抽搐、肌肉收缩。它还可以减少血小板聚集，使 DIC 的发生率降至最低。刚开始治疗时，给药剂量为 4g，20min 后，给予 1g/h 的量来维持血液中镁离子的水平。只有在出现明显的肾衰竭或抽搐复发时，才应测量血液中镁离子的水平。其治疗浓度范围为 2～4mmol/L，高于 5mmol/L 会导致腱反射消失，超过 6mmol/L 会使呼吸受抑制。硫酸镁可以通过肌内注射给药，但肌内注射通常很痛，有时还会导致脓肿形成。因此，首选给药途径是静脉注射。

In the past various drugs were used to control the fits:

- Eclamptic seizures are usually self-limiting. Acute management is to ensure patient safety and protect the airway.

- Magnesium sulphate is the drug of choice for the control of fits thereafter. The drug is effective in suppressing convulsions and inhibiting muscular activity. It also reduces platelet aggregation and minimizes the effects of DIC. Treatment is started with a bolus dose of 4 g given over 20 minutes. Thereafter blood levels of magnesium are maintained by giving a maintenance dose of 1 g/h. The blood level of magnesium should only be measured if there is significant renal failure or seizures recur. The therapeutic range is 2–4 mmol/L. A level of more than 5 mmol/L causes loss of patellar reflexes, and a value of more than 6 mmol/L causes respiratory depression. Magnesium sulphate can be given by intramuscular injection, but the injection is often painful and sometimes leads to abscess formation. The preferred route is therefore by IV administration.

在首次发生抽搐后，重要的是要防止再次发作，控制血压，严格监测液体平衡，并使尿量维持在 0.5～1.0ml/（kg·h）。为此，应与重症监护室医护人员共同监测患者状况。麻醉医生给予持续护理。一般治疗原则是总输液量应控制在 80～100ml/h。若尿流量降至 30ml/h 以下，应考虑测量中心静脉压。液体负荷过多可能会导致肺水肿和 ARDS，甚至危及生命。

After the first seizure, it is important to ensure that further fits are prevented, BP is well controlled, fluid balance is strictly monitored, and urine output is maintained at 0.5–1.0 mL/kg/h. To this end, the patient should be managed jointly with staff in an intensive care/high-dependency unit. Constant nursing attendance is essential by staff accustomed to managing patients with airway problems. As a general principle, total fluid input should be restricted to 80–100 mL/h. If the urine flow falls to below 30 mL/h, a central venous pressure measurement should be considered. Fluid overload in these women may induce pulmonary oedema and ARDS with lethal consequences.

2. 控制血压（Control of blood pressure）

因此，控制血压是降低产妇脑出血风险的关键。肼屈嗪是一种对于急性治疗的有效药物，每分钟静

> **! 注意**
>
> 一直检测血液中镁离子水平是不切实际的。重要的是避免镁中毒，因为镁中毒可能导致呼吸暂停。子痫与反射亢进有关，还可能与阵发性抽搐有关，因此可以通过腱反射来反映机体内镁离子水平。若腱反射消失，则应立即停用镁离子。在出现呼吸抑制的情况下，则应给予 10ml 的 10% 葡萄糖酸钙纠正，静推时间超过 2～3min。
>
> It is not always possible to monitor the blood levels of magnesium. It is, however, important to avoid toxic levels of magnesium, as they may result in complete respiratory arrest. Eclampsia is associated with hyper–reflexia and, on occasions, with clonus, so a guide to the levels of magnesium can be obtained by regular checks of the patellar reflexes. If patellar reflexes are absent, magnesium should be stopped. In the event of the suppression of respiration, the effects can be reversed by the administration of 10 mL of 10% calcium gluconate given intravenously over 2–3 minutes.

脉滴注 1 次，若血压未得到控制，15min 后重复注射。因孕妇处于妊娠状态，所以一定不要将舒张压降至 90mmHg 以下，以免影响子宫 – 胎盘之间的血流。

It is essential to control the BP to minimize the risk of maternal cerebral haemorrhage. Hydralazine is a useful drug in acute management and is given intravenously as a 5-mg bolus over an interval of 5 minutes and repeated after 15 minutes if the BP is not controlled. If the mother is still pregnant, it is important not to drop the BP below a diastolic BP of 90 mmHg in order not to compromise the uterine/placental blood flow.

另一种选择是静脉注射拉贝洛尔，开始剂量是 20mg，逐渐增加 40mg 和 80mg，最后达到 200mg。

An alternative is to use IV labetalol, starting with a bolus of 20 mg followed by further doses of 40 mg and 80 mg to a total of 200 mg.

随后可以持续注射 5～40mg/h 肼屈嗪或 20～160mg/h 拉贝洛尔来控制血压。

Subsequent BP control can be maintained with a continuous infusion of hydralazine at 5–40mg/h or labetalol at 20–160mg/h.

硬膜外麻醉：可以缓解分娩疼痛，并通过扩张下肢血管来控制血压。然而，在插入硬膜外导管之前需要监测凝血功能，若出现凝血障碍，可能会导致出血，进入硬膜外间隙。

Epidural analgesia relieves the pain of labour and helps to control the BP by causing vasodilatation in the lower extremities. However, it is essential to perform clotting studies before inserting an epidural catheter because of the risk of causing bleeding into the epidural space if there is a coagulopathy.

3. 终止妊娠（Delivery of the infant）

重度子痫前期 / 子痫的诊断表明，孕妇和胎儿继续妊娠的风险将超过分娩风险。如果妊娠不到 26 周，与早产相关的新生儿严重并发症及剖宫产的风险增加，需要在决定分娩时咨询新生儿和母胎医学专家。

A diagnosis of severe pre-eclampsia/eclampsia indicates that the risk to both the mother and the infant of continuing the pregnancy will exceed the risk of delivery. Where the gestation is less than 26 weeks, serious neonatal morbidity associated with prematurity and an increased risk for the requirement of a classical caesarean section necessitates that the decision to deliver includes consultation with neonatal and maternofetal medicine specialists.

由于干预本身可能会引发高血压危象，在分娩之前，对血压的合理控制是至关重要的。

It is essential to establish reasonable control of the BP before embarking on any procedures to expedite delivery, as the intervention itself may precipitate a hypertensive crisis.

如果宫颈充分扩张，孕妇和胎儿的条件允许，可以进行人工破膜，并使用催产素静脉滴注催产。若条件不允许，或者孕妇和胎儿的情况受到影响，最好通过剖宫产分娩，这种情况下需要及早联系麻醉医师。

If the cervix is sufficiently dilated and the conditions of the mother and the fetus allow, an artificial rupture of the membranes may be performed and labour induced with an oxytocin infusion. If this is not possible or the maternal or fetal condition is compromised, it is best to proceed to delivery by caesarean section, which requires early consultation with an anaesthetic colleague.

4. 产后护理（Management after delivery）

子痫的风险不会随分娩而停止，子痫前期和子痫的治疗应持续至分娩后 7 天，如果分娩后 48h 首次发生抽搐，则应考虑其他诊断，如癫痫或颅脑疾病（如静脉血栓形成）。高达 45% 的子痫发作发生在分娩后，其中 12% 发生在 48h 后。

The risks of eclampsia do not stop with delivery, and the management of pre-eclampsia and eclampsia continues for up to 7 days after delivery, although if a seizure occurs for the first time 48 hours after delivery, alternative diagnoses such as epilepsy or intracranial pathology such as cortical vein thrombosis must be considered. Up to 45% of eclamptic fits occur after delivery, including 12% after 48 hours.

应遵守以下治疗原则。

- 持续观察患者病情，保持环境安静。

- 适当镇痛，若孕妇已经给予硫酸镁治疗，在最后一次发作后继续输液 24h，直至达到利尿效果。

- 继续给予降压治疗，直至血压恢复正常。通常进行口服药物治疗，通常在第一周后会有显著改善，但高血压可能会持续 6 周。

- 应严格控制液体量，白天每小时观察 1 次血压和尿量，晚上每 2 小时观察 1 次。生化和血液学指标应每天监测，直到参数稳定或开始恢复正常。

The following points of management should be observed:

- Maintain the patient in a quiet environment under constant observation.

- Maintain appropriate levels of pain relief. If the mother has been treated with magnesium sulphate, continue the infusion for 24 hours after the last fit or until a diuresis is seen.

- Continue antihypertensive therapy until the BP has returned to normal. This will usually involve transferring to oral medication, and although there is usually significant improvement after the first week, hypertension may persist for the next 6 weeks.

- Strict fluid balance charts should be kept and BP and urine output observed on an hourly basis during the day and 2-hourly at night. Biochemical and haematological indices should be made on a daily basis until the values have stabilized or started to return to normal.

虽然大多数患有子痫前期或子痫的女性血压都会恢复正常，但在分娩后 6 周复查对于这些女性来说是非常重要的。若高血压或蛋白尿在这个阶段持续存在，应该对她们进行其他因素的调查，如潜在的肾脏疾病。她们也应该接受自身免疫性疾病、易栓症或抗磷脂综合征引起的疾病的筛查。长期以来，人们发现患有严重妊娠期高血压综合征的女性在晚年患高血压和心血管疾病的概率更高。

Although most mothers who have suffered from preeclampsia or eclampsia will completely recover and return to normal, it is important to review all such women at 6 weeks after delivery. If the hypertension or proteinuria persists at this stage, they should be investigated for other factors such as underlying renal disease. Women should also be investigated for the possibility of an autoimmune, thrombophilic or antiphospholipid cause of her disease. Long term, women with severe pregnancy-induced hypertension have been found to have a higher rate of hypertension and cardiovascular disease later in life.

二、产前出血（Antepartum haemorrhage）

各国对产前出血的定义各不相同。世界卫生组织（WHO）的将其定义为妊娠 24 周后阴道出血，这一定义被包括英国在内的许多国家所接受。在其他国家，如澳大利亚，产前出血的定义为 20 周；有的国家将其定义为 28 周。导致产前大出血的因素可能在 20 周之前就存在了，但先兆流产和产前大出血的区别取决于出血时胎儿是否有存活的可能性。产前出血仍然是导致围产期孕产妇并发症和死亡率的一

病例分析	Case study
T 女士是一名 28 岁的初产妇，是一名初级医务人员的妻子。她的妊娠过程一直顺利，直到 37 周，她查出高血压，住院卧床休息。血压维持在 140/90mmHg 左右，尿液中有微量蛋白质。妊娠 38 周时，经阴道分娩，她顺利产下一名健康男婴。	Mrs T was a 28-year-old primigravida and the wife of one of the junior medical staff. Her pregnancy was uneventful until 37 weeks, when she developed hypertension and was admitted to hospital for bed rest. Her BP stayed around 140/90 and there was a trace of protein in the urine. At 38 weeks' gestation, labour was induced and she had a normal delivery of a healthy male infant.
第二天她已经可以自由活动了，但告知医务人员有头痛、消化不良和上腹部不适等症状。服用了对乙酰氨基酚和抗酸药，但症状仍存在。高血压无改善，最高值为 145/98mmHg。傍晚时候，发生抽搐。不幸的是，她摔倒在床上，导致颧骨骨折。虽然在分娩前没有发作过，但需注意的是，产后产妇的重度子痫前期症状在分娩后和产前一样重要。	The following day she was fully mobile but complained to the midwifery staff that she had a frontal headache and indigestion, with epigastric discomfort. She was given paracetamol and an antacid, but the symptoms persisted. Her hypertension also persisted, with the highest reading being 145/98 mmHg. Later that day she had a seizure. Unfortunately, she fell against the side of her bed and fractured her zygoma. Although she had not had a fit before delivery, it is important to remember that symptoms of severe pre-eclampsia in a postnatal woman are as significant after delivery as they are antenatally.

个重要原因。

The definition of antepartum haemorrhage varies from country to country. The World Health Organization (WHO) definition, accepted by many countries including the UK, is haemorrhage from the vagina after the twenty-fourth week of gestation. In other countries, including Australia, the defined gestation is 20 weeks; however, a few use a 28-week definition. The factors that cause antepartum haemorrhage may be present before 20 weeks, but the distinction between a threatened miscarriage and an antepartum haemorrhage is based on whether the fetus is considered potentially viable at the time of the bleed. Antepartum bleeding remains a significant cause of perinatal and maternal morbidity and mortality.

阴道出血的原因如下。

- 胎盘及子宫出血：前置胎盘、胎盘早剥、子宫破裂。

- 生殖器病变：大量见红 / 临产（宫颈上皮出血）、宫颈外翻 / 癌、宫颈炎、息肉、外阴静脉曲张、创伤和感染。

- 胎儿血管出血，其中包括前置血管（非常罕见）。

Vaginal bleeding may be due to:

- haemorrhage from the placental site and uterus: placenta praevia, placental abruption, uterine rupture

- lesions of the lower genital tract: heavy show/onset of labour (bleed from cervical epithelium), cervical ectropion/carcinoma, cervicitis, polyps, vulval varices, trauma and infection

- bleeding from fetal vessels, including vasa praevia (very rare)

在吸烟或社会经济地位较低的女性中，产前出血率通常会增加。因此，通过对人群研究发现，这

一发病率为 2%～5%。对于任何入院治疗的女性来说，出血的原因往往不确定。在任何大型产科医院，入院后的诊断大致如下。

- 未分类 / 原因不明：50%。

- 前置胎盘：30%。

- 胎盘早剥：20%。

- 前置血管：罕见。

The rate of antepartum haemorrhage is generally increased in women who smoke or who have a lower socioeconomic status. The rate therefore varies from 2% to 5% depending upon the population studied. For any woman admitted with bleeding, the cause is often not immediately obvious. In any large obstetric unit, the diagnoses after admission are approximately:

- unclassified/uncertain cause: 50%

- placenta praevia: 30%

- placental abruption: 20%

- vasa praevia (rare)

（一）前置胎盘（Placenta praevia）

当全部或部分胎盘附着在子宫下段时，胎盘被称为前置胎盘，因此胎盘位于胎儿先露的旁边或前面（图 8-8）。

The placenta is said to be praevia when all or part of the placenta implants in the lower uterine segment and therefore lies beside or in front of the presenting part of the fetus (Fig. 8.8).

1. 发病率（Incidence）

前置胎盘发生率大概占全部妊娠的 1%，与胎盘

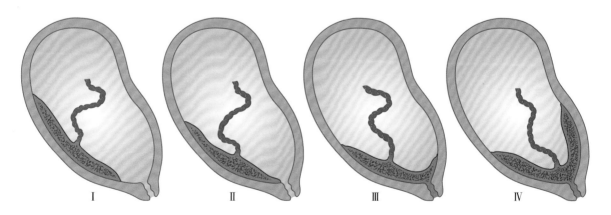

▲ 图 8-8 前置胎盘的胎盘位置，分别为Ⅰ级、Ⅱ级、Ⅲ级和Ⅳ级

Fig. 8.8 The placental siting for placenta praevia. Grade Ⅰ, Ⅱ, Ⅲ and Ⅳ, respectively.

早剥的发生率不同，胎盘早剥的发生率随社会和营养因素的不同而不同，前置胎盘的发生率非常稳定。

Approximately 1% of all pregnancies are complicated by clinical evidence of a placenta praevia. Unlike the incidence of placental abruption, which varies according to social and nutritional factors, the incidence of placenta praevia is remarkably constant.

前置胎盘在多胎妊娠、多孕产次和剖宫产史的经产女性中更为常见。

Placenta praevia is more common in multiparous women, in the presence of multiple pregnancy and where there has been one or more previous caesarean sections.

2. 病因（Aetiology）

前置胎盘被认为是由于受精卵着床延迟，以至于胎盘种植在子宫下段。

Placenta praevia is presumed to be due to a delay in implantation of the blastocyst so that implantation occurs in the lower part of the uterus.

3. 分类（Classification）

前置胎盘是通过超声诊断的。鉴于子宫下段形成于妊娠 24～28 周后，因此前置胎盘不能在这之前诊断。如果胎盘在 24 周前被检测到位于宫颈 2cm 以内，这被称为"低位"，95% 的胎盘在胎盘下段发育后完全脱离了宫颈。

Placenta praevia is diagnosed using ultrasound. Given that the lower segment forms at 24–28 weeks of pregnancy, a diagnosis of placenta praevia cannot be made before that gestation. If a placenta is detected to be within 2 cm of the cervix before 24 weeks, it is called 'low lying', with 95% of such placentas ending well clear of the cervix after the lower segment develops.

前置胎盘有多种分类。分级是提供最好解剖学描述和临床信息的分类。Ⅰ级，胎盘附着于子宫下段，但未覆盖宫颈内口；Ⅱ级，胎盘附着于子宫下段，下缘达到宫颈内口；Ⅲ级，胎盘组织部分覆盖宫颈内口，但是也可以看到一些胎盘组织附着在子宫上部；Ⅳ级，胎盘组织完全覆盖宫颈内口，胎盘的中心部分在宫颈上方（图 8-8）。胎盘附着子宫前壁Ⅰ级或Ⅱ级的孕妇在失血不多的情况下通常可以正常的阴道分娩。后壁Ⅱ级前置胎盘，胎盘位于母体骶骨前，可防止胎头下沉到骨盆；Ⅲ级和Ⅳ级前置胎盘，若出现早产或足月产分娩大出血则需紧急剖宫产。

There are numerous classifications of placenta praevia.

The classification that affords the best anatomical description and clinical information is based on grades. Grade Ⅰ is defined as a placenta with the lower edge implanted on the lower segment but not to or over the internal cervical os; grade Ⅱ is when the lower edge of the placenta reaches the internal os, but the bulk of the placenta is in the upper uterine segment; grade Ⅲ is determined when the placenta is covering the cervical os, but some placental tissue is also seen attached to the upper uterine segment; and grade Ⅳ is determined when all the placenta is in the lower segment with the central portion of the placenta over the cervical os (see Fig. 8.8). Women with a grade I or grade Ⅱ placenta on the anterior wall of the uterus will commonly achieve a normal vaginal delivery without excess blood loss. A posterior grade Ⅱ placenta praevia, where the placental mass is in front of the maternal sacrum, prevents the descent of the fetal head into the pelvis, and along with a grade Ⅲ and Ⅳ placenta praevia, it will necessitate delivery by caesarean section, either urgently if labour or significant bleeding commences pre-term or electively at or near term.

前置胎盘出血是由于子宫下段形成和宫颈消失时与胎盘分离所致。这种出血发生在子宫下段宫壁上的静脉窦，出血量可能较大，因此可能需要终止妊娠以确保产妇平安。若失血不多但出现胎盘剥离，可能会危及胎儿，可通过 CTG 监测胎儿情况，必要时选择剖宫产终止妊娠。极少数情况下，可能发生胎盘破裂引起胎儿失血，这将使 CTG 监测出现异常，需及时终止妊娠。基于上述情况，在任何出血发生时都必须进行密切的胎儿监护。如果胎儿和产妇的情况稳定，出血停止，妊娠可推迟到 35 周，可能的话，甚至可推迟到 37～38 周。

Bleeding in placenta praevia results from separation of the placenta as the formation of the lower segment occurs and the cervix effaces. This blood loss occurs from the venous sinuses in the wall of the lower uterine segment. Bleeding may be profuse and/or relentless, so fetal delivery may be required to ensure maternal wellbeing. If the blood loss is controlled but the separation of the placenta is significant, fetal compromise may result, which will be detected on the CTG tracing, and delivery will be required for fetal reasons. Very occasionally, fetal blood loss may occur at the time of maternal bleeding if the placenta is disrupted. This will result in anomalies on the CTG record allowing for a timely delivery. For these reasons, close fetal monitoring must be undertaken during any bleeding. Where the fetal condition and the maternal condition are stable and the bleeding settles, delivery is delayed at least to 35 weeks, but until 37–38 weeks if possible.

4. 临床表现（Symptoms and signs）

前置胎盘的主要症状是无痛性阴道出血。有时可能会出现下腹部不适，伴有轻度胎盘分离（胎盘早剥）。

The main symptom of placenta praevia is painless vaginal bleeding. There may sometimes be lower abdominal discomfort where there are minor degrees of associated placental separation (abruption).

前置胎盘体征如下。

- 阴道流血。

- 胎先露异常。

- 子宫收缩。

The signs of placenta praevia are:

- vaginal bleeding

- malpresentation of the fetus

- normal uterine tone

出血是不可预测的，可能是轻度的（最初出血常见）到大量的，甚至危及生命的出血。

The bleeding is unpredictable and may vary from minor-common with the initial bleed-to massive and life-endangering haemorrhage.

5. 诊断（Diagnosis）

(1) 临床表现（Clinical findings）

无痛性阴道出血发生得很突然，而且往往会反

复出现。分娩开始时，宫颈扩张，可能会出现大量流血。前置胎盘为Ⅰ级附着前壁或侧壁的前置胎盘，出血可能较少。随着分娩过程的进展，破膜过程可能是安全的，这将有助于头部下降，并进一步减缓失血。如果该过程是安全的，可以经阴道分娩。

Painless bleeding occurs suddenly and tends to be recurrent. If labour starts and the cervix dilates, profuse haemorrhage may occur. Where there is a grade I anterior or lateral placental praevia, the bleeding may be less profuse. As labour is establishing, it may be safe to rupture the fetal membranes, which may assist the descent of the head and slow the blood loss even further. If it is safe, the labour can be allowed to progress to a vaginal delivery.

(2) 腹部检查（Abdominal examination）

- **先露部分移位：** 出现无痛性阴道出血，并伴有胎先露高浮或横位或斜位常强烈提示前置胎盘的可能性。在这些情况下，有经验的产科医生可能会进行内检，以判断阴道失血量，出血是否源于阴道，但在进行超声检查之前，不得进行阴道检查。因为阴道检查可能会破坏胎盘，导致出血过多。

- Displacement of the presenting part: The finding

<table>
<tr><th>病例分析</th><th>Case study</th></tr>
<tr><td>

Jane T 在妊娠 28 周时因首次无痛性阴道流血约 100ml 而入院治疗。胎先露部位偏高但居中，子宫肌张力适中。超声提示Ⅲ级前置胎盘，胎儿没有任何窘迫迹象。考虑到胎盘的位置和进一步出血的风险，简被建议住院观察，直至分娩。随后出血止住了，在妊娠 32 周时，她要求回家举行婚礼。由于路上需要 1h 的飞行时间，医院强烈建议她不要这么做，因此她的丈夫飞往简的身边，婚礼安排在医院附近的一座教堂里。在婚礼上，简在走红毯时又出现一次大出血，随后被紧急送回医院。入院时，出血已止住，胎儿未受损。考虑到妊娠小于 35 周，医务人员决定观察并试图继续延长妊娠时间以改善新生儿预后。妊娠 35 周时，简在病房里再次大出血，血浸透了她的床单，流到了床边。医务人员开放两条静脉通路，她被紧急送往手术室。她出现休克、血压很低，医务人员很难维持她的血压。胎心率出现减速，最后出现心动过缓，并伴有胎盘灌注不良，随后立即进行了"剖宫产"，术中确诊为Ⅲ级前置胎盘，剖宫产获一健康男婴。为 Jane 输注 10 单位血液纠正了休克。若 Jane 在出血时在家，那么她和她的孩子很有可能活不下来。

</td><td>

Jane T was admitted to hospital at 28 weeks' gestation with a painless vaginal haemorrhage of approximately 100 mL in her first pregnancy. The presenting part was high but central, and the uterine tone was soft. A diagnosis of a grade III anterior placenta praevia was made on ultrasound, and the fetus showed no sign of compromise. Given the site of the placenta and the risk of a further and more substantial bleed, Jane was advised to stay in hospital under observation until delivery. The bleeding settled, and at 32 weeks' gestation, she asked to go home to marry her partner. As this necessitated a 1-hour flight, she was strongly advised against this action so her partner flew to Janet instead, and the wedding was arranged in a church close to the hospital. At the wedding, Janet had a further substantial bleed as she walked down the aisle and was rushed back into hospital. On admission the bleeding was found to be settling and the fetus was not compromised. Given the gestation was less than 35 weeks, management was to observe and attempt to prolong the gestation to improve neonatal outcome. At 35 weeks' gestation Janet had a massive haemorrhage in the ward to the extent that blood soaked her bed linen and flowed over the side of the bed. The resident staff inserted two IV lines and she was rushed to theatre. She was shocked and hypotensive, and it was extremely difficult to maintain her BP. The fetal heart showed hypoxic decelerations and finally a bradycardia associated with poor placental perfusion. A 'crash section' was performed, and the diagnosis of grade III placenta praevia was confirmed. A healthy male infant was delivered. Janet was resuscitated with over 10 units of blood and blood product. Had Janet been at home at the time of the bleed, it is possible that neither she nor her baby would have survived.

</td></tr>
</table>

of painless vaginal bleeding with a high central presenting part, a transverse or an oblique lie strongly suggests the possibility of placenta praevia. Although a speculum examination may be undertaken by a skilled obstetrician in these cases to check the amount of the blood loss in the vagina and that it is not of vaginal origin, a digital vaginal examination must not be undertaken until an ultrasound has been performed. A digital examination may disrupt the placenta and cause excessive bleeding.

- **子宫收缩力正常：** 与胎盘早剥不同，子宫张力通常是正常的，胎方位很容易触到。

- Normal uterine tone: Unlike with abruption, the uterine muscle tone is usually normal and the fetal parts are easy to palpate.

(3) 诊断（Diagnostic procedures）

- **超声：** 经腹超声，对后壁胎盘的经阴道超声可用于定位胎盘。胎盘在前壁时，膀胱为子宫下段提供了重要的标志，因此诊断更加准确。当胎盘在后壁时，骶骨角可用于子宫下段的标志。但当腹部扫描无法检查时，则使用经阴道扫描来确定从子宫颈口到胎盘下缘的距离。因为在孕 30 周时子宫下段的发育将导致胎盘明显向上移位，妊娠早期胎盘部位的定位可能会导致前置胎盘的诊断不准确。

- Ultrasound scanning: Transabdominal and, for posterior placentas, transvaginal ultrasound are used to localize the placenta where there is a suggestion of placenta praevia. Anteriorly, the bladder provides an important landmark for the lower segment, and diagnosis is more accurate. When the placenta is on the posterior wall, the sacral promontory is used to define the lower segment; however, if this cannot be seen with transabdominal scanning, a transvaginal scan is used to determine the distance from the cervical os to the lower margin of the placenta. Localization of the placental site in early pregnancy may result in an inaccurate diagnosis, as development of the lower segment will lead to an apparent upwards displacement of the placenta by 30 weeks.

- **磁共振：** 可以在胎盘附着于上次剖宫产切口的子宫下段时使用。尽管在这种情况下超声检查也是一种好的成像方式，但磁共振成像可能有助于确定胎盘组织是否通过子宫瘢痕植入或穿透进入了膀胱组织（见"胎盘植入疾病"）。

- Magnetic resonance imaging: This is used when the placenta is implanted on the lower uterine segment over an old caesarean scar. It may help to determine whether the placental tissue has migrated through the scar (placenta percreta) or even into the bladder tissue, although ultrasound is a better modality of imaging in this situation-see the Placenta accreta spectrum section.

6. 治疗（Management）

当出现产前出血时，应首先考虑前置胎盘，并建议入院治疗。建立静脉通道，并积极备血，根据需要对孕妇进行抢救。行 CTG 检查以确定胎儿状况。通过超声查找出血的原因，切记 50% 的产前出血病例中，无法找出明显的原因。在急性情况下，在没有超声诊断时，对产前出血的孕妇进行阴道检查只能在为紧急剖宫产做准备。

When antepartum haemorrhage of any type occurs, the diagnosis of placenta praevia should be suspected and hospital admission advised. An IV line should be established and the mother resuscitated as necessary after blood has been taken for full blood count and cross-match. A CTG should be performed to determine fetal status. A cause for the bleeding should be sought by ultrasound imaging, remembering that in up to 50% of cases of antepartum haemorrhage no obvious cause will be seen. In the acute setting, in the absence of an ultrasound diagnosis, a vaginal examination on a woman who has suffered an antepartum haemorrhage should be performed only in an operating theatre which is prepared for an emergency caesarean section and with cross-matched blood readily available.

行阴道检查唯一指征。

There is only one indication for performing a vaginal examination:

- 由于超声设备不足而对诊断有严重疑问时，产程已经开始，出血也已解决。资深的产科专家可以把患者送进手术室后进行阴道检查。先要通过阴道穹隆进行手指触诊，以确定先露的部位是否容易摸到。如果触诊胎儿头部有困难或有凹凸不平的肿物，则很可能是低处的胎盘。如果通过穹隆很容易感觉到先露的部分，表明下段没有胎盘，则可以通过子宫颈触诊，力求人工破膜分娩。

- When there is serious doubt about the diagnosis due to inadequate ultrasound facilities, labour appears to have commenced and bleeding has settled. The patient can be taken to theatre by a very senior obstetrician. First the examination has to be by digital palpation through the vaginal fornices to feel whether the presenting part can be felt easily. If there is difficulty in palpating the fetal head and/or a boggy mass is felt, then it is likely that that boggy mass is placenta that is low lying. If the presenting part is easily felt via the fornices suggesting that there is no placenta in the lower segment, careful digital examination through the cervix can occur with the intention of rupturing the membranes to induce labour.

在早产和出血不危及生命的情况下，应考虑保守治疗前置胎盘。让孕妇住院后备血，直到胎儿成熟，然后根据前置胎盘的等级可通过剖宫产分娩胎儿。出血后，孕妇应给予铁剂治疗，以维持足够的血红蛋白浓度。与所有产前出血一样，如果孕妇是 Rh 阴性血，就需要注射抗 D 免疫球蛋白。为了确定所需的剂量，需要采集血液进行 Kleihauer-Betke 试验，以确定母胎输血的程度。

Conservative management of placenta praevia should always be considered in the pre-term situation and where the bleeding is not life threatening. This involves keeping the mother in hospital with cross-matched blood until fetal maturity is adequate and then delivering the child by caesarean section depending on the grade of placenta praevia. After any bleed, the mother should be treated by oral iron or iron infusion where necessary so that an adequate haemoglobin concentration is maintained. As with any antepartum haemorrhage, anti-D immunoglobulin needs to be given if the mother is Rhesus negative. To ascertain the dose required, blood is taken for the Kleihauer-Betke test to determine the extent of any fetomaternal transfusion.

产后出血也是产前低位胎盘的一个危险因素，因为下段的收缩不如上段的收缩好，导致静脉窦出血得不到控制。

Postpartum haemorrhage is also a hazard of the antenatal low-lying placenta, as contraction of the lower segment is less effective than contraction of the upper segment, leaving bleeding from the venous sinuses uncontrolled.

在前置胎盘的情况下，胎盘植入发生在原来子宫瘢痕的位置上，这会增加胎盘植入的风险。

There is an increased risk of placenta accreta/increta/percreta (placenta accreta spectrum) where, in the situation of placenta praevia, placental implantation occurs over the site of a previous uterine scar.

7. 胎盘植入（Placenta accreta spectrum）

胎盘植入是用来描述胎盘异常附着于子宫壁的情况。这一术语包括胎盘粘连（附着于子宫肌层而不是蜕膜的胎盘）、胎盘植入（胎盘侵入肌层）和胎盘穿透（胎盘侵袭子宫壁和浆膜及周围结构），这种异常侵袭是由于滋养细胞附着时蜕膜基底层的缺失。以往的子宫创伤或手术，如剖宫产术、子宫内膜消

融术、子宫肌瘤切除术、子宫动脉栓塞术（治疗肌瘤）、扩张和刮宫术或手工摘除胎盘，可在瘢痕上发现蜕膜层缺失。

Placenta accreta spectrum is the term used to describe the condition where the placenta is abnormally adherent to the uterine wall. The term includes placenta accreta (placenta attached to the myometrium and not the decidua), placenta increta (placental invasion into the myometrium) and placenta percreta (placental invasion through the uterine wall and into the serosa and surrounding structures). The abnormal invasion is due to an absence of the normal decidual basalis at the time of trophoblast attachment. The absence of the decidual layer is found over scars associated with previous uterine trauma or surgery such as caesarean section, endometrial ablation, myomectomy, uterine artery embolization as a treatment for fibroids, dilatation and curettage or manual removal of placenta.

胎盘植入的主要问题是，在第三产程中，胎盘不会从子宫壁剥离，供给胎盘床的血管可能会破裂出血，甚至会大量出血。胎盘植入通常在第三产程中因胎盘滞留而试图手动剥除胎盘时而被诊断。无论是否使用宫内球囊导管，这个情况的出血通常可以通过缩宫素来抑制出血。有时出血得不到控制，需要行 B-Lynch 缝合，若缝合效果不佳，就需要摘除子宫。产前发现的子宫上段胎盘植入并不常见，因为通常植入的面积很小。

The primary issue with placenta accreta spectrum disorder is that the placenta does not separate from the uterine wall in the third stage of labour, and blood vessels feeding the placental bed can bleed-at times profusely. Placenta accreta spectrum in the upper segment of the uterus is usually diagnosed when a manual removal of the placenta is attempted for retained placenta in the third stage of labour. Bleeding at this time can usually be controlled with the use of oxytocic drugs with or without the use of an intrauterine balloon catheter. Occasionally bleeding is not controlled and a surgical procedure like a B Lynch suture or, if that fails, a hysterectomy is required. The antenatal detection of an upper-segment placenta accreta spectrum disorder is uncommon, as the area of the accreta is usually small.

前置胎盘植入是产科中最致命的疾病之一，前置胎盘存在且胎盘异常附着在先前剖腹产瘢痕区域。在这种情况下，滋养层细胞生长到瘢痕组织中，并可能侵入浆膜或上覆的膀胱。如果增生不止一小部分瘢痕，分娩时可能发生大出血。

The placenta praevia accreta, where there is a placenta praevia and the placenta is abnormally attached over the area of a previous caesarean section scar, is one of the most lethal conditions in obstetrics. In this condition, the trophoblast grows into the scar tissue and may invade the serosa or the overlying bladder. Where the accreta involves more than a small section

病例分析	Case study

J 夫人是一名 30 岁的孕妇，这是她第三次妊娠。她之前的 2 次妊娠都是因为难产通过剖宫产分娩的。在这次妊娠期间，12 周时超声显示正常，20 周的超声报告显示低置胎盘，覆盖宫颈内口和疑似覆盖在子宫瘢痕部位。24 周时，超声结果显示，确诊为胎盘植入，瘢痕上的胎盘上有多个低回声区域，存在血管陷窝，子宫浆膜 / 母体膀胱界面缺失（图 8-9），血管从膀胱植入到子宫边缘。

终止妊娠时间定于孕 35 周，以最大限度减少孕妇与胎儿的不良预后。对此进行了一次多学科会诊讨论手术方式，其中包括以下人员。

- 产科医生。

- 妇科肿瘤专家。

- 麻醉师。

- 泌尿科医生，考虑到可能存在胎盘侵入膀胱和骨盆侧壁的可能性，将输尿管支架置入输尿管。

- 介入放射学，讨论髂内动脉球囊减少辅助手术部位失血的效果。

在手术前 48h，血库通知患者备血，给予孕妇糖皮质激素促进胎儿肺成熟。

那位孕妇咨询专家后同意剖宫产。她了解到胎儿将通过剖宫产分娩，分娩后胎盘将被充分暴露。如果未见明显的穿孔层，且胎盘可以正常分离，则应将其剥除，并止血。如果胎盘根本没有分离，也没有出血，我们讨论结果时将胎盘留在原位、结束手术，然后在晚些时候取出胎盘；不过，这种情况可能发生延迟出血和败血症。第三种情况是，在手术中，打开腹腔发现植入明显，考虑到胎盘部位的血管异常，分娩后，则应由专业的外科医生（如妇科医生）行子宫切除术。由于缺乏强有力的证据证明髂内球囊的使用是有效的，所以其没有被使用。

手术时，输尿管支架放置在恰当的位置，其作用是在手术中识别输尿管。在打开腹腔时，确诊为大面积胎盘植入，胎儿通过剖宫产分娩，关闭子宫切口以恢复止血，并行子宫切除术。使用细胞回输器以减少输血的必要性；然而，胎盘侵入盆腔组织导致 7L 的血液流失。用血液制品替代血液以维持凝血功能，输血后产妇血红蛋白为 87g/L。分娩后，向产妇告知术中情况。产妇 5 天后出院，婴儿因早产及喂养迟缓问题 10 天后出院。

Mrs J is 30-year-old woman in her third pregnancy. Her two previous pregnancies were delivered by uncomplicated caesarean sections for obstructed labour on both occasions. In this pregnancy, she had a normal 12-week scan. The 20-week scan reported the presence of a low-lying anterior placenta which covered the cervical os and the presumed site of the uterine scar. At 24 weeks, she had an ultrasound scan that confirmed the signs of placenta accreta: multiple hypoechoic areas in the placenta overlying the scar, which represent vascular lacunae, and a loss of the uterine serosa/maternal bladder interface (Fig. 8.9) and maternal vessels passing from the bladder to the uterine margin.

Delivery was planned for 35 weeks, which is best to minimize pathology for both mother and fetus. A multidisciplinary meeting was held to plan surgery, which included:

- Obstetricians

- Gynaecology oncology specialist

- Vascular surgeon

- Anaesthetists

- Urologists-to place ureteric stents into the ureters, given the probable involvement of the placenta invasion into the bladder and the pelvic sidewall

- Interventional radiology-to discuss the benefits or otherwise of internal iliac artery balloons to help stem blood loss from the surgical site

The blood bank was alerted about the case 48 hours before the procedure, and blood was cross-matched and the mother was administered steroids to promote fetal lung maturation.

The mother was fully counselled and consented for a caesarean section. She was told the baby would be delivered through a classical caesarean incision and after delivery the placenta would be visualized. If obvious percreta was not seen and the placenta appeared to separate normally, it would be removed and haemostasis achieved if possible. If the placenta did not separate at all and there was no bleeding, the possibility of leaving it in situ, completing the operation and then removing the placenta at a later date was discussed; however, this scenario is associated with delayed bleeding and possible sepsis. The third scenario explained was that if at operation the percreta was obvious on opening the abdomen and after delivery of the baby, a hysterectomy would be performed with highly trained surgeons, such as a gynaecology oncologist, given the abnormal blood vessels feeding the placental site. The use of internal iliac balloons was not discussed due to the lack of strong evidence they are of benefit.

At operation, ureteric stents were put in place to aid the identification of the ureters at surgery. On opening the abdomen, a major degree of placenta accreta was diagnosed, the baby was delivered through a classical caesarean section incision, the uterine incision was closed to restore haemostasis and a difficult hysterectomy was performed. A cell saver was used to try to minimize the need for transfusion; however, the invasion of the placenta into the pelvic tissue resulted in the loss of 7 L of blood. Blood replacement with blood products to maintain clotting was transfused to the point that the maternal haemoglobin after operation was 87 g/L. Following delivery, the mother was debriefed and given counselling support. Mother was discharged on day 5, and baby was discharged after 10 days due to prematurity and slow feeding issues.

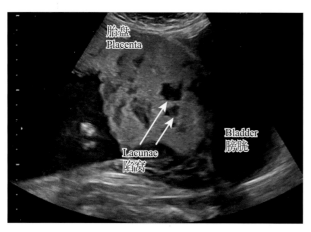

▲ 图 8-9　前置胎盘并植入的超声图像显示有胎盘陷窝

Fig. 8.9　Ultrasound picture of a placenta praevia accreta showing presence of placental lacunae.

of the scar, massive haemorrhage may occur at delivery.

（二）胎盘早剥（Abruptio placentae）

胎盘早剥或意外出血定义为胎盘过早剥离引起的出血。"意外"一词的意思是由于创伤而分离，但大多数病例并不涉及创伤，而是自发性的。

Abruptio placentae or accidental haemorrhage is defined as haemorrhage resulting from premature separation of the placenta. The term *accidental* implies separation as the result of trauma, but most cases do not involve trauma and occur spontaneously.

1. 病因（Aetiology）

胎盘早剥的发生率为 0.6%～7.0%，这取决于所研究的人群。在饮食缺乏，特别是叶酸缺乏和吸烟的社会因素下，更易发生。它还与高血压疾病、母体血栓史、胎儿生长受限和男性胎儿有关。虽然交通事故、跌倒、严重的家庭暴力和妊娠后期的腹部撞击，通常与胎盘早剥有关，但创伤是相对不常见的原因。大多数情况下，无法确定某一特定因素。若无分娩史，则在初次妊娠和以后的妊娠中复发率都很高。

The incidence of placental abruption varies from 0.6% to 7.0%, with the rate depending on the population studied. It occurs more frequently under conditions of social deprivation in association with dietary deficiencies, especially folate deficiency, and tobacco use. It is also associated with hypertensive disease, maternal thrombophilia, fetal growth restriction and a male fetus. Although motor vehicle accidents, falls, serious domestic violence and blows to the abdomen in later pregnancy are commonly associated with placental separation, trauma is a relatively uncommon cause. In the

majority of cases, no specific predisposing factor can be identified for a particular episode. There is a high recurrence rate both within a pregnancy if delivery is not required with the first episode and in subsequent pregnancies.

对胎儿的主要影响是围产期死亡率高。在美国，一项对 750 万例妊娠的研究中发现，胎盘早剥的发生率为 6.5‰，相关病例的围产期死亡率为 1.19‰。孕妇吸烟对胎儿预后最不利。

The main fetal effect is a high perinatal mortality rate. In one study of 7.5 million pregnancies in the United States, the incidence of placental abruption has been recorded as 6.5/1000 births with a perinatal mortality in associated cases of 119/1000 births. Fetal prognosis is worst with maternal tobacco use.

无论是什么因素导致胎盘早剥，其在胎盘早剥发生之前就已具备该条件了。

Whatever factors predispose to placental abruption, they are well established before the abruption occurs.

2. 临床类型和临床表现（Clinical types and presentation）

虽然已描述了 3 种类型的胎盘早剥，即显性的、隐匿性的或混合性的（图 8-10），但这种分类对临床没有帮助。通常在分娩后发现隐藏的血块时才进行分类。

Although three types of abruption have been described, i.e. revealed, concealed or mixed (Fig. 8.10), this classification is not clinically helpful. Commonly the classification is made after delivery when the concealed clot is discovered.

与前置胎盘不同，胎盘早剥表现为疼痛、阴道流血和子宫张力增高。

Unlike placenta praevia, placental abruption presents with pain, vaginal bleeding of variable amounts and increased uterine activity.

出血（Haemorrhage）

胎盘早剥涉及胎盘与子宫壁的分离以及随后的出血。显性的出血量取决于胎盘早剥的部位，胎盘下缘出血比上缘出血更容易通过宫颈口。宫腔内的血液导致子宫静息张力增加，可能引起宫缩，肌张力和血块的增加可能使胎儿触诊和听诊胎心变得困难。残留的血块也可能导致母体内凝血因子的异常消耗，甚至大量出血。

Abruption involves separation of the placenta from the uterine wall and subsequent haemorrhage. The amount of haemorrhage revealed will depend on the site of the abruption.

病例分析	Case study
Mandy 是一名 23 岁的初产妇，在妊娠 35 周时入院，她自诉自己有严重的腹痛，随后大量阴道流血。查体发现，患者有明显疼痛。血压为 150/90mmHg，子宫僵硬、触痛。脉搏率为 100/min，脸色苍白。子宫底可触及剑突水平。胎儿呈纵向横位，头部呈纵向。无法测到胎儿心搏，并且超声提示胎死宫内。紧急情况下，建立静脉通道，备血。给予 Mandy 镇痛药，并检查了她的血象和凝血功能。阴道检查显示子宫颈已消失，宫口扩张了 3cm，并且胎膜膨出。给予人工破膜，释放了血染的羊水。随后进行了分娩，3h 后 Mandy 分娩一死婴。大量的血凝块与胎盘一起被娩出，约有 50% 的胎盘已从子宫壁剥离。	Mandy, a 23-year-old primigravida, was admitted to hospital at 35 weeks' gestation with a complaint that she had developed severe abdominal pain followed by substantial vaginal bleeding. On examination, she was restless and in obvious pain. Her BP was 150/90 mmHg, and the uterus was rigid and tender. Her pulse rate was 100 beats/min, and she looked pale and tense. The uterine fundus was palpable at the level of the xiphisternum. The fetal lie was longitudinal, with the head presenting. The fetal heartbeat could not be detected, and the diagnosis of intrauterine fetal death was made using ultrasound. An IV line was established and blood cross-matched as a matter of urgency. Mandy was given pain relief, and her blood picture and clotting profile were examined. Vaginal examination showed that the cervix was effaced and 3 cm dilated and the membranes were bulging through the os. A forewater rupture was performed and blood-stained amniotic fluid was released. Labour ensued, and Mandy was delivered 3 hours later of a stillborn male infant. A large amount of clot was delivered with the placenta, and some 50% of the placenta appeared to have been avulsed from the uterine wall.

A bleed from the lower edge of the placenta will pass more easily through the cervical os than a bleed from the upper margin. Blood within the uterus causes an increase in the resting tone of the uterus and possibly the onset of contractions. The increased tone and blood clot may make palpation of the fetus and auscultation of the fetal heart difficult. The retained blood clot may also lead to abnormal consumption of maternal clotting factors and profuse bleeding.

在一些严重的病例中，出血穿透子宫壁，子宫表面出现出血点等，称为子宫卒中。在检查时，子宫会紧张和坚硬，子宫底会高于正常的胎龄。这种严重的胎盘早剥，通常会引起临产，并且约 30% 的病例胎儿心音会消失，胎死宫内。

In some severe cases, haemorrhage penetrates through the uterine wall and the uterus appears bruised. This is described as a Couvelaire uterus. On clinical examination, the uterus will be tense and hard and the uterine fundus will be higher than is normal for the gestational age. With this severe form of abruption, the mother will often be in labour and in approximately 30% of cases the fetal heart sounds will be absent and the fetus will be stillborn.

任何胎盘早剥的胎儿预后取决于胎盘分离的程度，与胎盘早剥和分娩之间的间隔时间成反比。这意味着在胎儿受损的情况下，及早评估和终止妊娠是至关重要的。

The prognosis for the fetus in any abruption is dependent

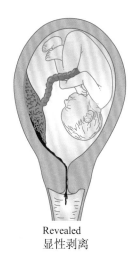 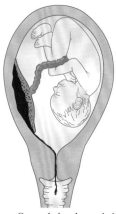

Revealed
显性剥离

Concealed
隐性剥离

Concealed and revealed
混合型剥离

▲ 图 8-10　胎盘早剥的类型

Fig. 8.10　Types of placental abruption.

！注意

重要的是要认识到，凡在 20 周后突然出现腹痛或子宫收缩并伴有或不伴有明显出血的孕妇都可能是胎盘早剥。需要对孕妇的血压、脉搏和氧合进行紧急评估，因为她可能存在大面积的隐性出血。如果患者脉率高于收缩压，如脉搏为 110/min，收缩压为 80mm/Hg，她可能会失血约 1L 甚至更多。若出血进一步加重，患者会因心动过速、低血压和少尿而休克。需要静脉补液、查血常规并备血、行胎儿 CTG 和（或）超声评估胎儿健康和胎盘状况，以及子宫内的出血情况。不幸的是，超声很难显示子宫内出血状况，因此对子宫早剥的处理应基于临床表现。

It is important to realize that any pregnant woman presenting after 20 weeks with the sudden onset of abdominal pain and/or uterine contractions with or without significant bleeding may have suffered a placental abruption. Urgent assessment of the mother's BP, pulse and oxygenation is warranted, as she may have a large concealed bleed. If her pulse rate is above the measure of her systolic BP, e.g. pulse is 110 beats per minute and systolic BP is 80 mmHg, she could have lost 1 L or more of blood. If she bleeds further, she will become shocked with the development of marked tachycardia, hypotension and oliguria. She requires IV fluids, blood for full blood count and cross-matching, fetal CTG and/ or ultrasound assessment of fetal welfare and placental status and possible visualization of blood in the uterus. Unfortunately, the visualization of fresh bleeding in the uterus can be difficult with ultrasound, so an abruption management should be based on clinical findings.

on the extent of placental separation and is inversely proportional to the interval between onset of the abruption and delivery of the baby. This means that early assessment and delivery in cases with fetal compromise are essential.

3. 临床评估 / 鉴别诊断(Clinical assessment/differential diagnosis）

诊断早剥的依据是阴道流血、腹痛、子宫张力增高，通常还有胎儿的纵产式。孕妇的状况可能比显性出血量应有的临床表现更糟。胎盘早剥必须与前置胎盘鉴别，前置胎盘表现为无痛性阴道流血，胎位不定、子宫张力正常，失血量与母体状况有关。然而，有时胎盘早剥的可能发生在胎盘位置较低的地方。换句话说，胎盘早剥也可能发生在低置胎盘的病例，在这种情况下，需要通过超声定位胎盘位置。

The diagnosis of abruption is made on the history of vaginal bleeding, abdominal pain, increased uterine tone and,

commonly, the presence of a longitudinal lie of the fetus. The condition of the mother may be worse than the revealed blood would indicate. This must be distinguished from placenta praevia, where the haemorrhage is painless, the fetal lie is unstable with the uterus having a normal tone and an amount of blood loss that relates to maternal condition. Occasionally, however, some manifestations of placental abruption may arise where there is a low-lying placenta. In other words, placental abruption can arise where there is low placental implantation and, on these occasions, the diagnosis can only really be clarified by an ultrasound scan localizing the site of the placenta.

胎盘早剥的诊断也应与其他急症（如急性羊水过多）相鉴别。急性羊水过多是指子宫体积增大、压痛、肌张力高，但无出血。其他急腹症，如溃疡穿孔、肠扭转和绞窄性腹股沟疝，可能会掩盖胎盘早剥征象，但这些问题在妊娠期罕见。

The diagnosis of abruption should also be differentiated from other acute emergencies such as acute hydramnios, where the uterus is enlarged, tender and tense but there is no haemorrhage. Other acute abdominal emergencies such as perforated ulcer, volvulus of the bowel and strangulated inguinal hernia may simulate concealed placental abruption, but these problems are rare during pregnancy.

4. 治疗（Management）

患者必须住院治疗，并根据病史、检查（图 8-11）和超声检查结果确定诊断。在早产情况下，轻度胎盘早剥（孕妇状况稳定且 CTG 正常）可以保守治疗。超声检查用于评估胎儿的生长和健康，以及胎盘定位。如果胎儿是早产，治疗的目的则是延长妊娠，若孕妇和胎儿条件允许，应先处理与胎盘早剥相关的疾病，如高血压。若出血严重，则先要对孕妇进行抢救，然后再处理胎儿问题。

.The patient must be admitted to hospital and the diagnosis established on the basis of the history, examination findings (Fig. 8.11) and ultrasound findings. In pre-term pregnancy, mild cases (mother stable and CTG normal) may be treated conservatively. An ultrasound examination should be used to assess fetal growth and wellbeing, and the placental site should be localized to confirm the diagnosis. If the fetus is pre-term, the aim of management is to prolong the pregnancy if the maternal and fetal conditions allow. Conditions that are associated with abruption, e.g. hypertension, should be managed appropriately. If the haemorrhage is severe, resuscitation of the mother is the first prerequisite, following which fetal condition can be addressed.

通常很难准确评估失血量，静脉滴注使用生理盐水、Hartmann 溶液或血液替代品，直到备血完成

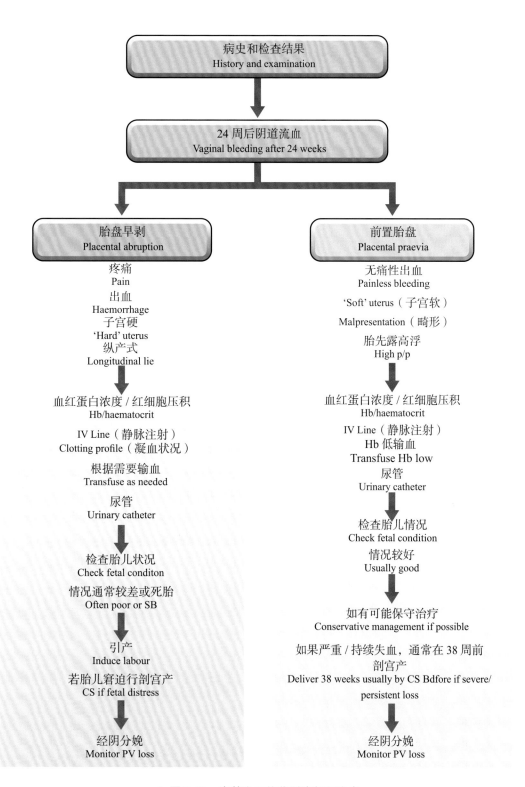

▲ 图 8-11　产前出血的鉴别诊断和治疗

Fig. 8.11　**Differential diagnosis and management of antepartum haemorrhage. CS, Caesarean section; IV, intravenous; Hb, Haemoglobin concentration; p/p, Presenting part; PV, per vaginum; SB, still birth.**

后可以开始输血。尿管对于监测尿量至关重要。

It is often difficult to assess the amount of blood loss accurately, and IV infusion should be started with normal saline, Hartmann's solution or blood substitutes until blood is cross-matched and transfusion can be commenced. A urinary catheter is essential to monitor the urine output.

如果是近足月活胎，且无不良临床迹象，或者胎死宫内，应尽快终止妊娠，必要时，静脉滴注缩宫素刺激子宫收缩。若胎儿有生命迹象，监测胎心，若出现胎儿受损的迹象，则尽快行剖宫产终止妊娠。如果由于宫颈口紧闭无法引产，持续出血导致产妇病情不稳定，或者产妇出现凝血障碍，则无论胎儿是否存活应在产科专家和麻醉人员在场的情况下行剖宫产术终止妊娠。可使用阿片类药物镇痛，在凝血功能结果未出前，禁止行硬膜外麻醉。

If the fetus is alive and close to term and there are no clinical signs of fetal compromise, or if the fetus is dead, induction of labour is performed as soon as possible and, where necessary, uterine activity is stimulated with an oxytocin infusion. Where the fetus is alive, the fetal heart should be monitored and caesarean section should be performed if signs of fetal compromise develop. If induction is not possible because the cervix is closed and maternal condition is unstable due to ongoing bleeding, or a maternal coagulopathy develops, delivery should be effected by caesarean section with senior obstetric and anaesthetic staff present, whether or not the fetus is alive. Pain relief is achieved by the use of opiates. Epidural anaesthesia should not be used until a clotting screen is available and is seen to be normal.

若出现先兆早产征象并且孕妇和胎儿的情况稳定，孕妇应该住院并密切监测，直至出血停止和疼痛消失，孕妇可在情况稳定 48h 后出院回家。若妊娠状态稳定，可在 37～38 周时引产。

If the fetus is pre-term and maternal and fetal conditions are stable, the mother should be admitted and monitored until all signs of bleeding and pain have settled. The mother may be discharged home 48 hours after blood loss has ceased and so long as any predisposing factors like hypertension have been adequately treated. Most units subsequently will induce labour at 37–38 weeks if the pregnancy remains stable.

5. 并发症（Complications）

胎盘早剥的并发症如图 8-12 所示。

The complications of placental abruption are summarized in Figure 8.12.

(1) 纤维蛋白原缺乏症（Afibrinogenaemia）

当发生严重胎盘早剥导致凝血活酶释放到母体循环中时，就会发生纤维蛋白原缺乏症。这可能导致弥散性血管内凝血和凝血因子（包括血小板）的消耗，并发展为低纤维蛋白原血症或纤维蛋白原缺乏症。发生这种情况可以在胎儿分娩后输注病毒灭活血浆、血小板和纤维蛋白原进行治疗。除非凝血功能得到纠正，否则可能会导致手术分娩时异常出血

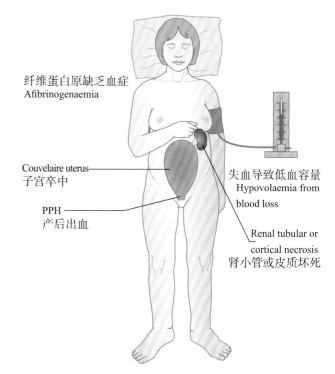

▲ 图 8-12　胎盘早剥并发症
PPH. 产后出血

Fig. 8.12　Complications of placental abruption.
PPH, Postpartum haemorrhage.

或无法控制的产后出血。考虑到胎盘剥离后组织物可能会快速产生纤维蛋白降解产物而使产妇凝血状况恶化，所以应在剖宫产胎盘娩出后及时给予治疗。

Afibrinogenaemia occurs when the clot from a severe placental abruption causes the release of thromboplastin into the maternal circulation. This in turn may lead to DIC and the consumption of coagulation factors, including platelets, with the development of hypofibrinogenaemia or afibrinogenaemia. The condition may be treated by the infusion of fresh frozen plasma, platelet transfusion and fibrinogen transfusion after delivering the fetus. It may lead to abnormal bleeding at operative delivery or uncontrolled postpartum haemorrhage unless the clotting defect has been corrected. Given that replacing products with the placenta in place may worsen the maternal clotting status through the rapid production of fibrin degradation products, replacement should be timed to be given after the placenta has been delivered at caesarean section.

(2) 肾小管或皮质坏死（Renal tubular or cortical necrosis）

这是未得到充分治疗的低血容量血症和 DIC 的并发症。评估尿量是至关重要的。孕妇发生无尿必须得到积极处理。如若不是，可能需要血液透析或腹膜透析。

This is a complication of undertreated hypovolaemia and DIC. A careful assessment of urinary output is essential. Anuria in a pregnant woman must be urgently and aggressively managed. If it is not, it may, on occasion, necessitate haemodialysis or peritoneal dialysis

（三）产前出血的其他原因（Other causes of antepartum haemorrhage）

这些在图 8-13 中进行了总结。

These are summarized in Figure 8.13.

1. 血管前置（Vasa praevia）

血管前置是一种非常罕见的情况，胎儿脐带血管的一个分支位于胎膜中并横跨宫颈口。当脐带和血管穿过胎膜到达胎盘时，或者胎盘有绒毛小叶，胎膜中的血管连接主要胎盘和分离的小叶时，就会发生这种情况。宫颈上的胎膜破裂可能会导致血管破裂，这将导致胎儿失血。多普勒超声可以诊断血管前置。

Vasa praevia is a very rare condition where one of the branches of the fetal umbilical vessels lies in the membranes and across the cervical os. This occurs when there is a membranous insertion of the cord and the vessels course through the membranes to the placenta, or if there is succenturiate lobe of the placenta and the vessels in the membrane connect the main placental mass and the separate lobe. Rupture of the membranes over the cervical os may cause a tear in the vessels, which will result in the rapid exsanguination of the fetus. Vasa praevia can be diagnosed with colour Doppler ultrasound at the fetal anatomy scan.

2. 原因不明的产前出血（Unexplained antepartum haemorrhage）

近 50% 的妊娠期间出现阴道出血的孕妇中，无法明确诊断为胎盘早剥或前置胎盘。

In almost 50% of cases of women presenting with vaginal bleeding in pregnancy, it is not possible to make a definite diagnosis of abruption or placenta praevia.

如果确认出血来自子宫腔，则认为病因是胎盘边缘出血。无论是什么原因导致，围产期死亡率都有显著增加，因此监测胎盘功能和胎儿在妊娠剩余时间的生长是很重要的。妊娠时间不应超过足月。

Where the bleeding is confirmed to be coming from the uterine cavity, it is proposed that the cause is bleeding from the edge of the placenta. Whatever the cause, there is a significant increase in perinatal mortality, and it is therefore important to monitor placental function and fetal growth for the rest of the

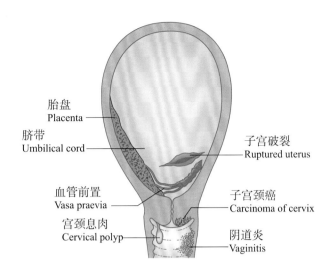

▲ 图 8-13　非胎盘原因引起产前出血

Fig. 8.13　Non-placental causes of antepartum haemorrhage.

pregnancy. The pregnancy should not be allowed to proceed beyond term.

3. 阴道炎（Vaginal infections）

阴道念珠菌病或滴虫病可能出现血性分泌物，一旦确诊，应采用恰当的治疗方法进行治疗。

Vaginal moniliasis or trichomoniasis may cause bloodstained discharge and, once the diagnosis is established, should be treated with the appropriate therapy.

4. 宫颈病变（Cervical lesions）

宫颈的良性病变，如宫颈息肉，可以通过切除息肉来治疗。宫颈柱状上皮异位不需要进一步治疗。

Benign lesions of the cervix, such as cervical polyps, are treated by removal of the polyp. Cervical erosions are best left untreated.

如在妊娠期间被确诊子宫颈癌，且妊娠时间短，则需要终止妊娠，然后进行癌症分期并进行明确的治疗。如果是在妊娠晚期确诊，则应进行活检来确定诊断，胎儿成熟后分娩，并根据病变分期进行治疗，包括行剖宫产术和在疾病早期行根治性子宫切除术。

Carcinoma of the cervix is occasionally found in pregnancy. If the pregnancy is early, termination is indicated followed by staging of the cancer and definitive therapy. If the diagnosis is made late in pregnancy, the diagnosis should be established by biopsy, the baby delivered when mature and the lesion treated according to the staging, including caesarean section and radical hysterectomy for early-stage disease.

三、多胎妊娠（Multiple pregnancy）

多胎妊娠是人类单腔子宫的一种反常妊娠现象，与许多其他物种不同的是，在其他物种中，孕妇的子宫是双角的，正常情况下可以孕育 2 个或多个后代。考虑到母婴发病率和死亡率的增加，双胎、三胞胎或胚胎数量较多的妊娠被认为是高风险妊娠。

Multiple pregnancy is an anomaly in the human with the single-cavity uterus, unlike many other species where the mother has a bicornuate uterus that allows for two or more offspring to be gestated as the norm. A pregnancy with twins, triplets or higher numbers of embryos is considered high risk given the increased risk of maternal and fetal morbidity and mortality.

（一）患病率（Prevalence）

多胎妊娠的发生率因种族和辅助生殖技术的使用而异。自然孪生的患病率在中非最高，每 1000 名活产婴儿中有多达 30 对双胎（60 对双胎），而在拉丁美洲和东南亚最低，每 1000 名活产婴儿中只有 6～10 对双胎。北美和欧洲的比例为每 1000 例中有 5～13 对双胎。1985—2005 年，由于生殖技术的发展，双胎的比例比以往增加了 1 倍多。双胎是由排卵诱导和体外受精（IVF）周期中 1 个以上受精胚胎的移植所致。考虑到多胎妊娠的风险，目前已摒弃通过移植多个胚胎来提高受孕率的技术，从而导致双胎率的下降。

The prevalence of multiple pregnancies varies with race and the use of assisted reproductive techniques. The prevalence of natural twinning is highest in Central Africa, where there are up to 30 twin sets (60 twins) per 1000 live births, and lowest in Latin America and Southeast Asia, where there are only 6–10 twin sets per 1000 live births. North America and Europe have intermediate rates of 5–13 twin sets per 1000 live births. Between 1985 and 2005 the rates of twins more than doubled due to reproductive technologies. The twins resulted from ovulation induction and the replacement of more than one fertilized embryo in the in vitro fertilization (IVF) cycle. Given the risks of multiple pregnancy, the technique of replacing multiple embryos to enhance the conception rate has been abandoned, resulting in a fall in the rates of twins.

三胎妊娠率的发生率在过去 30 年中有所增加。1985 年，英国的这一比例为 10.2/10 万，但在 2002—2006 年，这一比例接近 25/10 万，上升的原因尚不清楚。四胞胎和五胞胎等多胎出生率较高通常与药物的使用有关，但如果排除这一原因，英格兰和威尔士的数据显示发生率为 1.7/100 万。

The natural prevalence of triplet pregnancy rate appears to have increased over the past 30 years. In 1985, the rate in the UK was 10.2/100,000, but in 2002–2006, the rate was close to 25/100,000. The cause of this rise is unclear. Higher multiple births such as quadruplets and quintuplets are commonly associated with the use of fertility drugs, but if one excludes this cause, figures for England and Wales suggest a pregnancy rate of 1.7/1,000,000 maternities.

迄今为止，自然受孕最多的多胎妊娠是九胞胎。

The highest naturally occurring multiple pregnancy recorded so far is nonuplets.

（二）双胎的类型和绒毛膜性的测定（Types of twinning and determination of chorionicity）

任何多胎妊娠都可能是由排卵时释放一个或多个卵子造成的。

Any multiple pregnancy may result from the release of one or more ova at the time of ovulation.

1. 单卵多胎妊娠（Monozygotic multiple pregnancy）

如果一个卵子导致多胎妊娠，这些胚胎被称为单卵胚胎，也可以称为同卵胚胎。这两个婴儿的性别都是一样的。同卵双胎的发生率约为 1/280，不受种族的影响，由于辅助生殖技术导致其发生率增加。受精卵在受精后一段时间内分裂（图 8-14）。如果分裂发生在受精后，则会出现以下可能。

0～4 天会出现 2 个胚胎、2 个羊膜和 2 个绒毛膜（如同双卵双胎）：25%～30%。

4～8 天有 2 个胚胎、2 个羊膜和 1 个绒毛膜：65%～70%。

9～12 天有 2 个胚胎、1 个羊膜和 1 个绒毛膜：1%～2%。

13 天以上有 1 对双胎、1 个羊膜和 1 个绒毛膜：低于 1%。

If a single ova results in a multiple pregnancy, the embryos are called *monozygotic*, with alternative names of *uniovular* and *identical*. Both babies will have the same gender. The rate of monozygotic twins is approximately 1/280 pregnancies, is unaffected by race and is increased by reproductive technology for unknown reasons. The zygote divides some time after conception (Fig. 8.14). If the split postconceptually occurs at:

0–4 days there will be two embryos, two amnions and

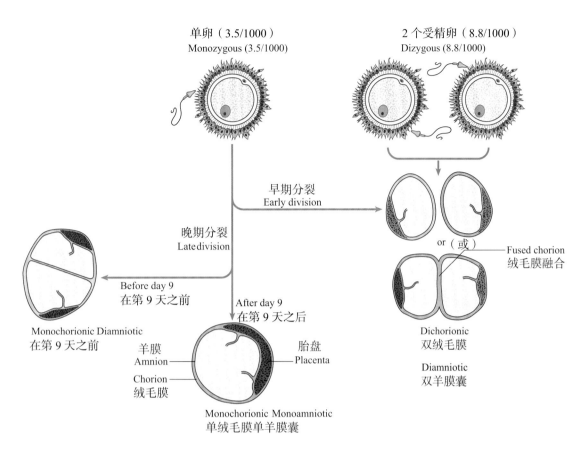

单卵（3.5/1000）
Monozygous (3.5/1000)

2 个受精卵（8.8/1000）
Dizygous (8.8/1000)

早期分裂
Early division

晚期分裂
Late division

Fused chorion
绒毛膜融合

or（或）

Before day 9
在第 9 天之前

After day 9
在第 9 天之后

Dichorionic
双绒毛膜

Diamniotic
双羊膜囊

Monochorionic Diamniotic
在第 9 天之前

羊膜
Amnion

胎盘
Placenta

Chorion
绒毛膜

Monochorionic Monoamniotic
单绒毛膜单羊膜囊

▲ 图 8-14　双胎的类型，显示了胎膜和胎盘的结构。请注意，不同性别的双胎是异卵双胎，而只有一个绒毛膜的双胎总是单卵双胎。同性双绒毛膜双胎可以是单合子的，也可以是异合子的

Fig. 8.14　Types of twinning, indicating the structure of the membranes and placentae. Note that twins of different sexes are always dizygous and those with a single chorion are always monozygous. Dichorionic twins of the same sex can be monozygous or dizygous.

two chorions (as for dizygotic twins): 25–30%

4–8 days there will be two embryos, two amnions and one chorion: 65–70%

9–12 days there will be two embryos, one amnion and one chorion: 1–2%

13+ days there will be conjoined twins, one amnion and one chorion: <1%

考虑到胚胎在某种未知的影响下分裂，单卵多胎妊娠被认为是生殖的异常。有时胚胎分裂成 3 个，形成单卵三胞胎。在三胞胎的情况下，分裂可能同时发生或顺序发生，从而导致在一个绒毛膜内形成独立的连体双胎。

Given that the embryo splits under some unknown influence, monozygotic multiple pregnancy is considered to be an anomaly of reproduction. Occasionally the embryo splits into three, resulting in monozygotic triplets. In the case of triplets, the splitting may occur at the same time or sequentially, resulting in conjoined twins with a separate singleton pregnancy all within one chorion!

早期行超声检查，最好是在 14 周之前确定单合子性。如果受精卵在 4 天后分裂，则两个胚胎和单一的胎盘块之间会有一层薄薄的膜（单绒毛膜双羊膜囊）或没有膜（单绒毛膜单羊膜囊）。如果胚胎在 4 天前发生分裂，可能出现两个分离的胎盘，超声显示更清楚，在胎膜和胎盘相交的地方有双峰征。此外观与双绒毛膜双胎相同，可见单一胎盘。早期确定合子性是很重要的，因为它可以让家人计划如何照顾孕妇。羊水、绒毛膜绒毛样本或产后获得的脐带血的遗传评估可用于确认合子性，这些技术在现代超声技术应用后很少使用。

The determination of monozygosity is undertaken at an early ultrasound scan, preferably before 14 weeks. A pregnancy where the zygote splits after 4 days will show a single thin membrane (monochorionic diamniotic) or no membrane (monochorionic monoamniotic) separating the two embryos and a single placental mass. If the split in the embryo was in the first 4 days, there may be two separate placental masses or a single mass with a membrane that is easier to visualize on ultrasound and which has a twin peak sign where the membrane and the placenta intersect. This appearance is the same as that for diamniotic dichorionic twins where there is a single placental mass. Early determination of zygosity is important, as it allows the caregiver to plan the management of the pregnancy. Genetic assessment of amniotic fluid, chorionic villous samples or postnatally obtained cord blood can be used to confirm zygosity. These techniques are seldom used in the face of modern ultrasound technology.

2. 异卵双胎（Dizygotic twins）

来自不同精子和不同卵子的受精。在这类妊娠中，50% 的胎儿是男性＋女性，25% 是男性＋男性，25% 是女性＋女性。所有患者都将在超声结果中看到有 2 个独立的胎盘，或者有 1 个带有厚膜的单胎盘，膜上有"双峰"征象。妊娠早期胎盘附着膜部位出现 λ 征（膜间绒毛）或 T 征（膜间无绒毛膜）具有重要判断价值，因为它可以确定一对双胎是单绒毛膜还是双绒毛膜（图 8–15）。单绒毛膜双胎风险较高，因为他们可能有胎盘血管吻合，这可能导致双胎输血综合征及其后续并发症的发生。胎儿畸形发生率也更高。

These come from the separate fertilization of separate ova by different sperm. In 50% of such pregnancies the fetuses are male-female, with 25% being male-male and 25% being female-female. All will have either two separate placentas on ultrasound or a single placenta with a thick membrane with a 'twin peak' sign. The presence of a lambda (chorion in between membranes) or T (absence of chorion in between membranes) sign at the site of membrane insertion of the placenta in the first trimester is valuable in that it allows for the determination of whether a set of twins is monochorionic diamniotic or dichorionic diamniotic (Fig. 8.15). Monochorionic diamniotic twins are higher risk, as they may have placental vascular anastomosis, which may give rise to complications of twin-to-twin transfusion and its consequent sequelae. They also have a higher rate of fetal anomaly.

异卵双胎的比例因以下因素而异。

- 家族因素：家族因素在异卵双胎倾向中很明显，这似乎只发生在母亲一方。在美国盐湖城的一项研究记录中表明，自己是异卵双胎的女性的双胎率为 17.1‰，而普通人群的双胎率为 11.6‰，自己是异卵双胎的男性的双胎率仅为 7.9‰。

- 产次和产妇年龄：来自 Aberdeen 的研究表明，初产妇的产次比例从 10.4‰ 上升到第四胎孕

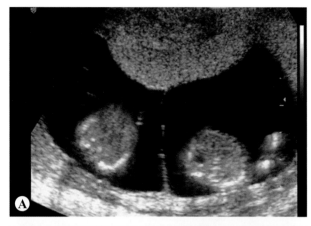

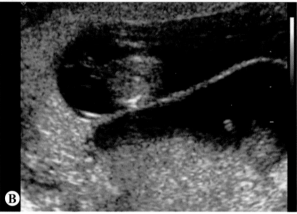

▲ 图 8–15 显示 T（A）和 λ（B）征的超声图像

Fig. 8.15　Ultrasound figure demonstrating (A) T and (B) lambda sign

妇的 15.3‰。高龄孕妇的双胎发生率也略有增加。

- 促排卵：在使用药物诱导排卵后，多胎妊娠就很常见了。值得注意的是，使用促性腺激素治疗会导致双胎、三胞胎甚至多胞胎的概率增加。在某种程度上，如果卵泡数量过多，可以通过监测卵巢卵泡发育和停止注射人绒毛膜促性腺激素（导致排卵）来避免这种情况。促排卵药物的使用占所有多胎妊娠的 10%～15%，因此显著改变了多胎妊娠的发生率。

The rate of dizygotic twins varies with:

- *Familial factors:* The familial tendency is apparent in dizygotic twinning, but this appears to be on the maternal side only. In a study of records at Salt Lake City, the twinning rates of women who were themselves dizygotic twins was 17.1/1000 maternities compared with 11.6/1000 maternities for the general population, but the rate for males who were themselves dizygotic twins was only 7.9/1000 maternities.

- *Parity and maternal age:* Studies in Aberdeen have shown that the rate increases from 10.4/1000 in primigravidae to 15.3/1000 in the para 4+ group. There is also a small increase in twinning in older mothers.

- *Ovulation induction:* Multiple pregnancy is common following the use of drugs to induce ovulation. It is important to note that the use of gonadotrophin therapy can result in twins, triplets or even higher-order pregnancies. To some degree, this can be avoided by monitoring ovarian follicular development and withholding the injection of human chorionic gonadotrophin (which causes ovulation) if excessive numbers of follicles develop. The use of fertility drugs accounts for 10–15% of all multiple pregnancies and has therefore significantly altered the incidence of multiple pregnancy.

如前所述，随着移植胚胎数量的限制，试管授精导致的多胎妊娠已呈降低趋势。

As mentioned earlier, the risk of multiple pregnancy as a result of IVF has decreased with the limitation of the number of embryos transferred.

（三）双胎妊娠的并发症（Complications of twin pregnancy）

在双胎（或多胞胎的妊娠）情况下，孕妇适应妊娠的正常生理过程会变得困难。与单胎妊娠相比，双胎孕妇体重平均多增加 3.5kg。红细胞数量虽然增加，但血容量较单胎妊娠增加 17%，因此仍然会出现贫血。使用血红蛋白来估算铁缺乏是不准确的，应使用血清铁蛋白来确定。与单胎妊娠相比，孕妇的心输出量增加了 20%，脑卒中发生率增加了 15%，心率增加了 3.5%。

The normal processes of maternal physiological adaptation to pregnancy are exaggerated in the presence of twins (or a higher-order pregnancy). Total weight gain is, on average, 3.5 kg greater than in singleton pregnancy. There is an increase in red cell mass as in singleton pregnancies. However, this does not match the expansion in plasma volume that exceeds that of a singleton pregnancy by 17% at term, and a relative anaemia develops. The use of haemoglobin estimation to determine iron deficiency is therefore flawed, and serum ferritin should be used. Compared with singleton pregnancies, maternal cardiac output was greater by 20% because of an increase in stroke volume by 15% and heart rate by 3.5%.

因此，可以预期的是，孕育 1 个以上胎儿给孕妇造成的压力会导致并发症的发生率更高（表 8-1）。

It is thus to be expected that the increased strain put on the mother by carrying more than one fetus will result in a higher incidence of complications (Table 8.1).

1. 与合子无关的并发症（Complications unrelated to zygosity）

(1) 恶心和呕吐（Nausea and vomiting）

在超声确诊之前，早期恶心和呕吐通常是双胎妊娠的征兆。双胎的呕吐发生率明显高于单胎妊娠。

Early onset of nausea and vomiting is often the sign that points to a twin pregnancy before ultrasound confirmation. The incidence of vomiting in twins is significantly higher compared with that of singletons.

(2) 贫血（Anaemia）

双胎与孕妇代谢需求有关。所有的孕妇都应该考虑在整个孕期补充铁和叶酸。

Twins are associated with extra metabolic demands on the mother. At a minimum, all mothers should consider iron and folate supplements throughout gestation.

(3) 流产（Miscarriage）

约 15% 的双胎妊娠会在 6～10 周内发生胎儿吸收，这被称为消失双胎综合征。双胎先兆流产和实

表 8-1　双胎妊娠的相关风险

Table 8.1　Risks associated with twin pregnancies

产科并发症 Obstetric complication	风险[*] Risk[*]
贫血 Anaemia	×2
子痫前期 Pre-eclampsia	×3
子痫 Eclampsia	×4
产前出血 Antepartum haemorrhage	×2
产后出血 Postpartum haemorrhage	×2
胎儿生长受限 Fetal growth restriction	×3
早产 pre-term delivery	×6
剖宫产 Caesarean section	×2

*. 与单胎妊娠相比的大概风险

*. Approximate risk compared with singleton pregnancies.

际流产的发生率更高。Aberdeen 的数据显示，26%的双胎孕妇和 20% 的单胎孕妇可能发生先兆流产，而 10～14 周的稽留流产是单胎孕妇的 2 倍。

Resorption of a fetus between 6 and 10 weeks occurs in over 15% of twin pregnancies and is referred to as the *vanishing twin syndrome*. The incidence of threatened and actual miscarriage is higher in twins. Evidence from Aberdeen has shown that threatened miscarriage occurs in 26% of twin pregnancies and 20% of singleton pregnancies, and missed miscarriage between 10 and 14 weeks is twice that of singletons.

(4) 产前出血（Antepartum haemorrhage）

双胎妊娠中因胎盘早剥和前置胎盘导致的产前出血发生率增加。

The incidence of antepartum haemorrhage as a result of abruption and placenta praevia doubles in twin pregnancies.

(5) 子痫前期（Pre-eclampsia）

双胎妊娠中妊娠期高血压，子痫前期和子痫的发生率增加。初产妇双胎妊娠的发生比例是单胎妊娠的 5 倍，而经产妇发生比例是单胎妊娠孕妇的 10 倍。

There is an increased incidence of gestational hypertension, pre-eclampsia and eclampsia in twin pregnancies. The rate in primigravidae is five times that of singletons, and in multigravidae, the rate is ten times that of women with singleton pregnancies.

(6) 胎儿生长受限（IUGR）（Intrauterine growth restriction (IUGR)）

在 20% 的双胎中，一胎儿明显小于另一个胎儿，其腹围的差异超过 20%。鉴于这种差异无法在临床上检测到，因此必须定期对双胎妊娠的生长和胎儿健康行超声检查。

In 20% of twins, one fetus is significantly smaller than the other as defined by a difference in the abdominal circumference of more than 20%. Given that this difference is impossible to detect clinically, regular ultrasound screening of growth and fetal wellbeing in twin pregnancies is mandatory.

(7) 早产（Pre-term labour）

早产是双胎妊娠最重要的并发症（表 8-2）。约 40% 的双胎妊娠在妊娠 37 周之前要终止妊娠。这种现象与子宫过度膨胀有关，子宫过度膨胀与多个胎儿的存在有关，若羊水容量增加，这种现象会进一

步增加。

The occurrence of pre-term labour is the most important complication of twin pregnancy (Table 8.2). The onset of labour before 37 weeks' gestation occurs in over 40% of twin pregnancies. The phenomenon appears to be associated with overdistension of the uterus associated with the presence of more than one fetus and is further increased if the amniotic fluid volume is increased.

表 8-2　按胎儿数分列的早产率

Table 8.2　Rates of pre-term delivery by fetal number

胎儿数 Number of fetuses	<28 周 <28 weeks
单胎 Singleton	0.7%
双胎 Twins	4.4%
三胎 Triplets	21.8%

2. 与合子相关的并发症（Complications related to zygosity）

同卵双胎的围产期死亡率比异卵双胎高，这是由于先天性异常、早产和胎盘血管异常（包括双胎输血综合征）的发病率较高引起的。

Monozygotic twins have a higher perinatal mortality rate than dizygotic twins. This is due to a higher incidence of congenital abnormalities, pre-term delivery and abnormalities of placental vasculature including the twin-twin (fetofetal) transfusion syndrome.

(1) 双胎输血综合征（TTTS）（Twin-to-twin transfusion syndrome (TTTS)）

10%～15% 的单绒毛膜双胎妊娠中会发生该综合征。在这种情况下，胎儿（供体）通过胎盘中相互连接的血管通道向另一个胎儿（受体）输血。往往发生在妊娠中期。供体双胎尿少，生长受限，伴有羊水过少，受体胎儿表现出羊水过多，有心脏肥大和胎儿水肿的风险。

This syndrome arises in 10–15% of all monochorionic diamniotic twin pregnancies. In this condition, one fetus (the donor) transfuses the other (the recipient) through interlinked vascular channels in the placenta. Presentation occurs in the second trimester. The donor twin is oliguric and growth-restricted with oligohydramnios, and the recipient fetus exhibits polyhydramnios and is at risk of cardiomegaly and hydrops fetalis.

若不进行治疗，TTTS 的围产期死亡率超过80%。治疗方案包括持续羊膜穿刺术以减少受体双胎周围的液体，通过胎儿镜，激光消融交互血管。激光治疗的存活率为 49%～67%。若一胎儿在激光治疗前发生宫内死亡，另一胎儿也将因急性血流动力变化而死亡。

Without treatment, the perinatal mortality in significant TTTS exceeds 80%. Treatment options include serial amniocenteses to remove fluid from around the recipient twin, selective feticide or laser ablation, via a fetoscope, of the communicating vessels. Laser treatment has survival rates of 49–67%. If one twin dies in utero before laser treatment, the other twin also often dies as a result of acute haemodynamic changes.

(2) 单胎和连体双胎（Monoamniotic and conjoined twinning）

1% 的单绒毛膜双胎出现单羊膜性，22 周的脐带缠绕是常见的并发症，存活率低至 50%。

Monoamnionicity occurs in 1% of monochorionic twins, and cord entanglement by 22 weeks is a common complication, such that survival rates are as low as 50%.

联体双胎的发生率为 1.3/10 万，融合发生在胎儿身体的不同部位。能否成功分离一对双胎，以及出生后是否能正常生活取决于融合部位，由妊娠 18～20 周的超声和磁共振（MRI）来确诊。如果存在主要的心血管融合或基本器官的融合（心脏、大脑），那么可以肯定的是，至少有 1 个胎儿在分离时会死亡。

Conjoined twinning occurs in 1.3/100,000 births, with fusion occurring at different sites on the bodies of the fetuses. Whether any set of twins can be successfully separated and the outlook for a normal life after birth depend on the site of fusion, which is determined with tertiarylevel ultrasound and magnetic resonance imaging (MRI) by 18–20 weeks' gestation. Where there is a major cardiovascular connection or a shared essential organ (heart, brain), perinatal death of at least one twin at separation is almost certain.

3. 产前诊断（Prenatal diagnosis）

多胎妊娠，特别是单卵多胎，会增加结构异常的风险，如无脑儿和先天性心脏病。绒毛膜性的确定、产前诊断和 TTTS 的评估尤为重要，可以在 12 周产检时进行。虽然双绒毛膜双胎的颈部透明度的增加更有可能与胎儿畸形 / 非整倍体有关，但单绒毛膜双胎之一的颈部透明度增加往往是发生 TTTS 的先

兆，因为两个双胎都由相同的基因构成。由于需要区分 2 个羊膜囊，因此筛查特别困难，所有此类筛查都应转至专业的产前诊断中心。

The risk of structural abnormalities such as anencephaly and congenital heart defects is increased in multiple pregnancies, particularly with monozygotic babies. Determination of chorionicity, prenatal diagnosis and assessment for impending TTTS is particularly important and can be performed at the 12-week scan. Whereas an increase in the nuchal translucency in a dichorionic twin is more likely associated with a fetal anomaly/aneuploidy, a raised nuchal translucency in one of a monochorionic twin pair is often a warning of possible TTTS, given both twins have the same genetic makeup. Screening for abnormalities presents particular difficulties because of the need to differentiate between the two sacs, and all such screening should be referred to a specialist obstetric scanning centre.

> **！注意**
>
> 在现代超声筛查技术出现之前，双胎和其他多胎妊娠的漏诊是常见的，常规检查如果没有超声检查仍会发生这种情况。过去对双胎的最初临床诊断以子宫异常增大为基础，但这种评估极不准确。没有及时确诊双胎的真正危险是，如果在第一个胎儿出生后使用缩宫素，会导致第二个胎儿被困住。之后即使再使用抑制宫缩的药物，这种情况也不能逆转，通常会导致第二个胎儿的损伤或死亡。若未确诊是否为双胎，也没有超声诊断，应禁用缩宫素；在第一个胎儿娩出后立即触诊产妇的腹部，以确认子宫中是否有第二个胎儿。
>
> The missed diagnosis of twins and other multiple pregnancies was relatively common before the advent of modern ultrasound screening techniques and still occurs where such facilities are not available on a routine basis. Although the initial clinical diagnosis of twins was always made in the past on the basis of an abnormally enlarged uterus, such assessments were notoriously inaccurate. The real danger of undiagnosed twins is that oxytocic drugs are administered after delivery of the first twin, leading to entrapment of the second twin. This situation cannot be reversed even with the use of tocolytic drugs and often results in the death of or damage to the second twin. If there is any suspicion of undiagnosed twins and ultrasound is not available, do not give oxytocic drugs; palpate the maternal abdomen immediately after delivery of the first twin to ensure there is not a second baby still in the uterus.

（四）双胎妊娠的处理（Management of twin pregnancy）

与单胎妊娠相比，多胎妊娠出现各种并发症的频率更高。因此，早期诊断是必要的，常规妊娠早

期超声会提供确切证据（图8-16）。

Multiple pregnancies exhibit every type of complication at a greater frequency than occurs in singleton pregnancy. Early diagnosis is therefore essential and provides a convincing argument for routine early-pregnancy ultrasound scanning (Fig. 8.16).

双胎妊娠最常见的临床症状是子宫较大，这在妊娠早期很容易发现，而不是在妊娠晚期。当然，子宫异常增大还有其他原因，如羊水过多和子宫肌瘤。

The commonest clinical sign of twin pregnancy is the greater size of the uterus, which is easier to detect in early, rather than late, pregnancy. There are, of course, other reasons why the uterus may be abnormally enlarged, such as hydramnios and uterine fibroids.

任何产前并发症的治疗都与单胎妊娠相同。谨记，特别是早产和子痫前期等并发症的发生，往往比单胎妊娠更早、更严重。过去一直主张从妊娠第28周开始常规入院卧床休息，但临床试验未能证明此疗效。每周进行2～4次产前监护和超声检查可以发现胎儿生长异常和TTTS发生。重要的是，多胎妊娠的孕妇终止妊娠时间的限定，可在一定程度上减轻并发症带来的风险。

Treatment of any antenatal complication is the same as in singleton pregnancies, but remember that the onset of complications, particularly pre-term labour and preeclampsia, tends to be earlier and of greater severity. Routine hospital admission from 28 weeks' gestation for bed rest has been advocated in the past, but clinical trials have failed to demonstrate efficacy. However, careful antenatal supervision and ultrasound examinations to detect fetal growth anomaly or TTTS should be undertaken 2 to 4-weekly. It is important that women with multiple pregnancies are booked for confinement where complications can be readily treated.

胎儿生长受限很常见，若出现，应考虑终止妊娠。一对或两对双胎的IUGR的发病率为29%，其中42%的单绒毛膜双胎和25%的双绒毛膜双胎会发生IUGR。

IUGR is common and, if detected, early induction of labour should be considered. The overall incidence of IUGR in one or both twins is 29%, involving 42% of monochorionic twins and 25% of dichorionic twins.

（五）分娩方式（Management of labour and delivery）

双胎妊娠分娩有许多困难，因为分娩的多样性和复杂性，以及第二个胎儿因胎盘分离和脐带脱垂

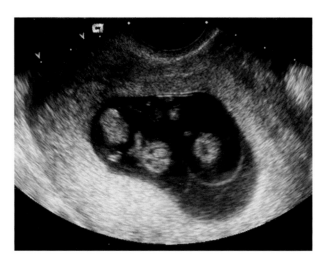

▲ 图 8-16　妊娠早期双胎超声扫描

经许可转载，引自 Leonard PC (2018) Building a Medical Vocabulary: With Spanish Translations, 10th edn. Elsevier, St Louis.

Fig. 8.16　Ultrasound scan of twins early in pregnancy.

(Reproduced with permission from Leonard PC (2018) Building a Medical Vocabulary: With Spanish Translations, 10th edn. Elsevier, St Louis.)

会导致胎儿窒息的风险明显增加。

Delivery poses many difficulties in twin pregnancy because of the variety and complexity of presentations and because the second twin is at significantly greater risk from asphyxia due to placental separation and cord prolapse.

1. 分娩胎位（Presentation at delivery）

双胎妊娠在分娩时的表现有许多变化，这部分会受到第二胎情况的影响。图8-17显示了汇总数据。

There are a number of permutations for presentation in twin pregnancy at delivery, which are partly influenced by the management of the second twin. Rounded-up figures for these presentations are shown in Figure 8.17.

到目前为止，最常见的胎位是头位（双胎1）/头位（双胎2）（50%），其次是头位/臀位（25%）、臀位/头位（10%）和臀位/臀位（10%）。其余5%包括头位/横位、横位/头位、臀位/横位、横位/臀位和横位/横位。

By far the commonest presentation is cephalic (twin 1)/cephalic (twin 2) (50%), followed by cephalic/breech (25%), breech/cephalic (10%) and breech/breech (10%). The remaining 5% consist of cephalic/transverse, transverse/cephalic, breech/transverse, transverse/breech and transverse/transverse.

2. 分娩方式（Method of delivery）

最好在分娩前就确定好采用何种分娩方式。

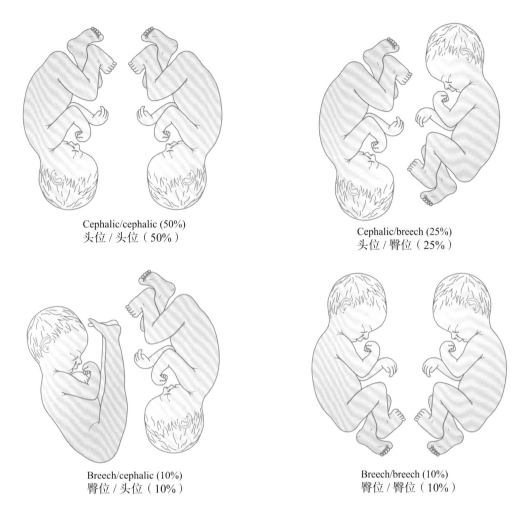

Cephalic/cephalic (50%)
头位 / 头位（50%）

Cephalic/breech (25%)
头位 / 臀位（25%）

Breech/cephalic (10%)
臀位 / 头位（10%）

Breech/breech (10%)
臀位 / 臀位（10%）

▲ 图 8-17　双胎妊娠的 4 种主要胎位，其他 5% 的异常表现没有列在这些主要表现中

Fig. 8.17　The four major presentations of twin pregnancy. The 5% of other variations are not listed in these major groups

A decision about the method of delivery should preferably be made before the onset of labour.

(1) 剖宫产（Caesarean section）

最近对足月双胎进行的试验研究了最安全的分娩方式，结果表明，当第一个胎儿胎位为头位时，行常规的剖宫产是没有指征的。选择剖宫产的原因与单胎妊娠相同。然而，行干预的指征通常较低。如果双胎存在其他并发症，如瘢痕子宫、长期的不孕史、重度子痫前期或妊娠期糖尿病，大多数产科医生会选择择期剖宫产终止妊娠。如果双胎中第一个胎儿胎位不正，那么妊娠 28～34 周的终止妊娠是剖宫产的一个指征，以确保第二个胎儿的安全分娩。此外，在决定最佳的分娩方式时，先露也起重要作用。在英国，双胎的剖宫产率从 1980—1985 年的 28% 上升到 1995—1996 年的 42%。一般来说，现在少有产科医生建议对双胎臀位或第一个双胎臀位

娩出时采用经阴道分娩，因为可能会出现双胎交锁现象。

The recent term twin trial looking at the safest way to deliver twins has shown that there is no indication for the routine delivery of twins by caesarean section when the first twin is presenting by the vertex. Delivery by elective caesarean section is indicated for the same reasons that exist for singleton pregnancies. However, the threshold for intervention is generally lower. Where an additional complication to the twinning exists, such as a previous caesarean scar, a long history of subfertility, severe pre-eclampsia or diabetes mellitus, most obstetricians will opt for elective caesarean section. Pre-term labour between 28 and 34 weeks' gestation is an indication for caesarean delivery to ensure the safe delivery of the second twin, as is malpresentation of the first twin. Furthermore, the presentation does have an important part to play in deciding the best method of delivery. Caesarean section rates for twins increased in the UK from 28% in 1980–1985 to 42% in 1995–1996, and in general, very few obstetricians now advise vaginal delivery for twin breech presentation or for a breech presentation of the first twin for fear of locked twins.

(2) 经阴道分娩（Vaginal delivery）

当正常经阴道分娩时，建议在早期建立静脉通道。产程与单胎分娩相同。

When labour is allowed to proceed normally, it is advisable to establish an IV line at an early stage. Labour normally lasts the same length of time as a singleton labour.

对胎儿行持续胎心监测，以确保两个婴儿的健康。第一个胎儿可以在 CTG 机上用头皮电极或腹部超声换能器进行监测，第二个胎儿则通过超声进行监测。重要的是要确保两次记录的不同，以确保两次胎心率都得到了准确的监测。当第一个胎儿娩出时，必须立即检查第二个双胎的胎位和临产状况，并记录胎心率。如果第二个双胎不是纵向的，有经验的助产师应该从外部进行胎儿头部固定以稳定胎儿，无论是臀位还是头位。

Continuous fetal monitoring is advised to ensure the wellbeing of both babies. The first twin can be monitored on the CTG machine either with a scalp electrode or by abdominal ultrasound transducer, with the second being monitored by ultrasound. It is important to ensure that both fetal heart rates are being accurately monitored by ensuring the two recordings differ. When the first twin is delivered, the lie and presentation of the second twin must be immediately checked and the fetal heart rate recorded. If the lie of the second twin is not longitudinal, an experienced assistant at delivery should perform an external cephalic version (ECV) to stabilize the fetus either as a breech or cephalic presentation.

对于第二胎的分娩，应保持胎膜完整，直到完全入盆，排除脐带脱垂情况。如果子宫在几分钟内没有宫缩，则应开始注射缩宫素。若出现胎心率异常，则应通过产钳加速分娩。因此，许多产科医生建议行硬膜外麻醉分娩。在特殊的情况下，可能需要剖宫产分娩第二个胎儿。由于产后出血的风险增加，第二胎分娩后催产素的使用很关键。

For delivery of the second twin, the membranes should be left intact until the presenting part is well into the pelvis and cord prolapse excluded. If the uterus does not contract within a few minutes, an oxytocin infusion should be started. If fetal heart rate anomalies occur, then delivery should be expedited by forceps delivery or breech extraction. For this reason, many obstetricians prefer an epidural anaesthetic to be placed in labour. Under very exceptional circumstances, it may be necessary to deliver the second twin by caesarean section. It is important to use oxytocic agents after the delivery of the second twin, as there is an increased risk of postpartum haemorrhage.

并不是所有的产科医生都提倡在第一胎分娩后立即按摩子宫。在胎心正常的情况下，可等待宫缩自行发生而无须进一步干预。然而，两次分娩的时间以 30min 为上限，由于第二个胎儿始终存在胎盘剥离和宫内窒息的风险，那么在较长的分娩间歇期内会使第二个分娩的胎儿发生窒息，这总会导致出现这样的疑问：为什么在早期没有采取干预措施？

Not all obstetricians advocate immediate stimulation of the uterus after delivery of the first twin. It is reasonable to wait for the spontaneous onset of further contractions without further intervention if the fetal heart rate is normal. However, because of the ever-present risk of placental separation and intrauterine asphyxia in the second twin, an upper limit of 30 minutes between the two deliveries is generally accepted as reasonable practice. The delivery of an asphyxiated second twin after a long birth interval will always lead to the question as to why intervention did not take place at an earlier stage.

多胞胎妊娠，如三胞胎或四胞胎，现在都是行剖宫产分娩的。在这些孕妇中，通常是因为早产、胎儿出生体重低、分娩不确定而进行终止妊娠。

Higher-order multiple births such as triplets or quadruplets are now delivered by caesarean section. In these pregnancies, the onset of labour is often pre-term, the birth weights are low and the presentations uncertain.

（六）分娩并发症（Complications of labour）

分娩有几种并发症，其中一些与胎位不正有关。胎儿娩出可能会受阻，如横位，这是剖宫产的指征。如果剖宫产是在横位娩出受阻的情况下进行的，下段切口可能会延伸到子宫血管和阔韧带，会导致大量出血，有时在子宫下段的上面或下面做垂直切口可能比横向切口更容易一些。

There are several complications of labour, some of which are associated with malpresentation. Babies may become obstructed, particularly where there is a transverse lie which is, in fact, an indication for delivery by caesarean section. If caesarean section is performed in the presence of an obstructed transverse lie, it may on occasions be preferable to make a vertical incision in the lower and upper segment rather than a transverse incision because of the possibility of extension of the lower segment incision into the uterine vessels and the broad ligaments, resulting in profuse haemorrhage.

正如前面提到的，双胎的经阴道分娩需要有经验的助产师操作。一旦第一个胎儿娩出，助产师需要通过腹部触诊稳定第二个胎儿的胎位，以确保它是纵向的。然后需要静脉滴注缩宫素，确保子宫收缩，使婴儿下降到骨盆。在整个过程中都会行胎心监测，以确保胎儿的健康。如果胎儿是枕先露，一旦头部进入骨盆，胎膜就会破裂。若胎儿是臀先露，在没有自然下降的情况下，助产师可能需要在将手放入子宫后握住胎儿的脚，子宫收缩至破裂胎膜，指引脚和臀部进入骨盆进行分娩（如果可能，可以用完整的膜抓住脚，以避免发生脐带下垂）。如前所述，该过程会使人不舒服，若孕妇同意的话，医护人员建议在双胎分娩期间放置硬膜外导管，以便在第二阶段变得复杂的情况下可以给予镇痛来减缓疼痛。极少情况下会出现在第一个胎儿出生后第二个胎儿娩出前，胎盘会先行分离，在这种情况下，若第二个胎儿未及时娩出，必须紧急行剖宫产娩出第二个胎儿。

As noted earlier, the vaginal delivery of twins requires the attendance of experienced practitioners. Once the first twin has been delivered, the attendant stabilizes the lie of the second twin via abdominal palpation to ensure it is longitudinal. An oxytocin infusion may then be needed to ensure the uterus contracts to cause the baby to descend into the pelvis. The fetal heart is auscultated throughout this process to ensure fetal welfare. If the baby presents by the vertex, the membranes are ruptured once the head is in the pelvis. If the baby is breech, in the absence of spontaneous descent, the attendant may need to hold the fetal foot after placing a hand into the uterus, rupture the membranes with a contraction and guide the foot and breech into the pelvis to effect delivery (if possible, the foot can be grasped with intact membranes to avoid cord prolapse). As this can be uncomfortable, as noted earlier, many attendants prefer, if the mother is agreeable, to have an epidural cannula in place during the labour of a twin pregnancy so adequate analgesia can be administered if the second stage becomes complicated. Very occasionally, after the delivery of the first twin, the placentae separate and attempt to deliver before the second baby. In this event, or in the event that the second baby cannot be delivered easily, a caesarean section must be urgently performed.

1. 双胎交锁（Locked twins）

这是一种非常罕见的并发症，第一个胎儿是臀位，第二个是头位。临床上，当第一个胎儿在分娩过程中下降时，这对双胎将下巴锁定在下巴上。这种情况通常直到第一个胎儿的一部分娩出后才被发现，除非紧急剖宫产，否则存活率较低。超声如显示第一胎位臀位，第二胎为头位，则通常选择择期剖宫产分娩。

This is a very rare complication, where the first twin is a breech presentation and the second is cephalic. Clinically, as the first twin descends during the delivery, the twins lock chin to chin. The condition is usually not recognized until delivery of part of the first twin has occurred and its survival is unlikely unless an urgent caesarean section is organized. Twins where ultrasound reveals the first is presenting by the breech and the second by the vertex are often delivered by elective caesarean section.

2. 连体双胎（Conjoined twins）

连体双胎是胚胎形成后分裂不完全的结果。联合可以发生在任何部位，但通常是头对头或胸对胸。在 20 周前用超声对双胎进行产前评估，可以确定预后及是否可以在出生后尝试手术分离。

The union of twins results from the incomplete division of the embryo after formation. Union may occur at any site but commonly is head-to-head or thorax-to-thorax. The antenatal assessment of the twins with tertiary-level ultrasound before 20 weeks allows for the prognosis to be determined and whether surgical separation may be attempted postnatally.

如果在终止妊娠前通过超声确认联合，那么双胎应该行剖宫产分娩。如果在终止妊娠前未发现异

病例分析	Case study
一名 22 岁的孕妇初次妊娠为双胎，妊娠 37 周时经阴道分娩。两个胎儿都是头位。放置硬膜外导管镇痛，产程进展顺利，第一个胎儿自然分娩。第二个胎儿的胎位被确认为头位，并为纵产式。由于先露部分仍在骨盆边缘以上，静脉滴注缩宫素以维持子宫收缩，胎膜完好，等待先露部分下降。不久，胎心监护显示胎心减慢，为 60/min。胎膜完好，在子宫内（内足型），定位胎儿的脚，将胎儿旋转至臀位，然后人工破膜，经臀位取出胎儿，以加快第二个胎儿的分娩过程。	A 22-year-old woman in her first pregnancy with twins presented at 37 weeks' gestation in spontaneous labour. The presentation of both babies was cephalic. An epidural catheter was sited for analgesia, and labour progressed uneventfully, with the first twin delivering spontaneously. The presentation of the second twin was confirmed as cephalic with a longitudinal lie. As the presenting part was still above the pelvic brim, an oxytocin infusion was commenced to maintain uterine contractions, and the membranes were left intact awaiting descent of the presenting part. Shortly afterwards, external monitoring of the fetal heartbeat showed a bradycardia of 60 beats/min. Delivery of the second twin was expedited by reaching inside the uterus with the membranes still intact (internal podalic version), locating the feet of the fetus and rotating the fetus to the breech presentation before rupturing the membranes and delivering the infant by breech extraction.

常，那么产程将会受阻。

If the union is recognized by ultrasound before the onset of labour, then the twins should be delivered by caesarean section. If the abnormality is not recognized before the onset of labour, then the labour will usually obstruct.

3. 围产期死亡率（Perinatal mortality）

与单胎妊娠相比，约 10% 的围产期死亡与多胎妊娠有关。死亡率随胎儿数量的增加而增加，即双胎 ×4（单绒双胎，其中第二胎 ×8 vs. 第一胎 ×1.5）和三胞胎 ×8。

Approximately 10% of all perinatal mortality is associated with multiple pregnancies. Compared with a singleton pregnancy, the mortality rate increases with the number of fetuses: twins ×4 (monochorionicity ×8, with the second twin vs. first twin ×1.5); triplets ×8.

双胎妊娠最常见的死亡原因是早产，约 50% 的双胎和 90% 的三胞胎在 37 周前终止妊娠。其中第二个胎儿有可能因分娩时窒息而死，这是由于在第一胎分娩后胎盘剥离，或者由于胎膜破裂时因胎位不正或胎先露高浮有关的脐带脱垂引起的。

The commonest cause of death in both twins is prematurity. Over 50% of twins and 90% of triplets deliver before 37 weeks. Second-born twins are more likely to die from intrapartum asphyxia with separation of the placenta following delivery of the first twin, or where cord prolapse occurs in association with a malpresentation or a high presenting part when the membranes are ruptured.

多胎妊娠的围产儿死亡率较高，需要高级护理，特别是单绒毛膜妊娠。总而言之，2010 年澳大利亚双胎、三胞胎和多胞胎的围产儿死亡率分别为 32.5‰、52‰ 和 23.1‰。与相同胎龄的单胎妊娠相比，双胎出生低出生体重（<2.5kg）婴儿的相对风险为 4.3。

Perinatal mortality rates for multiple pregnancy vary with access to high-level obstetric care, especially with monochorionic pregnancies. Overall, perinatal mortality rates in a multiple pregnancy in 2010 in Australia were 32.5, 52 and 231/1000 live and stillbirths for twins, triplets and higher multiple births, respectively. In comparison with singleton births of like gestational age, twins have a relative risk for low-birth-weight infants (<2.5 kg) of 4.3.

更令人担忧是，双胎妊娠分娩的脑瘫孩子的风险是单胞胎的 8 倍，三胞胎的风险是单胞胎的 47 倍。

Perhaps of greater concern is the fact that the risk of producing a child with cerebral palsy is 8 times greater in twins and 47 times greater in triplets compared with singleton pregnancies.

四、过期妊娠（Prolonged pregnancy）

"过期妊娠""延后妊娠"和"延期妊娠"这些术语都用来描述从一个周期为 28 天的女性且从末次月经第一天起超过 294 天的妊娠。

The terms *prolonged pregnancy, post-dates pregnancy and post-term pregnancy* are all used to describe any pregnancy that exceeds 294 days from the first day of the last menstrual period in a woman with a regular 28-day cycle.

"过成熟"一词指的是婴儿的状况，具有特征性（框 8-1）。这些都是宫内营养不良的指标，因此如果有胎盘功能障碍，在妊娠的任何阶段都可能发生。早产儿往往与羊水过少、羊水中胎粪污染发生率增加，以及宫内胎粪污染体液导致吸入性肺炎的风险增加有关。在 41 周的孕妇中有 2% 的人发生，在 42 周的孕妇中发现了高达 5% 的病例。对于该类孕妇来说，在如此漫长的妊娠期间胎儿意外死亡是一场惨痛悲剧，她和她的家人将永远愧疚，如果早点终止

框 8-1　过度成熟综合征	Box 8.1　Post-maturity syndrome
临床特征	**Clinical features**
• 皮肤干燥、脱皮和开裂，特别是手部和脚部	• Dry, peeling and cracked skin, particularly on the hands and feet
• 无胎儿皮脂和胎毛（细毛）	• Absence of vernix caseosa and lanugo (fine hair)
• 皮下脂肪的减少	• Loss of subcutaneous fat
• 皮肤的胎粪染色	• Meconium staining of the skin
并发症	**Complications**
• 围产期死亡率增加	• Increased perinatal mortality
• 产时胎儿窘迫	• Intrapartum fetal distress
• 手术分娩成功率提高	• Increased operative delivery rate
• 胎粪吸入	• Meconium aspiration

妊娠，孩子活下来的可能性很大。

The term *post-maturity* refers to the condition of the infant and has characteristic features (Box 8.1). These are all indicators of intrauterine malnutrition and may therefore occur at any stage of the pregnancy if there is placental dysfunction. Post-maturity is often associated with oligohydramnios, an increased incidence of meconium in the amniotic fluid, and an increased risk of intrauterine aspiration of meconium-stained fluid into the fetal lungs. It is found in 2% of pregnancies at 41 weeks and up to 5% of pregnancies at 42 weeks. Unexpected stillbirth in such prolonged pregnancies is a particular tragedy for the mother, and she and her carer will always live with the knowledge that the child would almost certainly have survived had action to deliver the baby been taken earlier.

过期妊娠的准确诊断因方法的不同而不同。根据末次月经计算，发病率为 10%，在妊娠最初 3 个月超声测定，这一数值可以降低到 1%。妊娠早期常规超声测定能提供有力的证据。

The accurate diagnosis of prolonged pregnancy varies with the method of dating. On the basis of the date of the last menstrual period, the incidence is about 10%, but by using accurate ultrasound dating in the first trimester this figure can be reduced to 1%. This provides a strong case for routine ultrasound dating in early pregnancy.

（一）病因（Aetiology）

过期妊娠可被视为正常妊娠的一种。然而，这种情况的发生可能是家族性的，有时与胎儿肾上腺 – 垂体轴的异常有关，如无脑儿。

Prolonged pregnancy can be considered one end of the spectrum of normal pregnancy. However, the condition may be familial and is sometimes associated with abnormalities of the fetal adrenal-pituitary axis, as in anencephaly.

（二）治疗（Management）

许多大型研究的数据表明，39 周后发生围产期死亡率会增加，因此要对每一位足月妊娠女性进行仔细评估，以确保妊娠超过 40 周对胎儿是安全的。为了做到这一点，许多机构采用了延期服务，即孕妇在 40~41 周进行 CTG 和羊水指数（AFI）评估。那些 AFI 较低（<5cm）的孕妇，胎儿患过熟综合征和缺氧发病率的风险更高。在咨询之后，孕妇将受到明确指导。大型研究表明，对于那些羊水量正常和 CTG 的人来说，无论是在 41~42 周时终止妊娠，都可以自然分娩，其剖宫产率是一致的。因此，许多医疗机构有一项政策，在 41+5 周前为所有孕妇提供健康指南。对那些拒绝终止妊娠的孕妇需要密切

监测，并行 CTG 和羊水量评估，直到分娩。该治疗方案实施的结果表明胎儿发病率几乎可以降为 0。

Evidence in many large studies suggests an increase in perinatal mortality after 39 weeks that necessitates a close appraisal of every pregnancy at term to ensure continuation beyond 40 weeks is safe for the fetus. To do this, many units employ a postdate service where women present between 40 and 41 weeks for a CTG and amniotic fluid index (AFI) assessment. Those with a low AFI, taken as less than 5 cm, are at increased risk of post-maturity syndrome and fetal hypoxic morbidity. They are offered induction after counselling. For those with normal liquor and CTG, large studies have shown that whether a woman is induced at 41–42 weeks or whether the labour is allowed to start spontaneously, the caesarean section rates are the same. Many units will therefore have a policy of offering induction to all women by 41+5 weeks. Those women who decline induction need careful monitoring with frequent CTG and liquor volume assessment until delivery. Management in this form has resulted in reported fetal morbidity of close to zero.

（三）成本管理（Labour management）

如果决定终止妊娠，可能会存在困难，因为出现该情况的妊娠女性子宫颈条件往往较差，Bishop 分数低于 3。在这种情况下，应尝试用前列腺素或机械方式对宫颈促成熟。如果失败或胎儿体重较大，最好选择剖宫产分娩。

Should the decision be made to induce labour, this may in itself prove difficult, as the cervix is often unfavourable, with a Bishop's score of less than 3. In these circumstances, cervical preparation with prostaglandins or mechanical methods should be attempted. If this fails and the infant is large, it may on occasions be preferable to deliver the child by elective caesarean section.

分娩过程必须谨慎，因为这是高危妊娠。

Careful observation during labour is mandatory, as these are high-risk pregnancies.

五、臀先露（Breech presentation）

臀位的发生率取决于开始分娩时的胎龄。32 周时，发病率为 16%，36 周时降至 7%，足月时降至 3%~5%。因此，很明显，胎儿通常会改变自己的胎位，一般情况下没有必要在 37 周之前纠正胎位。

The incidence of breech presentation depends on the gestational age at the time of onset of labour. At 32 weeks, the incidence is 16%, falling to 7% at 36 weeks and 3–5% at term. Thus it is clear that the fetus normally corrects its own presentation, and attempts to correct the presentation before 37 weeks are generally unnecessary.

（一）臀位的类型（Types of breech presentation）

臀位可能以下 3 种方式之一出现（图 8-18）。

The breech may present in one of three ways (Fig. 8.18).

- **Frank 臀位**：腿沿着胎儿躯干伸展，臀部弯曲，膝盖伸展。臀部将出现在骨盆入口处。这种先露也被称为延长臀位。

  - Frank breech: The legs lie extended along the fetal trunk and are flexed at the hips and extended at the knees. The buttocks will present at the pelvic inlet. This presentation is also known as an *extended breech*.

- **Flexed 臀位**：腿部在臀部和膝部弯曲，胎儿坐在腿上，这样两只脚就会出现在骨盆入口处。

  - Flexed breech: The legs are flexed at the hips and the knees with the fetus sitting on its legs so that both feet present to the pelvic inlet.

- **膝盖或足部先露**：胎儿的 1 条或 2 条下肢弯曲，胎儿的臀部在产妇骨盆上方，这样胎儿下肢的一部分（通常是脚）通过宫颈下降到阴道。

  - Knee or footling presentation: One or both of the lower limbs of the fetus are flexed and breech of the baby is above the maternal pelvis so that a part of the fetal lower limb (usually feet) descends through the cervix into the vagina.

臀位是以胎儿骶骨为界限来定义的。分娩开始时，臀位进入真骨盆边缘，双转子直径（小于 10cm）为下降直径。这个直径比足月胎儿的双顶颈直径略小。臀位呈现的类型对经阴臀位分娩的风险有重大影响。先露越不规则，发生肢体或脐带脱垂的风险越大。一只脚进入子宫颈以下的阴道可能会刺激产妇在子宫颈完全扩张之前向下继续分娩，导致头部嵌顿在子宫颈处（图 8-18）。

The position of the breech is defined using the fetal sacrum as the denominator. At the onset of labour, the breech enters the brim of the true pelvis with the bitrochanteric diameter (less than 10 cm) being the diameter of descent. This diameter is slightly smaller than the biparietal diameter in the full-term fetus. The type of breech presentation has a significant impact on the risk of vaginal breech delivery. The more irregular the presenting part, the greater the risk of a prolapsed cord or limb. A foot pressing into the vagina below the cervix may stimulate the mother to bear down before the

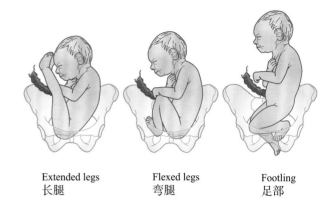

| Extended legs 长腿 | Flexed legs 弯腿 | Footling 足部 |

▲ 图 8-18　臀位类型

Fig. 8.18　Types of breech presentation.

cervix is fully dilated, which leads to entrapment of the head in the cervix (see Fig. 8.18).

（二）臀位的原因和危害（Causation and hazards of breech presentation）

臀位在妊娠 37 周之前是常见的，但大多数婴儿在足月前会自发转向（如前所述）。然而，臀位可能与多胎妊娠、孕妇子宫先天异常、胎儿畸形及药物继发的胎儿肌张力低下和胎盘位置（前置胎盘或宫角植入）等因素有关。

Breech presentation is common before 37 weeks' gestation, but most infants will turn spontaneously before term (as previously discussed). Breech presentation may, however, be associated with factors such as multiple pregnancy, congenital abnormalities of the maternal uterus, fetal malformation, fetal hypotonia secondary to medication use and placental location, either placenta praevia or cornual implantation.

也有证据表明，持续性臀位可能与胎儿不能从臀位转至头位有关，因可能存在一些下肢神经损伤（框 8-2）。

There is also evidence to suggest that persistent breech presentation may be associated with the inability of the fetus to kick itself around from breech to vertex and that there may therefore be some neurological impairment of the lower limbs (Box 8.2).

> **！注意**
>
> 即使剖宫产，臀位胎儿神经损伤的发生率也较高，尽管风险不到 1%。
>
> There is a higher incidence of neurological impairment in breech babies even when delivered by caesarean section, although the overall risk is still less than 1%.

与正常的头位分娩相比，臀位分娩对婴儿有一

框 8-2　臀位呈现的原因	Box 8.2　Causation of breech presentation
• 胎龄 • 胎盘位置 • 子宫异常 • 多胎妊娠 • 胎儿四肢神经损伤	• Gestational age • Placental location • Uterine anomalies • Multiple pregnancy • Neurological impairment of the fetal limbs

些特定的危害，特别是对早产儿和出生体重超过 4kg 的胎儿，具体如下。

Delivery by the breech carries some specific hazards to the infant compared with normal vertex presentation, particularly in pre-term infants and in infants with a birth weight in excess of 4 kg:

- 由于先露部分的不规则性，使得脐带压迫和脐带脱垂的风险增加，尤其是在腿弯曲或足先露的情况下。

- There is an increased risk of cord compression and cord prolapse because of the irregular nature of the presenting part. This is particularly the case where the legs are flexed or there is a footling presentation.

- 对于早产儿来说，头部卡在子宫颈是一个特殊的风险，在早产儿中，臀部大转子间的直径明显小于头部的双顶径。这意味着躯干可能需要通过不完全扩张的子宫颈口娩出，如头部较大可能被夹住。若分娩延迟，孩子可能会发生脑损伤，甚至因窒息而死。

- Entrapment of the head behind the cervix is a particular risk with the pre-term infant, in whom the bitrochanteric diameter of the breech is significantly smaller than the biparietal diameter of the head. This means that the trunk may deliver through an incompletely dilated cervix, resulting in entrapment of the larger head. If the delivery is significantly delayed, the child may be asphyxiated and either die or suffer brain damage.

- 胎儿颅骨在分娩过程中没有足够时间成形，因此，无论是早产儿还是足月儿，都有颅内出血的风险。

- The fetal skull does not have time to mould during delivery and therefore, in both pre-term and term infants, there is a significant risk of intracranial haemorrhage.

- 分娩过程中可能会对内脏造成损伤，如果产科医生过度抓紧胎儿腹部，会导致脾或肠道破裂。

- Trauma to viscera may occur during the delivery process, with rupture of the spleen or gut if the obstetrician handles the fetal abdomen.

（三）治疗（Management）

1. 产前治疗（Antenatal management）

由于臀位分娩对胎儿的风险，最好的选择是通过准确的产前诊断和外倒转术（ECV），避免经阴道臀位分娩。

Because of the risks to the fetus of breech birth, the best option is to avoid vaginal breech delivery through accurate diagnosis and performance of ECV.

2. 外倒转术（External cephalic version）

(1) 指征（Indication）

妊娠 36 周后持续臀位。

Breech presentation persisting after 36 weeks' gestation.

(2) 禁忌证（Contraindications）

凡是有产前大出血史、前置胎盘、脐带绕颈、CTG 异常、瘢痕子宫或多次妊娠史的，都不应进行 ECV。如果想通过剖宫产分娩，那么把胎儿转位也是没有意义的。

ECV should not be attempted where there is a history of antepartum haemorrhage, where there is placenta praevia, where there is a significant nuchal cord, where the CTG is abnormal, where there is a previous uterine scar or where the pregnancy is multiple. It is also pointless to turn the infant if the intention is to deliver the child by elective caesarean section for some other indication.

(3) 技术（Technique）

胸膝卧位。通过超声可以确认胎方位和胎盘的位置。检测胎心率，最好行 CTG。给予抑制宫缩药物（口服硝苯地平或皮下特布他林）放松子宫，因为这样可以提高成功率（图 8-19）。

The mother rests supine with the upper body slightly tilted down. The presentation of the fetus and placental position are confirmed by ultrasound. The fetal heart rate is checked, preferably with a small strip of CTG. A tocolytic agent (oral nifedipine or subcutaneous terbutaline SC terbutaline) is given to relax the uterus, as this improves the success rate (Fig. 8.19).

臀部从骨盆边缘分开，转移到下腹部，胎儿轻轻旋转，保持头部弯曲。在手术过程中应该监测胎心率。

The breech is disimpacted from the pelvic brim and shifted to the lower abdomen, and the fetus is gently rotated,

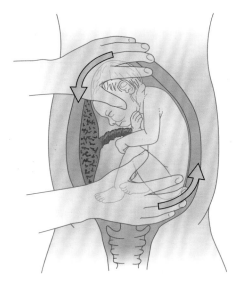

▲ 图 8-19 外倒转术：向相反方向施压于胎儿两个极点

Fig. 8.19 External cephalic version: pressure is applied in the opposite direction to the two fetal poles.

keeping the head flexed. The fetal heart rate should be checked during the procedure.

最重要的是不要过度用力，有迹象表明胎儿心动过缓时，如果心动过缓未超过中点，那么胎儿可能恢复到原来的样子，并持续对胎儿进行 CTG 监测。抗 D 免疫球蛋白应用于 Rh 阴性血型的患者。

It is essential not to use excessive force and, if there is evidence of fetal bradycardia, the fetus should be returned to the original presentation if the version is not past the halfway point and the fetus monitored with continuous CTG. Anti-D should be administered to the patient who has Rhesus-negative blood group.

（四）并发症（Complications）

手术的风险是脐带缠绕、胎盘早剥和胎膜破裂。持续性胎儿心动过缓的发生率约为 1%，这可能需要剖宫产紧急分娩。有一些证据表明，即使外倒转手术成功，由于难产和胎儿受损，剖宫产率也高于正常水平。ECV 在多达 50% 的案例中都是成功的。

The risks of the procedure are cord entanglement, placental abruption and rupture of the membranes. Persistent fetal bradycardia occurs in approximately 1%, and this may necessitate urgent delivery by caesarean section. There is some evidence to suggest that even where external version is successful, the section rate is higher than normal due to dystocia and fetal compromise. ECV is successful in up to 50% of cases in the best hands.

如果臀位在短期内持续存在，则应向孕妇提供有关其分娩方式的建议（请参阅下文）。若孕妇希望

经阴道分娩，重要的是要考虑可能出现阻碍分娩的问题，如产妇骨盆形状和巨大胎儿。

Where a breech presentation persists near term, the mother should be counselled about her delivery options (see later). If she wishes to consider a vaginal breech delivery, it is important to consider issues that may impede that delivery, like the size and shape of the maternal pelvis and a macrosomic fetus.

虽然母体骨盆的大小和形状可以通过盆腔检查或行 MRI 评估，但没有证据表明这两种技术是确定臀位分娩可能成功的准确方法。

Although the size and shape of the maternal pelvis can be assessed by pelvic examination or formally using MRI, neither technique has been shown to be accurate in determining the possible success of a breech delivery.

胎儿的大小可以通过超声来评估。如果胎儿胎龄大于 28 周、小于 32 周，胎儿体重小于 2kg，首先选择剖宫产。若在妊娠后期，胎儿体重超过 3.8kg，那么子宫下段剖宫产分娩是最好的选择，但须知道这种估计可能不可靠。臀位分娩的其他禁忌证包括胎儿畸形、足位臀位、胎儿头屈曲、胎盘低置、胎儿生物物理评分异常或急性母体疾病（如胎盘早剥 / 重度子痫前期）。

Fetal size can be assessed by ultrasound. If the fetal gestational age is less than 32 weeks and more than 28 weeks, the birth weight will be less than 2 kg, and delivery by caesarean section is the preferred option. If, later in pregnancy, the fetal weight is assessed to be in excess of 3.8 kg, then delivery by section is the preferred option, but it must be remembered that such estimates can be unreliable. Other contraindications for breech delivery are where there is fetal anomaly, a footing breech, a deflexed fetal head, a low-lying placenta, abnormal fetal welfare tests or an acute maternal condition like placental abruption/severe pre-eclampsia.

（五）分娩方式（Method of delivery）

2000 年，足月臀位临床试验表明臀位胎儿的分娩剖宫产最安全。因此，许多医疗机构现在不再对臀位进行经阴道分娩。大量文献表明，这项试验方法存在问题，结论可能并不合理。因此，一些医疗机构重新引入臀位经阴道分娩作为首选（见前述），但需具备协助分娩的专业产科医生，并且孕妇倾向这一选择。

In 2000, the term breech trial was published, which suggested that the delivery of the breech-presenting fetus was safest by caesarean section. As a result, many units now no longer perform vaginal delivery of the breech. Since that time, considerable literature has shown that the trial had methodological issues and the conclusions may not have been justified. Some units therefore reintroduced vaginal breech delivery as a safe option in selected cases (see earlier), where obstetricians with the appropriate expertise for assisting delivery are available and the mother is keen to pursue this option.

1. 经阴道分娩（Vaginal breech delivery）

第一产程和正常分娩没有什么不同。硬膜外麻醉是首选的镇痛方法，但不是必须的。一旦宫缩开始或胎膜破裂，应建议孕妇立即住院，入院时应进行阴道检查，以排除脐带先露或脐带脱垂。除第二产程以外，与头位分娩一样，当臀部下降导致胎粪排出时，胎粪污染同样具有重要意义。

The first stage of labour should be no different from labour in a vertex presentation. Epidural analgesia is the preferred method of pain relief but is not essential. The woman should be advised to attend hospital as soon as contractions commence or the membranes rupture, and vaginal examination should be performed on admission to exclude cord presentation or prolapsed cord. The presence of meconium-stained liquor has exactly the same significance as with a vertex presentation except in the second stage of labour, when descent of the breech will often result in the passage of meconium.

技术（Technique）如下。

当宫颈口完全扩张，且先露部分位于骨盆下方时，鼓励产妇呼吸，直到胎儿臀部和肛门出现（图8-20）。为了最大限度减少软组织阻力，除非盆底已松弛且阻力很小的情况，应考虑在局部或硬膜外麻醉下进行会阴侧切术。然后，通过胎儿的臀部和膝盖将腿从阴道中取出。产妇用力将胎儿娩出体外，产科医生触摸胎儿大腿上部，确保胎儿的背部保持在前部。一旦触摸躯干延伸到肩胛骨，可以将手指滑过肩膀并向下触摸胎儿头部轻松地传递一个手臂。如果手臂伸展造成分娩困难，握住婴儿的骨盆旋转胎儿的身体，直到后臂到达耻骨联合下方。手臂可以通过弯曲肘部和肩部来传递。通过旋转身体来传递另一只手臂（Loveset 手法），重复该过程。然后使躯干保持悬空约 30s，让头部进入骨盆，抓住腿，向上摆动 180°，直到看到胎儿的面部。此时，胎儿可能会自然分娩；使用产钳等的多种工具可确保头部的安全娩出。从腿部到头部的分娩时间不应超过 4min，以确保新生儿的安全。

When the cervix is fully dilated and the presenting part is

low in the pelvis, the mother is encouraged to bear down with her contractions until the fetal buttocks and anus come on view (Fig. 8.20). To minimize soft tissue resistance, an episiotomy should be considered under either local or epidural anaesthesia, unless the pelvic floor is already lax and offers little resistance. The legs are then lifted out of the vagina by flexing the fetal hip and knees. The baby is then expelled with maternal pushing, with the obstetrician only touching the upper thighs and then only to ensure that the fetal back remains anterior. Once the trunk has delivered as far as the scapula, the arms can usually be easily delivered one at a time by sliding the fingers over the shoulder and sweeping them downwards across the fetal head. If the arms are extended and pose difficulty in delivering, the body of the fetus is rotated by holding the baby's pelvis until the posterior arm comes under the symphysis pubis. The arm can then be delivered by flexing at the elbow and the shoulders. The procedure is repeated by rotating the body to deliver the other arm (Loveset's manoeuvre). The trunk is then allowed to remain suspended for about 30 seconds to allow the head to enter the pelvis and then the legs are grasped and swung upwards through an arc of 180 degrees until the child's mouth comes into view. At this point, the baby may spontaneously deliver; however, a number of techniques, including the use of forceps, can be used to ensure the safe delivery of the head. The time taken for the delivery from the legs to the head should be no more than 4 minutes to ensure neonatal wellbeing.

在胎儿娩出后，然后夹住脐带并将其断开，第三产程按常规的方式完成。

After the baby is delivered, the cord is then clamped and divided and the third stage is completed in the usual way.

良好的臀位分娩的本质是产程应该是连续的，处理胎儿的动作尽可能小且温和。

The essence of good breech delivery is that progress should be continuous and handling of the fetus must be minimal and as gentle as possible.

如果操作不当，让产妇在宫颈口完全扩张前用力，可能会出现并发症。

Possible complications occur with poor technique and allowing the mother to push before full dilatation of the cervix.

2. 剖宫产（Caesarean section）

剖宫产指征包括预估胎儿体重大于 3.8kg、足月分娩或头部偏转、无临床经验丰富的助产师接生、存在其他并发症（如重度子痫前期、胎儿生长受限、胎盘早剥、前置胎盘、既往剖宫产史）。若胎儿体重低于 700g，无论采用何种分娩方式，从死亡率和发病率来看，围产期结局都很差。

Delivery by caesarean section is indicated if the estimated birth weight is greater than 3.8 kg, for footling presentations or where the head is deflexed on ultrasound, where there is no obstetrician with available expertise in vaginal breech delivery

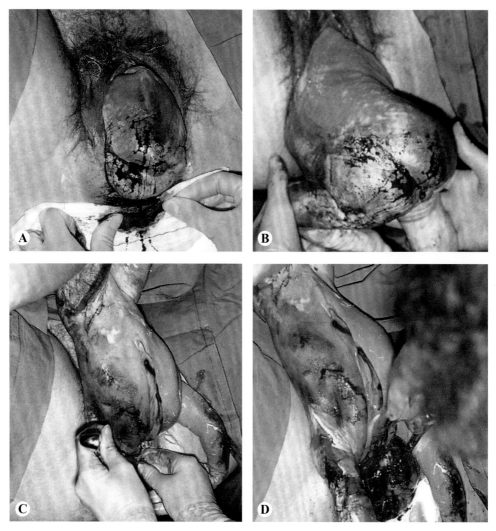

▲ 图 8-20　臀位。A. 暴露臀部；B. 避开的产道；C 和 D. 产钳应用于后脑

Fig. 8.20　Breech presentation. (A) Buttock on view. (B) Trunk expelled. (C) and (D) Forceps applied to aftercoming head.

or where there is an additional complication such as severe pre-eclampsia, fetal growth restriction, placental abruption, placenta praevia or a previous caesarean section. If the birth weight is calculated to be less than 700 g, the perinatal outcome both in terms of mortality and morbidity is poor irrespective of the method of delivery therefore.

虽然还没有大规模对体重极低的胎儿进行剖宫产的研究分析，但一些大的系列的描述性研究显示，以这种方式分娩的婴儿有良好预后。剖宫产是目前臀位极低出生体重儿的首选分娩方式。

Although there has been no large randomized trial of caesarean section for very-low-birth-weight infants, descriptive studies in some very large series show some improved outcome where the infant is delivered in this way. Caesarean section is currently the method of choice for delivery of very-low-birth-weight infants presenting as a breech.

通常，使用的技术是子宫下段剖宫产术。然而，对于早产儿，子宫下段可能没有形成，并且在这些情况下，优选的方法是通过形成下段部分的中线切口；子宫上部纵向切口有时可能是首选切口。在出生极低体重的新生儿中发现，臀部和躯干比头部窄得多，并且剖宫产分娩时可能会发生头部夹伤，除非切口适当。

Normally, the technique used is LUSCS. However, with a pre-term infant, the lower segment may not have formed, and, under these circumstances, the preferred method is a midline incision through that part of the lower segment that is formed; a classical (upper uterine longitudinal) incision may on occasions be the incision of choice. In very-low-birth-weight infants, the buttocks and trunk are substantially narrower than the head, and entrapment of the head may occur at the time of delivery through the uterine incision unless an adequate incision is made.

六、不稳定胎位、横位和肩位（Unstable lie, transverse lie and shoulder presentation）

不稳定的胎位是指不断变化的胎位。通常伴有多胎，如产妇腹壁松弛、胎盘附着位置低或异常子宫（如双角子宫、子宫肌瘤和羊水过多）。

An unstable lie is one that is constantly changing. It is commonly associated with multiparity, where the maternal abdominal wall is lax, low placental implantation or uterine anomalies such as a bicornuate uterus, uterine fibroids and polyhydramnios.

（一）并发症（Complications）

如果不稳定胎位持续到临产，可能会导致脐带脱垂或肩先露，当手臂和腿都娩出时，可能会导致手臂脱垂或复合先露（图 8-21）。

If an unstable lie resulting in a transverse lie persists until the onset of labour, it may result in prolapse of the cord or a shoulder presentation and a prolapsed arm or a compound presentation when both an arm and a leg may present (Fig. 8.21).

（二）治疗（Management）

在妊娠 37 周前，不稳定的胎位不需要采取任何措施，除非自然分娩。重要的是通过超声探查到胎盘、盆腔肿瘤（子宫肌瘤 / 低位胎盘 / 道格拉斯囊内卵巢囊肿）和胎儿异常的原因。大多数情况下，找不到明显原因。

No action is necessary in an unstable lie until 37 weeks' gestation unless the labour starts spontaneously. It is important to look for an explanation by ultrasound scan for placental localization, the presence of any pelvic tumours (fibroids/low-lying placenta/ovarian cyst in the pouch of Douglas) and the presence of fetal abnormalities. However, it must be remembered that, in most cases, no obvious cause is found.

37 周后，在没有任何原因的情况下，试图行 ECV 纠正这个胎位。如果不稳定的情况持续存在，建议在妊娠 39 周之前让孕妇住院，以防发生自发性胎膜破裂伴有脐带脱垂，入院将紧急行剖宫产分娩。

After 37 weeks, in the absence of any cause, an attempt should be made to correct the lie by ECV. It is advisable to admit the mother to hospital by 39 weeks' gestation if the unstable lie persists in case spontaneous rupture of the membranes occurs accompanied by a prolapse of the cord. Admission will allow for rapid delivery by caesarean section.

如果不能识别出胎盘低置等特殊因素，可采取

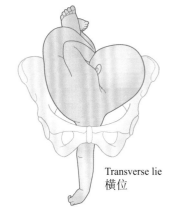

Transverse lie
横位

Shoulder presentation
肩先露

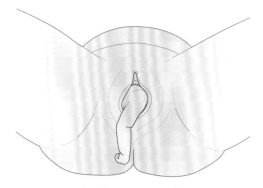

Anterior arm presentation
前肩先露

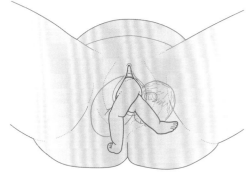

Anterior arm and leg presentation
前臂和前腿先露

▲ 图 8-21 脱垂手臂脱垂到阴道内，有时导致肩部脱垂

Fig. 8.21 **Prolapse of the arm into the vagina, sometimes resulting in a shoulder presentation.**

以下 3 种方法之一。

- 让孕妇住院，等待胎位自行纠正，或在分娩开始时纠正胎位。

- 稳定诱导，首先将胎位纠正为头位，然后在头部接近骨盆边缘时破膜，给予耻骨上施压，然后静脉滴注缩宫素。

- 足月剖腹产。

Assuming that no specific factor such as a low-lying placenta can be identified, the approach may take one of three courses:

- Keep the mother in hospital and await spontaneous correction of the lie, or correct the lie as labour starts spontaneously.
- Stabilize induction, performed by first correcting the lie to a cephalic presentation and then rupturing the membranes as the head approaches the pelvic brim assisted by gentle suprapubic pressure, followed by oxytocin infusion.
- Delivery by caesarean section at term.

如果有任何其他复杂的因素，在某些情况下，建议采用剖宫产终止妊娠（框 8-3）。

If there are any other complicating factors, it may on occasions be advisable to deliver the mother at term by planned elective section (Box 8.3).

如果孕妇在分娩时发生肩先露或手臂下垂，则

框 8-3 不稳定胎位的治疗	Box 8.3 Management of unstable lie
• 排除固定原因 • 妊娠 37 周时住院 • 足月稳定引产 • 为脐带脱垂做好准备	• Exclude causes that are fixed • Hospitalization at 37 weeks • Stabilizing induction at term • Be prepared for cord prolapse

应试图纠正这种情况或经阴道分娩；分娩应该行剖宫产术。若手臂楔入骨盆，通过传统或中线的上段切口分娩可能比下段切口更安全，因为在这种情况下，可能下段没有形成。

If the mother arrives in established labour with a shoulder presentation or prolapsed arm, no attempt should be made to correct the presentation or to deliver the child vaginally; delivery should be effected by caesarean section. Sometimes, if the arm is wedged into the pelvis, it may be safer to deliver the child through a classic or midline upper segment incision rather than through a lower segment incision as, in these cases, there may be little lower segment formed.

本章概览	Essential information

妊娠期高血压
• 发达国家最常见的妊娠并发症
• 妊娠期高血压：以前血压正常的孕妇在分娩 20 周或 24h 内出现高血压
• 子痫前期：20 周后出现高血压和蛋白尿
• 子痫：子痫前期抽搐，分娩后 48h 内发病
• 子痫前期的发病机制不确定：血管紧张素 II 受体增加、内皮功能障碍、抗氧化物质减少都是原因之一
• 子痫前期的治疗
  – 卧床休息
  – 抗高血压药物治疗
• 子痫的治疗
  – 控制发作
  – 控制血压
  – 经阴道分娩或剖宫产
 	
产前大出血
• 24 周后阴道流血
 	
前置胎盘
• 下段植入
• 发生率 1%
• 分类：边缘、中央和侧方
• 诊断：无诱因、无痛性阴道流血、子宫张力低
• 经超声或磁共振诊断
• 诊断：如果孕妇为瘢痕子宫，排除胎盘植入的风险
• 治疗：保胎至 37 周，排除胎盘植入可能
• 出现主要症状需住院治疗
• 备血
• 剖宫产，除 I 级外
	Hypertension in pregnancy
	• Commonest complication of pregnancy in the most developed countries
	• Gestational hypertension-hypertension alone after 20 weeks or within 24 hours of delivery in a previously normotensive woman
	• Pre-eclampsia-hypertension and proteinuria after 20 weeks
	• Eclampsia-pre-eclampsia plus convulsions, up to 48 hours after delivery
	• Pathogenesis of pre-eclampsia uncertain-increase in angiotensin II receptors, endothelial dysfunction, decreased antioxidants all contribute
	• Management of pre-eclampsia
	  – Bed rest
	  – Antihypertensive drug therapy
	• Management of eclampsia
	  – Control of fits
	  – Control of BP
	  – Deliver infant by induction of labour or caesarean section
	
	Antepartum haemorrhage
	• Vaginal bleeding after 24 weeks
	
	Placenta praevia
	• Lower segment implantation
	• Incidence 1%
	• Classification-marginal, central and lateral
	• Diagnosis-painless loss, unstable lie, soft uterus
	• Diagnosis confirmed by ultrasound or MRI
	• Diagnosis-rule out placenta accreta spectrum if mother has a caesarean section scar
	• Management-conservative until 37 weeks unless placenta accreta spectrum
	• Hospital admission for all major degrees
	• Blood held-cross-matched
	• Caesarean section unless grade 1

（续表）

本章概览	Essential information
• 胎儿预后：良好 • 若为瘢痕子宫，须排除胎盘植入的风险	• Prognosis for the fetus-good • Rule out placenta accreta spectrum if there is a previous caesarean scar
胎盘植入 • 胎盘异常粘连，通常附着在以前的剖宫产瘢痕上 • 妊娠 28 周后诊断 • 在高危中心接受护理 • 预计分娩时会大量失血 • 35 周终止妊娠 • 胎儿娩出后通常需要切除子宫	**Placenta accreta spectrum** • Abnormally adherent placenta usually onto a previous caesarean scar • Diagnosis made by 28 weeks' gestation • Care at high-risk centre • Anticipate massive blood loss at delivery • Deliver by 35 weeks • Commonly requires hysterectomy after delivery of the fetus
胎盘早剥 • 发病率 0.6%～7% • 诊断：子宫张力高、触痛 • 胎儿正常胎位 • 通常与产妇高血压有关 • 治疗：输血 　－ 检查 DIC 　－ 如果胎盘早剥严重，终止妊娠 　－ 胎儿预后不良 • 产妇并发症 　－ 纤维蛋白原缺乏症 　－ 肾小管坏死	**Placental abruption** • Incidence 0.6-7% • Diagnosis-uterus hypertonic, tender • Normal fetal lie • Commonly associated with maternal hypertension • Management-replace blood loss 　－ Check for DIC 　－ Deliver the infant if abruption severe 　－ Prognosis for fetus poor • Maternal complications 　－ Afibrinogenaemia 　－ Renal tubular necrosis
其他原因 • 宫颈和阴道病变 • 前置血管	**Other causes** • Cervical and vaginal lesions • Vasa praevia
多胎妊娠的患病率 • 单卵双胎比例恒定 • 双合子率增加	**Prevalence of multiple pregnancy** • Monozygous twin rates constant • Dizygous rates increasing
过期妊娠 • 与围产期死亡率增加有关 • 与胎粪的发病率增加相关 • 治疗方式 　－ 41 周后常规指引 　－ 加强监测	**Prolonged pregnancy** • Is associated with increase in perinatal mortality • Is associated with increased incidence of meconium • Management options are 　－ Routine induction after 41 weeks 　－ Increased monitoring
臀位 • 发生在 3% 的足月妊娠中 • 相关性 　－ 早产 　－ 多胎妊娠 　－ 胎儿异常 　－ 前置胎盘 　－ 异常子宫 • 37 周行臀位外倒转术 • 选择性剖宫产 • 阴道分娩的指征 　－ 胎儿体重超过 1.5kg，小于 4kg 　－ 屈曲或直臀 　－ 弯曲的头	**Breech presentation** • Occurs in 3% of pregnancies at term • Associated with 　－ Pre–term delivery 　－ Multiple pregnancy 　－ Fetal abnormality 　－ Placenta praevia 　－ Uterine abnormalities • ECV at 37 weeks • Elective caesarean section • Criteria for vaginal delivery are 　－ Fetal weight more than 1.5 kg, less than 4 kg 　－ Flexed or frank breech 　－ Flexed head
胎位不稳定 • 相关性 　－ 多胎次 　－ 羊水过多 　－ 异常子宫 　－ 低置胎盘	**Unstable lie** • Associated with 　－ High parity 　－ Polyhydramnios 　－ Uterine anomalies 　－ Low-lying placenta

第9章 母体医学
Maternal medicine

Suzanne V. F. Wallace　David James　著　　孟金来　译　　杨慧霞　校

学习目标	LEARNING OUTCOMES
学习本章后你应当能够:	After studying this chapter you should be able to:
知识标准	**Knowledge criteria**
• 描述：下面各疾病的病因、危险因素、风险及治疗方法：	• Describe the aetiology, risk factors, risks and management of:
－ 妊娠期贫血	－ Anaemia in pregnancy
－ 妊娠期糖尿病	－ Gestational diabetes
－ 妊娠期感染	－ Infections in pregnancy
－ 妊娠期血栓栓塞性疾病	－ Thromboembolic disease in pregnancy
－ 肝病	－ Liver disease
• 妊娠前合并症孕期的临床表现和处理方法，包括：	• Contrast the clinical presentation and management of pre-existing medical conditions in pregnancy, including:
－ 糖尿病	－ Diabetes
－ 肥胖	－ Obesity
－ 血栓形成	－ Thrombophilias
－ 癫痫	－ Epilepsy
－ 甲状腺疾病	－ Thyroid disease
－ 心脏病	－ Cardiac disease
－ 呼吸道疾病	－ Respiratory disease
－ 肾脏疾病	－ Renal disease
－ 血红蛋白病	－ Haemoglobinopathies
• 讨论对罹患疾病的女性进行孕前咨询的作用，及其妊娠风险和改进方法	• Discuss the role of pre-conceptual counselling for women with pre-existing illness and the risks and modifications required to continue drug treatment during pregnancy
临床能力	**Clinical competencies**
• 向孕妇说明妊娠期轻微不适的原因及管理计划，包括：	• Explain to the mother the causes and plan the management of minor complaints of pregnancy, including:
－ 腹痛	－ Abdominal pain
－ 胃灼热	－ Heartburn
－ 便秘	－ Constipation
－ 背痛	－ Backache
－ 晕厥	－ Syncope
－ 静脉曲张	－ Varicosities
－ 腕管综合征	－ Carpal tunnel syndrome

一、概述（Introduction）

母体医学涵盖了女性在妊娠期间可能出现的各种疾病。其中一些可能在妊娠前发生，另一些可能在妊娠期间发生。目前在英国，随着其他产科护理领域的改善，现在大多数产妇死亡都是由医疗条件造成的。在英国和爱尔兰最新一期的"2013—2015 年孕产妇死亡和发病率保密调查"中，每 10 万名产妇中有 1.13 人死于静脉血栓栓塞，2.34 人死于心脏病。

Maternal medicine encompasses the spectrum of medical conditions a woman can present with in pregnancy. Some of these may pre-date pregnancy and others may develop during pregnancy. Currently in the UK, with improvements in other areas of obstetric care, most maternal deaths are now caused by medical conditions. In the most recent edition of the *UK and Ireland Confidential Enquiries into Maternal Deaths and Morbidity 2013–15*, venous thromboembolism was responsible for maternal death in 1.13 per 100,000 maternities, whilst cardiac disease was responsible for maternal death in 2.34 per 100,000 maternities.

越来越多的女性妊娠期间存在合并症。罹患疾病导致自愿或非自愿不孕 [如囊性纤维化（cystic fibrosis，CF）]，现在这部分人妊娠数量正在增加。此外，更多的女性在开始妊娠时年龄较大，并有更多后天获得性的问题，如肥胖和高血压。

There are an increasing number of women with medical conditions in pregnancy. Women with significant pre-existing medical conditions that in the past may have led to voluntary or involuntary infertility (for example, cystic fibrosis (CF)) are now becoming pregnant in increasing numbers. In addition, more women are older when embarking on pregnancy and have more acquired problems such as obesity and hypertension.

无论一名女性是在妊娠前已明确患有疾病，还是在妊娠期间发生的疾病，成功治疗的关键是有一个框架来确保考虑到这种疾病存在的所有影响（图 9-1）。这使得无论疾病是常见还是罕见，都能制订强有力的妊娠计划。

Whether a woman is known to have a medical condition prior to pregnancy or develops one within pregnancy, the key to successful management is to have a framework to ensure that all the implications of the condition are considered (Fig. 9.1). This enables robust pregnancy plans to be made whether a disease is common or rare.

 经验 多学科和多专业的团队合作也是管理这些女性的基本要素。

Multidisciplinary and multi-professional teamworking are also essential elements in caring for these women.

二、妊娠期轻微症状（Minor complaints of pregnancy）

根据定义，轻微的症状不会造成重大的医疗问题。然而，受影响的女性通常认为轻微的症状并不轻微，并可能对女性妊娠期间的生活质量产生相当大的影响。此外，许多轻微症状与需要排除的重大病理疾病的症状相同。症状通常与身体对妊娠的生理适应有关，应该让女性放心（一旦排除了病理），这些症状代表着正常的妊娠变化。

Minor complaints of pregnancy, by definition, do not cause significant medical problems. However, minor medical complaints are often not perceived as minor by the women affected and can have considerable impact on a woman's quality of life in pregnancy. In addition, many of the symptoms of minor conditions of pregnancy are the same as those of significant pathological diseases that need to be excluded. Symptoms frequently relate to physiological adaptations of the body to pregnancy, and women should be reassured (once pathology has been excluded) that these symptoms represent normal pregnancy changes.

（一）腹痛（Abdominal pain）

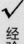 **经验** 腹部的疼痛或不适在妊娠中很常见，通常是短暂性和生理性的。然而，找出可能有病理原因的病例还是很重要的。

Abdominal pain or discomfort is common in pregnancy and is usually transient and physiological. However, it is important to identify cases where there may be a pathological cause.

生理性原因如下。

- 腹部韧带和肌肉的伸展。

- Braxton Hicks 宫缩（假性宫缩）。

- 妊娠子宫对腹部内容物的压力。

- 便秘。

The physiological causes include:

- stretching of the abdominal ligaments and muscles

- Braxton Hicks ('practice') contractions

- pressure of the gravid uterus on the abdominal contents

- constipation

在患有严重、不典型或复发性疼痛的女性中，很重要的一点是区分生理性腹痛和病理性。具体措

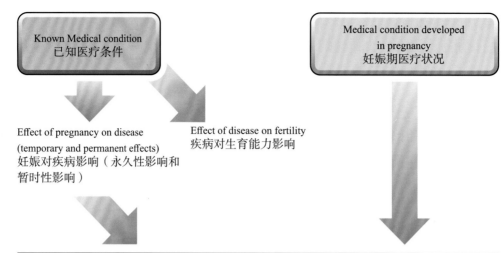

Effect of disease on pregnancy 疾病对妊娠期影响		
	Maternal risks/complications 孕妇风险 / 并发症	Fetal/neonatal risks/complications 胎儿 / 新生儿意外 / 并发症
First trimester 妊娠早期		
Second trimester 妊娠中期		
Third trimester 妊娠晚期		
Labour 临产		
Delivery 分娩		
Postnatal 产后		
Medication issues 用药问题		

▲ 图 9-1 孕期医学疾病框架

Fig. 9.1 Framework for medical disorders in pregnancy.

施如下。

- 早孕问题，如异位妊娠和流产。

- 妇科原因，如卵巢扭转。

- 尿路感染。

- 手术原因，如阑尾炎和胰腺炎。

- 产科原因，如胎盘早剥和分娩。

It is important to differentiate physiological abdominal pain from pathological causes in women with severe, atypical or recurrent pain. These include:

- early pregnancy problems such as ectopic pregnancy and miscarriage
- gynaecological causes such as ovarian torsion
- urinary tract infection
- surgical causes such as appendicitis and pancreatitis
- later obstetric causes such as placental abruption and labour

社会原因，特别是家庭暴力，应该被考虑到出现于反复发作腹痛的女性中，并且腹痛的器质性病理已被排除在外时。

Social causes, particularly domestic abuse, should be considered in women who present with recurrent episodes of abdominal pain where organic pathology has been excluded.

一旦病理原因被排除，安抚通常是一种有效的治疗方案，很少需要镇痛药。

Once a pathological cause has been excluded, reassurance is often a successful management option and analgesics are rarely required.

（二）胃灼热（Heartburn）

胃食管反流更容易发生在妊娠期，因为胃排空延迟，食管括约肌压力降低，胃内压升高。这种情况影响多达 80% 的孕妇，特别是在妊娠晚期，鉴别诊断如下。

- 引起胸痛的其他原因，如心绞痛、心肌梗死和肌肉痛。
- 引起类似反流的上腹部疼痛的原因，如先兆子痫、妊娠急性脂肪肝（acute liver of pregnancy，AFLP）和胆结石。

Gastro-oesophageal reflux is more likely to occur in pregnancy because of delayed gastric emptying, reduced lower oesophageal sphincter pressure and raised intragastric pressure. It affects up to 80% of pregnant women, particularly in the third trimester. The differential diagnoses are:

- other causes of chest pain such as angina, myocardial infarction and muscular pain
- causes of upper abdominal pain that can mimic reflux, for example, pre-eclampsia, acute fatty liver of pregnancy (AFLP) and gallstones

保守治疗包括饮食建议，避免辛辣和酸性食物，避免睡前进食。通过将睡姿改为更直立的姿势，症状可以得到改善。如果保守措施不成功，抗酸药在妊娠期间是安全的，可以随时使用。组胺受体拮抗药，如雷尼替丁和质子泵抑制药，在妊娠期间有良好的安全性，如果仅有抗酸药不足以改善症状时，可以使用。

Conservative management includes dietary advice to avoid spicy and acidic foods and to avoid eating just prior to bed. Symptoms can be improved by changing sleeping position to a more upright posture. If conservative measures are not successful, antacids are safe in pregnancy and can be used at any time. Histamine-receptor blockers, such as ranitidine, and proton pump inhibitors have a good safety profile in pregnancy and can be used if antacids alone are insufficient to improve symptoms.

（三）便秘（Constipation）

由于孕酮水平升高、结肠动力减慢及子宫对直肠的压力，便秘在妊娠期间很常见，特别是在妊娠早期。经常在妊娠期间服用的口服铁补充剂可能也会加剧这种情况。

Constipation is postulated to be more common in pregnancy because of both elevated progesterone levels slowing colonic motility and the pressure of the uterus on the rectum. It is particularly common in the first trimester. It can be exacerbated by oral iron supplements, frequently taken in pregnancy.

应该建议女性增加液体和膳食纤维的摄入量。大多数渗透性和刺激性泻药在妊娠期间是安全的，如果保守治疗不成功，可以考虑使用。罕见的是，严重的便秘会阻止胎头下降到骨盆，从而导致妊娠晚期不能平卧。

Women should be advised to increase their fluid and dietary fibre intake. Most osmotic and stimulant laxatives are safe in pregnancy and can be considered if conservative management is unsuccessful. Rarely, severe constipation can be a cause of unstable lie in late pregnancy by preventing the fetal head from descending into the pelvis.

（四）背痛（Backache）

背痛是一种非常常见的妊娠主诉，特别是在妊娠后期。最常见的原因是来自妊娠子宫的压力，导致腰椎前凸过大，以及激素对支撑软组织的影响。鉴别诊断包括尿路感染、肾盂肾炎和早产。

Backache is a very common pregnancy complaint, especially as pregnancy advances. The commonest cause is a combination of pressure from the gravid uterus causing an exaggerated lumbar lordosis and a hormonal effect on the supporting soft tissues. Differential diagnoses include urinary tract infection, pyelonephritis and early labour.

物理治疗方面可以通过身体姿势的改变、适当的伸展和锻炼来帮助女性。可能需要简单的镇痛药，虽然对乙酰氨基酚和可待因制剂在妊娠期间是安全的，但应该避免服用阿司匹林和非甾体抗炎药。可待因的一个缺点是它会导致便秘。

Physiotherapy review can help by advising on posture and appropriate stretches and exercises. Simple analgesics may be required. Whilst paracetamol and codeine formulations are safe in pregnancy, aspirin and non-steroidal anti-inflammatory medication should be avoided. One disadvantage of codeine is that it can cause constipation.

（五）晕厥（Syncope）

黄体酮对血管平滑肌的作用是产生生理性血管扩张，导致血液聚集，体位性低血压，可能导致晕厥。在妊娠后期（从妊娠 20 周左右）可能会发生腔静脉压迫，进一步减少静脉回流到心脏，并导致低血压。虽然妊娠期晕厥通常是良性的，但如果是复发性贫血，则应排除低血糖、脱水和心律失常。

Physiological vasodilatation from the effects of progesterone on the vascular smooth muscle causes a pooling of blood in dependent areas, causing postural hypotension that can lead to syncope. Later in pregnancy, caval compression from the gravid uterus can occur (from around 20 weeks' gestation), reducing further the venous return to the heart and precipitating hypotension. Whilst syncope in pregnancy is usually benign, if it is recurrent anaemia, hypoglycaemia, dehydration and arrhythmias should be excluded.

建议女性在从卧位站起来之前先坐一会儿，避免长时间站立；妊娠后期应避免仰卧，以减少下腔静脉压迫和仰卧位低血压。应避免脱水。

Women should be advised to sit for a while prior to standing when getting up from a lying position and to avoid prolonged standing; later in pregnancy, lying supine should be avoided to reduce caval compression and supine hypotension. Dehydration should be avoided.

（六）静脉曲张（Varicosities）

腿部或外阴静脉曲张可能会恶化或复发，这是由于妊娠子宫对盆腔静脉的压力，减少了下肢静脉回流，以及对血管平滑肌松弛的孕激素效应。这些表现通常被误诊，但如果疼痛，那么血栓性静脉炎和深静脉血栓（deep vein thrombosis，DVT）应该被排除。

Varicosities in the legs or vulva may worsen or appear de-novo because of a combination of pressure on the pelvic veins from the gravid uterus reducing venous return from lower limb veins and the progestogenic effect on relaxing the vascular smooth muscle. Their appearance is usually diagnostic but if painful then thrombophlebitis and deep vein thrombosis (DVT) should be excluded.

坐姿或卧位抬腿可能会改善症状。使用压力袜既可缓解症状，又可以降低扩张静脉内淤血导致静脉血栓栓塞的风险。如果存在严重的静脉曲张，并存在静脉血栓栓塞的其他危险因素，则可能需要考虑肝素预防。

Elevating the legs while sitting or lying may improve symptoms. The use of compression stockings can both alleviate symptoms and reduce the risk of venous thromboembolism from stasis in the dilated veins. If severe varicosities are present and there are other risk factors for venous thromboembolism, heparin prophylaxis may need to be considered.

（七）腕管综合征（Carpal tunnel syndrome）

妊娠期间由于毛细血管通透性增加而发生液体潴留。由于正中神经穿过腕管，这会压迫正中神经，从而导致或加重腕管综合征。

Fluid retention occurs in pregnancy due to increased capillary permeability. This can cause or worsen carpal tunnel syndrome through compression of the median nerve as it travels through the carpal tunnel.

在大多数病例中，减少手腕屈曲的手腕夹板通常是主要的治疗方法。在严重的情况下，偶尔需要注射类固醇激素，可以在妊娠期间注射。对于妊娠相关腕管综合征患者，很少需要手术松解腕管韧带，因为大多数患者在妊娠后腕管韧带就松解了。

Wrist splints that reduce wrist flexion are usually the mainstay of treatment in the majority of cases. In severe cases steroid injections are occasionally required and can be given in pregnancy. Surgical release of the carpal tunnel ligament is rarely required with pregnancy-related carpal tunnel syndrome, as most resolve post-pregnancy.

（八）骨盆环功能障碍（耻骨联合骨盆腔功能障碍，SPD）[Pelvic girdle dysfunction (symphyseal pelvic dysfunction, SPD)]

妊娠期间松弛素水平的升高可增加关节活动度，从而使骨盆环扩张以供胎儿出生。但是，在某些女性中，这种影响可能会被放大，并会导致骨膜、髋关节或骨盆周围其他部位的不适；这通常随着妊娠的增加而恶化。女性经常描述为行走或站立时骨盆环上有压痛的特征性疼痛。骨盆前方疼痛应排除尿路感染。

Raised levels of relaxin in pregnancy increase joint mobility to allow expansion of the pelvic ring for birth. However, in some women, this effect can be exaggerated and cause discomfort either at the symphysis, the hip or at other points around the pelvis; this usually worsens with increasing gestation. Women often describe characteristic pain on walking or standing with tenderness over the pelvic ring. Urinary tract infection should be excluded with anterior pain.

理疗师会建议通过锻炼来提高稳定性，并提供在日常活动中尽量减少症状的技巧，以及分娩时的体位。骨盆带支撑可以改善症状。与背部疼痛一样，可以使用简单的镇痛药。这个问题通常在分娩后就会消失。

Physiotherapists will advise on exercises to improve stability, techniques for minimizing symptoms during daily activities and positions for birth. A pelvic girdle support may improve symptoms. As with back pain, simple analgesics can be used. The problem usually resolves after pregnancy.

三、妊娠期间出现的医疗问题（Medical problems arising in pregnancy）

（一）贫血（Anaemia）

贫血通常发生在妊娠期间。虽然在许多发达国家，它是轻微的，并且可以快速而容易得到治疗，从而使并发症的发生率降至最低，但在某些国家，它是严重的，并且是孕产妇死亡的主要原因。

Anaemia commonly occurs in pregnancy. While in many developed countries it is mild and quick ly and easily treated, resulting in minimal complications, insome countries, it is severe and a major contributor to maternal death.

1. 病因学（Aetiology）

妊娠会引起血液系统的许多变化，其中包括血浆体积和红细胞数量的增加；如果前者大于后者，结果就经常发生"生理性贫血"。铁和叶酸的需求增加，以促进红细胞数量的增加和满足胎儿的需求，而母体饮食并不总是能满足这一需求。因此，缺铁性贫血是妊娠中常见的疾病，尤其是在妊娠晚期。表 9-1 显示了正常妊娠中血红蛋白和红细胞参数的变化。

Pregnancy causes many changes in the haematological system, including an increase in both plasma volume and red cell mass; the former is greater than the latter, with the result that a 'physiological anaemia' often occurs. There is an increased iron and folate demand to facilitate both the increase in red cell mass and fetal requirements, which is not always met by maternal diet. Iron-deficiency anaemia is thus a common condition encountered in pregnancy, particularly in the third trimester. Table 9.1 shows the changes in haemoglobin and red cell parameters in normal pregnancy.

2. 风险因素（Risk factors）

妊娠前的危险因素是与慢性贫血有关的因素。

- 饮食不良导致的铁缺乏。
- 月经过多。
- 妊娠间隔时间短。
- 贫血状况的存在，如镰状细胞疾病、地中海贫血和溶血性贫血。

妊娠期间的危险因素包括多胎妊娠，这是由于

表 9-1　血红蛋白和红细胞指数（平均值和计算的第 2.5 至第 97.5 百分位数参考范围）

Table 9.1　Haemoglobin and red cell indices (mean and calculated 2.5th—97.5th percentile reference ranges)

红细胞指数 Red cell indices	妊娠期 Gestation			
	18 周 18 weeks	32 周 32 weeks	39 周 39 weeks	产后 18 周 8 weeks postpartum
血红蛋白（Hb）g/L Haemoglobin (Hb) g/L	119（106～133）	119（104～135）	125（109～142）	133（119～148）
红细胞计数 ×10¹²/L Red cell count × 10^{12}/L	3.93（3.43～4.49）	3.86（3.38～4.43）	4.05（3.54～4.64）	4.44（3.93～5.00）
平均细胞体积（MCV）fl Mean cell volume (MCV) fL	89（83～96）	91（85～97）	91（84～98）	88（82～94）
平均细胞血红蛋白（MCH）pg Mean cell haemoglobin (MCH) pg	30（27～33）	30（28～33）	30（28～33）	30（27～32）
平均细胞血红蛋白浓度（MCH）g/dl Mean cell haemoglobin concentration (MCH) g/dL	34（33～36）	34（33～36）	34（33～36）	34（33～36）
血细胞比容 Haematocrit	0.35（0.31～0.39）	0.35（0.31～0.40）	0.37（0.32～0.42）	0.39（0.35～0.44）

经许可转载，引自 Shepard, MJ, Richards VA, Berkowitz RL,et al. (1982) An evaluation of two equations for predicting fetal weight by ultrasound. Am J Obstet Gynecol 142:47-54. ©1982 Elsevier.

Reproduced with permission from Shepard, MJ, Richards VA, Berkowitz RL, et al. (1982) An evaluation of two equations for predicting fetal weight by ultrasound. Am J Obstet Gynecol 142:47-54. © 1982 Elsevier.

多胎妊娠情况下对铁的需求增加。

Pre-pregnancy risk factors are those associated with chronic anaemia:

- iron deficiency secondary to poor diet
- menorrhagia
- short interval between pregnancies
- presence of anaemic conditions, such as sickle cell disease, thalassaemia and haemolytic anaemia

Risk factors within pregnancy include multiple pregnancy due to the increased iron demand in multiple pregnancy scenarios

3. 临床特征与诊断（Clinical features and diagnosis）

贫血通常通过常规全血细胞计数的结果被确定。一些女性会出现呼吸急促和嗜睡等症状。妊娠期正常血红蛋白水平有变化，并随着妊娠的进展逐渐下降。在妊娠早期血红蛋白水平低于 100g/L，妊娠中期和晚期血红蛋白水平低于 105g/L 可诊断为贫血。

Anaemia is often identified as the result of routine full blood count measurements. Some women will present with symptoms such as shortness of breath and lethargy. There is a variation in normal haemoglobin levels in pregnancy and a gradual fall as pregnancy progresses. Anaemia can be diagnosed with a haemoglobin level less than 100g/L in the first trimester and less than 105g/L in the second and third trimesters.

4. 对妊娠的影响（Implications for pregnancy）

缺铁性贫血主要影响母亲。患有轻度贫血时，尽管母亲的携氧能力降低，但胎儿通常不受影响。但是，由于子宫内胎儿铁的储存缺乏，婴儿在出生后的第一年内更容易缺铁。患有严重贫血时，早产和低出生体重儿的风险增加，分娩时失血可能性更大。

Iron-deficiency anaemia mainly affects the mother. With mild anaemia, the fetus is usually unaffected despite the reduced oxygen-carrying capacity of the mother. However, the baby is more likely to have iron deficiency in the first year of life because of a lack of development of fetal iron stores in utero. With severe anaemia, there is an increased risk of pre-term birth and low birth weight and possibly greater blood loss at delivery.

在整个妊娠期间，对母亲的影响是出现症状性贫血的风险，这种症状性贫血可能会导致疲劳、工作能力下降及增加感染的易感性。如果贫血持续到分娩时，如果发生大量失血，血液储备就会缺乏。严重贫血与孕产妇死亡率之间有很强的联系。围产

期需要输血的风险也增加。

The implications to the mother in all trimesters are the risk of developing symptomatic anaemia that can cause fatigue, reduced work performance and an increase in susceptibility to infections. If anaemia persists to the time of delivery, there will be a lack of reserve if significant blood loss occurs. There is a strong association between severe anaemia and maternal mortality. The risk of requiring blood transfusions peripartum is also raised.

5. 治疗方法（Management）

及时识别和治疗进行性贫血可优化孕妇的血红蛋白水平，并降低分娩时贫血的风险。

Prompt recognition and treatment of developing anaemia optimize a woman's haemoglobin levels in pregnancy and reduce the risk of commencing labour anaemic.

尽管妊娠期间的大多数贫血是由于铁缺乏引起的，但应考虑是否存在潜在的贫血状况或是否也可能涉及叶酸缺乏。

Although most anaemia in pregnancy is secondary to iron deficiency, consideration should be given as to whether there is an underlying anaemia condition or if folate deficiency could also be involved.

如果临床上怀疑缺铁不是导致贫血的原因，或者如果女性对补铁没有效果，则应通过铁蛋白或原卟啉锌水平评估铁的状态，测定叶酸并进行血红蛋白电泳以排除血红蛋白病。建议口服补铁作为一线治疗。如果与抗坏血酸（如橙汁）一起服用，并且在摄入时避免喝茶和咖啡，则可以更好地吸收。饮食建议也应给予补铁。由于便秘和胃刺激性的副作用，补充铁的依从性通常较差。如果铁不能耐受或铁治疗后血红蛋白没有改善，则可以考虑胃肠外铁剂治疗。有时，如果贫血很严重，并且在分娩前被诊断出，则需要输血。

If there is clinical suspicion that iron deficiency is not the cause of the anaemia or if a woman has failed to respond to iron supplementation, then the iron status should be assessed by either ferritin or zinc protoporphyrin levels, folate measured and haemoglobin electrophoresis performed to exclude haemoglobinopathies. Oral iron supplementation is recommended as first-line treatment. This is better absorbed if taken with ascorbic acid (for example, orange juice) and if tea and coffee are avoided at the time of ingestion. Dietary advice should also be given. Compliance with iron supplementation is often poor due to the side effects of constipation and gastric irritation. If iron is either not tolerated or if improvements in haemoglobin are not seen despite iron therapy, then parenteral iron can be considered. Sometimes a blood transfusion is considered if the anaemia is severe and it is diagnosed close to delivery.

充分持续的产后治疗对降低女性进一步妊娠贫血的风险至关重要。

Adequate continued postnatal treatment is essential to reduce the risk of a woman entering a further pregnancy anaemic.

维生素 B_{12} 缺乏症在妊娠中极为罕见，但如果确诊，可以通过口服或胃肠外补充维生素 B_{12} 进行治疗。

B_{12} deficiency is extremely rare in pregnancy, but if it is diagnosed, treatment is with oral or parenteral B_{12} supplementation.

6. 预防（Prophylaxis）

孕期常规补铁（通常与叶酸结合）可以降低缺铁的风险。由于缺乏改善结果的证据，目前在英国这不是常规建议。在其他一些普遍缺铁的国家，这是标准做法。

Routine iron supplementation (usually combined with folic acid) throughout pregnancy may reduce the risk of iron deficiency. This is currently not a routine recommendation in the UK due to the lack of evidence of improved outcomes. In some other countries where iron deficiency is common, this is standard practice.

（二）妊娠期糖尿病（Gestational diabetes）

在西方国家，妊娠期糖尿病是一种越来越常见的产科并发症，发生率高达9%。但是，高危人群（如亚洲或肥胖女性）的患病率更高。

Gestational diabetes is an increasingly common antenatal condition occurring in up to 9% of all pregnancies in Western countries. However, the prevalence is much higher in at-risk populations (e.g. Asian or obese women).

1. 病因学（Aetiology）

妊娠会诱发糖尿病。这主要是由于胎盘中产生的抗胰岛素激素（人胎盘泌乳素、胰高血糖素和皮质醇）而增加了对胰岛素作用的抵抗力，另外母体在妊娠期间糖皮质激素和甲状腺激素的增加也会造成这种情况。因此，母体胰腺必须增加胰岛素的分泌来对抗这种情况。在一些孕妇中，不能实现代偿性增加，结果就导致了妊娠期糖尿病。

Pregnancy induces a diabetogenic state. This is predominantly because of increased resistance to the actions of insulin due to the placental production of the anti-insulin hormones (human placental lactogen, glucagon and cortisol), though the increased production of maternal glucocorticoids and thyroid hormones during pregnancy also contributes to this. In response, the maternal pancreas must increase its production of insulin to combat this. In some women this is not achieved, and gestational diabetes is the result.

2. 高危因素（Risk factors）

高危因素与2型糖尿病相同，列在框9-1中。该清单摘自NICE临床指南"妊娠期糖尿病"（2008年、2015年修订）。该指南仅建议在实践中使用某些风险因素进行筛查。如果存在其中一种或多种危险因素，应进行75g口服糖耐量试验（OGTT）。然而，许多临床医生认为，任何风险因素的存在，而不是一个子集，都应进行OGTT。

Risk factors are the same as those for type 2 diabetes and are listed in Box 9.1. This list is taken from the NICE Clinical Guideline 'Diabetes in pregnancy' (2008, amended 2015). The guideline only recommends that some of the risk factors be used for screening in practice. The presence of one or more of these risk factors should lead to the offer of a 75-g oral glucose tolerance test (OGTT). However, many clinicians feel that the presence of any risk factor, rather than a subset, should trigger the offer of an OGTT.

3. 临床特征和诊断（Clinical features and diagnosis）

妊娠期糖尿病可能是无症状的，因此筛查就需要及时进行，糖尿病筛查可以是普遍性的也可以是选择性的。但出于实际和经济原因，大多数单位更喜欢采取选择性的筛查方法。框9-1中列出的高风险人群可以进行选择性筛查。如前所述，筛查是在孕中期28周通过75g OGTT进行的，如果风险很高，则可提前在孕中期进行筛查，然后在28周重复进行（如果第一次测试正常）。在OGTT中，首先测量空腹血糖水平，然后给予75g负荷剂量的葡萄糖，并在糖负荷后2h进一步测量葡萄糖水平。关于应诊断为妊娠期糖尿病的葡萄糖水平存在争议。表9-2列出了2种最常用的诊断标准。

Gestational diabetes may be asymptomatic. As such, a screening programme needs to be in place that can either be universal or selective. Most units prefer a selective approach for practical and financial reasons. Selective screening is offered to the at-risk groups listed in Box 9.1. As described earlier, screening is by a 75-g OGTT at 28 weeks, or if very high risk, early in the second trimester and then repeated at 28 weeks (if

框 9–1　妊娠期葡萄糖不耐受风险增加的孕妇	Box 9.1　Women at increased risk of glucose intolerance in pregnancy
• 既往分娩过巨大儿婴儿（4.5kg 及以上）* • 既往患过妊娠期糖尿病 * • 糖尿病患者一级亲属 * • 肥胖（BMI 大于 30kg/m²）* • 特定的糖尿病患病率高的种族 * 　– 南亚人（特别是家庭国籍为印度、巴基斯坦或孟加拉国的女性） 　– 加勒比黑种人 　– 中东地区（特别是家庭国籍为沙特阿拉伯、阿拉伯联合酋长国、伊拉克、约旦、叙利亚、阿曼、卡塔尔、科威特、黎巴嫩或埃及的女性） • 当前妊娠巨大儿（在不同的研究中有不同的定义，如用超声测量胎儿腹围＞第 90 百分位，或者使用基于超声测量公式估计胎儿体重） • 尿糖≥1+ 多于一次或≥2+ 一次 • 既往围产期胎儿意外死亡 • 多囊卵巢综合征病史 • 羊水过多 • 空腹血糖（FBG）≥6.0mmol/L 或随机血糖≥7.0mmol/L	• Previous macrosomic infant (more than 4.5 kg or above)* • Previous gestational diabetes* • First-degree relative with diabetes* • Obesity (BMI more than 30 kg/m²)* • Specific ethnic family origin with a high prevalence of diabetes*: 　– South Asian (specifically women whose country of family origin is India, Pakistan or Bangladesh) 　– Black Caribbean 　– Middle Eastern (specifically women whose country of family origin is Saudi Arabia, United Arab Emirates, Iraq, Jordan, Syria, Oman, Qatar, Kuwait, Lebanon or Egypt) • Macrosomia in current pregnancy (variably defined in different studies, e.g. fetal abdominal circumference measured with ultrasound >90th centile, or fetal weight estimated using formulae based on ultrasound measurements) • Glycosuria ≥ 1+ on more than one occasion or ≥ 2+ on one occasion • Previous unexpected perinatal death • History of polycystic ovary syndrome • Polyhydramnios • Fasting blood glucose (FBG) more than 6.0 mmol/L or random blood glucose more than 7.0 mmol/L

*. 标记的危险因素是 NICE 临床指南建议在妊娠期以 75g 口服糖耐量试验的形式进行筛查的危险因素。摘自 National Institutes for Health and Clinical Excellence（2008, amended and updated 2015）. *Diabetes in pregnancy: Management of diabetes and its complications from pre-conception to the postnatal period.* NICE Publication Guideline NG 63.

*. Risk factors in bold are those that the NICE Clinical Guideline recommends should be used for screening in practice during pregnancy in the form of a 75-g oral glucose tolerance test. From National Institutes for Health and Clinical Excellence (2008, amended and updated 2015). *Diabetes in pregnancy: Management of diabetes and its complications from pre-conception to the postnatal period.* NICE Publication Guideline NG 63.

表 9–2　75g 口服葡萄糖耐量试验诊断妊娠期糖尿病的标准

Table 9.2　Diagnostic criteria for gestational diabetes using a 75-g oral glucose tolerance test

诊断标准 Diagnostic criteria		空腹正常值（静脉血糖） Normal fasting value(venous plasma glucose)	正常 2h 值（静脉血糖） Normal 2–hour value(venous plasma glucose)
WHO 1999[a]	一个或多个异常值 One or more abnormal values required	＜7.0mmol/L	＜7.8mmol/L
IADPSG[b]	一个或多个异常值 One or more abnormal values required	＜5.1mmol/L	＜8.5mmol/L

IADPSG. 国际糖尿病和妊娠研究小组协会；WHO. 世界卫生组织

在特定人群中，使用 IADPSG 标准比使用 WHO 标准诊断更多的 "妊娠期糖尿病"

a. 引自 World Health Organization. Definition, Diagnosis and Classification of Diabetes Mellitus and Its Complications:Report of a WHO Consultation. Part 1: *Diagnosis and Classification of Diabetes Mellitus*. Geneva, World Health Organization, 1999.

b. 引自 Metzger BE, Gabbe SG, Persson B, et al. (2010) International association of diabetes and pregnancy study groups recommendations on the diagnosis and classification of hyperglycemia in pregancy.Diabetes Care 33:676-682.

IADPSG, International Association of Diabetes and Pregnancy Study Groups; WHO, World Health Organization.

In a given population, use of the IADPSG criteria results in more diagnoses of 'gestational diabetes' than using the WHO criteria.

a. World Health Organization. *Definition, Diagnosis and Classification of Diabetes Mellitus and Its Complications: Report of a WHO Consultation.* Part 1: Diagnosis and Classification of Diabetes Mellitus. Geneva, World Health Organization, 1999.

b. Metzger BE, Gabbe SG, Persson B, et al. (2010) International association of diabetes and pregnancy study groups recommendations on the diagnosis and classification of hyperglycemia in pregnancy. Diabetes Care 33:676-682.

normal at the first test). In the OGTT, a fasting glucose level is first measured, then a 75-g loading dose of glucose is given and a further glucose level taken at 2 hours post-sugar load. There is an ongoing debate as to the levels of glucose at which gestational diabetes should be diagnosed. Table 9.2 indicates the two most commonly used diagnostic criteria.

4. 对妊娠的影响（Implications for pregnancy）

妊娠期糖尿病主要发生在妊娠晚期，有时发生在妊娠中期（表 9–3）。在母体中，妊娠期糖尿病的存在增加了反复感染和先兆子痫发展的风险。对于胎儿而言，羊水过多和巨大儿的风险增加，后者与血糖控制的程度有关。死产的风险增加。考虑到分娩，患有妊娠期糖尿病的女性更有可能进行引产，如果进行阴道分娩，肩难产、器械分娩和会阴撕裂延长是很常见的。患有妊娠期糖尿病的女性进行剖宫产更常见。婴儿更有可能需要进入新生儿科病房。由于子宫内胎儿胰腺的相对过度活跃，新生儿患低血糖症的风险增加。如果母亲的血糖在分娩时得到很好的控制，这种情况就不太可能发生。孕妇的葡萄糖很容易通过胎盘，而胰岛素则不能。

Gestational diabetes is predominantly a disease of the third and sometimes second trimester (Table 9.3). In the mother, the presence of gestational diabetes increases the risk of recurrent infections and of pre-eclampsia developing.

表 9–3　妊娠期糖尿病对妊娠的影响

Table 9.3　Effect of gestational diabetes on pregnancy

	孕产妇风险 / 并发症 Maternal risks/complications	胎儿 / 新生儿的风险 / 并发症 Fetal/neonatal risks/complications
妊娠早期 First trimester	–	–
妊娠中期 Second trimester	子痫前期 Pre-eclampsia	巨大儿 Macrosomia
妊娠晚期 Third trimester	复发性感染 Recurrent infections	羊水过多 Polyhydramnios 死胎 Stillbirth
临产 Labour	引产 Induction of labour 分娩进展不佳 Poor progress in labour	
分娩 Delivery	器质性分娩 Instrumental birth 创伤性分娩 Traumatic delivery 剖宫产 Caesarean section	肩难产 Shoulder dystocia
产后 Postnatal		新生儿低血糖 Neonatal hypoglycaemia 新生儿科入院 Neonatal unit admission 呼吸窘迫综合征 Respiratory distress syndrome 黄疸 Jaundice
一段时间后 Longer term	日后生活出现 2 型糖尿病 Type 2 diabetes later in life	儿童及以后生活中出现肥胖和糖尿病 Obesity and diabetes in childhood and later life

For the fetus, there is increased risk of polyhydramnios and macrosomia, with the latter being related to the degree of glucose control. There is an increased risk of stillbirth. Considering birth, women with gestational diabetes are more likely to have an induction of labour. If vaginal birth occurs, shoulder dystocia, an instrumental birth and extended perineal tears are more common. Women with diabetes are more likely to have a caesarean section. Babies are more likely to need admission to the neonatal unit. They are at increased risk of neonatal hypoglycaemia due to the relative over-activity of the fetal pancreas in utero. This is less likely to occur if maternal blood sugars are well controlled around the time of birth. Maternal glucose readily crosses the placenta, whilst insulin does not.

> **！注意**
>
> 请记住，葡萄糖容易穿过胎盘，而母体高血糖会导致胎儿血糖水平升高。另一方面，胰岛素不会穿过胎盘，因此胎儿完全依靠自身胰岛素的供应来调节血糖水平。
>
> Remember that glucose crosses the placenta readily and that maternal hyperglycaemia results in elevated blood glucose levels in the fetus. Insulin, on the other hand, does not pass across the placenta, and therefore the fetus is entirely dependent on the supply of its own insulin production for the regulation of its blood sugar levels.

对于大多数女性来说，妊娠期糖尿病会在妊娠后消失，但在一些女性中，发现了患有 2 型糖尿病，并且糖尿病护理需要继续。

Whilst for the majority of women gestational diabetes will resolve post-pregnancy, in some women, this diagnosis is the unmasking of type 2 diabetes and diabetic care will need to continue.

> **✓ 经验**
>
> 患有妊娠期糖尿病的女性在以后的生活中罹患 2 型糖尿病的风险仍然较高。这些女性应定期进行某种形式的筛查，每年 1 次以排除糖尿病。
>
> Women who have had gestational diabetes remain at higher risk of developing type 2 diabetes later in life. These women should have some form of regular screening, such as annually, to exclude diabetes.

对于婴儿来说，胎儿远期效应会增加儿童后期肥胖和糖尿病的风险。

For the babies, fetal programming effects increase the risk of obesity and diabetes in later childhood.

5. 治疗方法（Management）

由妇产科医生、糖尿病医师、糖尿病专科护士、助产士和营养师组成的多学科团队应共同管理妊娠期糖尿病。

Multidisciplinary teams consisting of obstetricians, diabetic physicians, diabetic specialist nurses and midwives and dieticians should manage diabetes in pregnancy.

在产前，目的是通过实现良好的血糖控制来降低并发症的风险。最初，这是通过饮食措施来避免葡萄糖水平的大幅波动：摄入更多低血糖指数的糖类和瘦肉蛋白，避免高血糖指数的糖类食物。如果不成功，则可以使用药物。二甲双胍和格列本脲在孕妇中使用的越来越多，可能减少对胰岛素的需求，但许多妊娠期糖尿病女性将需要胰岛素更好地控制。血糖控制的目标是，餐前 / 空腹时的毛细血管葡萄糖水平应在 4.0～6.0mmol/L，餐后 2h 的血糖水平应在 6.0～8.0mmol/L。随机对照试验证据表明，以实现女性正常血糖为目标的妊娠期糖尿病治疗可改善结局。建议进行连续生长扫描，以警惕巨大儿的发生。

Antenatally, the aim is to reduce the risk of complications by achieving good glucose control. Initially, this is by dietary measures aiming to avoid large fluctuations in glucose levels: consuming increased amounts of low-glycaemic-index carbohydrate and lean protein and avoiding high-glycaemic-index carbohydrate foods. If this is unsuccessful then medication can be used. Metformin and glibenclamide are increasingly used in pregnancy and may reduce the need for insulin, but a number of women with gestational diabetes will need insulin to optimize control. The aim is that pre-prandial/fasting capillary glucose levels should be between 4.0 and 6.0 mmol/L and that the 2-hour post-prandial value should be between 6.0 and 8.0 mmol/L. Randomized controlled trial evidence has demonstrated that treatment of gestational diabetes with the aim of achieving normoglycaemia in the woman improves outcomes. Serial growth scans are advised to alert to increasing macrosomia.

> **！注意**
>
> 对于子痫前期的发生应保持警惕。
>
> Vigilance should be maintained for the development of pre-eclampsia.

建议足月分娩以减少胎儿死亡的风险，当然这可能需要根据糖尿病的控制程度，巨大儿的存在或是否出现其他情况（如先兆子痫）来最终确定。如果诊断为早产，则应考虑使用产前糖皮质激素来降低新生儿呼吸窘迫的可能性和严重程度。为了使血糖保持在正常范围内糖皮质激素的量可能短期内需要增加。在分娩中，应定期测量血糖并治疗高血糖症，以减少新生儿低血糖症的风险。并随时监测胎儿。胎盘分娩后可终止糖尿病治疗。对婴儿进行血糖测量以防止低血糖症，并尽早开始喂养以帮助婴儿维持其血糖水平。

Delivery at term is recommended to reduce the risk of stillbirth. This may need to be brought forward depending on the degree of diabetic control, the presence of macrosomia or if other conditions have arisen, such as pre-eclampsia. If preterm delivery is considered, antenatal corticosteroids should be considered to reduce the likelihood and severity of respiratory distress in the newborn. The corticosteroids may necessitate a short-term increase in diabetic treatment to keep blood glucose values in the normal range. In labour, blood glucose should be regularly measured and hyperglycaemia treated to reduce the risk of neonatal hypoglycaemia. The fetus should be continuously monitored. Diabetic therapy can be discontinued with the delivery of the placenta. The baby will need blood glucose measurements to look for hypoglycaemia, and feeding should be commenced early to assist the baby in maintaining its sugar level.

产后应停止所有糖尿病治疗，并继续进行毛细血管血糖监测。对于大多数女性，如血糖恢复正常，表明这是妊娠期糖尿病。如果血糖仍然升高，则怀疑是 2 型糖尿病，并建议转诊给糖尿病治疗组。应告知女性妊娠期糖尿病的长期影响，建议由全科医生每年进行 1 次 OGTT 定期筛查，并建议其改正增加糖尿病风险的生活习惯。

Postnatally, all diabetic treatment should be discontinued and capillary glucose testing continued. In the majority of women, these values will be normal, indicating that this was genuine gestational diabetes. If they remain elevated, then there is a suspicion of type 2 diabetes and referral to a diabetic team is indicated. Women should be advised of the long-term implications of gestational diabetes and the need for regular screening by, for example, an annual OGTT by their general practitioner. Advice on reducing other lifestyle risks associated with diabetes may also be appropriate.

（三）孕期感染（Infections acquired in pregnancy）

孕期女性和未妊娠女性被感染的风险是一样的，但是妊娠的相对免疫抑制状态会影响身体对感染的反应方式。

Women will encounter infections in pregnancy just as they would outside of pregnancy. However, the relative immunosuppressive conditions of pregnancy can affect the way the body responds to the infection.

1. 风险因素（Risk factors）

有孩子的孕妇或工作中接触孩子的孕妇更有可能感染许多传染病。

Pregnant women with small children or who work with children are more likely to come across many infectious conditions.

2. 对妊娠的影响及其管理（Implications on pregnancy and management）

不同的感染情况对孕妇的影响和治疗方法不同。需要重申的是，同时考虑对母亲和胎儿的影响很重要。当相同的感染在不同妊娠期发生时，对胎儿的影响可能会产生改变。

The implications on pregnancy and management vary depending on the specific infection. Once more, it is vital to consider both the impact on the mother and the fetus. The impact on the fetus can change when the same infection is contracted at different gestations.

3. 水痘（Chicken pox）

水痘是一种由水痘带状疱疹病毒引起的儿童期高传染性疾病。它对母亲和胎儿都有严重影响。孕妇特别容易患能引起产妇和胎儿高死亡率的水痘肺炎。如果在妊娠早期感染，胎儿发生先天性水痘综合征（眼缺陷、肢体发育不全和神经系统异常）的风险为 1%～2%。如果是近期感染的，则新生儿会因水痘有很大的死亡风险。

Chicken pox is a highly infectious childhood illness caused by *Varicella zoster* virus; it has significant implications on both the mother and fetus. Pregnant women are particularly at risk of developing a varicella pneumonia that has a high maternal and fetal mortality rate. If acquired early in pregnancy, there is a 1–2% risk to the fetus of congenital varicella syndrome (eye defects, limb hypoplasia and neurological abnormalities). If acquired near term there is a risk of neonatal varicella that has a significant mortality risk.

如果没有免疫能力的孕妇暴露于水痘病毒下，可以给其使用带状疱疹免疫球蛋白以减少感染的风险。如果产妇被感染，应给予阿昔洛韦以减少产妇出现并发症的风险。超声成像可以筛查先天性水痘综合征。如果是足月感染，最好推迟分娩，以便有时间将抗体被动转移给胎儿，注意避免与其他非免疫孕妇接触。

If a non-immune pregnant woman is exposed to chicken pox, she can be offered zoster immunoglobulin to reduce the risk of infection. If a woman becomes infected, acyclovir should be given to reduce the risk of maternal complications. Ultrasound imaging can screen for congenital varicella syndrome. With infection at term, delivery should ideally be delayed to allow time for passive transfer of antibodies to the fetus. Care should be taken to avoid contact with other non-immune pregnant women.

4. 微病毒 B19（Parvovirus B19）

微病毒 B19 感染也被称为感染性红斑、第五种疾病或面颊综合征，这是一种常见的儿童疾病，母体的症状包括发热、皮疹和关节病，但通常影响很小。但对于孕妇，微病毒感染迅速分裂的细胞并可能在妊娠初期引起流产，并在妊娠后期引起胎儿贫血和心力衰竭（"胎儿积水"），因此对胎儿有潜在的重大危害。

Infection with parvovirus B19 is also known as *erythema infectiosum, fifth disease or slapped cheek syndrome*. A common childhood illness, maternal symptoms can include fever, rash and arthropathy, but often effects are minimal. In contrast, there are potentially significant fetal effects as parvovirus infects rapidly dividing cells and can cause miscarriage in early pregnancy and fetal anaemia and heart failure ('fetal hydrops') later in pregnancy.

治疗方法包括使用简单的镇痛药和退热药来缓解孕产妇的症状，并避免与其他孕妇接触。如果是在妊娠 20 周后感染的，则对胎儿大脑中动脉血流进行多普勒超声扫描可以检测出是否为胎儿贫血（血流量增加），并可能需要宫内输血进行治疗。

Management includes the use of simple analgesics and antipyretic agents for the maternal symptoms and avoidance of contact with other pregnant women. If the infection is contracted after 20 weeks, serial Doppler ultrasound scanning of the blood flow in the fetal middle cerebral artery can detect fetal anaemia (blood flow increased) that may need to be treated with in utero blood transfusions.

5. H1N1 流感（Influenza H1N1）

甲型 H1N1 流感在 2009 年和 2010 年引起了世界范围的大流行性感染，现在已成为主要的季节性流感病毒株之一。孕妇出现发热和咳嗽的情况与未妊娠女性相似。然而，孕妇发生呼吸衰竭和继发性细菌感染等并发症的风险更大，死亡的风险明显高于未妊娠的人。此外，还可能使早产、死产和新生儿死亡的风险增加。

Influenza H1N1 caused a worldwide pandemic infection in 2009 and 2010 and is now one of the predominant seasonal influenza virus strains. Pregnant women present with fever and cough similar to non-pregnant individuals. However, pregnant women are at greater risks of complications such as respiratory failure and secondary bacterial infections and have a significantly higher risk of dying than non-pregnant individuals. In addition, implications include an increased risk of pre-term birth, stillbirth and neonatal death.

治疗方法有使用抗病毒药物（如奥司他韦或扎那米韦），并在必要时给予呼吸支持。应该建议所有孕妇都接种 H1N1 疫苗。

Management includes treatment with antiviral agents, such as oseltamivir or zanamivir, and respiratory support if necessary. All pregnant women should be advised to be immunized against H1N1.

6. 人类免疫缺陷病毒感染（Human immunodeficiency virus infection）

HIV 是一种会削弱免疫系统的病毒，随着时间的流逝，AIDS 可能会发展。HIV 还会增加感染其他传染病和罹患癌症的风险。但是，艾滋病病毒感染者可能多年没有症状。全世界感染艾滋病病毒的人数正在增加，其中很大一部分是育龄女性。随着疾病的研究，高活性抗反转录病毒疗法（HAART）已被证明可以降低 HIV 感染的发病率和死亡率。

HIV is a virus that weakens the immune system, and over time AIDS may develop. HIV also increases the risk of catching other infections and developing cancers. However, people with HIV infection may be asymptomatic for many years. The number of people living with HIV worldwide is increasing, and a significant proportion of these are women of reproductive age. With advancing disease, highly active antiretroviral therapy (HAART) has been shown to reduce morbidity and mortality from HIV infection.

(1) 妊娠对疾病的影响（Implications of pregnancy for the disease）

妊娠似乎并不能加快 HIV 感染的进程或增加 AIDS 发生的机会。

Pregnancy does not appear to accelerate the course of HIV infection or increase the chance of AIDS developing.

(2) 疾病对妊娠的影响（Implications of the disease for pregnancy）

HIV 对孕妇最主要的隐患是在没有医疗干预的情况下，艾滋病病毒从母亲垂直传播到婴儿的风险很高（高达 45%），甚至可以在产前、经阴分娩时通过胎盘发生和产后通过母乳喂养发生。在疾病晚期，血清转化和高病毒载量下，风险最高。在没有母乳喂养的女性中，传播率降至 25% 以下。通过采取多种抗反转录病毒疗法形式的医学干预，有可能进一步将垂直传播率降至小于 2%。

The main concern in pregnancy is the high risk of vertical transmission (up to 45%) of HIV from mother to baby without medical intervention. This can occur transplacentally in the antenatal period, during vaginal birth and postnatally through breast-feeding. The risk is highest in advanced disease, at seroconversion and with high viral loads. In women who do not breast-feed, transmission rates fall to less than 25%. With medical intervention in the form of multiple antiretroviral therapy, it is possible to reduce vertical transmission further to less than 2%.

此外，晚期 HIV 女性患者中，流产、胎儿生长受限、早产和死产的风险增加。

In addition there are increased risks of miscarriage, fetal growth restriction, prematurity and stillbirth in women with advanced HIV disease.

一些女性在妊娠前就已使用过 HAART 治疗，应对此进行权衡，以考虑孕妇服用个别药物的安全性。许多女性将不接受任何药物治疗。

Some women will already be on HAART prior to pregnancy, and this should be reviewed to consider the safety of individual medications in pregnancy. Many women will be treatment naïve.

使用 HAART 治疗且病毒载量低于 400 拷贝 /ml 的女性可以通过阴道进行分娩，因为垂直传播的风险非常低。但是，应建议那些未使用 HAART 治疗和（或）病毒载量≥400/ml 或更高的患者进行剖宫产以降低垂直传播的风险。

Women who are taking HAART and have viral loads less than 400 copies/mL can deliver vaginally, as there is a very low risk of vertical transmission. However, those who are not taking HAART and/or have viral loads of ≥400 copies/mL or more should be advised to have a caesarean section to reduce the risk of vertical transmission.

有一些证据表明，妊娠的激素效应可能增加女性抗反转录病毒治疗的毒性风险，特别是核苷反转录酶抑制药，据报道不良反应包括乳酸性酸中毒、肝衰竭，甚至产妇死亡。此外，一些抗反转录病毒药物被认为具有致畸性，在妊娠期间应避免使用。

There is some evidence that the hormonal effects of the pregnancy may increase the risk of toxicity of antiretroviral therapy in the woman, especially the nucleoside reverse transcriptase inhibitors. Side effects reported have included lactic acidosis, hepatic failure and even maternal death. In addition, some antiretroviral agents are thought to be teratogenic and should be avoided in pregnancy.

(3) 筛查（Screening）

尽管许多女性在妊娠时就会知道自己感染了艾滋病病毒，但由于长期处于无症状状态，一些女性并不重视艾滋病病毒。正因如此，由于高垂直传播率和干预措施的有效性，许多国家现在提倡孕期筛查。通常在妊娠初期进行此检查，但对于高危女性，在妊娠后期应进行重复检测。应向女性提供有关筛查艾滋病病毒原因的全面咨询，如果诊断出艾滋病，则可以尽早防控。

Although many women will know they have HIV when they become pregnant, some women will be unaware that they are HIV positive due to the long asymptomatic stage of the condition. In view of this, the high vertical transmission rate and the efficacy of intervention, many countries now advocate screening in pregnancy. This is usually performed early in pregnancy, but in high-risk women it may be appropriate to offer repeat testing later in pregnancy. Women should be fully counselled about the reason for screening for HIV and the improvements in outcome that can be achieved if HIV is diagnosed.

(4) 治疗方法（Management）

应定期对女性进行临床评估，并测量血液中的病毒载量和 CD4 计数。

Women should be regularly assessed clinically and with blood measurements of viral load and CD4 count.

> **！注意**
> 妊娠的 HIV 感染女性应由专科医生和 HIV 医师共同治疗。儿科团队应在产前进行诊断，以讨论新生儿的筛查和治疗方案。
> Women with HIV who become pregnant should be managed jointly by a specialist obstetrician and HIV physician. Input from the paediatric team should occur antenatally to discuss neonatal screening and treatment.

艾滋病病毒感染女性妊娠时的最基本治疗原则包括抗使用艾滋病病毒药物、剖宫产和避免母乳喂养。事实证明，对孕妇使用抗 HIV 药物可降低垂直传播的风险。一些女性已经因为自身健康需要而使用 HAART，如果后期没有证明这些药物对女性有任何毒性作用或对胎儿有致畸性，这种治疗可以一直持续。对于未接受过治疗的女性，抗 HIV 药物应在孕中期开始使用，并一直持续到分娩。使用的治疗方案包括齐多夫定单药治疗和 HAART（核苷酸类似物和蛋白酶抑制药似乎相对安全；应避免使用非核苷类反转录酶抑制药）。但是，仍然建议选择 HAART。虽然对疾病未抑制的女性仍然提倡剖宫产，但在妊娠期间使用 HAART 的且病毒载量 <400 拷贝 /ml 的女性现在可以选择经阴分娩而不会增加传播。妊娠和分娩时应避免侵入性操作，如羊膜穿刺术、使用胎儿头皮电极和胎儿头皮采血。

The initial package of care for women with HIV in pregnancy involves anti-HIV medication, caesarean section and avoiding breast-feeding. The use of anti-HIV drugs in pregnancy has been shown to reduce the risk of vertical transmission. Some women will already be taking HAART for their own health needs, and this should continue, provided the agents have not been reported to have any toxic effects in the woman or teratogenicity in the fetus. In treatment-naïve women, anti-HIV medication should commence in the second trimester and continue until birth. Regimes used include zidovudine monotherapy and HAART (nucleotide analogues and protease inhibitors appear relatively safe; non-nucleoside reverse transcriptase inhibitors should be avoided). However, HAART is the recommended treatment of choice. Whilst caesarean section is still advocated for women with non-suppressed disease, women with a viral load of <400 copies/mL who have taken HAART in pregnancy can now opt for vaginal birth without increasing transmission. Invasive procedures should be avoided in pregnancy and labour, for example, amniocentesis, the use of fetal scalp electrodes and fetal scalp blood sampling.

新生儿 HIV 感染筛查从出生，一直持续到 12 周。如婴儿暴露于病毒则数周内需要进行新生儿抗反转录病毒治疗。强烈建议病毒携带者女性不要母乳喂养。

Neonatal screening for HIV infection commences at birth and continues until 12 weeks. Babies require neonatal antiretroviral treatment as post-exposure prophylaxis for several weeks. Women should be strongly advised not to breast-feed.

对于某些家人可能不了解其状况的艾滋病病毒携带者女性来说，保密有时也是一个问题。应该向女性保证，尽管增加了医疗干预，但仍可为其保密。

Confidentiality is an issue for some women with HIV whose families may not know their status. Women should be reassured that confidentiality can and will be maintained despite the increased medical intervention.

（四）急性病毒性肝炎（Acute viral hepatitis）

目前已知的有 7 种肝炎病毒，最常见的是甲型、乙型和丙型肝炎。所有病毒的表现均相似，为全身不适、恶心、呕吐和发热，并伴有肝功能障碍。但是，在乙型和丙型肝炎中，很大一部分是无症状的（丙型肝炎女性患者中高达 80%）。甲型肝炎通过粪 –

口途径传播，而乙型和丙型肝炎则通过血液传播途径传播。它们可以通过血清学测试来区分。甲型肝炎通常在初次感染后免疫。乙型肝炎可以被清除，可以作为携带者持续存在，也可导致慢性感染；丙型肝炎通常会导致慢性感染，其长期存在有导致肝硬化和肝衰竭的风险。

Seven hepatitis viruses have been identified, the most common being hepatitis A, B and C. All can present similarly with general malaise, nausea, vomiting and pyrexia together with hepatic dysfunction; however, with hepatitis B and C, a significant proportion can be asymptomatic (up to 80% of women with hepatitis C). Hepatitis A is spread by the faeco-oral route, while B and C are transmitted by a blood-borne route. They can be differentiated by serological tests. Hepatitis A is usually cleared after the initial infection; hepatitis B can be cleared, can persist as a carrier state or can lead to chronic infection; and hepatitis C commonly leads to chronic infection and a long-term risk of cirrhosis and liver failure.

妊娠肝炎存在地理性差异。在英国，有 1%～4% 的女性会感染乙型或丙型肝炎。

The incidence of hepatitis in pregnancy has a wide geographical variation. In the UK, 1–4% of women will be infected with hepatitis B or C.

妊娠通常不会改变急性肝炎感染的过程。少数慢性乙型肝炎携带者在妊娠期间可能会重新出现疾病症状。有病例表明，丙型肝炎女性妊娠可能导致疾病更加严重。

Pregnancy does not usually change the course of an acute hepatitis infection. A small number of chronic hepatitis B carriers may suffer a reactivation of the disease state during pregnancy. There is some evidence that pregnancy in women with hepatitis C may cause acceleration of the disease progression.

肝炎通常不会影响孕妇本身。但在妊娠期间患有严重急性感染的女性中，自发性早产的发生率升高。主要影响是新生儿的风险。对于甲型肝炎，如果在分娩前的最后几周发生急性感染，可能会发生这种情况。对于慢性乙型和丙型肝炎，婴儿期感染可能发生在围产期，在患有慢性丙型肝炎的女性中，每 20 例分娩中就有 1 例发生垂直传播。

Hepatitis usually does not impact on the pregnancy itself. In women who have a severe acute infection during pregnancy, there is an increase in the incidence of spontaneous pre-term labour. The main concern is the risk of transmission to the neonate. With hepatitis A, this can happen if acute infection occurs in the last couple of weeks before delivery. With chronic hepatitis B and C, carriage transmission can occur perinatally.

In women with chronic hepatitis C, vertical transmission will occur in 1 in 20 births.

妊娠期间的治疗包括预防、识别和减少垂直传播的风险。在甲型肝炎流行地区，可以通过采取卫生措施和对女性进行免疫接种来降低感染甲型肝炎的风险。妊娠期间接种疫苗并非禁忌。应就冒险行为（特别是静脉注射毒品）向有可能感染乙型和丙型肝炎的女性提供劝阻建议。可以在妊娠之前和妊娠期间进行乙肝疫苗接种。但是目前尚无针对丙型肝炎的有效疫苗。

Management in pregnancy relates to prevention, identification and reduction of the risk of vertical transmission. The risk of hepatitis A infection can be reduced by hygiene measures and consideration of immunization for women in areas of endemic hepatitis A infection. Vaccination is not contraindicated during pregnancy. Women at risk of hepatitis B and C should be counselled regarding risk-taking behaviour (particularly intravenous drug use). Hepatitis B immunization can be offered before and during pregnancy; however, there is currently no effective immunization against hepatitis C.

孕妇可以进行乙型和丙型肝炎筛查。这可能是基于病史的普遍或选择性筛查。产前筛查对减少垂直传播具有重要意义。对于患有丙型肝炎的女性，应排除艾滋病病毒的合并感染。

Women can be screened for hepatitis B and C in pregnancy. This may be universal or selective screening based on a woman's history. Identification antenatally is important to reduce vertical transmission. In women with hepatitis C, co-infection with HIV should be excluded.

剖宫产或避免母乳喂养并不能降低乙型和丙型肝炎的垂直传播风险。因此，提倡阴道分娩（除非有剖宫产的其他产科指征），但要避免采取可能增加血液接触的干预措施，如胎儿头皮电极定位或采集胎儿血样。乙型肝炎患者母亲的婴儿可以接受乙型肝炎免疫球蛋白和早期乙型肝炎免疫治疗，从而将传播率降低至 5%～10%。降低丙型肝炎传播率的方法选择有限，但早期感染的新生儿应充分随访患慢性肝病的风险。

Vertical transmission of hepatitis B and C is not reduced by either caesarean delivery or avoidance of breast-feeding. Thus vaginal delivery is advocated (unless there are other obstetric indications for caesarean delivery) but with avoidance of interventions that may increase blood contact, such as fetal scalp electrode siting or fetal blood samples. Babies of mothers with hepatitis B can be treated with hepatitis B immunoglobulin and early hepatitis B immunization, which reduces transmission rates to 5–10%. There are limited options to reduce transmission rates with hepatitis C, but early identification of infected neonates ensures adequate follow-up for the risk of chronic liver disease.

1. 结核（Tuberculosis）

结核病仍然是世界卫生问题，每年至少有 800 万新病例，有 200 万人死亡。尽管发达国家的感染率很低，但往返于流行地区的难民和旅行者的感染率很高。结核病和艾滋病病毒具有协同作用。艾滋病病毒是导致结核病再度被激活的最常见诱因之一，而艾滋病病毒感染者死亡约 25% 的原因是因为结核。结核病对胎儿主要的两个风险是使用某些抗结核药及母亲患有严重的呼吸道疾病并持续缺氧。结核分枝杆菌很少能穿过胎盘。未经治疗的结核病对女性的风险与未妊娠女性患者相同。高危地区应进行常规结核菌素检测，特别是如果怀疑患者患有该病。呈阳性的患者应进行胸部 X 线检查和痰培养，如果确诊，则如非孕妇患者一样，应进行多种疗法治疗。患有结核病的女性也应接受艾滋病病毒筛查。链霉素是唯一在妊娠中绝对禁忌的药物，因为存在胎儿耳毒性的风险。

Tuberculosis (TB) remains a world health issue with at least 8 million new cases per year and up to 2 million deaths. Although the developed world has low rates of infection, higher rates are found in refugees and travellers to and from endemic areas. TB and HIV are synergistic. HIV is one of the commonest triggers for TB reactivation, and TB is responsible for about 25% of the deaths in people with HIV. The two main proven risks to the fetus are the use of certain anti-tuberculous drugs and if the mother has severe respiratory illness with sustained hypoxia. *Mycobacterium tuberculosis* rarely crosses the placenta. The risks to the woman from untreated TB are the same as in non-pregnant patients. Tuberculin testing should be undertaken routinely in high-risk areas and specifically if the disease is suspected in a patient. Chest X-ray and sputum culture should be performed in those who test positive. If the diagnosis is confirmed, then multiple therapy, as in the non-pregnant patient, is indicated. Women with proven TB should also be screened for HIV. Streptomycin is the only drug that is absolutely contraindicated in pregnancy because of the risk of fetal ototoxicity.

2. 疟疾（Malaria）

每年有 2 亿多人患疟疾，并导致超过 100 万人死亡。在该病流行国家，这是妊娠常见的并发症。妊娠似乎增加了感染的可能性。生活在流行地区的女性出现该疾病严重症状的概率增加。疾病的严重程度与寄生虫的种类、寄生虫血症的程度和个人的免疫状况有关。恶性疟原虫是攻击性最强的生物，因为它攻击所有形式的红细胞。寄生虫在胎盘中生长，15%～60% 的病例都有胎盘疟疾。先天性疟疾在具有免疫力的母亲所生的婴儿中很少见，因为保护性免疫球蛋白 G（IgG）可以穿过胎盘。

Malaria occurs in over 200 million people per year and results in more than 1 million deaths annually. It is a common complication of pregnancy in those countries where the disease is endemic. Pregnancy appears to increase the likelihood of infection. Women who live in endemic areas also show an increased prevalence of the severe forms of the disease. The severity of disease is related to the species of parasite, the level of parasitaemia and the immune status of the individual. *Plasmodium falciparum* is the most virulent of the organisms, as it attacks all forms of the erythrocyte. The parasite grows in the placenta, and placental malaria occurs in anywhere between 15% and 60% of cases. Congenital malaria is rare in infants born to mothers who have immunity, as protective immunoglobulin G (IgG) crosses the placenta.

对于女性而言，急性疟疾带来的主要后果是严重贫血及其他症状。在胎儿中，急性疟疾与生长、流产、早产、先天性感染和围产期死亡率增加有关。

The main risk of acute malaria to the woman is severe anaemia and its consequences. In the fetus, acute malaria is associated with an increased likelihood of growth restriction, miscarriage, pre-term birth, congenital infection and perinatal death.

前往流行地区的孕妇应采取预防措施，或者在妊娠结束之前不要去该地区。还应建议她们保护裸露皮肤，并使用杀虫剂以最大限度减少被蚊子叮咬的风险。

Mothers travelling to endemic areas should take prophylaxis or, preferably, not go to the area until the pregnancy is completed. They should also be advised to keep their skin covered and to use insecticides to minimize the risk of being bitten by mosquitoes.

急性发作时的药物治疗将取决于感染的性质。预防措施以磷酸氯喹为主，剂量为每周 300mg，从出行前 1 周开始，到离开该地区后持续 4 周。如果存在耐氯喹菌株，可以使用氯喹和乙胺嘧啶与磺胺多辛的组合，或者使用鸟嘌呤和甲氟喹。这些药物需要与叶酸补充剂一起服用。虽然大剂量的氯喹会在母亲和胎儿中引起视网膜和耳蜗前庭损害，但尚未证明预防性服用会使出生缺陷发生率增加。

Drug treatment of an acute attack will depend on the nature of the infection. Prophylaxis is given in the form of chloroquine phosphate at a dose of 300 mg each week, starting 1 week before travel and continuing for 4 weeks after leaving the area. Where chloroquine-resistant strains exist, a combination of chloroquine and pyrimethamine with sulfadoxine can be used or proguanil and mefloquine. These drugs need to be taken with a folic acid supplement. Although chloroquine can cause retinal and cochleovestibular damage in high doses in both the mother and the fetus, it has never been shown to be associated with an increased incidence of birth defects where it has been taken for prophylaxis.

3. 风疹感染（Rubella infection）

风疹（又称德国麻疹或 "第三种疾病"）是一种通过呼吸道飞沫传播感染的单链 RNA 病毒引起的发疹性疾病。经过 2～3 周的潜伏期，有症状的患者会出现皮疹、发热、关节痛和淋巴结肿大。50%～75% 的感染患者表现出临床特征。严重并发症（如脑炎和出血体质）很少见。

Rubella (German measles or 'third disease') is an exanthematous disease caused by a single-stranded RNA virus acquired via respiratory droplet exposure. After a 2-to 3-week incubation period, symptomatic patients develop a rash, fever, arthralgias and lymphadenopathy. Fifty to seventy-five percent of infected patients manifest clinical features. Severe complications such as encephalitis and bleeding diathesis are rare.

在成人和儿童中，风疹感染通常是一种轻度疾病。但是，胎儿感染造成的后果可能很严重。先天性风疹综合征（congenital rubella syndrome，CRS）可能产生短暂性异常（如紫癜、脾大、黄疸、脑膜脑炎和血小板减少症）或永久性异常（如白内障、青光眼、心脏病、耳聋、小头畸形和智力低下）。据报道远期后遗症包括糖尿病、甲状腺异常、性早熟和进行性风疹全脑炎。几乎每个器官都有因风疹造成缺陷的病例。

Rubella infection is usually a mild illness in adults and children. However, fetal infection can be severe. Congenital rubella syndrome (CRS) may produce transient abnormalities (e.g. purpura, splenomegaly, jaundice, meningoencephalitis and thrombocytopenia) or permanent abnormalities (e.g. cataracts, glaucoma, heart disease, deafness, microcephaly and mental retardation). Long-term sequelae reported include diabetes, thyroid abnormalities, precocious puberty and progressive rubella pan-encephalitis. Defects involving virtually every organ have been reported.

胎儿感染率最高的时期为 11 周和 36 周以后。然而，先天性缺陷的总发生率在孕中期最高（90%），并在孕中期和孕晚期稳步下降。

The rate of fetal infection is highest at 11 weeks and

>36 weeks. However, the overall rate of congenital defects is greatest in the first trimester (90%) and declines steadily in the second and third trimesters.

风疹疫苗的引入极大降低了 CRS 的发生率。可以通过儿童疫苗接种来预防风疹，麻疹、腮腺炎和风疹（mumps and rubella，MMR）也是针对十几岁女孩的疫苗接种计划的一部分。但是，零星的病例仍然发生，特别是在未接种疫苗的女性中。因此，理想情况下，女性应在妊娠前检查其血清状况，如果阴性，应接种疫苗。尽管建议在接种疫苗后至少 28 天避免受孕，但没有证据表明妊娠接种疫苗对胎儿有任何影响，并不建议近期接种孕妇终止妊娠。

The introduction of rubella vaccine has dramatically reduced the incidence of CRS. The problem should be prevented by childhood vaccination as part of the measles, mumps and rubella (MMR) programme backed up by vaccination rogrammes for girls in their early teens. However, sporadic cases still occur, especially in women who have not been vaccinated. Thus, ideally women should check their serological status before they conceive and, if negative, they should be offered vaccination. Though the advice is to avoid conception for at least 28 days after vaccination, there is no evidence that vaccination in pregnancy has any effect on the fetus and is not an indication for termination.

在许多国家，所有女性在第一次就诊时都会检查风疹免疫力（以血清 IgG 阳性为准）。但是在英国，由于风疹患病率较低，这种检查于 2016 年被叫停。如果风疹免疫的女性受到感染，在接触后 3 周内没有查到急性标志物（血清 IgM），这表明她没有被感染，可以放心。但是，如果风疹易感性女性暴露，则最重要的是要确定诊断，此后的治疗将取决于女性是否感染（通过 IgM 阳性诊断）、妊娠阶段及女性的意愿。

In many countries, rubella immunity (indicated by positive serum IgG) status is checked at the first clinic visit for all women. However, in the UK this practice stopped in 2016 because of the low population prevalence of rubella. If a rubella-immune woman is exposed to infection, the absence of the acute marker (serum IgM) by 3 weeks after exposure confirms that she has not been infected and can be reassured. However, if a rubella-susceptible woman is exposed, it is first important to confirm the diagnosis in the index case. The management thereafter will depend on whether the woman develops infection (diagnosed by becoming IgM positive), the stage of pregnancy and the woman's wishes.

4. 寨卡病毒感染（Zika virus infection）

寨卡病毒是由埃及伊蚊传播的蚊媒黄病毒，它也能传播登革热和基孔肯雅病毒。这种蚊子遍布非洲、亚洲、美洲和太平洋岛屿的大部分地区。自 2015 年以来，该病毒和相关疾病在人群中迅速传播，尽管第一次疫情是在 2007 年报道的。但是截至目前，该病毒及其危害仍然有很多未知的地方。

Zika virus is a mosquito-borne flavivirus transmitted by *Aedes aegypti* mosquitoes, which also transmits dengue and chikungunya virus. The mosquitoes are found throughout much of Africa, Asia, the Americas and the Pacific Islands. There has been a rapid spread of the virus and associated illness in humans since 2015, although the first outbreak was reported in 2007. Consequently, there is still much about the virus and its effects that is not understood.

2017 年，RCOG/RCM/PHE/HPS 联合发布了临床指南 "寨卡病毒感染和妊娠"，以帮助医疗保健专业人员。

In 2017, a joint RCOG/RCM/PHE/HPS clinical guideline, 'Zika Virus Infection and Pregnancy', was published to help health care professionals.

大多数寨卡病毒病例是从由感染的蚊虫叮咬引起的。然而，已经报道了一些性传播病例和一些通过输血传播的病例。大多数感染寨卡病毒的人（80%）没有症状。如果确实出现症状，通常会在暴露后 3～12 天出现。通常患者轻度感染会在 2～7 天出现的疾病症状包括皮疹、瘙痒、发热、头痛、关节痛、肌痛、结膜炎和下背部疼痛。这些症状与登革热和基孔肯雅热相似，应对患者进行所有这三种微生物的检测。孕妇既不容易受到感染，也没有更严重的疾病。据报道尽管发生 Guillain-Barré 综合征的可能性有所增加，但由于寨卡病毒感染而导致成年人出现严重并发症很少见。寨卡病毒可以在症状出现后 1 周内通过血液的聚合酶链反应（PCR）检测到，通常在国家专业实验室进行检测。除非怀疑胎儿有并发症，否则通常不建议对无症状的女性进行检查（见下述）。

The majority of cases of Zika virus are acquired from infected mosquito bites; however, a few cases of sexual transmission and some through blood transfusions have been reported. Most people (80%) infected with Zika virus have no symptoms. If symptoms do develop, these generally occur 3–12 days following the exposure. Those with symptoms have a mild, short-lived (2- to 7-day) illness comprising rash, pruritus, fever, headache, arthralgia, myalgia, conjunctivitis and lower back pain. These symptoms are similar to those of dengue fever and chikungunya, and patients should be tested for all three organisms. Pregnant women are not more vulnerable to infection, nor do they have a more serious illness. Serious complications in an adult from Zika virus infection are rare, although an increase in triggering of Guillain-Barré syndrome has been reported. Zika virus can be detected by polymerase chain reaction (PCR) of blood within 1 week of symptoms developing. This usually is performed at a national specialist laboratory. Testing of asymptomatic women is generally not recommended unless there are suspected fetal complications (see later).

寨卡病毒感染在孕期对胎儿的不良影响是主要问题。据报道有过一些母婴传播病例。在对截至 2016 年 5 月 30 日的文献数据进行系统分析之后，世界卫生组织（WHO）得出结论，妊娠期寨卡病毒感染是先天性脑畸形的原因。先天性寨卡病毒综合征（congenital Zika virus syndrome，CZVS）相关的异常包括各种颅骨异常（包括伴有脑萎缩的小头畸形、脑钙化、脑室扩大、脑室周围囊肿、小眼）和颅外异常（包括胎儿生长受限、羊水过少、胎儿缺足）。据报道，寨卡病毒阳性妊娠者中先天性寨卡病毒综合征的风险差异很大（6%～46%）。目前尚不清楚有症状女性的母婴传播风险是否更大。对于超声扫描上没有颅内异常证据的女性，目前尚不清楚阳性结果是否预示随后的胎儿异常，也不清楚感染后出生的新生儿有症状的比例。

The main concerns in pregnancy are the fetal implications of Zika virus infection. Some cases of maternal-fetal transmission have been reported. Following a systematic review of the literature up to 30 May 2016, the World Health Organization (WHO) concluded that Zika virus infection during pregnancy is a cause of congenital brain abnormalities. Abnormalities associated with congenital Zika virus syndrome (CZVS) include a variety of cranial abnormalities (including microcephaly with brain atrophy, cerebral calcification, ventriculomegaly, periventricular cysts, microphthalmia) and extra-cranial abnormalities (including fetal growth restriction, oligohydramnios, talipes). The reported risk of CZVS in Zika-positive pregnancies has varied widely (6–46%). It is not clear whether the risk of maternal-fetal transmission is greater in the symptomatic woman. In women with no evidence of cranial abnormalities on ultrasound scan, it is at present unclear if a positive result predicts a subsequent fetal abnormality or what proportion of neonates born after infection will have symptomatic disease.

目前没有针对寨卡病毒感染的抗病毒治疗方法。通常是支持性治疗，其中包括休息、补液、镇痛药和退热药。对于有实验室检测表明其血清或羊水中存在寨卡病毒的孕妇，应与胎儿医学专家和新生儿专家详细讨论选择方案。即使超声检查没有发现胎儿异常，有些女性还是选择终止妊娠，其他人则会选择继续妊娠，并通过连续的超声扫描来监测整个

妊娠剩余时间内胎儿解剖结构和生长情况。

No specific antiviral therapy is available for Zika virus infection. Treatment is generally supportive involving rest, fluids, analgesics and antipyretics. In a pregnant woman with laboratory evidence of Zika virus in her serum or amniotic fluid, the options should be discussed in detail with a specialist in fetal medicine and a neonatal specialist. Some women choose to terminate the pregnancy even if there are no fetal abnormalities on ultrasound examination. Others will opt for continuing the pregnancy and having serial ultrasound scans to monitor fetal anatomy and growth through the rest of the pregnancy.

尽管在母乳中发现了活病毒，但目前尚无证据表明寨卡病毒可通过母乳传播给婴儿，禁忌母乳喂养是不建议的。目前没有疫苗或药物可预防寨卡病毒感染。建议孕妇将去往寨卡病毒传播高风险地区的不必要旅行推迟，待产后再考虑，而对于寨卡病毒传播中风险地区也做相同建议。如果孕妇确实需要前往高风险或中风险地区，则应采取所有必要的防咬措施（着浅色、宽松的衣服，尽可能覆盖裸露的皮肤，使用以避蚊胺为基础的驱蚊剂，以及在蚊帐下睡觉 / 休息），并在其返回时进行监控和（或）检测。还建议女性在寨卡病毒传播高风险或中风险的地区旅行返回后至少 6 个月内，采用有效避孕措施避免妊娠。

Whilst viable virus has been detected in breast milk, there is currently no evidence that Zika virus can be transmitted to babies through breast milk, and mothers are advised that there is no contraindication to breast-feeding. There is currently no vaccine or drug available to prevent Zika virus infection. It is recommended that pregnant women postpone non-essential travel to areas with high risk of Zika virus transmission until after pregnancy and consider the same for areas with moderate risk of Zika virus transmission. If pregnant women travel to high- or moderate-risk areas, they should take all necessary bite-prevention measures (light-coloured, loose-fitting clothes that cover as much exposed skin as possible, DEET-based insect repellents and sleeping/resting under a mosquito net) and be monitored and/or tested on their return. It is also recommended that women avoid becoming pregnant by using effective contraception while travelling in an area with high or moderate risk of Zika virus transmission and for at least up to 6 months on her return.

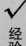

如果没有超声发现的胎儿小头症或其他相关颅内异常的情况，不建议对无症状孕妇进行检查，但建议进行对胎儿进行一系列超声检查。

Testing of asymptomatic pregnant women is not recommended in the absence of ultrasound–identified fetal microcephaly or other related intracranial abnormalities, but serial fetal ultrasound is recommended.

5. 急性肾盂肾炎和尿路感染（Acute pyelonephritis and urinary tract infections）

无症状菌尿症在所有性活跃女性中的发生率为 2%～10%。妊娠时，12%～30% 的女性会因结构和免疫功能的改变而上行性感染而发展为肾盂肾炎。如果用抗生素治疗细菌尿症，则可以将之后出现的急性上行尿路感染的风险降到最低。尽管如此，约有 1% 的孕妇并发急性肾盂肾炎。常见的微生物是大肠埃希菌，应根据已知的敏感性用抗生素积极治疗。大多数社区获得性感染通常对阿莫西林或头孢呋辛敏感。补充液体、缓解疼痛和卧床休息也会有益。妊娠期肾盂肾炎不能低估，因为超过 15% 的女性会发展为菌血症，其中一小部分会发展为败血性休克和（或）早产。

Asymptomatic bacteriuria occurs in 2–10% of all sexually active women. When pregnant, 12–30% of this group of women will develop pyelonephritis from ascending infection due to structural and immune changes to the renal tract. If the bacteriuria is treated with antibiotics, the risk of later development of acute ascending urinary tract infection can be minimized. Nevertheless, approximately 1% of all pregnancies are complicated by an episode of acute pyelonephritis. The common organism is Escherichia coli, and this should be treated aggressively with antibiotics according to known sensitivity. Most community-acquired infections are usually sensitive to amoxicillin or cefuroxime. Additional treatment with fluid replacement, pain relief and bed rest may also be of benefit. Pyelonephritis in pregnancy must not be underestimated, as over 15% of women will develop a bacteraemia, with a small proportion of these progressing to septic shock and/or pre-term labour.

（五）血栓栓塞性疾病（Thromboembolic disease）

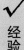

静脉血栓栓塞症（venous thromboembolism, VTE）是发达国家孕产妇死亡的主要原因之一。静脉血栓栓塞在妊娠期间的发病率是未妊娠时的 10 倍左右。

Venous thromboembolism (VTE) is one of the leading causes of maternal mortality in the developed world. VTE is around 10 times more common in pregnancy than when not pregnant.

1. 病因学（Aetiology）

妊娠时处于血栓形成状态。凝血因子增加，内源性抗凝物质减少，纤维蛋白溶解受到抑制。这些影响从妊娠早期开始，持续到出生后几周。此外，由于压迫盆腔血管，下肢出现静脉淤血，会进一步加剧这一问题。

Pregnancy is a prothrombotic state. Coagulation factors increase, endogenous anticoagulants decrease and fibrinolysis is suppressed. These effects commence in the first trimester and last until a few weeks following birth. In addition venous stasis occurs in the lower limbs from compression on the pelvic vessels, further exacerbating the problem.

2. 风险因素（Risk factors）

危险因素可能是早孕，也可能是由于产科情况而发生，也可能是暂时性的。具体如下。

- 预先存在的风险因素
  - 个人或家族静脉血栓栓塞病史。
  - 血栓形成、肥胖、吸烟、某些医疗状况（如镰状细胞病）、严重静脉曲张和产妇年龄增加。
- 一过性危险因素
  - 静止不动和脱水发作。
  - 卵巢过度刺激。
  - 外科手术。
- 产科危险因素
  - 多胎。
  - 子痫前期。
  - 手术分娩。

Risk factors can pre-date pregnancy, can occur as a result of obstetric conditions or can be transient. They include:

- pre-existing risk factors:
  - a personal or family history of VTE
  - thrombophilias, obesity, cigarette smoking, some medical conditions (such as sickle cell disease), gross varicose veins and increased maternal age
- transient risk factors:
  - episodes of immobility and dehydration
  - ovarian hyperstimulation
  - surgical procedures
- obstetric risk factors:
  - multiple pregnancy
  - pre-eclampsia
  - operative delivery

3. 临床特征和诊断（Clinical features and diagnosis）

静脉血栓栓塞的表现与非妊娠时相同。深静脉血栓形成伴腿部肿胀和压痛，肺栓塞（pulmonary embolism，PE）伴呼吸道症状（呼吸急促和胸膜炎性胸痛）或肺坍塌。妊娠期静脉血栓栓塞更容易发生在左侧（90%），因为右髂总动脉和卵巢动脉压迫左髂总静脉（右侧的静脉没有交叉）。妊娠期静脉血栓栓塞大部分发生在髂股静脉，因此下肢症状可能不那么明显。髂股静脉的血栓比小腿静脉的血栓更容易栓塞。

VTE presents as in non-pregnant individuals: DVT with swelling and tenderness of a leg and pulmonary embolism (PE) with respiratory symptoms (shortness of breath and pleuritic chest pain) or collapse. In pregnancy, DVT is more likely to occur on the left (90%) due to compression of the left common iliac vein by the right common iliac artery and ovarian artery (the vein is not crossed on the right). The majority of DVTs in pregnancy occur in the iliofemoral veins, so lower limb symptoms may not be as obvious. Clots in the iliofemoral veins are more likely to embolize than those in the calf.

D- 二聚体测定对妊娠的帮助有限；虽然阴性预测值很高，但阳性结果并不助于确定诊断，因为它会随着妊娠期凝血系统的生理变化而增加。

d-Dimer measurements are of limited help in pregnancy; although the negative predictive value is high, a positive result does not help to establish a diagnosis, as it can increase with the physiological changes in the coagulation system that occur in pregnancy.

放射学检查应该像对非妊娠个体一样进行。应进行下肢静脉多普勒超声检查或盆腔静脉磁共振成像（MRI）评估静脉血栓栓塞。用螺旋动脉计算机断层扫描（CT）或静脉灌注扫描诊断肺栓塞。在妊娠期间进行放射检查时必须小心，因为对胎儿有辐射风险，但最终如果需要进行检查才能确定诊断，就应该做。

Radiological investigations should be performed as in non-pregnant individuals. Doppler ultrasound of the lower limb veins or magnetic resonance imaging (MRI) of the pelvic veins should be performed to assess for DVT. Spiral artery computed tomography (CT) or venous perfusion scanning are used to diagnose PE. Although care must be taken when undertaking radiological examinations in pregnancy because of the radiation risk to the fetus, ultimately if an investigation needs to be done to establish a diagnosis, it should be done.

4. 对妊娠的影响（Implications for pregnancy）

在产前，如果对静脉血栓栓塞进行适当的治疗，

对母亲或胎儿的直接影响微乎其微。如果妊娠女性的静脉血栓未经治疗，那么孕产妇死亡的风险为30%。如果得到及时和适当的治疗，则死亡风险将降低至 3%～8%。用于治疗静脉血栓栓塞的药物还有其他风险（见后述）。出生后，风险仍然很高，治疗需要持续数周。

Antenatally, if VTE is adequately treated, there are minimal direct effects to mother or fetus. If a woman in pregnancy has a PE that is untreated, then there is a 30% risk of maternal death. However, if the woman receives prompt and appropriate treatment, that mortality risk reduces to 3–8%. There are additional risks from the medications used to treat VTE (see later). Postnatally, the risk remains high, and therapy will need to continue for a number of weeks.

5. 治疗方法（Management）

所有女性均应进行妊娠期静脉血栓栓塞的风险评估。根据风险评估，可以制订血栓预防计划以降低血栓形成的风险。对于低风险女性，可能不需要采取其他措施；对于某些女性，可能需要产后预防，而对于那些高风险女性，可以建议产前预防使用渐变弹性压缩袜和低分子肝素（low-mdecular-weight heparin，LMWH）。在最后一种情况下，血栓预防应在妊娠时尽早开始。

All women should have an individual risk assessment undertaken for VTE in pregnancy. Depending on the risk score, a plan for thromboprophylaxis can be made to reduce the risk of thrombosis occurring. For women with low risk, this may not require additional measures; for some women, postnatal prophylaxis may be required, and for those at highest risk antenatal prophylaxis may be recommended with graduated elastic compression stockings and low-molecular-weight heparin (LMWH). In this last scenario, thromboprophylaxis should be started as early as possible in pregnancy.

> **！注意**
>
> 如果妊娠期间怀疑急性静脉血栓栓塞，及时处理是至关重要的，肝素治疗应在等待调查期间开始经验性治疗。
>
> If acute VTE is suspected in pregnancy, prompt management is vital, and heparin therapy should be commenced empirically whilst awaiting investigations.

如果在随后的诊断测试中排除了 DVT 或 PE（见前述），则可以停用肝素。

If a DVT or PE is excluded on subsequent diagnostic testing (see earlier), then the heparin can be discontinued.

由于低分子肝素不穿过胎盘且具有良好的安全

性，因此已在妊娠中得到广泛使用。相反，华法林可穿过胎盘，如果在孕早期使用，可能致使胚胎病变，而在孕晚期使用，则可能致使胎儿颅内出血。大多数患有静脉血栓栓塞的女性可以接受低分子肝素的适当治疗，因此在这种情况下很少需要使用华法林。在大多数情况下，肝素治疗可在分娩时临时停止，以降低产后出血的风险，并在必要时进行局部麻醉（低分子肝素的使用与硬膜外血肿有关）。还应采用简单的措施，如避免脱水和使用渐变弹性压缩袜。

LMWH has been used extensively in pregnancy, as it does not cross the placenta and has a good safety profile. In contrast, warfarin crosses the placenta and is associated with an embryopathy if used in the first trimester and with fetal intracranial bleeding when used in the third trimester. Most women with VTE can be adequately managed on LMWH, so warfarin is rarely needed in this scenario. On most occasions, heparin therapy can be temporarily stopped around the time of birth to reduce the risk of postpartum haemorrhage and to enable regional anaesthesia to be given if required (LMWH use is associated with epidural haematoma). Simple measures such as avoiding dehydration and using graduated elastic compression stockings should also be employed.

产后，女性一般会继续进行肝素预防或治疗 6 周。如果在此妊娠中发生了急性静脉血栓栓塞事件，很可能需要在以后的妊娠中使用肝素预防。还应建议女性避免使用含雌激素的避孕药。

Postnatally, women traditionally continue on heparin prophylaxis or treatment for 6 weeks. If an acute venous thromboembolic event has occurred in this pregnancy, it is likely that heparin prophylaxis will be needed in future pregnancies. Women should also be advised to avoid oestrogen-containing contraceptives.

（六）肝病（Liver disease）

1. 产科胆汁淤积（Obstetric cholestasis）

（1）病因学（Aetiology）

产科胆汁淤积的病因尚不确切，但似乎存在对雌激素敏感的遗传易感性，这会引起肝功能异常。此外，据推测，这与激素、环境和饮食因素有关。

The exact aetiology of obstetric cholestasis is uncertain; however, there appears to be a genetic predisposition to sensitivity to oestrogen, which causes abnormalities in liver function. In addition, it has been speculated that hormonal, environmental and dietary factors are involved.

（2）风险因素（Risk factors）

某些种族（南美、南亚和北欧）和过去的产科胆汁淤积病史是产科胆汁淤积的主要危险因素。

Certain ethnicities (South American, South Asian and northern European) and a past history of obstetric cholestasis are the predominant risk factors for obstetric cholestasis.

（3）临床特征和诊断（Clinical features and diagnosis）

产科胆汁淤积症表现为强烈的瘙痒，尤其是在妊娠中期或晚期的手掌和脚底。很少有与瘙痒有关的皮疹，但抓痕经常出现。大便灰白、尿色深和黄疸少见。胆汁酸和（或）肝脏氨基转移酶升高，排除了其他病理（自身免疫性疾病、胆结石和病毒感染）后可确诊。

Obstetric cholestasis presents with intense itching, especially on the palms of the hands and soles of the feet in the second or third trimester. There is rarely a rash associated with the itching, but excoriation marks are frequently present. Rarely, pale stools, dark urine and jaundice are noted. The diagnosis is confirmed by a rise in bile acids and/or raised liver transaminases where other pathology (autoimmune disease, gallstones and viral infection) has been excluded.

一些女性在服用口服避孕药时或在月经周期的后半段会出现类似的症状。

Some women experience similar symptoms when taking the combined oral contraceptive pill or in the second half of the menstrual cycle.

（4）对妊娠的影响（Implications for pregnancy）

在产前，瘙痒会使人虚弱，影响夜间休息。对其他肝功能的影响可导致凝血时间延长。对于胎儿而言，死产的风险略有增加。早产的风险更高，但这主要是由于早期引产造成的。这对分娩的影响微乎其微，但胎粪更有可能在患有产科胆汁淤积的早产儿身上排出。

Antenatally, the pruritus can be debilitating, giving minimal rest, especially at night. The impact on other liver functions can result in a prolongation of blood clotting time. For the fetus, there is a small increase in the risk of stillbirth. The risk of pre-term birth is higher, but this is predominantly due to early induction of labour. The implications for labour and delivery are minimal, but meconium is more likely to be passed in pre-term fetuses with obstetric cholestasis.

产科胆汁淤积在以后的妊娠中有较高的复发率（超过 90%）。

Obstetric cholestasis has a high recurrence rate (over 90%) in future pregnancies.

（5）治疗方法（Management）

产科胆汁淤积性瘙痒很难治疗。妊娠期间使用局部润肤剂是安全的，但对症状的缓解作用不大。抗组胺药物有时用于镇静作用，但对瘙痒本身影响不大。熊去氧胆酸已被证明可以改善瘙痒和肝功能，但缺乏长期安全性数据。尽管如此，它还是产前治疗的主要手段。鉴于凝血异常的潜在风险，可以使用口服水溶性维生素 K 补充剂，特别是对那些凝血功能显示异常的女性。

The pruritus of obstetric cholestasis can be difficult to treat. Topical emollients are safe for use in pregnancy but provide little symptomatic relief. Antihistamines are sometimes used for their sedative ability but have little impact on the itch itself. Ursodeoxycholic acid has been shown to improve both pruritus and liver function, but long-term safety data are lacking. In spite of this, it is the mainstay of antenatal treatment. In view of the potential risk of clotting abnormalities, oral water-soluble vitamin K supplementation can be used, particularly for those women whose clotting tests suggest an abnormality.

对胎儿进行产前监测的最佳方法尚未确定。连续生长超声扫描和心电监护（cardiotocograph，CTG）等可以检测胎盘功能问题的方法并不能预测产科胆汁淤积的高危胎儿。因此，通常建议在胎儿成熟后分娩，以降低晚期死产的可能风险。

The best way to monitor the fetus antenatally has not yet been established. Methods such as serial growth ultrasound scans and cardiotocographs (CTGs) that can detect problems with placental function are not predictive of atrisk fetuses in obstetric cholestasis. Consequently, delivery once fetal maturation is reached is often recommended to reduce the small risk of late stillbirth.

产后，通常建议女性避免使用含雌激素的避孕药，因为避孕药可能导致症状复发。

Postnatally, women are usually advised to avoid oestrogen-containing contraceptives, which can precipitate a recurrence of symptoms.

2. 妊娠急性脂肪肝（Acute fatty liver of pregnancy）

(1) 病因学（Aetiology）

AFLP 是一种罕见但严重的妊娠反应。病因尚不清楚，但它具有严重子痫前期和 HELLP 综合征的许多特征（溶血、肝酶升高和血小板计数低），并被推测为先兆子痫的变种。最近有一种说法表明，在某些情况下，这种情况与隐性遗传性脂肪氧化紊乱有关。

AFLP is a rare but serious condition of pregnancy. The aetiology is uncertain, but it shares many characteristics with severe pre-eclampsia and HELLP syndrome (haemolysis, raised liver enzymes and a low platelet count) and is postulated to be a variant of pre-eclampsia. There has been a recent suggestion of an association of the condition with a recessively inherited fatty oxidation disorder in some cases.

(2) 风险因素（Risk factors）

初次妊娠，多胎妊娠和肥胖都是危险因素。

First pregnancy, multiple pregnancy and obesity are all risk factors.

(3) 临床特征和诊断（Clinical features and diagnosis）

AFLP 通常在妊娠晚期出现非特异性症状，其中包括恶心、呕吐、腹痛和全身不适。黄疸也可能出现，女性可能会随着肝衰竭、肾功能损害和凝血障碍而迅速恶化。肝肾功能检查结果通常是异常的，可能会出现低血糖。

AFLP usually presents in the third trimester with non-specific symptoms of nausea, vomiting, abdominal pain and general malaise. Jaundice may also be present, and women can rapidly deteriorate with liver failure, renal impairment and coagulopathy. Liver and renal function tests are usually abnormal, and hypoglycaemia may be present.

(4) 对妊娠的影响（Implications for pregnancy）

该病与产妇和胎儿高死亡率有关。产妇死亡继发于肝性脑病、出血和弥散性血管内凝血。

The condition is associated with high maternal and fetal mortality. Maternal death occurs secondary to hepatic encephalopathy, haemorrhage and disseminated intravascular coagulation.

(5) 治疗方法（Management）

应提醒曾经有 AFLP 病史的女性注意这些症状，并提供紧急联系电话，以便在症状复发时使用。应当定期进行肝功能监测和蛋白尿检测。

Women with a history of AFLP in a previous pregnancy should be reminded of the symptoms and given an emergency contact number to use if they recur; liver function monitoring and testing for proteinuria should be undertaken regularly.

诊治必须由多学科医生共同完成，并有重症护理专业人员参与。早期治疗有助于纠正存在的异常（电解质失衡、低血糖和凝血障碍）。一旦孕妇情况稳定后，应尽快分娩。产后可能需要透析；但很少需要进行肝移植。

Management must be multidisciplinary with support from critical care professionals. Initial management is supportive to correct the abnormalities present (electrolyte imbalance, hypoglycaemia and coagulopathy). Once the woman is stable, delivery should be expedited. Dialysis may be necessary postnatally; rarely, liver transplantation is required.

考虑该病的罕见性，有关复发率的信息很少，但一般认为复发的概率会有所增加。

Information regarding recurrence rates is sparse given the rarity of the condition but is suggestive of an increased chance of recurrence.

四、既往医疗状况和妊娠（Pre-existing medical conditions and pregnancy）

现在，越来越多的女性在妊娠前就有既往的健康状况。理想情况下，应该为这些女性提供孕前咨询，以便讨论妊娠对她们特定医疗状况的影响，并制订计划。这可能涉及推迟妊娠，直到达到疾病管理中的特定目标。然而，这个机会经常被错过。

An increasing number of women are now entering pregnancy with pre-existing medical conditions. Ideally, these women should be offered pre-conceptual counselling to allow the implications of pregnancy with their specific medical condition to be discussed and a plan put in place. This may involve deferring pregnancy until a specific target in the disease management is met. However, this opportunity is frequently missed.

（一）妊娠期肾病（Renal disease in pregnancy）

妊娠合并慢性肾脏疾病很少见（0.15%）；然而，它们与母婴结局不良的重大风险相关。在大多数病例中，风险和处理与肾脏损害的程度有关，而与肾

脏疾病的根本原因无关。

Pregnancies complicated by chronic renal disease are rare (0.15%); however, they are associated with a significant risk of adverse maternal and fetal outcomes. In the majority of cases, the risks and management relate to the degree of renal impairment and not to the underlying cause of the renal disease.

1. 妊娠对疾病的影响（Implications of pregnancy on the disease）

在患有慢性肾脏疾病的女性中，妊娠会导致肾功能恶化。大多数情况下，这种情况会在妊娠结束后恢复，但对于一些女性来说，这将导致肾功能的永久性下降，并缩短恶化至终末期肾衰竭的时间。肾脏恶化的可能性取决于肌酐水平（表 9-4）。

In women with chronic renal disease, pregnancy can cause a deterioration of renal function. Mostly this will recover after the end of the pregnancy, but for some women this will lead to a permanent reduction in renal functioning and a shorter time to end-stage renal failure. The likelihood of renal deterioration depends on baseline creatinine as shown in Table 9.4.

2. 疾病对妊娠的影响（Implications of the disease on pregnancy）

肾脏疾病与先兆子痫、胎儿生长受限、早产和剖宫产的风险增加有关。不良结局的风险与肾损害程度、高血压和蛋白尿的存在有关。大多数有轻度肾损害的女性都会有良好的结局。

Renal disease is associated with increased risks of preeclampsia, growth restriction, pre-term birth and a caesarean birth. The risks of an adverse outcome are related to the

表 9-4　妊娠期母体肾功能疾病与慢性肾脏疾病

Table 9.4　Maternal renal function and chronic renal disease in pregnancy

	血清肌酐（mmol/L） Serum creatinine (mmol/L)	妊娠期肾功能损失＞25%（%） Loss of ＞25% renal function in pregnancy (%)	产后肾功能恶化（%） Deterioration of renal function postpartum (%)
轻度肾损害 Mild renal impairment	＜125	2	0
中度肾损害 Moderate renal impairment	124～168	40	20
严重肾损害 Severe renal impairment	＞177	70	50

引自 Williams D, Davidson J. (2008) Chronic kidney disease in pregnancy. Br Med J 336:211-215.

Data from Williams D, Davidson J. (2008) Chronic kidney disease in pregnancy. Br Med J 336:211-215.

degree of renal impairment, the presence of hypertension and the presence of proteinuria. Most women with mild renal impairment will have good outcomes.

3. 治疗方法（Management）

理想情况下，患有慢性肾脏疾病的女性应该接受孕前咨询，讨论潜在妊娠的影响，以便做出明智的决定。对于一些女性来说，恶化至终末期肾衰竭的风险和透析的要求太大了，不能妊娠。

Women with chronic renal disease should ideally be seen for pre-pregnancy counselling to discuss the implications of a potential pregnancy so that informed decisions can be made. For some women, the risk of deterioration to endstage renal failure and a requirement for dialysis will be too great to undertake a pregnancy.

患有肾脏疾病的孕妇应由包括产科医生和肾脏或产科医师在内的多学科诊所提供护理。初步检查应包括评估肾功能、血压和蛋白尿。应该提供从 12 周到分娩的小剂量阿司匹林（75mg），以降低先兆子痫的风险。已接受抗高血压治疗的女性需要审查服用的药物，以确保其在妊娠期间使用对胎儿是安全的。妊娠期间需要仔细监测血压、肾功能和尿路感染。在妊娠晚期应安排生长扫描，以评估胎儿的生长情况。对于有蛋白尿的女性，应考虑预防性低分子肝素治疗，以降低静脉血栓栓塞的风险。孕期所有女性患尿路感染的风险都有所增加；对于患有慢性肾脏疾病且存在不止一种尿路感染的女性，可长期预防性使用抗生素。

Pregnant women with renal disease should be offered care in multidisciplinary clinics that include an obstetrician and a renal or obstetric physician. Initial review should involve assessment of baseline renal function, blood pressure and proteinuria. Low-dose aspirin (75 mg) from 12 weeks until delivery should be offered to reduce the risk of pre-eclampsia. Women already on antihypertensive treatment may need their medications reviewed to ensure that they are safe for use in pregnancy. Careful surveillance of blood pressure, renal function and for urinary tract infection is required throughout pregnancy. Growth scans should be arranged in the third trimester to assess fetal growth. For women with proteinuria, prophylactic LMWH should be considered to reduce the risk of VTE. All women are at increased risk of urinary tract infections; women with chronic renal disease and the presence of more than one confirmed urinary tract infection may benefit from the use of long-term prophylactic antibiotics.

4. 特殊情况（Special circumstances）

除一般情况外，一些肾脏疾病需要进一步诊断。

如多囊肾病是一种常染色体显性疾病，因此，应提前告知受这种疾病影响的女性其婴儿的遗传风险。

In addition to the general considerations, some renal conditions need further plans. For example, polycystic kidney disease is an autosomal-dominant condition, so women affected by this condition should be counselled about the inheritance risk to their baby.

行肾移植的女性通常在妊娠期间感觉良好。应避免在移植后立即受孕(在某些指南中长达 12 个月)，此时排斥反应风险最高，抗排斥药物正在稳定。许多免疫抑制药物在妊娠期间使用是安全的，但孕前咨询很重要，以便在有致畸风险的情况下有时间更换药物。

Women with renal transplants generally do very well in pregnancy. Conception should be avoided (for up to 12 months in some guidelines) in the immediate post-transplant period, when risks of rejection are highest and anti-rejection medications are being stabilized. Many immunosuppressive drugs are safe for use in pregnancy, but pre-pregnancy counselling is important to allow time for change in medications in those cases where teratogenicity is a risk.

5. 肾结石（Renal calculi）

与非妊娠期相比，妊娠期肾结石的发病率并不会更高。超声是诊断的第一线检查，但阳性预测值较低（60%）。MRI 更准确，并且可以在妊娠期安全使用。但是，患有肾结石的女性发生尿路感染的概率更高，相比没有肾结石的女性，这种感染的治疗时间要比单纯尿路感染的治疗时间更长。补液、尿液碱化和保守治疗的镇痛应该是一线治疗，因为这将有助于防止尿酸和胱氨酸结石的沉淀。多数（＞80%）结石经保守治疗后可以自然排出。如果这些疗法无效，则可以进行支架植入术。然而，在缺乏关于安全性的全面数据情况下，妊娠期禁忌使用体外碎石术。

Symptomatic renal stone disease is no more common in pregnancy than in the non-pregnant state. Ultrasound is the first-line investigation for diagnosis but it has low positive predictive value (60%). MRI is more accurate and is considered to be safe in pregnancy. However, women with renal calculi have an increased frequency of urinary tract infections, and such infections should be treated for longer than isolated urinary tract infections in women without renal stones. Fluid loading, alkalinization of the urine and pain relief with conservative management should be the first line of management, as this will tend to prevent the precipitation of uric acid and cystine stones. The majority (>80%) of stones pass spontaneously with conservative measures. In cases not responding to this approach, stenting has been performed successfully. However, in the absence of comprehensive data concerning safety, extracorporeal lithotripsy is contraindicated in pregnancy

（二）糖尿病（Diabetes mellitus）

糖尿病是女性妊娠期间最常见的既往疾病之一。既往患有糖尿病的孕妇的发病率约为 0.4%。其中大多数人患有 1 型糖尿病；然而，随着人口结构的变化，患有 2 型糖尿病的女性人数不断增加。患有 2 型糖尿病的女性往往比患有 1 型糖尿病的女性年龄更大，肥胖程度更高，意外妊娠的次数也更多。两组女性的妊娠并发症发生率相似。

Diabetes is one of the commonest pre-existing medical conditions women are seen with in pregnancy. The incidence of pregnant women with pre-existing diabetes is around 0.4%. The majority of these have type 1 diabetes; however, with changes in population demographics there are an increasing number of women with type 2 diabetes. Women with type 2 diabetes tend to be older, be more obese and have more unplanned pregnancies than women with type 1 diabetes. Rates of complications in pregnancy are similar in both groups of women.

1. 妊娠对疾病的影响（Implications of pregnancy on the disease）

- 胎盘激素的抗胰岛素作用导致妊娠期间需要更多的胰岛素。女性必须将胰岛素需求量提高到原来的 3 倍才能与之抗衡。这些变化在分娩后几小时内恢复到妊娠前的状态。

- The anti-insulin effects of placental hormones result in a larger insulin requirement in pregnancy. Women have to increase their insulin requirements up to threefold to combat this. These changes revert to the pre-pregnancy state within hours of birth.

- 妊娠初期呕吐会使饮食和药物平衡变得复杂。

- Vomiting in early pregnancy can complicate diet and medication balance.

- 妊娠可能减少低血糖的"警告信号"。

- Pregnancy can reduce the 'warning signs' of hypoglycaemia.

- 对于患有糖尿病并发症（如视网膜病和肾病）的女性，妊娠可以加速这些并发症发生的进程。

- In women with complications of diabetes, such as retinopathy and nephropathy, pregnancy can accelerate the progress of these complications.

2. 疾病对妊娠的影响（表 9-5）[Implications of the disease on pregnancy (Table 9.5)]

妊娠期糖尿病的许多并发症也出现在患有既往糖尿病的女性身上。然而，在围孕期和妊娠早期，还会发生其他与葡萄糖稳态异常有关的并发症，以及与女性长期潜在的血管疾病有关的并发症。

Many of the complications seen with gestational diabetes are also seen with women with pre-existing diabetes. However, there are additional complications related to abnormal glucose homeostasis in the periconception period and in the first trimester, as well as complications related to longstanding underlying vascular disease in women with preexisting disease.

患有糖尿病，特别是神经管缺陷和先天性心脏病的女性，胎儿先天畸形的风险会增加。发生这种情况的可能性与围产期和早孕期的血糖控制水平有关。糖化血红蛋白（HbA1c）高于 10% 的女性发生胎儿畸形的可能性高达 25%。女性在整个妊娠期间失去胎儿的风险增加，这也与血糖控制有关。

There is an increased risk of congenital abnormality in women with pre-existing diabetes, particularly neural tube defects and congenital heart disease. The likelihood of this occurring is related to the level of glycaemic control periconceptionally and in early pregnancy. Women with an HbA1c above 10% have up to a 25% chance of a fetal abnormality. Women are at an increased risk of fetal loss throughout pregnancy, which again is related to glycaemic control.

虽然巨大儿是糖尿病中最常见的胎儿生长模式，但在有血管疾病和早期先兆子痫的女性中，胎儿生长受限可能成为一个问题。

Although fetal macrosomia is the most common fetal growth pattern in diabetes, in women with pre-existing vascular disease and those who develop early pre-eclampsia, fetal growth restriction can be a problem

患有高血压和（或）糖尿病性肾病的女性发生先兆子痫的风险很高（约 30%）。

Women with hypertension and/or diabetic nephropathy are at high risk of developing pre-eclampsia (approximately 30%).

3. 治疗方法（Management）

对既往患有糖尿病的女性进行孕前管理咨询，使她们能够了解妊娠和糖尿病的情况。

Pre-conception counselling for women with pre-existing diabetes enables them to be informed about pregnancy and diabetes.

表 9-5　妊娠期既往糖尿病的风险

Table 9.5　Risks of pre-existing diabetes in pregnancy

	孕产妇风险 **Maternal concerns**	胎儿 / 新生儿的风险 **Fetal/neonatal concerns**
妊娠早期 First trimester	增加胰岛素的需求 Increased insulin requirements	流产 Miscarriage 胎儿畸形 Fetal abnormality
妊娠中期 Second trimester 妊娠晚期 Third trimester	子痫前期 Pre-eclampsia 复发性感染 Recurrent infections 血管疾病会加重视网膜病变 Worsening retinopathy if vascular disease	巨大儿 Macrosomia 羊水过多 Polyhydramnios 死胎 Stillbirth 生长受限 Growth restriction
临产 Labour	引产 Induction of labour 分娩进展不佳 Poor progress in labour	早产 Pre-term delivery
分娩 Delivery	器质性分娩 Instrumental birth 出生创伤 Birth trauma 剖宫产 Caesarean section	肩难产 Shoulder dystocia
产后 Postnatal	在分娩后几小时内恢复孕前控制 Return to pre-pregnancy control within hours of birth	新生儿低血糖 Neonatal hypoglycaemia 新生儿科入院 Neonatal unit admission 呼吸窘迫综合征 Respiratory distress syndrome 黄疸 Jaundice
一段时间后 Longer term	-	儿童糖尿病（若母亲患有 1 型糖尿病，概率为 2%～3%；若母亲患有 2 型糖尿病，则为 10%～15%） Diabetes in childhood (2–3% if mother has type 1;10–15% if mother has type 2)

　　孕前咨询也让女性考虑尝试妊娠的最佳时机。由于糖尿病的许多并发症与血糖控制水平有关，我们的目标是在妊娠前使糖化血红蛋白低于 6.1%。如果实现了这一点，糖尿病女性的妊娠并发症发生率并不会比正常人群高出多少。可以对药物进行审查。

胰岛素，无论是传统的还是新型的，都已被证明在妊娠期间是安全的。通常，二甲双胍可以持续服用，但其他口服降糖药通常要停用。因此，许多患有 2 型糖尿病的女性在妊娠期间需要胰岛素。然而，部分用于治疗糖尿病并发症的药物并不安全。如用于治疗糖尿病肾病的血管紧张素转化酶（angiotensin-converting enzyme，ACE）抑制药应在妊娠期停用。考虑到神经管缺陷的风险增加，患有糖尿病的女性应该服用更高剂量的叶酸（5mg/d，而不是正常的400µg/d）。

Pre-conception counselling also allows women to consider the best time to try to conceive. As many of the complications of diabetes relate to the level of glycaemic control, the aim is to get the HbA1c less than 6.1% before conception. If this is achieved, the complication rate of pregnancy in women with diabetes is not much greater than the normal population. Medications can be reviewed. Insulins, both traditional and the newer agents, have been shown to be safe in pregnancy. Metformin is usually continued, but other oral hypoglycaemic agents are usually stopped. Consequently, many women with type 2 diabetes will require insulin in pregnancy. However, some of the medications used to treat the complications of diabetes are not safe. For example, angiotensin-converting enzyme (ACE) inhibitors used in the treatment of diabetic nephropathy should be stopped in pregnancy. Women with diabetes should take a higher periconceptual dose of folic acid (5 mg/d rather than the normal 400 µg/d) in view of the increased risk of neural tube defects.

多科室团队合作是治疗女性糖尿病患者的关键。产科治疗糖尿病孕妇的团队通常由产科医生、内分泌科专家、糖尿病专科护士、营养师和专科助产士组成。在整个妊娠期间，该团队将定期观察女性。

Multidisciplinary team-working is key in managing women with diabetes. Obstetric diabetes clinics will often consist of an obstetrician, endocrinologist, diabetes specialist nurse, dietician and specialist midwife. Women will be seen regularly throughout pregnancy by this team.

妊娠期的代谢目标是将血糖维持在尽可能接近正常的非糖尿病范围，同时避免严重低血糖。这包括增加毛细血管血糖监测和比平时更严格的控制。目标水平与妊娠期糖尿病章中给出的目标水平相同（见前述）。由于鼓励女性严格控制血糖，因此她们会遭受低血糖并发症带来的不适。需要采取各种措施[口服葡萄糖制剂和（或）肌内注射胰高血糖素]来应对这种并发症。

The metabolic goal during pregnancy is to maintain blood glucose as close to the normal non-diabetic range as possible while avoiding severe hypoglycaemia. This involves increasing capillary blood glucose monitoring and tightening control more than is usual outside of pregnancy. The target levels are the same as given in the section on gestational diabetes (see earlier). Because women are encouraged to keep glucose control tight, they can experience unpleasant attacks of hypoglycaemia. Various measures (oral glucose preparations

and/or intramuscular (IM) glucagon) need to be in place to deal with this complication.

胎儿异常评估包括在妊娠早期对染色体问题（如果母亲愿意的话）进行综合测试，并在 20 周时进行常规解剖扫描。考虑先天性心脏病的风险增加，有时建议进行额外的扫描以查看心脏的解剖结构。定期进行连续生长扫描可检测出巨大儿和胎儿生长受限的情况。

Fetal assessment for abnormalities involves combined testing for chromosomal problems (if the mother wishes) in the first trimester and a routine anatomy scan at 20 weeks. Additional scanning to look at cardiac anatomy is sometimes recommended in view of the increased risk of congenital cardiac disease. Regular serial growth scans can detect both macrosomia and fetal growth restriction.

为了孕产妇的健康，从妊娠中期开始服用低剂量的阿司匹林可以降低先兆子痫的风险。在患有血管疾病的女性中，应注意保持血压得到良好控制，以降低疾病恶化的风险。所有既往患有糖尿病的女性每 3 个月都应进行眼科检查，以便尽早发现糖尿病性视网膜病恶化的迹象。

For maternal wellbeing, low-dose aspirin from the second trimester can reduce the risk of pre-eclampsia developing. In women with vascular disease, care should be taken to keep blood pressure well controlled to reduce the risk of disease deterioration. All women with pre-existing diabetes should have an ophthalmic assessment in each trimester for evidence of development of worsening of diabetic retinopathy.

糖尿病女性应在设有新生儿治疗设施的医院分娩。分娩计划将取决于妊娠期间糖尿病的稳定性、胎儿的大小及母婴健康状况；但是，通常建议在 38～39 周分娩。阴道分娩通常是有计划的，但是糖尿病女性的剖宫产率很高。如果预测胎儿的出生体重为 4.5kg 或更重，许多医生建议选择剖宫产。在分娩过程中应该持续监测胎儿。阴道分娩需警惕继发于胎儿巨大儿的肩难产。新生儿也有新生儿低血糖症的风险。可以通过在分娩中严格控制血糖来降低这种风险，并对患有糖尿病的女性按比例滴注胰岛素 – 葡萄糖来实现血糖控制。

Women with diabetes should give birth in a hospital with neonatal facilities. Delivery plans will depend on the stability of diabetes in pregnancy, fetal size and maternal and fetal wellbeing; however, delivery at around 38–39 weeks is usually recommended. Vaginal birth is often planned, but caesarean section rates are high in this group of women. If the estimated fetal birth weight is 4.5 kg or more, many recommend an elective caesarean section. The fetus should be monitored continuously in labour. Vigilance for shoulder dystocia secondary to fetal macrosomia is required with a vaginal delivery. The neonates are at risk of neonatal hypoglycaemia. This risk can be reduced by strict glycaemic control in labour, and a sliding-scale infusion of insulin-dextrose is often required to achieve this control in women with pre-existing diabetes.

产后，女性在进食和饮水后便立即采用孕前治疗方案。

Postnatally, women return to pre-pregnancy treatment regimens as soon as they are delivered and eating and drinking.

（三）妊娠甲状腺疾病（Thyroid disease in pregnancy）

各种类型的甲状腺疾病使 2%～5% 的妊娠复杂化。正常妊娠过程雌激素增加会导致甲状腺结合球蛋白增加，这需要增加甲状腺激素的分泌产生来维持游离 T_4 和 T_3 的水平。这些生理变化及由于肾脏负担增加而使孕妇血浆中的碘水平下降，导致甲状腺增大了 10%～20%。甲状腺刺激激素（TSH）水平的下降也是妊娠前半期的特征，这可能是由于人绒毛膜促性腺激素对甲状腺的刺激作用所致。

Thyroid disorders of various types complicate approximately 2–5% of pregnancies. Increased oestrogen in normal pregnancy leads to an increase in thyroid-binding globulin that necessitates an increased production of thyroid hormone to maintain free T_4 and T_3 levels. These changes, along with a fall in iodine levels in the maternal plasma due to increased renal loss, result in an enlargement of the thyroid gland of 10–20%. A fall in the thyroid-stimulating hormone (TSH) levels is also a feature of the first half of pregnancy, which may be explained by thyroid stimulatory effects of human chorionic gonadotrophin.

1. 甲状腺功能减退（Hypothyroidism）

甲状腺功能减退是妊娠中最常见的甲状腺问题，妊娠并发症多达 5%。大多数病例都有自身免疫性疾病的基础，在这类疾病中，甲状腺过氧化物酶等自身抗体以及与桥本病相关的抗体会导致腺体破坏和纤维化。甲状腺功能减退也可能是医源性的，一般是由甲状腺切除术、放射性碘消融或过量服用抗甲状腺药引起的。

Hypothyroidism is the commonest thyroid problem to occur in pregnancy and complicates up to 5% of pregnancies. Most cases have a basis in autoimmune diseases, where autoantibodies like thyroid peroxidase and those associated with Hashimoto's disease cause gland obstruction and fibrosis. Hypothyroidism may also be iatrogenic as the consequence of thyroidectomy, radio-iodine ablation or excessive doses of antithyroid drugs.

(1) 妊娠对疾病的影响（Implications of pregnancy on the disease）

妊娠对甲状腺功能减退的影响很小。通常替代疗法的量需要增加。

There are few effects of pregnancy on hypothyroidism. An increase in replacement therapy is usually required.

(2) 疾病对妊娠的影响（Implications of the disease on pregnancy）

明显甲状腺功能减退的孕妇和胎儿预后更差。未经治疗的甲状腺功能减退最严重且罕见的后果是黏液性水肿昏迷（包括体温过低、心动过缓、反射减弱和意识改变，并伴有低钠血症、低血糖症、低氧血症和高碳酸血症）。这是一种医疗紧急情况，死亡率为 20%，需要支持性治疗和甲状腺素替代治疗。更常见的是，自然流产、先兆子痫、妊娠高血压、产后出血和低出生体重儿的风险增加。然而，最近的一些研究怀疑其与妊娠高血压病的关系。婴儿的智商有轻微下降的风险，但先天性畸形的风险没有增加。如果有足够的替代治疗，妊娠结局是很好的。

Maternal and fetal outcomes are worse with overt hypothyroidism. The most serious but rare consequence of untreated hypothyroidism is myxoedema coma (comprising hypothermia, bradycardia, reduced reflexes and altered consciousness together with hyponatraemia, hypoglycaemia, hypoxia and hypercapnia). It is a medical emergency with a 20% mortality rate, requiring supportive therapy and thyroid replacement. More commonly, there are increased risks of spontaneous abortion, pre-eclampsia, pregnancyinduced hypertension, postpartum haemorrhage and low birth weight. However, some recent studies have questioned the association with hypertensive disease in pregnancy. There is a risk of a slight reduction in IQ in the infant but no increased risk in congenital malformations. With adequate replacement, pregnancy outcomes are excellent.

(3) 治疗方法（Management）

这些女性的甲状腺功能测试应该每 3 个月进行一次，使用妊娠期特定的参考范围，并应随着 T_4 水平的下降（由于孕妇细胞外液水平的增加而下降）进行调整。TSH 水平升高可以诊断为治疗不充分 / 甲状腺功能减退。

Thyroid function testing in these women should be performed every trimester using pregnancy-specific reference ranges, and replacement should be adjusted as T_4 levels fall due to the increase in maternal extracellular fluid levels. The diagnosis of inadequate treatment/hypothyroidism in the mother is made by a raised level of TSH.

如果甲状腺功能减退是母体甲状腺功能亢进治疗继发的，则应进行新生儿甲状腺功能障碍监测，因为甲状腺功能障碍本身是由胎盘传递 TSH 受体抗体引起的。

Where hypothyroidism is secondary to treatment for maternal hyperthyroidism, neonatal surveillance for neonatal thyroid dysfunction, itself secondary to transplacental transmission of TSH receptor antibodies, should be undertaken.

碘缺乏症在许多国家是地方性流行病。若未经治疗会导致孕妇流产、死产、新生儿死亡和新生儿先天性畸形（包括克汀病）。应建议所有孕妇在妊娠期间通过补充摄入足够的碘。如果母亲接受了适当的替代治疗，新生儿会很健康。

Iodine deficiency in many countries is endemic. Untreated, it is associated with poor fetal outcomes from miscarriage, stillbirth, neonatal death and congenital abnormalities, including cretinism. All pregnant women should be encouraged to ensure an adequate iodine intake in pregnancy, if necessary through supplementation. Where the mother is receiving adequate replacement therapy, the outcome for the infant is normal.

2. 甲状腺功能亢进（Hyperthyroidism）

甲状腺功能亢进在孕妇中的发病率约为 0.2%，其中 95% 是由于 Graves 病引起的。通过 T_4 和 T_3 的水平升高与 TSH 水平降低进行诊断。

Hyperthyroidism occurs in approximately 0.2% of pregnancies, 95% of which are due to Graves' disease. Diagnosis is made by the finding of elevated T_4 and T_3 levels associated with a lowered TSH level.

(1) 妊娠对疾病的影响（Implications of pregnancy on the disease）

妊娠通常引起甲状腺素需求增加。正在接受甲状腺功能亢进治疗的女性在妊娠期间通常不太需要治疗。但是，很容易产生产后发作。未经治疗的甲状腺毒症可导致甲状腺亢进危象和心力衰竭，死亡率约为 25%。

Pregnancy is usually associated with an increased requirement for thyroxine. Women being treated for hyperthyroidism often need less treatment in pregnancy; however, postpartum flares are common. Untreated thyrotoxicosis can result in a thyroid crisis and heart failure in pregnancy with a 25% mortality rate.

(2) 疾病对妊娠的影响（Implications of the disease on pregnancy）

不受控制的甲状腺功能亢进症与先兆子痫、胎儿生长受限、早产、死产和胎儿甲状腺功能亢进症等的发生率较高有关。

Uncontrolled hyperthyroidism is associated with higher rates of pre-eclampsia, fetal growth restriction, prematurity, stillbirths and thyrotoxicosis in the fetus.

新生儿甲状腺功能亢进症发生在 1% 的婴儿中。这是暂时性的，是由于 TSH 受体抗体通过胎盘转移的结果。

Neonatal thyrotoxicosis occurs in 1% of babies. This is transient and due to the transfer of TSH receptor antibodies across the placenta.

(3) 治疗方法（Management）

甲状腺功能测试应每 4～6 周进行一次，并相应调整治疗方法。甲状腺功能检查数据应使用参考妊娠的范围。大多数抗甲状腺药物在妊娠期间是安全的，但使用前需咨询内分泌学家的意见。

Thyroid function testing should be carried out every 4–6 weeks and therapy adjusted accordingly. Pregnancy-specific ranges for thyroid function tests should be used. Most antithyroid medications are safe in pregnancy, but specialist advice from an endocrinologist should be sought.

建议对胎儿甲状腺进行一系列生长测量和超声检查，并定期评估胎心率（寻找胎儿心动过速作为胎儿甲状腺功能亢进的标志）。

Serial growth measurements and ultrasound examination for fetal goitre, together with regular assessment of fetal heart rate (looking for fetal tachycardia as a marker of fetal hyperthyroidism), are advisable.

分娩后有必要调整孕妇甲状腺药物的使用。可能需要延长产后住院时间，评估新生儿是否有甲状腺功能亢进症的迹象。

Adjustment of maternal thyroid medication will be necessary after delivery. A prolonged postnatal hospital stay may be required to assess the neonate for signs of thyrotoxicosis.

（四）肥胖（Obesity）

肥胖对孕期带来的影响正在增加。患病率取决于所调查的人口，通过 2009 年英国的一项全国性调查发现，每 10 万名产妇中有 9.3 人的体重指数（BMI）超过 50（英国肥胖监测系统）。患有肥胖症的女性经常感到羞耻；然而，肥胖症与妊娠期间必须解决的重大医疗问题有关。肥胖女性更有可能患有高血压、睡眠呼吸暂停、糖尿病和心血管疾病等并发症，所有这些都会进一步增加妊娠的风险。

The impact of obesity in pregnancy is increasing. Prevalence is dependent on the population served, though a national survey in the UK in 2009 found that in 9.3 per 100,000 maternities women had a body mass index (BMI) of more than 50 (UK Obesity Surveillance System). Women with obesity often feel stigmatized; however, obesity is associated with significant medical problems in pregnancy that must be addressed. Obese women are more likely to suffer with co-morbidities such as hypertension, sleep apnoea, diabetes and cardiovascular disease, all of which can increase further the risks of pregnancy.

1. 妊娠对肥胖的影响（Implications of pregnancy on obesity）

目前尚未确定孕妇的最佳体重增加数值。但是，对于肥胖女性，谨慎的做法是在产前尽量减少体重增加。

The optimum weight gain in pregnancy has not been established. However, in obese women, it is prudent to minimize weight gain during the antenatal period.

2. 肥胖对妊娠的影响（表 9-6）[Implications of obesity on pregnancy (Table 9.6)]

产前肥胖与母婴并发症的数量有关。在妊娠早期，流产和先天畸形（特别是神经管缺陷）的风险增加，尽管其病因尚未确定。在整个孕期，静脉血栓栓塞的风险都会增加。在妊娠后期，肥胖女性更有可能患先兆子痫和妊娠期糖尿病。此外，许多轻微的妊娠并发症，如胃食管反流和骨盆带功能障碍，更有可能发生在 BMI 更高的女性身上。

Antenatally, obesity is associated with number of maternal and fetal complications. In the first trimester, the risk of miscarriage and congenital abnormality (especially neural tube defects) is increased, although the aetiology of this has not been established. Throughout pregnancy, there is an increased risk of VTE. Later in pregnancy, obese women are more likely to develop pre-eclampsia and gestational diabetes. In addition, many minor complications of pregnancy such as gastro-oesophageal reflux and pelvic girdle dysfunction are more likely to occur in women with a raised BMI.

肥胖与巨大儿有关；然而，无论是临床还是超声检查，母亲的肥胖都会对准确确定胎儿大小的能力产生影响。死产和新生儿死亡的风险增加。从长远来看，肥胖母亲的孩子更有可能患上儿童肥胖症和青少年糖尿病。

Obesity is associated with fetal macrosomia; however, maternal adiposity can have significant impact on the ability to accurately determine fetal size, both clinically and using ultrasound. There is an increased risk of stillbirth and neonatal death. In the long term, children of obese mothers are more likely to have childhood obesity and juvenile diabetes.

肥胖女性更有可能引产，分娩进展不佳，并进行剖宫产。肥胖女性较高的剖宫产率被认为是胎儿巨大儿、合并症及分娩时脂肪组织的激素作用共同引起的。

Obese women are more likely to have an induction of labour, to have poor progress in labour and to have a caesarean section. This higher rate of caesarean births in obese women is thought to be secondary to a combination of fetal macrosomia, co-morbid conditions and the hormonal effect of adipose tissue on labour.

BMI 较高的女性行剖宫产（包括麻醉和生产）的风险较高。如果是顺产，肩关节难产和会阴撕裂更常见。产后出血的风险较高。

The risks of caesarean section, both anaesthetic and obstetric, are higher in women with a higher BMI. If vaginal birth is achieved, shoulder dystocia and extended perineal tears are more frequent. There is a higher risk of postpartum haemorrhage.

3. 治疗方法（Management）

理想情况下，孕前咨询可以建议女性推迟妊娠直至达到接近正常的 BMI，但这种情况极少发生。

Ideally, pre-conceptual counselling would allow women to defer pregnancy until a nearer normal BMI is achieved, but this rarely occurs.

肥胖女性应接受医院的护理，因为这会给妊娠和分娩带来风险。营养师给予支持的目的是实现更健康的饮食，而不是减肥。叶酸应该服用到 12 周。考虑到神经管缺损的风险增加，一些权威人士建议使用更高的剂量（5mg），但尚无证据。应该对子痫前期和静脉血栓栓塞的其他危险因素进行彻底地评估。基于此，适当地使用阿司匹林降低先兆子痫的风险，或者作为血栓预防措施来降低静脉血栓栓塞的风险是可以的。妊娠中期晚期应进行妊娠期糖尿病筛查的 OGTT 试验。

Women with obesity should have hospital-based care because of the associated risks in pregnancy and at birth.

表 9-6　妊娠期间肥胖的风险

Table 9.6　Risks of obesity in pregnancy

	孕产妇风险 / 并发症 Maternal risks/complications		胎儿 / 新生儿的风险 / 并发症 Fetal/neonatal risks/complications
妊娠早期 First trimester	静脉血栓栓塞 Venous thromboembolism		流产 Miscarriage 胎儿畸形 Fetal abnormality
妊娠中期 Second trimester 妊娠晚期 Third trimester	子痫前期 Pre-eclampsia 妊娠期糖尿病 Gestational diabetes 静脉血栓栓塞 Venous thromboembolism		巨大儿 Macrosomia 死胎 Stillbirth 难以进行胎儿评估 Difficulty in performing fetal assessment
临产 Labour	引产 Induction of labour 分娩进展不佳 Poor progress in labour		—
分娩 Delivery	器质性分娩 Instrumental birth 剖宫产 Caesarean section 创伤性分娩 (阴道和剖宫产) Traumatic birth (vaginal and caesarean births) 麻醉并发症 (插管或硬膜外插入困难) Anaesthetic complications (difficulties with intubation or epidural insertion)		肩难产 Shoulder dystocia
产后 Postnatal	产后出血 Postpartum haemorrhage 静脉血栓栓塞 Venous thromboembolism		新生儿科入院 Neonatal unit admission 新生儿死亡 Neonatal death
一段时间后 Longer term	—		儿童肥胖 Childhood obesity 青少年糖尿病 Juvenile diabetes

Support from a dietician should be offered with the aim of achieving a healthier diet rather than weight reduction. Folic acid should be taken until 12 weeks. Some authorities recommend a higher dose (5 mg) in view of the increased risk of neural tube defects, but evidence for this is lacking. A thorough assessment for other risk factors for pre-eclampsia and VTE should be performed. Based on this, aspirin to reduce the risk of pre-eclampsia or as thromboprophylaxis to reduce the risk of VTE may be appropriate. An OGTT to screen for gestational diabetes should be offered in the late second trimester.

在肥胖女性中，常规超声筛查异常的效果会因

可视性差而降低。此外，尽管对胎儿生长的临床评估受到母体习惯的限制，但几乎没有证据表明超声波能提供更准确的评估，这也是因为可视化程度较差所致。

The efficacy of routine ultrasound screening for anomalies is reduced in obese women because of poor visualization. Furthermore, although clinical assessments of fetal growth are limited by maternal habitus, there is little evidence that ultrasound provides a more accurate assessment, again because of poor visualization.

考虑到分娩和分娩的潜在并发症，肥胖女性应

在医院分娩。如果没有其他顺产的禁忌证，可以考虑顺产。

In view of the potential complications of labour and birth, obese women should deliver in a hospital unit. If there are no other contraindications to vaginal birth, this should be the planned method.

（五）血栓性疾病（Thrombophilia）

血栓性疾病可以遗传或获得。遗传性血栓形成在约 15% 的高加索人群中被发现，最常见的是因子 V 和凝血酶原（因子 Ⅱ）基因突变。不太常见的遗传性疾病是蛋白 C、S 和抗凝血酶缺乏。最常见的获得性血栓形成症是抗磷脂综合征（antiphospholipid syndrome，APS），它与妊娠期间的并发症有关。其他获得性疾病还有阵发性夜间血红蛋白尿和原发性血小板减少症。妊娠期间 20%～50% 的静脉血栓形成事件与血栓性疾病有关。

Thrombophilia can be inherited or acquired. Inherited thrombophilias are found in approximately 15% of the Caucasian population, the most common being factor V Leiden and the prothrombin (factor 2) gene mutation. Less common inherited conditions are deficiencies of proteins C, S and anti-thrombin. The most common acquired thrombophilia is antiphospholipid syndrome (APS) that is associated with number of adverse outcomes in pregnancy. Other acquired conditions are paroxysmal nocturnal haemoglobinuria and essential thrombocytopenia. Thrombophilias are responsible for 20–50% of venous thromboembolic events in pregnancy.

1. 妊娠对疾病的影响（Implications of pregnancy on the disease）

妊娠是一种血栓前状态，因此患有血栓形成症的女性在这段时间内特别容易发生静脉血栓栓塞。不同的血栓形成与不同程度的凝血风险有关，因此治疗必须进行相应的个体化调整。

Pregnancy is a prothrombotic state, and as such women with thrombophilia are at particular risk of VTE during this time. Different thrombophilias are associated with differing levels of risk of clotting, and management must be individualized accordingly.

2. 疾病对妊娠的影响（Implications of the disease on pregnancy）

众所周知，除了患静脉血栓栓塞症的风险外，血栓性疾病（遗传和后天的）还与产科问题有关。例如，在有 V 因子突变的女性中，与胎儿丢失、先兆子痫、胎盘早剥和子宫内生长受限的关系都已被描述。不良

妊娠结局，其中包括反复流产、胎儿死亡和继发于胎盘疾病的早产，构成了 APS 定义的一部分。

Thrombophilias (both inherited and acquired) are known to be associated with obstetric problems in addition to their risks of VTE. For example, in women with factor V Leiden, associations with fetal loss, pre-eclampsia, placental abruption and in utero growth restriction have all been described. Adverse pregnancy outcomes, including recurrent miscarriage, fetal death and premature birth secondary to placental disease, form part of the definition of APS.

3. 筛选（Screening）

对于有静脉血栓栓塞史或家族史的女性，以及产科病史较差的女性，如反复流产、死产、早发性先兆子痫和早剥，应考虑筛查血栓形成。然而，由于造血系统的正常变化，在妊娠期间进行的筛查测试可能很难分辨。理想情况下，这些检查应在并发症发生后（为解决妊娠变化留出时间）或在孕前咨询时进行。

Screening for thrombophilias should be considered in women with a personal or family history of VTE and women with a poor obstetric history such as recurrent miscarriage, stillbirth, early-onset pre-eclampsia and abruption. However, screening tests performed in pregnancy can be difficult to interpret because of the normal changes in the haemopoietic system. Ideally, these should be performed either postnatally after an adverse event (allowing time for resolution of pregnancy changes to occur) or in the setting of pre-conceptual counselling.

4. 治疗方法（Management）

患有血栓性疾病的女性最好在产科和血液科联合就诊。在计划对具有不同血栓形成风险和妊娠相关发病率的大范围疾病进行护理时，血液学家的意见是关键。除了血栓性疾病外，对静脉血栓栓塞的所有危险因素进行全面评估将有助于做出适当预防措施的决定；无论是产前和（或）产后使用低分子肝素，还是避免脱水和使用渐变弹性压缩长袜。

Women with thrombophilia should be ideally seen in a combined obstetric-haematology clinic. Input from a haematologist is key when planning care for the large spectrum of disorders with their varying risks of thrombosis and pregnancy-related morbidity. A full assessment of all risk factors for VTE in addition to the thrombophilia will allow decisions about the appropriate prophylaxis to be made: whether this be antenatal and/or postnatal LMWH or avoiding dehydration and the use of graduated compression stockings.

如前所述，肝素在妊娠期间使用是安全的，但应谨慎计划在分娩前后减少或短暂停止使用，以最

大限度地减少出血的风险，并确保女性有各种可供选择的镇痛药物。关于除 APS 以外其他血栓形成的产科风险，尚不清楚阿司匹林或肝素治疗是否能改善妊娠结局。但是，对于患有 APS 的女性，有一些证据表明，使用阿司匹林（可能还有肝素）确实可以减少妊娠并发症的发生。

As previously discussed, LMWH is safe for use in pregnancy, but care should be taken to plan for reducing or briefly stopping its use around the time of birth to minimize the risks of bleeding and ensure that a woman has the full range of analgesic options available to her. In terms of the other obstetric risks of thrombophilias, except for APS, it is unclear if treatment with aspirin or heparin improves pregnancy outcome. However, for women with APS, there is some evidence that the use of aspirin (and possibly heparin) does reduce the incidence of pregnancy complications.

> **！注意**
>
> 妊娠期间的监测应包括警惕血栓和脑卒中，先兆子痫和胎儿生长的一系列评估和脐动脉多普勒记录。
>
> Surveillance during the pregnancy should include vigilance for thrombosis and stroke, pre-eclampsia and serial assessment of fetal growth and umbilical artery Doppler recordings.

（六）癫痫（Epilepsy）

癫痫症在约 100 个产科患者中有 1 人发生。

Epilepsy affects approximately 1 in 100 of the obstetric population.

1. 妊娠对疾病的影响（Implications of pregnancy on the disease）

妊娠对癫痫的影响是多种多样的。通常癫痫发作频率不变，但是少数女性的癫痫发作会增加。目前认为这是由多种因素引起的，其中包括不遵守药物治疗、压力和睡眠不足及血液稀释后继发的低惊厥药物水平。

The effect of pregnancy on epilepsy is variable. Usually the seizure frequency is unchanged, but a minority of women will have increased seizures. This is thought to be due to several factors, including non-compliance with medication, stress and sleep deprivation and lower anticonvulsant drug levels secondary to haemodilution.

有迹象表明，癫痫患者不明原因猝死的风险在妊娠期间会增加。然而，这也可能与不遵守药物治疗有关，而不是潜在的妊娠影响。

> **！注意**
>
> 抗癫痫药的水平通常在妊娠时下降而在产褥期上升，因此可能需要更改药物剂量以维持癫痫发作的控制。
>
> Often anti-epileptic drug levels fall in pregnancy and rise in puerperium, so drug doses may need to be altered to maintain seizure control.

There is a suggestion that the risk of sudden unexplained death in epilepsy is increased in pregnancy. However, again this may relate to non-compliance with medication rather than an underlying pregnancy effect.

2. 疾病对妊娠的影响（Implications of disease on pregnancy）

不同的抗癫痫药对胎儿有不同的影响。丙戊酸钠似乎风险最大，如果可能，在育龄女性中应避免使用。

Different anti-epileptic medications have different effects on the fetus. Sodium valproate appears to have the greatest risk and should be avoided if possible in women of reproductive age.

在患有癫痫病的女性中，先天畸形的风险更高（3%，而普通人群为 1%～2%）；如果女性正在服用抗癫痫药物，这一风险会进一步增加（4%～9%）。主要异常是神经管缺陷和心脏异常。

In women with epilepsy, there is a higher risk of congenital abnormalities (3% compared with 1–2% in the general population); this risk is increased further if a woman is taking anti-epileptic drugs (4–9%). The main abnormalities are neural tube defects and heart abnormalities.

其他增加的胎儿风险包括围产期死亡率、宫内生长受限及更微妙的长期神经发育影响。强直阵挛发作，尤其是癫痫持续状态，可增加胎儿死亡的风险。当服用 1 种以上的抗癫痫药时，这些胎儿风险会进一步增加。卡马西平、左乙拉西坦和拉莫三嗪被认为是妊娠期间使用的最安全抗癫痫药物。一些抗惊厥药会诱发维生素 K 缺乏症，这会导致新生儿出血性疾病的风险增加。

Other fetal risks that are increased include the perinatal death rate, in utero growth restriction and more subtle longterm neurodevelopmental effects. Tonic-clonic seizures and, in particular, status epilepticus contribute to the increased risk of fetal death. These fetal risks are increased further when more than one anti-epileptic drug is being taken. Carbamazepine, levetiracetam and lamotrigine are considered the safest anti-epileptic drugs for use in pregnancy. Some anticonvulsant medications induce vitamin K deficiency that can lead to an increased risk of haemorrhagic disease of the newborn.

如果父母双方中的任何一方患有癫痫病，则其患癫痫病的可能性会增加，为 4%～5%，但是如果父母双方均有，则该风险会增加至 20%。

The probability of having a child with epilepsy is increased if either parent has epilepsy, approximately 4–5%, but increases to up to 20% if both parents are affected.

3. 治疗方法（Management）

理想的情况是，患有癫痫的女性应预先就诊以寻求咨询，了解其妊娠的风险，并审查其药物治疗。药物可能需要改变，有时建议延迟妊娠，直至建立"更安全"的药物治疗方案。应建议女性不要因为担心胎儿而突然停止用药，并强调癫痫失控的风险大于服用药物的风险。妊娠前和妊娠期间的总体目标是在癫痫得到控制的情况下，以最低剂量服用最少的药物。由于神经管缺陷的风险增加，建议妊娠早期增加 5mg 的叶酸剂量。

Ideally women with epilepsy should be seen preconceptually for counselling about their risks in pregnancy and to review their medications. Medications may need to be altered, and sometimes it is appropriate to advise delaying pregnancy until a 'safer' drug regimen is established. Women should be advised not to abruptly stop their medication because of fears about the fetus, and it should be emphasized that the risk of uncontrolled epilepsy is greater than the risks of the medications being taken. The overall aim before and during pregnancy is to be on the fewest medications at the lowest dose commensurate with the epilepsy remaining controlled. A higher 5-mg dose of folic acid is recommended periconceptually and in the first trimester due to the increased risk of neural tube defects.

孕妇应该由多科室团队进行管理，避免妊娠期间的癫痫发作。染色体疾病的联合筛查和解剖扫描可以照常进行。可以多次进行生长扫描，特别是当一名女性正在服用多种药物时。如果正在服用导致维生素 K 缺乏的抗癫痫药物，可以在妊娠的最后几周给母亲服用维生素 K，婴儿出生后就可以肌内注射维生素 K，以降低新生儿患出血性疾病的风险。

Women should be managed by a multidisciplinary team with the aim of avoiding seizures in pregnancy. Combined screening for chromosomal disorders and anatomy scanning can be performed as normal. Serial growth scans may be required, particularly if a woman is on more than one medication. If anti-epileptic medication that induces vitamin K deficiency is being taken, vitamin K can be given to the mother in the last few weeks of pregnancy, and the baby can receive IM vitamin K just after birth to reduce the risk of haemorrhagic disease of the newborn.

尽管女性担心因为疲倦和压力分娩时会发生癫痫发作，但这种情况并不常见，建议在医院分娩。

Although women worry about seizures occurring in labour, given the associated tiredness and stress, this is uncommon, but giving birth in a hospital unit is advisable.

对患有癫痫的女性在产前和产后进行有关新生儿护理时安全措施的建议，如不要独自给婴儿洗澡，在地板上而不是高大的婴儿床上换尿布。

Women with epilepsy should be given advice antenatally and after birth regarding safe practices when looking after their newborn, such as not bathing the baby on their own and changing the baby on the floor rather than a high changing table.

对于服用大多数抗癫痫药物的女性来说，母乳喂养是安全的。

Breast-feeding is safe for women on most anti-epileptic medications.

4. 偏头痛（Migraine）

头痛在妊娠过程中很常见。最常见的是偏头痛和因紧张而引起的偏头痛。新出现的头痛，特别是与局部或异常神经体征、智力受损和影响睡眠的疼痛相关的头痛，需要专家评估。

Headaches are common in pregnancy. The most common are migraine and those due to tension. New-onset headaches, especially those associated with focal or abnormal neurological signs, impaired intellect and pain that impairs sleep, need specialist assessment.

在妊娠前患有偏头痛的女性中，妊娠期间发作的频率下降了 50%～80%，尤其是在孕晚期，但是在产褥期再次增加。如果真的发作了，则初始治疗包括简单的镇痛、避光、卧床休息和各种应对机制。如果这些简单的措施不起作用且偏头痛持续发作，那么更有效的镇痛药、β 受体拮抗药和（或）三环类抗抑郁药都可以使用。麦角衍生物通常用于妊娠外的预防 / 治疗，由于它们的血管收缩作用，在妊娠期间是禁忌的。

In women who suffer migraine before pregnancy, the frequency of attacks drops by 50–80% during pregnancy, especially in the third trimester, but increases again in the puerperium. If an attack does occur, the initial treatment comprises simple analgesia, avoidance of light, bed rest and various coping mechanisms. If these simple measures do not work and the migraine is persistent, then more potent analgesics, beta-blockers and/or tricyclic antidepressants have all been used with success. The ergot derivatives often used as prophylaxis/treatment outside pregnancy are contraindicated in pregnancy due to their vasoconstrictive effects.

（七）心脏疾病（Cardiac disease）

近年来，妊娠期间的心脏病患者人数大大增加。目前，美国妊娠合并慢性心脏病的总体患病率为1.4%。虽然有一部分原因是因为患有先天性心脏病的女性现在有了孩子，但大多数都是后天获得性的。在英国和美国，心脏病是导致产妇间接死亡的主要原因。妊娠期间可能会遇到多种心脏疾病，其中包括瓣膜病变、先天性心脏病、心肌病、心律不齐和局部缺血性心脏病。

There has been a large increase in cardiac disease in pregnancy in recent years. The overall prevalence of chronic cardiac disease complicating pregnancy in the United States currently is 1.4%. Although some of this is explained by women who themselves have had congenital heart disease now having children, the majority are acquired. Cardiac disease is now the main cause of indirect maternal death in the UK and the United States. A multitude of cardiac conditions can be encountered in pregnancy, including valvular lesions, congenital heart disease, cardiomyopathies, arrhythmias and ischaemic heart disease.

1. 妊娠对疾病的影响（Implications of pregnancy on the disease）

妊娠对孕妇的心血管系统造成了很大压力。心输出量增加会导致某些情况的恶化，如主动脉瓣狭窄，因为这些女性的心输出量固定。在其他情况下，如反流性病变，可以正常妊娠。

Pregnancy puts a great strain on the maternal cardiovascular system. The associated rise in cardiac output can result in deterioration of some conditions, such as aortic stenosis, as these women have a fixed cardiac output. In other conditions, such as regurgitant lesions, pregnancy can be well tolerated.

心脏病的许多症状也是妊娠的症状，如呼吸困难、心悸和晕厥；妊娠时也会出现心血管症状（脉搏跳动、收缩期杂音），因此很难诊断出新的心脏疾病或已知心脏疾病的恶化。

Many symptoms of cardiac disease are also symptoms of pregnancy, such as breathlessness, palpitations and syncope; cardiovascular signs are also mimicked by pregnancy (bounding pulse, systolic murmur), and as a result it can be difficult to diagnose a new cardiac condition or deterioration in a known cardiac condition.

根据潜在的心脏状况，女性在妊娠期间可能面临以下风险。

- 充血性心力衰竭。
- 恶化的缺氧。
- 心律失常和猝死。
- 细菌性心内膜炎。
- 静脉血栓栓塞。
- 心绞痛和心肌梗死。
- 主动脉夹层。

Depending on the underlying heart condition, women can be at risk in pregnancy for the following conditions:
- congestive cardiac failure
- worsening hypoxia
- arrhythmias and sudden death
- bacterial endocarditis
- VTE
- angina and myocardial infarction
- aortic dissection

2. 疾病对妊娠的影响（Implications of the disease on pregnancy）

同样，心脏病对妊娠的影响将取决于具体的心脏问题。但是，增加的风险包括先兆子痫、宫内生长受限、早产和胎儿流产。在这种情况下服用的某些药物（如 ACE 抑制药和华法林）具有致畸性，因此需要对它们的使用情况进行审查，以确定是否有合适的替代方法，或者是否应该继续服用该药物。在患有先天性心脏病的女性中，其子女患疾病的风险增加了高达 5%。

Again, the implications of cardiac disease on pregnancy will depend on the specific cardiac problem. However, increased risks include pre-eclampsia, intrauterine growth restriction, pre-term birth and fetal loss. Some medications taken in these conditions, such as ACE inhibitors and warfarin, are teratogenic, and their use will need to be reviewed as to whether there is a suitable alternative or if, on balance, the medication should be continued. In women with congenital heart disease, there is an increased risk of the condition in their children of up to 5%.

3. 治疗方法（Management）

产科医生、心脏病医生和产科麻醉师之间的多学科管理最好从妊娠前开始，仔细讨论对女性和胎儿的潜在风险。对于一些心功能状况不佳的女性来说，妊娠可能是不建议的。在某些情况下，产妇死亡的风险可能非常高；如在患有艾森门格综合征的女性中，产妇死亡率为 40%～50%。如果一个女性真的决定妊娠，在妊娠前尽量优化她的医疗状况非常重要。

Multidisciplinary management between obstetricians, cardiologists and obstetric anaesthetists should ideally start at the pre-conception phase with a careful discussion of the potential risks for the woman and the fetus. For some women with poor cardiac functional status, pregnancy may not be advisable. The risk of maternal death can be extremely high in some conditions; for example, in women with Eisenmenger's syndrome, maternal death rates of 40–50% are described. If a woman does decide to undertake pregnancy, it is important to optimize her medical status before she conceives.

尽管纽约心脏协会（NYHA）分类提供了一些可能的预后信息（框 9-2），但护理计划应该量身定制。产前应尽量减少贫血和感染等应激源。有些女性可能需要改变药物治疗，也可能需要抗凝治疗。胎儿监护应该包括连续生长扫描和多普勒测量，以及心脏缺陷的筛查。孕妇监护则包括定期的超声心动图检查。

Although the New York Heart Association (NYHA) classification provides some information about possible prognosis (Box 9.2), care plans should be individualized. Antenatally, stressors such as anaemia and infection should be minimized. Medication may need to be altered in some women, and anticoagulation may also be required. Fetal surveillance should include serial growth scans and Doppler measurements,

as well as screening for cardiac defects. Maternal surveillance may involve regular echocardiograms.

分娩是一个充满问题的时段，应尽力减少孕妇的痛苦并确保尽力保持体液平衡。产后即刻发生的血流动力学变化通常是心脏病女性的最危险时期，产科、心脏和麻醉小组的密切监视和联合管理至关重要。

Labour is a problematic time, and attempts should be made to minimize pain and ensure fluid balance is diligently maintained. The haemodynamic changes that occur in the immediate postpartum period mean that this is often the riskiest time for women with cardiac disease, and careful surveillance and joint management by the obstetric, cardiac and anaesthetic teams are vital.

（八）呼吸系统疾病（Respiratory disorders）

呼吸系统疾病，主要是哮喘，在妊娠期很常见。就像评估心脏病一样，区分生理变化和病理变化可能很困难，因为女性会感到呼吸困难（呼吸困难），这种感觉从妊娠早期开始增加，到 30 周时达到顶峰。

Respiratory disease, predominantly asthma, is common in pregnancy. As with the assessment of cardiac disease, differentiating physiological changes from pathological ones can be difficult as women experience a sense of breathlessness (dyspnoea) that increases from early pregnancy to peak at 30 weeks.

1. 哮喘（Asthma）

哮喘是一种越来越常见的疾病，预计会影响 5%～10% 的孕妇。

框 9-2　纽约心脏协会分类	Box 9.2　New York Heart Association classification
等级 1：正常运动耐力	Grade 1: Normal exercise tolerance
等级 2：中度运动时呼吸困难	Grade 2: Breathless on moderate exertion
等级 3：轻中度运动时呼吸困难	Grade 3: Breathless on less-than-moderate exertion
等级 4：休息时无明显活动时呼吸急促	Grade 4: Breathless at rest without significant activity
Ⅰ级	Class Ⅰ
无体力活动限制；一般体力活动不会引起过度疲劳、心悸、呼吸困难或心绞痛	No limitations on physical activity; ordinary physical activity does not cause undue fatigue, palpitation, dyspnoea or angina pain
Ⅱ级	Class Ⅱ
轻微限制体力活动；普通体力活动导致疲劳、心悸、呼吸困难或心绞痛	Slight limitation on physical activity; ordinary physical activity results in fatigue, palpitation, dyspnoea or angina pain
Ⅲ级	Class Ⅲ
明显限制体力活动；少于正常活动导致疲劳、心悸、呼吸困难或心绞痛	Marked limitation on physical activity; less-than-ordinary activity causes fatigue, palpitation, dyspnoea or angina pain
Ⅳ级	Class Ⅳ
无法无不适地进行任何身体活动；即使在休息时也可能出现心功能不全或心绞痛综合征的症状；任何身体活动都会增加不适	Inability to perform any physical activity without discomfort; symptoms of cardiac insufficiency or angina syndrome may be present, even at rest; any physical activity increases discomfort

Asthma is an increasingly common disorder and can be expected to affect 5–10% of pregnant women.

(1) 妊娠对疾病的影响（Implications of pregnancy on the disease）

妊娠对哮喘的影响是不可预测的，尽管约有 1/3 的女性会好转，1/3 的女性会恶化，而 1/3 的女性保持不变。约 10% 的患有哮喘的女性在妊娠期间会出现急性加重。

The effect of pregnancy on asthma is not predictable, although approximately one-third of women will improve, one-third will get worse and one-third stay the same. Approximately 10% of women with asthma will have an acute exacerbation in pregnancy.

(2) 疾病对妊娠的影响（Implications of the disease on pregnancy）

哮喘控制良好的女性妊娠结局良好，控制良好的哮喘对妊娠没有明确的不良影响。相比之下，哮喘控制不佳或妊娠期间严重恶化的女性患胎儿生长受限、早产和先兆子痫的风险更高。

Women with well-controlled asthma have good pregnancy outcomes, and there are no established adverse effects of well-controlled asthma on pregnancy. In contrast, women with poorly controlled asthma or those with severe exacerbations in pregnancy are at increased risk of fetal growth restriction, premature birth and pre-eclampsia.

(3) 治疗方法（Management）

应在妊娠初期进行基线峰值流量测量。应建议女性继续服用哮喘药物，避免由于担心药物对胎儿的影响而停止药物治疗导致病情加重。尽管有关某些新疗法的数据掌握较少，但大多数哮喘药物在妊娠中可以安全使用（包括类固醇疗法）。妊娠期间哮喘急性加重的治疗方法与非妊娠哮喘患者相同。

Baseline peak flow measurements should be taken at the start of pregnancy. Women should be encouraged to continue their asthma medication, as a significant number of exacerbations are caused by cessation of medication due to concerns about the possible effects on the fetus. Most asthma medications are safe in pregnancy (including steroid therapy), although there is less information about some of the newer therapies. The management of acute exacerbations of asthma is the same in pregnancy as in non-pregnant asthmatics.

2. 囊性纤维化（Cystic fibrosis）

尽管囊性纤维化是一种致命的疾病，但在过去的 30 年里，由于早期诊断和治疗方法的进步，囊性纤维患者的预期寿命显著增长。在高加索人群中，5% 的成年人携带隐性基因，囊性纤维化的发病率为 0.05%～0.1%。预期寿命的延迟为囊性纤维女性患者提供了考虑妊娠的机会。因此，在美国和英国，患有囊性纤维化的女性占妊娠总数的 0.4%～0.8%，其中高达 80% 实现了活产。

Although CF is ultimately a fatal disease, the life expectancy of someone with CF has markedly increased in the last 30 years due to early diagnosis and improvements in treatment. The incidence of CF is 0.05–0.1% of births in Caucasian populations in which 5% of adults carry the recessive gene. The increased life expectancy has provided opportunities for women with CF to consider pregnancy. As a result, women with CF account for 0.4–0.8% of pregnancies in United States and UK, with up to 80% achieving a live birth.

(1) 妊娠对疾病的影响（Implications of pregnancy on the disease）

尽管妊娠带来的不适可以忍受，但许多女性确实遇到了困难，因为它对肺功能的影响可能是不可预测的，保持足够的营养可能是有问题的。妊娠的风险与肺功能障碍的程度和相关的肺动脉高压有关。在最初肺功能较差（FEV1＜50%）的女性中，妊娠期间可能会出现明显的下降，这可能是不可逆转的。

Although pregnancy can be tolerated well, many women do experience difficulties as the effects on lung function can be unpredictable and maintaining adequate nutrition can be problematic. The risks of pregnancy relate to the degree of pulmonary dysfunction and associated pulmonary hypertension. In women with initial poor lung function (FEV_1 <50%), significant decline can occur in pregnancy that may be irreversible.

(2) 疾病对妊娠的影响（Implications of the disease on pregnancy）

作为常染色体隐性遗传病，存在将疾病遗传给婴儿的风险。可以进行产前诊断。由于胰腺纤维化，妊娠期糖尿病的风险增加。在患有囊性纤维化的女性中，约有 1/3 的胎儿将早产。对于营养状况较差的人来说，胎儿生长受限可能是一个问题。

As an autosomal-recessive condition, there is a risk of transmission of the disease to the infant. Prenatal diagnosis can be offered. There is an increased risk of gestational diabetes due to fibrosis in the pancreas. Around one-third of babies of women with CF will be born pre-term. Fetal growth restriction may be an issue in those with poor nutritional status.

(3) 治疗方法（Management）

理想情况下，计划妊娠前应进行孕前咨询。这包括遗传咨询、优化肺和胃肠功能的治疗，以及肺动脉高压评估。肺动脉压显著升高与产妇高死亡率有关，此时应避免妊娠。围产期应服用大剂量叶酸（5mg/d）以降低胎儿畸形的风险。

Ideally pregnancies should be planned and pre-pregnancy advice sought. This involves genetic counselling, the optimization of treatment of lung and gastrointestinal function and an assessment for pulmonary hypertension. Significantly raised pulmonary pressures are associated with a high maternal mortality, and pregnancy should be avoided. High-dose folate (5mg/day) should be taken periconceptually to reduce the risk of fetal anomaly.

包括产科医生、呼吸内科医生和产科麻醉师在内的多学科护理是很重要的。应在妊娠初期进行肺功能检查，并根据症状重复检查。必须提供营养支持，专业营养师应该能够就必要的补充剂提供建议。胸部感染应及时治疗。

Multidisciplinary care is essential, including obstetricians, respiratory physicians and obstetric anaesthetists. Pulmonary function tests should be performed at the start of pregnancy and repeated according to symptoms. Nutritional support is mandatory, and specialist dieticians should be able to advise on the necessary supplements. Chest infections should be treated promptly.

女性应通过 OGTT 试验进行妊娠期糖尿病筛查。应监测胎儿生长情况，保持对早产的警惕。

Women should be screened for gestational diabetes with an OGTT. Fetal growth should be monitored, and vigilance for pre-term labour should be maintained.

分娩应在可以获得高度依赖护理和呼吸护理（如果需要）的环境中进行。严重的呼吸损害可能需要在区域镇痛下剖宫产。

Delivery should occur in a setting with access to highdependency care and respiratory care if needed. Caesarean section under regional analgesia may be needed for severe respiratory compromise.

（九）自身免疫性疾病（Autoimmune disease）

自身免疫性疾病在女性中的发病率是男性的 5 倍。系统性红斑狼疮（systemic lupus erythematosus，SLE）、硬皮病、APS 和自身免疫性甲状腺疾病（见前述）都可以影响胎盘功能，导致流产、胎儿生长受限、早发性重度子痫前期、血栓形成和胎儿死亡。一些自身免疫状况，如类风湿关节炎和克罗恩病，在妊娠期的类固醇环境改变后有所改善，但产褥期复发的风险明显增加。

Autoimmune disease is five times more common in women than men. Systemic lupus erythematosus (SLE), scleroderma, APS and autoimmune thyroid disorders (discussed earlier) all can have an effect on placental function and result in miscarriage, fetal growth restriction, early-onset severe pre-eclampsia, thrombosis and fetal death. Some autoimmune conditions, such as rheumatoid arthritis and Crohn's disease, improve in the altered steroid environment of pregnancy, but there is a serious increased risk of relapse during the puerperium.

系统性红斑狼疮（Systemic lupus erythematosus）

系统性红斑狼疮是一种以复发和缓解期为特征的多系统疾病。系统性红斑狼疮的诊断依赖于血清中抗核抗体（antinuclear antibody，ANA）的血清学诊断，以及美国风湿病协会公布的其他 11 项临床或实验室标准中的至少 4 项，其中包括皮疹、肾脏损害、关节炎和血小板减少症。

SLE is a multisystem disorder characterized by periods of relapse and remission. The diagnosis of SLE is dependent on the serological finding of the antinuclear antibody (ANA) in the serum and at least 4 of 11 other clinical or laboratory criteria published by the American Rheumatology Association, including rash, renal impairment, arthritis and thrombocytopenia.

(1) 妊娠对疾病的影响（Implications of pregnancy on the disease）

有数据表明，妊娠期间复发更为频繁，并且在出生后肯定会出现"发作"或病情加重。约 75% 的患者患有肾脏疾病。狼疮性肾炎恶化的女性有可能在妊娠期间肾功能恶化，这可能是不可逆转的（见前述有关慢性肾脏疾病的内容）。

There is some evidence that relapses occur more frequently in pregnancy, and there certainly is an increase in 'flares' or exacerbations in the postnatal period. About 75% of patients have renal disease. Women with an exacerbation of lupus nephritis are at risk of deterioration in their renal function that may be irreversible during pregnancy (see the previous section on chronic renal diseases).

(2) 疾病对妊娠的影响（Implications of the disease on pregnancy）

患有系统性红斑狼疮的女性早产、死产、早发性先兆子痫、胎儿生长受限和早产的风险增加。如果她们有肾脏受累，或者如果她们也有抗磷脂综合征（APS），发生这种情况的可能性就会增加。

Women with SLE are at increased risk of early miscarriage,

stillbirth, early-onset pre-eclampsia, fetal growth restriction and pre-term birth. The likelihood of these occurring is increased if they have renal involvement or if they also have APS.

女性，特别是那些伴有系统性红斑狼疮的 APS 患者，患 VTE 的风险更高。

Women, especially those with APS alongside their SLE, are at increased risk of VTE.

婴儿有患新生儿狼疮和先天性心脏传导阻滞的风险。

Infants are at risk of neonatal lupus and congenital heart block.

(3) 治疗方法（Management）

女性应由多学科团队管理，有机会最好进行孕前咨询。如果在"发作"爆发后至少 6 个月内避免妊娠，效果会更好。

Women should be managed by a multidisciplinary team with the opportunity for pre-pregnancy counselling. Outcomes are better if pregnancy is avoided until at least 6 months after a 'flare'.

建议女性服用小剂量的阿司匹林以降低先兆子痫的风险；在 APS 并存的情况下，还应使用低分子肝素。

Women should be advised to take low-dose aspirin to reduce the risk of pre-eclampsia, and LMWH should be used in addition where APS co-exists.

应通过症状检查和定期评估疾病标志物（尤其是肾功能和抗磷脂抗体）来监测疾病。严重狼疮患者可以继续服用免疫抑制药，但如果有致畸作用，可能需要更换使用的药物。

The disease should be monitored by symptom review and regular assessment of disease markers, especially renal function and antiphospholipid antibodies. Immunosuppression can be continued in women with severe lupus, although the agents used may need to be changed if teratogenic.

通常在 37～38 周时引产，以避免妊娠晚期血栓并发症。

Labour is usually induced at 37–38 weeks to avoid latepregnancy thrombotic complications.

（十）血红蛋白病（Haemoglobinopathies）

1. 镰状细胞综合征（Sickle cell syndromes）

这些遗传性疾病涉及血红蛋白合成的异常，导致异常 S 血红蛋白的产生。疾病谱可以从相对无症

状的镰状细胞特征（女性是镰状基因的杂合子）到纯合子镰状细胞疾病（女性可能定期发生镰状细胞病）不等。尽管该疾病与某些种族有很强的关联性，特别是来自撒哈拉以南非洲和中东的种族，但现在镰状细胞综合征在世界各地都可以看到。

These genetic disorders involve abnormalities in haemoglobin synthesis resulting in abnormal S haemoglobin being produced. The disease spectrum can range from the relatively asymptomatic sickle cell trait, where women are heterozygous for the sickle gene, to homozygous sickle cell disease, where women can have regular sickle cell crises. Although there is a strong link with certain ethnicities, especially those from sub-Saharan Africa and the Middle East, sickle cell syndromes are now seen throughout the world.

(1) 妊娠对疾病的影响（Implications of pregnancy on the disease）

妊娠并发症，如恶心、呕吐、贫血和感染，都会增加患有镰状细胞病的女性发病的可能性，因此妊娠可能会导致更多的发病机会。

Pregnancy complications such as nausea and vomiting, anaemia and infection can all increase the likelihood of a sickle cell crisis occurring in women with sickle cell disease, and so pregnancy can result in an increased frequency of crises.

(2) 疾病对妊娠的影响（Implications of the disease on pregnancy）

镰状细胞综合征的遗传影响取决于伴侣的基因，因此建议及早对伴侣进行检测。根据这一结果，女性可能需要来自遗传学团队的意见，以确定她们是否希望继续进行产前诊断。

The genetic implications of the sickle cell syndromes depend on the status of the partner, and so early partner testing is recommended. Depending on the result of this, women may need input from the genetics team to determine if they wish to proceed with prenatal diagnosis.

具有镰状细胞综合征的女性通常在妊娠期间感觉良好，尽管贫血和感染可能是潜在的问题。相比之下，镰状细胞病与严重的产科并发症有关，包括流产、早产、胎儿生长受限和围产期死亡等的风险增加。母亲患静脉血栓栓塞、产前出血和先兆子痫的风险也会增加。

Women with the sickle cell trait generally do well in pregnancy, although anaemia and infections can be a problem. In contrast, sickle cell disease is associated with significant obstetric complications, including increased risks of miscarriage, pre-term birth, fetal growth restriction and perinatal mortality. There are also increased maternal risks of VTE, antepartum haemorrhage and pre-eclampsia.

(3) 治疗方法（Management）

备孕期女性及其伴侣应就妊娠风险进行咨询。在疾病管理得到优化之前，也应建议她们不要妊娠。

Pre-pregnancy women and their partners should be counselled about the risks for pregnancy. They should also be advised against conception until the disease management is optimized.

建议产科医生和血液科医生共同护理。如果可以，伴侣也携带镰状基因的女性可以接受产前诊断。所有患有镰状细胞综合征的女性都应该被建议服用更高剂量的叶酸（5mg），以降低神经管缺陷的风险，因为她们的溶血性贫血会增加她们叶酸缺乏的风险。对于患有镰状细胞病的女性，应该考虑服用小剂量的阿司匹林来降低先兆子痫的风险，并预防性使用抗生素来降低感染的风险。应该进行连续生长扫描，以观察胎儿生长过程中是否有问题。贫血可能会在妊娠期间恶化，可能需要输血来维持足够的血红蛋白水平。如果发生危险，应及时处理，以降低对胎儿的风险。

Joint care between obstetricians and haematologists is advised. Women whose partners also carry the sickle gene can be offered prenatal diagnosis if desired. All women with sickle cell syndromes should be advised to take a higher dose (5 mg) of folic acid to reduce the risk of neural tube defects, as their haemolytic anaemia increases their risk of folate deficiency. In women with sickle cell disease, low-dose aspirin should be considered to reduce the risk of pre-eclampsia and prophylactic antibiotics to reduce the risks of infection. Serial growth scans should be performed to look for evidence of growth problems. Anaemia can worsen during pregnancy, and blood transfusions may be required to maintain an adequate haemoglobin level. If crises occur, they should be treated promptly to reduce the risk to the fetus.

在妊娠和分娩期间，应避免脱水，并应根据是否其存在他危险因素，定期评估预防 VTE 的出现。

During pregnancy and labour, dehydration should be avoided, and the need for VTE prophylaxis should be regularly assessed depending on the presence of other risk factors.

2. 地中海贫血（The thalassaemias）

这些疾病与血红蛋白的 α- 和 β- 珠蛋白链的产生速度降低有关。在 α- 地中海贫血症中，损害的程度取决于缺失的 α- 珠蛋白基因的数量，其中 1 个缺失只会导致轻微的症状，4 个缺失会致命。大多数患有 α- 地中海贫血症的女性妊娠后会缺失 1～2 个 α- 基因，并会有轻度贫血。在 β- 地中海贫血患者中，个体可能是纯合子或杂合子，再次导致一系列症状。纯合子 β- 地中海贫血症女性很少妊娠；然而，杂合 β- 地中海贫血症女性症状轻微，对妊娠没有影响。

These disorders are associated with a reduction in the rate of production of the alpha- and beta-globin chains of haemoglobin. In alpha-thalassaemia, the degree of impairment depends on the number of alpha-globin genes absent, with one absent causing minimal symptoms and four being incompatible with life. Most of the women with alpha-thalassaemia who become pregnant will have one or two alpha genes missing and will have mild anaemia. In beta-thalassaemia individuals can be homozygous or heterozygous, resulting again in a spectrum of symptomatology. Women with homozygous beta-thalassaemia rarely become pregnant; however, women with heterozygous beta-thalassaemia have minimal symptoms and no impairment to pregnancy.

(1) 妊娠对疾病的影响（Implications of pregnancy on the disease）

妊娠可导致许多地中海贫血女性所表现的轻度贫血显著恶化。

Pregnancy can cause a significant worsening of the mild anaemia seen in many women with thalassaemias.

(2) 疾病对妊娠的影响和治疗（Implications of the disease on pregnancy and management）

地中海贫血病对妊娠的主要影响是遗传地中海贫血症基因的风险。伴侣检测将确定有可能怀上纯合子胎儿的女性，然后可以转介这些女性进行产前检测。有问题的贫血可能需要在妊娠期间输血治疗。由于女性有铁过载的危险，铁疗法必须谨慎使用。由于胎儿生长受限的风险，应该监测胎儿生长。

The main implication of the thalassaemias on pregnancy is the risk of inheriting the thalassaemia genes. Partner testing will identify women who are at risk of carrying a homozygous fetus, who can then be referred for prenatal testing. Problematic anaemia may need to be treated with transfusions in pregnancy. Iron therapy must be used cautiously, as women are at risk of iron overload. Fetal growth should be monitored because of the risk of fetal growth restriction.

五、结论（Conclusions）

构造具体框架来考虑妊娠期间的医疗状况对女性和胎儿的影响是至关重要的。现在，这种状况造成了越来越多的产妇死亡，要扭转这一趋势，就必须充分了解这一情况。

It is essential to have a framework for considering the implications of medical conditions in pregnancy on both the woman and the fetus. Such conditions now are responsible for an increasing number of maternal deaths, and adequate understanding is essential if this trend is to be reversed.

本章概览	Essential information

孕期轻微不适
- 这些通常是由于妊娠期间的生理变化引起的，但重要的是要确保没有病理原因贫血

贫血
- 在英国，血红蛋白水平<11g/dl（某些地区使用<10.5g/dl）被定义为贫血，尤其是在妊娠晚期
- 通常由以下原因引起
  - 膳食铁摄入不足
  - 铁吸收受损（胃酸缺乏症、营养不良、慢性腹泻、钩虫）
- 检查：平均红细胞体积（MCV）、平均红细胞血红蛋白浓度（MCHC）、血清铁和铁结合、铁蛋白、叶酸和维生素 B，有一些原因还不清楚
- 治疗，通常使用口服铁 / 叶酸

糖尿病
- 分类为 1 型、2 型或妊娠期糖尿病
- 需要严格管理，目的是将末梢血血糖保持在非糖尿病范围内
- 饮食和胰岛素管理（1 型）；饮食、口服降糖药 ± 胰岛素（2 型）；饮食 ± 口服降糖药 ± 胰岛素（妊娠期糖尿病）

孕期感染
- 妊娠期一些感染可对母亲和胎儿造成不利影响，但并不总是同等严重
- 可以通过在妊娠期间进行抗反转录病毒治疗将 HIV 的垂直传播降至最低风险。如果在妊娠末期可检测病毒，则建议通过剖宫产选择性分娩
- 甲型、乙型、丙型肝炎女性的主要治疗策略是采取各种措施来防止垂直传播，但是选择性剖宫产似乎没用
- 妊娠期间结核病的主要风险在于女性的健康。胎盘转移很少见。链霉素是唯一禁用的抗结核药
- 无症状和有症状的菌尿是妊娠期间的常见感染，为防止恶化为肾盂肾炎，必须及时诊断和治疗
- 有些感染可以事先通过免疫来预防（如风疹），有些可以在妊娠期间得到有效治疗。对于其他（如寨卡病毒感染）没有有效的治疗方法，避免在妊娠期间感染是最好的方法。

Minor complaints in pregnancy
- These are usually due to physiological changes in pregnancy, but it is important to ensure there is not a pathological cause

Anaemia
- In the UK, this is defined as a haemoglobin level <11 g/dL (some use <10.5 g/dL), especially towards the start of the third trimester
- Usually caused by:
  - Inadequate intake of dietary iron
  - Impaired absorption of iron (gastric achlorhydria, malnutrition, chronic diarrhoea, hookworm)
- Investigations-Mean Corpuscular Volume (MCV), Mean Corpuscular Haemoglobin Concentration (MCHC), serum iron and iron-binding, ferritin, folate and vitamin B; others if cause still obscure
- Management, usually with oral iron/folic acid

Diabetes
- Classified as type 1, type 2 or gestational
- Needs strict management, with the aim of keeping capillary glucose in the non-diabetic range
- Management by diet and insulin (type 1); diet, oral hypoglycaemic agents ± insulin (type 2); diet ± oral hypoglycaemic agents ± insulin (gestational diabetes)

Infections acquired in pregnancy
- Some infections in pregnancy can adversely affect the mother and the fetus, though not always equally seriously
- Vertical transmission of HIV can be reduced to a minimum by antiretroviral therapy during pregnancy. If virus is detectable at the end of pregnancy, elective delivery by caesarean section is recommended.
- The main management strategy in women with hepatitis, A, B or C is to implement a variety of measures to prevent vertical transmission, though an elective caesarean section does not appear to help this.
- The main risk of TB in pregnancy is on the health of the woman. Placental transfer is rare. Streptomycin is the only anti-tuberculous drug that is contraindicated.
- Asymptomatic and symptomatic bacteriuria are common infections in pregnancy, and prompt recognition and treatment are necessary to prevent progression to pyelonephritis.
- Some infections can be prevented by prior immunization (such as rubella), and some can be treated effectively during pregnancy. For others (such as Zika virus infection), there is no effective treatment, and avoidance of contracting the infection during pregnancy is the best approach.

（续表）

本章概览	Essential information
血栓栓塞 • 这是孕产妇死亡的主要原因之一 • 既往病史和可增加凝血性的遗传风险 • 应在产前、分娩期间和产后评估每个女性的潜在风险，并应采取预防措施（尤其是使用肝素） • 如果临床诊断怀疑有 DVT 或 PE 的可能，则应在检查结果出来之前开始全面抗凝治疗。如果诊断没有得到确认，则停止治疗	**Thromboembolism** • This is one of the major causes of maternal deaths. • A previous history of the condition and hereditary conditions with increased coagulability increase the risk. • Every mother should be assessed in the antenatal period, during labour and postpartum for the possible risk, and prophylactic measures (especially using LMWH) should be undertaken. • If a DVT or PE is suspected clinically, full anticoagulation should be commenced until the results of the investigations are available. If the diagnosis is not confirmed, the treatment is stopped.
肝病 • 产科胆汁淤积的病因尚不确定 • 该病会使女性的手掌和脚底产生剧烈的瘙痒 • 该病与胎儿死亡风险增加相关，因此通常主张在 37～38 周时择期分娩以降低该风险。	**Liver disease** • Obstetric cholestasis is of uncertain aetiology. • It produces intense itching of the woman's palms and soles of the feet. • It is associated with an increased risk of fetal death, and elective delivery at 37-38 weeks is often advocated to lessen that risk.
肾脏疾病 • 中度至重度的慢性肾脏疾病通常在妊娠期间恶化，分娩后可能无法改善。 • 肾脏疾病导致胎儿宫内生长受限、早产和围产儿受影响的发生率增加。 • 必须进行多学科管理，以优化女性和胎儿的结局。	**Renal disease** • Moderate-severe chronic renal disease usually worsens during pregnancy and may not improve after delivery. • Renal disease causes increased rates of intrauterine growth restriction, pre-term delivery and perinatal loss. • Multidisciplinary management is necessary to optimize the outcome for the woman and fetus.
甲状腺疾病 • 甲状腺功能减退最常见的原因是自身免疫性疾病或医源性疾病（甲状腺切除术后）。碘缺乏症较少见。TSH 水平升高是可以诊断的，应通过 TSH 水平监测甲状腺素治疗的有效性。 • 妊娠期甲状腺功能亢进症通常是由 Graves 病引起的。它可能导致低出生体重和早产。治疗方法是抗甲状腺药物	**Thyroid disease** • Hypothyroidism is most commonly due to autoimmune disease or iatrogenic (post-thyroidectomy). Iodine deficiency is less common. Raised levels of TSH are diagnostic, and the effectiveness of thyroxine treatment should be monitored with TSH levels. • Hyperthyroidism in pregnancy is usually due to Graves' disease. It can cause low birth weight and premature labour and birth. Treatment is with anti-thyroid drugs.
肥胖 • 理想情况下，肥胖女性应达到最佳 BMI 后再妊娠 • 由于肥胖风险增加，肥胖女性应接受基于医院的护理 • 应该对妊娠期糖尿病和胎儿过度生长进行筛查 • 剖宫产需要特殊准备（如大手术台）	**Obesity** • Ideally obese women should defer pregnancy until they reach their optimal BMI. • Obese women should have hospital-based care because of the increased risks. • Screening should be undertaken for gestational diabetes and excessive fetal growth. • Special preparation is necessary for a caesarean section (e.g. a large operating table).
癫痫 • 少数女性在妊娠期间癫痫发作频率增加 • 据报道，所有抗癫痫药物都具有致畸性，丙戊酸钠似乎风险最大。然而，癫痫的危害超过了治疗的风险 • 妊娠期间的首要任务是用最少的药物和最低的有效剂量预防癫痫发作	**Epilepsy** • A minority of women have an increase in seizure frequency in pregnancy. • All anti-epileptic drugs have been reported to be teratogenic, with sodium valproate appearing to have the greatest risk. However, the hazards of epilepsy exceed the risks of treatment. • The main priority in pregnancy is to prevent seizures with the fewest drugs and at the lowest effective dose.

（续表）

本章概览	Essential information
心脏疾病 • 女性和胎儿的风险因诊断而异 • 尽管心脏病的一些症状在妊娠期间也是正常的生理主诉，但 NYHA 的分类为女性心脏病的严重程度提供了一个指标 • 监督和管理应由多学科团队进行，治疗方案根据患者具体情况进行定制 呼吸系统疾病 • 哮喘 – 这在孕妇中很常见，通常不会因妊娠而加重 – 有些症状是妊娠期间的正常不适 – 基线峰值流量测量应在妊娠初期进行 – 急性发作和持续维持的治疗与未妊娠者相同，这对孕妇和胎儿是安全的 • 囊性纤维化 – 尽管情况不常见，但它与女性和胎儿的风险增加有关 – 监督和管理应由多学科团队进行，治疗方案根据患者具体情况进行定制	**Cardiac disease** • The risks for the woman and fetus vary with the diagnosis. • The NYHA classification gives an indication as to the severity of the cardiac disease in the woman, though some of the symptoms of cardiac disease are also normal physiological complaints in pregnancy. • Surveillance and management should be by a multidisciplinary team and individualized. **Respiratory disease** • Asthma – This is common in pregnancy and is not commonly exacerbated by the pregnancy. – Some symptoms are normal complaints in pregnancy. – Baseline peak flow measurements should be taken at the start of pregnancy. – Treatment for both acute attacks and ongoing maintenance is the same as for non-pregnant individuals and is considered safe. • Cystic fibrosis – Though an uncommon condition, it is associated with increased risk for the woman and fetus. – Surveillance and management should be by a multidisciplinary team and individualized.

第 10 章　胎儿先天性异常及健康评估

Congenital abnormalities and assessment of fetal wellbeing

David James　SuzanneV.F.Wallace 著　黄　薇　朱慧莉 译　杨慧霞 校

学习目标	LEARNING OUTCOMES
学习本章后，你应当能够：	• After studying this chapter you should be able to:
知识标准	**Knowledge criteria**
• 描述胎儿异常发育导致的常见结构异常	• Describe the common structural abnormalities resulting from abnormal development
• 列举导致常见胎儿异常的风险因素	• List the risk factors for the common fetal abnormalities
• 比较胎儿异常的诊断方法	• Compare the diagnostic tests for fetal abnormality
• 描述孕期超声检查在筛查、诊断和评估胎儿异常，以及评价胎儿发育和健康的作用	• Describe the role of ultrasound scanning in pregnancy in screening, diagnosis and assessment of fetal abnormalities and in assessing fetal growth and health
• 描述 Rh 同种免疫溶血的病因、风险因素及其管理	• Describe the aetiology, risk factors and management of Rhesus isoimmunization
临床能力	**Clinical competencies**
• 解读胎儿健康发育指标	• Interpret the results of investigations of fetal wellbeing
• 制订小于孕龄儿的监测和管理方案	• Plan the investigation and management of the small for gestational age baby
专业技能及态度	**Professional skills and attitudes**
• 审慎向家庭成员反馈胎儿异常的诊断	• Reflect on the impact on a family of a diagnosis of fetal abnormality
先天性异常	**Congenital abnormalities**
胎儿先天性异常见于：	Fetal abnormality is found in:
• 超过总妊娠的 50%	• over 50% of conceptions
• 约 70% 的流产	• about 70% of miscarriages
• 从孕 20 周至产后 1 年，有 15% 死亡	• 15% of deaths between 20 weeks' gestation and 1 year postnatal
• 有 1%～2% 新生儿出现严重畸形和轻微畸形（严重畸形是指导致婴儿死亡或重度残疾的异常）	• 1–2% of births, including major and minor anomalies (a major abnormality is an abnormality or abnormalities that result in the death of the baby or severe disability)
• 8% 的儿童需要特殊护理或残疾	• 8% of special needs register/disabled children

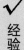

经验

过去 30 年，由于孕期筛查项目的推广，孕期诊断结果显成功提升，以及父母面对诊断严重畸形儿选择终止妊娠的态度，先天性异常在英国的总体发生率明显下降。

The overall incidence of congenital abnormalities in the UK has fallen over the past three decades due to the introduction of screening programmes in pregnancy, the resultant greater success at diagnosis during pregnancy and parents opting to terminate a pregnancy once a severe abnormality has been diagnosed.

最常见的 4 类先天性异常包括神经管缺陷（3‰～7‰）、先天性心脏病（6‰）、唐氏综合征（1.5‰）和唇裂 / 腭裂（1.5‰）（表 10-1）。

The commonest four groups of congenital abnormalities are neural tube defects (3–7/1000), congenital cardiac defects (6/1000), Down's syndrome (1.5/1000) and cleft lip/palate (1.5/1000) (Table 10.1).

一、神经管缺陷（Neural tube defects）

神经管缺陷是最为常见的严重先天性异常，其中包括先天无脑畸形、小头畸形、脊柱裂（伴或不伴脊髓脊膜膨出）、脑膨出、前脑无裂畸形和积水性无脑（图 10-1）。神经管缺陷的发生率约为 1/200；以往有异常孩子者，再次发生概率高达 1/20。

Neural tube defects are the commonest of the major congenital abnormalities and include anencephaly, microcephaly, spina bifida with or without myelomeningocele, encephalocele, holoprosencephaly and hydranencephaly (Fig. 10.1). The incidence is approximately 1/200, and the chance of having an affected child after one previous abnormal child is 1/20.

多数病例在中孕早期通过超声（ultrasound, US）诊断确诊。当存在开放性神经管缺陷时，孕妇血清甲胎蛋白（maternal serum alpha-fetoprotein, MSAFP）水平升高。超声还能诊断其他胎儿异常，必要时应进行染色体核型分析。

Commonly cases are identified by ultrasound (US) screening in the early second trimester. Where there is an open neural tube, maternal serum alpha-fetoprotein (MSAFP) levels are raised. US assessment for other abnormalities should be undertaken and karyotyping offered if they are found.

推荐多学科咨询和关爱。先天无脑或小头畸形的婴儿通常无法存活，大多会在分娩过程中死亡，其余的则会在产后第一周内死亡。患有开放性神经

表 10-1　严重先天性异常

Table 10.1　Major congenital abnormalities

异常 Abnormality	大致发生率 （每 1000 个新生儿） Approximate incidence (per 1000 births)
神经管缺陷 Neural tube defects	3～7
先天性心脏病 Congenital heart disease	6
唐氏综合征 Down's syndrome	1.5
唇裂 / 腭裂 Cleftlip/palate	1.5
马蹄足 Talipes	1～2
四肢畸形 Abnormalities of limbs	1～2
耳聋 Deafness	0.8
失明 Blindness	0.2
包括泌尿道异常在内的其他先天性异常 Others,including urinary tract abnormalities	2
合计 Total	15～30

经许可转载，引自 James DK, Weiner CP, Gonik B, Crowther CA, Robson SC, eds (2011) High Risk Pregnancy: Management Options, 4th edn. Saunders Elsevier, St Louis.

Reproduced with permission from James DK, Weiner CP, Gonik B, Crowther CA, Robson SC, eds (2011) High Risk Pregnancy: Management Options, 4th edn. Saunders Elsevier, St Louis.

管缺陷的婴儿往往可以存活，尤其是出生后通过皮肤手术修复病变的婴儿。但是，该缺陷可能导致截瘫和大小便失禁，需要反复多次手术。此类孩子通常具有正常的智力和领悟力，尤其能意识到自身缺陷给父母带来的困难。闭合的神经管缺陷通常不会引起注意，往往直到出生后才会被发现。

Multidisciplinary counselling and care are recommended. Infants with anencephaly or microcephaly do not usually survive. Many die during labour and the remainder within the first week of life. Infants with open neural tube defects often survive, particularly where it is possible to cover the lesion surgically with skin after birth. However, the defect may result in paraplegia and bowel and bladder incontinence and the

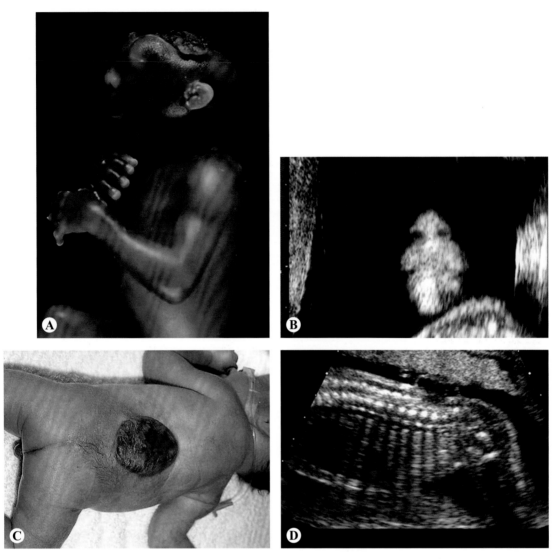

▲ 图 10-1　两种常见的中枢神经系统畸形

A. 新生的无脑儿；B. 无脑畸形儿的孕中期超声图像（可见脸部但无颅骨）；C. 脊柱裂，伴开放性神经管缺陷；D. 脊柱裂畸形的孕中期超声图像 [图片 A 由 Ed Uthman, MD 提供。https://commons.wikimedia.org/w/index.php?curid=1405306。图 C 经许可转载，引自 Lissauer T, Carroll W (2018) Illustrated Textbook of Paediatrics, 5th edn. Elsevier.]

Fig. 10.1　Two common abnormalities of the central nervous system.

(A) Anencephaly in a newborn. (B) Mid-trimester ultrasound image of anencephaly (face visualized but no cranium). (C) Spina bifida with open neural tube defect. (D) Mid-trimester ultrasound image of spina bifida. (A Courtesy Ed Uthman, MD. https://commons. wikimedia.org/w/index.php?curid=1405306. C Reproduced with permission from Lissauer T, Carroll W (2018) Illustrated Textbook of Paediatrics, 5th edn. Elsevier.)

need for repeated further surgery. The child often has normal intelligence and has insight, being particularly aware of the problems posed for the parents. Closed lesions generally do not cause problems and may escape detection until after birth.

> **！注意**
>
> 针对流产组织、死产或新生儿死亡，应寻求胚胎检测以排除其他异常。
>
> Permission for postmortem should be sought with abortuses, stillbirths or neonatal obeaths to exclude other abnormalities.

有充分证据表明，在孕前和围孕期补充叶酸（400μg/d）可以减少这些情况的发生。一旦女性妊娠后，重点是借助筛查技术及时发现胎儿异常，存在致命畸形时提供妊娠终止。

There is good evidence that pre- and periconceptual folic acid supplementation (400 μg/day) reduces the incidence of this condition. Once a woman is pregnant, the major effort is directed toward screening techniques that enable recognition of the abnormality and the offer of a termination of the pregnancy where there is a lethal abnormality.

对于有神经管缺陷妊娠史的女性应在孕前和孕期进行膳食补充叶酸，推荐服用更大剂量（5mg/d）叶酸预防措施。

Folic acid dietary supplementation is indicated both before and during pregnancy in those women who have experienced a pregnancy complicated by a neural tube defect. In these cases, a higher dose of folic acid prophylaxis (5 mg/day) is recommended.

> **！注意**　针对开放性神经管缺陷的胎儿手术已有开展，但此类手术目前仍应视为处于试验阶段。
>
> Fetal surgery for open neural tube defects has been undertaken but should be considered experimental at present.

二、先天性心脏病（Congenital cardiac defects）

孕妇出现胎儿先天性心脏病的可能性约为 0.6%。部分胎儿表现为宫内生长受限和羊水过少，但大多数是在出生后才被发现并诊断。随着实时超声影像的发展，许多心脏缺陷在孕期即有可能被发现。尽早发现此类缺陷对于采取相应措施至关重要，超声筛查是可行的。多数医院会在孕早期（约 11 周）进行胎儿颈项透明层检查，在孕中期（18～20 周）进行胎儿心脏四腔观察（图 10-2）。此外，部分医院会在孕 11 周检查静脉导管和三尖瓣的血流情况，并在 18～20 周检查左、右流出道的血流，以期发现更多异常。尽管采用了超声筛查，即使在最好的医院，也只有不到 50% 的先天性心脏病在产前确诊。

The likelihood of a pregnant woman having a fetus with a congenital cardiac defect is about 0.6%. Some of these infants present with intrauterine growth restriction and oligohydramnios, but in many cases the condition is only recognized and diagnosed after birth. With improvements in real-time US imaging, recognition of many cardiac defects has become possible. However, early recognition is essential if any action is to be taken. Screening is performed by US. Most centres would undertake nuchal translucency scanning in the first trimester (around 11 weeks) and a four-chamber view of the fetal heart in the second trimester (at 18–20 weeks) (Fig. 10.2). In addition, some centres are looking at blood flow in the ductus venosus and across the tricuspid valve at 11 weeks and the left and right outflow tracts at 18–20 weeks to try and identify more abnormalities. Despite this screening, even in the best centres less than 50% of congenital heart defects are

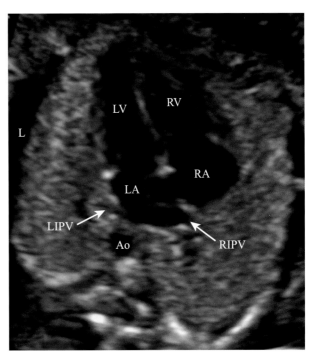

▲ 图 10-2　胎儿心脏超声四腔图像

Ao. 主动脉；L. 左；LA. 左心房；LIPV. 左肺静脉；LV. 左心室；RA. 右心房；RIPV. 右肺静脉；RV. 右心室

Fig. 10.2　Four-chamber ultrasound view of the fetal heart.

Ao, Aorta; L, Left; LA, Left atrium; LIPV, Left interstitial pulmonary vein; LV, Left ventricle; RA, Right atrium; RIPV, Right interstitial pulmonary vein; RA, Right atrium.

currently identified prenatally.

最常见的心脏缺陷为心室和房间隔缺损、肺动脉和主动脉狭窄，包括法洛氏四联症的主动脉缩窄和移位，这些病变通常是在孕 18～20 周的四腔筛查时发现。

The most common defects are ventricular and atrial septal defects, pulmonary and aortic stenosis, coarctation and transpositions of the great vessels, including the tetralogy of Fallot. These lesions can generally now be recognized on the four-chamber views recorded during detailed 18-to 20-week-gestation scans.

一旦确定胎儿有异常，应进行进一步的诊断性超声检查以确定胎儿缺陷的程度及有无其他胎儿异常（可能包括核型分析），并采取多学科咨询会诊。在预后不良的情况下，父母可选择终止妊娠。而在其他情况下，应选择在具备全面新生儿心脏疾病救治能力（包括心脏手术）的医院分娩。

Once an abnormality is identified, management comprises further diagnostic US examination to establish the extent of the defect and whether there are any other fetal abnormalities (this may include karyotyping) and multidisciplinary counselling and care. In some cases where the prognosis is poor, the parents may opt for a termination of pregnancy. In other cases, delivery should occur in a centre with full neonatal cardiological services, including cardiac surgery.

三、腹壁缺损（Defects of the abdominal wall）

超声影像能够诊断腹壁缺损。95% 以上于孕中期（18～20 周）在优秀的医院超声筛查确诊。腹壁缺损包括胎儿腹裂（图 10-3A）和脐膨出（图 10-3B），在这两种情况下，肠管突出于腹腔外，两者之间的主要区别在于：腹裂是一种与脐带无关的缺陷（通常位于脐带下方右侧 2～3cm 处），无腹膜覆盖，往往是独立的病症；而脐膨出实质上是一种大的脐带疝气，有腹膜覆盖，伴潜在的染色体异常（尤其是 18 三体综合征）风险增加。

Defects of the abdominal wall can be diagnosed by US imaging. US screening in the second trimester (18–20 weeks) in the best centres detects over 95% of cases. They include gastroschisis (Fig. 10.3A) and exomphalos (Fig. 10.3B). In both cases, the bowel extrudes outside the abdominal cavity. The main differences between the two are that a gastroschisis is a defect that is separate from the umbilical cord (usually 2–3 cm below and to the right), does not have a peritoneal covering and is usually an isolated problem. In contrast, an exomphalos is essentially a large hernia of the umbilical cord with a peritoneal covering and an increased risk of an underlying chromosomal abnormality, especially trisomy 18.

如果诊断为腹裂，可告知其父母预后很好，需要提供多学科护理，可以阴道分娩，但应在能够实施新生儿手术的医院分娩。所有婴儿需接受新生儿手术纠正缺陷，90% 以上的患儿可以存活。

If a gastroschisis is diagnosed, the parents can be told the prognosis is very good. Multidisciplinary care is needed. Delivery can be vaginal and should take place in a hospital with neonatal surgical facilities. All babies will require neonatal surgery to correct the defect; however, over 90% will survive.

相反，脐膨出的预后很差。除染色体异常因素外，复合结构缺陷风险增加（超过 60%），尤其是心脏结构缺陷。一旦诊断，应进行详细的超声检查和提供核型分析报告，同时提供多学科会诊。如果胎儿父母选择继续妊娠，则应在包括配备手术的综合新生儿设施医院分娩。

In contrast, exomphalos has a very poor prognosis. Apart from the association with chromosomal abnormality, there is an increased risk (over 60%) of co-existent structural defects, especially cardiac. Further careful detailed US examination of the fetus should be undertaken once the diagnosis is made and karyotyping offered. Multidisciplinary care is advisable. If the parents opt to continue with the pregnancy rather than have a termination of pregnancy, this should take place in a unit with comprehensive neonatal facilities, including surgery.

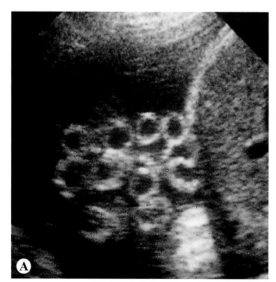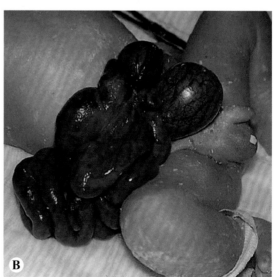

▲ 图 10-3　A. 腹裂肠管包在腹膜囊内；B. 脐膨出 - 肠管膨出

经许可转载，引自 Lissauer T & Carroll W (2018) Illustrated Textbook of Paediatrics, 5th edition, Elsevier.

Fig. 10.3　(A) Gastroschisis-bowel contained within peritoneal sac. (B) Exomphalos-bowel extrusion.

(Reproduced with permission from Lissauer T & Carroll W (2018) Illustrated Textbook of Paediatrics, 5th edition, Elsevier.)

四、染色体异常（Chromosomal abnormalities）

染色体异常较为常见，估计的发生率至少占所有妊娠的 7.5%。多数情况会导致流产，活产率低，约为 0.6%。染色体异常可通过培养羊水或绒毛膜中的胎儿 / 胎盘细胞并进行核型分析确诊。染色体异常包括核型结构异常和数量异常，最常见是 21 三体综合征或唐氏综合征（Down's syndrome，DS），此时，至少 92% 患儿的每个细胞的第 21 号染色体为 3 条而不是 2 条（约 8% 为易位，见后述），这将在后面进一步讨论。其次是性染色体异常（Klinefelter 综合征，表现为 2 条 X 染色体和 1 条 Y 染色体基础上多出 1 条性染色体；三 X 染色体综合征，多出 1 条性染色体，表现为 3 条 X 染色体；Turner 综合征，只有 1 条性染色体，即 1 条 X 染色体），然后是 13 三体综合征（Patau 综合征）和 18 三体综合征（Edwards 综合征）。

Chromosomal abnormalities are common, with an estimated incidence of at least 7.5% of all conceptions. However, many of these result in a miscarriage, and the liveborn incidence is much less than that, at about 0.6%. Chromosomal abnormalities can be identified from culturing and karyotyping fetal/placental cells in the amniotic fluid or from the chorionic plate. The chromosomal abnormalities include both structural and numerical abnormalities of the karyotype. The commonest abnormality is that associated with trisomy 21, or Down's syndrome (DS). In this condition, in at least 92% of cases the chromosomal abnormality is that each cell has three rather than two number 21 chromosomes (about 8% of cases are translocations-see later). This condition is discussed further later. The next most common are abnormalities of the sex chromosomes (Klinefelter's syndrome with one extra sex chromosome in the form of two X-chromosomes and one Y-chromosome; Triple-X syndrome with an extra sex chromosome in the form of three X-chromosomes; and Turner's syndrome with one only one sex chromosome, an X-chromosome), followed by trisomies 13 and 18 (Patau and Edwards syndromes, respectively).

唐氏综合征（Down's syndrome）

唐氏综合征特征是典型的异常面部特征（图 10-4）、不同程度的学习障碍和先天性心脏病。染色体异常核型包括第 21 对染色体中多出 1 条染色体（"21 三体综合征"；图 10-5），总体发病率为 1.5‰ 出生婴儿，随着母亲年龄增加而发生概率增高（见下述），被认为是减数分裂时染色体不分离的频率增加所致。

DS is characterized by the typical abnormal facial

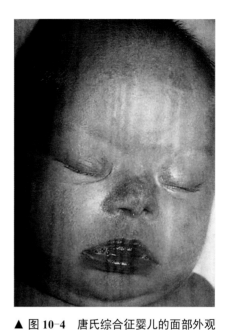

▲ 图 10-4　唐氏综合征婴儿的面部外观

Fig. 10.4　Facial appearance of infant with Down's syndrome.

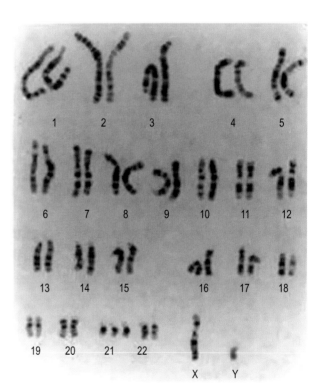

▲ 图 10-5　21 三体综合征的核型（男性）

Fig. 10.5　Trisomy 21 karyotype (male).

features (Fig. 10.4), learning disability of varying degrees of severity and congenital heart disease. The karyotype includes an additional chromosome in group 21 ('trisomy 21'; Fig. 10.5). The incidence overall is 1.5/1000 births. However, the chance increases with advancing maternal age (see later). The underlying reason is thought to be an increased frequency of non-disjunction at meiosis.

6%～8% 的婴儿由于染色体易位患病，此时多出的 21 号染色体与另一条染色体（通常是与第 13～15 号染色体）连接在一起，其母亲或者父亲是平衡异位携带者。

About 6–8% of affected infants have the disease as a result of a translocation and the extra 21 chromosome carried on to another chromosome, usually in group 13–15. The mother or the father will usually be a carrier of a balanced translocation.

五、评估胎儿正常（Assessing fetal normality）

（一）筛查（Screening）

此处的筛查是指从普通人群确认胎儿异常高风险孕妇的过程。通过确定临床危险因素、超声和母体血液检测进行筛查。尽管处理方案因胎龄而异，但整个孕期的临床风险因素均可确定，而超声和生化检查应在妊娠前半期进行。理想的筛查是在早孕末期联合筛查（超声和生化）非整倍体，以及孕 20 周详细的超声扫描。早期扫描还有助于确认胎龄。孕妇若错过孕早期非整倍体筛查，则应在孕 16 周进行生化筛查。

Screening in this context is the process whereby women with a higher chance of fetal abnormality are identified in the general population. This screening is undertaken using identification of clinical risk factors, US and biochemical testing of maternal serum. Clinical risk factors can be identified throughout pregnancy, though the options for management are different depending on the gestational age. US and biochemical screening are offered to women in the first half of pregnancy. Ideally women should be offered a combined screening test (using US and biochemistry) for aneuploidy towards the end of the first trimester and a detailed US scan at about 20 weeks. The early scan also allows gestational age to be confirmed. If a woman presents too late for the first-trimester aneuploidy screening, then she should be offered a biochemical screening test at about 16 weeks.

1. 临床危险因素：妊娠早期（Clinical risk factors: early pregnancy）

具体如下（These include: ）：

- 母亲年龄和非整倍体风险，尤其是唐氏综合征（表 10-2 和表 10-3）。

- 母体药物摄入

　- 抗惊厥类药物（如苯妥英、卡巴西平和丙

表 10-2　分娩时产妇年龄与发生妊娠唐氏综合征的概率

Table 10.2　The chance of having a pregnancy affected by Down's syndrome according to maternal age at the time of birth

分娩时产妇年龄（岁） Maternal age at delivery (years)	Chance of Down's syndrome 唐氏综合征概率
15	1 : 1578
20	1 : 1528
25	1 : 1351
30	1 : 909
31	1 : 796
32	1 : 683
33	1 : 574
34	1 : 474
35	1 : 384
36	1 : 307
37	1 : 242
38	1 : 189
39	1 : 146
40	1 : 112
41	1 : 85
42	1 : 65
43	1 : 49
44	1 : 37
45	1 : 28
46	1 : 21
47	1 : 15
48	1 : 11
49	1 : 8
50	1 : 6

经许可转载，引自 James DK, Weiner CP, Gonik B, Crowther CA, Robson SC, eds（2011）High Risk Pregnancy: Management Options, 4th edn. Saunders Elsevier, St Louis.

Reproduced with permission from James DK, Weiner CP, Gonik B, Crowther CA, Robson SC, eds (2011) High Risk Pregnancy: Management Options, 4th edn. Saunders Elsevier, St Louis.

表 10-3 孕 16 周行羊膜腔穿刺术时孕妇年龄与胎儿染色体异常（单位为每 1000 例的发生率）

Table 10.3 Chromosomal abnormalities by maternal age at the time of amniocentesis performed at 16 weeks' gestation (expressed as rate per 1000)

孕妇年龄（岁） Maternalage(years)	21 三体综合征 Trisomy 21	18 三体综合征 Trisomy 18	13 三体综合征 Trisomy 13	XXY	所有染色体异常 All chromosomal anomalies
35	3.9	0.5	0.2	0.5	8.7
36	5.0	0.7	0.3	0.6	10.1
37	6.4	1.0	0.4	0.8	12.2
38	8.1	1.4	0.5	1.1	14.8
39	10.4	2.0	0.8	1.4	18.4
40	13.3	2.8	1.1	1.8	23.0
41	16.9	3.9	1.5	2.4	29.0
42	21.6	5.5	2.1	3.1	37.0
43	27.4	7.6		4.1	45.0
44	34.8			5.4	50.0
45	44.2			7.0	62.0
46	55.9			9.1	77.0
47	70.4			11.9	96.0

戊酸钠）可能导致中枢神经系统缺陷，尤其是神经管缺陷。

- 癌症治疗或器官移植后免疫抑制的细胞毒性药物导致胎儿生长受限的风险增加。

- 孕早期使用华法林致畸，妊娠后期使用则可能导致胎儿出血性疾病。

• maternal age and risk of aneuploidy especially DS (Tables 10.2 and 10.3).

• maternal drug ingestion:

– anticonvulsant drugs (e.g. phenytoin, carbamazepine and sodium valproate) can produce defects of the central nervous system, especially neural tube defects.

– cytotoxic agents used in cancer therapy or for immunosuppression with organ transplantation are associated with an increased risk of fetal growth restriction.

– warfarin is teratogenic when used in the first trimester and can produce a fetal bleeding disorder when used later in pregnancy.

• 既往异常胎儿史

– 例如，如果一名女性过去分娩唐氏综合征的胎儿，其复发概率则会比单纯年龄因素可能性更大。

– 不过，并非所有胎儿异常都导致后续妊娠的复发风险增加。

• previous history of fetal abnormality:

– if, for example, a woman has had a DS baby in the past, she has a greater chance of recurrence than the likelihood given by her age alone.

– however, not all fetal abnormalities are associated with a greater risk of recurrence in a subsequent pregnancy.

• 母体疾病（见第 9 章）

– 糖尿病：报道的胎儿异常风险在 3%～8%。如果孕妇在孕前和孕早期控制好糖尿病，且在围孕期服用了叶酸，发生率则会显著降低。

– 先天性心脏病：患有先天性心脏病的女性，其胎儿心脏异常的风险为 1%～2%。

• maternal disease (see Chapter 9), including:

– diabetes: the reported risks of fetal abnormality vary between 3% and 8%. This figure is reduced

239

significantly if the diabetes is well controlled before and during the first trimester and the woman takes periconceptual folic acid.

- congenital cardiac disease: a woman who has a congenital cardiac defect has a 1–2% risk of a cardiac abnormality in her fetus.

2. 临床风险因素：妊娠晚期（Clinical risk factors: late pregnancy）

以下是与胎儿异常可能性上升相关的风险因素。

- 妊娠晚期持续性臀先露或异常胎位。

- 阴道出血，但是多数孕妇孕期阴道出血不是因为胎儿异常。

- 异常胎动（无论是增加还是减少），通常会注意到这种细微的差别的孕妇往往有过正常的妊娠史，并以此为参照。

- 羊水量异常：包括羊水过多（通常与胃肠系统异常尤其是梗阻相关）和羊水过少（通常与泌尿系统梗阻异常相关，如尿道瓣或肾发育不全）。

- 生长受限，尽管大多数生长受限的胎儿并未出现异常。

The following are risk factors associated with a higher likelihood of fetal abnormality:

- persistent breech presentation or abnormal lie in late pregnancy
- vaginal bleeding; however, the majority of pregnant women with vaginal bleeding in pregnancy do not have a fetal abnormality
- abnormal fetal movements, both increased and decreased, though for women to be aware of this perhaps subtle difference, they usually must have had a normal pregnancy previously, which they can use as a reference
- abnormal amniotic fluid volume: both polyhydramnios (which is commonly associated with abnormalities of the gastrointestinal system, especially obstruction) and oligohydramnios (which is commonly associated with obstructive abnormalities of the renal tract, such as urethral valves or renal agenesis)
- growth restriction, though most fetuses that are growth restricted do not have an abnormality

3. 超声（Ultrasound）

在英国，大多数孕妇会在孕早期去看医生。这就意味着她们在妊娠前半期可以获得 2 次超声扫描。

Most pregnant women in the UK present for their first visit to a health professional in the first trimester. This means that they can be offered two US scans in the first half of pregnancy.

首次检查在孕 11^{+0} 周至 13^{+6} 周进行最为理想。此次检查所记录的内容如下。

- 确认妊娠位置（如位于子宫内）。

- 通过胎心搏动确认胎儿存活。

- 确认胎儿数量。若为双胎，通过"驼峰征"（双绒毛膜）或 T 征（单绒毛膜）确定绒毛膜特征（图 10–6）。

- 测量顶臀长（crown-rump length，CRL）评估胎龄（见第 4 章）。

The first scan ideally is performed between $11w^{+0}d$ and $13w^{+6}d$. The features recorded at this examination are:

- Confirmation of the location of pregnancy (i.e. that it is in the uterus).
- Confirmation of fetal viability by the demonstration of cardiac activity.
- Establishing the number of fetuses. If there are twins, then the chorionicity should be determined by identifying either the 'lambda sign' (dichorionic) or 'T-sign' (monochorionic) (Fig. 10.6).
- Assessment of gestational age by measurement of crown-rump length (CRL) (see Chapter X).

如果孕妇希望筛查胎儿异常，则应进行以下检查。

- 测量胎儿颈项透明层（nuchal translucenc, NT）（图 10–7）作为"联合筛查"项目的一部分（见后述）。

- 胎儿解剖结构异常筛查。此孕期内并非所有的大的结构异常能够筛查出来，其中包括无脑儿、前脑无裂畸形和大的腹壁缺损。

If the woman wishes to have screening for fetal abnormality, she can have:

- Measurement of fetal nuchal translucency (NT) (Fig. 10.7) as part of the 'combined testing' programme (see next section).
- Fetal anatomical screening for malformations. Not all major structural anomalies are easily detectable at this gestation. Those that are include anencephaly, holoprosencephaly and major abdominal wall defects.

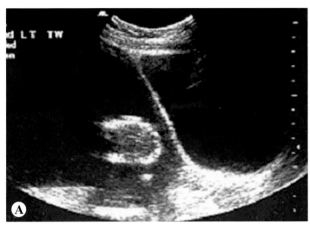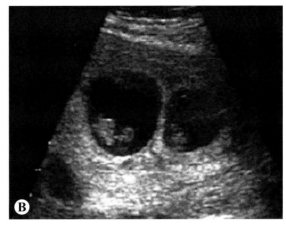

▲ 图 10-6　绒毛膜性

A. 单绒毛膜双胎（T 征）；B. 双绒毛膜双胎（驼峰征）

经许可转载，引自 Dodd JM, Grivell RM, Crowther CA (2011) Multiple pregnancy. In: James DK, Weiner CP, Gonik B, Crowther CA, Robson SC, eds. High Risk Pregnancy: Management Options, 4th edn. Saunders Elsevier, St Louis.

Fig. 10.6　Chorionicity.

(A) Monochorionic twins (T-sign). (B) Dichorionic twins (lambda sign).

(Reproduced with permission from Dodd JM, Grivell RM, Crowther CA (2011) Multiple pregnancy. In: James DK, Weiner CP, Gonik B, Crowther CA, Robson SC, eds. High Risk Pregnancy: Management Options, 4th edn. Saunders Elsevier, St Louis.)

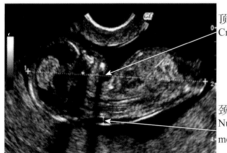

顶臀长
Crown-rump length

颈项透明层测量
Nuchal translucency measurement

▲ 图 10-7　当顶臀长（crown-rump length，CRL）= 45～84mm 时测量颈项透明层（nuchal translucency，NT）

NT 测量：精确在矢状位的顶臀长，适当放大（>70% 图像），远离羊膜，胎头居中，取 3～5 个测量值的最大值

Fig. 10.7　Nuchal translucency (NT) measurement (undertaken when crown-rump length (CRL) = 45–84 mm).

NT measurement: strict sagittal view appropriate for CRL, appropriate magnification (>70% image), away from the amnion, neutral position of the fetal head, biggest of three to five measurements.

　　第 2 次超声筛查在孕 18～20 周期间，多数在孕 20 周进行。此次检查所记录的内容如下。

- 确认胎儿存活。

- 确认胎儿数量。

- 测量胎儿的生物测量 [头围、腹围、双顶径（biparietal diameter，BPD）和股骨长度]。据

此确定或确认胎龄。多数医院仅测量双顶径，有的医院会采用多种测量。

- 评估羊水量。

- 评估胎盘位置和脐带附着点。

The second US scan is offered to women when they are between 18 and 20 weeks. Most are undertaken at 20 weeks. The features recorded at this examination are:

- Confirmation of fetal viability.

- Establishing the number of fetuses.

- Measurement of fetal biometry (head and abdominal circumferences, biparietal diameter (BPD) and femur length). From these, the gestational age can be established or confirmed. Most centres use the BPD only for this, though some use a combination of measurements.

- Assessment of amniotic fluid volume.

- Assessment of placental location and cord insertion.

- 为孕妇提供解剖学检查，以确认胎儿的下述器官系统是否正常。妊娠 20 周时检出下述系统中结构异常的成功率各异，据 2009 年相关超声筛查报告，近似检出率如下。

　– 所有大的异常：37%。

　– 中枢神经系统：84%。

– 脐膨出和腹裂：80%。

– 呼吸系统：75%。

– 大的心脏异常：63%（所有心脏异常的检出率＜50%）。

– 生殖器：58%。

– 膈疝：38%。

– 胃肠道：31%。

– 肾脏和泌尿道：31%。

– 肌肉骨骼系统：26%。

– 面裂：22%

- Offering the woman an anatomical survey which seeks to confirm a normal appearance in a number of organ systems listed next. The success at identifying structural abnormalities in these systems at about 20 weeks varies, and the approximate rates of detection with US reported in 2009 are:
  – All major malformations-37%
  – Central nervous system-84%
  – Exomphalos and gastroschisis-80%
  – Respiratory-75%
  – Major cardiac abnormalities-63% (all cardiac abnormalities have a detection rate of <50%)
  – Genitalia-58%
  – Diaphragmatic hernia-38%
  – Gastrointestinal-31%
  – Kidneys and urinary tract-31%
  – Musculoskeletal-26%
  – Facial clefts-22%

4. 生化（Biochemistry）

为孕 11^{+0} 周至 13^{+6} 周的孕妇提供胎儿非整倍体联合筛查。大多数医院的此项筛查内容包括评估 21 三体综合征风险，即 NT 测量（增厚）、孕妇年龄（年龄越大风险越高），以及 21 三体综合征时游离 β– 人绒毛膜促性腺激素（β-human chorionic gonadotrophin，β-hCG）升高和妊娠相关血浆蛋白 A（pregnancy-associated plasma protein A，PAPP-A）降低的孕妇血清标志物。对于上述三个参数中的每一个参数，基于孕妇年龄背景风险，在储存超过 200 000 已知 21 三体综合征胎儿妊娠数据库中计算出 21 三体综合征胎儿的似然比，将三个似然比合并

为一个风险值提供给每位孕妇，以 1 ∶ 150 为 21 三体综合征风险阈值的检出率为 90%，假阳性率为 5%。

Women should be offered combined fetal aneuploidy screening between $11w^{+0}$d and $13w^{+6}$d. In most centres, this comprises a risk estimate for trisomy 21 based on NT measurement (increased in trisomy 21), maternal age (increased chance of trisomy 21 with higher age) and maternal serum markers (free β-human chorionic gonadotrophin (β-hCG), which is higher with trisomy 21, and pregnancy-associated plasma protein A (PAPP-A), which is lower with trisomy 21). For each of these three parameters, the likelihood of a trisomy 21 fetus, given the background risk from the woman's age, is calculated against a database of over 200,000 pregnancies with known fetal trisomy 21 status. The three likelihood ratios can be merged into a single risk for the individual woman. Using a risk cut-off of 1:150 for trisomy 21, this screening approach has a detection rate of 90%, for a 5% false-positive rate.

该联合检查还可确定 90% 以上的其他染色体异常，其中包括 18 三体、13 三体、Turner 综合征和三倍体。增厚的 NT 即使核型正常也提示大的心脏缺陷及其他结构异常风险增高，罕见的遗传综合征和其他不可预测的结果。

This combined testing also identifies over 90% of other chromosomal abnormalities, including trisomies 18 and 13, Turner's syndrome and triploidy. Increased NT with a normal karyotype is at increased risk for major cardiac defects as well as other structural anomalies, rare genetic syndromes and other unfavourable outcomes.

如果 NT 和（或）联合检查提示高风险，则应对胎儿进行更为详尽的超声检查和染色体核型分析。

If the NT and/or the combined testing indicates a high risk, more detailed ultrasonic examination of the fetus should be undertaken and karyotyping offered.

如果 NT 增厚而核型正常，且孕 11^{+0} 周至 13^{+6} 周的超声检查也显示正常，建议分别在孕 14～16 周和 20～22 周进行重复超声检查以排除异常。胎儿异常的检出率取决于所涉及器官系统、超声医师的经验以及母亲的体质量指数（body mass index，BMI）。

If the NT is raised but the karyotype is normal and the 11^{+0} to 13^{+6} week anomaly scan is apparently normal, it is advisable to repeat the anomaly scan at 14–16 weeks and again at 20–22 weeks to exclude anomalies. Detection rates for fetal anomalies are dependent on the organ system involved, sonographer experience and the mother's body mass index (BMI).

尽管非整倍体筛查最好是在孕早期采取联合筛查进行（见前述），不过，如果孕早期未进行此项筛

查，则应在孕 14～17 周内为孕妇提供替代性的联合筛查，检测内容包括产妇年龄以及"四重检查"（β-hCG、游离雌三醇（unconjugated oestriol，uE3）、MSAFP 和抑制素 A）。考虑孕妇年龄背景风险，计算出 21 三体综合征胎儿的似然比，并将其合并为一个风险评估值给每个孕妇。此项孕中期筛查不如孕早期筛查，采用 1：150 风险阈值的检出率为 65%，假阳性率为 5%。如果综合风险增高，将进行核型分析。

Whilst aneuploidy screening is best performed by combined screening in the first trimester (see earlier), when this has not taken place, women should be offered an alternative combination screening test at 14–17 weeks comprising maternal age and the 'quadruple test' (β-hCG, unconjugated oestriol (uE3), MSAFP and inhibin-A). Again, individual likelihood ratios for a trisomy 21 fetus are calculated for each (given the background risk from the woman's age) and combined into a single risk estimate. This second-trimester screening test does not 'perform' as well as the firsttrimester test, having a detection rate (using a 1:150 risk threshold) of 65%, for a 5% false-positive rate. If the combined risk is raised, women should be offered karyotyping.

英国国家疾病筛查委员会的推荐是 21 三体风险阈值大于 1：150 则为"高"风险，应当和孕妇及其伴侣讨论在孕早期行绒毛取样（chorionic villus sampling，CVS）或孕中期羊膜腔穿刺以进一步评估。实际上，医生们会将风险评估呈现给孕妇本人，以供其自行决定。例如，一位年龄 40 岁的孕妇在孕 16 周进行了四联筛查，提示胎儿患 21 三体的风险为 1：130，而孕妇的背景年龄风险为 1：75，相比之下此风险值是可接受的（表 10-3），尤其是羊膜腔穿刺术存在 1：100 流产风险的情况下（见后述）。相反，一名 20 岁孕妇分娩 21 三体婴儿的风险值大于 1：1500（表 10-2），认为 1：180 的孕早期风险评估值过高，需要进行侵入性检查（CVS，见后述）。

The recommendation from the UK National Screening Committee is that a trisomy 21 risk of greater than 1:150 indicates a 'high' risk and that further assessment in the form of chorionic villus sampling (CVS) in the first trimester or amniocentesis in the second trimester should be discussed with the woman and her partner. In practice, many prefer to present the risk estimate to the woman and allow her to make her own decision. For example, a woman aged 40 years who has a trisomy 21 risk of 1 in 130 from a quadruple test undertaken at 16 weeks may consider that to be an acceptable risk compared to her background age risk of 1:75 at that stage of pregnancy (see Table 10.3), especially when there is a risk of 1:100 of losing the pregnancy from an amniocentesis (see later).

Conversely, a woman aged 20 years with a background risk of delivering a baby with trisomy 21 of over 1:1500 (see Table 10.2) may consider a 1:180 risk estimate in the first trimester to be too high and might want an invasive test (CVS, see later).

5. 非侵入性产前检查和诊断（Non-invasive prenatal testing and diagnosis (NIPT and NIPD)）

NIPT 和 NIPD 利用孕妇外周血样进行产前检查。

NIPT and NIPD allow women to have prenatal testing using a peripheral maternal blood sample.

尽管应用程度不一，这些技术已开始纳入临床实践，这项工作基于少量胎儿 DNA 通过胎盘循环进入到母体血中，提取和分析细胞游离胎儿 DNA（cell-free fetal DNA，cffDNA）的技术。cffDNA 在产后 1h 内就会被母体循环所清除，因此此项技术仅限于孕期。

These techniques are starting to be incorporated into clinical practice, though the degree they are used varies. They work on the basis that small quantities of fetal DNA derived from placental tissue circulate as cell-free fetal DNA (cffDNA) in the maternal plasma during pregnancy. Techniques have been developed to extract and analyze this cffDNA. The cffDNA is cleared from the maternal circulation within the first hour after birth, so it is specific to a woman's current pregnancy.

针对非整倍体的 NIPT 已经发展成熟，用于唐氏综合征、Edwards 综合征、Patau 综合征和 Turner 综合征的筛查。该技术对唐氏综合征的检出率近 98%，假阳性率低于 0.5%；对 Edwards 综合征（18 三体）和 Patau 综合征（13 三体）的敏感度稍差，因而检出率较低。不过，NIPT 仍可用作筛查检测手段，得到阳性结果后需要进行侵入性诊断检测（CVS 或羊膜腔穿刺术）以确认诊断。这项技术的价值在于很低的假阳性率，由此减少侵入性诊断检查的次数，以及由此导致的妊娠丢失风险。在美国，向有较高非整倍体风险的孕妇（无论是年龄因素还是前述的非整倍体联合筛查）推荐 NIPT，但并不作为低风险人群的常规初筛。在英国，该技术应用差异较大，期待推出全国性指南。

NIPT for aneuploidy is well established and can be used as a screening test for DS, Edwards syndrome, Patau syndrome and Turner's syndrome. The technology identifies approximately 98% of cases of DS, with a false-positive rate of less than 0.5%. It is less sensitive for Edwards syndrome (trisomy 18) and Patau syndrome (trisomy 13), with lower detection rates. However, NIPT is still a screening test, and when a positive result is obtained, an invasive diagnostic testing (by CVS or amniocentesis) is required to confirm the diagnosis. Its value is that it has a low false-positive rate and therefore has the potential to reduce the number of invasive diagnostic tests and pregnancy losses resulting from them. In the United States, NIPT is recommended where women have an increased prior risk of aneuploidy (either because of their age or combined aneuploidy screening as described earlier). However, it is not used for routine primary screening in low-risk populations. In the UK, the way in which these tests are used varies; however, national guidance is anticipated.

在临床实践中，目前 NIPD 用于以下情况。

- 已知母亲是严重的 X 性联锁疾病基因携带者时，用于确定婴儿性别。仅在胎儿为男性时才进行侵入性诊断。

- 协助管理存在常染色体隐性遗传性疾病（如先天性肾上腺皮质增生风险）的妊娠。因该病可导致女胎男性化风险，予以孕妇地塞米松。

- 在 Rh 自体免疫和部分其他红细胞抗体疾病确定胎儿基因表型。

In clinical practice, NIPD is currently offered:

- To determine the sex of a baby when the mother is known to be a carrier of a serious X-linked condition. An invasive diagnostic procedure will only be necessary if the fetus is male.

- To aid in the management of pregnancies at risk of the autosomal-recessive condition congenital adrenal hyperplasia. Dexamethasone may be given to women carrying affected female fetuses who are at risk of virilization.

- To determine the fetal genotype in Rhesus disease and some other red cell antibody disorders.

最后，若超声确定有胎儿结构异常，这些技术不能替代侵入性检测。

Finally, these techniques are not an alternative to invasive testing when a fetal structural abnormality is identified on US scan.

6. 超声和生化检测前咨询（ Counselling in advance of US and biochemical testing ）

孕妇在接受检测胎儿异常的任何筛查项目之前，有必要进行适当的筛查前咨询，应涵盖以下内容。

- 强调绝大多数新生婴儿是很正常的，异常的仅占很小一部分。

- 保证理解筛查项目涉及的内容。

- 了解项目如下。

  - 筛查项目的局限性，其中包括漏检异常的概率。

  - 筛查检测为"正常"或"阴性"的含义是什么。

  - 筛查结果为"异常"或"阳性"的含义是什么。

  - 若筛查结果为"异常"或"阳性"，实际的选择是什么。

Before a woman participates in any screening programme aimed at detecting fetal abnormalities, it is imperative that she has appropriate pre-test counselling. This should cover the following:

- emphasizing that the great majority of newborn babies are normal and that only a very small minority have an abnormality

- ensuring an understanding of the condition(s) that might be detected with the screening programme

- understanding:
  - the limitations of the screening programme, including the chances of missing an abnormality
  - what a 'normal' or 'negative' screening test means
  - what an 'abnormal' or 'positive' screening test means
  - what are the practical options if the screening test is 'abnormal' or 'positive'

（二）"异常"或"阳性"筛查结果的管理选择 (Management options with an 'abnormal' or 'positive' test)

1. 进一步咨询（ Further counselling ）

检测结果为异常 / 阳性的孕妇（及其伴侣）应尽可能接受专业的咨询和管理服务，其中包括关注胎儿问题的产科医生或胎儿医学专家。优先为孕妇及其伴侣提供非指令性咨询，包括如下内容。

- 他们被告知什么内容。

- 他们对检测结果为异常 / 阳性含义的理解。

- 检测结果为异常 / 阳性的实际含义是什么。

- 有哪些选择。

Women (with their partner) with an abnormal/positive test should be seen as soon as possible by a health professional with the appropriate expertise and training for ongoing counselling and management. This will either be an obstetrician with a special interest in fetal problems or a fetal medicine subspecialist. The priority is for the woman and her partner to have non-directive counselling covering:

- what they have been told
- what they think the abnormal/positive test means
- what the abnormal/positive test actually means
- what the options are

2. 进一步评估（Further assessment）

对于检测呈异常/阳性的夫妇而言，应考虑接受进一步评估。

- 对于染色体异常风险增加的孕妇，提供侵入性检查，其中包括孕早期绒毛活检/取样（图 10–8）或孕中期羊膜腔穿刺术（图 10–9）。操作前，孕妇应该知晓操作是无菌的，检查将提供染色体数目和结构的信息，但存在流产的风险（约为 1%）。

It may be appropriate for the couple to consider further assessment in the form of:

- For women with an increased risk of a chromosomal abnormality, an invasive test such as a chorionic villus biopsy/sampling (Fig. 10.8) if the woman presents in the first trimester or an amniocentesis (Fig. 10.9) if the woman presents in the second trimester. Before undertaking the procedure, the woman should be informed that it is undertaken aseptically and will provide information about chromosome number and structure but that it carries a risk of miscarriage (about 1%).

- 对于疑有胎儿结构异常的孕妇，需要进一步的影像检查明确诊断，1～2 周后再次超声检查（胎儿生长，以便更好地看清其解剖），或者进行核磁共振成像（magnetic resonance imaging，MRI）扫描（特别适用于中枢神经系统异常）。如果解剖显示胎儿有染色体异常，应进行绒毛取样（此妊娠阶段更准确的术语为胎盘活检）或羊膜腔穿刺术。

- For women suspected to have a structural fetal abnormality, further imaging to clarify the diagnosis either in the form of further US examinations after 1–2 weeks (to allow for fetal growth and better visualization of fetal anatomy) or a magnetic resonance imaging (MRI) scan (especially useful with abnormalities of the central nervous system). If the anatomical appearances suggest that the fetus has a chromosomal abnormality, a CVS (which is more accurately termed *placental*

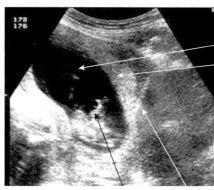

羊水
Amniotic fluid

Chorionic plate
(early placenta)
绒毛膜板
（早期胎盘）

Fetus　Needle in chorionic plate
胎儿　在绒毛膜板的针

▲ 图 10–8　绒毛取样（要求超声可视化，操作类似于羊膜穿刺术；图 10–9A）

Fig. 10.8　Chorionic villus sampling (ultrasound visualization is mandatory and undertaken in a similar way to that shown for amniocentesis; see Fig 10.9A).

biopsy at this stage of pregnancy) or amniocentesis could be offered.

3. 妊娠选择（Options for pregnancy）

一旦诊断有胎儿异常导致死亡或严重残疾的概率很大，在接受咨询后，有的父母认为不希望继续妊娠，选择终止妊娠；但是，有的父母可能会决定继续妊娠。决定是由父母而非他人做出，因此需要"非指令性"咨询。

Once a fetal abnormality is diagnosed with a high chance of death or serious disability, after counselling, the parents may feel that they do not wish to continue with the pregnancy and opt for a termination. However, faced with the same facts, other parents may decide to continue with the pregnancy. The decision is for the parents to make and no one else, hence the need for 'non-directive' counselling.

4. 可能的干预措施（Possible interventions）

对于某些胎儿异常问题，可为孕妇及其伴侣提供改善胎儿状况的干预措施。具体如下。

- 孕妇服用抗心律不齐类药物以治疗胎儿心律不齐。

- 针对尿道瓣膜疾病，将膀胱引流管插入胎儿膀胱以绕过尿道阻塞，预防后续的肾后压和损害。

With some fetal abnormalities, a woman and her partner may be offered interventions aimed at improving or ameliorating the fetal condition. Examples include:

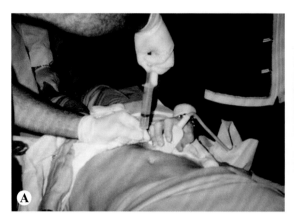 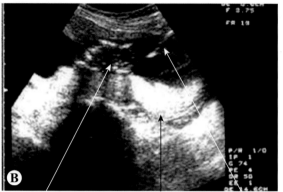

Fetus (transverse section)　Posterior placenta　Needle in amniotic fluid
胎儿（横切面）　　　　　后壁胎盘　　　　羊水里的针

▲ 图 10-9　羊膜腔穿刺术

A. 同步超声可视；B. 显示穿刺针的超声图像（箭）[A 经许可转载，引自 Chabner D-E. (2017) The Language of Medicine, 11th edn. Elsevier, St Louis.]

Fig. 10.9　Amniocentesis.

(A) Simultaneous ultrasound (US) visualization. (B) US image with needle *(arrows)*. (A Reproduced with permission from Chabner D-E. (2017) The Language of Medicine, 11th edn. Elsevier, St Louis.)

- Maternally administered anti-arrhythmic drugs to treat fetal cardiac arrhythmias.
- Insertion of a vesicoamniotic drain into the fetal bladder to by-pass urethral obstruction in cases of urethral valves to prevent further renal back-pressure and damage.

5. 孕期监测（Surveillance in pregnancy）

所有查出胎儿存在异常但又决定继续妊娠的孕妇均需定期接受专业支持和咨询，此类支持与咨询由少部分知悉该诊断的健康专业人士提供。在特定情况下，有必要定期进行超声检查，以评估异常引起的并发症是否需要干预（见前述）。

All women who decide to continue with the pregnancy with a fetal abnormality will need to be seen regularly for support and counselling by a small number of health professionals who are aware of the diagnosis. In specific cases, there will be a need to undertake regular US examinations to assess whether complications of the abnormality are developing and warrant intervention (see earlier).

6. 分娩问题（Delivery issues）

分娩问题如下。

- 分娩之前，基于婴儿出生后可能的资源需求，如新生儿重症监护或外科手术决定分娩地点，并安排相关的新生儿医护专业人员与父母沟通。
- 为保证完善的新生儿管理资源，工作日分娩

更可行。

- 对于某些异常的胎儿，如受损风险高的脑积水胎儿，最好避免阴道分娩。

Delivery issues may include:

- In advance of the delivery deciding on the place of birth based on the baby's likely need of resources after birth, e.g. neonatal intensive care or surgery, and arranging for the relevant neonatal medical professionals to meet the parents.
- Arranging elective delivery if it is considered desirable that the baby would benefit from delivery during the working day and week when full neonatal resources are available.
- With some fetal abnormalities, it is preferable to avoid a vaginal birth, e.g. where there may be a greater risk of fetal trauma, such as in a case of fetal hydrocephalus.

六、正常胎儿的健康评估（Assessing the health of a normally formed fetus）

（一）胎儿健康筛查（Screening for fetal health）

经验

相对于为孕妇提供的用于评估胎儿异常风险的筛查，用于确定不健康胎儿的方法是有限的。

In contrast to the screening offered to pregnant women to assess their risk of fetal abnormality, what is offered to identify the unhealthy fetus is limited.

首先依赖于确定高危胎儿窘迫的临床风险因素，对于没有胎儿窘迫风险因素（"低风险"）的孕妇。

- 母亲对妊娠后半期的胎动保持警觉。

- 每次产检时进行宫高测量，即耻骨联合与子宫底的距离（图 6-12），测量时将卷尺翻转为空白，测量后翻转卷尺读数（cm）。孕 16～36 周的宫高正常范围为孕周 ±3cm，因此，孕 32 周的正常范围为 32±3cm。

It relies initially on identification of clinical risk factors associated with a greater risk of fetal compromise. Women with no risk factors for fetal compromise ('low risk') have:

- Maternal vigilance for fetal activity over the second half of pregnancy.

- Fundal height measurement at every antenatal clinic visit. This involves measuring the distance between the maternal symphysis pubis and uterine fundus (see Fig. 6.12). The reverse blank side of tape measure uppermost and the distance (in cm) is read after it has been determined by turning the tape measure over. The normal range between 16 and 36 weeks is gestational age in weeks ±3 cm. Thus at 32 weeks the normal range is 32 ± 3 cm.

- 每次产检时进行胎心听诊。胎心听诊可使用 Pinard 听诊器（图 10-10A）或手持式 Doppler 超声设备（图 10-10B）。常规操作中并不记录心率，而只是记录胎儿心脏在搏动。因此，可能会漏诊胎心率基线异常。

- Auscultation of the fetal heart at every antenatal

clinic visit. This is undertaken either using a Pinard stethoscope (Fig. 10.10A) or a handheld Doppler US device (Fig. 10.10B). In routine practice, the rate is not recorded but just a note that the fetal heart is beating. Thus, abnormalities of the fetal baseline heart rate may be missed.

存在危险因素的孕妇（"高风险"）根据假定的潜在病理生理过程而决定个性化监测。更多常见示例见表 10-4。

Women with risk factors ('high risk') have customized surveillance that is determined by the presumed underlying pathophysiological process. The more common examples are shown in Table 10.4.

（二）高危妊娠胎儿健康监测（Surveillance of fetal health in at-risk pregnancies）

基于临床风险评估筛查结果（见前述），将为"高危"孕妇提供孕期个性化的胎儿监护方案。在此讨论最常用的方法。

Based on the clinical risk assessment screening (see earlier), an individualized programme of fetal surveillance will be offered to 'at-risk' women during their pregnancy. The most commonly used methods are discussed here.

1. 胎儿多普勒记录（Fetal Doppler recordings）

在未发现胎儿异常的情况下，胎儿多普勒记录目前是评估"高危"妊娠胎儿健康的最佳工具。

Fetal Doppler recordings are currently the best tools for fetal assessment in 'at-risk' pregnancies in the absence of fetal abnormality.

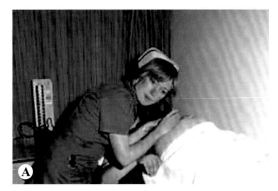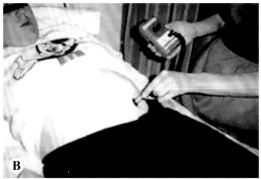

▲ 图 10-10　胎心脏听诊（将听诊器 / 传感器尽可能靠近胎儿心脏。如果胎儿背部在前，最佳听诊位则位于胎儿左肩胛骨上方。如果胎儿背部在后，最佳听诊位则位于孕妇肚脐周围

A. 使用 Pinard 听诊器；B. 使用手持式多普勒超声记录仪

Fig.10.10　Auscultation of the fetal heart (the aim is to place the stethoscope/transducer as close to the fetal heart as possible. If the fetal back is anterior, the best site is over the left fetal scapula. If the fetal back is posterior, the best site is around the maternal umbilicus.

(A) Using the Pinard stethoscope; (B) using a handheld Doppler ultrasound recording device.

表 10-4 胎儿窘迫的危险因素

Table 10.4 Risk factors for fetal compromise

危险类型 Type of risk	危险因素 / 问题 Risk factor/problem	假定的病理生理 Presumed pathophysiology	监测措施 Surveillance
	母体血管疾病，如高血压（已有高血压、严重的妊娠期高血压疾病、先兆子痫）、抗磷脂抗体狼疮抗体和肾病 Maternal vascular disease, e.g. hypertension (pre-existing, severe pregnancy-induced hypertension, pre-eclampsia), antiphospholipid or lupus antibodies, renal impairment	子宫胎盘血管疾病（uteroplacental vascular disease, UPVD），即供给胎盘及胎盘内血供不足，气体交换和营养交换下降 Uteroplacental vascular disease (UPVD), i.e. poor blood flow to and within the placenta with associated reduced gaseous and nutritional transfer	孕妇对胎动保持警惕 Maternal vigilance for fetal movements 脐动脉（umbilical artery, UA）多普勒记录；若不正常，则记录大脑中动脉和静脉导管（ductus venosus, DV）多普勒 Umbilical artery (UA) Doppler recordings; if this is abnormal, record middle cerebral artery (MCA) and ductus venosus (DV) Doppler 超声监测胎儿发育 US monitoring of fetal growth 若发现任何异常，则进行生物物理学评分 Biophysical assessment if any of these not normal
特异性 Specific	孕妇患有糖尿病，尤其是有血管病变者 Maternal diabetes, especially if associated with vascular disease	不确定的胎儿病理生理风险 The pathophysiology of fetal risk is uncertain	患有子宫胎盘血管疾病的孕妇用相同的监测，但在预测胎儿死亡方面的效果较差 The same package of surveillance is used as in women with UPVD, but it is less effective at predicting fetal death
	双胎 Twins	主要风险有： 对于所有双胎：因子宫胎盘血管疾病而胎儿生长受限 For all twins: fetal growth restriction from UPVD 对于单绒毛膜双胎（除上述风险之外）：双胎输血综合征（twin-twin transfusion syndrome, TTTS），即共享胎盘循环，其中一个胎儿成为"供体"，而另一个则成为"受体" For monochorionic twins (in addition): the twin-twin transfusion syndrome (TTTS), i.e. shared placental circulation with risk of one fetus being the 'donor' and the other being the 'recipient'	对于胎儿生长受限： For fetal growth restriction: • 有子宫胎盘血管疾病的高危孕妇进行胎儿监测（见前） • Fetal surveillance as in women at risk of UPVD (see earlier) 对于双胎输血综合征，监测单绒毛膜双胎的输血综合征征兆： For TTTS, monitoring of monochorionic twins to look for signs of TTTS: • 一胎（受体）的羊水量（Amniotic fluid volume, AFV）增加，而另一胎（供体）的羊水量减少 • Amniotic fluid volume (AFV) raised in one twin (recipient) and reduced in the other (donor) • 胎儿膀胱无尿 • Absence of urine in fetal bladders • 任一胎儿的脐动脉多普勒记录异常 • Abnormal umbilical artery Doppler recording in either fetus

（续表）

危险类型 Type of risk	危险因素 / 问题 Risk factor/problem	假定的病理生理 Presumed pathophysiology	监测措施 Surveillance
特异性 Specific	Rh 抗体引起的同种免疫 Isoimmunization due to Rhesus antibodies	经胎盘途径的母源抗体（抗 D 或抗 Kell 或抗 Duffy）导致胎儿重度贫血 Transplacental passage of maternal antibodies (anti-D or Kell or Duffy) causing severe fetal anaemia	胎儿重度贫血情况下，胎儿大脑中动脉多普勒血流量增加，经胎儿血液采样（fetal blood sampling，FBS）确认 With severe fetal anaemia, the fetal MCA Doppler recording of blood flow is raised and confirmed by fetal blood sampling (FBS)
	死胎史		
	胎儿生长受限史 Previous fetal growth restriction		
	母亲或父亲出生时为小于胎龄儿 Mother or father was small for gestational age when born		
	PAPP-A <0.4 MoM（孕早期非整倍体生化筛查检测） PAPP-A <0.4 MoM (a firsttrimester biochemical aneuploidy screening test)		对高危子宫胎盘血管疾病孕妇的胎儿监测（见前）
	孕妇感觉胎动减少 Maternal perception of reduced fetal movements	多种病理会导致胎儿死亡，胎儿生长受限，胎动减少，阴道出血和腹痛。除非已知原因，初步判定是子宫胎盘血管疾病 A variety of pathologies result in fetal death, fetal growth restriction, reduced movements, vaginal bleed and abdominal pain. Unless the cause is known, the normal approach initially is to assume it is UPVD	对于胎动（fetal movement，FM）减少的孕妇，持续监测到胎动恢复正常
	阴道出血 Vaginal bleeding		对于阴道出血或腹痛的孕妇，在症状持续的情况下需要持续监测
	腹痛 Abdominal pain Previous fetal death		Fetal surveillance as in women at risk of UPVD (see earlier)
非特异性主要危险因素 Non-specific major risk factors			In women with reduced fetal movement (FM), ongoing surveillance is only needed where the FM does not return to normal
	其他：孕妇年龄>40 岁，吸烟>10 支／天，使用可卡因 Others: maternal age >40 yr, smoking >10/day, cocaine use		In women with vaginal bleeding or abdominal pain, ongoing surveillance is needed only where the symptoms persist

249

（续表）

危险类型 Type of risk	危险因素 / 问题 Risk factor/problem	假定的病理生理 Presumed pathophysiology	监测措施 Surveillance
非特异性主要危险因素 Non-specific major risk factors	通过耻骨联合与子宫底间高度图表确定异常子宫大小和（或）生长（大于或小于正常） Abnormal uterine size and/or growth (larger or smaller than normal) identified from abnormal symphysiofundal height charts/graphs	多数为临床怀疑胎儿发育异常未被超声检查证实。如果得到证实，胎儿生长受限则可能由多种病理导致。除非已知原因，否则，初步判定为子宫胎盘血管疾病 Many cases of clinically suspected abnormal fetal growth are not confirmed with US. If confirmed, a variety of pathologies result in fetal growth restriction. Unless cause is known, the normal approach is to assume it is UPVD	在高危子宫胎盘血管疾病的孕妇超声测量确定胎儿大小 / 生长异常（见前述） If abnormal fetal size/growth confirmed with US fetal assessment as in women at risk of UPVD (see earlier)
非特异性次要风险因素；三个或更多风险因素视为孕 20—24 周进行子宫动脉多普勒检查的指征 Non-specific minor risk factors; three or more are considered an indication for uterine artery Doppler at 20-24 wk	孕妇年龄 35—39 岁 Maternal age 35–39 未产妇 Nulliparity BMI<20 或 >30 BMI <20 or 30 or more 吸烟小于或等于 10 支 / 天 Smoking <=10/day 体外受精（invitro fertilization, IVF）单胎妊娠 Invitro fertilization (IVF) singleton pregnancy 先兆子痫史 Previous pre-eclampsia	这些导致胎儿生长受限的次要风险因素假定为子宫胎盘血管疾病 These are minor risk factors for fetal growth restriction presumed to be due to UPVD	妊娠 20—24 周进行子宫动脉 Doppler 检查，对高危子宫胎盘血管疾病孕妇，若异常常需要详细的超声胎儿评估（见前） Uterine artery Doppler at 20–24 wk-if abnormal for detailed US fetal assessment as in women at risk of UPVD (see earlier)

2. 脐动脉（umbilical artery，UA）血流多普勒记录（Doppler recordings of blood flow in the umbilical artery (UA)）

这项检查显著改善高危妊娠胎儿结局。图 10-11A 显示 1 例正常记录。

This investigation has been shown to significantly improve fetal outcome in high-risk pregnancies. Figure 10.11A shows a normal recording.

图 10-11B 显示了一例"舒张末期血流缺失"（absent end-diastolic flow，AEDV）的病例。最常见的解释是胎盘血管阻力增大（记录起点的"下游"），是典型的脐带胎盘血管疾病（umbilical placental vascular disease，UPVD）。AEDV 的胎儿预后较差，发育受限、缺氧和死亡均较为常见。不过，通常情况下，上述危险并非突发，管理选择包括连续的生物物理试验监测直至可存活的胎龄，或出现生物物理试验异常，如果这种异常情况发生在孕 34 周或以上孕周，多数医生会建议孕妇择期早产分娩（产前使用类固醇药物提高胎儿的肺成熟度），而不是继续妊娠面临胎儿死亡的可能。AEDV 出现前先表现为舒张压逐渐下降 [导致收缩压与舒张压比值（systolic to diastolic，S/D）升高]。收缩压与舒张压比值升高可视为疾病的较轻和较早阶段，存在产生最终不良后果的风险相同。

Figure 10.11B shows an example of 'absent end-diastolic flow' (AEDV). The commonest explanation is an increase in placental vascular resistance ('downstream' from the point of recording), which is typical of umbilical placental vascular disease (UPVD). The prognosis for the fetus with AEDV is worse, with growth restriction, hypoxia and death all being commoner. However, the risk is not usually immediate, and management options include continued close surveillance with biophysical testing until a viable gestational age is reached or the biophysical testing is abnormal. If this abnormality occurs at 34 weeks or beyond, most would offer the woman elective pre-term delivery (with pre-delivery maternal steroids to enhance fetal lung maturation) rather than continuing the pregnancy and the possibility of fetal death. The appearance of AEDV is preceded by the gradual reduction in the diastolic recording (and associated increase in 'systolic to diastolic (S/D) ratio'). A raised S/D ratio can be considered a milder and earlier stage of the same pathology with the same risk of eventual adverse outcome.

图 10-11C 显示了 1 例"逆向舒张期血流"的病例。这是一个更需要警惕的特征，与胎儿立即死亡有非常高的相关性。处理方案取决于孕龄，如果孕

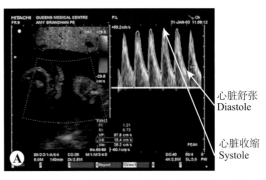
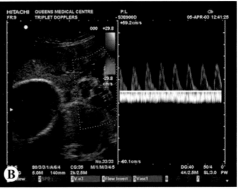
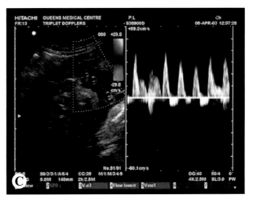

心脏舒张 Diastole
心脏收缩 Systole

▲ 图 10-11　脐动脉血流的多普勒超声记录

A. 正常。注意左侧超声图像显示脐动脉，红色和蓝色表示血流。右侧超声图像为脐动脉的多普勒记录。波峰、波谷分别表示胎儿心动周期的收缩期峰值和舒张期。在正常的胎儿胎盘循环中，心脏不收缩时，也一直存在前向血流，这是因为胎盘循环内的低阻力。B. 异常：舒张末期血流缺失。注意，在多数心动周期中，舒张期没有前向血流。C. 异常：舒张期血流逆向。注意，收缩期脐动脉中有前向血液流动，但舒张期血液流动是反向

Fig. 10.11　Doppler ultrasound (US) recording of umbilical artery blood flow.

(A) Normal. Note: The left US image shows the umbilical artery (UA) with red and blue colours indicating blood flow. The right US image is the Doppler recording taken from that UA. The peak of the wave represents the peak of the systolic phase and the trough the diastolic phase of the fetal cardiac cycle, respectively. In the normal fetoplacental circulation, there is always forward flow even when the heart is not contracting because there is a low resistance to flow within the placental circulation. (B) Abnormal-absent end diastolic flow. Note: There is no forward flow during diastole for most of the cardiac cycles. (C) Abnormal-reversed diastolic flow. Note: There is forward flow of blood in the UA during systole but the direction of flow reverses in diastole.

期达到 26 周或以上，则须与胎儿父母讨论是选择择期早产（面临早产儿的相关风险）还是继续妊娠（胎儿死亡的高风险）。如果孕周不到 26 周，这种讨论更困难，父母可能会选择不干预。

Figure 10.11C shows an example of 'reversed diastolic flow'. This is an even more ominous feature and is associated with a much higher chance of imminent fetal death. Management will depend on gestational age. If the pregnancy is at 26 weeks or more, elective pre-term delivery (with the attendant risks of prematurity) compared with continuing the pregnancy (and the high risk of fetal death) must be discussed with the parents. If the pregnancy is less than 26 weeks, the discussions are more difficult and the parents may opt for no intervention.

3. 胎儿大脑中动脉（middle cerebral artery, MCA）血流多普勒记录（图 10–12）（Doppler recordings of blood flow in the fetal middle cerebral artery (MCA) (Fig. 10.12)）

超声多普勒检查记录的异常血流类型可能与胎儿血流的重新分配较多的氧到重要器官如大脑和心脏有关，从而达到"大脑保护"效果，通过降低胎儿大脑中动脉血流阻力及增加收缩压值实现。这是妊娠晚期与脐带胎盘血管疾病有关的非对称性胎儿生长受限（fetal growth restriction, FGR），即胎儿头部发育保持正常而身体其他部位的生长受到限制（见后述）。

An abnormal flow pattern in the UA Doppler may be associated with redistribution of blood flow in the fetus to allow better oxygenation to vital organs such as the brain and heart, leading to the 'brain-sparing' effect. This is demonstrated by a reduced resistance to blood flow in the MCA and an increase in systolic values. This is the reason for asymmetrical fetal growth restriction (FGR) being associated with UPVD in late pregnancy where head growth can remain normal whilst growth of the rest of the body can be restricted (see later).

MCA 还作为评估胎儿贫血程度的非侵入性方法，最常用于患有 Rh 同种免疫疾病的孕妇（孕妇是 Rh 阴性，她们产生的抗 D 抗体穿过胎盘，导致 Rh 阳性胎儿发生溶血性贫血）。此类情形下，胎儿贫血的超声证据有助于选择侵入性胎儿检测和胎儿输血的最佳时机（图 10–13）。

The MCA also can be used as a non-invasive method of assessing the degree of fetal anaemia. This is most commonly used in women with Rhesus disease (where the women are Rhesus-negative and they are producing anti-D antibodies that can cross the placenta causing a haemolytic anaemia in a Rhesus-positive fetus). In those cases, US evidence of fetal anaemia allows optimization of the timing of invasive fetal testing and fetal blood transfusion (Fig. 10.13).

4. 胎儿静脉导管（ductus venosus, DV）血流多普勒记录（图 10–14）（Doppler recordings of blood flow in the fetal ductus venosus (DV) (Fig. 10.14)）

胎儿体内血流的重新分配与子宫胎盘血管疾病相关，原因是右心的后负荷增加导致静脉循环阻力增大，以及胎儿酸中毒导致的胎儿心肌缺氧，引起心室内压升高。最常用的静脉多普勒仪是静脉导管（DV），四相波形对调节氧气和营养的分配非常重要，"a"波为胎儿心房收缩同步，是用于监测胎儿生长受限的常用参数；随着胎儿生长受限的加剧，不断增加的心脏后负荷会减少右房收缩期间的静脉前向流量，从而导致"a"波波形变深；反向的"a"波意味着心力衰竭和心脏失代偿。脐静脉应有恒定流速的血液流向胎儿，在缺氧的胎儿，脐静脉出现逆向搏动，通常见于一定程度的缺氧，此时 DV 出现反向"a"波。这些发现是死亡前兆，表明必须立即分娩。

This redistribution of blood flow within the fetus in association with UPVD is reflected in higher resistance in venous circulation due to an increasing afterload of the right heart and increasing intraventricular pressure caused by hypoxia of the fetal myocardium correlating with fetal acidosis. The most commonly used venous Doppler is the DV, which is a four-phase waveform that is important in regulating distribution of oxygen and nutrition. The 'a' wave, synonymous with atrial contraction of the fetal heart, is the common parameter used for monitoring in FGR. As FGR progresses, the rising cardiac afterload reduces forward venous flow during right atrial contraction, causing the 'a' wave to become progressively deeper. A reversed 'a' wave signifies heart failure and cardiac decompensation. The umbilical vein should have a constant velocity of flow to the fetus. In a compromised fetus, there may be retrograde pulsatility in the umbilical vein, which is commonly seen at the same degree of compromise when there is reversed 'a' wave in the DV. These findings are pre-terminal, indicating a need for immediate delivery.

5. 母体子宫动脉内血流（图 10–15）多普勒记录（Doppler recordings of blood flow in the maternal uterine artery (Fig. 10.15)）

子宫动脉多普勒记录是胎盘功能的生物物理标志。在孕早期和孕中期胎盘受损出现的胎盘血管不正常的血流和阻力 [表现为 S/D 比值升高和（或）子宫动脉波形的"凹痕"]，与孕妇胎儿并发症如早发的子痫前期和 FGR 有关。总部位于伦敦的英国

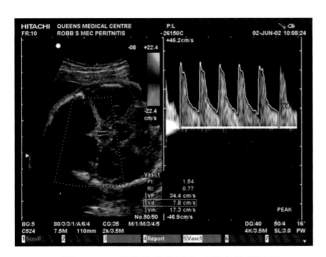

▲ 图 10-12　正常胎儿大脑中动脉多普勒波形

Fig. 10.12　Normal fetal middle cerebral artery Doppler waveforms.

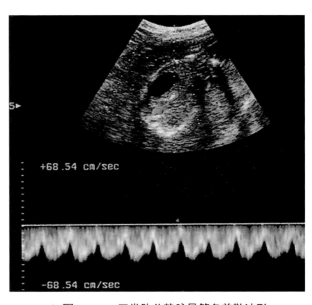

▲ 图 10-14　正常胎儿静脉导管多普勒波形

Fig. 10.14　Normal fetal ductus venosus Doppler waveforms.

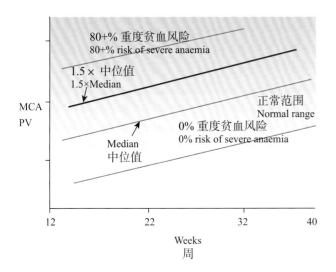

▲ 图 10-13　大脑中动脉的收缩期峰值血流可预测胎儿贫血

绿线表示正常范围和中值；红色实线表示（1.5×中位值）的阈值。在胎儿溶血性疾病，低于该阈值的胎儿没有重度贫血，而高于该阈值的胎儿 80% 风险患有重度贫血，需要子宫内输血。MCA. 大脑中动脉；PV. 峰值流速

Fig. 10.13　Peak systolic blood flow in the middle cerebral artery as a predictor of fetal anaemia.

Green lines indicate the normal range and median values; the solid red line indicates the threshold for the [1.5 × median] value. In cases of fetal haemolytic disease, fetuses with values below that line do not have severe anaemia, whilst those fetuses with values above the line have an 80% risk of severe anaemia requiring intrauterine transfusion. MCA, Middle cerebral artery; PV, peak velocity.

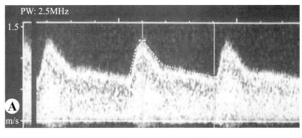

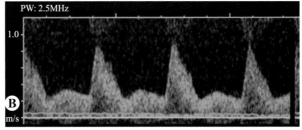

▲ 图 10-15　孕妇子宫动脉多普勒波形

A. 显示子宫动脉正常波形，高容积舒张期血流表明滋养细胞植入成功；B. 显示异常的子宫动脉波形，低容积舒张期血流，凹槽表明滋养细胞植入失败，胎盘阻力增加 [经许可转载，引自 Baschat AA (2011) Fetal growth disorders. In: James DK, Weiner CP, Gonik B, Crowther CA, Robson SC, eds. High Risk Pregnancy: Management Options, 4th edn, Saunders Elsevier, St Louis.]

Fig. 10.15　Maternal uterine artery Doppler waveforms.

The upper image (A) shows a normal uterine artery wave form with high-volume diastolic flow indicating successful trophoblastic implantation. The lower image (B) shows an abnormal uterine artery wave form with low-volume diastolic flow, with notching indicating unsuccessful trophoblastic implantation with increased placental resistance. (Reproduced with permission from Baschat AA (2011) Fetal growth disorders. In: James DK, Weiner CP, Gonik B, Crowther CA, Robson SC, eds. High Risk Pregnancy: Management Options, 4th edn, Saunders Elsevier, St Louis.)

皇家妇产科学会（Royal College of Obstetricians and Gynaecologists，RCOG）是致力于胎儿生长受限风险筛查的学会，会员包括拥有或无医学学位的从业于妇产科的人们，即妊娠、分娩及女性性健康和生殖健康领域。该学会会员多达 16 000 多名，分布于 100 多个国家 / 地区，其中近 50% 的会员居住在不列颠群岛以外的地区。2014 年，RCOG 推荐在高风险人群进行孕 20~24 周的子宫动脉多普勒检查，对预测严重小于胎龄（severely small for gestational age，SGA）者具有中等预测价值；确定有 SGA 的孕妇在分娩时应提供子宫动脉多普勒；在 20~24 周出现异常子宫动脉多普勒的孕妇，应连续超声检查评估胎儿大小和健康，并在孕 26~28 周开始子宫动脉多普勒检查。

Uterine artery Doppler is a biophysical marker of placental function. Impaired placentation with abnormal blood-flow velocity and resistance in the placental vessels (indicated by a rise in the ratio of S/D values and/or 'notching' in the uterine artery waveform) in the first and second trimesters is associated with maternal fetal complications such as early-onset pre-eclampsia and FGR. In screening for fetuses at risk of growth restriction, the Royal College of Obstetricians and Gynaecologists (RCOG) is a professional association based in London. Its members, including people with and without medical degrees, work in the field of obstetrics and gynaecology, that is, pregnancy, childbirth and female sexual and reproductive health. The college has over 16,000 members in over 100 countries with nearly 50% of those residing outside the British Isles. In 2014, the RCOG recommended that in high-risk populations UA Doppler recordings at 20–24 weeks of pregnancy have a moderate predictive value for a severely small for gestational age (SGA) neonate. Women who are identified to have risk factors for delivery of an SGA neonate should be offered uterine artery Doppler. Women with an abnormal uterine artery Doppler at 20–24 weeks should be referred for serial US measurement of fetal size and assessment of wellbeing, with UA Doppler commencing at 26–28 weeks.

6. 胎儿生长（Fetal growth）

孕期连续超声测量头围（head circumference，HC）和腹围（abdominal circumference，AC）是最好的胎儿生长记录。

Fetal growth is best documented in pregnancy using serial US measurements of head (HC) and abdominal (AC) circumferences.

(1) 小胎儿（Small fetuses）

胎儿生长不足有 3 种类型。一旦胎儿的腹围仅达到或低于最低的百分位，则称为小胎儿。

Three patterns of suboptimal fetal growth are recognized. Once the AC is on or below the lowest centile, the fetus is termed *small-for-dates*.

图 10-16A 展示了 1 例先天小胎儿的数据。遗传因素导致这一类型，通常母亲个子比较矮小和（或）亚裔。若为经产妇，她之前的孩子可能也小。即使此类胎儿没有病理性小胎儿的并发症风险高（见后述），但与正常发育胎儿相比，仍有风险。

Figure 10.16A illustrates a constitutionally small fetus. Genetic factors contribute to this pattern. Typically, the mother will be short and/or of Asian ethnicity. If multiparous, her previous baby(ies) may have been small. Whilst this fetus is not at such a high risk of complications as in the pathologically small fetus (see later), those risks are still greater compared to a normally grown fetus.

图 10-16B 和 C 描述了由于病理原因导致的胎儿发育类型，这代表胎儿生长受限谱的不同点。非对称型倾向于发生在妊娠晚期，更常见于孕晚期的子宫胎盘血管疾病；而对称型则倾向于表现为妊娠早期的病理性后果，如胎儿异常和严重的早发型先兆子痫。两种情况均存在胎儿死亡和缺氧、早产和胎盘出血高风险。

Figure 10.16B and C represents fetal growth patterns that are due to a pathological cause. They represent different points on the spectrum of FGR. The asymmetrical type tends to occur later in pregnancy and is more commonly associated with conditions such as UPVD in the last trimester, whereas the symmetrical type tends to represent a pathological insult that operated from an early point in pregnancy, e.g. fetal abnormality and severe early-onset preeclampsia. Both are associated with a higher risk of fetal death and hypoxia, pre-term delivery and placental bleeding.

(2) 巨大儿（Big fetuses）

相对于小胎儿，巨大儿具有以下特点。

- 先天型大（"大于胎龄儿"），其头围和腹围增长曲线均达到高百分位线。通常母亲的个子高和（或）属于非洲 – 加勒比种族。

- 病理学意义上的大（"巨大儿"），头围增长曲线处于百分位的正常范围，但腹围增长曲线显示越过百分位的加速增长，这种发育类型最常见于糖尿病孕妇的胎儿。

In an analogous way to small fetuses, large fetuses can either be:
- Constitutionally large ('large-for-dates') with the HC and AC growth trajectories both following the top

centile line. Typically, the woman would be tall and/or of Afro-Caribbean ethnicity.

- Pathologically large ('macrosomia') with the HC growth trajectory following a centile in the normal range but the AC growth trajectory demonstrates accelerated growth upwards across centiles. This pattern of growth is most commonly seen in fetuses of diabetic women.

7. 羊水量 [Amniotic fluid volume (AFV)]

最准确评估羊水量的方法是超声，有两种方法。

- 单一最大羊水深度（正常范围是 2～8cm）。

- 羊水指数（amniotic fluid index，AFI）系子宫 4 个象限（右上、左上、右下和左下）的各羊

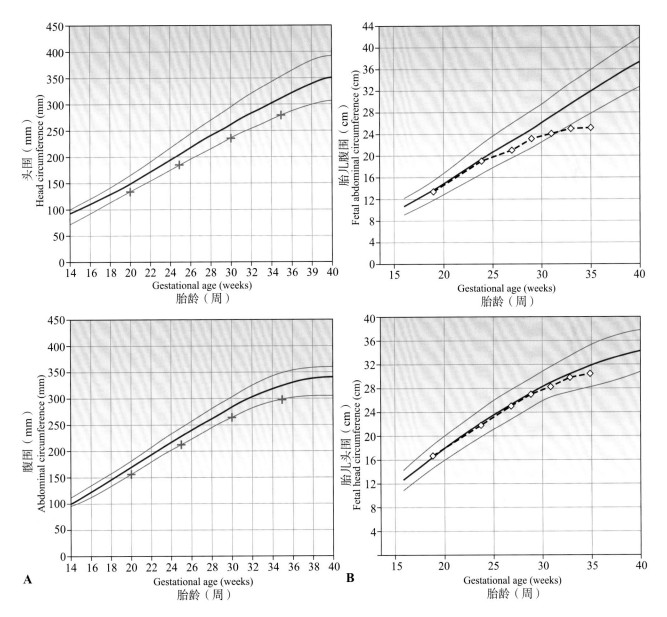

▲ 图 10-16　超声检测的胎儿生长类型

A. 先天性小胎儿。注意，其头围和腹围在最低的增长曲线。B. 非对称型小胎儿。注意，头围增长符合正常曲线，而腹围增长则越过正常曲线并最终落在正常范围外。下方和上方蓝线分别代表正常群体生长的第 5 和第 95 百分位，红线代表第 50 百分位

Fig. 10.16　Fetal growth patterns detected using ultrasound.

(A) Constitutionally small fetus. Note: Both head circumference (HC) and abdominal circumference (AC) follow the lowest growth trajectories. (B) Asymmetrically small fetus. Note: The HC follows a normal trajectory, whilst the AC crosses trajectories and eventually falls outside the normal range. The lower and upper blue lines are the 5th and 95th growth centiles respectively and the red line is the 50th growth centile for the normal population.

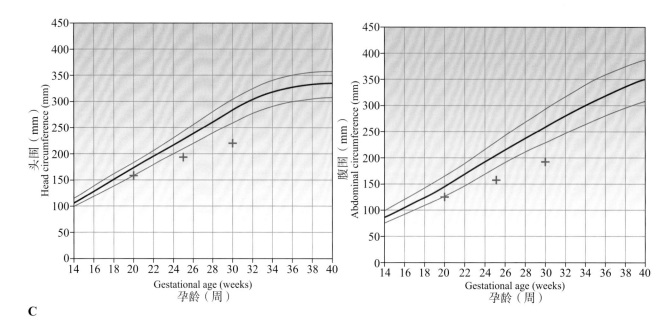

C

▲ 图 10-16（续）　C. 对称型小胎儿。注意，头围和腹围均脱离正常生长轨迹，这种头部发育障碍会增加儿童发育迟缓的可能性

Fig. 10.16, cont'd.　(C) Symmetrically small fetus. Note: Both HC and AC fall away from the normal growth trajectories. Such head growth compromise carries a greater likelihood of developmental delay in childhood.

水池深度的总和。图 10-17 显示了孕期羊水指数的正常范围。

羊水减少和增多的原因在第 4 章讨论。

The most accurate estimate of AFV is with US. Two methods are used:

- Single deepest pocket (the normal range is 2–8 cm).
- Amniotic fluid index (AFI), which is the sum of the depths of the pools of amniotic fluid in each of the four quadrants of the uterus (top right and left and bottom right and left). Figure 10.17 shows the normal range of the AFI during pregnancy.

Causes of reduced and increased amniotic fluid are discussed in Chapter X.

8. 生理物理评分（Biophysical measurements）

胎儿行为是显示其即时健康状态的有用指标。对于多数胎儿病理而言，这些参数受累相对晚于过程。临床实践中使用的 5 个指标如下。

- 胎心率（fetal heart rate，FHR）：用胎心监护仪（cardiotocograph，CTG）记录（如在分娩时）。最长记录时间为 40min，在此时间内，胎心率至少应有 2 次加速，幅度为 15/min 或以上，持续至少 15s。心率变化模式与分娩时相似（见第 11 章），不同之处在于子宫活动微

弱，重点在基线心率的解释。图 10-18 显示胎心基线变化大于 5/min 伴加速，且无减速。图 10-19 显示一例正常的基线心率，但其基线变异降低。

- 胎动：在 40min 的超声观察中，胎儿至少应有 3 次单独 / 不显眼的动作。

- 胎儿张力：这些胎动中至少有一次应体现出一个完整的 90° 屈 – 伸 – 屈周期。

- 胎儿呼吸：在 40min 的观察期内，胎儿应有一个持续 30s 的规律胎儿呼吸动作。

- 羊水量：至少应有一个羊水池垂直深度为 2～8cm。

The behaviour of a fetus is a useful indicator of his or her immediate wellbeing. With most fetal pathologies, these parameters are affected relatively late in the process. The five observations used in practice are:

- Fetal heart rate (FHR): this is recorded with a cardiotocograph (CTG) (as in labour). The maximum recording time is 40 minutes and in that time, there should be at least two accelerations of the FHR by 15 beats/min or more and lasting for at least 15 seconds. The patterns of heart rate change are similar to those described in labour (see Chapter 11), with the difference that uterine activity is minimal and more emphasis is therefore placed on the

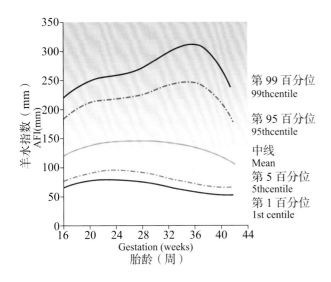

▲ 图 10-17　羊水指数

Fig. 10.17　Amniotic fluid index.

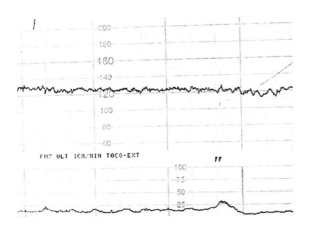

▲ 图 10-19　产前胎心监护显示该心率正常但基线变异减小

Fig. 10.19　Antenatal cardiotocograph showing a normal heart rate but reduced baseline variability.

interpretation of baseline heart rate. An example of a normal antenatal CTG is shown in Figure 10.18. This shows a baseline variability of more than 5 beats/min with accelerations and no decelerations. Figure 10.19 shows a normal baseline rate but reduced baseline variability.

- Fetal movements: there should be at least three separate/discreet movements in 40 minutes of fetal observation with US.
- Fetal tone: at least one of these fetal movements should demonstrate a full 90-degree flexion-extension-flexion cycle.
- Fetal breathing: there should be a sustained 30-second period of regular fetal breathing movements during the 40-minute observation period.
- AFV: there should be at least one vertical pool measuring between 2 and 8 cm.

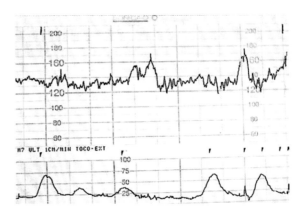

▲ 图 10-18　正常产前胎心监护，该记录显示 >5/min 的基线变化和心搏加速

Fig. 10.18　Normal antenatal cardiotocograph. The recording shows a baseline variability of >5 beats/min and episodes of accelerations.

所有 5 个参数综合起来即为生物物理评估（biophysical profile，BPP）或生物物理评分（biophysical score，BPS）。胎儿在 40min（或者更短时间）内表现出至少 4 个上述参数为正常反应。最初的生物物理评分记录时间为 30min，但该时长未考虑到胎儿正常"睡眠"的可能性，而胎儿睡眠时间可能会长达 40min，期间观察不到胎动、心搏加速或呼吸动作，为此，观察窗改为 40min。

The use of all five parameters in combination is called *the biophysical profile* or *biophysical score* (BPP or BPS). A normal response is for the fetus to exhibit at least four of these parameters in a period of up to 40 minutes (they may be seen in a much shorter period). The original BPS was recorded over 30 minutes but that did not take account of the possibility of normal fetal 'sleep', which can last up to 40 minutes and during which no movements, accelerations or breathing may be seen, hence the change to an observation window of 40 minutes.

七、干预（Interventions）

（一）非特异性风险（For non-specific risk）

胎儿监测证实胎儿的理论风险后，仅 3 种有效干预措施。

- 择期分娩：如果确定风险在孕 34 周或以上，通常需要立即分娩。如果在 34 周前确定风险，则通过评估胎儿死亡的即时风险来确定处理方案，因此，如果生物物理评分或胎心监护记录（紧急监护措施）异常和（或）子宫动脉中舒张末期血流逆向，应与胎儿父母讨论即时分娩问题。如果上述参数未见异常，则可继续密切监护，以"争取"更多妊娠时间，并为孕妇应用类固醇激素。

- 早产前应用类固醇：选择性早产可能发生在高危妊娠中，仅胎儿健康的长期监测是异常的，如未达标的胎儿发育、无子宫动脉舒张多普勒记录，则建议该孕妇服用 1 个疗程的倍他米松。

- 早产前使用硫酸镁：早产与新生儿脑损伤和随后的神经发育障碍的风险增加相关，损伤可能表现为以下 1 种或多种形式：弥散性白质损伤、脑室内出血和（或）脑实质出血，以及囊性和脑室周围白质软化。新生儿最易感的孕期为 24～34 周。但是，孕妇产前使用硫酸镁对极早早产儿（尤其 30 周前）具有神经保护作用，但是硫酸镁的神经保护作用详细机制尚不清楚。

When a theoretic risk to the fetus is proven to be real by fetal surveillance, the only three interventions of value are:

- Elective delivery: if the risk is identified at 34 or more weeks, there is usually no reason to delay the delivery. Where the risk is identified before 34 weeks, the management is determined by the assessment of immediate risk of fetal death. Thus, if the BPS or CTG (acute measures of health) are abnormal and/or there is reversed end diastolic flow in the UA, then delivery without delay is discussed with the parents. Where there is no abnormality in these parameters, continued close monitoring could continue to 'gain' time in the pregnancy and allow the maternal administration of steroids.

- Steroids administered to a woman before pre-term birth: if it is clear that elective pre-term delivery is likely to occur in an at-risk pregnancy but only the chronic measures of fetal health are abnormal, e.g. suboptimal growth and absent UA Doppler diastolic recordings, the woman would be advised to have a course of betamethasone.

- Magnesium sulphate administered to woman before preterm birth: pre-term birth is associated with an increased risk of brain injury in the newborn and subsequent neurodevelopmental disability. The injury can be in the form of one or more of the following: diffuse white matter injury, intraventricular and/or intraparenchymal haemorrhage and cystic and periventricular leukomalacia. The gestation when newborns are most susceptible is between 24 and 34 weeks. However, prenatal administration of magnesium sulphate to extremely pre-term infants (especially before 30 weeks) has been shown to have neuroprotective effects. The detailed mechanisms for this neuroprotective effect of magnesium sulphate are unknown.

（二）特异性风险（For specific risk）

这些相对不常见的风险如下。

- 孕妇服用药物治疗胎儿心律不齐。

- 为严重的 Rh 同种免疫胎儿宫内输血。

- 双胎输血综合征的胎盘血管循环激光消融术。

These are relatively uncommon and include:

- maternal drugs for fetal cardiac arrhythmias
- intrauterine blood transfusion for fetuses with severe Rhesus isoimmunization
- laser ablation of placental vascular communications in twin-to-twin transfusion syndrome

八、结论（Conclusions）

- 目前的筛查项目可在孕期内发现大部分（尽管并非全部）的胎儿结构或染色体异常。

- 对于正常孕育的胎儿，一旦确定了风险，无论是特异性还是非特异性风险，在确定胎儿处于死于宫内"危险"时，目前的监测措施是孕妇服用类固醇以及择期分娩相结合。

- 对于正常孕育的无明显风险的胎儿，现有的孕期常规监测方法（孕妇感知胎动、宫高测量和胎心听诊）是有限的，无法识别所有真正有风险的胎儿。

- Most, though not all, fetuses with structural or chromosomal abnormality are identified during pregnancy with current screening programmes.

- In normally formed fetuses, once risk is identified, both specific and non-specific, the current methods of surveillance coupled with the judicious use of maternal steroid administration and elective delivery are effective in the sense that most fetuses identified to be 'at risk' will not die in utero.

- In normally formed fetuses that are apparently at no risk, the current method of routine surveillance during pregnancy (maternal perception of fetal movements, fundal height measurement and auscultation of the fetal heart) is limited and does not identify all fetuses that are genuinely at risk.

本章概览	Essential information

先天性异常

- 胎儿先天性异常常见于
  - 50% 以上妊娠
  - 约 70% 的流产
  - 孕 20 周至产后 1 年死亡的 15%
  - 1%～2% 的新生儿异常（包括严重畸形和轻微畸形）
  - 8% 的特殊需求儿童 / 残疾儿
- 过去 30 年，英国总体发生下降，这得益于
  - 引入孕期筛查流程
  - 孕期诊断成功率的提高
  - 胎儿父母选择终止妊娠
- 最为常见的四类缺陷为
  - 神经管缺陷（3～7/1000 个新生儿）
  - 先天性心脏病（6/1000 个新生儿）
  - 唐氏综合征（1.5/1000 个新生儿）
  - 唇裂 / 腭裂（1.5/1000 个新生儿）
- 筛查胎儿异常采取
  - 妊娠早期的临床情况（包括孕妇年龄、某些药物、异常胎儿妊娠史和糖尿病）
  - 妊娠晚期的临床情况（包括异常子宫大小、胎动异常和胎位异常）
  - 使用超声设备（包括在孕早期末期的 NT 和孕 20 周的系统解剖检查）
  - 生化检测（测量生化标志物，结合 NT 评估染色体异常风险）
  - 超声和生化筛查前适度的咨询非常重要
- 在异常 / 阳性筛查检测非指令性咨询后建议
  - 进一步评估（包括间隔一段时间后重复超声扫描、羊膜腔穿刺术或绒毛取样以明确染色体核型，其他影像包括 MRI）
  - 特定的干预措施（如抗心律不齐药物、胎儿积液引流）
  - 终止妊娠
  - 继续妊娠并提供持续监护，并制订分娩时间、方式和地点的计划

评估正常孕育胎儿的健康

- 低危妊娠的胎儿健康监测内容包括
  - 孕妇在妊娠后半期的关注胎动
  - 测量宫高并用图表表示
  - 听诊胎心
- 高危妊娠的胎儿健康监测内容包括
  - 检测取决于假定的潜在病理生理 [如孕妇子宫动脉多普勒、胎儿多普勒（子宫动脉、大脑中动脉和静脉导管血流）、疑似受脐带胎盘血管疾病影响的胎儿生长情况，以及针对胎儿贫血风险的大脑中动脉血流多普勒记录]
  - 对于大多数胎儿，包括存在病理生理不确定性的胎儿，将对其以下参数进行联合连续测量
    - 胎儿多普勒记录（子宫动脉、大脑中动脉和静脉导管血流）
    - 胎儿生长（尤其是头围和腹围）
    - 羊水量
    - 生物物理参数（胎心率、胎动、张力和呼吸）

Congenital abnormalities

- Fetal abnormality is found in:
  - over 50% of conceptions
  - about 70% of miscarriages
  - 15% of deaths between 20 weeks and 1 year postnatal
  - 1–2% of births, including major and minor anomalies
  - 8% of special needs register/disabled children
- The overall UK incidence has fallen over the past 30 years due to:
  - Introduction of screening programmes in pregnancy
  - Greater success at diagnosis during pregnancy
  - Parents choosing pregnancy termination
- The commonest four groups of defects are
  - Neural tube defects (3/7/1000 births)
  - Congenital cardiac defects (6/1000 births)
  - Down's syndrome (1.5/1000 births)
  - Cleft lip/palate (1.5/1000 births)
- Screening for fetal abnormality can be undertaken
  - Clinically in early pregnancy (including maternal age, certain drugs, previous abnormal baby, diabetes)
  - Clinically in late pregnancy (including abnormal uterine size, abnormal fetal movements, abnormal fetal lie)
  - Using US (including measurement of NT at the end of the first trimester and an anatomical survey at 20 weeks)
  - Biochemically (measurement of biochemical markers which in combination with NT measurement estimate chromosomal abnormality risk)
  - Balanced pre-test counselling is important with US and biochemical screening
- Options following non-directive counselling with an abnormal/positive screening test include
  - Further assessment (such as repeat US scan after an interval, amniocentesis or CVS to establish the felt karyotype, other imaging including MRI)
  - Specific interventions (such as anti-arrhythmic drugs, drainage of fetal fluid collections)
  - Termination of pregnancy
  - Continuation of pregnancy with ongoing surveillance and specific plans for timing, mode and place of delivery

Assessing the health of a normally formed fetus

- Surveillance of fetal health in a low–risk pregnancy comprises
  - Maternal vigilance for fetal activity in the latter half of pregnancy
  - Fundal height measurement and charting
  - Auscultation of the fetal heart
- Surveillance of fetal health in a high-risk pregnancy comprises
  - Tests used will depend on the presumed underlying pathophysiology (such as maternal uterine artery Doppler, fetal Dopplers (UA, MCA and DV blood flow) and fetal growth for suspected UPVD and Doppler recordings of MCA blood flow if fetal anaemia is a risk)
  - The majority of fetuses, including those where there is uncertainty about the pathophysiology, will have combined serial measurements of
    - Fetal Doppler recordings (UA, MCA and DV blood flow)
    - Fetal growth (especially HC and AC)
    - Amniotic fluid volume
    - Biophysical parameters (FHR, movements, tone and breathing)

（续表）

本章概览	Essential information
• 干预 　– 非特定或未知的病理生理 • 择期分娩：时间选择取决于胎儿风险程度 • 若已计划早产，孕妇则应服用类固醇 　– 特定或已知病理生理（罕见） 　– 孕妇服用抗心律不齐类药物治疗胎儿心律不齐 　– 重度贫血胎儿的胎儿输血 　– 双胎输血综合征胎儿实施胎盘血管循环的激光消融术	• Interventions 　– Non-specific or unknown pathophysiology • Elective delivery-the timing, depending on the degree of fetal risk • Maternal administration of steroids if a pre-term delivery is planned 　– Specific or known pathophysiology (rare) 　– Maternal anti-arrhythmic drugs for fetal cardiac arrhythmias 　– Fetal blood transfusion(s) for severe fetal anaemia 　– Laser ablation of placental vascular anastamoses with twin-twin transfusion syndrome

（续表）

第 11 章　分娩机制管理
Management of labour

Sabaratnam Arulkumaran　著　　王　珊　译　　杨慧霞　校

学习目标	LEARNING OUTCOMES
学习本章后，你应当能够：	After studying this chapter you should be able to:

知识标准

- 描述正常分娩和异常分娩的机制、诊断和管理
- 描述引产和促进分娩的方法，其中包括适应证、禁忌证和并发症
- 描述脐带脱垂的病因和处理
- 讨论早产、胎膜早破和早产的影响和处理
- 总结分娩中使用的胎儿健康评估方法，如胎粪、胎心率监测和胎儿头皮采血
- 解释分娩镇痛和麻醉的选择

临床能力

- 参与正常分娩的管理
- 分析分娩中胎心率监测的结果
- 评估分娩的进展，包括使用产程图，并向产妇解释产程进展

专业技能和态度

- 尊重分娩中的文化和宗教差异
- 有效沟通、安慰产妇，表现出同理心
- 重视产妇护理工作中的多专业合作（与助产士和医生交流产程进展和管理计划）

Knowledge criteria

- Describe the mechanisms, diagnosis and management of normal and abnormal labour
- Describe the methods of induction and augmentation of labour, including the indications, contraindications and complications
- Describe the aetiology and management of cord prolapse
- Discuss the impact and management of pre-term labour, pre-labour rupture of membranes and precipitate labour
- Summarize the methods of assessment of fetal wellbeing used in labour, e.g. meconium, fetal heart rate monitoring and fetal scalp blood sampling
- Explain the options available for pain relief and anaesthesia in labour

Clinical competencies

- Participate in the management of normal labour
- Interpret the results of fetal heart rate monitoring in labour
- Assess the progress of labour, including the use of partograms, and explain the findings to the labouring woman

Professional skills and attitudes

- Demonstrate respect for cultural and religious differences in attitudes to childbirth
- Demonstrate empathy by effective communication and providing reassurance to women in labour
- Demonstrate awareness of importance of multiprofessional working in the care of women in labour (communicate findings and management plans with midwives and doctors)

分娩是指妊娠 24 周后，妊娠产物从子宫腔排出的过程。有 93%～94% 在足月分娩，即 37～42 周，而 7%～8% 在足月前分娩，即在 24～37 周分娩。早产指在妊娠 37 周前发生的分娩。24 周前，胎儿娩出不能存活，称为流产。产程延长指初产妇分娩持续 24h 以上或经产妇分娩持续 16h 以上。产程延长会增加母胎发病率和死亡率。

Labour, or *parturition*, is the process whereby the products of conception are expelled from the uterine cavity after the twenty-fourth week of gestation. About 93–94% deliver at term, i.e. between 37 and 42 weeks, while about 7–8% develop pre-term labour and deliver pre-term from 24 to 37 weeks. *Pre-term labour* is defined as labour occurring before the commencement of the thirty-seventh week of gestation. Prior to 24 weeks, this process results in a pre-viable fetus and is termed *miscarriage*. *Prolonged labour* is defined as labour lasting more than 24 hours in a primigravida and 16 hours in a multigravida. Prolonged labour is associated with increased fetal and maternal morbidity and mortality.

一、产程（Stages of labour）

先兆临产（分娩前阶段）可持续数天或数周，而疼痛性的宫缩发动和分娩时间较短，这一过程称为产程或分娩。随着子宫收缩，宫颈进行性变软、宫颈管消退、宫口扩张。

The early preparation (pre-labour phase) goes on for days and weeks, while the onset of painful uterine contractions and delivery is shorter and the process is called *parturition or labour*. The cervix ripens by becoming softer, shorter and dilated, which takes a greater speed with onset of uterine contractions.

为了便于临床管理，连续的"观察"总产程分为如下 3 个过程。

For purposes of clinical management, the 'observed' labour, which is a continuum, is divided into three stages:

第一产程从规律宫缩开始、宫颈管进行性消退、宫口扩张到宫口开全。第一产程分为潜伏期和活跃期。早期缓慢的潜伏期，宫颈管从长度 3cm 开始消退至宫口扩张至 5cm。根据最近的研究，潜伏期被定义为宫口开大至 5cm，活跃期为宫口开大 5cm 至宫口开全（10cm）。最新研究证据描述了大量自然分娩中初产妇和经产妇的宫口开大率。初产妇宫口从 3cm 开大至 4cm 的中位时间为 1.8h，4cm 开大至 5cm 为 1.3h，5cm 开大至 6cm 为 0.8h，6cm 开大至 7cm 为 0.6h，7cm 开大至 8cm 为 0.5h，8cm 开大至 9cm 为 0.5h，9cm 开大至 10cm 为 0.5h。基于此，可以认为活跃期从宫口开大 5cm 开始。

The first stage commences with the onset of regular painful contractions and cervical changes until it reaches full dilatation and the cervix is no longer palpable. The first stage is divided into an early slow latent phase when the cervix becomes effaced and shortens from 3 cm in length and dilates up to 5 cm. Following recent studies, the latent phase has been defined to continue to 5 cm, and an active phase when the cervix dilates from 5 cm to full dilatation or 10 cm. The evidence comes from recent studies that have described rates of cervical dilatation in a large number of nulliparous and multiparous women admitted in spontaneous labour. Median time in nullipara for cervical change of 3–4 cm was 1.8 hours, 4–5 cm was 1.3 hours, 5–6 cm was 0.8 hours, 6–7 cm was 0.6 hours, 7–8 cm was 0.5 hours, 8–9 cm was 0.5 hours and 9–10 cm was 0.5 hours. Based on this, one could state that the active phase starts from 5 cm cervical dilatation.

第二产程从宫口开全到胎儿娩出。这一过程又分为胎头在骨盆下降的骨盆期（被动期）和产妇有更强的推动力、胎儿随宫缩和产妇用力娩出的会阴期（主动期）。

The second stage is the duration from full cervical dilatation to delivery of the fetus. This is subdivided into a pelvic or passive phase, when the head descends in the pelvis, and an active or perineal phase, when the mother gets a stronger urge to push and the fetus is delivered with the force of the uterine contractions and the maternal bearing-down effort.

第三产程为从胎儿娩出到胎盘胎膜娩出的时间。

The third stage is the duration from the delivery of the newborn to delivery of the placenta and membranes.

二、分娩发动（Onset of labour）

一般很难确定分娩发动的确切时间，因为宫缩可能是不规律的，可能在没有宫颈变化的情况下开始和停止，即"假临产"。为了临床管理，临产判断是基于观察宫缩情况、宫颈变化及胎头下降。这一概念必须根据各地实际情况来判断，因为在一些偏远地区，产妇可能在临产后 1 天产程没有任何进展而就诊，应根据产妇的一般状况和胎儿情况指导治疗。在宫颈手术后出现宫颈狭窄的罕见病例中，正常的临产宫缩可能会导致宫颈变薄却不扩张。

It is often difficult to be certain of the exact time of onset of labour because contractions may be irregular and may start and stop with no cervical change, i.e. 'false labour'. The duration of labour for management purposes is based on the observed progress of the contractions and cervical changes along with the descent of the head. This concept may have to be judged based on the place of practice, as in some remote areas a mother may be brought in after a day of labour with no progress. Her general condition and findings of the maternal and fetal conditions should dictate management. In the rare cases of cervical stenosis that can occur after surgery to the cervix, normal contractions of labour may produce thinning of the cervix without cervical dilatation.

分娩发动的临床标志如下。

The clinical signs of the onset of labour are:

频率、持续时间和强度增加的规律、疼痛宫缩，伴随进行性宫颈管消失、宫口扩张和胎先露部下降。

Regular, painful uterine contractions that increase in frequency, duration and intensity that produce progressive cervical effacement and dilatation and descent of the fetal presenting part.

宫颈流出带血的宫颈黏液，即所谓的"先兆"，与分娩发动有关，但其本身并不是分娩发动的标志。

The passage of blood-stained mucus from the cervix, called the *show*, is associated with but is not on its own an indicator of the onset of labour.

同样，胎膜破裂可发生在分娩发动时，但这是可变的，胎膜破裂可在无宫缩的情况下发生。若胎膜破裂（rupture of membranes，ROM）到疼痛的宫缩开始的潜伏期大于 4h，则称为胎膜早破（prelabour ROM，PROM），发生在足月前称为未足月胎膜早破（preterm pre-labor ROM，PPROM）。

Similarly, rupture of the fetal membranes can be at the onset of labour, but this is variable and may occur without uterine contractions. If the latent period between rupture of membranes (ROM) to onset of painful uterine contractions is greater than 4 hours, it is called *prelabour rupture of membranes (PROM)*, and this can occur at term or in the pre-term period, when it is called *preterm pre-labour rupture of membranes (PPROM)*.

临产是最常见的临床症状之一，但诊断可能需要时间和不断的阴道检查来评估宫颈变化，除非产妇在临产晚期入院。临产的准确诊断很重要，可避免不必要的干预，如人工破膜或催产素的使用。

Labour is one of the commonest clinical conditions, and yet the diagnosis may need time and sequential vaginal examination to assess cervical changes unless the mother is admitted in advanced labour. Accurate diagnosis of labour is important to avoid unnecessary interventions such as artificial rupture of membranes (ARM) or the use of oxytocin infusion.

临产（Initiation of labour）

分娩的开始包括黄体酮的撤退以及雌激素和前列腺素作用的增加。调节这些变化的机制尚不清楚，很可能涉及胎盘产生的肽类激素促肾上腺皮质激素释放激素（corticotrophin-releasing hormone，CRH）。妊娠期出现无痛性不规则子宫收缩。CRH 在妊娠早期最少，随着妊娠进展增多。一系列事件由胎儿 – 胎盘单位调节和控制。在妊娠结束时，保持子宫和子宫颈静态的因素逐步下调，促进收缩的因素逐步上调。

The onset of labour involves progesterone withdrawal and an increase in oestrogen and prostaglandin action. The mechanisms that regulate these changes are unresolved but are likely to involve placental production of the peptide hormone corticotrophin-releasing hormone (CRH). During pregnancy, painless irregular uterine activity is present. It is minimal in early pregnancy and greater with advancing gestation. A cascade of events is regulated and controlled by the feto-placental unit. At the end of gestation, there is gradual downregulation of those factors that keep the uterus and cervix quiescent and an upregulation of pro-contractile influences.

妊娠期间胎盘的发育导致合体滋养层细胞核数量呈指数增长、CRH 基因转录。这一过程导致母体和胎儿血浆 CRH 水平呈指数增长。CRH 对胎盘增加雌激素合成、减少孕酮合成有直接作用。在胎儿中，CRH 直接刺激肾上腺的胎儿区产生脱氢表雄酮（dehydroepiandrosterone，DHEA），这是胎盘雌激素合成的前体。CRH 还通过细胞膜刺激前列腺素的合成。孕酮的下降和雌激素及前列腺素的增加导致连接蛋白43 的增加，连接蛋白43 促进子宫肌细胞的偶联并改变子宫肌细胞的电兴奋性，从而导致宫缩增强。

Placental development across gestation leads to an exponential increase in the number of syncytiotrophoblast nuclei in which transcription of the *CRH* gene occurs. This maturational process leads to an exponential increase in the levels of maternal and fetal plasma CRH. The CRH has direct actions on the placenta to increase oestrogen synthesis and reduce progesterone synthesis. In the fetus, the CRH directly stimulates the fetal zone of the adrenal gland to produce dehydroepiandrosterone (DHEA), the precursor of placental oestrogen synthesis. CRH also stimulates the synthesis of prostaglandins by the membranes. The fall in progesterone and increase in oestrogens and prostaglandins lead to increases in connexin 43 that promote connectivity of uterine myocytes and change uterine myocyte electrical excitability, which in turn lead to increases in generalized uterine contractions:

子宫肌细胞收缩过程不同于横纹肌，横纹肌细胞收缩后能恢复到原来的长度。

The uterine myocytes contract and shorten, unlike the process in striated muscle, where cells contract but then return to their pre-contraction length.

子宫肌内的离子通道影响钙离子内流并促进子宫肌细胞的收缩。

Ion channels within the myometrium influence the influx of calcium ions into the myocytes and promote contraction of the myometrial cells.

胎盘产生的其他激素（如松弛素、激活素 A、卵泡抑素、人绒毛膜促性腺激素和 CRH）通过影响环磷酸腺苷的产生导致子宫肌细胞松弛，从而直接或间接影响子宫收缩力。

Other hormones produced in the placenta directly or indirectly influence myometrial contractility (e.g. relaxin, activin A, follistatin, human chorionic gonadotrophin (hCG) and CRH) by influencing the production of cyclic adenosine monophosphate (cAMP) that causes relaxation of myometrial cells.

子宫颈的完整性对保留胎儿至关重要。它包含肌细胞和成纤维细胞，由于白细胞浸润的增加和随着蛋白水解酶活性的增加胶原量的减少，它变得柔软和可拉伸。透明质酸生成的增加降低了纤连蛋白对胶原蛋白的亲和力，透明质酸对水的亲和力使子宫颈变得柔软和可拉伸，即子宫颈成熟。

The integrity of the cervix is essential to retain the products of conception. It contains myocytes and fibroblasts, and towards term becomes soft and stretchable due to an increase in leucocyte infiltration and a decrease in the amount of collagen with the increase in proteolytic enzyme activity. Increased production of hyaluronic acid reduces the affinity of fibronectin for collagen. The affinity of hyaluronic acid for water causes the cervix to become soft and stretchable, i.e. ripening of the cervix.

产程进展需要降低宫颈阻力（就像松开汽车的刹车）和增加子宫收缩的频率、持续时间和强度（就像汽车的油门）。第一产程从疼痛的规律宫缩发动开始到宫口开全，分为宫颈管消退的缓慢潜伏期和活跃期，潜伏期即颈管消失到宫口开大至 5cm（初产妇平均为 6～8h，经产妇为 4～6h），活跃期即宫颈以平均每小时 1cm 的速度从 5cm 至宫口开全。

Reduced cervical resistance (i.e. release of the brakes in a car) and increasing frequency, duration and strength of uterine contractions (i.e. accelerator of the car) are needed for the progress of labour. The first stage of labour that starts from onset of painful uterine contractions to full dilatation is divided into a slow latent phase when the cervix becomes shorter,

i.e. effaced and dilated to 5 cm (an average of 6–8 hours in nulliparae and 4–6 hours in a multiparae) and an active phase of labour when the cervix dilates at an average of 1 cm per hour from 5 cm to full cervical dilatation.

三、分娩期子宫活动：产力（Uterine activity in labour: the powers）

子宫在整个妊娠过程中表现出偶发的、低强度的收缩。随着足月的临近，子宫活动的频率、持续时间和收缩强度均增加。通过触诊或外部宫缩描记法可以确定宫缩的频率和持续时间，但需要宫内压力导管来评估宫缩的强度。如果以常规方式在 10min 内观察到两次持续时间超过 20s 的宫缩，则可能将分娩。分娩时的正常静息压在 10～20mmHg 开始，分娩时略有增加（图 11-1）。宫缩强度随着产程进展增加，在某些时候表现为宫缩持续时间的延长。世界卫生组织（WHO）建议根据宫缩的频率和持续时间在产程图上记录宫缩。

The uterus exhibits infrequent, low-intensity contractions throughout pregnancy. As full term approaches, uterine activity increases in frequency, duration and strength of contractions. By palpation or external tocography one can identify the frequency and duration of contractions, but intrauterine pressure catheters are needed to assess the strength of contractions. It is likely that labour would be established if two contractions each lasting for >20 seconds are observed in 10 minutes in a regular manner. Normal resting tonus in labour starts at around 10–20 mmHg and increases slightly during labour (Fig. 11.1). Contractions increase in intensity with progress of labour, which in some ways is characterized by the increasing duration of contractions. The World Health Organization (WHO) recommends contraction recording on the partograph based on the frequency and duration of contractions.

> **！注意**
>
> 在妊娠晚期，有时可触摸到不造成宫口扩张的强烈宫缩，这不是真正的临产。
>
> In late pregnancy, strong contractions can sometimes be palpated that do not produce cervical dilatation, and hence do not constitute true labour.

由于进行性子宫收缩，子宫上段肌层纤维的缩短和子宫下段的拉伸和变薄，导致宫颈管消退和宫口开大（图 11-2），这个过程被称为缩复作用。随着产程进展，子宫下段被拉长变薄，子宫上段和下段之间的交界处在腹部隆起。当产程受阻时，上段和

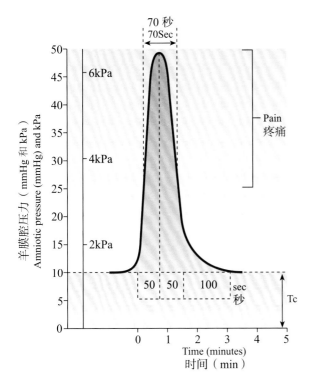

▲ 图 11-1　第一产程子宫收缩达到 50mmHg (6.5kPa) 的压力，当羊水压力超过 25 mmHg (3.2kPa) 时，宫缩会产生痛感

Fig. 11.1　Uterine contractions reach pressures of 50mmHg (6.5kPa) with first stage of labour. Contractions become painful when amniotic pressure exceeds 25mmHg (3.2kPa).

and thinned as labour progresses, and the junction between the upper and lower segment rises in the abdomen. Where labour becomes obstructed, the junction of the upper and lower segments may become visible at the level of the umbilicus; this is known as a *retraction ring* (also known as *Bandl's ring*).

子宫起搏点从未通过解剖学、药理学、电学或生理学研究得到证实。电收缩脉冲从一侧或两侧宫底部区域开始，并通过子宫肌层向下扩散。宫缩在宫底和上段比下段更强，持续时间更长。这种优势对宫颈管消退和宫口扩张至关重要。随着子宫和圆韧带的收缩，子宫的轴线变直，并将胎儿的纵轴拉向前腹壁，与真骨盆入口对齐。

A pacemaker for the uterus has never been demonstrated by anatomical, pharmacological, electrical or physiological studies. The electrical contraction impulse starts in one or the other uterine fundal region and spreads downwards through the myometrium. Contractions are stronger and last longer in the fundus and upper segment than in the lower segment. This *fundal dominance* is essential for progressive effacement and dilatation of the cervix. As the uterus and the round ligaments contract, the axis of the uterus straightens and pulls the longitudinal axis of the fetus towards the anterior abdominal wall in line with the inlet of the true pelvis.

当胎儿被直接向下推入盆腔时，子宫轴重新对准促进了先露部的下降（图 11-3）。

The realignment of the uterine axis promotes descent of the presenting part as the fetus is pushed directly downwards into the pelvic cavity (Fig. 11.3).

四、产道（The passages）

骨盆的形状和结构见前述（见第 1 章）。骨盆的

下段的交界处可能在脐水平处观察到，这被称为缩复环（也称为 Bandl 环）。

Progressive uterine contractions cause effacement and dilatation of the cervix as the result of shortening of myometrial fibres in the upper uterine segment and stretching and thinning of the lower uterine segment (Fig. 11.2). This process is known as *retraction*. The lower segment becomes elongated

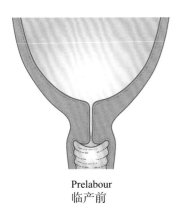

Prelabour
临产前

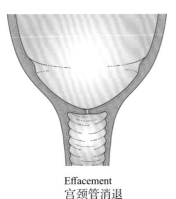

Effacement
宫颈管消退

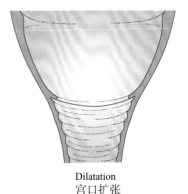

Dilatation
宫口扩张

▲ 图 11-2　伴随子宫下段的形成，临产时宫颈管消退和宫口开大

Fig. 11.2　Effacement and dilatation of the cervix in labour with formation of the lower uterine segment.

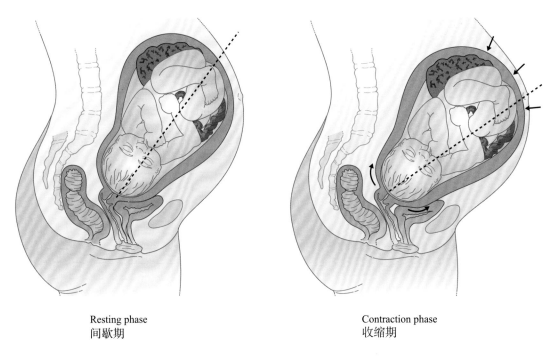

Resting phase
间歇期

Contraction phase
收缩期

▲ 图 11-3　宫缩时胎儿和子宫轴线的变化

Fig.11.3　Change in direction of the fetal and uterine axis during contractions in labour.

大小和形状因人而异，并非所有女性都有女型骨盆；有些人可能有扁平骨盆、类人猿骨盆或男型骨盆，从而影响分娩结局。骶髂韧带和耻骨联合的软化允许盆腔扩张，这一特征及由俯屈、旋转和塑形引起的头径的动态变化，有助于产程正常进展和阴道自然分娩。

The shape and structure of the bony pelvis have already been described (see Chapter 1). The size and shape of the pelvis vary from woman to woman. Not all women have a gynaecoid pelvis; some may have a platypelloid, anthropoid or android pelvis, thus influencing the outcome of labour. Softening of the sacroiliac ligaments and the pubic symphysis allows expansion of the pelvic cavity, and this feature, along with the dynamic changes of the head diameter brought about by flexion, rotation and moulding, facilitates normal progress and spontaneous vaginal delivery.

骨盆的软组织比非妊娠状态下更容易拉伸。盆底和阴道口的实质性扩张发生在胎头下降和娩出期间。骨盆软组织、阴道和会阴的扩张有助于降低胎头下降和胎头娩出时会阴和阴道壁撕裂的风险。

The soft tissues of the pelvis are more distensible than in the non-pregnant state. Substantial distension of the pelvic floor and vaginal orifice occurs during the descent and birth of the head. The distensible nature of the pelvic soft tissues, vagina and perineum helps to reduce the risk of tearing of the perineum and vaginal walls during descent and birth of the head.

五、分娩机制（The mechanism of labour）

骨盆入口的横径大于前后径，这促使胎头在横径上衔接入骨盆入口。胎头和躯干通过骨盆的通道遵循既定模式，因为骨盆入口平面是横向的，中骨盆平面是圆形的，骨盆出口平面是纵向的。95% 的胎儿为头先露，称为正常先露。头先露中，90% 的胎儿俯屈良好，头部旋转至枕前位，并以最短径线衔接，即枕下前囟径（9.5cm）和双顶径（9.5cm）；因此，枕骨位于骨盆前半部的枕前位为正常位置。俯屈或仰伸的枕后位和枕横位，作为临时性胎位，可进一步仰伸为额先露或面先露，枕后位时，以枕臀至前囟径或枕额径（11.5cm）衔接入骨盆，分娩时间延长。

The pelvic inlet offers a larger lateral than an anteroposterior diameter. This promotes the head to normally engage in the pelvis in the transverse position. The passage of the head and trunk through the pelvis follows a well-defined pattern because the upper pelvic strait is transverse, the middle pelvic strait is circular and the outer pelvic strait is anteroposterior. The fetal head presents by the vertex in 95% of the cases, and hence is called *normal presentation*. With the vertex presentation, the head is well flexed in 90% of the cases and the head rotates to an occipitoanterior position and presents the shortest diameters, i.e. anteroposterior suboccipitobregmatic

(9.5 cm) and lateral biparietal (9.5 cm) diameters; hence, the occipitoanterior position where the occiput is in the anterior half of the pelvis is called the *normal position*. A deflexed or extended head presents as an occipitoposterior or transverse position and with further extension as a brow or face presentation. Labour with an occipitoposterior position is prolonged as a larger anteroposterior diameter of occipitobregmatic or occipitofrontal diameter (11.5 cm) presents to the pelvis.

额先露时，胎头很难以最大的枕颏径（13.5cm）入盆。额先露预示可以俯屈为顶先露或仰伸为面先露。如果产程停滞，额先露的胎儿最好剖宫产分娩。

With the brow presentation, entry of the head into the pelvic brim is difficult, as it presents the largest anteroposterior mentovertical diameter (13.5 cm). The brow presentation can flex to a vertex or extend to a face presentation. If there is no progress of cervical dilatation, the baby is best delivered by caesarean section in a term brow presentation.

因此，正常分娩的过程包括胎头为适应母亲骨盆的不同节段和径线，会发生以下过程（图 11-4）。

The process of normal labour therefore involves the adaptation of the fetal head to the various segments and diameters of the maternal pelvis, and the following processes occur (Fig. 11.4):

1. 胎头下降贯穿整个分娩过程，这既是胎儿分娩的一个特征，也是胎儿分娩的先决条件。在大多数初产妇中，胎头衔接通常发生在分娩发动之前，但经产妇分娩发动后胎头才开始衔接。胎头下降是评估产程进展的一个标志。

1. Descent occurs throughout labour and is both a feature and a prerequisite for the birth of the baby. Engagement of the head normally occurs before the onset of labour in most primigravid women but may not occur until labour is well established in a multipara. Descent of the head provides a measure of the progress of labour.

2. 胎头下降至骨盆中部和前倾的盆底时发生俯屈，使胎儿下颏靠近胸部。俯屈能使枕额径变为更小的径线枕下前囟径。

2. Flexion of the head occurs as it descends and meets the medially and forward-sloping pelvic floor, bringing the chin into contact with the fetal thorax. Flexion produces a smaller diameter of presentation, changing from the occipitofrontal diameter, when the head is deflexed, to the suboccipitobregmatic diameter, when the head is fully flexed.

3. 内旋转：胎头到达骨盆底时旋转，枕骨通常从侧方向耻骨联合前方旋转。这是由于胎头到达盆底

最低位置，盆底肌收缩力在胎儿脊椎与头骨的交界处通过脊椎传递到头部。有时，它会向后朝骶骨旋转，以面先露的方式分娩。

3. Internal rotation: The head rotates as it reaches the pelvic floor, and the occiput normally rotates anteriorly from the lateral position towards the pubic symphysis. This is due to the force of contractions being transmitted via the fetal spine to the head at the point the spine meets the skull, which is more posterior and due to the medially and forward-sloping pelvic floor. Occasionally, it rotates posteriorly towards the hollow of the sacrum, and the head may then deliver as a face-to-pubis delivery.

4. 仰伸：完全俯屈的胎头下降并扩张盆底和外阴，胎儿枕骨与耻骨下支相接。胎头逐渐仰伸直至娩出。会阴和阴道口的最大扩张发生在头部最后娩出之前，当胎头出现在阴道口，并且在宫缩间歇不再回缩，这一过程称胎头着冠。

4. Extension: The acutely flexed head descends to distend the pelvic floor and the vulva, and the base of the occiput meets the inferior rami of the pubis. The head now extends until it is delivered. Maximal distension of the perineum and introitus occurs just prior to the final expulsion of the head, a process that is known as *crowning* when the head is seen at the introitus but does not recede in between contractions.

5. 复位：胎头娩出后旋转，使胎头和胎肩恢复正常的关系。恢复后的枕骨方向指向娩出前的位置。

5. Restitution: Following delivery of the head, it rotates back to be in line with its normal relationship to the fetal shoulders. The direction of the occiput following restitution points to the position of the vertex before the delivery.

6. 外旋转：当胎肩到达盆底时，它们旋转成与骨盆出口前后径一致的方向，伴随胎头的旋转，胎儿面部对向产妇的大腿。

6. External rotation: When the shoulders reach the pelvic floor, they rotate into the anteroposterior diameter of the pelvis. This is accompanied by rotation of the fetal head so that the face looks laterally at the maternal thigh.

7. 双肩娩出：双肩娩出后，胎体最终随之娩出。前肩首先通过向后牵引胎头的方式从耻骨弓下方露出，后肩是通过将头向前抬娩出会阴，随后躯干和下肢快速娩出。

7. Delivery of the shoulders: Final expulsion of the trunk occurs following delivery of the shoulders. The anterior shoulder is delivered first by traction posteriorly on the fetal head so that the shoulder emerges under the pubic arch. The posterior shoulder is delivered by lifting the head anteriorly over the perineum, and this is followed by rapid delivery of the

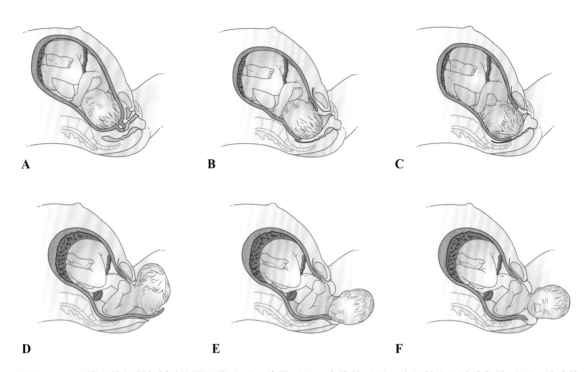

▲ 图 11-4 正常分娩机制包括胎先露下降（A）、俯屈（B）、内旋转（C）、会阴扩张和胎头仰伸（D）、胎头娩出（E）、胎肩娩出（F）

Fig. 11.4 The mechanisms of normal labour involve (A) descent of the presenting part; (B) flexion of the head; (C) internal rotation; (D) distension of the perineum and extension of the fetal head; (E) delivery of the head; (F) delivery of the shoulders.

remainder of the trunk and the lower limbs.

枕骨通常向前旋转，但如果向后旋转，俯屈就会造成更大的径线通过骨盆，造成第二产程延长，增加会阴和阴道损伤的风险。

The occiput normally rotates anteriorly, but if it rotates posteriorly, it deflexes and presents a larger diameter to the pelvic cavity. As a result, the second stage may be prolonged and the damage to the perineum and vagina is increased.

六、第三产程（The third stage of labour）

第三产程从胎儿娩出开始到胎盘和胎膜的娩出（图 11-5）。

The third stage of labour starts with the completed expulsion of the baby and ends with the delivery of the placenta and membranes (Fig. 11.5).

胎儿娩出后，子宫收缩促使胎盘剥离，并将胎盘推入子宫下段和阴道穹隆。

Once the baby is delivered, the uterine muscle contracts, shearing off the placenta and pushing it into the lower egment and the vault of the vagina.

胎盘剥离的典型症状包括少量鲜血流出、脐带延长和腹腔内宫底升高。当宫底随着胎盘下降到子宫下段，宫底变硬、变小、变圆不再是宽的球形。

The classic signs of placental separation include trickling of bright blood, lengthening of the umbilical cord and elevation of the uterine fundus within the abdominal cavity. The uterine fundus becomes firm to hard and smaller and rounded instead of being broad and globular and sits on top of the placenta as it descends into the lower segment.

在前肩娩出时可以使用催产药物来缩短胎盘剥离的时间。

The duration of placental separation may be compressed using oxytocic drugs administered at the delivery of the anterior shoulder.

胎膜伴随胎盘娩出，尽管胎膜经常撕裂，可能需要使用卵圆钳钳夹，但很少需要子宫探查才能完整娩出。检查脐带、胎盘、羊膜和绒毛膜后，应记录胎盘和胎膜的完整性。

As the placenta is expelled, it is accompanied by the fetal membranes, although the membranes often become torn and may require additional traction by using a sponge forceps to grasp them. Uterine exploration is rarely needed to complete their removal. The completeness of the placenta and membranes should be recorded after checking the cord, placenta and membranes from the amniotic as well as the chorionic sides.

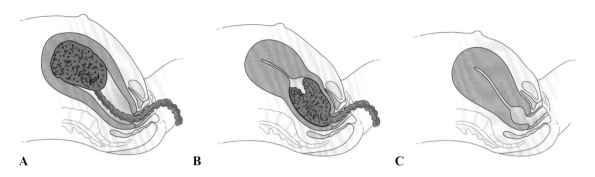

▲ 图 11-5　正常的第三产程：**A.**胎盘从子宫壁剥离；**B.**排入子宫下段和阴道上部；**C.**胎盘和胎膜从阴道完全排出

Fig.11.5　The normal third stage: (A) separation of the placenta from the uterine wall; (B) expulsion into the lower uterine segment and upper vagina; (C) complete expulsion of the placenta and membranes from the genital tract.

整个过程持续 5～10min，如果超过 30min 仍未娩出胎盘，则可诊断为胎盘滞留和第三产程异常。

The whole process lasts between 5 and 10 minutes. If the placenta is not expelled within 30 minutes, a diagnosis of retained placenta is made and the third stage considered abnormal.

大多数的分娩并发症，如产后出血，骨盆或会阴血肿及任何产妇或新生儿状况的恶化，都在分娩后最初几小时内发生，因此大多数情况下，需要在产房密切观察产妇和新生儿 2h 再送回病房。如果产妇分娩后想出院，应密切观察 6h 后出院。

Most complications of labour and delivery such as postpartum haemorrhage, pelvic or perineal haematoma and any deterioration of the maternal or newborn condition take place within the first few hours of delivery and hence in most settings the mother and baby are closely examined with periodic observations in the delivery unit for up to 2 hours before the mother and baby are sent to the postnatal ward. The observations are continued for 6 hours if the mother is to be discharged home from the delivery unit.

七、分娩疼痛（Pain in labour）

分娩时宫缩都伴随着疼痛，随着分娩的进行，宫缩的强度、频率和持续时间增加。疼痛的原因尚不清楚，可能是由于宫颈神经纤维受压或肌细胞受压缺氧所致。当宫内压超过 25mmHg 时，可感到下腹部疼痛及腰背痛。

Contractions in labour are invariably associated with pain, particularly as they increase in strength, frequency and duration with progress of labour. The cause of pain is uncertain, but it may be due to compression of nerve fibres in the cervical zone or to hypoxia of compressed muscle cells. Pain is felt in the lower abdomen and as lumbar backache when the intrauterine pressure exceeds 25mmHg.

八、正常分娩的管理（The management of normal labour）

产时管理的主要目的是保证健康的产妇顺利分娩健康的孩子。产妇为分娩过程做准备早在临产前就开始了。对于产妇和她的伴侣来说，了解在分娩的各个阶段发生了什么是很重要的。应在产前培训中加入应对分娩疼痛的策略，包括通过控制呼吸进行心理准备，并对产妇进行教育，使其了解在第二产程中如何用力。

The primary aim of intrapartum care is to deliver a healthy baby to a healthy mother. The preparation of the mother for the process of parturition begins well before the onset of labour. It is important for the mother and her partner to understand what happens during the various stages of labour. Strategies to deal with pain in labour, including mental preparation with controlled respiration, should be introduced during antenatal classes, as well as educating the mother about the regulation of expulsive efforts during the second stage of labour.

产前培训课程还应包括有关新生儿护理和母乳喂养的指导，尽管这是一个需要在产后加强的过程。

Antenatal classes should also include instructions about neonatal care and breast-feeding, although this is a process that requires reinforcement in the postdelivery period.

当规律宫缩间隔 10～15min、有产兆或胎膜破裂时，应该建议产妇住院；如果在家里分娩，应打电话给助产士。在产妇分娩的早期阶段，应该鼓励她洗澡并排空肠道和膀胱。现代观点认为没有必要剃去阴毛或腹部毛发，因为剃毛引起擦伤和出血可能成为引起细菌增殖和感染的病灶。

The mother should be advised to come into hospital, or to call the midwife in the event of a home birth, when contractions are at regular 10- to 15-minute intervals, when there is a show or when the membranes rupture. If the mother is in early labour, she should be encouraged to take a shower and to empty her bowels and bladder. Shaving of the pubic hair or abdomen is no longer considered necessary and is likely to cause abrasions with some bleeding that may become the nidus for bacterial proliferation and subsequent infection.

在英国，在家分娩率为 2%~3%，但通常的做法是采用"多米诺骨牌"（日间）分娩，即产程顺利的情况下，产妇在分娩 6h 后就出院回家，这证明分娩并不复杂。

The home birth rate in the UK is about 2–3%, but it is common practice to organize 'domino' (*domiciliary* in and out) deliveries, whereby the mother is discharged home 6 hours after delivery, provided that the delivery is uncomplicated.

（一）分娩发动时所需要的检查（Examination at the commencement of labour）

入院时，应进行以下检查。

On admission, the following examination should be performed:

- 一般检查，其中包括体温、脉搏、呼吸、血压（BP）和水合状态，并检测尿液中的葡萄糖、酮体和蛋白质。

- Full general examination, including temperature, pulse, respiration, blood pressure (BP) and state of hydration; the urine should be tested for glucose, ketone bodies and protein.

- 腹部产科检查：先视诊，再触诊以确定胎儿的胎产式、胎先露、胎方位，可触及头部的 20% 位置判断胎先露部分。使用多普勒设备听胎心，可使产妇及其伴侣听见。

- Obstetrical examination of the abdomen: Inspection is followed by palpation to determine the fetal lie, presentation and position and the station of the presenting part by estimating fifths of head palpable. Auscultation of the fetal heartbeat is by a stethoscope or by using a Doptone device, which enables the mother and her partner to hear.

- 阴道检查应在清洁外阴和阴道后进行，并遵循无菌原则使用无菌手套和消毒乳膏。一旦检查开始，在检查完成之前，手指不应该从

阴道中抽出。应注意使拇指远离阴蒂和前庭区域。

- Vaginal examination in labour should be performed only after cleansing of the vulva and introitus and using an aseptic technique with sterile gloves and an antiseptic cream. Once the examination is started, the fingers should not be withdrawn from the vagina until the examination is completed. Care should be taken to deflect the thumb away from the clitoral and vestibular area.

应注意以下因素。

The following factors should be noted:

- 宫颈的位置、硬度、颈管消退和宫口扩张。

- The position, consistency, effacement and dilatation of the cervix

- 胎膜是否完整，如果破裂，注意羊水的颜色和流出量。

- Whether the membranes are intact or ruptured and, if ruptured, the colour and quantity of the amniotic fluid

- 胎先露（如头位、臀位）和先露部分的胎方位 [如左枕前位（LOA）、右枕前位（ROA）、右枕后位（ROP）等] 及先露部分与坐骨棘水平的关系（如 S–1 或 S+1 等）。

- The fetal presentation (e.g. vertex, breech) and position (e.g. left occipito anterior (LOA), right occipito anterior (ROA), right occipito posterior (ROP), etc.) of the presenting part and its relationship to the level of the ischial spines (e.g. station −1 or +1, etc.).

- 在头位分娩时，应注意头部软组织肿胀、颅骨变形（0、+1、+2、+3）和均倾位（矢状缝平分骨盆）的程度。

- In vertex presentation, the degree of caput (soft tissue scalp swelling), moulding (0, +1, +2 and +3) and synclitism (sagittal suture bisects the pelvis) should be noted.

- 评估骨性骨盆的上、中、下三个平面及骨盆出口。

Assessment of the bony pelvis at the upper, middle and lower pelvic strait and the pelvic outlet.

（二）第一产程管理的一般原则（General principles of the management of the first stage of labour）

管理的指导原则如下。

The guiding principles of management are:

- 观察产程进展，如果产程缓慢则进行干预。

  - Observation of the progress of labour and intervention if it is slow

- 监测胎儿和产妇状况。

  - Monitoring the fetal and maternal condition

- 分娩期间缓解产妇疼痛和对其情感支持。

  - Pain relief during labour and emotional support for the mother

- 整个分娩过程中充足的水分和营养。

  - Adequate hydration and nutrition throughout labour

1. 观察：使用产程图（Observation: the use of the partogram）

引入宫口扩张和胎头下降的图形记录，是对产程管理的一大进步。它使人们能够及早发现到产程停滞。产程图（图 11-6）是一张纸，上面有产程进展的图形表示。在同一张纸上，可以记录与产程有关的其他观察结果。有几个部分可以输入宫缩的频率和持续时间、胎心率（fetal heart rate，FHR）、羊水的颜色、胎头受压情况、胎头的位置或下降、母亲的心率、血压和体温。产程图应在产妇进入产房后立即开始记录，无论宫缩何时开始，进入产房时间记录为零。产程图上的切入点取决于入院时阴道检查的评估。这种记录系统的价值在于，它能在视觉上引起人们对正常产程中的任何异常情况的注意。

The introduction of graphic records of progress of cervical dilatation and descent of the head was a major advance in the management of labour. It enables the early recognition of a labour that is non-progressive. The partogram (Fig. 11.6) is a single sheet of paper on which there is a graphic representation of progress in labour. On the same sheet, other observations related to labour can be recorded. There are sections to enter the frequency and duration of contractions, fetal heart rate (FHR), colour of liquor, caput and moulding, station or descent of the head, maternal heart rate, BP and temperature. The partogram should be started as soon as the mother is admitted to the delivery suite, and this is recorded as zero time, regardless of the time at which contractions started. However, the point of entry on the partogram depends on a vaginal assessment at the time of admission to the delivery suite. The value of this type of record system is that it draws attention visually to any aberration from normal progress in labour.

产程图的应用首先是在非洲偏远的产科病房引入的，在那里，早期认识到产程进展异常能够在发生严重滞产前及早转移到专科医院。

The use of partograms at an applied level was first introduced in remote obstetric units in Africa, where recognition that progress in labour is becoming abnormal enables early transfer to specialist units before serious obstruction occurs.

由于避免了子宫破裂、脓毒症和产后出血，并降低了膀胱或直肠阴道瘘的发病率，大大降低了孕产妇死亡率。提早发现产程停滞，及时采取剖宫产术终止妊娠可防止此类悲剧的发生。

This has led to a major reduction in maternal mortality due to avoidance of uterine rupture, sepsis and postpartum haemorrhage and reduction in severe morbidity of vesico or recto vaginal fistula. Earlier recognition of obstructed labours and immediate attention by caesarean delivery where indicated prevents such tragedies.

2. 胎儿情况（Fetal condition）

胎心率（FHR）在第一产程宫缩间歇每隔 15 分钟进行一次听诊，持续时间为 1min，在第二产程宫缩间歇每隔 5 分钟或每隔一次宫缩 1 分钟后进行一次听诊。计数 15s 并乘以 4 或计数 30s 并乘以 2 会导致 FHR 测量错误。胎心率在产程图中的指定空白处以次 / 分表示，在宫缩后不久听到的胎心减速通过向下箭头记录最低心率。

The FHR is auscultated every 15 minutes for a duration of 1 minute soon after a contraction in the first stage of labour and after every 5 minutes or after every other contraction for a duration of 1 minute in the second stage of labour. Counting for 15 seconds and multiplying by 4 or counting for 30 seconds and multiplying by 2 lead to error in the FHR observation. The FHR is charted as beats/min in the designated space in the partogram, and decelerations of heart rate that are heard soon after contractions are recorded by an arrow down to the lowest heart rate recorded on the partogram.

这些记录是实际听诊 FHR 的记录和（或）通过持续心电监护（CTG）记录的胎儿电子监护（EFM）的辅助记录。

These records are an adjunct to the actual recording of auscultated FHR in the notes and/or electronic fetal monitoring (EFM) by continuous cardiotocography (CTG).

同时记录胎膜破裂（ROM）的时间、羊水的性质（即羊水是透明的还是羊水粪染的），以及羊水的量。同时注意胎头的形状和受压情况，因为它们往往反映了头盆不称。矢状缝闭合为变形 +，矢状缝颅骨重叠且轻压可还原为 ++，矢状缝颅骨重叠轻压不可还原为 +++。头皮的软组织肿胀称为头皮水肿，也被标记为 + 至 +++，这基于临床医生的相对经验判断。

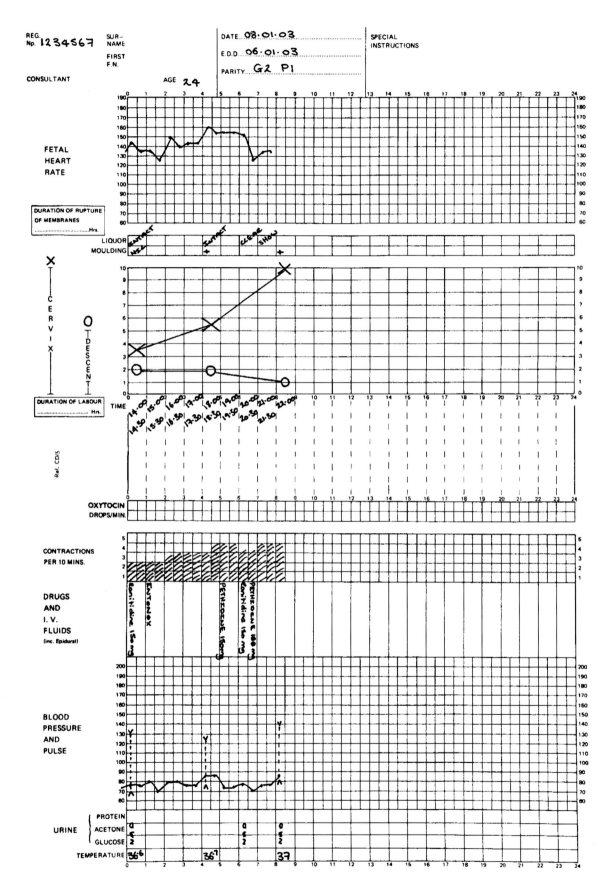

▲ 图 11-6　产程图是分娩过程中测量结果的完整可视记录（图片由 Catherine Tamizian. 提供）

Fig.11.6　The partogram is a complete visual record of measurements made during delivery. (Courtesy Catherine Tamizian.)

The time of ROM, the nature of the amniotic fluid, i.e. whether it is clear or meconium stained, and quantity are also recorded. Moulding of the fetal head and the presence of caput are also noted, as they provide an indicator of cephalopelvic disproportion. The suture lines meeting is moulding +, overriding but reducible with gentle pressure is ++ and overriding and not reducible with gentle pressure is +++. The soft tissue swelling of the scalp called caput is also marked from + to +++ but is based on the relative impression formed by the clinician.

3. 产程进展（Progress in labour）

分娩的进展是通过评估宫口扩张和先露部下降的速度来衡量的。入院时通过阴道检查评估进展，在第一产程后每 3～4 小时检查 1 次。宫口扩张是沿着宫颈描记器 0～10 的刻度以厘米（cm）为单位绘制的。经产妇在 6～8h、初产妇在 8～10h 内宫颈消退并扩张至 5cm（潜伏期），随后，宫颈扩张以每小时约扩张 1cm 的速度从 5cm 扩张到 10cm（活跃期），经产妇比初产妇扩张更快。在活跃期，产程图上以每小时 1cm 的速率描记预想曲线被称为警戒线，这有助于识别出进展缓慢的产妇。与警戒线平行 2h 的称为行动线，可用于确定在没有胎儿畸形、头盆不称或胎儿窘迫的情况下何时进行人工破膜或催产素输注以加速分娩。

Progress in labour is measured by assessing the rate of cervical dilatation and descent of the presenting part. The progress is assessed by vaginal examination on admission and every 3 to 4 hours afterwards during the first stage of labour. Cervical dilatation is plotted in centimetres along the scale of 0–10 of the cervicograph. The cervix is expected to efface and dilate from 0 to 5 cm (latent phase) in 6–8 hours in a multipara and 8–10 hours in a nullipara, followed by approximately 1 cm per hour from 5 to 10 cm dilatation (active phase) in nulli and multipara, although multipara tend to dilate faster. The expected progress recorded on the chart at a rate of 1 cm per hour from admission dilatation in the active phase of labour is called the *alert line*, which helps to identify those who are progressing slowly. A line 2 hours parallel with the alert line called the *action line* can be drawn to decide on when to actively intervene with artificial ROM or oxytocin infusion to augment labour in the absence of malpresentation, disproportion or concern for fetal condition.

如果宫口扩张的进展滞后于预期的扩张速度 2h 以上，就会与行动线交叉，说明活跃期进展不良。英国国家健康与临床卓越研究所指南建议，当 3h 内宫口扩张＜1cm 且无其他变化（如宫颈消退或胎膜破裂时胎头下降），应在排除头盆不称的情况下先用人工破膜助产，如无进展或进展缓慢可输注催产素。

在产程图上描述胎头下降是根据在骨盆边缘上方的可触摸的胎头占五分之几，也就是它需要 5、4、3、2 或 1 个手指来覆盖头部。

If the progress of cervical dilatation lags more than 2 hours behind the expected rate of dilatation, it will cut the action line, indicating the poor progress in the active phase of labour. The UK National Institute for Health and Clinical Excellence guidelines suggest that when encountered with slow progress of <1 cm in 3 hours with no other changes such as cervical effacement or descent of the head in the presence of ruptured membranes, cephalopelvic disproportion should be excluded and labour augmented first by artificial ROM, and if there is no or slow progress, with an oxytocin infusion. Descent of the station of the head is charted on the partogram based on the palpable portion of the head above the pelvic brim in fifths, i.e. whether it needs 5, 4, 3, 2 or 1 finger to cover the head.

在产程图上胎头的位置显示为 0～5 级。

The station of the head is plotted on the 0–5 gradation of the partogram.

也可以通过评估先露部在坐骨棘水平上下几厘米来记录下降情况，在坐骨棘的上方标记为 –1、–2 和 –3，在坐骨棘的下方标记为 +1、+2 和 +3。

Descent is also recorded by assessing the level of the presenting part in centimetres above or below the level of the ischial spines and marked as −1, −2 and −3 when it is above the spines and +1, +2 and +3 if it is below the spines.

宫缩的特征和频率是每 10 分钟收缩次数以阴影的形式记录在产程图上，虚线方格表示宫缩持续时间小于 20s，交叉方格为宫缩持续时间在 20～40s，而持续时间超过 40s 的宫缩则以方格的完全阴影表示。宫缩的频率和持续时间可以通过临床触诊或体外产力描记法来测量。宫缩的强度不能通过产妇感觉到的疼痛程度或腹部触诊子宫来评估，只能通过宫内压力导管来确定。然而，在分娩过程中并不常规使用宫内导管，因为使用宫内导管并不能改善分娩进程。

The nature and frequency of the uterine contractions are recorded on the chart by shading in the number of contractions per 10 minutes. Dotted squares indicate contractions of less than 20 seconds' duration, cross-hatched squares are contractions between 20 and 40 seconds' duration, while contractions lasting longer than 40 seconds are shown by complete shading of the squares. Frequency and duration of contractions can be measured by clinical palpation or external tocography. The intensity of contractions cannot be assessed by the degree of pain felt by the mother or by palpating the uterus abdominally and can only be determined by intrauterine pressure catheters. However, intrauterine catheters are not used routinely in the management of labour because their use has been shown not to improve the outcome.

4. 分娩过程的液体和营养（Fluid and nutrition during labour）

目前在发达国家中大多数产科病房剖宫产率超过 20%，因此，饮食问题就变得尤为重要。如果产妇有可能需要在全身麻醉下进行手术分娩，那么在第一产程要禁食水，因为如果手术分娩需要全身麻醉时，会使胃排空延迟，可能导致呕吐和误吸。不过，现在大多数手术分娩都是在局部麻醉下完成的，因此如果分娩进展正常，预期能阴道分娩，可以给予一些液体和少量营养。最近的临床试验表明，除了液体以外，不考虑给产妇喂软的、易消化的固体营养物质。如果分娩不是迫在眉睫，应在分娩 6h 后给予静脉补充液体，因为酮症酸中毒的主要原因是脱水，产妇排尿时除了检查尿糖和尿蛋白外，还应检查尿液中是否有酮体。在静脉补液时最好使用生理盐水或 Hartmann 溶液，并监测液体的输入和输出，以免母亲水分过多或过少。

In most maternity units in the developed world, caesarean section rates now exceed 20%. The issue of what can be taken by mouth therefore becomes particularly important. If there is a likelihood that the mother will need operative delivery under general anaesthesia, then it is clearly important to avoid oral intake at any significant level during the first stage of labour. Delayed gastric emptying may result in vomiting and inhalation of vomitus if general anaesthesia for operative delivery is needed. On the other hand, most operative deliveries are now achieved under regional anaesthesia, and therefore there is a case for giving some fluids and light nutrition orally if labour is progressing normally and a vaginal delivery can be anticipated. Recent clinical trials have suggested little concern with feeding the mother with soft, easily digestible, solid nutrition in addition to fluids. Intravenous (IV) fluid replacement should be considered after 6 hours in labour if delivery is not imminent. The major cause of acidosis and ketosis is dehydration, and urine should be checked for ketones in addition to sugar and protein whenever the mother passes urine. Administration of normal saline or Hartmann's solution is preferred, and the fluid input and output should be monitored so not to over- or under-hydrate the mother.

九、分娩镇痛（Pain relief in labour）

在分娩中有许多镇痛的方法，这些方法应该在产前告知孕妇。从本质上讲，这些技术旨在减少分娩时的疼痛程度，同时将母婴的风险降到最低。

> 分娩时脱水的典型症状包括心动过速、轻度发热和组织肿胀消失。请记住，分娩是一项繁重的体力劳动，提高产房的环境温度往往是为了满足新生儿的需要，而不是产妇的需要，这会导致产妇大量的液体不自觉地流失。
>
> The classic signs of dehydration in labour include tachycardia, mild pyrexia and loss of tissue turgor. Remember that labour can be hard physical work and that the environmental temperature of delivery rooms is often raised to meet the needs of the baby rather than the mother, leading to considerable insensible fluid loss.

A number of strategies are used in labour for the relief of pain, and these should be discussed with the pregnant mother in the antenatal period. Essentially, these techniques are aimed at reducing the level of pain experienced in labour whilst invoking minimal risk for the mother and baby.

分娩时的疼痛程度差别很大，有些人几乎感觉不到疼痛，而有些人则会在整个分娩过程中经受腹背部的疼痛，而且疼痛程度越来越高。因此，任何减轻疼痛的方案都必须适应个体的需要。医务人员可以根据产妇是初产妇还是经产妇、目前宫口扩张的情况、产程进展的速度，以及产妇对疼痛的耐受程度，给出最佳的止痛方式。减轻疼痛的方式最好由产妇根据医务人员给予的建议来决定，通常是多种方法的结合，从最少的到最有效的方法来减轻她的疼痛。唯一能完全缓解疼痛的技术是硬膜外麻醉镇痛。

The level of pain experienced in labour varies widely-some experience very little, whilst others suffer from abdominal and back pain of increasing intensity throughout their labour. Thus, any programme for pain relief must be tailored to the needs of the individual. The caregiver may be able to advise the best mode of pain relief based on whether the mother is nulliparous or multiparous, the current cervical dilatation, the rate of progress of labour and the extent to which the mother is feeling the pain. The mode of pain relief is best decided by the mother based on the advice given. Often this may result in a combination of methods, starting from the least to most effective method to alleviate her pain. The only technique that can provide complete pain relief is epidural analgesia.

（一）麻醉镇痛（Narcotic analgesia）

传统上哌替啶是使用最广泛的麻醉药，但在英国和澳大利亚的许多中心哌替啶已被吗啡取代。所有阿片类药物的常见不良反应是产妇的恶心和呕吐，以及婴儿的呼吸抑制，并且通常在分娩后 2h 内给药对新生儿的影响尤为重要，所以阿片类药物常与止吐药配合使用以减轻产妇恶心。

Pethidine has traditionally been the most widely used narcotic agent but has been replaced in many centres in the UK and Australia by morphine. The common side effects for all the opiates are nausea and vomiting in the mother and respiratory depression in the baby. The effect on the neonate is particularly important when the drug is given within 2 hours of delivery. Opiates are often administered with anti-emetics to reduce nausea.

一些中心使用瑞芬太尼，因为这是一种超短效阿片类药物，其镇痛效果优于哌替啶，对新生儿呼吸的影响较小。

Remifentanil is used in some centres, as this is an ultra-short-acting opioid that produces superior analgesia to pethidine and has less of an effect on neonatal respiration.

由于一些产妇不适合局部镇痛，如那些使用抗惊厥药物的产妇，阿片类药物可能继续在分娩镇痛中发挥重要作用。

Because some mothers are unsuitable for regional analgesia, e.g. those on anticonvulsants, opiates are likely to continue to play a significant role in pain relief in labour.

（二）吸入麻醉镇痛（Inhalational analgesia）

这些药物用于分娩早期，直到产妇改用更强的镇痛药。最适合在第一和第二产程后期的短期镇痛，最广泛使用的是笑气，它是氧化亚氮（笑气）和氧气各占 50% 的混合物。这种气体为自动给药，以避免在摘下面罩时过量释放，并在宫缩开始后立即吸入。笑气是英国使用最广泛的分娩镇痛药，可缓解大多数人的疼痛。

These agents are used in early labour until the mother switches to much stronger analgesics. It is best for shortterm pain relief in the late first and second stage of labour. The most widely used agent is Entonox, which is a 50/50 mixture of nitrous oxide and oxygen. The gas is self-administered to avoid overdosing when they drop the mask off and is inhaled as soon as the contraction starts. Entonox is the most widely used analgesic in labour in the UK and provides sufficient pain relief for the majority.

研究表明，如果长时间接触氧化亚氮，会对助产护士产生不良影响；这些影响包括生育力下降、骨髓改变和神经改变。每 6～10 小时强制换气一次可以有效降低氧化亚氮的含量，故所有产房都应强制换气。

Nitrous oxide has been shown to have adverse effects on birth attendants if exposure is prolonged; these effects include decreased fertility, bone marrow changes and neurological changes. Forced air change every 6–10 hours is effective in reducing the nitrous oxide levels and should be mandatory in all delivery rooms.

（三）非药物方法（Non-pharmacological methods）

经皮电神经刺激（TENS）包括在脊柱背面的 T10～L1 和 S2～S4 水平上每侧放置 2 对 TENS 电极，电流为 0～40mA，频率为 40～150Hz。这在产程早期是有效的，但在产程晚期中通常是不够的。为了使这项技术有效，对产妇的产前培训是必不可少的。

Transcutaneous electrical nerve stimulation (TENS) involves the placement of two pairs of TENS electrodes on the back on each side of the vertebral column at the levels of T10–L1 and S2–S4. Currents of 0–40 mA are applied at a frequency of 40–150 Hz. This can be effective in early labour but is often inadequate by itself in late labour. For the technique to be effective, antenatal training of the mother is essential.

其他无创方法包括针灸、皮下无菌水注射、按摩和放松技术，这些方法的有效性还存在争议。

Other non-invasive methods include acupuncture, subcutaneous sterile water injections, massage and relaxation techniques, the effectiveness of which is debated.

（四）局部镇痛（Regional analgesia）

硬膜外镇痛是最有效、应用最广泛的局部镇痛方式。它为 95% 的产妇提供了完全的镇痛。这一方法可以在任何时候开始，并且不会影响子宫收缩力，但可能在第二产程中由于降低会阴部的压力感，减少了 Ferguson 反射从而减少子宫活动。Ferguson 反射是指由于临产部位挤压扩张宫颈和阴道上部而产生的催产素反射性释放所导致的子宫活性增加。

Epidural analgesia is the most effective and widely used form of regional analgesia. It provides complete relief of pain in 95% of labouring women. The procedure may be instituted at any time and does not interfere with uterine contractility. It may reduce the desire to bear down in the second stage of labour due to lack of pressure sensation at the perineum and reduced uterine activity due to loss of 'Ferguson's reflex', which is an increased uterine activity due to reflex release of oxytocin due to the presenting part stretching the cervix and upper vagina.

将细导管置入腰椎硬膜外间隙，并注射局部麻醉药，如丁哌卡因（图 11-7）。在局部使用阿片类药物麻醉大大减少了丁哌卡因的用量，从而保留下肢的运动功能，并减少了低血压和胎心率异常的典型并发症。

A fine catheter is introduced into the lumbar epidural space, and a local anaesthetic agent such as bupivacaine is injected (Fig. 11.7). The addition of an opioid to the local anaesthetic greatly reduces the dose requirement of bupivacaine, thus sparing the motor fibres to the lower limbs and reducing the classic complications of hypotension and abnormal FHR.

该程序包括以下步骤。

The procedure involves:

- 留置静脉导管，并用不超过 500ml 的生理盐水或 Hartmann 溶液预负荷。

- Insertion of an IV cannula and preloading with no more than 500 mL of saline or Hartmann's solution.

- 在 $L_3 \sim L_4$ 间隙置入硬膜外导管，并以有效镇痛所需的最小剂量注射局部麻醉药。

- Insertion of the epidural cannula at the L_3–L_4 interspace and injection of the local anaesthetic agent at the minimum dose required for effective pain relief.

- 监测血压、脉搏和胎心率，调整产妇姿势，以达到预期的镇痛效果。

- Monitoring BP, pulse rate and FHR and adjusting maternal posture to achieve the desired analgesic effect.

硬膜外镇痛的并发症包括以下几种情况。

The complications of epidural analgesia include:

- 低血压：可以通过预负荷和使用小剂量麻醉药和阿片类药物来避免。

- Hypotension: this can be avoided by preloading and the use of low-dose anaesthetic agents and opioid solutions.

- 意外硬膜刺穿：在硬膜外麻醉中发生率不到 1%。

- Accidental dural puncture: occurs in fewer than 1% of epidurals.

- 硬膜外麻醉后头痛：使用 16 号或 18 号针头，约 70% 的产妇会出现头痛。持续 24h 以上的硬膜外麻醉后头痛应该用硬膜外填充治疗。

- Postdural headache: about 70% of mothers will develop a headache if a 16- or 18-gauge needle is used. A postdural headache that persists for more than 24 hours should be treated with an epidural blood patch.

局部麻醉的禁忌证包括以下几种情况。

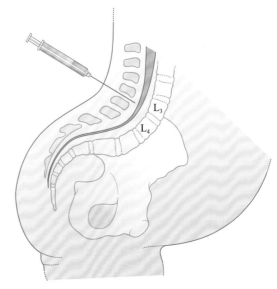

▲ 图 11-7 腰椎硬膜外间隙注射局部麻醉药引起的硬膜外麻醉

Fig.11.7 Epidural anaesthesia is induced by injection of local anaesthetic agents into the lumbar epidural space

Contraindications to regional anaesthesia include:

- 产妇拒绝。

- maternal refusal

- 凝血功能障碍。

- coagulopathy

- 局部或全身感染。

- local or systemic infection

- 未纠正的低血容量。

- uncorrected hypovolaemia

- 工作人员或设施不足或缺乏经验。

- inadequate or inexperienced staff or facilities

> ! 注意
>
> 许多女性在临产时没有要求任何形式的止痛。然而，随着产程进展，产妇意识到分娩是痛苦的，产妇将改变要求。因此，能够随时提供硬膜外镇痛服务非常重要，是分娩管理水平先进的表现。
>
> Many women set out in labour without requesting any form of pain relief. However, as labour progresses, the realization that labour can be painful will change the requirements of the mother. It is therefore essential to have an epidural service that can be readily available so that the labour is not too far advanced before the epidural can become established.

（五）其他形式的局部麻醉（Other forms of regional anaesthesia）

腰麻通常用于手术分娩，特别是作为独立手术。它不用于分娩镇痛，因为硬膜外镇痛具有极高的安全性，而且可以补充适当的剂量或持续输注，以较长时间缓解疼痛。剖宫产通常采用腰硬联合麻醉，脊髓提供快速有效的麻醉，而硬膜外麻醉可以在接下来的 24h 内继续起效，以达到良好的止痛效果。

Spinal anaesthesia is commonly used for operative delivery, particularly as a single-shot procedure. It is not used for control of pain in labour because of the superior safety of epidural analgesia and the ability to top up with suitable doses or as continuous infusion to get pain relief over a long period. Often a 'spinal–epidural' combination is used for caesarean section, with the spinal providing quick and effective anaesthesia whilst the epidural can be continued over the next 24 hours for good pain relief.

宫颈旁阻滞包括局部麻醉药渗入宫颈旁组织。这很少用于产科手术，如果麻醉药物进入血管，对胎儿产生不良反应的可能性更大。

Paracervical blockade involves the infiltration of local anaesthetic agents into the paracervical tissues. This is rarely used for obstetric procedures and has the greater chance of side effects to the fetus should it enter a vessel.

阴部神经阻滞麻醉包括出会阴神经管的阴部神经和直肠下神经周围浸润麻醉（图 11-8）。它是过去阴道分娩手术的一种广泛使用的局部麻醉，现在已被硬膜外麻醉所取代而不再常用了。

Pudendal nerve blockade involves infiltration around the pudendal nerve as it leaves the pudendal canal and the inferior haemorrhoidal nerve (Fig. 11.8). It was a widely used form of local anaesthesia for operative vaginal deliveries in the past but is now less frequently used, as it has been replaced by epidural anaesthesia.

在会阴切开部位直接浸润麻醉仍被广泛用于缝合会阴伤口。此操作必须非常小心，避免在局部浸润时将麻醉药直接注入静脉。意外将麻醉药注入静脉，特别是在剂量较大的情况下可能会导致心律失常和抽搐等中毒症状。

Infiltration directly into the perineal tissues over the episiotomy site is still widely used for the repair of perineal wounds. Great care must be taken to avoid direct IV injection of the drug at the time of local infiltration. Toxic symptoms such as cardiac arrhythmias and convulsions may result from accidental injection of the anaesthetic drug, especially with larger dosages.

十、分娩姿势（Posture in labour）

在分娩的第一产程，有些孕妇喜欢持续走动或

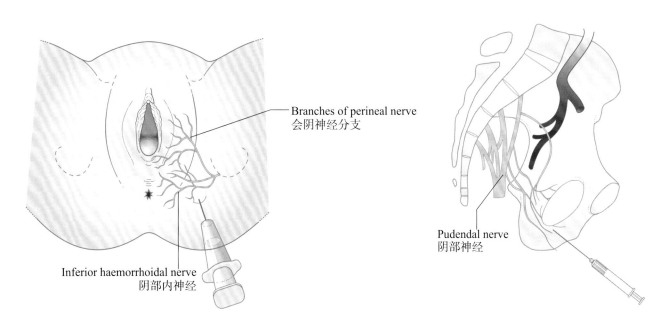

▲ 图 11-8　阴部神经阻滞是通过在坐骨水平的阴部神经周围注射局部麻醉药来实现的。额外的浸润被用来阻滞直肠下神经和会阴神经的分支

Fig. 11.8　Pudendal nerve blockade is achieved by injection of local anaesthetic around the pudendal nerve at the level of the ischial spine. Additional infiltration is used to block branches of the inferior haemorrhoidal and perineal nerves.

277

坐在椅子上；当进入第二产程时，大多数孕妇喜欢躺着，而一些孕妇更喜欢蹲下利用重力来帮助生产。在过去，硬膜外麻醉的孕妇由于暂时性运动障碍，必须保持仰卧位。联合阿片类药物的低剂量麻醉法已解决了这一问题，有了这样的混合硬膜外麻醉，使孕妇可以随意四处走动。

Some women prefer to remain ambulant or to sit in a chair during the first stage of labour. However, most women prefer to lie down as labour advances into the second stage, although some will prefer to squat to use the forces of gravity to help expel the baby. In the past, women who had epidural anaesthesia had to remain supine because of temporary motor impairment. This has been overcome using low-dose anaesthesia combined with opiates. With such mixed epidurals, women can move about and often ambulate.

水中分娩（Water births）

有些孕妇喜欢浸泡在水中以减轻疼痛，浮力可更好的支撑妊娠的子宫，因此大多数孕妇更喜欢在水中分娩。但水中分娩有一个弊端：婴儿可能会在第一次呼吸时吸入浴水，如果浴水被母亲的粪便污染，这可能会给婴儿造成麻烦。浴缸的温度也必须定期检查，并且不要将孕妇独自留在水中。

Some mothers prefer immersion in a water bath for pain relief. Flotation improves support of the pregnant uterus. Most women prefer to deliver outside water. There is a possibility of the baby inhaling the bath water with the first breath, which can cause problems to the baby if the bath is contaminated with maternal faeces. The temperature of the bath must be regularly checked, and the mother should not be left alone in the water bath.

十一、胎儿监测（Fetal monitoring）

胎心率的变化或新的粪染的羊水（胎儿排便）可能提示胎儿缺氧。这些征象可在正常的分娩中发生，但更多发生在高危孕妇中，必要时，需对胎儿的头皮采血（scalp blood sampling，FBS）进行辅助检查，以确定胎儿情况。入院时胎动（fetal movement，FM）减少可能提示胎儿处于危险之中，而胎动停止可能表明死亡，因此应在入院时仔细询问胎动情况。

Changes in the FHR or the passage of new meconiumstained liquor (fetal bowel motion) may suggest possibility of fetal hypoxia. These signs can occur in normal labour but more so in high-risk pregnancies and need to be studied to determine the fetal condition, if necessary, with the adjunct use of fetal scalp blood sampling (FBS). Diminution of fetal movements

(FMs) on admission may indicate fetal jeopardy, and cessation of movements may indicate death and hence enquiry about FM should be made on admission in labour.

（一）间歇听诊（Intermittent auscultation）

在第一产程，使用手持式多普勒超声换能器或 Pinard 胎儿听诊器在宫缩间歇每隔 15 分钟监测胎心率，持续 1min。在第二产程，每隔 5 分钟或每隔 1 次宫缩后就进行胎心率的听诊。通过人工触诊监测宫缩，持续 10min，以确定频率和持续时间。推荐进行间歇性听诊（IA）的频率，是因为在随机对照研究中，胎儿和新生儿结局无差异：该研究比较了第一产程用胎心听诊器每 15 分钟听诊 1 次胎心，持续 1min，第二产程每隔 5 分钟。理想的听诊应该在入院时听取并记录胎心基线（对照母体脉率进行交叉检查），然后胎动时予以听诊以证实胎心有加速，并确认在收缩后不久没有减速。技术的进步使得手持多普勒可以显示胎动为数字并转换信息以在发光二极管（LED）屏幕上生成 CTG，可以看到该图像，并将其存储在设备中，如有需要可重复查看。

The FHR is monitored every 15 minutes for a period of 1 minute soon after a contraction using a handheld Doppler ultrasound transducer or Pinard fetal stethoscope in the first stage of labour. In the second stage, the FHR is auscultated every 5 minutes or soon after every other contraction. Contractions are monitored by manual palpation over a period of 10 minutes to determine the frequency and duration. The frequency of intermittent auscultation (IA) was recommended on the basis that there was no difference in fetal and neonatal outcome in randomized studies that compared IA every 15 minutes for 1 minute after a contraction in the first stage and every 5 minutes in the second stage with EFM. Ideal auscultation practice should be listening and recording the baseline FHR on admission (cross-checked against the maternal pulse rate) followed by auscultation with the FMs to demonstrate an acceleration and soon after a contraction to confirm that there are no decelerations. Technological advances have made it possible for a hand-held Doptone to display the digital FHR and convert the information to produce a CTG on a light-emitting diode (LED) screen, which can be seen, stored within the device and reviewed later if the need arises (Fig. 11.9).

电子胎心监护的临床使用指南已由英国国家卫生与临床卓越研究所、澳大利亚和新西兰妇产科学院，以及美国和加拿大的类似机构，如国际妇产科医生联合会（FIGO）等制定。这些机构的指南具有很大的相似性和微小的差异，不太可能影响临床结果。不建议低风险孕妇使用电子胎心监护或持续电子监护。但是，经过适当的建议后，还是应该尊重女性的意愿。这取决于该孕妇入院后是否希望使用电子胎心监护仪或持续电子胎心监护仪。持续电子胎心监护仪的具体适应证见表 11-1。

The clinical guidelines for the use of EFM have been produced by the National Institute for Health and Clinical Excellence in the UK, Australia and New Zealand College of Obstetricians and Gynaecologists and by similar bodies in the United States and Canada, as well as by the International Federation of Gynaecologists and Obstetricians (FIGO). They have great similarities and minor differences that are unlikely to influence clinical outcome. Admission CTG or routine CTG using electronic monitoring is not recommended for women classified as low risk. However, the woman's wishes should be respected after appropriate counselling. This may be that the woman wishes or not the use of admission CTG or continuous CTG. The specific indications for continuous EFM are listed in Table 11.1.

（二）胎儿心动图（Fetal cardiotocography）

电子胎心监护能够连续监测胎心率及子宫收缩的频率和持续时间。胎儿的心率通常是使用多普勒超声换能器计算的，该换能器从外部应用于产妇腹部。检测到的信号是心脏运动的信号，测量的是心动周期之间的时间间隔，这会转换为心率，也可以通过将电极直接施加到提示部位上，根据从胎儿心电图（ECG）获得的 RR 波间隔来测量心率。

EFM enables continuous monitoring of the FHR and the frequency and duration of uterine contractions. The heart rate of the fetus is usually calculated using a Doppler ultrasound transducer, which is applied externally to the maternal abdomen. The signals that are detected are those of cardiac movement, and what is measured is the time interval between cardiac cycles. Traditionally, this is converted to heart rate. The heart rate can also be measured from the RR wave intervals obtained from the fetal electrocardiogram (ECG) by direct application of an electrode to the presenting part.

可以在上腹壁上（宫底和脐之间的位置）应用一个压力传感器或应用将充满液体的导管或压力传感器经宫颈管插入子宫腔来记录子宫活动（图 11-10）。外部层析成像可以准确测量宫缩频率和持续时间，但只显示宫内压信息。准确的宫压测量需要子宫内导管或换能器，但由于缺乏临床益处的证据，大多数医疗中心并不将其作为常规。

Uterine activity is recorded either with a pressure transducer applied over the anterior abdominal wall between the fundus and the umbilicus or by inserting a fluid-filled catheter or a pressure sensor into the uterine cavity through the cervical canal (Fig. 11.10). External tocography gives an accurate

表 11-1　使用连续胎儿电子监护的适应证

Table 11.1　Indications for the use of continuous electronic fetal monitoring

孕产妇 Maternal	胎儿 Fetal
既往剖宫产 Previous caesarean section	胎儿生长受限 Fetal growth restriction
子痫前期 Pre-eclampsia	早产 Prematurity
过期妊娠 Post-term pregnancy	羊水过少 Oligohydramnios
长时间胎膜破裂 Prolonged rupture of the membranes	多普勒动脉血流异常 Abnormal Doppler artery velocimetry
引产 Induced labour	多胎妊娠 Multiple pregnancy
糖尿病 Diabetes	胎粪污染 Meconium-stained liquor
产前出血 Antepartum haemorrhage	臀先露 Breech presentation
其他孕产妇疾病 Other maternal medical diseases	

measurement of the frequency and duration but only relative information of intrauterine pressure. Accurate measurements of pressure need an intrauterine catheter or transducer, and this is not used as a routine in most centres due to lack of evidence of its clinical benefit.

1. 基线心率（Baseline heart rate）

定义 FHR 的正常模式比定义什么是异常要容易。正常心率在 110～160/min 波动（图 11-11）。心率超过 160/min 为胎儿心动过速，小于 110/min 为胎儿心动过缓。

The definition of normality in the pattern of the FHR is easier than defining what is abnormal. The normal heart rate varies between 110 and 160 beats/min (Fig. 11.11). A rate faster than 160 is defined as *fetal tachycardia*, and a rate less than 110 is *fetal bradycardia*.

基线变化（Baseline variability）

胎心率出现与基线不同的变化，称为基线变异。尽管在每一次跳动的基础上有可变性，标准胎儿监护仪取 3～5 次跳动的平均数，并将其作为基线变异记录在标准 CTG 上。因此，我们将其称为基线变异，而不是每次跳动的变化，这可在计算机化系统中实

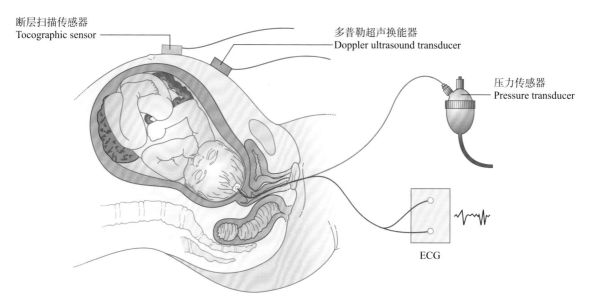

▲ 图 11-9　分娩过程监测。宫缩可通过宫内和宫外扫描成像记录；胎心率可通过外部多普勒超声记录或直接在胎先露部位应用 ECG 电极记录

Fig. 11.9　Monitoring during labour. Contractions are recorded by intrauterine and extrauterine tocography; the fetal heart rate is recorded externally by Doppler ultrasonography or by direct application of an ECG electrode to the presenting part.

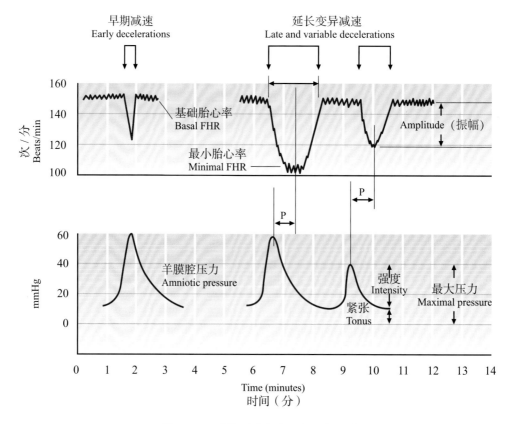

▲ 图 11-10　分娩时胎心率和宫压变化模式

FHR. 胎心率

Fig. 11.10　Patterns of fetal heart rate change and amniotic pressure change in labour.

FHR, Fetal heart rate.

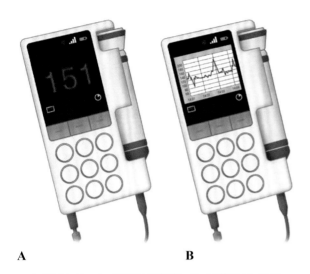

A　　　　　　　　　　**B**

▲ 图 11-11　A. 屏幕显示数字；B. 屏幕显示 CTG

Fig.11.11　**(A) Doptone showing digital display. (B) Doptone showing a CTG display.**

现。纸速，无论是 1cm/min、2cm/min 还是 3cm/min，都会影响基线变异的外在表现。基线变异是胎心率在基线率附近的振荡记录，通常在 5～25/min 变化。基线变异是由于交感神经和副交感神经活动对心脏的毫秒级的反应，反映了自主神经系统的完整性，在胎儿睡眠时期会减少。缺氧、感染和药物治疗可减少基线变异。FHR 变异小于 5/min 持续＞90min 是不正常的，可能提示胎儿危险。

The heart rate exhibits variations from the baseline, which is known as *baseline variability*. Although there is variability on a beat-to-beat basis, the standard fetal monitor averages 3–5 beats and records it as *baseline variability* on the standard CTG. Hence, we term it as *baseline variability* rather than beat-to-beat variation, which is possible with computerized systems. The paper speed, whether it is 1 cm, 2 cm or 3 cm/min, will affect the appearance of the baseline variability. Baseline variability is a record of the oscillations in heart rate around the baseline rate and normally varies between 5 and 25 beats/min. Baseline variability is due to the millisecond-to-millisecond reaction of the sympathetic and parasympathetic activity on the heart and reflects the integrity of the autonomic nervous system. It is reduced during the fetal sleep phase. Hypoxia, infection and medication can reduce baseline variability. An FHR with a variability of less than 5 beats/min for >90 minutes is abnormal and may indicate fetal jeopardy.

2. 胎心率的短暂变化(表 11-2)[Transient changes in fetal heart rate (Tables 11.2)]

(1) 加速（Accelerations）

胎心率一过性增加超过 15/min 续时间超过 15s

称为加速，与 FM 有关。加速反映了躯体神经系统的活动，是胎儿没有缺氧的安全征象。

Accelerations are defined as transient abrupt increases in heart rate of more than 15 beats/min for more than 15 seconds and are associated with FMs. Accelerations reflect the activity of the somatic nervous system and are a reassuring sign of a fetus that is not hypoxic.

(2) 减速（Decelerations）

胎心率下降超过 15/min 持续时间超过 15s 称为减速。各种减速由它们与子宫收缩的关系或由引起它们的病理生理机制来分类。一些变化模式通常被认为与缺氧有关，具有临床意义。

Decelerations are defined as decreases in heart rate of more than 15 beats/min for more than 15 seconds. These are defined by their relationship to uterine contractions or by the pathophysiological mechanism that causes them. Some patterns of change are generally considered to have clinical significance in relation to hypoxia.

(3) 早期或胎头受压减速（Early or head compression decelerations）

这种减速与子宫收缩是同步的。FHR 有一个逐渐下降和上升的过程。最低点出现在宫缩的高峰，胎心率下降通常小于 40/min。这种减速通常是由于胎头受压产生的，是生理性的，出现在第一产程后期和第二产程。

These decelerations are synchronous with uterine contractions. There is a gradual fall and rise of the FHR. The nadir occurs at the peak of the contraction, and the decrease in heart rate is generally less than 40 beats/min. These decelerations are generally due to head compression and are physiological. Hence, they are seen in the late first and second stages of labour.

(4) 晚期减速或胎盘功能不全减速（Late or placental insufficiency decelerations）

胎心率减慢开始于子宫在收缩开始 20s 后，并且直到宫缩结束不能恢复到基线水平。

The onset of the slowing of heart rate occurs >20 seconds after the contraction commences and does not return to the normal baseline rate until after the contraction is completed.

晚期减速是由于胎盘功能不全，反复出现这种减速时，基线升高，基线变异减少可能提示胎儿缺氧。

Late decelerations are due to placental insufficiency, and with repeated such decelerations, rise in the baseline rate

表 11-2 正常、可疑和病理胎心率（FHR）轨迹的定义及推荐措施 [NICE（2017）分娩护理：NICE 指南 CG190, 2017 年 2 月]

Table 11.2 Definition of normal, suspicious and pathological fetal heart rate (FHR) traces and recommended actions (NICE (2017) Intrapartum Care: NICE guideline CG190, February 2017)

类别 Category	定义 Definition	行动 Action
正常的 Normal	所有 4 种特征都被归类为安全的 FHR 轨迹 An FHR trace in which all four features are classified as reassuring	根据风险因素继续进行间歇或连续监测 Continue intermittent or continuous monitoring as indicated by risk factors.
可疑的 Suspicious	FHR 轨迹的一个特征为不安全的，其余的特征为安全的 An FHR trace with one feature classified as non-reassuring and the remaining features classified as reassuring	排除需要立即结束分娩的因素（脐带脱垂、子宫破裂、胎盘早剥）。治疗脱水、过度应激、低血压及改变体位。继续 CTG Exclude factors indicating need for immediate delivery (cord prolapse, uterine rupture, abruption). Treat dehydration, hyperstimulation, hypotension and change position. Continue CTG.
病理 Pathological	具有 2 个或 2 个以上不安全特征或 1 个及 1 个以上异常特征的 FHR 轨迹 An FHR trace with two or more features classified as non-reassuring or one or more classified as abnormal	排除需要立即分娩的因素（脐带脱垂、子宫破裂、胎盘早剥）。治疗脱水、过度应激和改变体位。如果长时间胎心过缓应结束分娩。通过采集胎儿头皮血液获得进一步信息或结束分娩 Exclude factors indicating need for immediate delivery (cord prolapse, uterine rupture, abruption). Treat dehydration, hyperstimulation and change position. Deliver if prolonged bradycardia. Either obtain further information on fetal status by fetal blood scalp sampling or deliver.

and reduction in baseline variability may be indicative of fetal hypoxia.

(5) 变异或脐带压缩减速（Variable or cord compression decelerations）

变异减速在时间、形状和幅度上各不相同而得名。它们的基线频率开始短暂的轻度上升，然后急剧下降，然后迅速恢复到正常的基线，并稍高于这一水平。在突然减速之前的轻微加速和恢复时的轻微增加被称为肩征。胎心率下降通常在 40/min 以上，是由于脐带受压，脐带受压随每次宫缩变化，导致形状、大小和减速时间变化，在 CTG 描记中被认为是不安全的特征。减速深度和持续时间增加，减速间隔时间缩短，基线率增加和基线变异减少均提示缺氧加重。单纯变异减速的额外变化，以缓慢恢复到基线率的形式，或以联合出现的形式，即变异减速紧跟着晚期减速，称为非典型变异减速或带有"可关注特征"的变异减速，是异常表现。

Variable decelerations vary in timing, shape and amplitude-hence their name. They have an initial slight transitory rise in the baseline rate followed by a precipitous fall followed by a quick recovery to the normal baseline rate and slightly beyond. The slight increase just before the sudden decline and the slight increase in the recovery is termed *shouldering*. The heart rate usually falls by more than 40 beats/min and is due to cord compression, which varies with each contraction, giving rise to variable shapes, sizes and timing of decelerations, and are considered non-reassuring features in a CTG trace. Increase in the depth and duration of the decelerations, reduction of interdeceleration intervals, rise in baseline rate and reduction in baseline variability suggest worsening hypoxia. Additional changes to simple variable decelerations in the form of slow recovery to baseline rate or a combined, i.e. variable followed immediately by late decelerations are called *atypical variable decelerations* or variable decelerations with 'concerning features' and are abnormal features.

(三) 胎儿心电图（The fetal electrocardiogram）

胎儿心电图可以通过头皮电极或放置孕妇腹部电极来记录。进行 ECG 波形分析，需要胎儿头皮电极和母亲皮肤对照电极。一些单位使用特殊设备（STAN，Neoventa Ltd.，Sweden）和 FHR 一起使用计算机分析 ST 波形来检测缺氧。即使有 ST 波形分析，临床决策也需要人工解释 CTG。

The fetal ECG can be recorded from scalp electrodes or by the placement of maternal abdominal electrodes. For ECG waveform analysis a scalp electrode and a maternal skin reference electrode are necessary. Some units use computerized analysis of the ST waveform with the use of special equipment (STAN, Neoventa Ltd., Sweden) along with FHR to detect hypoxia (Fig. 11.12). Even with ST waveform analysis, manual interpretation of CTG is needed for clinical decision-making.

（四）胎儿的酸碱平衡（Fetal acid-base balance）

分娩时胎心率异常可能是胎儿酸中毒的表现，应检查胎儿酸碱状态以验证这些表现。

Where abnormalities of FHR occur in labour, they may provide an indication of fetal acidosis, but to confirm these findings, the fetal acid-base status should be examined.

胎儿血液通过羊膜镜直接从头皮获得。宫颈必须至少扩张 2cm，以使仪器通过宫颈插入，要求母亲以侧卧位躺卧。侧卧位比仰卧位或截石位更合适，因为这样可以避免引起仰卧位低血压。在胎儿头皮上切一小口，将血液收集到肝素化的毛细管中，然后，在血气分析仪中分析样本。

Fetal blood is obtained directly from the scalp through an amnioscope. The instrument is inserted through the cervix, which must be at least 2 cm dilated. The mother is requested to lie in the lateral position. The latter is preferable to a dorsal or lithotomy position, as it will avoid the risk of inducing supine hypotension. A small stab incision is made in the fetal scalp, and blood is collected into a heparinized capillary tube. The sample is then analyzed in a blood gas analyzer.

正常的 pH 在 7.25～7.35。第一产程的 pH 在 7.20～7.25，提示轻度酸中毒，应在 30min 后重复取样。如果小于 7.20，建议结束分娩，除非胎儿将立即娩出。如果有足够的样本，应进行完整的血气分析，因为 pH 正常时 CO_2 分压升高可能提示可随母亲状态改变而自行纠正的呼吸性酸中毒。胎儿代谢性酸中毒的程度也可以通过测量胎儿头皮血液乳酸水平来评估，通常仅需少量血液（5μl）并且可以使用便携式手持设备完成。用于确定临床措施需要的确切值/截断值需根据所使用的设备的正常值而变化。

Normal pH lies between 7.25 and 7.35. A pH between 7.20 and 7.25 in the first stage of labour indicates mild acidosis, and sampling should be repeated within the next 30 minutes. If it is <7.20, delivery is recommended unless spontaneous delivery is imminent. If there is sufficient sample, a full blood gas analysis should be performed, as a raised $P\text{co}_2$ with a normal base excess may indicate a respiratory acidosis that may correct itself if the posture of the mother is changed. The degree of metabolic acidosis in the fetus may also be assessed from fetal scalp blood by measuring lactate levels. This generally requires smaller blood volumes (5 μL) to measure and can be done using portable handheld devices. The exact values/cut-off used to determine the need for clinical action vary according to the normal values established using the device used.

十二、早产（Pre-term delivery）

在英国，24 周至 36^{+6} 周的分娩被认为是早产。发病率各国不同，甚至在同一国家的不同种族和社会经济群体中也不相同。文献报道发病率为 6%～12%。其中，近 75% 在 34～37 周，通常这些婴儿很少有短期或长期并发症。在资源充足的国家，高水平的围产期护理可给予良好的生存照顾，包括小于妊娠 32 周的婴儿或出生体重超过 1500g 的婴儿。在妊娠不足 32 周出生的婴儿中，约有 1/3 是未足月胎膜早破，1/3 是由于自发早产，剩下的 1/3 是由于因医疗或产科疾病导致的医源性干预，如先兆子痫、产前出血或宫内生长受限。

Delivery from 24 completed weeks (in the UK) up to 36 weeks and 6 days is considered a pre-term birth. The incidence varies from country to country and even within different ethnic and socioeconomic groups in the same country. The literature suggests an incidence of 6–12%. Of this, nearly 75% are between 34 and 37 weeks, and generally these infants suffer few short- or long-term complications. The high standards of perinatal care in well-resourced countries can care for babies with good intact survival at even less than 32 weeks or any infant with a birth weight more than 1500 g. Of those born at less than 32 weeks' gestation, about a third follow pre-labour ROM, a third are due to spontaneous pre-term labour and the remaining third are due to iatrogenic intervention where delivery is indicated for a medical or obstetric condition such as pre-eclampsia, antepartum haemorrhage or intrauterine growth restriction.

（一）自发早产（Spontaneous pre-term labour）

1. 病因学（Aetiology）

尽管许多病例原因不明，但已知有许多因素与自发早产有关。

A number of factors are known to be associated with spontaneous pre-term labour, although in many cases the cause is unknown.

与早产有关的一些主要因素见图 11–13。它与社会条件差、营养状况、产前出血、多胎妊娠、子宫畸形、宫颈机能不全和常与感染相关的胎膜早破有关。既往的早产史是最好的单一预测因素。相对危险度约为 3，如果有一次以上的早产，风险更高。妊娠期间的并发症也可能导致早产；这包括子宫过度膨胀，如多胎妊娠和羊水过多。其他因素，如早期妊娠和中期妊娠早期阶段的出血，增加了早产的风

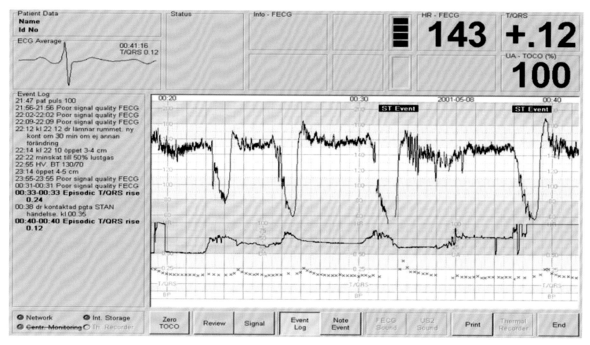

▲ 图 11-12　显示胎心率、胎儿心电图及计算的 T/QRS 比的胎儿心电图仪屏幕

Fig.11.12　Screen of a fetal electrocardiogram (ECG) monitor that displays the fetal heart rate, fetal ECG and the calculated T/QRS ratio.

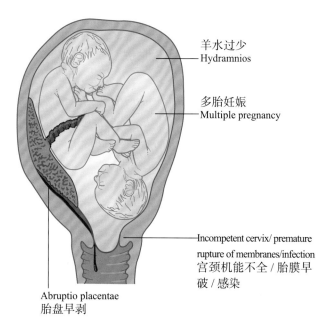

羊水过少
Hydramnios

多胎妊娠
Multiple pregnancy

Incompetent cervix/ premature rupture of membranes/infection
宫颈机能不全 / 胎膜早破 / 感染

Abruptio placentae
胎盘早剥

▲ 图 11-13　早产的诱因

Fig. 11.13　Factors predisposing to premature labour.

险。严重的母体疾病，特别是发热性疾病，也可促进分娩过早发动。

Some of the major factors associated with pre-term labour are shown in Figure 11.13. There is an association with poor social conditions, nutritional status, antepartum haemorrhage, multiple

pregnancy, uterine anomalies, cervical incompetence and PROM, which is often associated with infection. A previous history of pre-term delivery is the best single predictor. The relative risk is about 3, and the risk increases if there has been more than one pre-term delivery. Complications during a pregnancy may also precipitate pre-term labour; these includes over-distension of the uterus, such as multiple pregnancy and polyhydramnios. Other factors, such as haemorrhage in either the first or early second trimester, increase the risk of subsequent pre-term labour. Severe maternal illness, particularly febrile illness, may also promote the early onset of labour.

社会因素包括产妇年龄（20 岁以下或 35 岁以上）、首次妊娠、种族、婚姻状况、吸烟、药物滥用和繁重、工作压力大（框 11-1）。早期研究认为积极的社会干预似乎可以降低早产的发生率，但由于缺

框 11-1　早产：社会因素	Box 11.1　Pre-term labour: social factors
• 贫困 • 产妇年龄（<20 岁，>35 岁） • 工作压力大 • 婚姻状况 • 吸烟 • 滥用药物	• Poverty • Maternal age (<20 and >35 years) • Heavy stressful work • Marital status • Cigarette smoking • Substance abuse

乏良好的科学证据，尚未得到一致认可。最近，已在那些有可能早产的人身上鉴定出基因标记。

Social factors involve maternal age (under 20 or over 35 years), first pregnancy, ethnicity, marital status, cigarette smoking, substance abuse and heavy, stressful work (Box 11.1). Active social intervention appeared to reduce the incidence of pre-term labour in early studies but has not received unanimous support due to lack of good scientific evidence. Very recently, genetic markers have been identified in those who are likely to go into pre-term labour.

2. 生殖道感染的作用（The role of genital tract infection）

生殖道感染可能通过促进子宫肌层活动或引起胎膜早破而起作用。已发现与绒毛膜羊膜炎和早产发病有关的微生物包括淋病奈瑟菌、B 族溶血性链球菌、沙眼衣原体、人型支原体、解脲支原体、阴道加德纳菌和拟杆菌等。在这些细菌中，B 族链球菌可能是最重要的。

Genital tract infection may act either through promoting myometrial activity or by causing pre-labour rupture of the fetal membranes. Organisms that have been found to be associated with chorioamnionitis and the onset of pre-term labour include *Neisseria gonorrhoeae*, group B haemolytic streptococci, *Chlamydia trachomatis*, *Mycoplasma hominis*, *Ureaplasma urealyticum*, *Gardnerella vaginalis*, *Bacteroides* spp. and *Haemophilus* spp. Of these, group B streptococci are probably the most sinister.

穿过黏液栓的细菌产生蛋白酶，导致组织破坏和胎膜早破。生物体也可能释放磷脂酶 A_2 和磷脂酶 C，磷脂酶 A_2 和磷脂酶 C 从羊膜中释放花生四烯酸，导致前列腺素的释放。细菌毒素的释放也可能启动蜕膜和胎膜的炎症过程，导致前列腺素和细胞因子的产生，特别是白介素（IL-1、IL-6）和肿瘤坏死因子。

The bacteria that have penetrated the mucus plug produce proteases, resulting in tissue destruction and PROM. Organisms may also release phospholipase A_2 and phospholipase C, which releases arachidonic acid from the amnion, causing the release of prostaglandins. Release of bacterial toxins may also initiate an inflammatory process in the decidua and membranes, resulting in the production of prostaglandins and cytokines, particularly interleukins (IL-1, IL-6) and tumour necrosis factor.

（二）早产儿（The pre-term infant）

1. 存活率（Survival）

如果病因是感染，可能会影响母亲，但主要影响的是胎儿。新生儿服务的提高给健康状况良好和出生体重合理的新生儿提供了良好存活率。24 周后每推迟一天分娩，存活率就会增加 3%～6%，因此尽可能延长妊娠期。出生体重不足 500g 的婴儿存活的概率很小，而出生体重 1500g 的婴儿几乎和足月婴儿有一样的存活率。在 500～1000g，每增加 100g，存活率显著增加（图 11-14）。极低出生体重儿死亡的主要原因是感染、呼吸窘迫综合征（respiratory distress syndrome，RDS）、坏死性小肠结肠炎和心室周围出血。

If the cause is of infective origin, it may affect the mother, but the effect is predominantly on the fetus. Improvements in neonatal services provide good chance of intact survival if the newborn is in good condition and is of reasonable birth weight. Each day of delay in birth after 24 weeks increases the chance of survival by 3–6%, and hence the need to conserve the pregnancy as long as possible. An infant born with a birth weight of less than 500 g has little chance of survival, whereas one born weighing 1500 g is nearly as likely to survive as a full-term infant. Between 500 and 1000 g, every 100-g increment produces a significant increase in survival (Fig. 11.14). The major causes of death in very-low-birth-weight infants are infection, respiratory distress syndrome (RDS), necrotizing enterocolitis and periventricular haemorrhage.

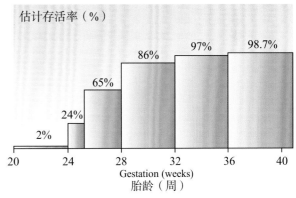

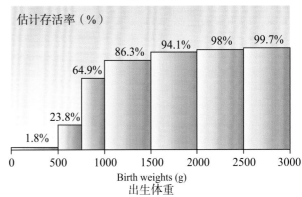

▲ 图 11-14 出生体重、胎龄和围产儿结局

Fig. 11.14 Birth weight, gestational age and perinatal outcome.

2. 早产的并发症（Complications of pre-term birth）

直接并发症有呼吸窘迫、黄疸、低血糖和体温过低。长期并发症包括肺发育不良和神经发育迟缓。

Immediate complications are respiratory distress, jaundice, hypoglycaemia and hypothermia. Long-term complications include pulmonary dysplasia and neurodevelopmental delay.

（三）早产的管理（The management of pre-term labour）

早产的诊断是基于有疼痛的规律子宫收缩伴进行性宫颈缩短和扩张。孕期子宫收缩是常见的、正常的，不一定会导致分娩。30% 以上因疑似早产而入院的产妇可能未分娩就出院回家。24 周后超声评估宫颈长度小于 2.5cm 是预测早产的有用指标。宫颈内胎儿纤维连接蛋白的出现可用于评估早产的风险，如果胎膜完好，且在过去 24h 内没有性交或阴道检查，可以从子宫颈取拭子进行检测。阴性结果表示不太可能在 7 天内分娩（＜3%），阳性结果的预测价值较小，只有 20% 的女性会在 7 天内分娩。超声检查的宫颈缩短联合纤维连接蛋白阳性在预测有宫缩的女性早产临产更有价值。

The diagnosis of pre-term labour is based on the onset of regular painful uterine contractions associated with progressive cervical effacement and dilatation. Uterine contractions are common and a normal occurrence during pregnancy and do not always progress to established labour. Over 30% of hospital admissions for suspected pre-term labour may be discharged home undelivered. Ultrasound assessment of the length of the cervix of <2.5 cm after 24 weeks is a useful predictor of possible pre-term labour. The presence of the protein fetal fibronectin in the cervix can be used in the assessment of the risk of pre-term delivery. The test can be performed by taking a swab from the cervix, provided that the membranes are intact and the woman has not had intercourse or a vaginal examination within the previous 24 hours. A negative result makes delivery within the next 7 days unlikely (<3%), although a positive test result is of less value, as only 20% of such women will deliver in the same period. A combination of short cervix on ultrasound and positive fibronectin is more useful in predicting impending pre-term labour in a woman with pre-term contractions.

1. 预防（Prevention）

预防工作已从不同的方面进行，一些有效，一些效果并不确切。对于已确诊的早产，很难证明任何干预的有效性，因为许多分娩不论治疗与否都会自行停止。预防的干预主要基于孕期应尽量减少繁重的工作和过度的体力活动。巴黎 Papiernik 的研究强烈建议社会干预以降低早产的发生率。其他研究并没有支持这些研究结果。然而，有早产史的女性在妊娠期间应注意生活方式和饮食，避免繁重或压力大的工作，这似乎是合理的。用抗生素治疗无症状菌尿已被证明可降低早产的发生率。当宫颈拭子中检测到 β– 溶血链球菌，抗生素治疗有可能可降低胎膜早破的发生率。最近的随机对照试验研究了超声下宫颈缩短的女性和 17α– 羟孕酮己酸酯的作用。24 周后宫颈缩短小于 2.5cm 的女性中，使用孕酮可降低分娩的发生率。大量随机对照研究显示超声下宫颈缩短的孕妇进行预防性宫颈环扎没有任何益处。既往提倡使用子宫托，可改变宫颈与宫体的角度，但是文献研究结果尚无定论。

Prevention has been approached from different directions, some of which appear to have been effective, while others have not been convincing. It has been difficult to prove efficacy with any interventional therapy for established preterm labour because many labours stop spontaneously irrespective of treatment. Interventional studies have been based on the concept that heavy work and excessive physical activity should be kept to a minimum during pregnancy. Studies by Papiernik in Paris strongly supported social intervention programmes as the way to reduce the incidence of pre-term labour. Other studies have not supported these observations. However, it appears logical to suggest that those women who have a history of pre-term labour should be advised concerning lifestyle and diet and that they should avoid heavy or stressful work during pregnancy. The treatment of asymptomatic bacteriuria with antibiotics has been shown to reduce the likelihood of pre-term labour and, where β-haemolytic streptococci are detected in cervical swabs, antibiotic treatment appears to reduce the incidence of PROM. Recent randomized controlled trials investigated women with short cervical length on ultrasound and the role of 17-alpha-hydoxyprogesterone caproate. In women who have a short cervix of <2.5 cm beyond 24 weeks, the use of progesterone reduced the incidence of delivery. Large randomized trials which studied the role of prophylactic cervical cerclage for women with short cervix on ultrasound did not show any benefit. The Arabin cervical pessary, which changes the angulation of the cervix to the body of the uterus, and other pessaries have been advocated, but results from studies show different outcomes-some supporting its use whilst others do not.

2. 治疗（Treatment）

孕妇因早产住院，需决定处理方法。尽管在极早的早产期每延迟一天分娩会提高胎儿生存率、减少发病率和对重症监护的依赖，防止早产的远期益处并不确定。延迟分娩为使用糖皮质激素争取时间，使 II 型肺细胞释放胎儿肺表面活性物质，以减少透明膜病（HMD）和 RDS 的发生（图 11–15），这是没有争议的。

Once the woman is admitted to hospital in established preterm labour, a decision must be made as to the approach to management. The long-term advantages of preventing pre-term labour are uncertain, although every day of delay in the early pre-term period increases the chance of survival and reduces morbidity and more dependence on intensive care. There is no controversy in postponing delivery long enough for the administration of corticosteroids to enable the release of fetal lung surfactant from type II pneumocytes with the aim of reducing the chance of hyaline membrane disease (HMD) and RDS (Fig. 11.15).

决定是否继续分娩或抑制子宫收缩取决于孕周，无感染、出血或胎儿窘迫，胎膜完整、宫颈扩张小于 5cm。如果超声测定胎龄小于 34 周，可以使用药物抑制宫缩，以给母亲使用糖皮质激素来促进胎儿肺成熟。硫酸镁 4g 静脉注射（其后继续每小时输注 1g，持续 24h）已被证明具有神经保护作用，专业机构推荐用于 32 周之前的早产。

The decision on whether labour should be allowed to proceed or to inhibit uterine activity depends on the period of gestation, absence of infection, bleeding or fetal compromise, intact membranes and the cervix being less than 5 cm dilated. In cases where gestational age by ultrasound dating is less than 34 weeks, it is appropriate to inhibit uterine activity pharmacologically until corticosteroids can be administered to

> **! 注意**
> 由于存在产妇血流动力学改变及感染的风险，因此，在存在出血的情况下禁忌使用宫缩抑制药，因为延迟分娩可能会损害母亲和胎儿的健康。
>
> Tocolysis is contraindicated in the presence of bleeding, because of the risk of maternal haemodynamic compromise, and with infection, as delay may compromise the health of mother and fetus.

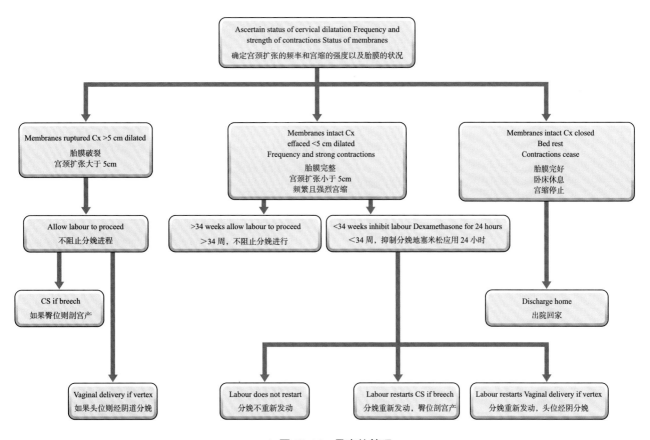

▲ 图 11-15　早产的管理

CS. 剖宫产；Cx. 宫颈

Fig. 11.15　Management of pre-term labour.

CS, Caesarean section; Cx, cervix.

the mother to enhance fetal lung maturity. Magnesium sulphate 4 g IV (in some series followed by 1 g hourly for 24 hours as an infusion) has been shown to be neuroprotective, and its use is now recommended by professional organizations for use in pre-term labour less than 32 weeks.

推迟分娩的药物治疗可根据作用的不同原理分组（框 11–2）。

Drug therapy to delay the delivery can be divided into groups operating on different principles (Box 11.2).

(1) β 肾上腺素受体激动药（β-Adrenergic agonists）

这些药物作用于子宫肌细胞膜上的 $β_2$ 肾上腺素受体，激活腺苷酸环化酶，导致细胞内 cAMP 增加。通过抑制肌动蛋白 – 肌球蛋白相互作用抑制子宫活动。

These drugs act on the β-2-adrenergic receptor sites on the membranes of the myometrial cells, with the activation of adenyl cyclase resulting in an increase in intracellular cAMP. Action is by inhibition of actin-myosin interaction, which inhibits uterine activity.

> **！注意**
>
> 这些药物具有潜在危害母体的不良反应，因此必须谨慎使用。不良反应包括心悸和震颤、缺血性心律不齐、体液潴留、肺水肿，偶见猝死。
>
> These drugs have potentially dangerous maternal side effects and hence must be used with caution. The side effects include palpitations and tremor, ischaemic arrhythmias, fluid retention, pulmonary oedema and sometimes sudden death.

框 11–2 早产的药物治疗	Box 11.2 Drug treatment for pre–term labour
• β 肾上腺素受体激动药 • 前列腺素合成酶抑制药 • 硫酸镁 • 缓释的钙通道阻滞药 • 皮质类固醇 • 催产素拮抗药	• β-Adrenergic agonists • Prostaglandin synthetase inhibitors • Magnesium sulphate • Slow calcium channel blockers • Corticosteroids • Oxytocin antagonists

最常用的药物是利托君、沙丁胺醇和特布他林。已知有心血管疾病或高血压病史的患者不应使用该类药物。

The most commonly used drugs are ritodrine, salbutamol and terbutaline. The drugs should not be used where there is a known history of cardiovascular disease or hypertension.

药物以 5% 葡萄糖或葡萄糖 / 生理盐水稀释后给药，输注速率应每 10～20 分钟递增 1 次，直到宫缩

减至每 15 分钟一次，或直到产妇心律达到 140/min 为止。仔细监测产妇脉搏、血压、液体出入量和血液电解质是必不可少的。静脉输液引起的液体超负荷和药物引起抗利尿激素增加导致液体潴留是肺水肿和心衰的主要原因，在多胎妊娠中发生的可能性更大。

The drugs are administered diluted in 5% dextrose or dextrose/saline, and the infusion rate should be incrementally increased every 10–20 minutes until contractions are reduced to one every 15 minutes, or until the maternal heart rate has reached 140 beats/min. Careful monitoring of maternal pulse rate, BP, fluid input/output and plasma electrolytes is essential. Fluid overload due to IV fluids and drug action increasing antidiuretic hormone causing retention of fluids is the main cause of pulmonary oedema and heat failure, and this may be greater in multiple pregnancy.

> **！注意**
>
> 长时间使用 β 肾上腺素受体激动药可引起低钾血症、高血糖症（糖尿病患者酮症酸中毒）和肺水肿。
>
> β-Adrenergic drugs can cause hypokalaemia, hyperglycaemia (ketoacidosis in diabetics) and pulmonary oedema with prolonged use.

给孕妇应用皮质类固醇后，可缓慢降低剂量。如果胎龄超过 34 周，对胎儿不会产生任何明显益处。如果孕妇需转诊至具有新生儿重症监护设施的三级医疗中心，可继续治疗。口服维持疗法尚未得到证实，不建议使用。

The dosage can be reduced slowly after the administration of corticosteroids to the mother. It is unlikely that any major benefit will accrue to the fetus if the gestational age exceeds 34 weeks. It is necessary to continue treatment until the mother is transferred to a tertiary care centre with neonatal intensive care facilities. Oral maintenance therapy remains unproven and is not recommended.

(2) 前列腺素合成酶抑制药（Prostaglandin synthetase inhibitors）

孕妇以 1～3mg/kg 的剂量服用吲哚美辛(Indocin) 等药物 24h，可抑制前列腺素的产生，从而抑制子宫活性。这类药物在预防分娩方面非常有效，但有可能导致宫内动脉导管早闭而对胎儿循环产生不利影响。在某些情况下，可能会选择此类药物，如当婴儿的早产比动脉导管早闭所带来的危害更大时。该药物还会增加肺和肾动脉的阻力，并可能引起羊水

过少。以最小有效剂量使用 1～3 天，可以很好地避免此类后果，通常以 100mg 栓剂的形式给药。

Drugs such as Indocin (indomethacin) given at a dose of 1–3mg/kg maternal body weight for 24 hours inhibit prostaglandin production and thus uterine activity. These drugs are very effective in preventing the progression of labour. However, they may result in in-utero closure of the ductus arteriosus and therefore adversely affect the fetal circulation. There may be occasions when they are the drug of choice and where the pre-term delivery of the infant constitutes a greater risk than the not-invariable early closure of the ductus. This drug also increases pulmonary and renal artery resistance and can cause oligohydramnios. Such consequences are best avoided by using the drug for 1–3 days at the minimum required dose. Usually it is given as 100-mg suppositories.

 经验　吲哚美辛还通过影响胎儿肾功能而减少羊水量，在羊水过多的病理中可能还有其他正向作用。
Indomethacin also reduces liquor volume by its effect on fetal renal function and may be of additional benefit in cases of polyhydramnios.

(3) 钙通道阻滞药（Calcium antagonists）

缓释钙离子通道阻滞药在抑制子宫活性方面的作用不容置疑。动物实验表明，在器官形成期间大剂量使用此类药物（尤其是硝苯地平），可能会引起胎儿肋骨融合。但是，如果在中、晚期妊娠此类用药，远远超过了这个时期，没有证据表明可构成威胁。

The effect of slow calcium channel blockers in inhibiting uterine activity is not in doubt. There has been some evidence in animal studies using very large doses of these compounds, particularly nifedipine, that they may cause rib fusions in the fetus if given during the period of organogenesis. However, if the drugs are administered in the late second and third trimesters, this is well past this period and there is no evidence that they pose a threat.

硝苯地平的初始口服剂量为 20mg，此后每 4～6 小时服用 10～20mg。严重的不良反应很少。

Nifedipine is administered with a starting oral dose of 20 mg followed by 10–20 mg every 4–6 hours thereafter. Severe side effects are rare.

(4) 皮质类固醇（Corticosteroids）

皮质类固醇在预防呼吸窘迫中的用途是基于这些化合物增强 II 型肺细胞表面活性物质释放的作用，从而使肺泡在分娩时迅速膨胀并建立正常的呼吸功

！注意　钙通道阻滞药要尽管在英国未获准用于妊娠，但由于其效果好且价格低廉，因此被皇家妇产科学院推荐作为抑制子宫活性的首选药物。
Calcium antagonists, although not licensed for use in pregnancy in the UK, are recommended by the Royal College of Obstetricians and Gynaecologists as the drug of choice to inhibit the uterine activity because of its efficacy and low cost.

能。皮质类固醇在早产儿产前应用的对照试验表明，RDS、脑室周围出血和坏死性小肠结肠炎显著减少。

The use of corticosteroids in the prevention of respiratory distress is based on the action of these compounds in enhancing the release of surfactant from type II pneumocytes, thus enabling rapid expansion of the alveoli at the time of delivery and the establishment of normal respiratory function. Controlled trials on the antenatal effects of corticosteroids in pre-term infants have shown that there are significant reductions in RDS, periventricular haemorrhage and necrotizing enterocolitis.

倍他米松的剂量为 2 次，每次 12mg，间隔 24h 肌内注射。地塞米松是给药 4 次，每次肌内注射 6mg，每 12 小时 1 次。如果分娩可以延迟至少 24h 至 7 天，可以达到最佳效果。妊娠 34 周以上，不应使用皮质类固醇。母体给予促甲状腺激素释放激素（TRH）也可以促进磷脂酰胆碱的生成。

The dosage of betamethasone is two doses of 12 mg given intramuscularly 24 hours apart. Dexamethasone is given as four 6 mg doses intramuscularly 12 hours apart. Optimal benefit can be achieved if delivery is postponed for at least 24 hours and up to 7 days. Over 34 weeks' gestation, the administration of corticosteroids is not justified. The production of phosphatidylcholine can also be enhanced by the administration of thyrotropin-releasing hormone (TRH) to the mother.

！注意　目前，28～34 周分娩的未给予皮质类固醇治疗可被视为疏忽。
Failure to prescribe corticosteroids before delivery between 28 and 34 weeks may now be considered egligent.

(5) 硫酸镁的神经保护作用（Neuroprotection by magnesium sulphate）

由于效果差，已广泛放弃使用硫酸镁作为宫缩抑制药。但是，大量的随机对照研究显示，早产前使用对新生儿具有神经保护作用。它可以稳定毛细

血管膜并减少脑室内和脑室周围出血的发生。单次静脉注射 4 克 MgSO$_4$，接下来的 24h 每小时 1g。但是，有一项对照试验表明，即使不进行后续连续给药也可以有效，并且 24h 后即可发挥神经保护作用。如果分娩没有立即发生并且孕妇再次发动早产，是否可以重复这种方案的信息很少。一种实用的方法是，如果间隔时间大于 1 周，则应再给予一次治疗。

The use of magnesium sulphate as a tocolytic has largely been abandoned because of its low efficacy. However, large randomized studies have shown a neuroprotective effect in the neonate with its use prior to pre-term delivery. It stabilizes capillary membranes and reduces the incidence of intraventricular and periventricular haemorrhage. An IV dose of 4 g MgSO$_4$ is given followed by 1 g every hour for the next 24 hours. However, there is a trial that suggests that even a bolus dose of 4 g without subsequent continued dosing is effective and offers neuroprotection after 24 hours. Little information is available as to whether this regimen could be repeated if the delivery does not ensue and the mother restarts in pre-term labour. A pragmatic approach is to give another dose if the interval was greater than 1 week.

3. 分娩方式（Method of delivery）

在许多情况下，抑制分娩是不可能或没有希望的。妊娠期超过 34 周很少会抑制分娩，因为干预的益处不会比允许分娩继续进行的益处多。如果子宫收缩力强且频繁，并且宫颈在入院时扩张超过 5 厘米，则成功阻止早产的可能性很低。如果胎膜破裂并且没有感染的迹象，短期抑制宫缩以争取皮质类固醇给药时间是值得的。如果有产前出血、不安全的 FHR 或可疑宫内感染，允许分娩进展和胎儿分娩可能更安全，有时可能需要促进分娩。

On many occasions, it may not be either possible or desirable to inhibit labour. It is rare to inhibit labour when the gestation is over 34 weeks because the benefits of intervention do not outweigh those of allowing the labour to proceed. If the contractions are strong and frequent and the cervix is more than 5 cm dilated on admission, the likelihood of successfully stopping pre-term delivery is low. If the membranes have ruptured and there is no sign of infection, short-term inhibition of contractions to enable the administration of corticosteroids is worthwhile. If there is any antepartum bleeding, non-reassuring FHR or suspicion of intrauterine infection, it may be safer to allow progress of labour and for the fetus to be delivered, and at times the delivery may need to be expedited.

尽管重要的是尽可能轻柔地控制分娩，但并没

有证据表明使用产钳或扩大的会阴切开术可以改善头位胎儿的结局。如果会阴过紧，长时间压迫早产儿的较软的颅骨是不明智的，突然的娩出可能由于突然的减压而导致颅内出血，常规产钳助产不是常态，可取的是温柔且可控的分娩。

There is no proven evidence that the use of forceps or a wide episiotomy improves fetal outcome in the presence of a vertex presentation, although it is important that delivery be as gentle and controlled as possible. If the perineum is tight, it is not sensible to allow the soft, pre-term skull to be battered on the perineum for a long period. A sudden expulsive delivery may produce intracranial bleeding due to sudden decompression. Routine forceps delivery is not the norm, and a gentle controlled delivery is preferred.

如果是臀位，除非妊娠大于 34 周，否则最好采用剖宫产。尽管没有随机对照研究，但由于围生期死亡率降低和长期神经功能缺损，一些比较臀位经阴分娩和剖宫产分娩结果的大型研究绝大多数都主张剖宫产分娩。原因是 34 周之前，头部相对于躯干较大，胎儿躯干可能经未完全扩张的宫颈娩出而头部被卡住，用力分娩会导致头部突然受压和减压而导致颅内出血。因此，在早产臀位剖宫产时，需要仔细规划切口。例如，可向上延伸的下段中部切口或使用宫缩抑制药使子宫松弛以防止胎头卡住。

In the presence of a breech presentation, delivery by caesarean section is the preferred option unless the gestation is greater than 34 weeks. Although there are no randomized studies, several large studies on the outcome comparing vaginal breech delivery and delivery by caesarean section overwhelmingly favour delivery by caesarean section because of lower perinatal mortality and longterm neurological deficits. The reason for this is that up to 34 weeks, the head is relatively larger than the trunk and the fetal trunk may be pushed through an incompletely dilated cervix and the head may get stuck. Forceful delivery causes sudden compression and decompression of the head and possible intracranial haemorrhage. Hence with caesarean section to deliver a pre-term breech, the incision type needs to be carefully planned, such as a lower segment midline incision extending upwards or use of a tocolytic to relax the uterus to prevent entrapment of the after-coming head.

十三、胎膜早破（Pre-labour rupture of the membranes）

早产可能与 PROM 有关，但自然的破膜可能在足月或早产时单独发生而没有分娩。与胎膜早破相关的因素具体如下。

Pre-term labour may be associated with PROM, but spontaneous ROM may occur in isolation at term or pre-term without the onset of labour. Factors that are associated with pre-labour ROM are:

- 胎膜的抗拉强度，可能会因感染而减弱。

- 周围组织的支撑，体现在宫颈扩张时；宫颈扩张越大，破膜的可能性就越大。

- 羊水压力。

- The tensile strength of the fetal membranes, which may be weakened by infection.

- The support of the surrounding tissues, which is reflected in the dilatation of the cervix; the greater the dilatation of the cervix, the greater the likelihood that the membranes will rupture.

- The intra-amniotic fluid pressure.

（一）发病机制（Pathogenesis）

胎膜早破没有已知的主要危险因素，但与孕早期和孕中期出血有关，而与吸烟有关的可能性较小。但是，最常见的因素是感染，在这方面已描述了各种病原微生物。其中包括 B 族溶血性链球菌、沙眼衣原体和引起细菌性阴道病的微生物。

Pre-labour ROM has no known major risk factor but is associated with first- and second-trimester haemorrhage and, less predictably, with smoking. However, the most common factor is infection. Various organisms have been described in this context; these include group B haemolytic streptococci, C. trachomatis and those organisms causing bacterial vaginosis.

（二）处理（Management）

母亲会有突然阴道流出羊水的病史。尽管有时难以确诊，入院时应行窥器检查以确认羊水的存在。硝嗪拭子可随 pH 的变化而变换颜色，但其使用价值有限。使用基于 α– 甲胎蛋白和胰岛素样生长因子（IGF）的更特异性的检测更未精确，但由于其成本而未得到广泛使用。

The mother will come with a history of sudden loss of amniotic fluid from her vagina. On admission to hospital, a speculum examination should be performed to confirm the presence of amniotic fluid, although sometimes it can be difficult to confirm the diagnosis. The use of nitrazine sticks, which shows colour change with pH, is of limited value. Tests using more specific markers based on the presence of α-fetoprotein and insulin-like growth factor (IGF) are more accurate but not widely used because of their cost.

对母亲和婴儿的风险主要是感染的风险。长期排出羊水可能导致胎儿肺发育不全。困难在于决定何时分娩胎儿及分娩方式，因为子宫可能对催产素敏感性差，尤其是极早期的早产。

The risks to the mother and baby are those of infection. Long-term drainage of amniotic fluid may result in fetal pulmonary hypoplasia. The difficulty is to decide when to deliver the fetus and how to effect delivery, as the uterus may not respond adequately to the action of oxytocic agents, especially in the very pre-term period.

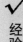

> 经验
>
> 如果不准备立即发动分娩，应避免指检以减少外源性感染的风险。
>
> If the plan was not to stimulate labour immediately, avoid digital examination to reduce the risk of introducing infection.

如果 PROM 不能确诊，最好继续观察所穿的卫生垫的湿润程度，以协助诊断。超声检查显示羊水量正常，在胎先露和宫颈之间有液体，且没有阴道流液，这强烈提示胎膜完整。

Where there is doubt about PROM, it is better to continue observation to look for wetness of a sanitary pad worn to assist in the diagnosis. An ultrasound examination that shows the presence of normal quantities of amniotic fluid with a pocket of fluid between the presenting part and the cervix with no fluid escaping into the vagina is highly suggestive of intact membranes.

如果有明显的证据表明阴道中有羊水，则应使用拭子取羊水进行培养。产妇感染可能导致子宫压痛，胎儿和（或）产妇心动过速和发热，以及脓性白带。最好通过检测血白细胞计数和 C 反应蛋白（CRP）来监测母体是否有败血症。连续监测 CRP 水平升高提示存在感染。

If there is clear evidence of amniotic fluid in the vagina, swabs should be taken for culture. Maternal infection may result in uterine tenderness, fetal and/or maternal tachycardia and pyrexia, as well as the presence of a purulent vaginal discharge. Monitoring for the presence of maternal sepsis is best performed by the measurement of blood white cell count and C-reactive protein (CRP). Increasing levels of CRP on subsequent estimations suggest the presence of infection.

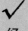

> 经验
>
> 皮质类固醇可能会导致孕妇白细胞数量增加，以及 CTG 基线变异减少。
>
> Corticosteroids may cause an increase in maternal white blood count and reduction in baseline variability in the CTG trace.

如果存在细菌培养阳性或母亲感染的征象，应使用适当的抗生素。如果有感染的迹象，为了胎儿和母亲着想，应使用催产素输注发动分娩引产。如果没有感染的证据，应采取保守治疗并加用红霉素治疗。如果宫缩已经很好地发动，在胎膜破裂的情况下，宫缩抑制药通常是无效的，应该考虑潜在的诱发因素是否是感染。妊娠超过 28 周分娩，婴儿可能会有更好的存活率。大多数 PROM 的孕妇会在 48h 内自然分娩。

If there is a positive culture or evidence of maternal infection, the appropriate antibiotic should be administered. If there is evidence of infection, labour should be induced using an oxytocic infusion and delivery expedited in the interest of the fetus and the mother. If there is no evidence of infection, conservative management with erythromycin cover should be adopted. Tocolysis is generally ineffective in the presence of ruptured membranes if contractions are already well established, and one should consider whether the underlying triggering factor may be infection. If gestation is over 28 weeks, the infant probably has a better chance of survival if delivered. Most women with PROM will deliver spontaneously within 48 hours.

妊娠足月，PROM 的女性在入院时或破膜 24h 后用前列腺素或合成催产素引产。未足月，采取保守治疗，并告知可能存在感染、胎盘早剥、脐带脱垂、肺发育不全或死产的风险，保守治疗是为了使胎儿更成熟以提高存活率和改善结局。

At term, women with PROM are induced with prostaglandins or Syntocinon on admission or after 24 hours of PROM. In the pre-term period, conservative management is adopted with the warning that there may be risks of infection, abruption, cord prolapse, pulmonary hypoplasia or stillbirth, but the need for conservatism is to advance to a mature gestation for better survival and outcome.

十四、引产（Induction of labour）

当母亲或孩子继续妊娠的风险超过引产的风险时，就会引产。这是人为启动子宫的活动以达到经阴道分娩的目的。引产的发生率在各个国家之间及各个医学中心之间差异很大，取决于医学中心内管理的高风险人群，引产的发生率可能在 5%~25%。

Labour is induced when the risk to the mother or child of continuing the pregnancy exceeds the risks of inducing labour. It is the act of artificially initiating uterine activity with the aim of achieving vaginal delivery. The incidence of induction varies widely from country to country and centre to centre and can be from 5 to 25% depending on the highrisk population managed in the centre.

（一）适应证（Indications）

引产的主要适应证如下。

The major indications for induction of labour are:

- 过期妊娠（妊娠超过 42 周）。

- 先兆子痫。

- 胎盘功能不全和宫内生长受限。

- 产前出血：胎盘早剥及来源不明的产前出血。

- Rh 血型不合。

- 糖尿病。

- 慢性肾脏疾病。

- prolonged pregnancy (more than 42 weeks' gestation)
- pre-eclampsia
- placental insufficiency and intrauterine growth restriction
- antepartum haemorrhage: placental abruption and antepartum haemorrhage of uncertain origin
- Rhesus isoimmunization
- diabetes mellitus
- chronic renal disease

月经周期为 28 天的女性，从末次月经期的第一天开始，妊娠超过 294 天，定义为过期妊娠。与妊娠 40 周相比，围产期死亡率在 42 周后翻了 1 倍，在 43 周后翻了 3 倍。尽管常规引产对总的围产期死亡率的影响很小，但要在 41 周以上才应用，因为不良结局对于个体而言是不可接受的。某些人更倾向于保守治疗过期妊娠，需要至少每周 2 次对胎儿进行超声评估羊水量和使用产前 CTG 进行无应激试验（NST）。如果可疑胎儿胎盘功能减退，需进行引产。然而，许多女性会因妊娠引起的身体不适而要求引产。应根据胎次和宫颈评分为孕妇分析成功经阴分娩的概率。刚过 40 周应用人工破膜术减少了 41 周后可能需要引产的人数。

Prolonged pregnancy is defined as pregnancy exceeding 294 days from the first day of the last menstrual period in a woman with a 28-day cycle. The perinatal mortality rate doubles after 42 weeks and trebles after 43 weeks compared with 40 weeks' gestation. Although routine induction of labour has a minimal effect on the overall perinatal mortality rate, it is offered after 41+ weeks, as an adverse outcome is not an acceptable option for the individual mother. Conservative management of prolonged pregnancy is preferred by some, and it involves at least twice-weekly monitoring of the fetus with ultrasound assessment of liquor volume and non-stress test (NST) by antenatal CTG. Induction is undertaken if there is suspicion of fetoplacental compromise. However, many women request induction of labour based on the physical discomfort of the continuing pregnancy. The chance of successful vaginal delivery should be considered and explained to the mother based on parity and cervical score. Artificial separation of membranes just past 40 weeks reduces the number who may need induction after 41 weeks.

（二）宫颈评估（Cervical assessment）

宫颈的临床评估可以预测引产的可能结果。最常用的评估方法是 Bishop 评分或改良的该评分。该宫颈评分需要对宫颈进行临床检查，以根据宫颈在骨盆中的位置、韧度、容受性、宫口扩张、先露位置来给予数字评分。

Clinical assessment of the cervix enables prediction of the likely outcome of induction of labour. The most commonly used method of assessment is the Bishop score or by modification of this score. This cervical score involves clinical examination of the cervix to formulate a numerical score based on the features of the position of the cervix in the pelvis, consistency, effacement, dilation and station of the head.

Bishop 得分超过 6 分可以高度预测容易发动分娩，正常进展并经阴分娩的成功率很高。分数低于 5 分提示不满意，提示需要促宫颈成熟。

A Bishop score of more than 6 is strongly predictive of easy initiation of labour with successful clinical outcome of normal progress and vaginal delivery. A score of less than 5 is not that favourable and indicates the need for cervical ripening.

（三）引产方法（Methods of induction）

引产方法取决于胎膜是否完整及宫颈评分。

The method of induction will be determined by whether membranes are still intact and the score on cervical assessment.

1. 前羊膜囊破膜（Forewater rupture of membranes）

破膜应在产房完全无菌的条件下进行。理想的情况下，宫颈应柔软，容受并至少扩张 2cm，胎头先露部应衔接固定在骨盆中。实际上，这些条件常常不能完全满足，其遵守的程度取决于发动分娩的紧迫性。孕妇取仰卧位或截石位，擦拭并覆盖外阴后，一根手指插入宫颈，并将胎膜与子宫下段分开：这一过程称为剥膜。然后用 Kocher 钳、Gelder 前羊膜

切开钳或破膜钩刺破膨出的胎膜（图 11-16）。羊水缓慢流出，注意防止脐带先露或脱垂。在破膜前后，应监护 FHR 30min。

ROM should be performed under conditions of full asepsis in the delivery suite. Under ideal circumstances, the cervix should be soft, effaced and at least 2 cm dilated. The head should be presenting by the vertex and should be engaged in the pelvis. In practice, these conditions are often not fulfilled, and the degree to which they are adhered to depends on the urgency of the need to start labour. The mother is placed in the supine or lithotomy position and, after swabbing and draping the vulva, a finger is introduced through the cervix, and the fetal membranes are separated from the lower segment: a process known as *stripping the membranes*. The bulging membranes are then ruptured with Kocher's forceps, Gelder's forewater amniotomy forceps or an amniotomy hook (Fig. 11.16). The amniotic fluid is released slowly, and care is taken to exclude presentation or prolapse of the cord. The FHR should be monitored for 30 minutes before and following ROM.

2. 后羊膜囊破膜（Hindwater rupture of membranes）

另一种手术引产的方法是在先露上方进行破膜，这叫后羊膜囊破膜。将 Drew-Smythe 导管插入宫颈并刺破先露上方的胎膜（图 11-17），这项技术的理论优势是能够降低脐带脱垂的风险。在临床实践中，前羊膜囊破膜的风险甚至比自发破膜更低，后羊膜囊破膜技术现在很少使用。

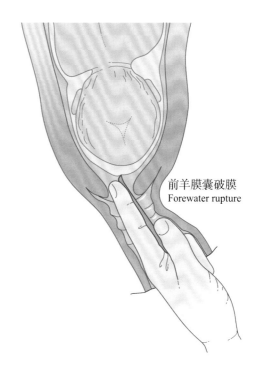

前羊膜囊破膜
Forewater rupture

▲ 图 11-16　前羊膜囊破膜引产

Fig. 11.16　Induction of labour by forewater rupture.

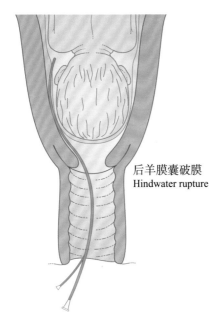

▲ 图 11-17 后羊膜囊破膜引产

Fig. 11.17 Induction of labour by hindwater rupture.

An alternative method of surgical induction involves ROM behind the presenting part. This is known as *hindwater rupture*. A sigmoid-shaped metal cannula known as the *Drewe-Smythe catheter* is introduced through the cervix and penetrates the membranes behind the presenting part (Fig. 11.17). The theoretical advantage of this technique is that it reduces the risk of prolapsed cord. In reality, the risk is even lower with forewater rupture than with spontaneous ROM, and the technique of hindwater rupture is now rarely used.

3. 破膜术后的药物引产（Medical induction of labour following amniotomy）

多种药物可用来刺激子宫活动。通常的做法是手术引产和合成催产素滴注联合应用。合理的方案是从 1mU/min 开始，每 30 分钟增加 3mU/min，直到形成每 10 分钟 3~4 次、每次持续 40s 的宫缩。

Various pharmacological agents can be used to stimulate uterine activity. It is common practice to combine surgical induction with a Syntocinon infusion. A suitable regimen would begin at 1 mU/min and increase by 3 mU/min every 30 minutes until three to four uterine contractions, each lasting >40 seconds, every 10 minutes become established.

手术和药物联合应用引产的主要危险如下。

The principal hazards of combined surgical and medical induction of labour are:

- 过度刺激：宫缩过频、持续时间过长，减少子宫血流，导致胎儿窘迫，即宫缩不应超过每 2 分钟一次，持续时间不应超过 1min。如果发生过度的子宫活动或出现病理性 FHR 模式，应停止输注催产素。

- Hyper-stimulation: Excessive or too frequent and prolonged uterine contractions reduce uterine blood flow and result in fetal asphyxia, i.e. contractions should not occur more frequently than every 2 minutes and should not last more than 1 minute. The Syntocinon infusion should be discontinued if excessive uterine activity occurs or if there are signs of a pathological FHR pattern of concern.

- 脐带脱垂：应在前羊膜囊破膜时予以排查，随后，如果胎心监护出现严重的变异减速，应予以排查。

- Prolapse of the cord: This should be excluded by examination at the time of forewater ROM or, subsequently, if severe variable decelerations occur on the FHR trace.

- 感染：引产到分娩时间间隔过长可增加羊膜腔感染的风险，从而增加婴儿和母体的风险。羊水性状恶化和（或）发生生产妇发热，应终止分娩，除非胎儿将在短时间内娩出。

- Infection: A prolonged induction-delivery interval increases the risk of infection in the amniotic sac, with consequent risks to both infant and mother. If the liquor becomes offensive and/or maternal pyrexia occurs, the labour should be terminated unless the delivery is imminent and the infant delivered.

4. 药物引产和促宫颈成熟（Medical induction of labour and cervical ripening）

这是一种选择的方法，当膜是完整的或宫颈不适合手术诱导。最常用的医疗诱导形式如下。

This is the method of choice where the membranes are intact or where the cervix is unsuitable for surgical induction. The most commonly used forms of medical induction are:

- 通过不同途径给予前列腺素。

- administration of prostaglandins by various routes

- 宫颈机械扩张。

- mechanical dilation of the cervix

英国国家卫生和临床优化研究所推荐包括宫颈条件满意时所有引产使用前列腺素 PGE_2 栓剂或凝胶每 6 小时 1 次，或长效、缓释、以 PGE_2 聚合物为基础的控释分娩系统。

The National Institute for Health and Clinical Excellence recommends the use of prostaglandins PGE_2 pessaries or gel every 6 hours or a long-term, slow-release, PGE₂ polymer-based control release delivery system over 24 hours for all inductions of labour, including when the cervix is favourable.

前列腺素（Prostaglandins）

最广泛使用的是前列腺素 E_2（PGE_2）制剂，用来促宫颈成熟，可以用以下方法给药。

The most widely used form is prostaglandin E_2 (PGE_2). This is used to ripen the cervix and may be administered:

- 口服：剂量从 0.5mg 增加到 2mg/h，直到产生宫缩。然而，由于呕吐和腹泻的不良反应，这在目前的实践中并不使用。

- Orally: Doses of 0.5 mg are increased to 2 mg/h until contractions are produced. However, this is not used in current practice due to the side effects of vomiting and diarrhoea.

- 经阴道途径：最常用的方法是将前列腺素栓剂或木糖凝胶置入后穹隆。宫颈成熟不佳的初产妇（Bishop 评分小于 4 分）初始剂量为 2mg 凝胶。Bishop 评分大于 4 的经产妇和初产妇初始剂量为 1mg。如果有必要，在 6h 后重复使用，第二天再重复一次，最大剂量为 4mg，直到临产或可以破膜，并继续输注催产素引产。栓剂剂量是 3mg。如果第一次栓剂在 6h 内没有起效，没有出现规律宫缩或者宫颈的改变，可放入第二个栓剂。如果母亲没有临产或宫颈没有改变，第二天将再次置入一个栓剂。

- By the vaginal route: The most commonly used method is to insert prostaglandin pessaries or xylose gel into the posterior fornix. Nulliparous women with an unfavourable cervix (Bishop score of less than 4) are given an initial dose of 2 mg gel. Multiparous women and nulliparae with a Bishop score of more than 4 are given an initial dose of 1 mg. This is repeated if necessary after 6 hours and again the following day up to a maximum dose of 4 mg until labour is established or the membranes can be ruptured and the induction continued with oxytocin infusion. The pessaries come as 3-mg doses. If there is no response to the first pessary in 6 hours in the form of regular contractions or cervical changes, a second pessary is inserted. If the mother does not start labour or there is no cervical change, another pessary is inserted the next day.

随着技术进步已研制出聚合的、不可生物降解的、控释给药系统其中含有 10mg PGE_2，可在 24h 内均匀地少量释放药物（https://www.medicines.org.uk/emc/product/135/smpc）。使用这种系统引起宫缩过强的可能性很低。如果发生这种情况，可以通过拉动附着在上面的带子将其移除。一旦去除，过度宫缩就会稳定下来；如果没有，可以使用短效的 β 受体激动剂，如 0.25mg 特布他林皮下注射。这种长效置入器还有一个优点，就是避免了因使用 PGE2 凝胶或栓剂而在 24h 内反复进行阴道检查（图 11-8）。

Recent technological advances have allowed polymeric, non-biodegradable, controlled-release delivery systems to have 10 mg of PGE_2 which can be released in small amounts uniformly over 24 hours (https://www.medicines. org.uk/emc/product/135/smpc). The chance of hyper-stimulation is low with such a system. Should it happen, it can be removed by pulling on the tape attached to the delivery system. Once removed, the hyper-stimulation settles, and if not, a short-acting beta mimetic drug such as terbutaline 0.25 mg subcutaneously can be used. Such long-acting inserts also have the advantage of avoiding repeated vaginal examination within 24 hours to insert repeated doses of PGE_2 gel or pessaries (Fig. 11.18).

世界卫生组织（2011）引产指南建议每 2～4 小时口服 25µg 米索前列醇。米索前列醇（前列腺素 E_1）在许多国家未获许可用于产科，25µg 或 50µg 配方也并非在所有国家均可获得。有人把 200µg 的制剂分成 4 份或 8 份，得到 50µg 或 25µg 的剂量。有人将 200µg 片剂溶解成 20ml，取少量溶液使用。既往有子宫瘢痕的患者禁用前列腺素。人们谨慎使用前列腺素 E_2 栓剂或凝胶而不是前列腺素 E_1（即米索前列醇），因为（前列腺素 E_2 栓剂或凝胶）会增加子宫破裂的发生率，危及胎儿和母亲。在使用这类药物之前，产妇应进行充分的咨询。

The WHO (2011) guidelines on induction of labour recommend oral misoprostol 25 µg every 2–4 hours. Misoprostol (prostaglandin E_1) is not licensed in many countries for use in obstetrics, and the 25- or 50-µg formulations are not available in all countries. Some take a 200-µg formulation and divide it into four or eight segments to get 50-µg or 25-µg doses. Some dissolve a 200-µg tablet in 20 mL, and small aliquots of dissolved solution are taken as appropriate. The use of prostaglandins is contraindicated in the presence of a previous uterine scar. Some use the prostaglandin E_2 pessaries or gel with caution but not prostaglandin E_1 (i.e. misoprostol), as there is increased incidence of uterine rupture that will compromise the fetus and the mother. The mother should be properly counselled before these drugs are used.

5. 机械促宫颈成熟（Mechanical cervical ripening）

这通常包括经宫颈插入球囊导管。用 40～80ml

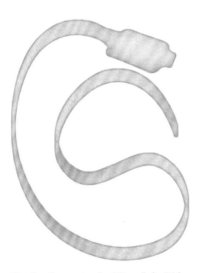
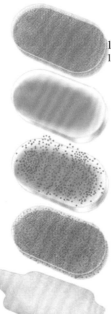

1. 聚乙烯的长链交联产生一种聚合物
1. Long chains of polyethylene oxide are cross-linked to produce a polymer.

2. 聚合物水化形成水凝胶
2. Hydration of polymer to form hydrogel

3. 装填地诺前列酮（10mg 储存）
3. Loading of dinoprostone (10-mg reservoir).

4. 干燥聚合物以固定地诺前列酮
4. Drying of polymer to trap dinoprostone.

Steady release rate of ~ 0.3 mg/h for 24 hours.
稳定释放速率约为 0.3mg/h，持续 24h

5. 聚合物插入物被放置在一个 30cm 长的编织可回收带中
5. Polymer insert is placed into a woven 30-cm long retrieval tape.

▲ 图 11-18　控释型前列腺素 E_2 释放系统
Fig.11.8　Controlled-release prostaglandin E_2 delivery system.

无菌水或生理盐水填充球囊，用于机械扩张宫颈管，持续 12h。有些可能会在此期间临产。有时，球囊会随着宫颈扩张而排出，否则，12h 后将取出球囊，如果宫颈条件良好，则可以进行人工破膜术。如果 4h 后宫缩没有进展到临产，就可以开始滴注催产素。目前，有单囊和双囊的 Foley 导管用于促宫颈成熟。另外，人工合成渗透扩张器（如：Dilapan http://www.dilapan.com/）可以吸收宫颈中的水分并膨胀，从而扩张宫颈。

Commonly this involves the insertion of a balloon catheter through the cervix. The balloon is used to mechanically distend the cervical canal by inflating the balloon with 40 to 80 mL of sterile water or saline over a 12-hour period. Some may go into labour during this period. In a few, the balloon would be expelled with cervical dilatation, and in the others, the balloon could be removed after 12 hours, and if the cervix is favourable, an amniotomy could be performed. If they do not progress to established labour with uterine contractions in the next 4 hours, an oxytocin infusion could be commenced. Currently Foley catheters with a single balloon as well as a specially designed double balloon catheter are available for cervical ripening. Alternatively, synthetically manufactured osmotic dilators (e.g. Dilapan-http://www.dilapan.com/) can be used which absorbs the water content in the cervix and swells, thereby dilating the cervix.

十五、急产（Precipitate labour）

少数情况下，正常或轻微增加的子宫活动可引起快速宫颈扩张和早产。分娩持续时间少于 2h 的经阴分娩被归类为急产。这类分娩的危险在于，胎儿可能会以迅速、不受控制的方式分娩在一个不适宜的环境下（如分娩到厕所）！

Occasionally, at one end of the spectrum of normal labour, normal or slightly increased uterine activity may produce rapid cervical dilatation and an early delivery. A labour lasting less than 2 hours resulting in vaginal delivery is classified as precipitate. The hazards of such labours are that the child may be delivered in a rapid and uncontrolled manner and in an inconvenient environment such as into a toilet!

胎儿病率和死亡率与缺乏复苏设施有关。产妇病率可由严重的会阴损伤和产后出血导致。急产往往会复发，如果有急产史，母亲最好在近预产期住院等待临产或有计划的引产。

Fetal morbidity and mortality may be related to the lack of resuscitation facilities. Maternal morbidity may arise from severe perineal damage and from postpartum haemorrhage. Precipitate labour tends to repeat itself with subsequent labours, and where there is such a history, the mother is best admitted to hospital near term to await the onset of labour or to have a planned induction.

子宫过度刺激（Uterine hyper-stimulation）

目前子宫过度刺激最常见的原因是过量使用促宫缩药物。在极端情况下，这可能导致子宫强直收缩。此时，会有频繁的强烈的宫缩，并且宫缩之间没有足够的时间恢复正常的基线宫腔压力。这种情况可以通过停止催产素输注迅速得到纠正。事实上，如果适当使用外部或内部的宫缩描记法进行宫缩活动监测，这种情况就不会发生。宫缩在 10min 内不应超过 5 次，10min 内超过 5 次宫缩称为宫缩过频，可能影响胎儿胎盘灌注和氧合，从而引起 FHR 变化。

The commonest contemporary cause of uterine hyperstimulation is the uncontrolled use of excessive amounts of oxytocic drugs. In extreme cases, this may result in uterine tetany with a continuous contraction. Leading up to this state, there will be frequent strong contractions and insufficient time between contractions to allow a return to normal baseline pressures. The condition can be rapidly corrected by turning off the oxytocin infusion. In fact, the condition should not arise if uterine activity is properly monitored by external or internal tocography. Contractions should not occur more frequently than five in 10 minutes. More than five contractions in 10 minutes is called *polysystole* and is likely to affect the placental perfusion and oxygenation of the fetus that can give rise to FHR changes.

随着宫颈扩张的进展，子宫对相同剂量的催产素变得越来越敏感。因此，需严密监测宫缩，当宫缩频率在 10min 内达到 5 次以上时，应减少或停止催产素输注。

The uterus becomes more and more sensitive to the same dose of oxytocin with advance in cervical dilatation. Hence, it is important to carefully monitor the contractions and reduce or stop the oxytocin infusion should the contraction frequency increase to more than five in 10 minutes.

子宫过度收缩可以发生于前列腺素使用的各种形式，这是由于药物可从阴道快速吸收，吸收速度受阴道温度和 pH 及是否存在感染 / 炎症的影响。最好的方法是取出 PG 栓剂，并使用短效抗宫缩药，如 0.25mg 特布他林皮下注射或加入 5ml 生理盐水缓慢静脉注射大于 5min。

Uterine hyper-stimulation can occur with the use of prostaglandins in various forms. This is due to rapid absorption of the drug from the vagina, as the rate of absorption is affected by the temperature and pH of the vagina and the presence of infection/inflammation. This is best managed by removal of the PG pessary and the use of a bolus dose of a short-acting tocolytic such as 0.25 mg terbutaline as a subcutaneous dose or in 5 mL saline as a slow IV over 5 minutes.

宫缩过强也可能导致子宫破裂，尤其是在以前的剖宫产或子宫肌瘤切除术后留下的瘢痕部位。这种破裂有时甚至在正常的宫缩时也会发生。

Hyper-stimulation may also lead to uterine rupture, particularly where there is a uterine scar from a previous section or myomectomy. Such a rupture may sometimes occur even in the presence of normal uterine activity.

十六、产程延长（Delay in progress in labour）

在过去的 20 年里，关于什么样的产程延迟是异常分娩的观点发生了明显的变化。现在，产程延长的定义更多地依赖于产程进展的速度，而不是绝对时间。然而，必须记住的是，90% 的初产妇在 16h 内分娩，90% 的经产妇在 12h 内分娩。现在，分娩时间超过 24h 的情况已经很少见了。当产程延长而进展异常缓慢时，必须考虑到头盆不称的可能性，但在大多数情况下进展缓慢与有效宫缩欠佳有关。

The view of what constitutes an abnormal labour has changed substantially over the last two decades. The definition of prolonged labour now relies more on the rate of progress than on absolute times. Nevertheless, it must be remembered that 90% of primigravid women deliver within 16 hours and 90% of multigravid women deliver within 12 hours. It is now rare to see a labour that lasts more than 24 hours. When labour becomes prolonged and progress is abnormally slow, the possibility of cephalopelvic disproportion must be considered, but in most cases slow progress is associated with inefficient uterine activity.

十七、有效宫缩（Efficiency of uterine activity）

宫缩效率是通过宫颈的消退和扩张以及胎头的下降的程度来判断的。有些不频繁的宫缩可能对某些女性有良好的作用（有效），相反，规律且频繁的宫缩反而不能获得良好的宫颈扩张（无效）。过去曾使用过张力过强和张力减低宫缩这两个术语，但由于没有明确的标准来定义，且诊断困难，在临床实践中很少使用。在胎盘早剥等病理情况下，血液渗入子宫肌层可能导致子宫张力增加（高张）和非常频繁的低幅度收缩（宫缩过频 / 频发宫缩缩）。触诊子宫感到"质硬""质软""敏感"。

Efficiency of uterine activity is judged by the desired result of effacement and dilatation of the cervix and descent of the head. Few infrequent contractions may result in good progress in some women (efficient), whilst good frequent uterine contractions may not result in good cervical dilatation (inefficient). In the past, the terms *hypertonic* and *hypotonic* uterine activity were used, but they are hardly used in clinical practice during physiological labour because there are no specific criteria to define and they are difficult to diagnose. In pathological conditions such as abruptio placenta, the blood seeping into the myometrium may cause increased tone of the uterus (hypertonicity) and very frequent low-amplitude contractions (hypersystole/polysystole). On palpation, the uterus would be 'woody hard', tender and 'irritable'.

子宫没有解剖或生理起搏点，但子宫收缩通常是协调的、有规律的间隔，随着分娩的进展，宫缩的频率、持续时间和幅度都在增加。在一些临产的女性中，2 次或 3 次宫缩可能会接连出现，然后一小段时间没有宫缩，接着又连续出现 2 次或 3 次宫缩，这称为不协调性子宫收缩。如果达到了预期的宫颈消退、扩张和胎头下降，不协调的宫缩并不意味着宫缩效率低下。

Despite the absence of an anatomical or physiological pacemaker in the uterus, contractions are usually coordinated and come at regular intervals increasing in frequency, duration and amplitude with progress of labour. In some women in labour, two or three contractions may come together followed by a small period of no activity, followed by another bout of two or three contractions. This is called *incoordinate uterine contractions*. Incoordinate contractions do not mean inefficient uterine activity if the desired progress of cervical effacement, dilatation and descent of the head is achieved.

处理措施（Management）

通常根据产程进展确认宫缩的效率。评估产力（子宫收缩）、胎位（胎儿）和产道（产妇骨盆）非常重要。仔细评估宫缩强度、产妇骨盆的大小和形状以及胎儿的大小来指导正确的处理。

宫缩乏力的一般处理原则如下。

- 安慰产妇及家属并解释情况。

- 充分缓解疼痛，主要采用硬膜外镇痛。

- 静脉输注葡萄糖生理盐水或 Hartmann 溶液以补充足够的液体。

- 加大催产素的剂量以刺激宫缩。

Efficiency of uterine activity is usually recognized by the progress in labour. It is essential to evaluate the power (uterine contractions), passenger (fetus) and passage (maternal pelvis). Careful assessment of uterine activity, size and shape of the maternal pelvis and size of the fetus will guide the proper management.

The general principles of management of inefficient uterine activity involve:

- Reassurance to the mother and partner and explanation of the situation

- Adequate pain relief, principally with epidural analgesia

- Adequate fluid replacement by IV infusion of dextrose saline or Hartmann's solution

- Stimulation of uterine activity using an escalating dose infusion of oxytocin

用 EFM 持续严密监护母亲和胎儿能保证母亲和胎儿的健康。

Careful continuous monitoring of the mother and fetus with EFM should reassure maternal and fetal health.

可以通过鼓励母亲活动来刺激子宫活性，如果胎膜完整，可以通过人工破膜来刺激。如果采取简单措施产程没有进展，可开始滴注催产素以加速产程和分娩。如果进展仍缓慢，或根据 CTG 显示有胎儿窘迫征象，或有宫颈扩张缓慢、胎头下降不良及胎头变形等提示的头盆不称征象，应剖宫产分娩。

Uterine activity may be stimulated by encouraging mobilization of the mother and, if the membranes are intact, by artificial ROM. If no progress is seen with the simple measures, an oxytocic infusion is commenced to augment labour and delivery. If progress continues to be slow, or there is evidence of fetal distress based on the CTG or there are signs of cephalopelvic disproportion as identified by poor progress of cervical dilation and descent of the head and increasing caput and moulding, delivery should be effected by caesarean section.

持续的宫缩不协调有可能导致"缩复环"，胎儿应在使用 – 拟交感神经药物、乙醚或氟烷麻醉放松缩复环后剖宫产分娩。

Continued uterine activity despite disproportion may lead to 'constriction ring'. The fetus is best delivered by caesarean section after relaxing the constriction ring using beta-sympathomimetic agents, or ether or halothane anaesthesia.

病例分析	Case study
一位 23 岁的初产妇因腹痛及规律宫缩入院，没有产前出血，宫颈扩张 2cm。4h 后，宫颈扩张 4cm，进展速度缓慢。宫口扩张记录如图 11-19 所示。置入硬膜外导管并开始硬膜外镇痛。人工破膜，流出清澈的羊水。产程仍进展缓慢，3h 后，宫颈扩张 5cm，开始滴注稀释的催产素，产程进展迅速，约 4h 后宫口开全经阴分娩。	A 23-year-old primigravida was admitted to hospital in labour with regular and painful contractions. There was no evidence of antepartum haemorrhage. The cervix was found to be 2 cm dilated. Four hours later, the cervix was 4 cm dilated and the rate of progress was delayed. The cervicogram is shown in Figure 11.19. An epidural catheter was inserted and epidural analgesia commenced. The membranes were ruptured artificially, and clear amniotic fluid was released. Progress in labour continued to be slow-3 hours later, the cervix was 5 cm dilated. A dilute oxytocin infusion was started. This resulted in rapid progress to full dilatation and vaginal delivery some 4 hours later.

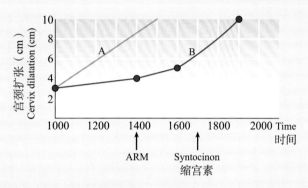

▲ 图 11-19　第一产程进展缓慢。A 线为行动线，B 线为实际宫颈扩张

ARM. 人工破膜

Fig. 11.19　Slow progress in the first stage of labour. The action time is line A, and line B is the actual cervical dilatation.

ARM, Artificial rupture of membranes.

十八、头盆不称（Cephalopelvic disproportion）

这可能是因为胎儿大，或者骨盆因素（特别是骨盆入口狭窄），或者这两种因素都有。产程开始时胎头不能衔接，但随着胎头俯屈和旋转、骨盆的重塑径线增大可能衔接。只有在没有胎儿窘迫和头盆不称征象的情况下，强烈宫缩足够长时间，才能真正检验骨盆情况。

This may arise because the fetus is large or where the pelvis, and especially the pelvic inlet, is small, or a combination of both factors. The head may not be engaged at the onset of labour but may engage with flexion and rotation of the head, moulding and progressive increase in pelvic dimensions. The pelvis can only be truly tested in the presence of strong uterine contractions over an adequate length of time in the absence of fetal compromise and signs of cephalopelvic disproportion.

处理（Management）

当可疑头盆不称时，产程中应严密监护。定期观察宫缩情况、宫颈扩张速度、先露下降、胎方位、囟门位置和形状，以及母亲和胎儿的情况。

When the possibility of cephalopelvic disproportion is suspected, labour should be carefully monitored. Regular observations must be recorded of uterine activity; the rate of cervical dilatation; the descent of the presenting part; the position, station and caput and moulding; and the condition of both the mother and the fetus.

初产妇的子宫在第一阶段晚期可能会变得乏力，宫缩可能会停止或减弱，宫颈扩张可能没有进展。如果超过 4～6h 宫颈扩张没有变化，胎头没有下降，胎头上升并且变形，应放弃经阴试产。同样，如果出现胎儿窘迫或产妇衰竭的临床症状，应通过剖宫产结束分娩。

In primigravid women, the uterus may become exhausted late in the first stage and contractions may cease or become attenuated, and there may be no progress in cervical dilatation. If there is no change in cervical dilatation over a period of 4–6 hours, with no descent of head, increasing caput and moulding, the trial of labour should be abandoned. Similarly, if clinical signs of fetal distress or maternal exhaustion develop, the labour should be terminated by caesarean section.

> **!注意**
>
> 如果产程受阻，经产妇发生子宫破裂的风险会增加。多产患者的产程延长应谨慎对待，因为这很可能与胎位不正或头盆不称有关，不恰当地使用催产素有更大的子宫破裂风险。
>
> Multiparous women are at increased risk of uterine rupture if the labour becomes obstructed. Delay in progress in a multigravid patient should always be treated with caution, as it is likely to be associated with malposition or cephalopelvic disproportion and there is a greater risk of uterine rupture with the injudicious use of oxytocic agents.

十九、脐带先露和脐带脱垂（Cord presentation and cord prolapse）

脐带先露是指脐带的任意部分位于先露部前方或者一侧。诊断通常是胎膜未破时阴道检查感受到脐带搏动，当胎膜破裂时，脐带脱垂，脐带可出现在外阴，或者可在先露前面触摸到。

Cord presentation (Fig. 11.21) occurs when any part of the cord lies alongside or in front of the presenting part. The diagnosis is usually established by digital palpation of the pulsating cord, which may be felt through the intact membranes. When the membranes rupture, the cord prolapses and may appear at the vulva or be palpable in front of the presenting part.

（一）诱发因素（Predisposing factors）

任何胎头移位或先露部分远离宫颈或先露部不规则并与宫颈衔接不良的情况都容易导致脐带先露或脱垂。在这种情况下，如果人工破膜引产，脐带可能会脱垂。在正常分娩时，子宫收缩会促使先露部下降并与盆腔衔接入盆，自然破膜发生在产程较晚期。应在人工破膜前排除脐带先露，以减少脐带脱垂的可能性。先露位置高时应使羊水缓慢流出，以使先露部缓慢下降并紧贴骨盆，避免脐带脱垂。人工破膜引产时，胎头可能较高，脐带脱垂的发生率略有增加。因此，手术应该在与手术室（OT）邻近的产房进行，当脐带脱垂发生时，婴儿可以迅速娩出。

Any condition that displaces the head or presenting part away from the cervix or where the presenting part is irregular and forms poor contact with the cervix will predispose to cord presentation or prolapse. Under these circumstances, if the membranes are ruptured artificially to induce labour, the cord may prolapse. In normal labour, the uterine contractions are likely to cause descent of the presenting part and fix it to the pelvic brim, and spontaneous ROM is much later in labour. The possibility of cord prolapse should be reduced by excluding cord presentation before artificial ROM. Slow release of amniotic fluid should be practised with high presenting part

病例分析	Case study
一名 38 岁的经产妇在足月准备经阴分娩。在分娩初期进展良好后，在宫口扩张 8cm 时出现明显的产程阻滞（图 11-20）。阴道检查证实存在枕后位伴相对头盆不称。宫颈最终开全，旋转胎头，用产钳助产分娩。	A 38-year-old multigravid woman was admitted in labour at term. After good initial progress in labour, significant arrest occurred at 8 cm dilatation (Fig. 11.20). Vaginal examination confirmed the presence of an occipitoposterior position associated with marginal cephalopelvic disproportion. The cervix eventually became fully dilated, and the head was rotated and delivered with forceps.

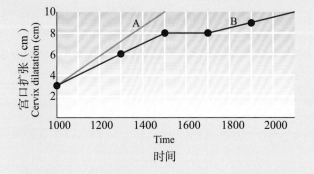

▲ 图 11-20　宫口扩张 **8cm** 时二次停滞，与枕后位有关

Fig. 11.20　Secondary arrest of cervical dilatation at 8 cm associated with the occipitoposterior position.

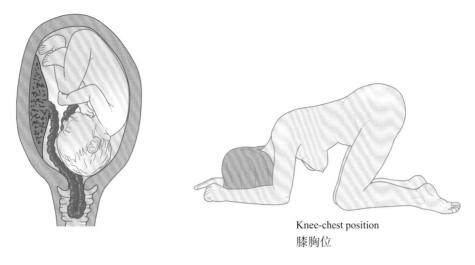

Knee-chest position
膝胸位

▲ 图 11-21　脐带脱垂（左）；产妇取膝胸位，可以将脐带受压降至最低

Fig. 11.21　Cord prolapse (left); pressure on the cord can be minimized by placing the mother in the knee-chest position.

to allow the presenting part to slowly descend and snugly fit into the pelvis to avoid cord prolapse. With artificial ROM for induction of labour, the head may be higher with slightly increased incidence of cord prolapse. Hence, the procedure should be done in the labour room that is near an operating theatre (OT) so that the baby can be delivered rapidly should cord prolapse occur.

（二）处理（Management）

脐带先露的诊断有时在破膜和脐带脱垂之前，但这是例外并不会经常发生。如果脐带通过未完全扩张的宫颈脱出，应该尽快娩出胎儿，因为先露部分会压迫脐带，或者暴露在冷空气中可能导致脐动脉痉挛，还纳脐带可能会产生同样的后果，脐带痉挛或受压会导致胎儿窘迫。

The diagnosis of cord presentation is sometimes made prior to ROM and prolapse of the cord, but this is the exception rather than the rule. If the cord prolapses through a partially dilated cervix, delivery should be effected as soon as possible, as the presenting part will compress the cord or the cord arteries may go into spasm on exposure to cold air. Handling of the cord may cause the same effect. Cord spasm or compression leads to fetal asphyxia.

脐带脱垂是产科急症，应立即召集高级产科医生、助产士、麻醉师、儿科医生和 OT 人员协助。

Prolapse of the cord is an obstetric emergency. Immediate assistance of a senior obstetrician, midwife, anaesthetist, paediatrician and OT staff should be summoned.

减少进入阴道的脐带并在阴道入口处擦拭可以帮助保持脐带的温度和水分，从而减少脐动脉痉挛的概率。

Reduction of the loops of cord into the vagina and swab at the introitus may help to preserve the warmth and moisture content of the cord, thus reducing the chance of cord arterial spasm.

除非胎儿可立即娩出，否则产妇应膝胸位置，或用枕头抬高臀部，或者在推车上放低头部，以减少对脐带的压力。膀胱充盈可能有助于减轻先露部对脐带的压迫。尽管有些报道，但将脐带还纳子宫很困难。

Unless spontaneous delivery is imminent, the woman should be placed in the knee-chest position, or the buttocks elevated by pillows or head tilt in a trolley to reduce pressure on the cord. Filling the urinary bladder may help to reduce pressure on the cord by the presenting part. It is difficult to replace the cord into the uterus, although there have been a few reports about this possibility.

阴道检查和用手指移动胎头缓解胎头对脐带的压迫是可行的，但尽管有遮挡，很难沿着走廊将有一只手插在阴道的女性转移到手术室。每次宫缩都可能进一步压迫骨盆边缘的脐带，单次大剂量的宫缩抑制剂（特布他林 0.25mg 皮下注射或加入 5ml 生理盐水缓慢静脉注射注射时间超过 5min）可能有助于缓解这种间歇性压迫。

Vaginal examination and digital displacement of the head to alleviate pressure of the head on the cord are a possibility, but it is difficult to transfer the woman to the theatre along the corridors with a hand in the vagina, although she would be covered. Each uterine contraction may further compress the cord at the pelvic brim against the presenting part, and a bolus dose of tocolytic (terbutaline 0.25 mg subcutaneously or slow IV in 5 mL saline over 5 minutes) may be of help to relieve this intermittent compression.

除非宫口开全，且在产妇用力的协助下，产钳或真空胎头吸引器可迅速娩出胎儿，否则应采用剖宫产。

Delivery should be effected by caesarean section unless the cervix is fully dilated and delivery can be achieved rapidly by forceps or vacuum with the assistance of the maternal expulsive efforts.

尽管胎儿会受到急性窒息损伤，出生时可能会

出现呼吸抑制（因此需要儿科医生待命），但这些婴儿的长期预后良好。如果没有原发的换气障碍，胎儿可以有效地承受急性窒息，而不会发生远期损害。

Despite the acute asphyxial insult to the fetus, which is likely to be depressed at birth (hence the need for paediatrician to be on stand-by), the long-term prognosis in these infants is good. Provided there is no pre-existing impairment to gaseous transfer, the fetus can effectively withstand an acute asphyxial episode without suffering long-term damage.

本章概览	Essential information
正常分娩 • 初产妇<24h • 经产妇<16h	**Normal labour** • Labour resulting in vaginal delivery • <24 hours in a primigravida • <16 hours in multigravida
产程 • 第一产程：分娩发动至宫口开全 • 第二产程：宫口开全至胎儿娩出 • 第三产程：胎儿娩出至胎盘胎膜娩出	**Stages of labour** • First stage-onset of labour to full dilatation • Second stage-full dilatation to delivery of the baby • Third stage-delivery of the baby to delivery of the placenta and membranes
分娩发动 • 腹痛及规律宫缩伴随宫颈变化	**Onset of labour** • Regular painful contractions with cervical changes

分娩开始
• 胎儿和母体因素的复杂相互作用
• 主要因素
  ➢ 孕酮 / 雌二醇的相互作用
  ➢ 胎儿皮质醇增加
  ➢ 前列腺素的局部活性
• 松弛素、激活素 A、卵泡抑素、绒毛膜促性腺激素和 CRH 对子宫肌的影响
• 见红
• 胎膜破裂
	Initiation of labour
	• Complex interaction of fetal and maternal factors
	• Principal components
	  – Interaction of progesterone/oestradiol
	  – Increased fetal cortisol
	  – Local activity of prostaglandins
	• Effects on myometrium of relaxin, activin A, follistatin, hCG and CRH
	• A 'show'
	• Rupture of fetal membranes

子宫活动 • 增加宫缩的频率、强度和持续时间 • 分娩时正常的静息张力略有增加 • 收缩引起子宫肌层细胞缩短 • 宫颈消退及扩张 • 宫底优势是产程进展所必需的	**Uterine activity** • Increasing frequency, 'intensity' and duration of contractions • Normal resting tonus increases slightly during labour • Contractions cause shortening of myometrial cells • Effacement and dilatation of the cervix • Fundal dominance necessary for progression
产道 • 骨盆韧带软化 • 盆底延展性增强	**The passages** • Softening of pelvic ligaments • Increased distensibility of pelvic floor
正常分娩机制 胎头通过以下方式适应： • 分娩过程中下降 • 俯屈 – 尽量减小先露径线 • 内旋转 – 当胎头到达盆底时 • 仰伸 – 伴随胎头娩出 • 外旋转 – 胎肩下降到骨盆 • 胎肩娩出后身体的其他部位娩出	**The mechanism of normal labour** The fetal head adapts by: • Descent throughout labour • Flexion-to minimize diameter of presentation • Internal rotation-as head reaches pelvic floor • Extension-with delivery of head • Restitution-head in line with shoulders • External rotation-shoulders descend into pelvis • Delivery of shoulders followed by rest of the body

（续表）

本章概览	Essential information
第三产程 胎儿娩出后 • 胎盘自子宫壁剥离 • 子宫将胎盘和胎膜排入下段 • 前肩娩出后给予宫缩药物 • 辅助胎盘和胎膜娩出 • 检查胎盘胎膜完整性 以下现象代表胎盘剥离： • 脐带延长 • 子宫底隆起，子宫变硬呈球形 • 流出鲜血 产程处理措施 • 用产程图观察宫颈扩张及胎头下降 • 产程中的液体平衡与营养 　– 镇痛 　– 麻醉药物 　– 吸入镇痛 　– 非药物方法 　– 局部镇痛 产时胎儿监护 • 酌情定期听诊或胎儿心电监护 　– 注释 (DrCBra VADO) 　　➤ Dr：评估风险 　　➤ C：宫缩 　　➤ Bra：基线率 　　➤ V：变异 　　➤ A：加速 　　➤ D：减速 　　➤ O：整体分类及意见 • 胎儿心电图 ST 段波形改变 • 采集胎儿头皮血液检测酸碱平衡 早产 • 37 周之前的分娩 • 发生在 6%～12% 的妊娠，每个地区各不相同 • 原因如下 　– 产前出血 　– 多胎妊娠 　– 感染 　– 羊水过多 　– 社会因素 • 妊娠 34 周之后存活率相同 • 预防措施包括治疗感染、使用孕酮栓剂和对某些病例施行宫颈环扎术 • 处理措施是使用糖皮质激素以及抑制宫缩 　– 34 周之后不需要使用 　– 产前出血（APH）、感染者禁用 　– 宫颈扩张超过 5cm，保胎药物可能无效。 　– 延迟分娩 48h 　– 有时间转院或注射类固醇 　– 可能引起产妇肺水肿 • 使用硫酸镁 4g，然后每小时静脉注射 1g，持续 24 小时，用于 <32 周胎儿的神经保护。 • 与臀位发生率升高有关 • 足月前臀位考虑剖宫产分娩	The third stage Following delivery: • Placenta shears off uterine wall • Uterus expels placenta and membranes into lower segment • Oxytocic drugs given with delivery of the anterior shoulder • Assisted delivery of placenta and membranes Check placenta and membranes Separation of the placenta is associated with: • Lengthening of cord • Elevation of uterine fundus and becoming hard and globular • Trickling of fresh blood Management of labour • Observe cervical dilatation and descent of the head with the use of partogram • Fluid balance and nutrition in labour 　– Pain relief 　– Narcotic agents 　– Inhalation analgesia 　– Non–pharmacological methods 　– Regional analgesia Fetal monitoring in labour • Regular intermittent auscultation or fetal cardiotocography as appropriate 　– Interpretation (DrCBraVADO) 　　➤ Dr: Define risks 　　➤ C: Contractions 　　➤ Bra: Baseline rate 　　➤ V: Variability 　　➤ A: Accelerations 　　➤ D: Decelerations 　　➤ O: Overall classification and Opinion • The fetal electrocardiogram for changes in the ST waveform • Fetal scalp blood sampling for acid-base balance Pre-term labour • Labour occurring prior to 37 weeks • Occurs in 6–12% of pregnancies-varies from centre to centre • Causes are: 　– Antepartum haemorrhage 　– Multiple pregnancy 　– Infection 　– Polyhydramnios 　– Socioeconomic • Chances of survival same as at term by 34 weeks • Prevention is by treatment of infection, use of progesterone pessaries and in selected cases cervical cerclage • Management is by administration of corticosteroids and tocolysis that 　– Is not needed after 34 weeks 　– Contraindicated in cases of antepartum haemorrhage (APH), infection 　– Tocolytics may not be effective if cervix more than 5 cm 　– Delays delivery by 48 hours 　– Allows time to transfer or give steroids 　– May cause maternal pulmonary oedema • Use of $MgSO_4$-4 g followed by 1 g IV per hour for 24 hours for neuroprotection for fetuses <32 weeks • Is associated with an increased incidence of breech presentation • Delivery by caesarean section considered in a pre–term breech presentation

（续表）

本章概览	Essential information
胎膜早破 • 足月或早产临产前胎膜破裂 • 原因有 　– 感染 　– 多胎妊娠 　– 羊水过多 　– 吸烟 • 通常 48 小时内分娩 • 如果早产，36 周前可在监测感染的情况下保守治疗	**Pre–labour rupture of membranes** • Rupture of membranes before onset of labour at term or pre–term period • Causes are: 　– Infection 　– Multiple pregnancy 　– Polyhydramnios 　– Smoking • Usually followed by labour within 48 hours • If it occurs in the pre–term period, can be managed conservatively by monitoring for signs of infection before 36 weeks
子宫活动的效率 • 90% 的初产妇在 16 小时内分娩 • 有效的宫缩的诊断基于产程记录 • 处理措施 　– 安抚产妇并解释情况 　– 缓解疼痛 　– 补液 　– 如果宫缩不频繁且乏力，则促进宫缩 　– 破膜 　– 增加催产素输注 　– 如果进展缓慢、头盆不称或胎儿窘迫，则应手术助产	**Efficiency of uterine activity** • 90% of primigravidae deliver within 16 hours • Diagnosis of efficient action is based on partogram • Management 　– Reassurance and explanation of the situation 　– Pain relief 　– Fluid replacement 　– Mobilize if infrequent, weak contractions 　– Rupture membranes 　– Augment with oxytocin infusion 　– Operative delivery if lack of progress, cephalopelvic disproportion or fetal distress
脐带脱垂 • 诱发因素 　– 多胎妊娠 　– 羊水过多 　– 先露高浮 • 处理措施 　– 将脐带推回阴道 　– 用 500ml 盐水 / 无菌水填充膀胱 　– 膝胸位 　– 剖宫产紧急分娩；如果宫口开全和先露低，用产钳或负压胎头吸引器助娩	**Cord prolapse** • Predisposing factors 　– Multiple pregnancy 　– Malpresentation 　– Polyhydramnios • Anticipation where presenting part is high Management 　– Reduction of cord into the vagina 　– Fill bladder with 500 mL saline/sterile water 　– Knee-chest position 　– Urgent delivery by caesarean section; if fully dilated and low station, by forceps or vacuum delivery

第 12 章　分娩处理

Management of delivery

Sabaratnam Arulkumaran　著　　王　珊　译　　杨慧霞　校

| 学习目标 | LEARNING OUTCOMES |

学习本章后，你应该能够：

知识标准

- 概述自然经阴分娩的机制
- 描述产程中常见胎位不正的病因、诊断及处理
- 会阴裂伤的不同类型的定义
- 描述经阴分娩和剖宫产的适应证、方法和并发症
- 列出肩难产的危险因素及处理的初步步骤
- 描述第三产程的并发症，其中包括产后出血、会阴裂伤、血肿和羊水栓塞

临床能力

- 指导正常的经阴分娩
- 用模型进行会阴切开术缝合
- 解释剖宫产和手术助产的程序

专业的技能及态度

- 考虑与母亲合作选择分娩方式的重要性，并尊重其他保健工作者的意见
- 考虑生育对女性、家庭和工作人员的情感影响

After studying this chapter you should be able to:

Knowledge criteria

- Outline the mechanism of spontaneous vaginal delivery
- Describe the aetiology, diagnosis and management of the common malpresentations and malpositions in labour
- Define the different types of perineal trauma
- Describe indications, methods and complications of vaginal delivery and caesarean section
- List the risk factors and initial steps in management of shoulder dystocia
- Describe the complications in the third stage of labour, including postpartum haemorrhage, perineal trauma, haematoma and amniotic fluid embolism

Clinical competencies

- Conduct a normal vaginal delivery
- Carry out an episiotomy repair on a practice mannequin
- Explain the procedures of caesarean section and instrumental delivery

Professional skills and attitudes

- Consider the importance of choice of mode of delivery in partnership with the mother and respect the views of other health care workers
- Consider the emotional implications of birth for the woman, family and staff

一、正常阴道分娩（Normal vaginal delivery）

正常经阴分娩标志着第二产程的结束。

Normal vaginal delivery marks the end of the second stage of labour.

第二产程定义为从宫颈完全扩张到胎儿娩出的时期。将第二产程分为两个阶段实用性强：在骨盆内下降，即骨盆期（或叫"被动"阶段），以及会阴期（或叫"主动"阶段）。在下降阶段，产妇通常不会有下降的感觉，从产科处理的角度来看，这一阶段可被视为第一产程的延续。在会阴期，有压迫感，给产妇使用硬膜外麻醉镇痛，这种压迫感可能会被掩盖或削弱。因此，除非宫缩时可见胎头，否则宫颈扩张和先露的位置应经阴道检查确认，然后才能鼓励产妇向下用力。

The second stage of labour is defined as the period from the time of complete cervical dilatation to the baby's birth. It is convenient to consider the second stage in two phases: the descent in the pelvis, i.e. the pelvic or 'passive' phase, and the perineal, or 'active', phase of the second stage. During the descent phase the mother does not normally experience the sensation of bearing down and, from a management point of view, this phase may be regarded as an extension of the first stage of the labour. In the perineal phase the urge to bear down is present, although this may be masked or diminished if epidural analgesia has been provided for the woman. Therefore, unless the head is visible with contractions, the dilatation of the cervix and the station of the presenting part should be confirmed by vaginal examination before encouraging the woman to bear down.

如果没有不良的临床因素，通常认为初产妇第二产程正常持续时间最长为 2h，经产妇为 1h。如果产妇接受了硬膜外镇痛，此时间分别延长 1h。第二产程的进展是通过腹部和阴道检查评估胎头下降来监测的。当腹部触及不到头的 20%，先露的骨质部分已经下降到坐骨棘的水平时，胎头衔接，有利于产妇向下用力。

Provided no adverse clinical factors are present, a normal duration of the second stage is commonly regarded as lasting up to 2 hours in the nulliparous woman and 1 hour in the multipara. If the woman has received epidural analgesia, these times are extended by 1 hour for each group, respectively. Progress in the second stage is monitored by descent of the fetal head assessed by an abdominal and vaginal examination. The fetal head is engaged and it is favourable for mother to bear down when no more than one-fifth of the head is palpable abdominally and the bony part of the vertex has descended to the level of the ischial spines.

如果产程正常，产妇可选择多种体位分娩，但不鼓励仰卧位分娩，因为仰卧位有发生低血压综合征的危险。许多女性采用半卧位，其优点是降低仰卧位低血压的风险，而且这是进行手术助产或会阴缝合的合适体位。

If the labour is normal, women may choose a variety of positions for delivery, but the supine position should be discouraged because of the risk of supine hypotensive syndrome. Many women adopt a semi-reclining position, which has the advantage of reducing the risk of supine hypotension and is a suitable position for assisted delivery or perineal repair should these procedures be required.

二、会阴切开或会阴损伤缝合（Repair of episiotomy or perineal injury）

应尽快对产妇的会阴进行仔细检查，以确定分娩过程中会阴或生殖道损伤的程度。由会阴切开术或撕裂引起的会阴创伤可分为一度、二度、三度和四度裂伤。一度伤仅为阴道和会阴皮肤裂伤，二度裂伤伤及阴道后壁和其下方的会阴肌肉，但不伤及肛门括约肌，三度裂伤伤及括约肌复合体，四度裂伤损伤包括肛门 / 直肠黏膜。

A careful examination of the mother's perineum should be made as soon as possible to identify the degree of perineal or genital tract trauma sustained during the birth. Perineal trauma caused either by episiotomy or tearing may be classified as first-, second-, third- or fourth-degree tears. A first-degree tear describes laceration to vaginal and perineal skin only. A second-degree tear involves the posterior vaginal wall and underlying perineal muscles but not the anal sphincter. Third-degree injury to the perineum is damage that involves the anal sphincter complex, and a fourthdegree laceration is injury to the perineum that includes the ano/rectal mucosa.

会阴一度裂伤，如果皮肤边缘对合，只要伤口不出血，就不需要缝合。会阴侧切和二度裂伤应缝合，以减少出血和加快愈合。三度和四度会阴裂伤应在硬膜外 / 脊髓或全身麻醉下由有经验的外科医生在光线良好的手术室进行修复缝合。这将在后述详细讨论。

In the case of a first-degree perineal tear, there is no need for suturing if the skin edges are already apposed, provided the wound is not bleeding. Episiotomies and second-degree lacerations should be sutured to minimize bleeding and to expedite healing. Third- and fourth-degree perineal lacerations should be repaired under epidural/spinal or general anaesthesia by an experienced surgeon

正常阴道分娩
Normal vaginal delivery

产妇应以自己的向下用力的欲望为指导，向下用力应缓慢地、轻柔地娩出胎头，可将短时用力和喘歇结合，从而使阴道和会阴组织有时间随着下降的胎头充分放松和扩张（图 12-1），着冠前可能会有几次宫缩，然后娩出。对于胎头位的娩出，无论是"托举"法（支撑会阴部和协助胎头俯屈）或"手平衡"法（手离开会阴部但做好准备）均可促进自然分娩。

Women should be guided by their own urge to push. Pushing effort should allow for an unhurried, gentle delivery of the fetal head, and this can be achieved by combining short pushing spells with periods of panting, thus giving the vaginal and perineal tissues time to relax and stretch over the advancing head (Fig. 12.1). Several contractions may occur before the head crowns and is delivered. For the delivery of the head, either the 'hands-on' technique-supporting the perineum and flexing the baby's head-or the 'handspoised' method-with the hands off the perineum but in readiness-can be used to facilitate spontaneous birth.

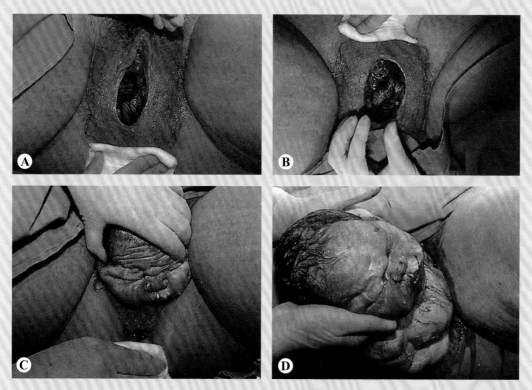

▲ 图 12-1　自然经阴道分娩

A. 第二产程，随着宫缩和母亲的用力可见胎头。B. 胎头着冠；C. 娩出时，胎头处于前后位；D. 胎头和胎肩的娩出

Fig. 12.1　Spontaneous vaginal delivery.

(A) The second stage of labour, the scalp becomes visible with contractions and expulsive efforts by the mother. (B) Crowning of the head. (C) At delivery, the head is in the anteroposterior position. (D) Delivery of the head and shoulders.

自然经阴道分娩通常不需要会阴切开，但如果会阴开始撕裂，或者会阴阻力妨碍胎头娩出，或者考虑胎儿健康需要加快分娩，则可能需要会阴切开术。在实施会阴切开术的地方，推荐的方法是在着冠时的斜外侧切口，从会阴后联合处开始，取 60° 的角度切开，当胎头娩出后，该角度变成 45° 的切口（图 12-2）。

Episiotomy is not routinely required for spontaneous vaginal birth but may be indicated if the perineum begins to tear, if the perineal resistance prevents delivery of the head or if concern for the wellbeing of the fetus requires that the birth be expedited. Where an episiotomy is performed, the recommended technique is a mediolateral incision at the time of crowning, originating at the vaginal fourchette and directed usually to an angle of 60 degrees, which becomes a cut of 45 degrees when the head is delivered (Fig. 12.2).

随着后续宫缩，头部沿着婴儿的纵轴被轻轻地向下推，直到前肩被推送到耻骨下弓下，然后婴儿被向前拉，以娩出后肩和躯干的其余部分，同时保护会阴以免娩出后肩时会阴撕裂。

With the next contraction, the head is gently pulled downwards along the longitudinal axis of the baby until the anterior shoulder is delivered under the sub-pubic arch, and then the baby is pulled anteriorly to deliver the posterior shoulder and the remainder of the trunk whilst protecting the perineum from tearing by the emerging posterior shoulders.

（续表）

正常情况下，婴儿出生后会立即啼哭，但如果呼吸延迟，应予鼻管吸氧，如果需要，使用面罩吸氧使婴儿肺充满氧气。如果呼吸建立时间进一步推迟，可能需要插管和机械通气。使用阿普加评分系统（表 12-1）在 1min 和 5min 评估婴儿状况，如果婴儿呼吸抑制，则在 10min 时再次评估。如果婴儿出生状态差（1min 时 Apgar 评分低于 4 分，5min 时低于 7 分），应双钳钳夹脐带进行脐带血气分析。

The infant will normally cry immediately after birth, but if breathing is delayed, the nasopharynx should be aspirated and, if needed, the baby's lungs inflated with oxygen using a face mask. If the onset of breathing is further delayed, intubation and ventilation may become necessary. The condition of the baby is assessed at 1 and 5 minutes using the Apgar scoring system (Table 12.1) and again at 10 minutes if the baby is depressed. If the baby is born in poor condition (Apgar score of less than 4 at 1 minute and less than 7 at 5 minutes), the cord should be double-clamped for paired cord blood gas analysis.

表 12-1　第 1 分钟和第 5 分钟的 Apgar 评分评估

Table 12.1　Evaluation of Apgar score at 1 and 5 minutes

	0	1	2
皮肤颜色 Colour	苍白 White	四肢青紫 Blue	全身红润 Pink
肌张力 Tone	松弛 Flaccid	僵硬 Rigid	正常 Normal
脉搏 Pulse	几乎触摸不到 Impalpable	<100 次 / 分 <100 beats/min	>100 次 / 分 >100 beats/min
呼吸 Respiration	无 Absent	不规则 Irregular	规则 Regular
反应 Response	无 Absent	欠佳 Poor	正常 Normal

第三产程的处理（Management of the third stage）

对第三产程进行积极的处理，其中包括肌内注射催产素（10U）给母亲，随后晚夹闭（>2min）和剪断脐带。当胎盘剥离的迹象出现时，即脐带延长、阴道流血和子宫因收缩变硬变成球形，并将胎盘挤压到下段时，胎盘采用可控脐带牵引（一种通常称为 Brandt-Andrews 技术的方法）（图 12-3）。

Active management of the third stage of labour is recommended, which includes the administration of oxytocin (10 I/U) intramuscularly to the mother, followed by late clamping (>2 minutes) and cutting of the cord. When the signs of placental separation are seen, i.e. the lengthening of the cord, trickle of blood and the uterus becoming globular and hard due to contraction and extruding the placenta into the lower segment, the placenta is delivered by controlled cord traction, a method commonly referred to as the *Brandt-Andrews technique* (Fig. 12.3).

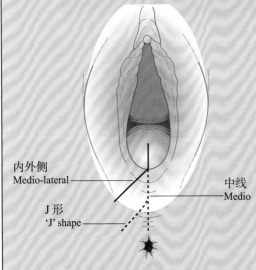

▲ 图 12-2　会阴切开术切口的位置：目的是避免切口延伸或撕裂肛门括约肌或直肠

Fig. 12.2　Sites for episiotomy incisions: the object is to avoid extension f the incision or tear into the anal sphincter or rectum.

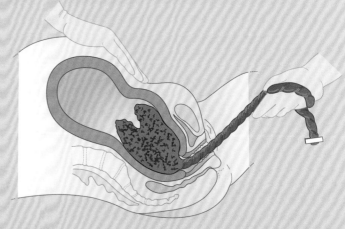

▲ 图 12-3　**Brandt-Andrews** 胎盘辅助分娩技术：在尝试这项技术之前，子宫底部必须收缩，并有胎盘剥离的迹象（流血、脐带延长）

Fig. 12.3　**Brandt-Andrews** technique for assisted delivery of the placenta: the uterine fundus must be contracted with signs of placental separation (trickle of blood, lengthening of the cord) before this technique is attempted.

<table>
<tr><td>会阴切开修复术
Episiotomy repair</td><td>知识链接
ABC</td></tr>
</table>

对于会阴切开术的修复缝合，产妇应取截石位，以获得伤口及其周围良好的视野（图 12-4）。须在使用局部麻醉药浸润或硬膜外或脊髓麻醉的有效镇痛的情况下进行修复缝合。闭合阴道伤口需要清楚地看到切口的顶点。推荐使用可吸收的合成缝合材料进行缝合，阴道壁和肌层使用连续缝合，连续皮内缝合皮肤。

For episiotomy repair, the woman should be placed in the lithotomy position so that a good view of the extent of the wound can be obtained (Fig. 12.4). Repair should only be undertaken with effective analgesia in place using either local anaesthetic agent infiltration or epidural or spinal anaesthesia. Closure of the vaginal wound requires a clear view of the apex of the incision. It is recommended that an absorbable synthetic suture material be used for the repair, using a continuous technique for the vaginal wall and muscle layer and a continuous subcuticular technique for the skin.

手术完成后，重要的是要确保阴道不缩窄，并能容易地容纳两个手指。此外，应进行直肠检查，确认没有缝线穿透直肠黏膜。如果出现这种情况，必须拆除缝线，否则可能会导致直肠阴道瘘的形成。

On completion of the procedure, it is important to ensure that the vagina is not constricted and that it can admit two fingers easily. In addition, a rectal examination should be performed to confirm that none of the sutures have penetrated the rectal mucosa. If this occurs, the suture must be removed, as it may otherwise result in the formation of a rectovaginal fistula.

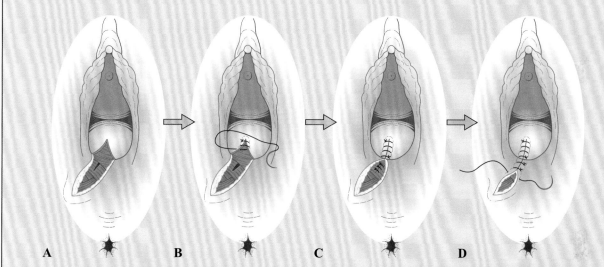

▲ 图 12-4　会阴切开术的修复缝合：阴道后壁可以连续或间断缝合封闭；将切开的肌肉对合并确保皮肤缝合前充分止血
A. 会阴伤口。B. 阴道后壁连续缝合。C. 在会阴肌切缘边缘间断缝合。D. 间断缝合会阴皮肤。目前的证据建议可吸收线皮内连续缝合皮肤。
Fig. 12.4　Repair of the episiotomy: the posterior vaginal wall may be closed with continuous or interrupted sutures; apposition of the cut levator muscle ensures haemostasis before skin closure.
(A) Episiotomy wound. (B) Continuous suture of posterior vaginal wall. (C) Interrupted sutures into the cut edge of the levator. (D) Interrupted suture into the perineal skin. Current evidence suggests subcuticular absorbable continuous suture for the skin.

in an operating theatre under good lighting conditions. This is discussed in more detail in the next section.

> **!注意**
> 会阴切开术的准确修复很重要。伤口缝合过度或阴道缩短可能会导致性交困难和与伴侣的性生活不和谐。未能识别以及修复肛门括约肌的损伤可能会导致不同程度的大便失禁。
>
> Accurate repair of an episiotomy is important. Overvigorous suturing of the wound or shortening of the vagina may result in dyspareunia and sexual disharmony with the partner. Failure to recognize and repair damage to the anal sphincter may result in varying degrees of incontinence of flatus and faeces.

（一）三度和四度裂伤（Third- and fourth-degree injuries）

产科肛门括约肌损伤是经阴分娩的并发症，可导致远期后遗症：大便失禁和肛门失禁（25%）、会阴不适、性交困难（10%）和罕见的直肠阴道瘘。三度裂伤是外括约肌和内括约肌的部分或完全断裂，累及 1 种或 2 种都有可能。这些裂伤常被细分如下。

• 3a：不到 50% 的外括约肌断裂。

• 3b：超过 50% 的外括约肌断裂。

- 3c：内外括约肌均断裂。

Obstetric anal sphincter injuries are a complication of vaginal deliveries and lead to long-term sequelae: faecal and flatus incontinence (up to 25%), perineal discomfort, dyspareunia (up to 10%) and rarely rectovaginal fistulas. A third-degree tear is a partial or complete disruption of the external and internal sphincter; either or both of these may be involved. These tears are often subclassified as:

- 3a: less than 50% of the external sphincter is disrupted
- 3b: more than 50% of the external sphincter is disrupted
- 3c: both the external and internal sphincters are disrupted

四度裂伤除了括约肌断裂外，还包括裂伤肛门和（或）直肠上皮。许多危险因素已经确定，尽管它们在预测或预防括约肌损伤方面的价值有限（框 12-1）。分娩后仔细检查会阴裂伤非常重要，以免遗漏括约肌损伤。这可能会增加括约肌损伤率，但有助于降低远期发病率。

Fourth-degree tears involve tearing the anal and/or rectal epithelium in addition to sphincter disruption. A number of risk factors have been identified, though their value in prediction or prevention of sphincter injury is limited (Box 12.1). It is important to examine a perineal injury carefully after delivery so as not to miss sphincter damage. This may increase the rate of sphincter damage, but it will help to reduce the rate of long-term morbidity.

框 12-1 肛门括约肌损伤的危险因素	Box 12.1 Risk factors for anal sphincter damage
• 巨大儿（>4kg）	• Large baby (>4 kg)
• 初次经阴分娩	• First vaginal delivery
• 手术助产（产钳多于胎吸）	• Instrumental delivery (more with forceps than with ventouse)
• 枕后位	• Occipitoposterior position
• 第二产程延长	• Prolonged second stage
• 引产	• Induced labour
• 硬膜外麻醉	• Epidural anaesthesia
• 肩难产	• Shoulder dystocia
• 混合痔切除术	• Midline episiotomy

数据引自 Robson S, Higgs P（2011）Third- and fourth-degree injuries.RANZCOG 13(2); 20-22.

Data from Robson S, Higgs P (2011) Third- and fourth-degree injuries. RANZCOG 13(2); 20-22.

（二）三度和四度撕裂的修复和处理（Repair and management of third-and fourth-degree tears）

应该请有经验的产科医生实施或监督修复。良好的暴露、照明和麻醉是先决条件，该过程应包括

修复后使用广谱抗生素和口服药物治疗至少 5 天。有 2 种公认的修复方式，其中包括端对端法和括约肌端部重叠法。详细记录描述撕裂程度、缝合方法，以及护理水平是至关重要的。修复后，应立即向产妇解释情况，并推荐她们进行理疗，还应使用大便软化剂。在产后 6 周复查时，需要特别询问产妇对粪便、胀气和排便的控制，以及尿急和性功能障碍，对于所有有括约肌损伤的产妇，如果仍然有症状，应在以后分娩时选择剖宫产。如果物理疗法没有缓解症状，建议尽早转诊到结肠直肠外科医生那里进行诊疗。

An experienced obstetrician should be performing or supervising the repair. Good exposure, lighting and anaesthesia are prerequisites. The procedure should be covered with broad-spectrum antibiotics and an oral regimen carried on for at least 5 days following the repair. There are two recognized forms of repair that include the end-to-end method and overlapping of the sphincter ends. Documentation describing the extent of the tear, the method of repair, as well as the level of supervision is vital. Immediately after the repair, the women should be debriefed and referred for physiotherapy and stool softeners should be prescribed. At the 6-week postnatal appointment, women need to be specifically asked about control of faeces, flatus and bowel movements, as well as urgency and sexual dysfunction. An elective caesarean section for subsequent deliveries should be offered to all women who have sustained a sphincter injury if they remain symptomatic. Early referral to a colorectal surgeon is advised if physiotherapy has not relieved her symptoms.

三、胎位不正（Malpresentations）

超过 95% 的胎儿为枕先露，称为正常。那些身体其他部位（臀部、面部、眉毛、肩膀、脐带）先露在下段和宫颈的称为胎位不正。胎位不正可能有其原因，但是在大多数情况不能明确原因，在分娩和生产过程中会出现特殊问题。现代产科，先露部位需要在分娩早期诊断，并采取适当的处理理措施以防止产妇或胎儿受伤。臀先露在第 8 章讨论。

More than 95% of fetuses present with the vertex and are termed *normal*. Those presenting with other parts of the body (breech, face, brow, shoulder, cord) to the lower segment and cervix are known as *malpresentations*. There may be a reason for malpresentation, although in most instances there is no identifiable cause. They also present with specific problems in labour and during delivery. In modern obstetrics, the presentation needs to be diagnosed early in labour and appropriate management instituted to prevent maternal or fetal injury. Breech presentation is discussed in Chapter 8.

（一）面先露（Face presentation）

在面先露中，胎儿的头部过度仰伸，使得头部在下巴和眼眶之间的部分，即眼睛、鼻子和嘴，可以用检查手指触及，是先露部分。发病率约为 500 次分娩中有 1 次。在大多数情况下原因不明，但与多产和胎儿畸形有关，特别是无脑儿。在现代产科实践中，大多数孕妇都进行了胎儿畸形的超声检查，因此很少看到这种情况导致的面先露。

In face presentation, the fetal head is hyperextended so that the part of the head between the chin and orbits, i.e. the eyes, nose and mouth, that can be felt with the examining finger is the presenting part. The incidence is about 1 in 500 deliveries. In most cases, the cause is unknown but is associated with high parity and fetal anomaly, particularly anencephaly. In modern obstetric practice where most pregnant women have an ultrasound scan for fetal abnormalities, it is rare to see such conditions as a cause of face presentation.

1. 诊断（Diagnosis）

面先露很少在产前诊断，通常在分娩过程中通过阴道检查来识别，此时宫颈充分扩张，可以触诊到特征性的面部特征。然而，可能由于水肿的进展，可能会模糊这些标志。如怀疑，可使用超声检查确认或排除诊断。面先露的位置是以下颏为标志点定义的，因此被记录为颏前位、颏横位和颏后位（图 12-5）。

Face presentation is rarely diagnosed antenatally, but rather is usually identified during labour by vaginal examination when the cervix is sufficiently dilated to allow palpation of the characteristic facial features. However, oedema may develop that may obscure these landmarks. If in doubt, ultrasound

will confirm or exclude the diagnosis. The position of a face presentation is defined with the chin as the denominator and is therefore recorded as mentoanterior, mentotransverse and mentoposterior (Fig. 12.5).

2. 处理措施（Management）

如果是颏前位，可以观察产程进展，期待自然阴道分娩。但是，如果产程进展异常缓慢，最好进行剖宫产。持续性颏后位，没有手工或产钳协助旋转，经阴分娩是不可能的，因需要考虑这些方法对孕妇和胎儿的安全，大部分产科医生会实施剖宫产。

If the position is mentoanterior, progress can be followed normally with the expectation of spontaneous vaginal delivery. However, if progress is abnormally slow, it is preferable to proceed to caesarean section. In cases of persistent mentoposterior positions, vaginal delivery is not possible without manual or forceps rotation. Because the risk associated with these manoeuvres to the mother and infant is considerable, most obstetricians will perform a caesarean delivery.

（二）额先露（Brow presentation）

当胎儿头部的姿态介于枕先露和面先露之间时，称为额先露（图 12-6），这是所有头先露中最不利的。这种情况很少见，每 1500 个新生儿中有 1 个。如果头部以额头径线枕额径（13cm）作为先露直径，不可经阴道分娩。

A brow presentation is described when the attitude of the fetal head is midway between a flexed vertex and face presentation (Fig. 12.6) and is the most unfavourable of all cephalic presentations. The condition is rare and occurs in 1 in 1500 births. If the head becomes impacted with a brow as the presenting diameter, the mentovertical diameter (13 cm), this is incompatible with vaginal delivery.

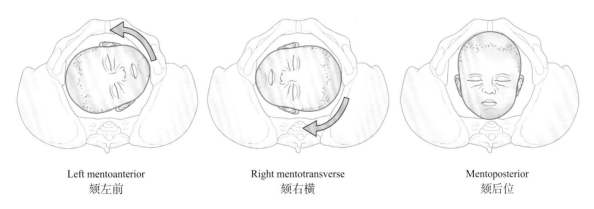

Left mentoanterior　颏左前　　Right mentotransverse　颏右横　　Mentoposterior　颏后位

▲ 图 12-5　面先露的位置，标志点是下颏

Fig. 12.5　Position of the face presentation. The denominator is the chin.

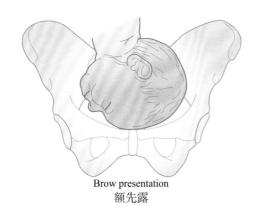

Brow presentation
额先露

▲ 图 12-6　额先露阻碍分娩

Fig. 12.6　Brow presentation preventing delivery.

诊断和治疗（Diagnosis and management）

在分娩时可以触及胎儿的前囟、鼻根以及鼻根内测的眼眶才可以诊断为额先露。正常生长的胎儿，额先露是不可能经阴分娩的，因为先露的部位是胎头最大的径线，因此，在绝大多数的额先露病例中，剖宫产是分娩的首选方法。

The diagnosis is almost always made in labour when the anterior fontanelle, supraorbital ridges and root of the nose are palpable. In the normally grown term fetus, vaginal delivery is not possible as a brow because of the large presenting diameters. Therefore in the vast majority of cases with brow presentation, caesarean section is the method of choice for delivery.

四、胎头位置不正（Malposition of the fetal head）

胎头的位置定义为胎头径线与母体骨盆固定点的关系。头部的标志点是先露部最明确可定义的突出点。在 90% 的病例中颅顶（枕部）出现在骨盆前半部分，因此被定义为"正常"或"枕前"（OA）位置。约 10% 的病例，胎头可能位置不正，即枕部位于骨盆后半部分，枕部面向骶骨或两个骶髂关节之一 [枕后（OP）位置] 或矢状缝沿骨盆横径方向 [枕横（OT）位]。顶骨位置不正常与胎头的俯屈或不同程度的倾斜有关，即一个顶骨，通常是前顶骨，在骨盆较低位置，使顶骨明显在不同水平。前不均倾导致胎头较大的先露径线，从而使正常分娩更加困难。

Position of the fetal head is defined as the relationship of the denominator to the fixed points of the maternal pelvis. The denominator of the head is the most definable prominence at the periphery of the presenting part. In 90% of cases, the vertex presents with the occiput in the anterior half of the pelvis in late labour, and hence is defined as the 'normal' or 'occipitoanterior' (OA) position. In about 10% of cases, there may be malposition of the head; i.e. the occiput presents in the posterior half of the pelvis with the occiput facing the sacrum or one of the two sacroiliac joints-the occipitoposterior (OP) position-or the sagittal suture is directed along the transverse diameter of the pelvis-the occipitotransverse (OT) position. Malposition of the vertex is frequently associated with deflexion of the fetal head or varying degrees of asynclitism, i.e. one parietal bone, usually the anterior, being lower in the pelvis with the parietal eminences at different levels. Asynclitism is most pronounced in the OT position. Deflexion and asynclitism are associated with larger presenting diameters of the fetal head, thereby making normal delivery more difficult.

（一）枕后位（The occipitoposterior position）

10%～20% 的头先露是在分娩开始时是 OP 位，要么是正 OP，要么是更常见的偏向右或左的 OP 位。在产程中，头部通常经横径向 OA 位进行长时间的旋转，但有少数（约 5%），保持在 OP 位置。当 OP 位持续存在时，由于头部的转动姿态导致较大的先露径线（11.5cm×9.5cm）大于 OA 位（9.5cm×9.5cm），这可能导致产程停滞。与背痛有关的产程延迟和分娩疼痛是胎儿枕后位的一个特征（图 12-7）。

Some 10–20% of all cephalic presentations are OP positions at the onset of labour, either as a direct OP or, more commonly, as an oblique right or left OP position. During labour, the head usually undertakes the long rotation through the transverse to the OA position, but a few, about 5%, remain in the OP position. Where the OP position persists, progress of the labour may be arrested due to the deflexed attitude of the head that results in larger presenting diameters (11.5 cm × 9.5 cm) than are found with OA positions (9.5 cm × 9.5 cm). Prolonged and painful labour associated with backache is a characteristic feature of a posterior fetal position (Fig. 12.7).

诊断与治疗（Diagnosis and management）

诊断通常是在产程中阴道检查时确认，当宫颈充分扩张，可以触诊矢状缝，后囟位于骨盆后方。在大多数情况下，产程将正常进展，胎头向前旋转并自然分娩。少数情况下，头部可以向后旋转，以持续性 OP 位分娩。

The diagnosis is usually made or confirmed on vaginal examination during labour when the cervix is sufficiently dilated to allow palpation of the sagittal suture with the posterior fontanelle situated posteriorly in the pelvis. In many cases, labour will progress normally, with the head rotating

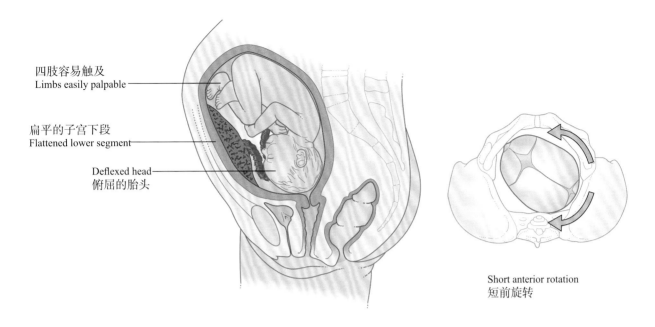

四肢容易触及
Limbs easily palpable

扁平的子宫下段
Flattened lower segment

Deflexed head
俯屈的胎头

Short anterior rotation
短前旋转

▲ 图 12-7　枕后位（A）的临床表现；胎头可向前后方旋转，也可在枕后位（B）停滞

Fig. 12.7　Clinical findings in the occipitoposterior position (A); the head may rotate anteriorly or posteriorly or may arrest in the occipitoposterior position (B).

anteriorly and delivering spontaneously. Occasionally the head may rotate posteriorly and deliver in a persistent OP position.

> **！注意**
>
> 由于胎头的俯屈和相对较大的先露直径，在后位分娩可能导致会阴过度扩张，导致三度或四度裂伤。
>
> Because of the deflexed head and the relatively large presenting diameters, delivery in the posterior position may result in over-distension of the perineum, resulting in third- or fourth-degree tears.

应为母亲充分缓解疼痛和补充液体，如果由宫缩乏力引起的分娩的进展慢于平均水平且无禁忌证，则应考虑采用输注催产素。如果产程进展缓慢，或者有其他需加速分娩的指征，进一步的处理将取决于胎头部位置、宫颈扩张程度和手术者实施产钳旋转或胎头负压吸引器手术助产的能力。

Adequate pain relief and fluid replacement should be provided for the mother, and if progress of the labour is slower than average, the introduction of an oxytocin infusion should be considered, provided there are no other contraindications to its use and contractions were thought to be inadequate. If progress is judged to be slow or if there are other indications to expedite delivery, further management will depend on the station of the head, the dilatation of the cervix and the competence of the operator to perform rotational forceps or vacuum-assisted delivery.

如果宫口未开全或胎头未衔接，剖宫产将是娩出婴儿的唯一选择。另一方面，如果头部衔接，宫口开全，可选择剖宫产、产钳或负压胎吸助产分娩，这取决于产科情况（枕部位置和姿态以及胎儿的状况）及操作者实施旋转器械分娩的能力。

If the cervix is not completely dilated or the head is not engaged, caesarean section will be the only option for delivery of the baby. On the other hand, if the head is engaged and the cervix is fully dilated, the choice of method will be between caesarean section and forceps or vacuum-assisted delivery, depending on the obstetric circumstances (station and position of the vertex and fetal condition) and the skill of the operator in performing rotational instrumental deliveries.

> **！注意**
>
> 当因 OP 位行剖宫产时，胎头有时会受到骨盆的阻碍而很难取出，在这种情况下，可取的做法是在将胎头从腹部取出之前，先从阴道将胎头推出骨盆。偶尔通过子宫切口行臀位娩出。
>
> When performing caesarean section for OP position, the head sometimes becomes impacted in the pelvis and may be difficult to dislodge. In such cases, it may be advisable to disimpact the head vaginally before extracting it abdominally. Occasionally a breech extraction is performed through the uterine incision.

（二）持续性枕横位（Deep transverse arrest）

胎头通常以 OT 或 OP 位置下降入骨盆，然后枕骨向前旋转，在耻骨弓下出现。有时，枕骨没能向前旋转，或者在 OP 位置无法旋转越过骨盆横径。由于胎儿 OT 位特征性的头不均倾产生的较大先露直径，将导致产程停滞，这种临床情况称为持续性枕横位。

The head normally descends into the pelvis in the OT or OP position and then the occiput rotates anteriorly to emerge under the pubic arch. Occasionally this anterior rotation of the occiput fails to occur or, in an OP position, fails to rotate beyond the transverse diameter of the pelvis. Labour will then become arrested due to the large presenting diameters resulting from asynclitism of the head that characterizes a fetal OT position. This clinical situation is referred to as *deep transverse arrest*.

诊断与治疗（Diagnosis and management）

在分娩过程中，当第二产程延长，宫颈完全扩张时，可通过阴道检查来诊断持续性枕横位。与 OP 滞产一样，分娩方式可选择剖宫产或器械助产。如果胎头与骨盆衔接，并且位置低于或位于坐骨棘水平，通常可以徒手或旋转产钳或负压胎吸（随着下降自动旋转）旋转到前位，并经阴道分娩。已没有地方应用 "heroic" 方法使用过度的力量旋转和牵拉胎头，这种方法可能导致胎儿颅内损伤和主要脑血管撕裂。如果胎头不容易旋转并下降，应放弃此法助产，使用剖宫产结束分娩。

The diagnosis of deep transverse arrest is made during labour by vaginal examination when the second stage is prolonged and the cervix is fully dilated. As with OP arrest, the choice of method of delivery will be between caesarean section and instrumental delivery. However, provided the head is engaged in the pelvis and the station is at or below the spines, it can usually be rotated to the anterior position, either manually or by rotational forceps or vacuum extraction (auto-rotation with descent) and delivered vaginally. There is no longer any place for 'heroic' procedures using excessive force to rotate and extract the head. Such procedures may result in fetal intracranial injury and laceration of major cerebral vessels. If the fetal head does not rotate and descend easily, the procedure should be abandoned and delivery completed by caesarean section.

五、器械助产（Instrumental delivery）

阴道助产主要采用两类仪器：产钳（图 12-8 和图 12-9）和产科真空负压吸引器（吸引器；图 12-10）。产钳在约 18 世纪被引入产科实践，而真空吸引器作为一种实用的产钳替代品在过去半个世纪才开始流行。

Two main types of instruments are employed for assisted vaginal delivery: the obstetric forceps (Fig. 12.8) and the obstetric vacuum extractor (ventouse; Fig. 12.10). The forceps were introduced into obstetric practice some three centuries ago, whereas the vacuum extractor as a practical alternative to the forceps only became popular over the past half-century.

（一）器械助产的适应证（Indications for instrumental delivery）

除了少数例外，这两种仪器都用于类似的适应证，但产钳技术完全不同于真空胎吸。

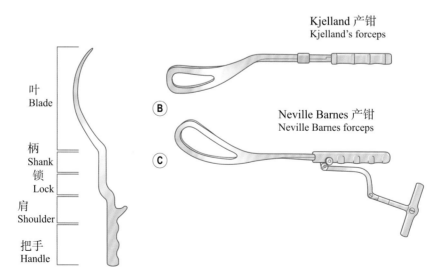

▲ 图 12-8 产钳部位（A）和常用钳（B 和 C）；Kjelland 产钳中没有骨盆曲线可使胎头旋转

Fig. 12.8 Forceps parts (A) and commonly used forceps (B, C); the absence of the pelvic curve in Kjelland's forceps enables rotation of the fetal head.

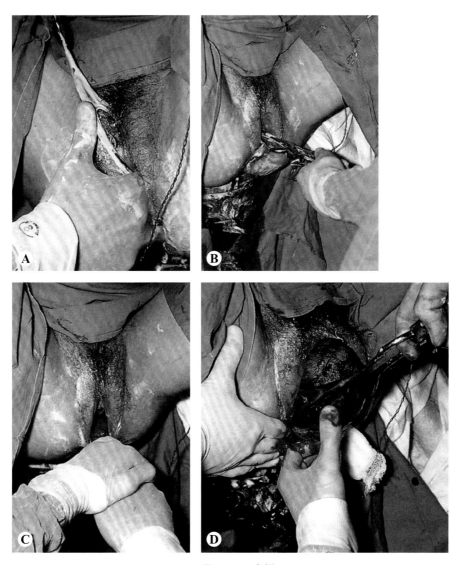

▲ 图 12-9　产钳

A. 骨盆左侧的左叶；B. 叶片之间的固定锁；C. 在产道方向间歇性牵引；D. 向前仰伸娩出胎头

Fig. 12.9　Forceps

(A) Left blade for left side of pelvis. (B) Fixed lock between blades. (C) Application of intermittent traction in direction of pelvic canal. (D) Delivery of head by anterior extension.

With few exceptions, both instruments are used for similar indications, but the technique with the forceps differs completely from that of vacuum extraction.

产钳或真空胎吸的常见指征如下。

- 第二产程延迟。

- 不安全胎儿状态（"胎儿窘迫"）。

- 产妇衰竭和医学疾病。

The common indications for forceps or vacuum-assisted delivery are:

- delay in the second stage of labour

- non-reassuring fetal status ('fetal distress')

- maternal exhaustion and medical disorders

可能影响需要阴道助产的临床因素包括盆底和会阴阻力、子宫收缩乏力、产妇耐受力差、胎位异常、头盆不称和硬膜外镇痛。

Clinical factors that may influence the need for assisted vaginal delivery include the resistance of the pelvic floor and perineum, inefficient uterine contractions, poor maternal expulsive effort, malposition of the fetal head, cephalopelvic disproportion and epidural analgesia.

（二）器械助产的先决条件（Prerequisites for instrumental delivery）

产妇取改良截石位，大腿、外阴及会阴部进行

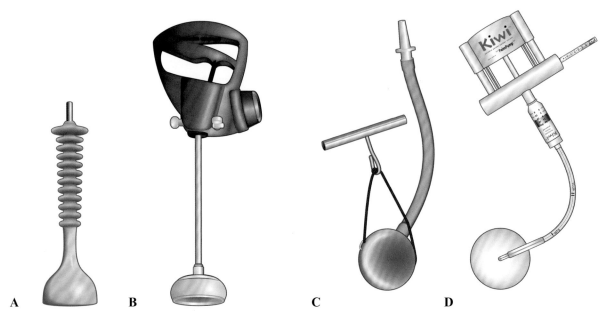

▲ 图 12-10　真空胎吸助娩装置

A 和 B. 用于非旋转（枕前）真空胎吸的前杯；C 和 D. 用于旋转（枕横和枕后）的真空胎吸的后杯

Fig. 12.10　Vacuum-assisted delivery devices

(A, B) Anterior cups for use in non-rotational (occipitoanterior) vacuum deliveries. (C, D) Posterior cups for use in rotational (occipitoposterior and occipitotransverse) vacuum deliveries.

冲洗、铺单。开始之前，应确认下列先决条件。

- 宫口开全。

- 枕先露。

- 胎头衔接，腹部触不到，位于或低于坐骨棘。

- 已知的胎头位置和姿态。

- 排空膀胱。

- 充分镇痛。

The mother should be placed in a modified lithotomy position, and the thighs, vulva and perineum should be washed and draped. The following prerequisites should be confirmed before proceeding:

- full cervical dilatation

- vertex presentation

- head engaged, not palpable abdominally and station at or below the spines

- known position and attitude of the head

- empty bladder

- adequate analgesia

（三）器械助产的方法（Method of instrumental delivery）

习惯上根据胎头的位置将器械助产分为三个级别，即出口、低位和中骨盆分娩，根据胎头的位置分为 2 种类型，即非旋转和旋转分娩。

It is customary to classify instrumental deliveries into three categories according to the station of the fetal head, i.e. outlet, low and midpelvic deliveries, and into two types according to position of the fetal head, i.e. non-rotational and rotational deliveries.

1. 非旋转工具分娩（Non-rotational instrumental delivery）

(1) 产钳（Forceps）

不需要头部向前旋转使用的产钳类型，如 NevilleBarnes 和 Simpson 产钳（图 12-8）。这两个钳都有胎头和骨盆弧度。产钳的两个叶是根据骨盆的侧面设计以使其适应骨盆。因此，左叶被应用到骨盆的左侧（图 12-9A）。两叶之间有一个固定的锁（图 12-9B）。产钳的两叶应在柄部牢牢锁定。矢状缝应垂直于柄部，枕骨在柄部 3～4cm 以上，胎头与两侧叶根部之间仅余一个手指间隙。随诊子宫收缩和产妇在产道方向上的用力，间歇性牵拉（图 12-9C），直到看见枕部，然后胎头向前仰伸娩出（图 12-9D）。

Examples of the types of forceps used when no anterior rotation of the head is required are the Neville Barnes and Simpson's forceps (see Fig. 12.8). Both of these forceps have cephalic and pelvic curves. The two blades of the forceps are designated according to the side of the pelvis to which they are applied. Thus the left blade is applied to the left side of the pelvis (Fig. 12.9A). There is a fixed lock between the blades (Fig. 12.9B). The two sides of the forceps should lock at the shank without difficulty. The sagittal suture should be perpendicular to the shank, the occiput 3–4 cm above the shank and only one finger space between the heel of the blade and the head on either side. Intermittent traction is applied coinciding with the uterine contractions and maternal bearing-down efforts in the direction of the pelvic canal (Fig. 12.9C) until the occiput is on view, and then the head is delivered by anterior extension (Fig. 12.9D).

(2) 真空胎吸（Vacuum delivery）

所有的真空吸引器都由一个附着在婴儿的头上的罩杯组成，一个真空源使罩杯附着，还有和牵引系统或手柄，使术者能够协助分娩（图 12-10）。与产钳一样，真空装置有两种主要的设计类型：所谓的前杯用于非旋转 OA 牵引和后杯用于需旋转 OP 和 OT 分娩。罩杯放置在胎头枕部（弯曲处）（图 12-11A），沿骨盆轴线方向牵引（图 12-11B），直到胎头下降到会阴（图 12-11C）。着冠后，向上牵拉，胎头娩出（图 12-11D）。

All vacuum extractors consist of a cup that is attached to the baby's head, a vacuum source that provides the means of attachment of the cup and a traction system or handle that allows the operator to assist the birth (see Fig. 12.10). As with forceps, there are two main design types of vacuum devices: the so-called *anterior* cups for use in non-rotational OA extractions and the *posterior* cups for use in rotational OP and OT deliveries. The cup is applied to the baby's head at a specific point on the vertex (the flexion point) (Fig. 12.11A), and traction is directed along the axis of the pelvis (Fig. 12.11B) until the head descends to the perineum (Fig. 12.11C). With crowning, traction is directed upwards and the head is delivered (Fig. 12.11D).

2. 可旋转器械助产（Rotational instrumental delivery）

如果胎儿头部的位置是 OP 或 OT，则必须使用专门设计用于这些胎位的产钳和真空胎吸器来实现头部的向前旋转。例如，Kjelland 产钳（图 12-8）有滑锁和最小的骨盆曲线，以便胎头随产钳旋转时能够避免产钳损伤阴道。对于旋转真空吸引器助产，一个"后"杯（图 12-10）将允许术者将杯子向俯屈点移动并越过俯屈点，从而促进胎头在分娩时俯屈和自动旋转到 OA 位。

If the position of the fetal head is OP or OT, forceps and vacuum extractors specifically designed for use in these positions must be used to achieve anterior rotation of the head. For example, Kjelland's forceps (see Fig. 12.8) has a sliding lock and minimal pelvic curve so that rotation of the fetal head with the forceps can be achieved without causing damage to the vagina by the blades. For rotational vacuum-assisted delivery, a 'posterior' cup (see Fig. 12.10) will allow the operator to manoeuvre the cup towards and over the flexion point, thereby facilitating flexion and *auto-rotation* of the head to the OA position at delivery.

（四）器械助产的步骤（Trial of instrumental delivery）

当产钳或真空胎吸转位有一定困难时，如怀疑头盆不称，应在手术室进行器械助产尝试，并做好剖宫产准备。如果每次牵拉无明显下降，则应放弃助产改行剖宫产手术。这样，可避免对婴儿和母亲造成重大创伤。

Where some difficulty with a forceps or vacuum delivery is anticipated, e.g. if there is a suspicion of borderline disproportion, the procedure should be attempted in the operating room as a 'trial' of instrumental delivery, with preparation made to proceed to caesarean section. If some descent is not evident with each traction, the procedure should be abandoned in favour of caesarean section. In this way, significant trauma to the infant and mother should be avoided.

六、剖宫产术（Caesarean section）

剖宫产是通过腹壁和子宫的切口分娩婴儿的方法。剖宫产主要有两种类型，即较常见和首选的子宫下段剖宫产术（图 12-12）和罕见的包括切开子宫上段的"经典"剖宫产术。

Caesarean delivery is the method by which a baby is born through an incision in the abdominal wall and uterus. There are two main types of caesarean section, namely, the more common and preferred lower uterine segment operation (Fig. 12.12) and the much less common 'classical' caesarean section that involves incising the upper segment of the uterus.

（一）剖宫产的适应证（Indications for caesarean section）

尽管剖宫产率因而异，但近年来这种分娩方式持续增长，以至于在许多发达国家，25%～30% 甚至更高的剖宫产率并不少见。剖宫产的常见指征如下。

• 不安全胎儿状态（"胎儿窘迫"）。

• 第一或第二产程的进展异常（难产）。

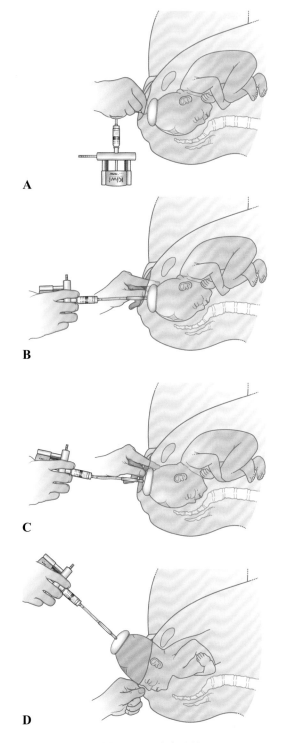

▲ 图 12-11 真空助娩

A. 将杯子置于俯屈点，以利于进行俯屈；B. 向下牵引，一个手指放在杯子上，另一个手指放在颅骨上，以检查并避免杯子移位；C. 随着胎头下降，拉力方向由下向水平的变化；D. 向上牵拉并保护会阴

Fig. 12.11　Vacuum-assisted delivery.

(A) Application of the cup over the flexion point to achieve a flexing median application. (B) Traction downwards with a finger on the cup and anther on the skull to detect and avoid any cup displacement. (C) Change of direction of pull from downwards to horizontal with descent of head. (D) Traction upwards with the protection of the perineum.

- 由于胎盘功能差而导致的宫内生长受限。
- 胎先露异常：臀、横、额位。
- 前置胎盘出血和（或）严重产前出血，如胎盘早剥。
- 剖宫产史，特别是多次。
- 重度子痫前期和其他母体医学指征。
- 脐带先露和脱垂。
- 各种不常见的指征。

Although caesarean section rates show considerable variation from place to place, there has been a consistent increase in this method of delivery over recent years to such an extent that in many developed countries, rates of 25–30% or even higher are not unusual. Common indications for caesarean section are:

- non-reassuring fetal status ('fetal distress')
- abnormal progress in the first or second stages of labour (dystocia)
- intrauterine growth restriction due to poor placental function
- malpresentations: breech, transverse lie, brow
- placenta praevia and/or severe antepartum haemorrhage, e.g. abruptio placentae
- previous caesarean section, especially if more than one
- severe pre-eclampsia and other maternal medical disorders
- cord presentation and prolapse
- miscellaneous uncommon indications

根据临床指征的紧迫性，将剖宫产依据手术时间分为四级。最紧急的，1 级，有即刻威胁孕妇或胎儿生命的情况；2 级，产妇或胎儿有不良状况，但没有立即危及生命的情况；3 级，没有产妇或胎儿不良，但需要提前结束分娩；4 级，指选择性计划剖宫产。

Depending on the urgency of the clinical indication, caesarean sections have been classified into four categories based on time limits within which the operation should be performed. The most urgent, *category* 1, describes indications where there is immediate threat to the life of the woman or fetus; *category* 2, where maternal or fetal compromise is present but is not immediately life threatening; *category* 3, where there is no maternal or fetal compromise but early delivery is required; and *category* 4 refers to elective planned caesarean section.

有过一次单纯子宫下段剖宫产史的女性，如果

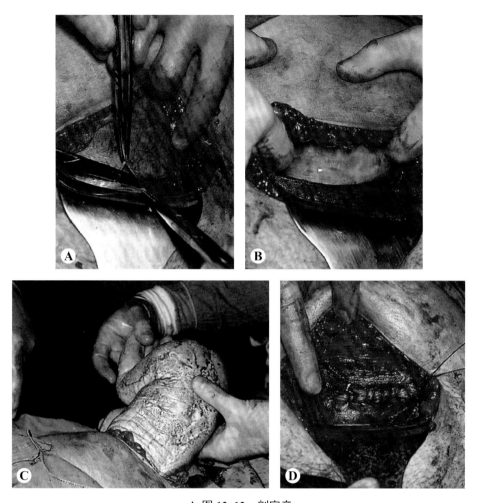

▲ 图 12-12　剖宫产

A. 膀胱从下段反折上来；B. 下段的切口；C. 先露部分娩出；D. 关闭切口

Fig. 12.12　Caesarean section.

(A) Bladder is reflected from the lower segment. (B) Incision made in lower segment. (C) Presenting part delivered. (D) Wound closure

没有其他不良的临床因素，可以尝试经阴道分娩。风险主要是子宫瘢痕开裂，但发生在前次子宫下段切口的概率较低。自然分娩子宫破裂的概率为 5‰，使用催产素为 8‰，使用前列腺素为 25‰。曾行经典（上段）剖宫产术的产妇子宫破裂发生率高并可能发生在临产之前。子宫破裂的临床表现包括耻骨上疼痛和压痛、胎儿窘迫、孕妇心动过速、阴道出血和衰竭。因此，剖宫产后经阴试产的女性应在医院分娩，医院有密切监测产妇和胎儿健康的设施，随时可进入手术室，具有有经验的产科、麻醉和儿科团队，能及时输血。

Women who have had one previous uncomplicated, lower segment caesarean section for a non-recurrent indication may attempt a vaginal delivery in a subsequent labour provided no other adverse clinical factors are present. The major concern is risk of dehiscence of the uterine scar, but this is low with a previous lower uterine segment incision. The figures quoted are 5/1000 with spontaneous labour, 8/1000 with the use of oxytocin infusion and 25/1000 with the use of prostaglandins. The risk is higher and may occur before the onset of labour where a classical (upper segment) caesarean section has been performed. Signs of impending or actual scar dehiscence include suprapubic pain and tenderness, fetal distress, maternal tachycardia, vaginal bleeding and collapse. Thus, women attempting a vaginal birth after caesarean section should deliver in a hospital where there are facilities for close monitoring of maternal and fetal wellbeing; ready accessibility to an operating theatre; an experienced obstetric, anaesthetic and paediatric team; and blood transfusion services.

（二）并发症（Complications）

尽管与大部分外科手术一样，剖宫产术的风险已显著降低，但术时和远期并发症与这种分娩方式有关。主要的直接并发症是围术期出血，这有时会导致休克。在手术过程中很少损伤膀胱或输尿管。剖宫产术后晚期并发症包括伤口或宫腔感染、晚期产后出血，少见深静脉血栓形成和肺栓塞。

Although the risks of caesarean delivery for a woman have decreased significantly, as with all major surgical operations, immediate and late complications are associated with this method of delivery. The main immediate complication is perioperative haemorrhage, which may occasionally result in shock. Rarely injury to the bladder or ureters may occur during the procedure. Late complications of caesarean section include infection of the wound or uterine cavity, secondary postpartum bleeding and, less commonly, deep vein thrombosis and pulmonary embolus.

七、肩难产（Shoulder dystocia）

肩难产是一种严重的情况，发生在胎头娩出，但肩部不能自然娩出或常规牵引不能娩出。胎头缩向在产妇的会阴部，形成所谓的海龟征。如果分娩延迟，婴儿可能会窒息，除非助产时恰当保护，否则用力过度可能发生臂丛神经麻痹或上肢骨折。肩难产与巨大儿（>4500g）有关，特别是如果母亲患有糖尿病。其他易发因素是第二产程延长和阴道助产分娩。

Shoulder dystocia is a serious condition that occurs when the fetal head has delivered but the shoulders fail to deliver spontaneously or with the normal amount of downward traction. The head recoils against the mother's perineum to form the socalled *turtle sign*. If delivery is delayed, the baby may become asphyxiated and, unless care is exercised when assisting the birth, may suffer brachial plexus palsy or limb fractures from over-vigorous manipulations. Shoulder dystocia is associated with the birth of macrosomic infants (>4500 g), especially if the mother has diabetes. Other predisposing factors are prolonged second stage of labour and assisted vaginal delivery.

不幸的是，肩难产是不可预测的，只有少数巨大儿会经历肩难产，大多数病例发生在正常分娩时，体重小于 4000g 的婴儿。因此，所有助产士都应熟悉识别这一严重急症和熟练掌握处理这一潜在的严重的急症的具体步骤。

Unfortunately, shoulder dystocia is unpredictable; only a minority of macrosomic infants will experience shoulder dystocia, and the majority of cases will occur in normal labours with infants weighing less than 4000 g. For this reason, all birth attendants should be skilled in the recognition and the specific steps in the management of this potentially serious emergency.

通常，前肩的分娩是通过柔和地向下牵引来实现的（图 12-13），然后向上牵引以娩出后肩（图 12-14）。如果不成功，推荐的肩难产一线治疗是 McRobert 的手法（框 12-2）。产妇取仰卧位，臀部屈曲，膝盖向胸部紧靠，同时，1 名助手在耻骨上方施加压力，以帮助移动前肩，并使其位于骨盆入口的斜径。

Normally, delivery of the anterior shoulder is achieved with gentle downward traction (Fig. 12.13) and then followed by upward traction to deliver the posterior shoulder (Fig. 12.14). If this is not successful, the recommended first-line treatment for shoulder dystocia is McRobert's manoeuvre (Box 12.2). The woman is placed in the recumbent position with the hips slightly abducted and acutely flexed with the knees bent up towards the chest. At the same time, an assistant applies directed suprapubic pressure to help dislodge the anterior shoulder and for it to be in the oblique diameter of the pelvic inlet.

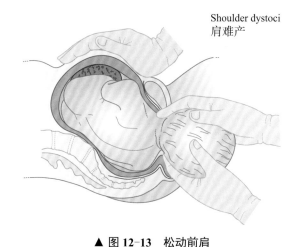

Shoulder dystoci
肩难产

▲ 图 12-13　松动前肩

Fig 12.13　Disimpaction of the anterior shoulder.

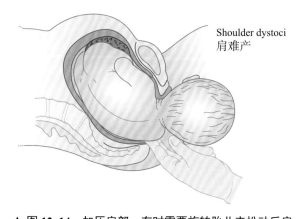

Shoulder dystoci
肩难产

▲ 图 12-14　加压肩部，有时需要旋转胎儿来松动后肩

Fig 12.14　Impacted shoulders. It is sometimes necessary to rotate the fetus to disimpact the posterior shoulder.

框 12-2　肩难产：应采取的措施	Box 12.2　Difficulty delivering shoulders: actions to be taken
• 召集帮助，其中包括资深产科医生、儿科医生和麻醉师 • 孕妇取仰卧位，臀部和膝盖完全弯曲并轻微外展（McRobert 动作） • 在耻骨上向前肩施加压力，使其向下和横向移位 • 行会阴切开术或延长切口 • 将一只手插入阴道，并将胎儿的肩膀旋转到骨盆的斜径 • 通过弯曲后臂的肘部并将手臂扫过胸部来娩出后臂	• Summon help, including senior obstetrician, paediatrician and anaesthetist • Place mother in recumbent position with the hips and knees fully flexed and slightly abducted (McRobert's manoeuvre) • Apply suprapubic pressure on the anterior shoulder to displace it downwards and laterally • Make or extend an episiotomy • Insert a hand into the vagina and rotate the fetal shoulders to the oblique pelvic diameter • Deliver the posterior arm by flexing it at the elbow and sweeping the arm across the chest

McRobert 动作和耻骨上加压在大多数肩难产中是成功的。还有其他更复杂的内部手法，如将整个手插入骨盆，将胎儿肩部旋转到骨盆某个斜径上，或者手动娩出后臂，以将较大的双肩径减少到略小的肩峰 - 腋下径，可以通过适当的中外侧斜会阴切开术来辅助以上步骤实施。

McRobert's manoeuvre and directed suprapubic pressure are successful in the majority of cases of shoulder dystocia. Other more complex internal manoeuvres are described, such as rotation of the fetal shoulders to one or another oblique pelvic diameter by inserting the whole hand into the pelvis, or manual delivery of the posterior arm to reduce a larger bi-acromial diameter to a slightly smaller acromio-axillary diameter. These steps may be facilitated by a generous mediolateral episiotomy.

八、第三产程异常（Abnormalities of the third stage of labour）

第三产程是指从胎儿娩出到胎盘娩出，通常在 10～15min 内完成，并应在 30min 内完成。

The third stage of labour lasts from the delivery of the infant to delivery of the placenta. This is normally accomplished within 10–15 minutes and should be complete within 30 minutes.

（一）产后出血（Postpartum haemorrhage）

原发性产后出血被定义为分娩后 24h 内生殖道出血超过 500ml（图 12-15）。

Primary postpartum haemorrhage is defined as bleeding from the genital tract in excess of 500 mL in the first 24 hours after delivery (Fig. 12.15).

晚期产后出血是指分娩后 24h 后至产后 6 周产褥期内任何时间发生的异常阴道出血。

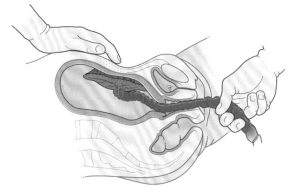

▲ 图 12-15　胎盘滞留时可能发生原发性产后出血

Fig. 12.15　Primary postpartum haemorrhage may occur in the presence of a retained placenta.

Secondary postpartum haemorrhage refers to abnormal vaginal bleeding occurring at any subsequent time in the puerperium up to 6 weeks after delivery.

1. 原发性产后出血（Primary postpartum haemorrhage）

（1）前因后果（Predisposing causes）

出血可能发生在生殖道的任何部位（原因见后述），但最常见的是胎盘部位。胎盘低置出血可能与胎盘植入部位子宫血管收缩不足有关。

Haemorrhage may occur from any part of the genital tract for reasons listed next but arises most commonly from the placental site. Low implantation of the placenta appears to be associated with inadequate constriction of the uterine blood vessels at the placental implantation site.

原发性产后出血的原因可概括为四 "T" ——收缩力、胎盘因素、裂伤或血凝块（指凝血功能障碍）。

Causes of primary haemorrhage are due to one of four 'Ts'-tone, tissue, trauma or thrombin (referring to clotting problems).

子宫收缩乏力占产后出血原因的 75%～90%。诱发因素如下。

- 子宫过度扩张，如多胎妊娠、羊水过多。

- 产程延长、器械助产。

- 产前出血：前置胎盘和胎盘早剥。

- 多产。

- 多发子宫肌瘤、子宫畸形。

- 全身麻醉。

- 生殖道损伤。

- 会阴切开术。

- 会阴、阴道和宫颈裂伤。

- 子宫破裂和剖宫产瘢痕裂开。

- 外阴、阴道和阔韧带血肿。

- 组织：胎盘滞留或胎盘植入。

- 凝血异常：妊娠期获得性，如 HELLP 综合征、脓毒症或弥散性血管内凝血（DIC）。

Uterine atony accounts for 75–90% of all causes of postpartum haemorrhage. Predisposing factors include:

- uterine over-distension, e.g. multiple pregnancy, polyhydramnios
- prolonged labour, instrumental delivery
- antepartum haemorrhage: placenta praevia and abruption
- multiparity
- multiple fibroids, uterine abnormalities
- general anaesthesia
- genital tract trauma
- episiotomy
- lacerations to perineum, vagina and cervix
- uterine rupture and caesarean scar dehiscence
- haematomas of the vulva, vagina and broad ligament
- tissue: retained placenta or placental tissue
- thrombin: acquired in pregnancy, e.g. HELLP syndrome, sepsis or disseminated intravascular coagulation (DIC)

(2) 处理（Management）

产后出血可能是突发和持续的，并可能迅速导致心血管衰竭。治疗目标是控制出血以及补充血液和体液流失（图 12–16）。

Postpartum bleeding may be sudden and profound and may rapidly lead to cardiovascular collapse. Treatment is directed towards controlling the bleeding and replacing the blood and fluid loss (Fig. 12.16).

(3) 控制出血（Controlling the haemorrhage）

简单的视诊就足以估计失血量和胎盘是否排出。

A brief visual inspection will suffice to estimate the amount of blood loss and whether the placenta has been expelled.

若胎盘残留，则做以下处理。

- 按摩子宫，确保子宫收缩良好。

- 尝试通过牵拉脐带娩出胎盘。

- 如果失败，在母亲充分复苏后，在脊髓、硬膜外或全身麻醉下进行徒手剥离胎盘。

If the placenta is retained:

- Massage the uterus to ensure it is well contracted.
- Attempt delivery of the placenta by controlled cord traction.
- If this fails, proceed to manual removal of the placenta under spinal, epidural or general anaesthesia when the mother is adequately resuscitated.

如胎盘已排出，则做以下处理。

- 按摩和按压子宫以排出所有残留的血凝块。

- 立即静脉注射催产素 5U，然后将 40U 溶于 500ml Hartmann 液中静脉滴注。

- 如果仍不能控制出血，静脉注射 0.2mg 麦角新碱（高血压或心脏病女性除外）。如果出血仍在继续，米索前列醇舌下含服 800μg[世界卫生组织（WHO）和国际妇产科联合会（FIGO）推荐]。

- 肌内注射或子宫肌内 15– 甲基前列腺素 F2α 0.25mg，每 15 分钟重复 1 次，最多 8 次。

- 氨甲环酸（抗纤溶剂）1g 缓慢静脉注射，如果出血继续，30min 可重复使用。如果出血在 24h 内复发，可重复使用氨甲环酸 1g。产后出血 3h 内使用氨甲环酸可使产后出血导致的死亡率降低 30%。

- 应用两个 14mm 口径（橙色，240ml/min）或 16mm 口径（灰色，180ml/min）静脉输液管充分注入液体或输血。

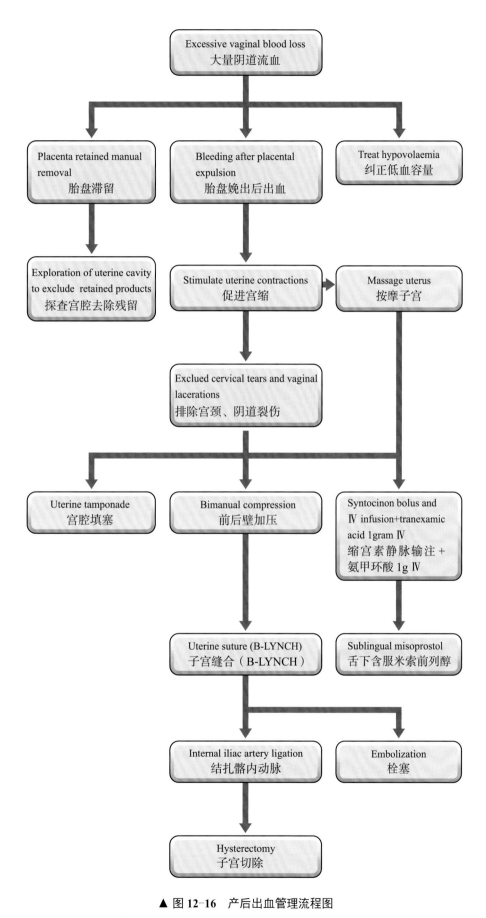

▲ 图 12-16 产后出血管理流程图

Fig. 12.16 Flow chart showing management of postpartum haemorrhage.

- 收集血液样本，检查 Hb%、凝血障碍和交叉配血。

- 检查胎盘和胎膜是否完整，如果不完整，应手工探查宫腔并取出胎盘胎膜。

- 同时，应在良好的照明下用窥器检查阴道和宫颈，缝合裂伤。

- 补充失血和复苏：必须在控制子宫出血的整个过程中补充失血。低血容量应积极静脉注射晶体、胶体、血和血制品治疗。已证实血细胞和血浆（1～2）：1 输注可以降低病死率并提高生存率。

If the placenta has been expelled:

- Massage and compress the uterus to expel any retained clots.

- Inject IV oxytocin 5 units immediately and commence an IV infusion of 40 units in 500 mL of Hartmann's solution.

- If this fails to control the haemorrhage, administer ergometrine 0.2 mg by IV injection (other than those women with hypertension or cardiac disease).

- If bleeding continues, administer misoprostol 800 µg sublingually (recommended by the World Health Organization (WHO) and the International Federation of Gynecology and Obstetrics (FIGO)).

- Intramuscular or intramyometrial injection of 15-methyl prostaglandin $F_{2\alpha}$ 0.25 mg can be given and repeated every 15 minutes for up to a maximum of eight doses.

- Tranexamic acid (anti-fibrinolytic agent) 1 g should be given by slow IV and, if bleeding continues, the dose should be repeated in 30 minutes. If bleeding restarts within 24 hours the tranexamic acid 1 g could be repeated. Administration of tranexamic acid within 3 hours of postpartum haemorrhage reduces maternal mortality due to bleeding by 30%.

- Two size 14-gauge (orange-240 mL/min) or 16-gauge (grey-180 mL/min) IV cannulas should be used to adequately infuse fluids or transfuse blood.

- Collect blood sample to check for Hb%, coagulation disorders and for cross-matching.

- Check that the placenta and membranes are complete. If they are not, manual exploration and evacuation of the uterus are indicated.

- At the same time, the vagina and cervix should be examined with a speculum under good illumination and any laceration should be sutured.

- Replacement of blood loss and resuscitation: It is essential to replace blood loss throughout attempts to control uterine bleeding. Hypovolaemia should be actively treated with IV crystalloid, colloid, blood and blood products. One or two packed cell volumes to one pack of plasma is shown to reduce morbidity and improve survival.

如果这些措施失败，可以实施一些外科手术，具体如下。

- 双手压缩子宫，应该保持 8～10min，以使血液在子宫血管内凝固。

- 子宫填塞球囊。

- 子宫压迫缝合（B-Lynch 或改良压迫缝合）。

- 髂内和子宫动脉结扎。

- 血管栓塞，有侵入性放射设施和专业知识。

- 主要血管栓塞，有放射介入设施和专家。

- 全子宫切除术或次全子宫切除术。

If these measures fail, a number of surgical techniques can be implemented, including:

- bimanual compression of the uterus-should be maintained for 8–10 minutes to allow clotting within the intramyometrial blood vessels

- uterine tamponade with balloon catheters

- uterine compression sutures (B-Lynch or modified compression suture)

- internal iliac and uterine artery ligation

- major vessel embolization where invasive radiological facilities and expertise are available

- total or subtotal hysterectomy

2. 晚期产后出血（Secondary postpartum haemorrhage）

(1) 病因和诱发因素（Causes and predisposing factors）

晚期产后出血的病因如下。

- 胎盘组织残留。

- 宫内感染。

- 罕见的原因，如滋养细胞疾病或异常血管，如宫内动静脉畸形。

Causes of secondary postpartum haemorrhage includes:

- retained placental tissue

- intrauterine infection

- rare causes, e.g. trophoblastic disease or abnormal vasculature like intrauterine arteriovenous malformation

(2) 治疗（Management）

治疗取决于出血程度，以及是否与可能的脓毒症表现有关。如果出血较少，子宫不软，且没有其他感染迹象，可使用一个疗程抗生素观察。然而，如果出血严重，特别是如果有感染的迹象，推荐静脉注射应用广谱抗生素（覆盖需氧菌和厌氧菌）并于麻醉下探查子宫。

Treatment will depend on whether the bleeding is mild or heavy and whether it is associated with signs of possible sepsis. If the bleeding is slight, the uterus is not tender and there are no other signs of infection, observation with a course of antibiotics is justified. However, if the bleeding is heavy and particularly if there are signs of infection, IV broad-spectrum antibiotics (to cover aerobes and anaerobes) and uterine exploration under anaesthesia are indicated.

（二）阴道壁血肿（Vaginal wall haematomas）

大量出血有时发生在阴道和会阴裂伤情况下，这些部位的出血应尽快控制。静脉出血可仅通过压迫止血，动脉出血需要结扎血管。阴道壁血肿可能发生的两个部位之一见下述（图 12–17）。

Profuse haemorrhage may sometimes occur from vaginal and perineal lacerations, and bleeding from these sites should be controlled as soon as possible. Venous bleeding may be controlled by compression alone, but arterial bleeding will require vessel ligation. Vaginal wall haematomas may occur in one of two sites (Fig. 12.17):

- 浅表：出血发生在肛提肌下方，扩开会阴能够看到血肿，导致产妇剧烈的疼痛。血肿必须引流并结扎所有出血的血管，但这些血管很难辨别。因此，在伤口重新缝合之前，应该放入引流。

- Superficial: The bleeding occurs below the insertion of the levator ani, and the haematoma will be seen to distend the perineum, causing the mother considerable pain. The haematoma must be drained and any visible bleeding vessels ligated, although they are rarely identified. For this reason, a drain should be inserted before the wound is re-sutured.

- 深部：出血发生在提肛肌上方，外部不可见。器械辅助分娩中比自然分娩更常见，并伴有持续盆腔疼痛、尿潴留和不明原因贫血的症状。通常可以通过阴道检查诊断出阴道壁上部的凸起物，或者超声检查确诊。如果脉搏和血压（BP）稳定在正常范围内，并且没有

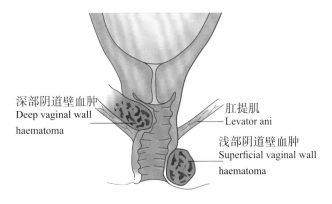

▲ 图 12-17　阴道壁血肿的部位
Fig. 12.17　The sites of vaginal wall haematomas.

深部阴道壁血肿
Deep vaginal wall haematoma

肛提肌
Levator ani

浅部阴道壁血肿
Superficial vaginal wall haematoma

血肿增大的迹象，即具有自限性，可以保守治疗。如果疼痛随着脉率的增加和血压的下降而增加，或者血肿增大，应行血肿切开和较大的腔内引流治疗。阴道应充分填塞，留置导尿。应进行抗生素治疗，必要时输血。

- Deep: The bleeding occurs deep to the insertion of the levator ani muscle and is not visible externally. It is more common after instrumental delivery than after spontaneous birth and presents with symptoms of continuous pelvic pain, retention of urine and unexplained anaemia. It can usually be diagnosed by vaginal examination as a bulge into the upper part of the vaginal wall. Alternatively, ultrasound examination will confirm the diagnosis. If the pulse and blood pressure (BP) are stable and within the normal range and there are no signs of increase in the size of the haematoma, i.e. self-limiting, then the management can be conservative. If there is increasing pain with rise in pulse rate and drop in BP or there is increase in size of the haematoma, the haematoma should be evacuated by incision and a large drain inserted into the cavity. The vagina should be firmly packed and an indwelling catheter inserted into the bladder. Antibiotic therapy should be administered and, if necessary, a blood transfusion is instituted.

（三）子宫外翻（Uterine inversion）

这是一种罕见的并发症，通常发生在试图分娩胎盘，其中宫底通过宫颈倒置并外翻。这种情况更易发生在胎盘在宫底部并粘连的时候。表现为剧烈的下腹痛和产妇休克和出血。处理是将胎盘保留在子宫，启动液体复苏，并尝试徒手或使用压力将宫底推回宫颈。如果不能立即做到，将有必要在全麻情况下使用子宫松弛剂进行治疗。如果这些措施失败，可能需要开腹和外科手术来纠正外翻。

This is a rare complication usually occurring during attempted delivery of the placenta, where the uterine fundus inverts and protrudes through the cervix. The condition is more likely to occur when the placenta is fundal and adherent. The symptoms are severe lower abdominal pain and maternal shock with haemorrhage. The management is to leave the placenta attached to the uterus, initiate fluid resuscitation and attempt to push the fundus back through the cervix manually or using hydrostatic pressure. If this cannot be accomplished immediately, it will be necessary to perform replacement under general anaesthesia in theatre with the use of uterine relaxants. If these measures fail, laparotomy and a surgical procedure may be needed to correct the inversion.

（四）会阴伤口裂开（Perineal wound breakdown）

会阴切口或会阴裂伤缝合后裂开可能因伤口感染或血肿导致。小面积的裂开可以通过定期清洁和抗生素治疗，并保留创面，直到愈合。更广泛的伤口裂开需应用抗生素、清洁、清创坏死组织来治疗。当感染活动期过后，可进行二次缝合。对于三度和四度裂伤的伤口开裂，应在二次缝合之前进行肠道准备，最好由经验丰富的手术者在手术室进行。

Breakdown of episiotomy or perineal wound repairs may occur due to infection or haematoma in the wound. Small areas of breakdown can be treated by regular cleaning and antibiotics and left to granulate until healed. More extensive wound breakdowns should be treated by antibiotics and cleansing and debridement of sloughing tissues. When signs of active infection have subsided, a secondary repair can then be performed. With third- and fourth-degree-tear wound breakdown, bowel preparation should precede the secondary repair, which is best undertaken in the operation room by an experienced operator.

（五）羊水栓塞（Amniotic fluid embolism, AFE）

羊水栓塞（AFE）是一种潜在的灾难性并发症，通常是致命的，常发生在分娩和娩出过程中。临床诊断是基于患者在产程中或分娩后不久突然发生和进展的急性呼吸窘迫和心血管衰竭。羊水进入母体循环，引发类似于过敏性休克的综合征。如果孕产妇在最初的事件中幸存下来，将有很高的概率发展成严重 DIC。因此，有效的复苏和治疗需要一个具有产科、重症监护、麻醉和血液学领域专家的多学科团队。尽管 AFE 是一种非常罕见的情况，发生率为妊娠的 1/80 000，但此病具有极高的孕产妇死亡率。

Amniotic fluid embolism (AFE) is a potentially catastrophic and often fatal complication that usually occurs suddenly during labour and delivery. The clinical diagnosis is based on the sudden development of acute respiratory distress and cardiovascular collapse in a patient in labour or who has recently delivered. Amniotic fluid enters the maternal circulation and triggers a syndrome like that seen with anaphylactic shock. If the woman survives the initial event, she has high chances of developing severe DIC. Therefore, effective resuscitation and treatment require a multidisciplinary team with expertise in the fields of obstetrics, intensive care, anaesthesia and haematology. Although AFE is a rare condition, that occurs in about 1/80,000 pregnancies, it has a disproportionately high maternal mortality rate.

本章概览	Essential information
第二产程的管理	**Management of the second stage**
• 胎头的娩出	• Delivery of the head
– 控制下降	– Controlled descent
– 尽量减少会阴损伤	– Minimize perineal damage
• 延迟断脐	• Delayed clamping of the cord
• Apgar 评分	• Evaluation of Apgar score
第三产程的管理	**Management of the third stage**
• 确认胎盘剥离	• Recognition of placental separation
• 牵拉脐带协助胎盘娩出	• Assisted delivery of the placenta with cord traction
• 胎头着冠或前肩娩出时常规使用催产素	• Routine use of oxytocic agents with crowning of the head or delivery of the anterior shoulder
少见先露	**Rare presentations**
• 面先露: 1/500	• Face presentation: 1/500
• 额先露: 1/1500	• Brow presentation: 1/1500
• 产式不稳定因素:	• Unstable lie associated with:
– 多胎次	– High parity
– 羊水过多	– Polyhydramnios
– 子宫异常	– Uterine anomalies
– 胎盘低置	– Low-lying placenta

（续表）

本章概览	Essential information

枕后位
- 头先露的 10%～20%
- 与背痛和产程延长有关
  治疗：
  - 足够的镇痛
  - 缩宫素
  - 剖宫产
  - 旋转产钳或真空胎吸

产后出血的处理
- 按摩和按压子宫以排出所有血凝块
- 立即静脉注射催产素 5U，并开始静脉输注催产素
- 麦角新碱 0.2mg 静脉注射，禁忌证为高血压和心脏病
- 肌内或子宫肌内注射 15– 甲基前列腺素 $F_{2\alpha}$ 0.25mg
- 氨甲环酸 1g 缓慢静脉注射超过 10min，如果出血继续或在 24h 内复发，则在 30min 内重复应用；越早越好，产后出血 3h 后效果降低
- 收集血样检查 Hb%、凝血障碍和交叉配血
- 如果有指征须徒手探查并排空子宫
- 寻找下生殖道创伤，如果存在，及时适当地治疗
- 纠正失血及呼吸

会阴损伤的修复
- 四度会阴损伤
- 三度和四度裂伤应由经验丰富的工作人员修复缝合，保证良好镇痛，通常在手术室进行
- 缝合后需检查：
  - 没有残留拭子
  - 没有直肠缝线
  - 阴道没有异常缩窄

Occipitoposterior position
- 10–20% cephalic presentations
- Associated with backache and prolonged labour
  Treatment:
  - Adequate analgesia
  - Syntocinon
  - Caesarean section
  - Rotational forceps or posterior cup vacuum extraction

Management of postpartum haemorrhage
- Massage and compress the uterus to expel any retained clots
- Inject IV oxytocin 5 units immediately and commence an IV infusion of oxytocin
- Ergometrine 0.2 mg by IV injection once hypertension and cardiac disease are excluded
- Intramuscular or intramyometrial injection of 15-methyl prostaglandin $F_{2\alpha}$ 0.25 mg
- Tranexamic acid 1 g slow IV over 10 minutes and repeat in 30 minutes if bleeding continues or recurs within 24 hours; the earlier, the better-less beneficial after 3 hours of onset of postpartum haemorrhage
- Collect blood sample to check for Hb%, coagulation disorders and for cross-matching
- Manual exploration and evacuation of the uterus if indicated
- Look for lower genital tract trauma and, if present, treat promptly and appropriately
- Replacement of blood loss and resuscitation

Repair of perineal damage
- Four degrees of perineal damage
- Third- and fourth-degree tears should be repaired by experienced staff with good analgesia and usually in theatre
- Following repair, check:
  - No retained swabs
  - No rectal suture
  - Vagina not abnormally constricted

第 13 章　产后及早期新生儿护理
Postpartum and early neonatal care

Shankari Arulkumaran　著　　吕　鸿　译　　杨慧霞　核

学习目标	LEARNING OUTCOMES
学习本章后，你应当能够：	After studying this chapter you should be able to:

知识标准

- 描述产妇在产褥期的正常变化
- 描述产后常见异常情况 / 急症的病因、诊断及处理，其中包括孕产妇衰竭、血栓栓塞、产褥感染、贫血和哺乳问题
- 讨论产科并发症（如早产）的后遗症
- 描述新生儿复苏的原则
- 描述新生儿期的正常变化

临床能力

- 进行常规产后临床复查
- 为产后女性避孕提供建议
- 进行新生儿检查

专业技能及态度

- 考虑母乳喂养对儿童健康的重要性

Knowledge criteria

- Describe the normal maternal changes in the puerperium
- Describe the aetiology, diagnosis and management of the common abnormalities/emergencies in the postpartum period, including maternal collapse, thromboembolism, puerperal infections, anaemia and problems with lactation
- Discuss the sequelae of obstetric complications (e.g. pre–term delivery)
- Describe the principles of resuscitation of the newborn
- Describe the normal changes in the neonatal period

Clinical competencies

- Carry out a routine postnatal clinical review
- Provide contraceptive advice to a woman in the postnatal period
- Carry out a newborn baby examination

Professional skills and attitudes

- Consider the importance of breast–feeding on childhood health

一、正常产后期（The normal postpartum period）

产褥期在拉丁语中是分娩的意思，所以我们用它来表示产后从婴儿出生到子宫复旧 6 周的这一时期。婴儿和胎盘娩出是泌乳或生育力恢复所必需的。

Puerperium is the Latin word for childbirth, so we use it with license to mean the postpartum period from the birth of the baby through to involution of the uterus at 6 weeks. Delivery of the baby and the placenta is necessary for lactation or a return to fertility.

二、生理变化（Physiological changes）

（一）生殖道（Genital tract）

分娩结束时子宫重 1 kg，产后 6 周不足 100g。子宫肌纤维发生自溶和萎缩，产后 10 天内腹部不再能扪及子宫（图 13-1）。到产褥期结束时，子宫已基本恢复到未孕时大小。子宫内膜在 6 周内再生，如果停止哺乳，这段时间内月经会复潮。如果继续哺乳，月经复潮可能会推迟 6 个月甚至更长时间。

The uterus weighs 1 kg after birth but less than 100 g by 6 weeks. Uterine muscle fibres undergo autolysis and atrophy, and within 10 days the uterus is no longer palpable abdominally (Fig. 13.1). By the end of the puerperium, the uterus has largely returned to the non-pregnant size. The endometrium regenerates within 6 weeks, and menstruation occurs within this time if lactation has ceased. If lactation continues, the return of menstruation may be deferred for 6 months or more.

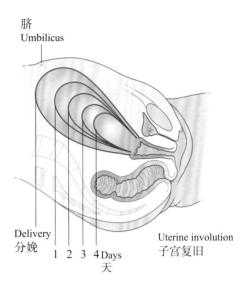

脐
Umbilicus

Delivery
分娩

1 2 3 4 Days
天

Uterine involution
子宫复旧

▲ 图 13-1　产褥期子宫复旧使子宫体积迅速缩小
Fig. 13.1　Uterine involution in the puerperium results in a rapid reduction in size.

子宫排出的分泌物称为恶露。起初包括新鲜或变质的血液（血性恶露），持续 2～14 天。随后转变为浆液性分泌物（浆液恶露），最后变为微白色分泌物（白色恶露）。这些变化在分娩后可持续 4～8 周。血性恶露持续时间延长可能提示有胎盘组织或胎膜残留。

Discharge from the uterus is known as *lochia*. At first this consists of blood, either fresh or altered (lochia rubra), and lasts 2–14 days. It then changes to a serous discharge (lochia serosa) and finally becomes a slight white discharge (lochia alba). These changes may continue for up to 4–8 weeks after delivery. Abnormal persistence of lochia rubra may indicate the presence of retained placental tissue or fetal membranes.

（二）心血管系统（Cardiovascular system）

心输出量和血浆容量约在产后 1 周内恢复正常。在第一周有 2L 的液体流失，在接下来的 5 周内又损失 1.5L。这种损失导致红细胞压积和血红蛋白浓度明显增加。血清钠、血浆碳酸氢盐以及血浆渗透压升高。产后 10 天内凝血因子的增加导致深静脉血栓和肺栓塞的风险增加。另外，血小板数量增加，黏附性也更强。纤维蛋白原水平在分娩过程中下降，但在产褥期升高。

Cardiac output and plasma volume return to normal within approximately 1 week. There is a fluid loss of 2 L during the first week and a further loss of 1.5 L over the next 5 weeks. This loss is associated with an apparent increase in haematocrit and haemoglobin (Hb) concentration. There is an increase of serum sodium and plasma bicarbonate as well as plasma osmolality. An increase in clotting factors during the first 10 days after delivery is associated with a higher risk of deep vein thrombosis (DVT) and pulmonary embolism. There is also a rise in platelet count and greater platelet adhesiveness. Fibrinogen levels decrease during labour but increase in the puerperium.

（三）内分泌变化（Endocrine changes）

内分泌系统的各个方面都在迅速变化。血清雌激素和孕激素水平迅速下降，产后第 7 天降至未孕水平。这与哺乳女性的血清催乳素水平升高有关。到产后第 10 天，人绒毛膜促性腺激素（hCG）已经检测不到了。

There are rapid changes in all facets of the endocrine system. There is a rapid fall in the serum levels of oestrogens and progesterone, and they reach non-pregnant levels by the seventh postnatal day. This is associated with an increase in serum prolactin levels in those women who breast-feed. By the tenth postnatal day, human chorionic gonadotrophin (hCG) is no longer detectable.

三、母乳喂养的重要性（The importance of breast-feeding）

（一）初乳（Colostrum）

初乳是妊娠 12～16 周出现于乳房中的第一批乳汁。它在产后 5 天内产生，6～13 天演变为过渡乳，自 14 天后演变为成熟乳。因含有 β- 胡萝卜素，初乳色黄质稠，平均能量值为 67kcal/dl，而成熟乳的平均能量值为 72kcal/dl。根据新生儿胃的大小，每次喂食的初乳量为 2～20ml。

Colostrum is the first milk and is present in the breast from 12 to 16 weeks of pregnancy. Colostrum is produced for up to 5 days following birth before evolving into transitional milk, from 6 to 13 days, and finally into mature milk from 14 days onwards. It is thick and yellow in colour due to β-carotene and has a mean energy value of 67 kcal/dL, compared to 72 kcal/dL in mature milk. The volume of colostrum per feed varies from 2 to 20 mL in keeping with the size of the newborn's stomach.

婴儿出生后与母亲皮肤接触与将初乳作为婴儿第一食物同样重要。这有利于婴儿被母亲的细菌定植。阴道分娩的婴儿，细菌定植在分娩过程中就开始了，而剖宫产分娩的婴儿更容易定植空气中的细菌。早期母乳喂养还能促进对抗原的耐受性，从而减少母乳喂养婴儿的食物过敏数量。健康肠道菌群的发育还可降低婴儿过敏性疾病、炎症性肠道疾病和轮状病毒腹泻的发生率。

Linked with the importance of the baby having colostrum as its first food is the importance of the baby being skin to skin with its mother after birth. This has the benefit of the baby being colonized by its mother's bacteria. Colonizing starts during the birth process for vaginally born infants, while those born via caesarean section are more likely to colonize bacteria from the air. Early breast-feeding also promotes tolerance to antigens, thus reducing the number of food allergies in breast-fed babies. The development of healthy intestinal flora also reduces the incidence of allergic disease, inflammatory gut disease and rotavirus diarrhoea in infants.

虽然母乳喂养是可取的，应该鼓励，但不应忽视女性的总体愿望。女性之所以选择不进行母乳喂养有其社会和情感上的原因。在某些情况下，母乳喂养是不可能，甚至是不可取的，如乳头内陷、既往乳房手术史、乳房假体、乳头皲裂、疼痛或者母亲患有某种疾病（如艾滋病）或可能正在接受母乳喂养禁用的药物治疗（如化疗药物）。

While breast-feeding is desirable and women should be encouraged, the overall wishes of the woman should not be ignored. There are social and often emotional reasons why a woman may choose not to breast-feed. In some cases, it is not possible or even advisable, such as inverted nipples, previous breast surgery, breast implants, cracked or painful nipples or the mother may have a condition (e.g. HIV) or may be on medical treatment (e.g. chemotherapeutic agents) that serve as a contraindication to breast-feeding.

（二）母乳喂养（Breast-feeding）

应定期清洗乳房和乳头。乳房应得到舒适的支撑，可使用水性润肤乳来软化乳头，从而避免在哺乳期间皲裂。哺乳初期每侧限制在 2～3min，随后这个时间可延长。母亲舒服地坐好，将整个乳头放入婴儿口中，注意保持呼吸道畅通（图 13-2）。婴儿正确地含接乳房是母乳喂养成功的关键。常见的问题，如乳头疼痛、乳房充血和乳腺炎，通常是由于婴儿含接姿势不正确或喂养次数不够导致的。母乳喂养大多是按需喂养，乳汁流量将满足吸吮刺激的需求。一旦婴儿正确地含接到乳头，吮吸的模式就会从短促的吮吸变为长而深的吮吸，并有停顿。有时由于乳房不适、乳头皲裂或婴儿生病，可能需要挤出乳汁并储存。可以手动或使用手泵 / 电动泵来挤出乳汁。母乳可以在 2～4℃的冰箱中安全储存 3～5 天，也可以冷冻储存 3 个月。

The breasts and nipples should be washed regularly. The breasts should be comfortably supported and aqueousbased emollient creams may be used to soften the nipple and thus avoid cracking during suckling. Suckling is initially limited to 2–3 minutes on each side, but subsequently this period may be increased. Once the mother is comfortably seated, the whole nipple is placed in the infant's mouth, taking care to maintain a clear airway (Fig. 13.2). Correct attachment of the baby to the breast is essential to the success of breast-feeding. The common problems such as sore nipples, breast engorgement and mastitis usually occur because the baby is poorly attached to the breast or is not fed often enough. Most breast-feeding is given on demand, and the milk flow will meet the demand stimulated by suckling. Once the baby is attached correctly to

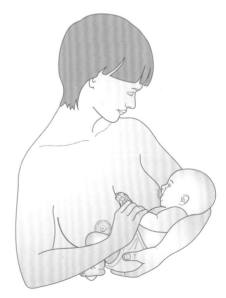

▲ 图 13-2　母亲保持舒适，婴儿正确含乳，以确保充分哺乳

Fig. 13.2　**The mother should be comfortable and the child placed well on to the breast to ensure adequate suckling.**

the nipple, the sucking pattern changes from short sucks to long deep sucks with pauses. It may, on occasions, be necessary to express milk and store it, either because of breast discomfort or cracked nipples or because the baby is sick. Milk can be expressed manually or by using hand or electric pumps. Breast milk can be safely stored in a refrigerator at 2–4°C for 3–5 days or frozen and stored for up to 3 months in the freezer.

对于选择不进行母乳喂养、死产、胎死宫内或有母乳喂养禁忌证的女性，可通过保守方法或药物治疗来抑制泌乳。牢牢支撑乳房，限制液体摄入，避免乳汁分泌和镇痛可能足以抑制泌乳。服用雌激素可有效抑制泌乳，但有发生血栓栓塞性疾病的风险。目前首选的治疗药物是多巴胺受体激动药卡麦角林，可单次服用，通过抑制催乳素释放从而抑制泌乳。溴隐亭也是有效的，但产生这种效果所需的剂量往往会产生相当大的不良反应。

In women who choose not to breast-feed, have suffered a stillbirth or intrauterine death or where there is a contraindication to breast-feeding, suppression of lactation may be achieved by conservative methods or by drug therapy. Firm support of the breasts, restriction of fluid intake, avoidance of expression of milk and analgesia may be sufficient to suppress lactation. The administration of oestrogens will effectively suppress lactation but carries some risk of thromboembolic disease. The preferred drug therapy is currently the dopamine receptor agonist cabergoline. This can be given as a single dose and will inhibit prolactin release and hence suppress lactation. Bromocriptine is also effective, but the dosage necessary to produce this effect tends to create considerable side effects.

四、产后并发症（Complications of the postpartum period）

（一）产褥感染（Puerperal infections）

早在公元前 5 世纪就有产后脓毒血症的报道。据英国 2016 年《降低母婴风险的秘密调查审计报告》（MBRRACE-UK）报道，脓毒血症是导致孕产妇发病和死亡的主要原因。尽管在 2009—2014 年期间英国脓毒血症的直接死亡率从 0.67/10 万下降到 0.29/10 万，但脓毒血症仍然是英国第二大死亡（包括直接和间接）原因。2016 年，在伦敦，脓毒血症是直接导致孕产妇死亡的主要原因。一旦怀疑患有脓毒血症，应建立脓毒血症集束化护理措施。前瞻性分析表明，立即采取这些护理路径可降低脓毒血症的死亡率。英国脓毒症信托基金会在 2013 年推出了这样一个集束化护理措施，即"脓毒血症六大护理组合"，并建

议在脓毒血症诊断后 1h 内完成（表 13–1）。

Puerperal sepsis has been reported as far back as the 5th century BC. Sepsis is a leading cause of maternal morbidity and mortality according to the Mothers and Babies: Reducing *Risk through Audits and Confidential Enquiries across the* UK (MBRRACE-UK) report in 2016. Despite the UK direct death rate from sepsis falling from 0.67 to 0.29 per 100,000 maternities between 2009 and 2014, it remains the second commonest cause of total (combined direct and indirect) deaths

表 13–1　脓毒血症六大护理组合

Table 13.1　Sepsis Six Care Bundle

通知产科和麻醉科会诊医师
Inform consultant obstetrician and consultant anaesthetist
1. 测量动脉血气，必要时给予高流量氧气
1. Take an arterial blood gas and give high–flow oxygen if required
旨在保持 $SpO_2 > 94\%$
Aim to keep $SpO_2 > 94\%$
2. 进行血培养
2. Take blood cultures
并考虑其他培养物，如尿液、阴道拭子
And consider other cultures, e.g. urine, vaginal swabs
3. 开始静脉注射抗生素
3. Start IV antibiotics
根据当地的治疗方案
According to local protocol
4. 开始静脉输液复苏
4. Start IV fluid resuscitation
如果低血压或乳酸≥4，立即给予 30ml/kg 晶体溶液
if hypotensive or lactate ≥4, give 30 ml/kg of crystalloid immediately
5. 抽血检测血红蛋白和乳酸水平
5. Take blood for haemoglobin and lactate levels
如果乳酸超过 4mmol/L，咨询重症监护室的意见
If lactate is over 4mmol/L, obtain critical care/intensive treatment unit advice
6. 测量每小时尿量
6. Measure hourly urine output.
必要时插导尿管
Insert a urinary catheter if needed

改编自 The UK Sepsis Trust. ED/AMU Maternal Sepsis Tool. Available at:https://sepsistrust.org/Professional-resources/clinical/（accessed 7 November 2018）.

Adapted from The UK Sepsis Trust. ED/AMU Maternal Sepsis Tool. Available at: https://sepsistrust.org/professional-resources/clinical/(accessed 7 November 2018).

in the UK. However, in London, it was the leading cause of direct maternal deaths in 2016. Once a diagnosis of sepsis is suspected, a sepsis care bundle should be instituted. Prospective analyses have indicated that immediate of these care pathways reduces mortality from sepsis. The UK Sepsis Trust produced one such care bundle in 2013, the 'Sepsis Six Care Bundle', and recommend that this be completed within an hour of diagnosis of sepsis, as shown in Table 13.1.

脓毒血症的常见原因包括尿路感染（UTI）、伤口感染（会阴或剖宫产瘢痕）和乳腺炎（框 13-1 和图 13-3）。

Common causes of sepsis include urinary tract infections (UTIs), wound infections (perineum or caesarean section scar) and mastitis (Box 13.1 and Fig. 13.3).

框 13-1　产褥期并发症	Box 13.1　Complications of the puerperium
• 生殖道感染 • 尿路感染 • 伤口感染 • 乳腺炎 • 血栓栓塞 • 尿失禁 / 尿潴留 • 肛门括约肌功能障碍 • 会阴切口裂开 • 产后抑郁症	• Genital tract infections • Urinary infection • Wound infection • Mastitis • Thromboembolism • Incontinence/urinary retention • Anal sphincter dysfunction • Breakdown of episiotomy wound • Postnatal depression

（二）子宫内膜炎（Endometritis）

在产褥期，子宫内胎盘附着面容易受到感染。它暴露在含有需氧菌和厌氧菌的阴道中。围产期事件，如长时间的胎膜破裂、绒毛膜羊膜炎、反复阴道检查、个人卫生不良、导尿、侵入性胎儿监护、器械分娩、剖宫产、会阴外伤和人工剥离胎盘，会使病原体进入子宫，从而导致产褥期感染。

In the puerperium, the placental surface in the womb is vulnerable to infection. It is exposed to the vagina, which harbours aerobic and anaerobic bacteria. Peripartum events, such as prolonged rupture of membranes, chorioamnionitis, repeated vaginal examinations, poor personal hygiene, bladder catheterization, invasive fetal monitoring, instrumental deliveries, caesarean sections, perineal trauma and manual removal of the placenta, lead to introduction of pathogens into the uterus and thus contribute to puerperal infections.

子宫内膜炎患者通常表现为发热、下腹痛、继发性产后出血（PPH）和阴道分泌物异味。所涉及的微生物包括 A 族 β- 溶血性链球菌、需氧革兰阴性杆菌和厌氧菌。检查时患者常有发热、心动过速和下腹压痛，可有恶臭的阴道分泌物，出血和宫颈刺激等症状。白细胞计数和 C 反应蛋白也会升高。阴道分泌物或血培养可确定致病的微生物。广谱抗生素是一线治疗方法，应在最初 48h 内开始使用。子宫内

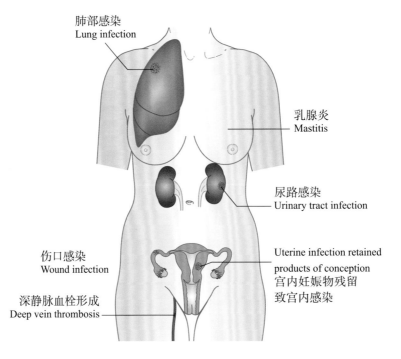

肺部感染
Lung infection

乳腺炎
Mastitis

尿路感染
Urinary tract infection

伤口感染
Wound infection

Uterine infection retained products of conception
宫内妊娠物残留致宫内感染

深静脉血栓形成
Deep vein thrombosis

▲ 图 13-3　产褥期发热的发病机制

Fig. 13.3　The pathogenesis of puerperal pyrexia.

膜炎的并发症有宫旁组织炎、腹膜炎、化脓性盆腔血栓性静脉炎、盆腔脓肿，以及罕见的中毒性休克综合征。

The patient with endometritis usually presents with fever, lower abdominal pain, secondary postpartum haemorrhage (PPH) and foul-smelling vaginal discharge. The organisms involved are group A β-haemolytic streptococci, aerobic Gram-negative rods and anaerobes. On examination, the patient often has a fever, is tachycardic and is tender on palpation of the lower abdomen. There may be foul-smelling vaginal discharge, bleeding and cervical excitation. The white cell count and C-reactive protein may be raised. Vaginal or blood cultures may identify the organism responsible. Broad-spectrum antibiotics are the first-line treatment, and resolution should start to occur within the first 48 hours. The complications of endometritis are parametritis, peritonitis, septic pelvic thrombophlebitis, pelvic abscesses and, rarely, toxic shock syndrome.

（三）尿路感染（Urinary tract infections）

尿路感染是产褥期感染最常见的原因。易感因素包括既往尿路感染史、多囊肾、先天性肾尿路畸形、神经源性膀胱和尿路结石，但大多数是特发性的。患者出现排尿异常（如尿急、尿频）、排尿困难、发热和肾角疼痛。尿液分析蛋白质和白细胞可呈阳性，不过亚硝酸盐更敏感。应在开始抗生素治疗前进行尿液培养。大肠杆菌、肠球菌、克雷伯菌、变形杆菌和表皮葡萄球菌是最常见的微生物。

UTIs are the most common cause of puerperal infections. The predisposing factors include a history of previous UTIs, polycystic kidneys, congenital abnormalities of the renal tract, neuropathic bladder and urinary tract calculi, but most are idiopathic. Patients present with voiding difficulties (e.g. urgency and frequency), dysuria, fever and pain in the renal angle. Urine analysis may be positive for protein and leucocytes, though nitrites are more sensitive. Urine should be sent for culture before commencing antibiotic treatment. The commonest organisms are *Escherichia coli*, *Enterococcus*, *Klebsiella*, *Proteus* and *Staphylococcus epidermidis*.

（四）乳腺炎和乳房脓肿（Mastitis and breast abscess）

症状包括乳房疼痛、发热和红斑。最常见的微生物是金黄色葡萄球菌、表皮葡萄球菌或 A 族、B 族和 F 族链球菌。通常口服抗生素足以治疗乳腺炎，但脓肿则需要静脉输液治疗。如果脓肿出现波动，可能需要手术引流。

Presenting symptoms include breast pain, fever and erythema. The commonest organisms are S. *aureus*; S.

epidermidis; or group A, B and F streptococci. Oral antibiotics are usually sufficient for mastitis, but intravenous treatment is required for an abscess. In the case of an abscess, fluctuance will be elicited and surgical drainage may be warranted.

（五）剖宫产伤口感染和会阴感染（Caesarean wound infections and perineal infections）

产褥感染在剖宫产中比在阴道分娩中更常见。术中使用抗生素有助于降低发病率。最常见的细菌包括金黄色葡萄球菌、耐甲氧西林金黄色葡萄球菌（MRSA）、皮肤菌群及子宫内膜炎相关细菌。并发症包括伤口裂开和坏死性筋膜炎。感染也可能发生在会阴切口或会阴撕裂处，由于会阴血供抗感染力强，这些感染相对少见。会阴变软发红，可见脓性分泌物渗出。当伤口破裂时，应保持伤口清洁，以使其二期愈合。除非伤口干净且创缘没有残余炎症，否则不应重新缝合。

Puerperal infection is more common in caesarean sections than vaginal deliveries. Intraoperative antibiotics have helped reduce the incidence. The commonest organisms involved are S. *aureus*, methicillin-resistant S. *aureus* (MRSA), skin flora and those involved with endometritis. Complications include wound dehiscence and necrotizing fasciitis. Infection may also occur in episiotomy wounds or perineal tears, although these infections are relatively uncommon because the vascularity of the perineum provides a higher resistance to infection. The perineum becomes tender and reddened and may be seen to exude purulent discharge. Where wound breakdown occurs, the wound should be kept clean and allowed to heal by secondary intention. Resuturing should not be performed unless the wound is clean and there is no residual inflammation around the wound margins.

（六）其他感染（Other infections）

一旦排除了常见部位的感染，就必须考虑其他部位感染或脓毒血症，其中包括肺炎、脑膜炎、细菌性心内膜炎，甚至是流感、疟疾和 H1N1。剖宫产胸腔感染的发生率高于阴道分娩，这是由于疼痛或病人全身麻醉后活动能力降低、空气进入减少所致。在英国，2006—2010 年，脓毒症死亡病例中几乎一半是由流感引起的，另有 10% 继发于肺炎。2006—2010 年，H1N1 流感大流行在全球造成 17 000 人死亡。H1N1 是 2009 年初在墨西哥发现的一种甲型流感病毒，在全球范围内传播，直到 2010 年 8 月才引起疫情暴发。在此期间，孕妇和产褥期女性尤其容易受到感染，住院率是普通人群的 4 倍，重症率是普通人群（ITU）的 7 倍。后来人们认识到，因为通常要等流感拭子结果，对这些女性开始适当治疗的时间有所延误。

Once more common sites of infection have been excluded, one must consider other sites of infection or sepsis. These include pneumonia; meningitis; bacterial endocarditis; or even influenza, malaria and H1N1. The incidence of chest infection is greater in caesarean sections than vaginal births due to reduced mobility and reduced air entry secondary to pain or if the patient has had a general anaesthetic. Between 2006 and 2010 in the UK, almost half of the deaths from sepsis were from influenza and another 10% were secondary to pneumonia. The period 2006–2010 covered the H1N1 influenza pandemic, which caused 17,000 deaths worldwide. H1N1 is a strain of influenza A that was discovered in Mexico in early 2009 and spread globally, causing outbreaks up until August 2010. During this period, it became apparent that pregnant women and those in the puerperium were particularly vulnerable, with a four times greater admission rate to hospital and seven times greater admission rate to an intensive treatment unit (ITU) than the general population. It has subsequently been recognized that there was a delay in starting appropriate treatment for these women, as it was frequently delayed until the influenza swab results were available.

（七）血栓栓塞（Thromboembolism）

1. 血栓性静脉炎（Thrombophlebitis）

这是最常见的血栓栓塞性疾病，往往在产后 3～4 天内出现。小腿浅静脉出现局部炎症、压痛和增厚。虽然该病痛苦，并可能沿腿部静脉蔓延，但它很少导致严重的栓塞疾病，也不需要抗凝治疗。应使用抗炎药物，以及局部应用甘油和鱼石脂。

This is the commonest form of thromboembolic disease and tends to arise within the first 3–4 days after delivery. Localized inflammation, tenderness and thickening occur in the superficial leg veins. Although the condition is painful and may spread along the leg veins, it rarely leads to serious embolic disease and does not require anticoagulant treatment. Anti-inflammatory drugs and local applications of glycerine and ichthyol should be used.

2. 静脉血栓（见第 9 章）（Phlebothrombosis (see also Chapter 9)）

深静脉血栓是一种更为严重的并发症，通常发生在产后 7～10 天，尤其在手术分娩或长时间制动后更容易发生。深静脉血栓的发生可能是悄无声息的，只有当血栓松动并以肺栓塞（PE）的形式滞留在肺部时才会出现症状，伴随胸痛、呼吸困难和咯血。临床症状包括听诊时的局部干啰音和胸膜摩擦音及扣诊实音。通气扫描或胸部计算机断层扫描（CT）

有助于确认或反驳诊断。如果不及时进行手术治疗，大面积肺栓塞会导致猝死。已有使用抗血栓药物和经皮动脉导管破碎血栓治疗成功的报道。

DVT is a much more serious complication that tends to arise 7–10 days after delivery and is particularly likely to occur after operative delivery or prolonged immobilization. Clotting occurring in deep veins may be silent and presents only when the clot breaks loose and lodges in the lung as a pulmonary embolus (PE), with consequent chest pain, dyspnoea and haemoptysis. Clinical signs include local rhonchi and pleural rub on auscultation and a pulmonary perfusion. A ventilation scan or chest computed tomography (CT) scan should help to confirm or refute the diagnosis. Massive PE results in sudden death unless treated by prompt surgical management. Successful treatments with antithrombolytic agents and fragmenting the clots with percutaneous arterial catheters have been reported.

3. 产后抗凝（Postnatal anticoagulation）

英国国家指南建议，对于非妊娠患者，如果发生瞬时危险因素相关的静脉血栓栓塞（VTE），小腿静脉血栓应持续抗凝治疗 6 周，对于近端深静脉血栓或肺栓塞应持续抗凝治疗 3 个月，对于首次发作的特发性 VTE，应持续抗凝治疗 6 个月。鉴于持续危险因素的存在和低分子肝素（LMWH）的安全性专家建议在妊娠期间和产后至少 6 周内持续抗凝治疗，并允许总疗程至少 3 个月。肝素和华法林产后使用效果均令人满意。

National guidelines in the UK recommend that in nonpregnant patients, anticoagulant therapy should be continued for 6 weeks for calf vein thrombosis and 3 months for proximal DVT or PE when venous thromboembolism (VTE) has occurred in relation to a temporary risk factor and 6 months for a first episode of idiopathic VTE. The presence of continuing risk factors and the safety of lowmolecular-weight heparin (LMWH) have led authorities to propose that anticoagulant therapy be continued for the duration of the pregnancy and until at least 6 weeks postpartum, and to allow a total duration of treatment of at least 3 months. Both heparin and warfarin are satisfactory for use postpartum.

肝素和华法林都不是母乳喂养的禁用药。如果女性选择在产后继续使用低分子肝素，可以继续产前使用的剂量，也可以使用厂家为非妊娠患者推荐的剂量。如果女性选择在产后开始使用华法林，则至少产后 3 天内应避免使用。在低分子肝素向华法林过渡期间，建议每日检测国际标准化比值（INR），以避免过度抗凝。有产后出血风险的女性应推迟使用华法林。

Neither heparin nor warfarin is contraindicated in breast-feeding. If the woman chooses to continue with LMWH postnatally, then either the doses that were employed antenatally can be continued or the manufacturers' recommended doses for the non-pregnant patient can be employed. If the woman chooses to commence warfarin postpartum, this should be avoided until at least the third postnatal day. Daily testing of the international normalized ratio (INR) is recommended during the transfer from LMWH to warfarin to avoid over-anticoagulation. Warfarin administration should be delayed in women with risk of PPH.

妊娠期或产褥期发生静脉血栓栓塞的女性，最好在产科诊所或产科血液科联合诊所进行产后复查。在产后复查时，应评估血栓形成的持续风险，其中包括回顾静脉血栓栓塞的个人史、家族史及易栓症筛查结果。应就未来妊娠和其他风险增加时期的血栓预防必要性提供建议。还应讨论激素避孕。

Postnatal clinic review for women who develop VTE during pregnancy or the puerperium should ideally be at an obstetric medicine clinic or a joint obstetric haematology clinic. At the postnatal review, the continuing risk of thrombosis should be assessed, including a review of personal and family history of VTE and any thrombophilia screen results. Advice should be given on the need for thromboprophylaxis in any future pregnancy and at other times of increased risk. Hormonal contraception should be discussed.

（八）原发性和继发性产后出血（Primary and secondary postpartum haemorrhage）

请参阅第 12 章。

Please see Chapter 12.

（九）贫血（Anaemia）

如果产后血红蛋白低于 7～8g/dl，在没有持续出血或出血危险的情况下，应在患者知情的基础上决定是否输血。在健康、无症状的患者中，几乎没有证据表明输血有益。如果遇到严重出血，怀疑有出血性疾病时，应进行适当的检查。应在分娩后至少 3～6 个月，当与妊娠相关的凝血改变已恢复时，非紧急地重复这些检查。

If the Hb is less than 7–8 g/dL in the postnatal period, where there is no continuing or threat of bleeding, the decision to transfuse should be made on an informed individual basis. In fit, healthy, asymptomatic patients, there is little evidence of the benefit of blood transfusion. If severe bleeding was encountered and if bleeding disorders were suspected, appropriate investigations should be made. These investigations should be repeated on a non-urgent basis at least 3–6 months after delivery when pregnancy-related coagulation changes have settled.

口服铁剂应是缺铁的首选一线治疗方法。当口服铁不能耐受、吸收，或者患者依从性有问题时，应肠外补铁。与口服治疗相比，肠外治疗疗程短，起效快，但更具侵入性且成本昂贵。蔗糖铁多次给药，而右旋糖酐铁可单次总剂量注射。重组人促红细胞生成素（rHuEPO）主要用于终末期肾病贫血患者。

Oral iron should be the preferred first-line treatment for iron deficiency. Parenteral iron is indicated when oral iron is not tolerated or absorbed or patient compliance is in doubt. Parenteral therapy offers a shorter duration of treatment and a quicker response than oral therapy. It is, however, more invasive and expensive to administer. Iron sucrose is given in multiple doses, whereas iron dextran may be given as a single total-dose infusion. Recombinant human erythropoietin (rHuEPO) is mostly used in the anaemia of end-stage renal disease.

（十）孕产妇衰竭（Maternal collapse）

孕产妇衰竭的定义为涉及循环呼吸系统和（或）大脑的急性事件，导致在妊娠任何阶段及产后 6 周内意识水平降低或丧失（甚至可能死亡）。所有女性应常规使用产科预警评分表，以便及早发现危重患者。尽管危险因素的存在使孕产妇发生衰竭的可能性增大，但在某些情况下，孕产妇衰竭的发生事先没有任何预警。对患严重疾病，有发生孕产妇衰竭风险的女性产前保健应包括多学科团队的参与，并制订妊娠和分娩管理计划。

Maternal collapse is defined as an acute event involving the cardiorespiratory systems and/or brain, resulting in a reduced or absent conscious level (and potentially death) at any stage in pregnancy and up to 6 weeks after delivery. An obstetric early-warning score chart should be used routinely for all women to allow early recognition of the woman who is becoming critically ill. In some cases, maternal collapse occurs with no prior warning, although there may be existing risk factors that make this more likely. Antenatal care for women with significant medical conditions at risk of maternal collapse should include multidisciplinary team input with a pregnancy and delivery management plan in place.

衰竭的原因有很多，可能与妊娠有关，也可能由孕前就存在的与妊娠无关的情况导致。用英国复苏委员会使用的 4Ts 和 4Hs 表可记住衰竭的常见可逆原因。在孕妇中，子痫和颅内出血应添加到该列表中。

There are many causes of collapse, and these may be pregnancy related or result from conditions not related

335

to pregnancy and possibly existing before pregnancy. The common reversible causes of collapse in any woman can be remembered using the 4 Ts and the 4 Hs employed by the Resuscitation Council (UK) . In the pregnant woman, eclampsia and intracranial haemorrhage should be added to this list.

出血是孕产妇衰竭最常见的原因。大多数大出血导致衰竭的病例，病因很明确，但不应忽视隐匿性大出血，其中包括剖宫产后的出血。其他罕见的隐匿性出血原因包括脾动脉破裂和肝破裂。

Haemorrhage is the most common cause of maternal collapse. In most cases of massive haemorrhage leading to collapse, the cause is obvious, but concealed haemorrhage should not be forgotten, including following caesarean section. Other rare causes of concealed haemorrhage include splenic artery rupture and hepatic rupture.

在英国，血栓栓塞是直接导致孕产妇死亡的最常见原因，可表现为孕产妇衰竭。适当预防血栓可降低孕产妇发病率和死亡率，但临床风险评估和预防措施仍需要改进。

In the UK, thromboembolism is the most common cause of direct maternal death and may present as maternal collapse. Appropriate use of thromboprophylaxis has improved maternal morbidity and mortality, but improvements in clinical risk assessment and prophylaxis are still required.

羊水栓塞（amniotic fluid embolism，AFE）表现为分娩过程中或分娩后 30min 内发生衰竭，出现急性低血压、呼吸窘迫和急性缺氧，可能发生抽搐和心搏骤停。疾病进展有不同的阶段；最初，肺动脉高压可能继发于碎片或血管收缩引起的血管闭塞。这种情况通常可缓解，并发展为左心功能不全或衰竭。常发生凝血障碍，导致产后大出血。其潜在的病理生理过程被比作过敏反应或严重脓毒血症。临床上可以怀疑 AFE，但只有尸检才能做出明确的诊断。

Amniotic fluid embolism (AFE) presents as collapse during labour or delivery or within 30 minutes of delivery in the form of acute hypotension, respiratory distress and acute hypoxia. Seizures and cardiac arrest may occur. There are different phases to disease progression; initially, pulmonary hypertension may develop secondary to vascular occlusion either by debris or by vasoconstriction. This often resolves, and left ventricular dysfunction or failure develops. Coagulopathy often occurs, resulting in massive PPH. The underlying pathophysiological process has been compared to anaphylaxis or severe sepsis. Clinically, an AFE can be suspected, but a definitive diagnosis can only be made on postmortem.

在英国，心脏病是目前间接导致孕产妇死亡的

主要原因。多数死于心脏问题的女性没有既往病史。导致死亡的心脏问题主要是心肌梗死、主动脉夹层和心肌病。妊娠期原发性心搏骤停很少见，多数心脏事件均有前驱症状和体征。主动脉根部夹层可表现为胸部中央或肩胛间区疼痛和脉压大，主要继发于收缩期高血压。出现新的心脏杂音必须立即转诊给心脏病专家并进行适当的影像学检查。随着先天性心脏病治疗水平的提高和移民的增多，妊娠期先天性心脏病和风湿性心脏病的发病率不断增加。其他的心脏问题包括冠状动脉夹层、急性左心室衰竭、感染性心内膜炎和肺水肿。

Cardiac disease is currently the leading cause of indirect maternal death in the UK. The majority of deaths secondary to cardiac causes occur in women with no previous history. The main cardiac causes of death are myocardial infarction, aortic dissection and cardiomyopathy. Primary cardiac arrest in pregnancy is rare, and most cardiac events have preceding signs and symptoms. Aortic root dissection can present with central chest or interscapular pain and a wide pulse pressure, mainly secondary to systolic hypertension. A new cardiac murmur must prompt referral to a cardiologist and appropriate imaging. The incidence of congenital and rheumatic heart disease in pregnancy is increasing secondary to improved management of congenital heart disease and increased immigration. Other cardiac causes include dissection of the coronary artery, acute left ventricular failure, infective endocarditis and pulmonary oedema.

菌血症可不出现发热或白细胞计数升高，继而迅速发展为严重脓毒血症和脓毒血症性休克，导致孕产妇衰竭。产科中最常见的微生物是 A 族、B 族、D 族链球菌；肺炎球菌和大肠埃希菌。

Bacteraemia, which can be present in the absence of pyrexia or a raised white cell count, can progress rapidly to severe sepsis and septic shock leading to collapse. The most common organisms implicated in obstetrics are the streptococcal groups A, B and D; *Pneumococcus*; and *E. coli.*

所有衰竭病例都应该考虑药物中毒 / 用药过量，应记住毒品过量是院外衰竭的潜在原因。就治疗性药物毒性而言，产科中常见的是在肾功能损害时应用硫酸镁和意外静脉注射局麻药。最初的影响包括醉酒和头晕目眩的感觉，随后出现镇静、口周感觉异常和抽搐；毒性严重时可能发生惊厥。静脉注射时，可迅速出现惊厥和心血管衰竭。局部麻醉剂全身吸收引起局麻药毒性可在首次注射后出现。严重中毒迹象包括突然的意识丧失，伴或不伴强直 - 阵挛性抽搐，以及心血管意外。

Drug toxicity/overdose should be considered in all cases of collapse, and illicit drug overdose should be remembered as a potential cause of collapse outside of hospital. In terms of therapeutic drug toxicity, the common sources in obstetric practice are magnesium sulphate in the presence of renal impairment and local anaesthetic agents injected intravenously by accident. Effects initially include a feeling of inebriation and light-headedness followed by sedation, circumoral paraesthesia and twitching; convulsions can occur in severe toxicity. On intravenous injection, convulsions and cardiovascular collapse may occur very rapidly. Local anaesthetic toxicity resulting from systemic absorption of the local anaesthetic may occur sometime after the initial injection. Signs of severe toxicity include sudden loss of consciousness, with or without tonic-clonic convulsions, and cardiovascular collapse.

子痫作为导致孕产妇衰竭的原因通常在住院患者中显而易见，因为通常已诊断为先兆子痫，并目睹癫痫发作。颅内出血是未控制的高血压，尤其是收缩期高血压的重要并发症，但也可由动脉瘤破裂和动静脉畸形引起。可能开始就表现为衰竭，但在此之前通常会出现严重的头痛。

Eclampsia as the cause of maternal collapse is usually obvious in the inpatient setting, as often the diagnosis of pre-eclampsia has already been made and the seizure witnessed. Intracranial haemorrhage is a significant complication of uncontrolled, particularly systolic, hypertension but can also result from ruptured aneurysms and arteriovenous malformations. The initial presentation may be maternal collapse, but often severe headache precedes this.

过敏反应引起血容量的重新分布，从而导致心输出量减少，并且可能引发急性心力衰竭和心肌缺血。继发于血管性水肿、支气管痉挛和小气道黏液堵塞的上呼吸道阻塞均导致明显缺氧和通气困难。常见的诱因是各种药物、乳胶、动物变应原和食物。

Anaphylaxis causes a significant intravascular volume redistribution, which can lead to decreased cardiac output. Acute ventricular failure and myocardial ischaemia may occur. Upper airway occlusion secondary to angioedema, bronchospasm and mucous plugging of smaller airways all contribute to significant hypoxia and difficulties with ventilation. Common triggers are a variety of drugs, latex, animal allergens and foods.

导致孕产妇衰竭的其他原因包括低血糖、其他代谢/电解质紊乱和其他原因导致的缺氧，如误吸/异物引起的气道阻塞，空气栓塞、创伤引起的张力性气胸和心脏压塞及罕见的低体温。

Other causes of maternal collapse include hypoglycaemia and other metabolic/electrolyte disturbances, other causes of hypoxia such as airway obstruction secondary to aspiration/foreign body, air embolism, tension pneumothorax and cardiac tamponade secondary to trauma and, rarely, hypothermia.

英国对孕产妇衰竭的管理遵循复苏委员会（英国）的指南，采用标准化 ABC 方法，即气道、呼吸和循环。应尽快用袖套式气管导管插管保护气道，并补充氧气。完成插管前应进行气囊和面罩通气。如果呼吸道畅通，但没有呼吸，应立即开始胸外按压。应尽快建立 2 个大的血管通路，以积极补充血容量。熟练的操作人员进行腹部超声检查有助于诊断隐匿性出血。除颤能量水平应与非妊娠患者相同。通常不应该改变药物或剂量算法。在整个复苏过程中应考虑孕产妇心肺骤停的常见可逆原因。如果孕妇实施心肺复苏（cardiopulmonary resuscitation，CPR）3min 后心输出量仍未恢复，则应实施剖宫产，这将提高母体复苏效果，并可能挽救婴儿。在产科会诊医生和会诊麻醉师与心搏骤停小组达成共识、做出决定之前，复苏工作应持续进行。具有相关经验的资深专业人员应尽早参与。无论复苏成功与否，准确记录所有孕产妇衰竭的病例都是至关重要的。建议向该女性及其家人和参与的工作人员介绍情况。所有病例都应生成临床事件表，并通过临床管理程序进行护理审查。所有孕产妇死亡病例均应向 MBRRACE-UK（英国降低母婴风险的秘密调查审计）报告。

The management of maternal collapse in the UK follows the Resuscitation Council (UK) guidelines using the standard A, B, C approach: airways, breathing and circulation. The airway should be protected as soon as possible by intubation with a cuffed endotracheal tube, and supplemental oxygen should be administered. Bag and mask ventilation should be undertaken until intubation can be achieved. In the absence of breathing despite a clear airway, chest compressions should be commenced immediately. Two wide-bore cannulae should be inserted as soon as possible to enable an aggressive approach to volume replacement. Abdominal ultrasound by a skilled operator can assist in the diagnosis of concealed haemorrhage. The same defibrillation energy levels should be used as in the non-pregnant patient. There should normally be no alteration in algorithm drugs or doses. Common reversible causes of maternal cardiopulmonary arrest should be considered throughout the resuscitation process. If cardiac output is not restored after 3 minutes of cardiopulmonary resuscitation (CPR) in a woman who is still pregnant, the fetus should be delivered by caesarean section, as this will improve the effectiveness in maternal resuscitation efforts and may save the baby. Resuscitation efforts should be continued until a decision is taken by the consultant obstetrician and consultant anaesthetist in consensus with the cardiac arrest team. Senior staff with appropriate experience should be involved at an early stage. Accurate documentation in all cases of maternal collapse, whether or not resuscitation is successful, is essential. Debriefing is recommended for the woman, her family and the staff involved in the event. All cases of maternal collapse should generate a clinical incident form, and the care should be reviewed through the clinical governance process. All cases of maternal death should be reported to MBRRACE-UK (Mothers and Babies: Reducing Risk through Audits and Confdential Enquiries across the UK).

五、产后避孕（Contraception in the postnatal period）

最好在女性出院前就避孕问题进行交谈，但进一步的随访是必不可少的。讨论最好涵盖所有的选择方案，其中包括哺乳期闭经、避孕套、阴道隔膜、纯孕激素避孕药、孕激素植入物或注射剂（Depo-Provera）和宫内节孕器（IUCD），如铜圈或左炔诺孕酮释放器（Mirena）。该咨询应包括适应证和禁忌证，以及每种方法的风险和益处。

A conversation regarding contraception is best before the woman leaves hospital, but further follow-up is essential. Discussion should ideally cover all options, including lactational amenorrhoea, condoms, diaphragm, progestogenonly pills, progestogen implants or injection (Depo-Provera) and an intrauterine contraceptive device (IUCD) such as a copper coil or levonorgestrel-releasing device (Mirena). This consultation should include the indications and contraindications, as well as the risks and benefts of each.

避孕套是不错的首选。它价格低廉，不太可能出现不良反应，而且在伴侣的配合下，避孕成功率高达 95%，同时可以提供保护，防止感染性传播疾病。铜制的宫内节育器很受欢迎，因为它的使用寿命为 10 年。那些有月经过多病史的女性可能会从曼月乐中获益。曼月乐可在胎盘娩出后立即放置，也可在产后 48h 内或产后 6 周子宫复旧后放置。

Condoms are a good first option. They are low cost, unlikely to have side effects and, with partner compliance, have a 95% success rate in preventing pregnancy whilst offering protection from sexual health infections. The copper IUCD is popular, as it has a lifespan of 10 years. Those women who have a history of menorrhagia may benefit from a Mirena. These can be inserted immediately after delivery of the placenta or within 48 hours, or after the uterus has involuted at 6 weeks.

由于雌激素会抑制泌乳，复合口服避孕药不能

用于纯母乳喂养的女性。纯母乳喂养的女性可以安全地使用纯孕激素避孕药和注射 / 植入式孕激素避孕药。由于可能出现不良反应或不规则出血，通常在产后 6 周开始使用，但如果意外妊娠风险高，可在分娩后立即使用。

The combined oral contraceptive pill cannot be used in fully breast-feeding women because the oestrogen will suppress lactation. The progesterone-only pill and injectable/implantable progestogenic contraceptives can be safely given to the fully breast-feeding woman. These are normally started 6 weeks postpartum because of the potential for side effects or irregular bleeding, but where the risk of unplanned pregnancy is high can be commenced immediately after delivery.

六、新生儿问题（Neonatal problems）

对于胎儿来说，通过产道是一种缺氧的经历。因为在平均 50～75s 的宫缩时间里，胎盘上重要的气体交换被阻断。虽然大多数婴儿都能很好地耐受这种情况，但少数不能耐受的婴儿可能需要帮助才能在分娩时建立正常呼吸。新生儿生命支持旨在提供这种帮助，其中包括以下内容，即擦干并包裹新生儿以保存热量、评估干预的必要性、打开气道、肺通气、人工呼吸、胸外按压，以及在极少数情况下使用药物。

Passage through the birth canal is a hypoxic experience for the fetus, since significant respiratory exchange at the placenta is prevented for the 50- to 75-second duration of the average contraction. Though most babies tolerate this well, the few who do not may require help to establish normal breathing at delivery. Newborn life support is intended to provide this help and comprises the following elements: drying and covering the newborn baby to conserve heat, assessing the need for any intervention, opening the airway, aerating the lung, rescue breathing, chest compression and, rarely, the administration of drugs.

如果胎儿在宫内严重缺氧，他将尝试呼吸。如果缺氧持续，胎儿最终会失去意识。不久之后，控制这些呼吸运动的神经中枢将因为缺氧而停止工作，胎儿随之进入原发性呼吸暂停时期。在此之前，心率保持不变，但随着心肌恢复为无氧代谢（一种低效产能机制），心率很快降至正常的 50% 左右。非重要器官循环减少，以维持重要器官灌注。乳酸是无氧代谢的副产物，它的释放会导致体内生化环境的恶化。

If subjected to sufficient hypoxia in utero, the fetus

will attempt to breathe. If the hypoxic insult is continued, the fetus will eventually lose consciousness. Shortly after this, the neural centres controlling these breathing efforts will cease to function because of lack of oxygen. The fetus then enters a period known as *primary apnoea*. Up to this point, the heart rate remains unchanged but soon decreases to about half the normal rate as the myocardium reverts to anaerobic metabolism: a less fueleefficient mechanism. The circulation to non-vital organs is reduced in an attempt to preserve perfusion of vital organs. The release of lactic acid, a by-product of anaerobic metabolism, causes deterioration of the biochemical environment.

如果这种损害持续，原始的脊髓中心就会引发颤抖（全身喘息）。如果这些喘息由于某种原因不能使肺通气，就会消失，新生儿进入一个被称为继发性或终末期呼吸暂停的时期。到此时为止，循环还一直得到维持，但随着终末期呼吸暂停的进展，心功能受损，导致心脏最终衰竭。如果没有有效的干预，胎儿就会死亡。

If the insult continues, shuddering (whole-body gasps) is initiated by primitive spinal centres. If for some reason these gasps fail to aerate the lungs, they fade away and the neonate enters a period known *as secondary* or *terminal apnoea*. Until now, the circulation has been maintained, but as terminal apnoea progresses, cardiac function is impaired. The heart eventually fails, and without effective intervention, the baby dies.

因此，在窒息的情况下，婴儿可以在整个原发性呼吸暂停期、整个喘息期，甚至在终末期呼吸暂停发作后的一段时间内保持有效的循环。对于出生时窒息的婴儿来说，最迫切的需求就是肺部有效地通气。如果婴儿的血液循环充足，含氧血液就会从充气的肺部输送到心脏。心率会加快，大脑会灌注含氧血液。随后，负责正常呼吸的神经中枢，在许多情况下会再次发挥作用，使婴儿恢复正常。在绝大多数情况下，仅仅肺通气就足够了。但在少数情况下，虽然肺通气仍然至关重要，但心功能恶化到循环不足的程度，无法将含氧的血液从充气的肺部输送到心脏。在这种情况下，可能需要短暂的胸外按压。在极少数情况下，肺通气和胸外按压是不够的，可能需要药物来恢复循环。后一组婴儿的预后不佳。

Thus, in the face of asphyxia, the baby can maintain an effective circulation throughout the period of primary apnoea, through the gasping phase, and even for a while after the onset of terminal apnoea. The most urgent requirement for any asphyxiated baby at birth is that the lungs be aerated effectively.

Provided the baby's circulation is sufficient, oxygenated blood will then be conveyed from the aerated lungs to the heart. The heart rate will increase, and the brain will be perfused with oxygenated blood. Following this, the neural centres responsible for normal breathing will, in many instances, function once again and the baby will recover. Merely aerating the lungs is sufficient in the vast majority of cases. Although lung aeration is still vital, in a few cases cardiac function will have deteriorated to such an extent that the circulation is inadequate and cannot convey oxygenated blood from the aerated lungs to the heart. In this case, a brief period of chest compression may be needed. In a very few cases, lung aeration and chest compression will not be sufficient, and drugs may be required to restore the circulation. The outlook in the latter group of infants is poor.

大多数足月出生的婴儿无须复苏，他们通常可以从胎盘"呼吸"非常平稳地过渡到肺呼吸。只要注意防止热量流失并且延迟剪断脐带，很少需要干预。但有些婴儿在分娩过程中会受到压力或损伤，则需要进行复苏。值得注意的是，早产儿，特别是孕周小于 30 周的婴儿情况就不同了。这类婴儿大多数在分娩时都是健康的，不过所有婴儿都有望从帮助过渡中获益。通常在这种情况下进行干预仅限于在过渡期间维持婴儿的健康，这被称作稳定。

Most babies born at term need no resuscitation, and they can usually stabilize themselves during the transition from placental to pulmonary respiration very effectively. Provided attention is paid to preventing heat loss and a little patience is exhibited before cutting the umbilical cord, intervention is rarely necessary. However, some babies will have suffered stresses or insults during labour, and resuscitation is then required. Significantly, pre-term babies, particularly those born below 30 weeks' gestation, are a different matter. Most babies in this group are healthy at the time of delivery and yet all can be expected to benefit from help in making the transition. Intervention in this situation is usually limited to maintaining a baby's health during this transition and is called stabilization.

七、进行常规产后临床检查（Conducting a routine postnatal clinical review）

产后是女性生命中一个重要的转折点。产后护理从住院延伸到社区和家庭，并由多名护理人员提供。产后母婴护理的目标包括提供产后的休息和恢复，支持母子依恋及协助发展产妇自尊。应支持家庭单位，并适当地识别和管理风险。如果母亲希望母乳喂养，就应该提倡和鼓励。应采取措施预防、

新生儿检查 **Examination of the newborn**	知识链接 **ABC**

检查的目的是查明父母的担忧，识别风险（如围产期病史 / 家族史），尽可能安抚父母，并就健康促进提供建议 [如预防婴儿猝死综合征（SIDS）、免疫接种]。虽然可在出生 6h 后，最迟不超过 7 天进行检查，但理想检查时间是出生后 24～72h。

The purpose of the examination is to ascertain parental concerns, identify risks (e.g. perinatal/family history), reassure parents where possible and offer advice on health promotion (e.g. prevention of sudden infant death syndrome (SIDS), immunizations). The ideal time for this is between 24 and 72 hours, though it may be undertaken after 6 hours of age and no later than 7 days of age.

对婴儿应该脱衣检查，观察他们的一般外貌、警觉度及面部特征和颜色。听诊心脏，触摸前囟和骨缝。检查耳 / 眼、鼻 / 口（包括腭部检查）、颈部（包括锁骨）、胳膊和手、腿和脚及生殖器和肛门。触诊腹部并感觉股动脉搏动。将婴儿转向俯卧位，检查背部和脊柱。让婴儿仰卧，检查臀部，测量头围并清楚记录。

Babies should be examined undressed. Look at their general appearance and alertness as well as facial features and colour. Listen to their heart and feel the anterior fontanelle and sutures. Examine their ears/eyes, nose/mouth (including palatal sweep), neck (including clavicles), arms and hands, legs and feet, as well as genitalia and anus. Palpate the abdomen and feel for femoral pulses. Turn the baby to the prone position and examine their back and spine. Place the baby supine and examine their hips. Measure the head circumference and clearly document.

识别和管理产后抑郁症。

The postnatal period marks a significant transition point in a woman's life. The period of postnatal care extends from the hospital stay to the community and home and is provided by multiple caregivers. The objectives of care of mother and baby in the postnatal period include provision of rest and recovery following birth, supporting maternal attachment and assisting in the development of maternal self-esteem. The family unit should be supported, and risks need to be identified and managed appropriately. If the mother wishes to breast-feed, this should be initiated and encouraged. Steps should be taken to prevent, identify and manage postnatal depression.

女性在社区中的大部分护理工作由社区助产士和全科医生负责。如果女性要返回医院进行临床复查，则是为了对孕期、产时或产后发生的并发症进行随访，或者是对糖尿病或高血压等疾病进行医学管理。应该利用这一机会来讨论计划生育、避孕及进行宫颈筛查。有关女性妊娠和产后需求的信件应及时寄出，因为它们对全科医生有帮助，而且在许多情况下是服务与服务之间的唯一联系。理想的产妇保健模式应力求最大限度地提高女性在整个生育期的健康水平，而不是只关注一次妊娠。

Most of a woman's care in the community is conducted by the community midwives and general practitioners. If a woman is returning for a clinical review in the hospital, it is either for debriefing following a complication during her pregnancy, labour, delivery or postnatal period or for the medical management of medical conditions such as diabetes or hypertension. The opportunity should be utilized to discuss family planning and contraception, as well as cervical screening. Letters regarding the woman's pregnancy and postnatal needs should be sent out in a timely fashion, as they are helpful to general practitioners and in many cases are the only link between the services. An ideal model of maternity care should seek to maximize the health of women across their reproductive life rather than focus on a single pregnancy.

本章概览	Essential information
生理变化 • 子宫复旧 • 恶露排出 • 子宫内膜再生 • 心输出量减少 • 第 1 周液体流失 2L	**Physiological changes** • Uterine involution • Lochial loss • Endometrial regeneration • Reduction of cardiac output • Fluid loss 2 L first week
内分泌变化 • 雌激素 / 孕酮降低，催乳素升高 • 产后 10 天检测不到 hCG	**Endocrine changes** • Oestrogen/progesterone falls, prolactin rises • hCG undetectable 10 days
泌乳和母乳喂养 • 初乳 • 2～3 天乳汁流量 • 哺乳过程、抑制泌乳	**Lactation and breast-feeding** • Colostrum • Milk flow 2–3 days • Suckling process, lactation suppression

（续表）

本章概览	Essential information
心理变化 • 产后抑郁症（见第 14 章）	**Psychological changes** • Puerperal depression (see Chapter 14)
产褥热 • 生殖道感染 • 尿路感染 • 乳腺感染 • 伤口感染	**Puerperal pyrexia** • Genital tract infection • Urinary tract infection • Breast infection • Wound infection

第 14 章　心理健康与分娩

Mental health and childbirth

Jo Black　著　　杨一华　译　　杨慧霞　校

学习本章后，你应当能够：

知识要点

- 认识围产期可能发生的各种心理障碍
- 了解采集心理健康病史的重要性，以积极预防的方式对待有患病风险的女性
- 阐述围产期精神疾病的症状
- 了解和处理围产期风险
- 了解围产期错误归因的风险
- 描述围产期用药原则
- 讨论围产期精神疾病的能力问题

临床能力

- 采集完整心理健康病史
- 制订精神疾病患者的临床治疗计划
- 评估和处理精神疾病患者的躯体健康
- 评估、沟通和处理围产期风险

专业技能及态度

- 培养积极倾听的能力
- 培养专业关注所有孕产妇心理健康的能力
- 了解患有心理障碍的女性在医疗保健方面可能会遇到的困难
- 在为存在心理健康问题或心理健康状况较差的人提供护理时，表现出尊重和包容的言语、态度和决策方面的领导力

After studying this chapter you should be able to:

Knowledge relating to mental disorders

- Demonstrate an awareness of the range of possible mental health disorders in the perinatal period
- Understand the importance of identification of mental health history and working in a proactive and preventative way with women at risk of illness
- Identify of symptoms of mental illness in the perinatal period
- Understand and manage risk in the perinatal period
- Understand the risk of misattribution in the perinatal period
- Describe the principles of prescribing in the perinatal period
- Discuss capacity issues in perinatal mental illness

Clinical competencies

- Take an adequate mental health history
- Make a clinical management plan for someone with a mental health diagnosis
- Assess and manage physical health for those with a mental health diagnosis
- Assess, communicate and manage risk in the perinatal period

Professional skills and attitudes

- Develop of active listening skills
- Develop professional curiosity about the mental wellbeing of all expectant and new mothers
- Understand the barriers women with mental health disorders may have and can experience in health care
- Show leadership in respectful and inclusive use of language, attitude and decision-making when offering care to those at risk of or experiencing poor mental health

理解孕产妇心理健康的重要性是每位产科医生的核心知识。而这要求必须对成人心理健康、婴儿心理健康、心理药理学、胚胎学、心理学、内分泌学、法医学框架及妊娠期和产后的特定心理健康问题有所了解。

Understanding the importance of good maternal mental health is expected core knowledge of every obstetrician. Knowledge of adult mental health, infant mental health, psychopharmacology, embryology, psychology, endocrinology, medicolegal frameworks and pregnancy- and postnatal-specific mental health issues is necessary.

本章旨在作为一个实用的入门指南，以更好地了解孕产妇在妊娠期间和产后可能遇到的常见心理健康问题，产科医生对孕产妇的心理问题应具备预防、发现、早期干预、评估风险和提供安全、循证的诊疗等的能力。

This chapter is designed to be a practical introductory guide to achieve a better understanding of common mental health problems which women can experience during and after pregnancy. The role of the obstetrician is prevention, detection, early intervention, assessing risk and providing safe, evidence-based care.

孕产妇心理障碍可使人虚弱并同时影响母亲和孩子健康。未经治疗的精神障碍是孕产妇发病和死亡的主要原因之一。2009—2013 年，有 161 名孕产妇死于心理健康因素。这表明在英国和爱尔兰，2009—2013 年期间每 10 万名孕产妇中有 3.7 人在妊娠期间或产后 1 年内死于心理健康相关原因（95%CI 3.2～4.4）（MBRACCE-UK）。

Mental health disorders can be debilitating and can affect both mother and child. Untreated they are a common cause of morbidity and are one of the leading causes of maternal deaths. One hundred sixty-one women died from mental health-related causes between 2009 and 2013. This represents a rate of 3.7 deaths from mental health-related causes during or up to 1 year after the end of pregnancy per 100,000 maternities in the UK and Ireland for 2009–2013 (95% CI 3.2–4.4) (MBRACCE-UK).

孕产妇不良心理状态增加了子代在婴儿期和儿童期的健康状况不佳的风险，同时增加了语言发育迟缓和更低受教育程度的可能性（引自 Avon 对父母和婴儿的纵向研究）。

Poor maternal mental health increases the risk to the infant of poorer health during infancy and childhood, the possibility of speech and language delay or lower educational attainment (Avon Longitudinal Study of Parents and Infants).

我们必须认识到，改善孕产妇心理健康的措施可以直接提高下一代的生存概率。

It is important to recognize that measures which improve the mental health of mothers can directly improve the life chances of the next generation.

助产士和产科医生处于独特位置，利于帮助孕产妇在整个妊娠期间保持良好的心理健康，并能快速发现新出现的心理健康问题并确保其能获得适当的治疗。要有效地做到这一点，最重要的是要全面地考虑你所负责的孕产妇的需求，尊重她们的长处、喜好、态度和文化传统。有心理健康病史的孕产妇会提出各种有关其妊娠、分娩和产褥期的看法、意见和要求。女性，也包括有心理健康问题的女性，需要获得准确、可理解和全面的信息，以帮助她们考虑自主的选择并做出知情的决定。

Midwives and obstetricians are uniquely placed to support women to stay mentally well throughout their pregnancies and to identify emerging mental health issues quickly and ensure access to appropriate treatment. To do this effectively, it is crucial to take a holistic view of the needs of women in your care, respecting strengths, preferences, attitudes and cultural heritage of women. Women with mental health histories will bring a range of views, opinions and wishes to decisions with regard to their pregnancy, birth and postnatal period. Women, including women with mental health issues, need to have access to accurate, understandable and comprehensive information in order to help them consider their options and make informed decisions.

这并不是指产科医生或助产士需要成为心理健康专家。你不用掌握有关心理健康的每一项诊断、每一种治疗、每一种处理，也不需要对疾病作出诊断或进行治疗。但是，产科医生要能获得足够的病史和评估当前的心理健康状况，并确保女性在需要时能够获得有用的信息以及进一步的评估和治疗。医疗制度各不相同。而在你所工作的体系中，你应该让有需要的孕产妇能够获得准确的信息、建议和治疗。基层医疗、可靠的在线资源、志愿者、助产士、随访人员、咨询和治疗服务都可以发挥作用。对于那些有最复杂或最严重心理健康问题的女性，建议接受心理健康专家的诊疗服务（最好是围产期心理健康诊疗服务）。

No one expects an obstetrician or midwife to be a mental health expert. You are not expected to know about every diagnosis, every therapy or every treatment in mental health. You are not expected to diagnose a disorder or initiate treatment. However, an obstetrician needs to be able to take an adequate history and assess current mental health and to ensure women have access to high-quality information, further assessment and treatment if required. Health care systems vary. Within the system in which you work, it is necessary to have measures in place for women to be able to access accurate information, advice and treatment. Primary care, reliable online resources, the voluntary sector, midwives, health visitors, counselling and therapy services all have a part to play. For those women with the most complex or serious mental health issues, access to a specialist mental health service (preferably a perinatal mental health service) is recommended.

一、产科医生在心理疾病与分娩的作用（The role of the obstetrician as relates to mental illness and childbirth）

在产前和产后检查中，需要注意以下与精神疾病有关的三个问题。

- 孕妇是否有精神病史？
- 孕妇目前是否有精神障碍的症状？
- 孕妇是否接受过任何精神障碍的治疗？

In antenatal clinic or at a postnatal review, there are three specific questions to consider in relation to mental illness

- Does the expectant mother have a <u>history</u> of mental illness?
- Does the expectant mother have any <u>current symptoms</u> of a mental illness or disorder?
- Does the expectant mother use any <u>treatment</u> for a mental illness or disorder?

二、采集心理健康病史（Taking a basic mental health history）

和任何医学分支领域一样，您的职责是采集完整病史和执行必要的检查。采集基础心理健康病史是产科医生应具备的能力（框 14-1）。

As in any branch of medicine, your role is to take an adequate history and perform the necessary examination. Taking a basic mental health history is an expected competency of an obstetrician (Box 14.1).

要与孕产妇进行有关她心理健康的有效对话，应该考虑自己是否擅长沟通心理健康主题。要始终

框 14-1 基础心理健康病史	Box 14.1 A basic mental health history
问题示例 1. 过去您的心理健康是否有任何问题？ 2. 您有过几次发作？ 3.（针对经产妇）您之前妊娠期间和之后的心理健康状况如何？ 4. 您能详细告诉我最糟糕时的情况吗？ 5. 您是否被确诊过精神疾病？如果有，是什么？ 6. 您接受了什么治疗？ 7. 您接受的治疗有效吗？ 8. 还有什么措施对您的心理健康有帮助？ 9. 您曾经需要住院治疗吗？您是否接受过住院治疗或因"心理健康法"入院？ 10. 您曾经是否感到人生毫无意义？ 11. 您曾经是否想过或试图结束自己的生命？如果有，能否详细说明？ 12. 您是否使用药物，或者正在接受治疗或心理健康方面的支持？您能详细说明吗？ 13. 如果已经停止服用药物，什么时候停止的呢？为什么？ 14. 您的家族中是否有人诊断出患有严重的精神疾病？ 15. 您在妊娠期间或产后是否担心心理健康问题？ 16. 您目前的心理健康状况如何？ 17. 关于你的心理健康情况我还有什么没问及但你觉得我应该知道或有必要让我了解的问题吗？	Suggested questions 1. Have you had any issues with your mental health in the past? 2. How many episodes have you had? 3. (For multiparous women) What was your mental health like during/after your previous pregnancies? 4. Can you tell me a bit more about what that was like for you when things were at their worst? 5. Were you given a diagnosis? What was it? 6. What treatment did you receive? 7. Did the treatment you received work? 8. What else helped with your mental health? 9. Did you ever need hospital care? Did you accept hospital care or was admission under the Mental Health Act? 10. Have you ever felt life was not worth living? 11. Have you ever thought about or tried to end your life? Can you say a bit more about that? 12. Do you use medication or are you engaged in treatment or receive ongoing support for your mental health? Can you describe these? 13. If not using medication (and you have used it previously), when did you stop and why? 14. Does anyone else in your family have a diagnosis of significant mental illness? 15. Are you worried about mental health in this pregnancy or after childbirth? 16. How are things currently with your mental health? 17. Is there anything I haven't asked you about in relation to your mental health that you think I should have or that you think it's important for me to know?

使用礼貌的语言进行开放式提问，并注意谈话中的语言和非语言提示，保持主动倾听，以及准备足够的时间。

To have a productive conversation with a woman about her mental health, you should consider whether you are at ease talking about mental health. Always use respectful language and open questioning and take notice of verbal and non-verbal cues in the conversation; actively listen; and allow adequate time.

2017 年，皇家妇产科学院邀请孕产妇分享她们的经验。这些论题在 2017 年的"女性之声"出版物中进行了整理。她们得出的结论如下。

In 2017, the Royal College of Obstetricians and Gynaecologists invited women to share their experiences. The themes were collated in their *Women's Voices Publication 2017.* They concluded:

"目前的体系过于依赖孕产妇站出来公开自己的情况。而对围产期各种心理健康状况的缺乏了解意味着，如果没有孕产妇站出来公开，症状将完全被忽略，这会使她们对体系失去信心。许多孕产妇提出逃避医疗人员的问题和隐藏自己的症状非常容易。还有许多孕产妇不愿谈论自己的感受和心理健康史，简单的勾选'是'和'否'的问题不能让她们打开心扉。这意味着只有那些有自信并能说出来的人才敢这样做，从而使许多弱势孕产妇陷入困境。

"The current system relies too heavily on women coming forward and disclosing their own conditions. The lack of understanding of various perinatal mental health conditions means that, without women coming forward and disclosing, symptoms are being completely missed and are damaging women's confidence in the system. A number of women reported how it was all too easy to evade healthcare professionals' questions and hide symptoms. Many women are reluctant to talk about how they are feeling and about their history of mental health, and simple tick box "yes" and "no" questions do not encourage a dialogue that allows a woman to open up. This means that only those who are confident and able to speak up are doing so, leaving many vulnerable women to fall through the gaps.

一些孕产妇着重强调了求助医疗专业人员失败的经历，从没有被倾听的糟糕经历，到多次求助后被告知正在处理却得不到任何帮助。她们感到沮丧的是自己的诉求没有得到认真对待，许多人只有在找到愿意倾听的医疗专业人员后才能获得帮助。

A number of women highlighted incidents of failings by healthcare professionals, ranging from bad experiences of not being listened to after repeatedly asking for help to being told that they were being referred but with no support then ever materialising. Women felt frustrated that their concerns had not been taken seriously and many only had access to support once they had found a healthcare professional who was willing to listen.

许多受访者认为没有足够的时间与医疗专业人员讨论他们的心理健康问题或者诊疗过于仓促。很多评论认为这是由于提供的服务超负荷，而不是因为医疗专业人员不关心。那些关于心理健康的谈话通常不是以个人或公开的方式进行的，感觉就像简单的'打钩'测试。"

——摘自 2017 年"产妇心理健康，女性之声 RCOG"

A lot of respondents commented that they did not feel that they had had enough time with healthcare professionals to discuss their mental health, or that appointments had been rushed. Many of these commented that they felt had been due to an overstretched service, not because the healthcare professional did not care. Where conversations about mental health were being had, they were often not held in a personal or an open way, or felt like simple "tick box" exercises.' Maternal Mental Health-Women's Voices RCOG 2017

如果一位孕产妇向你透露自己的心理健康有关的病史或担忧，对于她提供的情况，你和她就下一步诊疗计划达成一致很重要。制订计划应包括所有在围产期帮助她的人。

If you do enable a woman to disclose a mental health history or concern, it is important you and she have a shared understanding about what will happen with the information she has given. Making a plan undoubtedly involves including all those who work with her in the perinatal period.

始终要求她与其他医疗专业人员保持联系。原因如下。

Always ask for a woman's consent to liaise with other health care professionals with whom she may be involved. Why?

"有证据表明，在 57 名既往有心理健康问题的自杀孕产妇中，至少有 16 名孕产妇基层医疗和产科护理之间没有沟通其重要的精神病史。有时候是产妇护理部门未获悉该名女性既往精神病史，有时候是全科医生不知道该名孕产妇预约了产科护理。"

——摘自 2015 年"拯救生命，改善母亲护理"

"In at least 16 of the 57 women with a prior history of mental health problems, who died by suicide, there was evidence that significant aspects of the woman's past psychiatric history were not communicated between primary care and maternity services. In several instances, maternity services had not been informed of a woman's past psychiatric history and in some circumstances the GP was unaware that the women had booked for maternity care."

Saving Lives, Improving Mothers' Care 2015

！注意

有女性提出，很多时候由于她们在工作和固定关系中表达清晰、仪表整洁，医疗专业人员便认为她们不存在心理健康问题，于是没有提出询问，从而失去了进行干预的机会。

Frequently, women report that because they were articulate, well groomed, in employment and/or in a committed relationship, health care professionals made assumptions that mental health issues would not be present, so did not ask, and an opportunity to intervene was lost.

来自不同社会经济和文化背景的女性也提出，她们认为有关自己的心理健康、适应能力、支持网络所做出的猜想是没有任何证据的。

Similarly other women from a range of socioeconomic and cultural backgrounds report they felt assumptions were made about their mental health, their resilience and their support network without any evidence to support these views.

重要的是要认识到心理健康方面的无意识偏见。

It is important to be aware of unconscious bias with regard to mental health.

无意识的偏见是我们的大脑在对人和情况进行快速判断和评估时产生的。这受我们的背景、文化环境和个人经验的影响。我们甚至可能意识不到这些观点，或者它们的全部影响或含意。

Unconscious bias happens by our brains making quick judgements and assessments of people and situations. Our biases are influenced by our background, cultural environment and personal experiences. We may not even be aware of these views or aware of their full impact or implication.

三、制订心理健康计划（Making a mental health plan）

经确诊精神疾病的女性在妊娠、分娩和产后期间需要一份心理健康计划，计划包括她们的心理健

康以及精神障碍的治疗方案（包括药物治疗）。

Women with established mental health diagnoses need a mental health plan for their pregnancy, delivery and postnatal period which takes into account their mental health and the treatment (including medication) that they use for their mental health disorder.

四、制订妊娠、分娩和产后的心理健康计划（Making a mental health plan for pregnancy, birth and the postnatal period）

（一）什么是心理健康计划（What is a mental health plan?）

心理健康计划让有心理健康相关担忧或既往史的孕产妇在妊娠时得到有计划的综合护理。它考虑了她及她未出生的胎儿在妊娠、分娩和产后的需求，同时考虑到了她的保护网络、她的支持网络、她的文化和宗教信仰及她的选择。

A mental health plan enables a mother with a mental health concern or history to have planned, joined-up care when she is pregnant. It considers her and her unborn baby's needs in pregnancy, during delivery and during the postnatal period. It takes into account her protective factors, her support network, her cultural and religious beliefs and her choices.

它可以识别任何与她的心理健康相关的风险或潜在挑战，并通过制订计划将其降到最低，或者制订出现严重心理问题发作时的治疗方案。

It recognizes any risks or potential challenges related to her mental health and creates with her a plan of what can minimize these, or in the event of a significant mental health episode, what the plan of treatment will be.

（二）创建心理健康计划（Creating a mental health plan）

- 应当在妊娠 32 周之前完成一份健全的心理健康计划。

- 应准备足够的时间来完成全面的计划。

- 应邀请与孕产妇及其家庭有关的所有医疗专业人员参与计划。

- 该计划应考虑孕产妇、婴儿和其他家庭成员的需求。

- 该计划应指出当前的所有心理健康症状和推

病例分析 1	Case study 1
Sarah 今年 24 岁，是天体物理学博士。她患有双相情感障碍，并从 2 年前的最后一次急性发作开始使用锂剂，治疗效果良好。 发现妊娠后，她立刻停止了锂剂治疗。而妊娠并不在计划之中。 她和她的伴侣对妊娠这件事非常高兴。Sarah 的家人住在海外，她伴侣的家人则在当地。他们对她过去的心理状况一无所知。	Sarah is 24 years old and a PhD student in astrophysics. She has a diagnosis of bipolar affective disorder and used lithium since her last acute episode 2 years ago to good effect. She stopped her lithium abruptly on discovering her pregnancy. The pregnancy was not planned. She and her partner are happy to be expecting a baby. Sarah's family lives overseas, and her partner's family is local. They do not know anything about her past mental health.

病例分析 2	Case study 2
Thelma 今年 29 岁，从事零售业。她正处于第一次妊娠最初的 3 个月。Thelma 的体重指数（body mass index，BMI）在低或正常范围内，并在最近 4 周内有所下降。她有神经性厌食症的病史，并曾 2 次住院治疗。2 次入院都是遵循"心理健康法"转诊而非自愿，且 2 次都进行鼻饲（nasogastric，NG）。她已恢复健康，这次是有计划的妊娠。她因乳房增大而感到恐惧，并且害怕她的身体进一步变化。她承认有限制热量摄入的想法。	Thelma is 29 years old and works in retail. She is in the first trimester of her first pregnancy. Thelma's body mass index (BMI) is in the low/normal range and has fallen in the last 4 weeks. She has a history of anorexia nervosa and has had two hospital inpatient spells for treatment. Both admissions were involuntary under the Mental Health Act, and nasogastric (NG) feeding was administered on both occasions. She has been well for over a year, and this pregnancy was planned. She is horrified by her enlarging breasts and is dreading her body changing further. She admits to some temptation to restrict calories.

病例分析 3	Case study 3
Angela 今年 34 岁，是当地的一名全科医生。她在部门社交中认识几位产科医生。在她 10 多岁和 20 岁早期时曾患有抑郁症。妊娠 28 周，她提到自己情绪低落，后悔妊娠，并因背部和臀部疼痛及持续的恶心而对胎儿感到不满。同时她睡眠欠佳，有时觉得继续下去太难了。她不希望你和任何人分享这个信息也不希望你把它写进她的临床记录里。	Angela is 34 years old and works as a local general practitioner. She knows several obstetricians in the department socially. Angela has had episodes of depression throughout her teenage years and early twenties. She discloses at 28 weeks she is low in mood, regrets being pregnant and feels resentful of the baby, as she blames it for her sore back and hips and her ongoing nausea. She is not sleeping well and sometimes thinks it is too hard to go on. She does not want you to share this information with anyone or to include it in her clinical record.

病例分析 4	Case study 4
Selma 今年 30 岁，妊娠 28 周，正在接受第一次产前检查。她患有精神分裂症，每月看一次社区精神科护士。她住在具有看护的住所中，并且多次因心理健康入院。她说她目前没有服用任何药物。她似乎心不在焉，回答问题也很谨慎。同时她提了一些使您感到奇怪的问题和言论，如"你怎么知道这是人类胎儿？""被选中的孩子必将保护我免受痛苦"。	Selma is 30 years old, is 28 weeks' pregnant and is attending her first antenatal contact. She has a diagnosis of schizophrenia and sees a community psychiatric nurse monthly. She lived in supported accommodation and has had frequent hospital admissions for her mental health. She says she is not currently taking any medication. She seems distracted and guarded in her responses. She asks some questions and makes some remarks which strike you as odd. 'How do you know it's a human baby?' and 'The baby is chosen and will protect me from the pain.'

荐的治疗方案。

- 计划应说明妊娠期间使用的所有药物及用药后母婴的产后监测。

- 该计划需要提出发生心理健康危机时应采取的措施和应有的职责。

- 孕产妇的所有相关记录中都应包括这份计划。

- 该计划必须例明确保优先考虑母婴关系的因素。

- 该计划将详细介绍如何喂养婴儿以及早期发现产妇使用药物后关于母乳喂养的问题和担忧。

  - A robust mental health plan should be completed before the thirty-second week of pregnancy.
  - Adequate time is needed to complete a thorough plan.
  - All health care professionals involved with the mother and family should be invited to contribute.
  - The plan should include the needs of the mother, the infant and the rest of the family.
  - The plan should identify any current mental health symptoms and any treatment/therapy which is recommended.
  - The plan should describe any medication used in pregnancy and any monitoring recommended for the mother and baby postdelivery because of this.
  - The plan needs to address actions and responsibilities should a mental health crisis occur.
  - A copy of the plan should be included in all copies of the mother's notes.
  - The plan must identify factors to ensure priority is given to the relationship between the mother and baby.
  - The plan will detail how the baby will be fed and identify early any questions or concerns with breast-feeding if the mother uses medication.

五、妊娠期和产后特殊精神疾病诊断（Specific mental health diagnoses in pregnancy and the postnatal period）

（一）双相情感障碍（Bipolar affective disorder）

双相情感障碍是一种严重情绪波动（躁狂或重度抑郁发作）为特征并具有缓解和复发倾向的严重情感障碍（ICD 10）。

Bipolar affective disorder is a major affective disorder marked by severe mood swings (manic or major depressive episode) and a tendency to remission and recurrence (ICD 10).

双相情感障碍在成年人中患病率约为 1%。

Bipolar affective disorder has a lifetime prevalence of approximately 1% of the adult population.

在预约就诊时，患有双相情感障碍的孕产妇如果处于缓解期，那她可能表现完全正常，因此很容易认为她没有严重精神疾病。然而产后发作的风险仍然存在，因此和她公开沟通此类情况非常重要。

At booking, a woman with bipolar affective disorder may be completely well if in remission, and it is tempting to assume she does not have a major mental illness. Nonetheless, the risk of a postnatal episode is real, and it is crucial you and she can discuss this openly.

双相情感障碍是产后精神病的一个非常重要的高危因素和预测因素（见后述）。如果你在一个提供围产期精神病服务的医疗体系工作，那么对于所有被诊断患有双相情感障碍的孕产妇来说，必须优先考虑转诊这项服务。

Bipolar affective disorder is a highly significant risk factor and predictor for postpartum psychosis (see later). If you work in a health care system where a perinatal psychiatry service is available, it is imperative that a referral to this service is prioritized for all women with a diagnosis of bipolar affective disorder.

患有这种情况的孕产妇会使用情绪稳定类药物来保持良好状态，在计划妊娠时则需要考虑药物的风险和益处。理想情况下，这应该在围产期精神科医生和专科药剂师合作下完成。不建议突然停止任何精神药物治疗（NICE CG192）。

Women with this condition may use mood stabilizers to stay well and at booking of pregnancy are highly likely to want to consider the risks and benefits of medication options. Ideally this should be done in collaboration with a consultant perinatal psychiatrist and a specialist pharmacist. A sudden discontinuation of any psychotropic medication is not advisable (NICE CG192).

（二）产后（产褥期）精神病（Postpartum (puerperal) psychosis）

产后精神病是最复杂和最严重的产后并发症，在世界上不同年龄、背景、国家和文化的产妇中发病率为 2‰。危险因素包括有双相情感障碍的家族史，母系产后精神病家族史，以及既往有双相情感障碍、分裂情感性障碍或产褥期精神病的发作。

Postpartum psychosis is the most florid and often the most serious of the postpartum conditions, occurring in 2/1000 deliveries in women of all ages, backgrounds and cultures and countries in the world. Risk factors include a family history of bipolar illness; a maternal family history of postpartum psychosis; and previous episodes of bipolar illness, schizo-affective disorder or postpartum psychosis.

约 50% 曾患有双相情感障碍或产后精神病的产

妇会再次发病。这一风险证明在妊娠期间进行评估和监测是正确的，在产妇同意的情况下，产后应进行预防性干预。

Approximately 50% of women with a previous bipolar illness or postpartum psychosis will become ill. This risk justifies assessment and monitoring during pregnancy, and with the woman's consent, prophylactic intervention following delivery.

这种疾病的特点如下。

- 分娩后不久突然发作，病情每日恶化。

- 50% 的概率将在产后第 1 周内出现，多数会在 2 周内出现，几乎全部在分娩后 3 个月内出现。

- 表现为精神障碍、妄想、恐惧和困惑、意识混浊和躁动，有时可出现幻觉。

- 可出现激越行为和严重的不适。

The illness is characterized thus:
- Sudden onset in the early days following delivery, deteriorating on a daily basis.
- Half will present within the first postpartum week, the majority within 2 weeks and almost all within 3 months of delivery.
- Psychosis, delusions, fear and perplexity, confusion and agitation and sometimes hallucinations are apparent.
- Agitation and severe disturbance may also manifest.

在疾病的早期，情况经常发生变化，这通常被称为急性未分化型精神病。发展到后期，它更明显是一种双相障碍。1/3 将表现为躁狂，其余通常表现为抑郁为主，同时伴随有一些躁狂症状。

In the early days of the illness, the picture changes frequently and is often called *an acute undifferentiated psychosis*. Later it is more clearly a bipolar illness. A third will be manic and the rest usually mixed with some symptoms of mania but a predominantly depressive content.

（三）治疗（Management）

患者通常有必要紧急收入母婴病房住院治疗。这些孕产妇不该收入普通的成人精神病科，她们需要专门的诊疗和护理。婴儿与母亲同住不仅符合人性，而且有利于母亲的治疗及确保与婴儿良好关系的维系。

Urgent admission to an inpatient mother and baby unit is usually necessary. These women should not be admitted to a general adult psychiatric unit. Specialized medical and nursing care is required. The admission of the baby with the mother is not only humane but will facilitate the mother's treatment and ensure a good relationship with her infant.

这些疾病对治疗反应迅速。可以使用抗癫痫药、抗抑郁药和情绪稳定药，有时还可以使用电休克疗法（electroconvulsive therapy，ECT），完全康复的预后良好。

These illnesses respond rapidly to treatment. Antipsychotics, antidepressants and mood stabilizers may be used and, on occasion, electroconvulsive therapy (ECT). The prognosis for a full recovery is good.

产后精神病可以危及生命，产妇自杀和因失常行为造成的意外伤害的风险较高。不进食和不就医也会危害身体健康，而且患病的产妇会暂时无法照料婴儿。

Postpartum psychosis can be a life-threatening condition with an elevated risk of suicide and accidental harm from disturbed behaviour. There is risk to physical health from not eating and drinking and not accessing medical care, and the woman may be temporarily unable to care for the baby.

康复后需要继续治疗一段时间，因为早期几周内的复发率很高，尤其是当她已经出现躁狂并可能再次陷入抑郁状态。

Treatment needs to be continued for some time after recovery because the risk of relapse in the early weeks is high, particularly if she has been manic and may relapse into a depressive state.

患者在此后的妊娠出现复发的风险至少为 50%。因此，她应在下一次妊娠早期接受转诊，并制订治疗计划。

The risk of recurrence following all future pregnancies is at least 1 in 2. She should therefore be referred early in her next pregnancy and a management plan put into place.

（四）产前和产后抑郁症（Antenatal and postnatal depression）

- 采集病史（见前述）至关重要。患有轻度、自限性抑郁症的孕产妇与患有严重、使人衰弱且难以治疗症状的孕产妇需要不同的谈话和治疗计划。

- 服用抗抑郁药后保持良好状态的孕产妇可能会的情况下被建议停药没有充分考虑风险和益处。保持状态良好胜于应对复发。

- 心理疗法是有效的，如果孕产妇有症状并希望避免药物治疗，它可用于治疗妊娠期的抑郁症和焦虑症。

- 如果您记录了既往心理健康史，请注意不要将身体症状错误归因于"心理健康"。

  - 患有焦虑和抑郁的孕产妇可以因为自己的心理健康问题或躯体疾病而出现疲劳、头痛、心悸、恶心或头晕。关键要认真进行病史记录和检查。将症状错误归因于"心理健康"可导致孕产妇死亡（CEMACE），因此保持关注、开放的心态和全面的思考非常重要。

- 严重的产前或产后抑郁症是妊娠严重但可治疗的并发症。抑郁症状可能与其他任何时候的抑郁相似。所以医护人员通常会忽视围产期抑郁症的严重程度，并将症状归因于孕产妇的疲惫。孕产妇有时可以成功掩盖症状。

- Taking a history (see previous section) is crucial. A woman with a mild, self-limiting depression will need a different conversation and management plan from a woman with severe, debilitating and hard-to-treat symptoms.

- Women who use antidepressants to stay well may have been advised to discontinue medication without full consideration of the risks and benefits. Staying well is preferable to having to deal with relapse.

- Psychological therapies are effective and can be used for depression and anxiety in pregnancy if women are symptomatic and wish to avoid medication.

- Take care not to misattribute physical symptoms to 'mental health' if you note a past mental health history.

  - Women with anxiety and depression can have fatigue, headaches, palpitations, nausea or dizziness as a manifestation of their mental health problem or as a symptom of a physical illness. Being thorough in history taking and examination is key. Misattribution of symptoms to 'mental health' has contributed to maternal death (CEMACE), so it is essential to remain curious, open minded and thorough.

- A significant antenatal or postnatal depression is a serious and treatable complication of pregnancy. Depressive symptoms can be similar to depression at any other time. It is common for health care professionals to miss the severity of a perinatal depression and attribute the symptoms to exhaustion of motherhood. Women sometimes can and do successfully mask symptoms.

！注意

以下是及产妇严重精神疾病的"危险信号"表现，需要紧急的高级精神病学专家评估：

- 近期显著变化的精神状态或出现新症状。

- 新出现的暴力自残行为或想法。

- 新出现或持续出现作为母亲能力的缺失或与婴儿疏远的表现。

The following are 'red flag' signs for severe maternal illness and require urgent senior psychiatric assessment:

- recent significant change in mental state or emergence of new symptoms

- new thoughts or acts of violent self-harm

- new and persistent expressions of incompetency as a mother or estrangement from the infant

当孕产妇具有以下任一情况，则应考虑进入母婴病房：

- 精神状态改变迅速。

- 自杀意念（尤其是暴力性质）。

- 普遍内疚或绝望。

- 与婴儿的疏远。

- 作为母亲信念不足。

- 有患精神病的证据。

Admission to a mother and baby unit should always be considered where a woman has any of the following:

- rapidly changing mental state

- suicidal ideation (particularly of a violent nature)

- pervasive guilt or hopelessness

- significant estrangement from the infant

- beliefs of inadequacy as a mother

- evidence of psychosis

（五）进食异常（Eating disorders）

相对健康但有神经性厌食症或神经性贪食症病史的女性在妊娠期间和产后很可能出现特定问题。

- 对于患有神经性贪食症的孕妇来说，晨吐可能更具有挑战。

- 妊娠期间身体的变化可能会让人很难忍受。

- 即使是"健康"的女性在妊娠前也可能有明显的饮食限制情况，在妊娠期间尝试"健康饮食"通常会让人非常不舒服。

- 其他人注意甚至触摸女性不断变化的身体都会感到非常痛苦。

- 产后身体状态可能会让产妇感到震惊和痛苦，即使妊娠期间平安无事，也有可能出现严重产后发作。

Women who are relatively well but have a history of anorexia nervosa or bulimia nervosa may well have specific issues in pregnancy and postnatally.

- Morning sickness may well be more challenging for women with bulimia nervosa.
- Bodily changes in pregnancy may be very uncomfortable to tolerate.
- Even 'well' women may still have significant restriction pre-pregnancy, and trying to 'eat well' in pregnancy is often highly uncomfortable.
- Others noticing or even touching a woman's changing body can be deeply distressing.
- Her postpartum body can be shocking and distressing to the mother, and even if pregnancy was uneventful, a significant postpartum episode is a possibility.

患有活动性进食障碍的女性在妊娠期间会表现出心理和生理问题，如果没有主动管理，则存在重大风险。

- 活动性神经性贪食症可导致严重的血液生化异常，特别是临床上严重的低钾血症。

- 对于那些有限食、暴泻、全身不适和活动能力下降的孕产妇，应考虑高凝血症的可能。

- 已发现厌食症和低出生体重或早产有关，但并非在所有研究都得到重复。

- 产妇和胎儿之间的关系很容易受到影响。对于妊娠期间有矛盾或后悔情绪的产妇更有可能难以与宝宝建立亲密关系。

- 产后进食障碍行为很可能会进一步发展。

- 患有活动性进食障碍的母亲很可能隐瞒了她们病情的严重程度。

- 孕妇体重和 BMI 反映孕妇进食障碍的严重程度的价值有限，但 BMI 不变或下降具有临床意义。

Women with active eating disorders present both psychological and physical issues in pregnancy which, without active management, present significant risk.

- Active bulimia nervosa can contribute to grossly abnormal blood biochemistry, specifically clinically significant hypokalaemia.
- Hypercoagulability is a concern for those with restriction, binge-purging, general malaise and reduced mobility.
- Some associations with anorexia and low birth weight or prematurity have been found, but these findings have not been reproduced in all studies.
- The relationship between mother and her unborn is often affected. Mothers who have ambivalent or regretful emotions about being pregnant are more likely to have difficulty establishing a warm relationship with their baby.
- It is highly likely that postnatally, the eating disorder behaviours will escalate further.
- It is probable that mothers with active eating disorders may be concealing the extent of their illness.
- Maternal weight and BMI have limited use as a measure of severity of eating disorder in pregnancy, but a static or falling BMI is significant.

（六）边缘性人格障碍或情绪不稳型人格障碍（Borderline personality disorder/emotionally unstable personality disorder）

这是一个会引起担忧或困惑的诊断。

This is a diagnosis which can cause concern or confusion.

患有边缘型人格障碍 / 情绪不稳定型人格障碍（borderline personality disorder/emotionally unstable personality disorder，EUPD）的人很可能在早期经历过情感无效。他们经常遭遇忽视或虐待，可能包括性虐待。因此，他们通过各种方式与一系列情感创伤做斗争。

Someone who has an established diagnosis of borderline personality disorder/emotionally unstable personality disorder (EUPD) is likely to have experienced an emotionally invalidating early life. They have often experienced neglect or abuse, including possibly sexual abuse. As a result, they struggle with a range of emotional scars which can manifest in a variety of ways.

患有 EUPD 的孕产妇可能很难建立和维持关系，特别是在不确定或有分歧的时候。她们对威胁高度敏感，并经常在感知威胁时做出反应。她们经常经历快速变化和难以预测的极端情绪。有时她们会感到强烈的无助、愤怒和绝望。一些复杂行为会用来应对这些难以抗拒的情绪。而这些行为可以针对她们自己（自我伤害，其中包括用药过量、割伤、暴饮暴食、滥用毒品或酒精）或是其他方面（人际冲突、攻击性、依赖性、人际关系问题）。

Women with EUPD may struggle to form and maintain relationships, particularly in times of uncertainty or disagreement. They are highly attuned to threat and often respond when threat is perceived. They often experience rapidly changing and hard-to-predict extremes of emotion. At times they can experience strong senses of hopelessness, rage or desperation. Some difficult behaviours can be used to cope with these overwhelming emotions. These can be directed towards themselves (self-harm, including overdoses, cutting, binging/purging, substance or alcohol misuse) or others (interpersonal conflict, aggression, dependency, relationship issues).

医疗工作者可能会觉得为那些有人格障碍的人提供尊重的和持续的照顾是一种挑战。对任何有心理健康问题的人使用贬低、轻率、不尊重或居高临下的语言都是不可取的，这包括跟其他同事说“她是人格障碍、控制欲强、不理性、令人痛苦、忘恩负义或者噩梦”等词汇。你需要负责任地遵循范例处理，并认识早期创伤带来的所有挑战。

Staff can feel really challenged to provide respectful and consistent care for those with personality disorder. It is never acceptable to use demeaning, flippant, derogatory or patronizing language to or about anyone with a mental health problem. This could include using terms such as 'she's a PD/manipulative/irrational/a pain/ungrateful/a nightmare' to other colleagues. You have a responsibility to lead by example and recognize all the challenges presented as a result of earlier trauma.

值得注意的是，如果她是被虐待，特别是童年受到性虐待的幸存者，阴道检查、无法动弹、经历无法控制的疼痛、被触摸及无助感都可能对她造成同样的创伤和再次刺激。

It is worth considering for a moment that if she is a survivor of abuse, particularly childhood sexual abuse, vaginal examinations, being immobile, experiencing pain beyond her control, being touched and feeling powerless could all be very traumatic and retriggering for her.

在孕期考虑到孩子的健康，她很可能会避免采取以往的应对方案，如过量服药、酗酒或割伤，但这可能会使她的情感上更为痛苦。

She may well be avoiding previous coping strategies such as overdosing, binge drinking or cutting in her pregnancy for the wellbeing of her child but, in avoiding these, her emotional pain may feel even more acute.

她会很难想象，面对这样一个充满敌意的世界，她如何才能照顾孩子并保证他的安全。如果她没有感受过和善且充分的养育经历，她可能会害怕自己缺乏为人父母的技能。也可能她会过于担心其他人会认为她能力不够，在出生时就带走她的孩子。

She is likely to be struggling to imagine how she can parent and keep her baby safe in the face of such a hostile world. If she did not experience kind and adequate parenting, she may be terrified that she lacks the skills to parent. Or she may be so fearful that others will see her as inadequate that they will remove her baby at birth.

综合这些，我们可以看到妊娠和即将到来的分娩是如何使一个有人格障碍的母亲感到极度焦虑、警惕和防御性，在医疗保健系统中这被认为是“具有挑战性的”或者“困难的”。

In light of all this, one can begin to see how this pregnancy and imminent birth could cause a mother with personality disorder to feel extremely anxious, vigilant and defensive, and so may be seen within the health care system as 'challenging' or 'difficult'.

这类母亲需要友好、真诚、尊重和主动的照顾。她需要理解你和你的团队是专业的、人性化的，并且遵循循证医学。她需要知道，与任何其他女性一样，在有行为能力的情况下，她可以接受或拒绝调查、检查和干预。任何关于她的心理健康或孩子的问题都需要与她进行开诚布公的讨论。

This mother needs kind, truthful, respectful, proactive care. She needs to understand you and your team are professional and human and practise evidence-based medicine. She needs to know that, as with any other woman, in the presence of capacity, she can accept or decline investigations, examinations and interventions. Any concerns about her mental health or about her baby's welfare need to be discussed with her openly and honestly.

（七）强迫症（Obsessive-compulsive disorder）

强迫症（OCD）的特征是要么存在强迫观念，要么存在强迫行为，但通常两者都存在。这些症状可导致严重的功能损害和痛苦。强迫观念被定义为一种反复进入人的大脑的不想要的、侵入性想法、图像或冲动。强迫行为是一种被迫执行的重复行为或心理行为。强迫行为可以是明显的能被他人察觉到的行为，如检查门是否上锁，也可以是隐蔽的心理行为不被发现，如在脑海中重复某句话。

Obsessive-compulsive disorder (OCD) is characterized by the presence of either obsessions or compulsions, but commonly both. The symptoms can cause significant functional impairment and/or distress. An obsession is defined as an unwanted intrusive thought, image or urge that repeatedly enters the person's mind. Compulsions are repetitive behaviours or mental acts that the person feels driven to perform. A compulsion can either be overt and observable by others, such as checking that a door is locked, or a covert mental act that cannot be observed, such as repeating a certain phrase in one's mind.

通常我们认为 1%～2% 的人中患有强迫症，还有一些研究认为是 2%～3%。

It is thought that 1–2% of the population have OCD, although some studies have estimated 2–3%.

围产期强迫症更为严重。一个母亲反复经历与她的婴儿有关的侵入性想法或图像，可能会过于惊吓以至于难以求助，所以她会默默忍受。有些仪式会非常耗时，而这种强迫的想法或行为都会极大影响母亲日常照顾婴儿的舒适度。

Perinatal OCD can be particularly problematic. A mother experiencing a recurrent intrusive thought or image relating to her baby can be so horrified by its content that asking for help is exceptionally difficult, so she suffers in silence. Some rituals can be incredibly time consuming, and either the obsessional thought or the compulsion can dramatically interfere with the mother's comfort in carrying out day-to-day baby care tasks.

心理疗法和药物疗法在治疗强迫症方面是有效的，而且是首选方案，因为母亲和婴儿能舒适地在一起并享受彼此，这对婴儿的健康成长非常重要。关键是应尽快进行治疗，最大限度地减少母亲心理健康对婴儿的影响。

Psychological therapy and pharmacotherapy are effective in the treatment of OCD and are a priority as a mother's and baby's ability to be comfortable together and to enjoy one another are very important for the healthy development of the infant. Treatment as soon as possible minimizes the impact the mother's mental health has on the infant, which is critical.

（八）创伤后应激障碍（Post-traumatic stress disorder）

创伤后应激障碍（PTSD）在妊娠期间经常被漏诊，或被误诊为广泛性焦虑症、惊恐发作或抑郁症。

Post-traumatic stress disorder (PTSD) is frequently missed in pregnancy or misdiagnosed as a generalized anxiety disorder, panic attacks or depression.

创伤后应激障碍的症状包括幻觉重现、噩梦、过度警觉和严重焦虑的身体症状。

Symptoms of PTSD include flashbacks, nightmares, hypervigilance and physical symptoms of significant anxiety

创伤后应激障碍可导致围产期严重心理健康问题。

PTSD can contribute to significant mental health problems in the perinatal period.

高危人群包括避难者、难民、服务行业人员和那些最近经历过创伤的人，如经历过格伦费尔（Grenfell）灾难或曼彻斯特（Manchester）爆炸案的人群。应时刻注意你负责的社区和需要关注的特定群体。

High-risk groups include asylum seekers, refugees, services personnel and those who have been exposed to recent trauma, such as those involved in the Grenfell disaster or Manchester bombings. It is always advisable to be mindful of the communities who use your service and any specific groups you need to be aware of.

非高危人群也会经历创伤后应激障碍，因此需要对创伤史有更广泛的认识，其中包括之前的出生创伤。

PTSD is also experienced by those not from these highrisk populations, so broader awareness is necessary for a history of trauma, including previous birth trauma.

心理治疗是有效的，并且孕产妇应优先考虑心理治疗。

Psychological therapy is effective and should be prioritized in the pregnant and postnatal population.

对于患有明显创伤后应激障碍的孕妇，一份详细的分娩计划也有助于确保她的产时护理可以减少带来痛苦的触发或刺激。经历过生育创伤的女性在随后的妊娠中会遇到一些非常特殊的挑战。再次进入产房，同样的灯光、噪音和气味可能非常具有挑战性，这些需要事先仔细考虑。因以前的护理事件提出过投诉或担忧的孕产妇可能会担心接受不够满意的治疗，这可能需要高级医务人员保证不会再出现类似情况。

For antenatal women with marked PTSD, a careful birth plan can also be helpful to ensure her intrapartum care is designed specifically to reduce triggers or stimuli which could be distressing. Women who have experienced previous birth trauma can have some very specific challenges in subsequent pregnancies. Re-entering the delivery suite, the same lighting, noises and smells can be very challenging and need to be thought about carefully in advance. Women who have raised complaints or concerns about previous episodes of care may fear less favourable treatment and may need reassurance from senior staff that this will not be the case.

六、妊娠期精神科药物使用原则（Principles of prescribing psychotropic medication in pregnancy）

在教科书中特定药物的建议也存在问题。由于证据基础在不断发展和演变，使用这类已出版多年的参考资料可能会导致读者使用不再有效的或已被更新的建议和处方指南。

Including medication-specific advice in a textbook is problematic. The evidence base continues to grow and evolve, and using this resource years after publication could result in the reader using data which are no longer valid or that have been superseded by more up-to-date research and prescribing guidance.

妊娠期精神科药物使用原则见框 14–2。

Prescribing psychotropic medication in pregnancy follows the principles outlined in Box 14.2.

作为临床医生和处方者，重要的是要获取最新信息，以确保自己的知识和建议是最新的。英国术语学信息服务（The UK Teratology Information Service，UKTIS）和 2017 年英国心理药物学协会围产期指南是非常有用的资源。

As a clinician and a prescriber, it is important to access up-to-date information to ensure your knowledge and advice is current. The UK Teratology Information Service (UKTIS) and the British Association of Psychopharmacology Perinatal Guideline 2017 are helpful resources.

！注意 丙戊酸钠注意事项

Special mention of sodium valproate

妊娠期间服用含有丙戊酸钠的药物可导致 11% 的新生儿出现畸形，以及 30%～40% 的新生儿出现发育障碍。

Medicines containing valproate taken in pregnancy can cause malformations in 11% of babies and developmental disorders in 30–40% of children after birth.

除非不适合使用替代疗法或有避孕计划，女性，其中包括在青春期前的年轻女孩不得使用丙戊酸钠治疗。孕妇不得使用丙戊酸钠。另请参照 MHRA 工具包，以确保女性患者更好地了解孕期服用丙戊酸钠的风险（NICE CG192 2014）。

Valproate treatment must not be used in girls and women, including in young girls below the age of puberty, unless alternative treatments are not suitable and unless the conditions of the pregnancy prevention programme are met. Valproate must not be used in pregnant women. See also the MHRA toolkit to ensure female patients are better informed about the risks of taking valproate during pregnancy (NICE CG192 2014).

七、心理健康与行为能力（Capacity and mental health）

具有行为能力的女性有权决定自己的护理和治疗。能力评估是每个临床医生必须具备的核心技能，他或她必须准确保存医疗记录，以确保考虑了能力

框 14–2　妊娠期精神科药物使用原则
1. 使用最少药物的最低有效剂量
2. 如果可以，使用过去成功使用过的药物
3. 不要在发现妊娠后突然停止用药
4. 孕产妇需要能够与处方者或药剂师及时进行有关风险利益处的沟通
5. 考虑给孕妇用药时，应与其讨论母乳喂养问题
6. 鉴于孕妇循环血量的增加，在妊娠期间可能需要增加药物剂量
7. 如果使用了精神类药物，应考虑在产前、围产期和产后阶段对母婴进行必要的监测

Box 14.2　Prescribing psychotropic medication in pregnancy
1. Use the lowest effective dose of the minimum number of medications.
2. If possible, use what has been used successfully in the past.
3. Do not abruptly stop medication on discovery of pregnancy.
4. Women need to be able to have a timely risks/benefits conversation with a prescriber or pharmacist.
5. Breast-feeding should be discussed when thinking about medication with any pregnant woman.
6. Medication may need to be increased during pregnancy given the increasing maternal circulating volume.
7. Consider the monitoring needed for both mother and infant during the antenatal, perinatal and postnatal phases if psychotropic medication has been used.

问题并且进行了评估。

Women have the right to make decisions about their care and treatment if they have the capacity to do so. Capacity assessment is a core skill every clinical practitioner must have, and she or he must keep the medical records accurately to give assurance that capacity was considered and an assessment was done.

即使患有精神疾病的女性也应被认为具有行为能力。为特定决定而进行全面的能力评估至关重要。依照《精神健康法》被拘留且持续出现精神病症状的孕产妇，仍被认为具有决定其治疗方案的能力。

Women with mental illness must be assumed to have capacity, even when mentally ill. A thorough capacity assessment for a specific decision is essential. Women detained under the Mental Health Act with ongoing symptoms of psychosis must still be assumed to have capacity to make decisions about their medical treatment.

如果确定精神疾病影响了行为能力（如下例），你应咨询你所在医院的法律团队，考虑是否需要向法院提出申请。

If it is established that a mental illness has affected capacity (see the following example), you should consult the legal team for your hospital to consider the need for an application to a court to proceed.

因为 Mary 不相信自己怀孕了，所以她不会谈论胎儿的活动。

Because Mary does not believe she is pregnant, she will not engage in a conversation about the baby's movements.

你认为她的子痫前期有恶化的风险并希望她入院接受评估和治疗，但她拒绝了。

You believe she is at risk of worsening pre-eclampsia and would like to admit her for assessment and treatment. She refuses.

思考你认为接下来应该怎么办。

Consider what you think needs to happen next.

你还需要知道什么信息？

What additional information do you need to know?

还有谁需要参与进来？

Who else needs to be involved?

八、总结（Summary）

孕产妇心理健康与躯体健康同样重要。早期发现和预防可能的心理健康问题总是优于治疗。为高危孕产妇提供建议和支持来帮助她们保持良好的妊娠状态需要时间、专业知识、耐心、求知欲和善意。对心理健康问题的治疗是有效的，我们都应该努力让我们帮助的女性达到完全康复。

Maternal mental health is as important as maternal physical health. Early detection and prevention of possible poor mental health are always preferable to treatment. To advise and support a woman at risk to stay well in pregnancy takes time, expertise, patience, curiosity and kindness. Treatment of mental health problems are effective, and we should all be ambitious for the full recovery of the women with whom we work.

围产期心理健康问题影响不同行业、不同社会经济背景和不同种族的女性。它很常见，并且严重情况可导致孕产妇死亡。针对它的治疗是有效的，并且可以达到治愈效果。对于那些有严重心理健康问题的孕产妇，最好是由围产期心理健康治疗团队协调治疗，合适的话可以在社区进行，但如果急性发作时发现风险，则应寻求母婴病房治疗。

Perinatal mental health problems affect women from every walk of life, every socioeconomic background and every ethnicity. They are common, and at the severe end of the spectrum are a leading cause of maternal death. Treatments are effective, and recovery is absolutely achievable. Ideally for those with serious mental health problems, treatment should be coordinated by perinatal mental health teams, if suitable in the community, but where risk is identified in the acute episode, an admission to a mother and baby unit should be sought.

病例分析	Case study
Mary 今年 44 岁，被诊断为偏执型精神分裂症。她认为自己并没有妊娠，她的腹部隆起是因为她在接受情报局的实验后得了癌症。她已经妊娠 35 周合并有高血压，但她认为降压药是毒药，所以没有人确定她是否服药。她自诉最近经常出现头痛，而且你注意到她脚踝有肿胀。	Mary is 44 years old and has a diagnosis of paranoid schizophrenia. She believes she is not pregnant and her abdominal swelling is because she has cancer after being experimented on by the Secret Services. She is 35 weeks' pregnant and has high blood pressure, but she thinks the antihypertensive treatment is poison, so no one is sure if she is taking it or not. She admits to frequent headaches which have started recently, and you note ankle swelling.

本章概览	Essential information
• 精神疾病是孕产妇死亡的主要原因之一 • 重要的既往病史是预测围产期严重精神疾病最可靠的指标 • 产科医生和助产士具有独特的作用，可以让孕产妇分享她们的病史而不用担心评价、震惊、过度反应或排斥 • 围产期采集精神病史与采集心脏病史、糖尿病史或癫痫病史同等重要 • 围产期精神病是可以治愈的，良好的临床护理应包括为那些心理健康状况不佳的人传递希望	• Deaths related to mental illness remain a leading cause of maternal deaths. • A significant past history is the most reliable predictor of serious mental illness in the perinatal period. • Obstetricians and midwives are uniquely positioned to enable women to share their histories, without fear of judgement, shock, overreaction or rejection. • Obtaining a history of mental illness is as important as obtaining a history of heart disease, diabetes or epilepsy in the perinatal period. • Mental illness is treatable in the perinatal period. Instillation of hope for those experiencing poor mental health is part of good clinical care.

第三篇 妇科学基础
Essential gynaecology

第 15 章 妇科基础临床技能
Basic clinical skills in gynaecology

Ian Symonds 著 杨 欣 译 颜 磊 校

<table>
<tr><td>

学习目标

学习本章后，你应该能够：

知识标准

- 认识到引出妇科病史和体征的逻辑顺序
- 描述产科和妇科（O&G）症状和体征的病理生理学基础
- 列出在 O&G 常见情况管理中使用的相关调查

临床能力

- 从妇科患者获得病史
- 对非妊娠状态和妊娠早期（20 周以下）的女性进行腹部检查，识别出正常表现和常见异常
- 进行阴道检查（双合诊，双叶窥器），识别正常发现和常见异常
- 识别妇科患者的急性不适（疼痛、出血、低血容量、腹膜炎）
- 进行、介绍和解释以下相关检查：生殖器拭子（高位阴道拭子、宫颈内拭子）和子宫颈筛查试验
- 总结、整合病史、查体、检查结果；以清晰和合乎逻辑的方式制订管理计划；并在病历上做清楚记录

专业技能和态度

- 根据专业指导进行私密检查 [如英国皇家妇产科学院（RCOG），英国医学总会（GMC）]
- 进行私密检查时要有女性行为监督人在场
- 认识到同理心的重要性
- 承认和尊重文化多样性
- 表现出对社会因素与患者疾病相互作用的认识
- 维护患者的隐私
- 用患者能理解的语言向他们解释

</td><td>

LEARNING OUTCOMES

After studying this chapter you should be able to:

Knowledge criteria

- Recognize the logical sequence of eliciting a history and physical signs in gynaecology
- Describe the pathophysiological basis of symptoms and physical signs in obstetrics and gynaecology (O&G)
- List the relevant investigations used in the management of common conditions in O&G

Clinical competencies

- Elicit a history from a gynaecology patient
- Perform an abdominal examination in women in the non-pregnant state and in early pregnancy (under 20 weeks) and recognize normal findings and common abnormalities
- Perform a vaginal examination (bimanual, bivalve speculum) and recognize normal findings and common abnormalities
- Recognize the acutely unwell patient in gynaecology (pain, bleeding, hypovolaemia, peritonitis)
- Perform, interpret and explain the following relevant investigations: genital swabs (high vaginal swab, endocervical swab) and cervical screening test
- Summarize and integrate the history, examination and investigation results; formulate a management plan in a clear and logical way; and make a clear record in the case notes

Professional skills and attitudes

- Conduct an intimate examination in keeping with professional guidelines (e.g. Royal College of Obstetricians and Gynaecologists [RCOG], General Medical Council [GMC])
- Have a chaperone present when undertaking intimate examination
- Demonstrate an awareness of the importance of empathy
- Acknowledge and respect cultural diversity
- Demonstrate an awareness of the interaction of social factors with the patient's illness
- Maintain patient confidentiality
- Provide explanations to patients in language they can understand

</td></tr>
</table>

妇科学是对女性生殖道和生殖系统疾病的研究。妇科学和产科学之间是一个连续统一体，所以这种划分是多少有些武断的。早期妊娠（少于 20 周）的并发症，如流产和异位妊娠，通常被认为是妇科的范畴。

The term *gynaecology* describes the study of diseases of the female genital tract and reproductive system. There is a continuum between gynaecology and obstetrics so that the division is somewhat arbitrary. Complications of early pregnancy (less than 20 weeks) such as miscarriage and ectopic pregnancy are generally considered under the title of gynaecology.

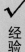
经验

在接受妇科服务的患者中，有精神疾病者高达 30%，不良生活事件、抑郁和妇科症状之间存在显著关联。请记住，目前的症状可能并不总是与患者的主要焦虑有关，可能需要一些时间和耐心来发现使患者就医咨询的各种问题。

Up to 30% of patients presenting to gynaecological services have psychiatric morbidity, and there is a significant association between adverse life events, depression and gynaecological symptoms. Remember, the presenting symptom may not always be related to the main anxiety of the patient and that some time and patience may be required to uncover the various problems that bring the patient to seek medical advice.

一、病史（History）

询问病史从介绍自己和解释你是谁开始。患者的姓名、年龄和职业的详细信息应该在问诊开始时就记录下来，除非这些信息已经提供（如在转诊信中）。患者的年龄将影响对许多现存问题的可能诊断。

When taking a history start by introducing yourself and explaining who you are. Details of the patient's name, age and occupation should always be recorded at the beginning of a consultation unless this information has already been provided (e.g. in a referral letter). The age of the patient will influence the likely diagnosis for a number of presenting problems.

病史应是全面的，但不是用一种与患者问题无关的具有打扰性方式提问。例如，从患有生殖道感染的年轻女性那里获得详细的性生活史是必要的，但有些女性可能会觉得讨论性生活史令她不舒服。无论年龄、宗教或社会状况如何，在研究临床病史时都要尊重患者，并根据每个患者的情况进行调整。

The history should be comprehensive but not intrusive in a manner that is not relevant to the patient's problem. For example, whilst it is essential to obtain a detailed sexual history from a young woman presenting with a genital tract infection, some women may find the discussion of sexual history uncomfortable. It is important to approach the clinical history with respect, regardless of age, religion or social situation, and tailor this approach to each individual patient.

（一）存在的问题 [The presenting problem(s)]

我们应要求患者描述她的问题的性质，并在病历记录中简单陈述其目前的症状。通过使用患者应用的实际词汇可以获得很多东西。重要的是确定问题的时间范围，并在适当情况下确定出现症状的情

境及其与月经周期的关系。发现任何由所提供症状导致患者的功能受到影响的严重程度也很重要。

The patient should be asked to describe the nature of her problem, and a simple statement of the presenting symptoms should be made in the case notes. A great deal can be learnt by using the actual words employed by the patient. It is important to ascertain the time scale of the problem and, where appropriate, the circumstances surrounding the onset of symptoms and their relationship to the menstrual cycle. It is also important to discover the degree of disability experienced for any given symptom.

更详细的问诊将依赖于当前问题的性质。月经紊乱是转诊妇科的最常见原因，所有育龄女性都应该有完整的月经史（见后述）。另一个常见的症状是腹痛，病史必须包括详细的起病时间和诱因，如性交、相关症状、疼痛的部位、放射部位及与月经周期的关系。

More detailed questions will depend on the nature of the presenting problem(s). Disorders of menstruation are the commonest reason for gynaecological referral, and a full menstrual history should be taken from all women of reproductive age (see later). Another common presenting symptom is abdominal pain, and the history must include details of the time of onset and precipitants, i.e. intercourse, associated symptoms, the distribution and radiation of the pain and the relationship to the menstrual cycle.

如果出现的症状是阴道分泌物，应该注意其颜色、气味及和月经的关系，也要注意任何用于治疗这些的非处方药的使用情况。它也可能与外阴瘙痒或皮肤改变有关，即皮疹 / 病变，特别是存在特定感染的情况下。

If vaginal discharge is the presenting symptom, the colour, odour and relationship to the periods should be noted, as well as any over-the-counter medications used to treat this. It may also be associated with vulval pruritus or skin changes, i.e. rash/lesions, particularly in the presence of specific infections.

腹部肿块的存在可能由患者自己发现，也可能在常规检查中发现。肿块压迫邻近盆腔脏器，如膀胱和肠道，均可引起症状。

The presence of an abdominal mass may be noted by the patient or may be detected during the course of a routine examination. Symptoms may also result from pressure of the mass on adjacent pelvic organs, such as the bladder and bowel.

阴道和子宫脱垂与肿块从阴道开口突出或排尿和排便困难的症状有关。常见的尿路症状包括尿频、尿疼或排尿困难、尿失禁、尿中带血或血尿。

Vaginal and uterine prolapse is associated with symptoms of a mass protruding through the vaginal introitus or difficulties with micturition and defecation. Common urinary symptoms include frequency of micturition, pain or dysuria, incontinence and the passage of blood in the urine, or haematuria.

在适当的情况下，性生活史应包括性交频率、有无性交痛（性交困难），以及与性欲、性满意度和性问题有关的性功能细节（见第 19 章）。

Where appropriate a sexual history should include reference to the coital frequency, the occurrence of pain during intercourse-*dyspareunia*-and functional details relating to libido, sexual satisfaction and sexual problems (see Chapter 19).

（二）月经史（Menstrual history）

关于月经史的第一个问题是末次月经的日期（LMP）。有关月经周期，你应确定她正常的月经周期长度、流血持续时间、月经周期是否规律，以及是否使用激素类避孕药。现在，女性通过手机应用程序跟踪月经周期也很常见，尤其是在试图妊娠的情况下。

The first question that should be asked in relation to the menstrual history is the date of the last menstrual period (LMP). In relation to the menstrual cycle, you should ascertain her normal cycle length, duration of bleeding, regularity/irregularity of cycle and whether any hormonal contraception is being used. It is also very common for women to now track their menstrual cycle with phone applications, especially if attempting to conceive.

第一次月经来潮，即月经初潮，通常发生在 12 岁，晚于 16 岁或早于 8 岁都为异常。在其他方面发育正常的女孩到 16 岁时月经未来潮被称为原发性闭经。

The time of onset of the first period, the menarche, commonly occurs at 12 years of age and can be considered to be abnormally delayed over 16 years or abnormally early at 8 years. The absence of menstruation in a girl with otherwise normal development by the age of 16 is known as primary amenorrhoea.

该术语应与阴毛初现区分开来，后者是性成熟的第一个迹象的开始。典型的情况是，乳房和乳头的发育比月经初潮早约 2 年（见第 16 章）。

The term should be distinguished from the pubarche, which is the onset of the first signs of sexual maturation. Characteristically, the development of breasts and nipple enlargement predate the onset of menstruation by approximately 2 years (see Chapter 16).

> **！注意**
> 没有成功获得末次月经的日期，可能会导致后续管理出现严重错误。
>
> Failure to check the date of the last period may lead to serious errors in subsequent management.

月经周期的长度是指月经第一天（即出血的第一天）到下一个月经第一天之间的时间。虽然月经周期的间隔通常是 28 天，但正常女性的周期长度可能在 21～42 天变化，可能只有在月经模式发生变化时才重要。

The length of the menstrual cycle is the time between the first day of one period (i.e. first day of bleeding) and the first day of the following period. Whilst there is usually an interval of 28 days, the cycle length may vary between 21 and 42 days in normal women and may only be significant where there is a change in menstrual pattern.

重要的是，要确保患者描述的不是从经期最后一天到下一个月经第一天之间的时间，因为这可能会给人一种月经频发的错误印象。

It is important to be sure that the patient does not describe the time between the last day of one period and the first day of the next period, as this may give a false impression of the frequency of menstruation.

以前有月经，超过 6 个月没有月经没有妊娠的女性为继发性闭经。月经稀发是指在 12 个月内月经来潮≤5 次。

Absence of menstruation for more than 6 months in a woman who is not pregnant and has previously had periods is known as secondary amenorrhoea. Oligomenorrhea is the occurrence of five or fewer menstrual periods over 12 months.

经期出血量和持续时间可能随年龄而改变，但也可能是疾病进程的一个有用的指示。正常的月经持续 4～7 天，正常的失血量为 30～40ml（6～8 汤匙）。

The amount and duration of the bleeding may change with age but may also provide a useful indication of a disease process. Normal menstruation lasts from 4 to 7 days, and normal blood loss varies between 30 and 40 mL (6–8 teaspoons).

月经形式的变化往往比实际失血量和出血时间更明显、更重要。在实践中，评估月经过多最好的方法是根据月经期间使用的卫生巾或卫生棉条的数量、有无血块和贫血症状。

A change in pattern is often more noticeable and significant than the actual time and volume of loss. In practical terms, excessive menstrual loss is best assessed on the history of the number of pads or tampons used during a period and the presence or absence of clots and symptoms of anaemia.

异常子宫出血（AUB）是指在月经间期出血紊乱，或出血过多、经期延长或不规则的子宫出血。经间期出血是指在明确的、周期性的、规律的月经期之间发生的任何出血。性交后出血是发生在性交过程中或之后的非月经性出血。AUB 总是需要检查，因为它可能是潜在疾病的首要症状。

Abnormal uterine bleeding (AUB) is any bleeding disturbance that occurs between menstrual periods or is excessive, prolonged or irregular. Intermenstrual bleeding is any bleeding that occurs between clearly defined, cyclical, regular menses. Postcoital bleeding is non-menstrual bleeding that occurs during or after sexual intercourse. AUB always requires investigation, as it may be the first symptom of an underlying potential medical condition.

月经过多（HMB）现在用来描述月经量过多或经期延长，指出血量大于 5～6 汤匙（>80ml），无论月经周期是规律的（月经过多）还是不规则的（不规则子宫出血）。

The term heavy menstrual bleeding (HMB) is now used to describe any excessive or prolonged menstrual bleeding which is greater than 5–6 tablespoons of blood (>80 mL), rrespective of whether the cycle is regular (menorrhagia) or irregular (metrorrhagia).

绝经是月经的终止，出血发生在绝经超过 12 个月后，为绝经后出血。应注意性交后或经期之间不规则阴道出血或失血的病史。

The cessation of periods at the end of menstrual life is known as *menopause*, and bleeding which occurs more than 12 months after this is described as postmenopausal bleeding. A history of irregular vaginal bleeding or blood loss that occurs after coitus or between periods should be noted.

（三）既往妇科病史（Previous gynaecological history）

必须详细记录以往任何妇科问题和治疗史。同样重要的是，在可能的情况下，应获得以往妇科手术的任何记录。患者常常不能确定手术的精确内容。需要多少关于之前妊娠的详细信息取决于目前的问题。

A detailed history of any previous gynaecological problems and treatments must be recorded. It is also important, where possible, to obtain any records of previous gynaecological surgery. Patients are often uncertain of the precise nature of their operations. The amount of detail needed about previous pregnancies will depend on the presenting problem.

多数情况下，需要了解之前妊娠的次数和他们的结局（流产、宫外孕或 20 周后分娩、剖腹产）。如果以前有过分娩，了解分娩方式很重要，即正常的阴道分娩、剖宫产或借助产钳、胎头吸引器等辅助器械分娩。此外，应该注意会阴裂伤或会阴切开术对会阴的任何损伤。

In most cases the number of previous pregnancies and their outcome (miscarriage, ectopic or delivery after 20 weeks, caesarean section delivery) is all that is required. If previous births have occurred, it is important to know the mode of delivery, i.e. normal vaginal delivery, caesarean section or assisted instrumental delivery via forceps or vacuum. Furthermore any injury to the perineum either via tear or episiotomy should be noted.

对所有性行为活跃的育龄女性来说，询问有关避孕和任何性传播疾病筛查的问题都是至关重要的。这不仅对确定妊娠的可能性很重要，而且因为所使用的避孕方法本身可能与目前的症状有关（如使用避孕药或宫内节育器时可能会发生不规则出血）。

For all women of reproductive age who are sexually active, it is essential to ask about contraception and any screening for sexually transmitted infections. This is important not only to determine the possibility of pregnancy but also because the method of contraception used may itself be relevant to the presenting complaint (e.g. irregular bleeding may occur on the contraceptive pill or when an intrauterine device is present).

对于年龄超过 25 岁的女性，应询问上次子宫颈筛查试验的日期及结果。澳大利亚最近对子宫颈筛查的更改意味着女性现在从 25 岁开始，每 5 年进行一次检查，而不是以前的间隔 2 年。新的子宫颈筛查方案在适当的情况下结合了人类乳头瘤病毒（HPV）基因型测试和液基细胞学检查（LBC）。

For women over the age of 25, ask about the date and result of the last cervical screening test. Recent changes to cervical screening in Australia mean that women now begin testing at the age of 25 and every 5 years instead of the previous 2-year interval. The new cervical screening test combines human papilloma virus (HPV) genotype testing and liquid-based cytology (LBC) where appropriate.

（四）既往内科及外科病史（Previous medical and surgical history）

对任何病史，全面的内科和外科病史都是至关重要的，妇科也不例外。这应该特别考虑到任何慢性肺部疾病病史、心血管系统疾病病史、既往的手术和麻醉史，这些都与可能需要手术密切相关。

A comprehensive medical and surgical history is vital to any medical history, and gynaecology is no different. This should take particular account of any history of chronic lung disease, disorders of the cardiovascular system and previous surgeries and anaesthetics, as these are highly relevant where any surgical procedure is likely to be necessary.

应记录所有目前的药物（包括非处方和非处方治疗）和任何已知的过敏药物。如果她正在计划近期妊娠，须检查她是否服用叶酸补充剂。

A record of all current medications (including nonprescription and over-the-counter treatments) and any known drug allergies should be made. If she is planning a pregnancy in the near future, check if she is taking folic acid supplements.

（五）社会心理病史（Psychosocial history）

社会心理病史对所有的医学诊断都很重要，而在涉及流产或绝育相关困难时尤其重要。例如，一名要求终止妊娠的 15 岁女性可能在父母的巨大压力下来流产，但可能她并不真正乐意遵循这一做法。

A psychosocial history is important with all medical presentations but is particularly relevant where the presenting difficulties relate to abortion or sterilization. For example, a 15-year-old female requesting a termination of pregnancy may be put under substantial pressure by her parents to have an abortion and yet may not really be happy about following this course of action.

询问有关吸烟、饮酒和其他娱乐药物（毒品）使用。重要的是询问精神健康史，其中包括焦虑、抑郁，以及他们目前是否正在接受治疗或看过精神卫生专业人员。家庭暴力是一个重大的社会问题，对女性的保健尤其重要，在诊所诊治女性时应重视。

Ask about smoking, alcohol and other recreational drug use. It is important to ask about mental health history, including anxiety, depression and if they are currently being treated or seen by a mental health professional. Domestic violence is a significant issue for society and is particularly important in women's health care and should be kept in mind when seeing women in clinic.

现在在澳大利亚，医疗保险要求对妊娠女性进行家庭暴力和性虐待筛查。在接受健康女性检查的女性中，有高达 40% 的人有家庭暴力史，不过妇科诊所的这一数字要低一些。

In Australia, screening in pregnancy for domestic violence and sexual abuse is now a Medicare requirement. Up to 40% of women presenting for a well-woman check will give a history of domestic violence, although the figure is lower in gynaecology clinics.

二、查体（Examination）

第一次就诊时应进行全面查体，其中包括评估脉搏、血压和体温。应仔细注意贫血的任何迹象。面部和身体毛发的分布通常很重要，因为多毛症可能是各种内分泌失调的一个表现症状。还应记录体重和身高，以计算身体质量指数（BMI）。

A general examination should always be performed at the first consultation, including assessment of pulse, blood pressure and temperature. Careful note should be taken of any signs of anaemia. The distribution of facial and body hair is often important, as hirsutism may be a presenting symptom of various endocrine disorders. Body weight and height should also be recorded to calculate a body mass index (BMI).

由于妇科检查的私密性，特别重要的是要确保尽一切努力确保隐私，确保查体时不被电话、呼机或关于其他患者的信息打断。检查最好在单独的就诊区域进行。

The intimate nature of gynaecological examination makes it especially important to ensure that every effort is made to ensure privacy and that the examination is not interrupted by phone calls, pagers or messages about other patients. The examination should ideally take place in a separate area to the consultation.

应该允许患者在隐蔽处脱衣服，必要时先排空膀胱（除非现在的问题是尿失禁，在这种情况下，排空膀胱可能掩盖压力性尿失禁的迹象）。在患者为检查脱衣后，一定要给患者提供一条毯子，让她们盖住自己，并尽快给患者检查。

The patient should be allowed to undress in privacy and, if necessary, empty her bladder first (unless the presenting problem is incontinence, in which case an empty bladder may mask signs of stress incontinence). Always offer a blanket for the patient to cover herself after undressing for the examination. After undressing there should be no undue delay prior to examination.

在开始查体前，并且在女性穿着完整的时候，向她解释阴道检查的内容，在获得患者口头同意后记录在案。应告知该患者，在接受检查过程中，她可以随时要求停止检查。无论妇科医生的性别，检查时通常都要有一名行为监督人。

Before starting the examination and whilst the woman is fully dressed, explain what will be involved in the vaginal examination, and verbal consent should be obtained and documented. The woman should be informed that she can ask for the examination to be stopped at any stage and that she is in control. A chaperone should generally be present, irrespective of the gender of the gynaecologist.

（一）乳房检查（Breast examination）

对有症状的或 45 岁以上女性第一次就诊时应进行乳房检查。有时出现与妊娠无关的乳汁分泌，称为溢乳症，可能表明内分泌异常或服用多巴胺拮抗药，如治疗精神疾病的药物。应采用手掌平部系统触诊，以排除乳房或腋窝内存在任何结节（图 15-1）。

The breast examination should be performed if there are symptoms or at the first consultation in women over the age of 45. The presence of the secretion of milk at times not associated with pregnancy, known as galactorrhoea, may indicate abnormal cndocrine status or medication with dopamine antagonists such as psychotropic medication. Systematic palpation with the flat of the hand should be undertaken to exclude the presence of any nodules in the breast or axillae (Fig. 15.1).

（二）腹部检查（Examination of the abdomen）

腹部检查可发现肿块的存在。应注意体毛的分布及瘢痕、妊娠纹和疝的存在。触诊腹部时要考虑到肌紧张和反跳痛。重要的是要让患者描述腹部疼痛的部位和有无放射性，还要进行肝、脾和肾的触诊。

Inspection of the abdomen may reveal the presence of a mass. The distribution of body hair should be noted, and the presence of scars, striae and hernias. Palpation of the abdomen should take account of any guarding and rebound tenderness. It is important to ask the patient to outline the site and radiation of any pain in the abdomen, and palpation for enlargement of the liver, spleen and kidneys should be carried out.

如果有肿块，试着确定它是固定的还是活动的，平滑的或规则的，以及它是否来自骨盆（你在耻骨上方不能触到包块的下缘）。检查疝孔，触诊腹股沟有无肿大的淋巴结。

If there is a mass, try to determine if it is fixed or mobile, smooth or regular, and if it arises from the pelvis (you shouldn't be able to palpate the lower edge above the pubic bone). Check the hernial orifices and feel for any enlarged lymph nodes in the groin.

叩诊腹部可勾勒出肿瘤的范围、检查膀胱是否充盈或识别是否存在鼓胀的肠襻。腹膜腔内的游离液体可以通过侧腹叩诊浊音和腹中部鼓音来识别（图 15-2）。

Percussion of the abdomen may be used to outline the limits of a tumour, to detect the presence of a full bladder or to recognize the presence of tympanitic loops of bowel. Free fluid in the peritoneal cavity will be recognized by the presence of dullness to percussion in the flanks and resonance over the central abdomen (Fig. 15.2).

当患者术后腹胀或急性腹痛，并怀疑有梗阻或肠梗阻时，应进行肠音听诊。

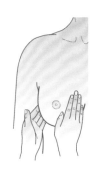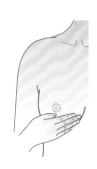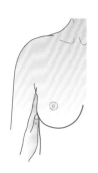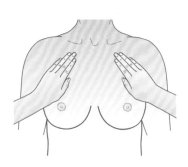

▲ 图 15-1　乳腺四象限的系统检查
Fig. 15.1　Systematic examination of the four quadrants of the breasts.

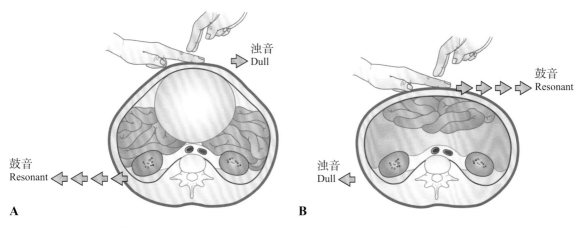

A   B

▲ 图 15-2　**A.** 巨大卵巢囊肿上方叩诊，可闻及中部浊音，两侧鼓音；**B.** 腹水时叩诊，可闻及侧腹叩诊的浊音和腹中部鼓音

Fig. 15.2　**(A)** Percussion over a large ovarian cyst-central dullness and resonance in the flanks. **(B)** Percussion in the presence of ascites-dullness in the flanks and central resonance.

Auscultation of bowel sounds is indicated in patients with postoperative abdominal distension or acute abdominal pain where obstruction or an ileus is suspected.

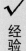 **经验**　要特别注意以往腹腔镜手术留下的脐部瘢痕，以及剖宫产和大多数妇科手术留下横切口的耻骨上区域。

Remember to look in particular in the umbilicus for scars from previous laparoscopies and in the suprapubic region where transverse incisions from caesarean sections and most gynaecological operations are found.

（三）盆腔检查（Pelvic examination）

并不是每次妇科就诊都必然做盆腔检查。应该考虑通过检查可以获得什么信息，这是一个筛查还是诊断程序，以及在这个时候是否有必要。

The pelvic examination should not be considered an automatic or inevitable part of every gynaecological consultation. You should consider what information will be gained by the examination, whether this is a screening or diagnostic procedure and whether it is necessary at this time.

患者应采取仰卧休息体位，膝盖向上并分开，或蹬脚截石位，特别是对于髋关节屈肌无力或关节炎继发关节疼痛的老年女性（图 15-3）。在进行阴道检查和窥器检查时，应双手戴手套。

The patient should be examined resting supine with the knees drawn up and separated or in stirrups in the lithotomy position, especially for older women with weak hip flexors or painful joints secondary to arthritis (Fig. 15.3). Gloves should be worn on both hands during vaginal and speculum examinations.

用左手分开小阴唇，观察尿道外口，检查外阴有无分泌物、红肿、溃疡和陈旧瘢痕。指诊前应进行窥器检查，以避免润滑油污染。最常用的是双叶形/鸭嘴形或 Cusco 窥器，可以获得各种大小的宫颈清晰视图。

Parting the lips of the labia minora with the left hand, look at the external urethral meatus and inspect the vulva for any discharge, redness, ulceration and old scars. Speculum examination should be performed before digital examination to avoid any contamination with lubricant. A bivalve/duckbill or Cusco's speculum is most commonly used and enables a clear view of the cervix to be obtained, with a variety of sizes available.

用左手撑开双侧的小阴唇，将窥器以器械尺寸最宽的横位方式插入阴道口，因为阴道在这个方向最宽大。当窥器到达阴道顶部时，轻轻打开双叶，观察宫颈（图 15-4）。记录是否有子宫颈分泌物或出血、息肉或溃疡面。

Holding the lips of the labia minora open with the left hand, insert the speculum into the introitus with the widest dimension of the instrument in the transverse position, as the vagina is widest in this direction. When the speculum reaches the top of the vagina, gently open the blades and visualize the cervix (Fig. 15.4). Make a note of the presence of any discharge or bleeding from the cervix and of any polyps or areas of ulceration.

记住，子宫颈的外观在分娩后发生了变化，外口更不规则，呈水平缝状。所谓的"糜烂"或外翻最常见。这是宫颈口周围的宫颈上皮区域，与宫颈其

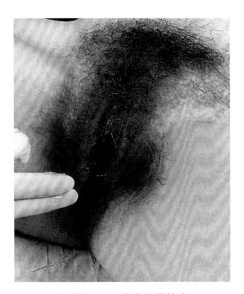

▲ 图 15-3 外生殖器检查

Fig. 15.3 Inspection of the external genitalia.

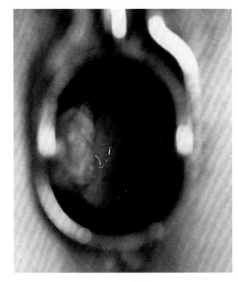

▲ 图 15-4 窥器检查正常子宫颈图

Fig. 15.4 View of normal cervix on speculum examination.

余部分的光滑粉色相比，它呈现出更深的红色。它不是糜烂，而是正常柱状上皮，从宫颈管延伸到子宫颈外。

Remember that the appearance of the cervix is changed after childbirth, with the external os more irregular with a horizontal slit. The commonest finding is of a so-called erosion or ectropion. This is an area of cervical epithelium around the cervical os that appears a darker red colour than the smooth pink of the rest of the cervix. It is not an erosion at all but normal columnar epithelium extending from the endocervical canal onto the ectocervix.

如果临床病史表明可能有感染，取阴道后穹隆和宫颈口拭子，放入运输培养基中寻找念珠菌和滴虫，取宫颈内不含培养基的拭子，进行聚合酶链反应核酸扩增检测（PCR NAAT）衣原体或淋球菌。用于宫颈筛查的样本，如果该样本是使用细胞刷收集用来进行液基细胞学检查的，也可进行 PCR 检测衣原体和奈瑟菌。

If the clinical history suggests possible infection, take swabs from the posterior vaginal fornices and cervical os and place in transport medium to look for *Candida* and *Trichomonas* and a separate swab without culture medium from the endocervix for polymerase chain reaction nucleic acid amplification testing (PCR NAAT) for *Chlamydia/Gonorrhoea*. PCR testing for *Chlamydia* and Neisseria can also be performed on the same sample used for cervical screening if this is collected using the cytobrush for liquid-based cytology.

当怀疑阴道壁脱垂时，可能需要使用 Sim 窥

器，因为这样可以更清楚地看到阴道壁。当使用 Sim 窥器时，患者最好采取半俯卧位或 Sim 体位（图 15–5 ）。

Where vaginal wall prolapse is suspected, a Sims' speculum might be required, as it often provides a clearer view of the vaginal walls. Where the Sims' speculum is used, it is preferable to examine the patient in the semi-prone or Sims' position (Fig. 15.5).

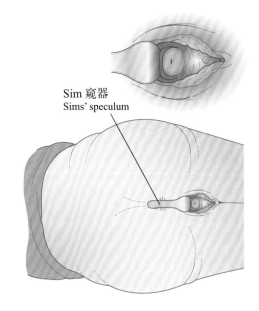

Sim 窥器
Sims' speculum

▲ 图 15-5 侧卧的 Sim 体位使用 Sim 窥器可以检查阴道壁

Fig. 15.5 Examination in the lateral semi-prone position with a Sims' speculum enables inspection of the vaginal walls.

进行子宫颈筛查试验（图 15-6）
Performing a cervical screening test (Fig. 15.6)

应该按照当地的指南进行，至少在妊娠 3 个月后进行，不在正常的月经期间做检查，以免血液污染。解释检查的目的，并告知患者，她可能会注意到有一些点滴出血。

This should be done in accordance with local guidelines and at least 3 months after pregnancy and not during normal menstruation due to contamination by blood. Explain the purpose of the test and warn the patient that she may notice some spotting afterwards.

在合适的玻片上记录日期、患者姓名和医院编号或出生日期。患者同意并摆好体位后，如前所述，轻轻插入窥器，并擦去任何分泌物或血液。注意子宫颈的外观。将中央的刷毛牢牢地压入宫颈口，外刷毛紧贴子宫颈口，进行 360 度扫刷。顺时针方向旋转细胞刷五次。

Record the date, patient's name and hospital number or date of birth on a suitable slide. After consent and appropriate positioning, insert the speculum gently, as noted earlier, and wipe away any discharge or blood. Note the appearance of the cervix. A 360-degree sweep should be taken with the central bristles of the cervical brush pressed firmly into the cervical os and the outer bristles against the ectocervix. Rotate the brush in a clockwise direction five times.

液基筛查试验（LBT，在大多数地区已取代了子宫颈细胞学）中，取样器被转移到保存溶液中，并剧烈搅动（避免溢出），以将细胞从取样器中分离出来。在实验室里，溶液要通过一个过滤器，这个过滤器会阻隔大的鳞状细胞，但允许小的红细胞、碎片和细菌通过。

In liquid-based screening tests (LBT-which has in most jurisdictions replaced cervical cytology) the sampling device is transferred into the preservative solution and agitated vigorously (avoiding spillage) to separate the cells from the device. In the laboratory, the solution is passed through a filter, which traps the large squamous cells but allows smaller red cells, debris and bacteria to pass through.

对鳞状细胞进行 HPV DNA 复制分析，在某些情况下，细胞也可以转移到玻片上进行常规细胞学检查（"巴氏涂片"）。如果是这样，标本会立即被薄而均匀地涂布于玻片上。载玻片用 95% 乙醇单独固定或联合 3% 冰醋酸固定。需要固定在液体中 30min。

The squamous cells are analyzed for HPV DNA replication, and in some circumstances cells might also be transferred to a glass slide to perform conventional cytology ('Pap smear'). If so, the specimen is spread immediately onto a clear glass slide in a thin, even layer. The slide is fixed with 95% alcohol alone or in combination with 3% glacial acetic acid. Fixation requires 30 minutes in solution.

LBT 涂片不满意的概率较低，而 LBT 的准确性似乎不受血液存在的影响。在澳大利亚，LBT 和高危 HPV 分型替代传统细胞学检查，有望将侵袭性宫颈癌的发病率降低 15%。LBT 还允许基于聚合酶链反应的衣原体和淋病检测。

The rate of unsatisfactory smears is lower in LBT, and LBT accuracy appears unaffected by the presence of blood. In Australia, the replacement of conventional cytology by LBT and high-risk HPV typing is anticipated to reduce the incidence of invasive cervical cancer by 15%. LBT also allows for PCR-based testing for *Chlamydia* and gonorrhoea.

最后，请填妥子宫颈筛查申请表。一般情况下，有关资料会在为集中筛选登记单位而订定的表格内列明；另外，确保测试的临床指征和任何相关的历史记录，如以前的测试结果、LMP 的日期。

Finally, complete the cervical screening test request form. Required details are usually specified in bespoke forms produced for centralized screening registration units; otherwise, ensure that clinical indications for the test and any relevant history, e.g. previous test results, date of LMP, is recorded.

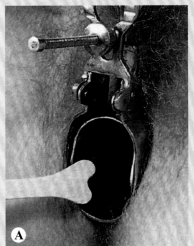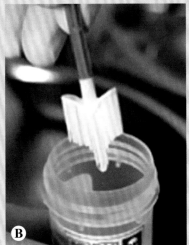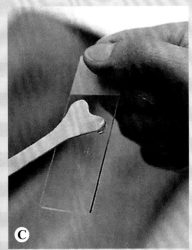

▲ 图 15-6　**A.** 使用刮板进行子宫颈涂片检查；**B.** 使用扫帚状装置进行液基细胞学取样；**C.** 将获得的组织涂抹在玻璃载玻片上并固定

Fig. 15.6　(A) A cervical smear is taken using an Ayres spatula. (B) A sample being taken for liquid-based cytology using the broom-like device. (C) The material obtained is plated onto a glass slide and fixed.

做阴道拭子 Taking vaginal swabs	知识链接 ABC

指征为阴道分泌物异常、不规则出血、盆腔炎等症状。拭子也可用于筛查无症状女性的性传播感染。

The indications are for symptoms of vaginal discharge, irregular bleeding and pelvic inflammatory disease. Swabs may also be taken to screen for sexually transmitted infection in asymptomatic women.

高位阴道拭子作为阴道窥器检查的一部分，将在培养基中浸湿的培养拭子的尖端在阴道后穹隆取样，然后立即将拭子放回合适的培养基中。主要用于鉴定微生物，如念珠菌或毛滴虫，并用于评估细菌性阴道病。

A high vaginal swab is taken as part of a speculum examination by dipping the tip of a culture swab moistened in culture media in the posterior vaginal fornix and then placing the swab immediately back into a suitable culture medium. This is used mainly to identify organisms such as *Candida* or *Trichomonas* and in the assessment of bacterial vaginosis.

宫颈管内拭子需要首先使用棉签清洁宫颈腔内区域，然后可以丢弃棉签。随后，将拭子的尖端插入子宫颈外口并旋转 2～3 次。使用标准培养基处理高位阴道拭子，这可以用于检测真菌感染如念珠菌种，或细菌感染如大肠埃希菌、解脲支原体或肺炎支原体。

Endocervical swabs need preparation of the endocervical area by first using a cotton swab to clean the area, which can then be discarded. Following this, the tip of the swab is placed into the external cervical os and rotated two or three times. Using standard culture media as for the high vaginal swab, this can be used to test for fungal infections such as Candida species or bacterial infections such as *Escherischia coli*, Ureaplasma urealyticum or *Mycoplasma pneumoniae*.

（四）双合诊（Bimanual examination）

双合诊是妇科系列检查的重要组成部分，但并非必需的常规检查或适合每位患者。通过将检查手的中指插入阴道口，并对直肠施加压力（图 15-7）。随着阴道口的打开，示指也放入阴道内。

The bimanual examination is an important part of the gynaecological series of examinations but is not necessarily routine or indicated for every patient. It is performed by introducing the middle finger of the examining hand into the vaginal introitus and applying pressure towards the rectum (Fig. 15.7). As the introitus opens, the index finger is introduced as well.

可以摸到子宫颈和鼻尖软骨一样的感觉。通过推动宫颈运动 / 摩擦来评估是否引起疼痛称为宫颈兴奋试验，阳性提示可能有盆腔疾病，特别是继发于感染或周围血液的炎症。

The cervix is palpated and has the consistency of the cartilage of the tip of the nose. Assessment of the cervix for elicitation of pain through its movement/rubbing is called *cervical excitation* and suggests possible pelvic pathology, particularly inflammation secondary to infection or surrounding blood.

必须记住，腹部的手是用来把盆腔器官压在检查阴道的手上的。必须注意子宫的大小、形状、连续性和位置。子宫通常为前位或前倾，但约 10% 的女性为后位或后倾。

It must be remembered that the abdominal hand is used to compress the pelvic organs onto the examining vaginal hand.

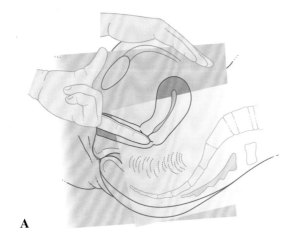

A

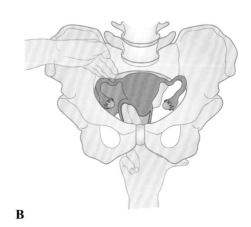

B

▲ 图 15-7　A. 双合骨盆检查；B. 检查双附件

Fig. 15.7　(A) Bimanual examination of the pelvis. (B) Examination of the lateral fornix.

The size, shape, consistency and position of the uterus must be noted. The uterus is commonly pre-axial or anteverted but will be postaxial or retroverted in some 10% of women.

如果后倾的子宫活动度很好，子宫后位很少有诊断意义。重要的是要先摸道格拉斯陷凹否有增厚或结节，然后再摸两侧穹隆是否可及卵巢或输卵管肿块。应该尝试区分附件包块和子宫包块，虽然这通常是不可能的。

Provided the retroverted uterus is mobile, the position is rarely significant. It is important to feel in the pouch of Douglas for the presence of thickening or nodules and then to palpate laterally in both fornices for the presence of any ovarian or tubal masses. An attempt should be made to differentiate between adnexal and uterine masses, although this is often not possible.

例如，带蒂肌瘤可能与卵巢肿瘤相似，而实性卵巢肿瘤，如果黏附在子宫，可能无法与子宫肌瘤区分。在正常骨盆内，如果患者较瘦，可触及卵巢；但只有当输卵管明显增大时，才能触及输卵管。

For example, a pedunculated fibroid may mimic an ovarian tumour, whereas a solid ovarian tumour, if adherent to the uterus, may be impossible to distinguish from a uterine fibroid. The ovaries may be palpable in the normal pelvis if the patient is thin, but the Fallopian tubes are only palpable if they are significantly enlarged.

对于处女膜完好的儿童或女性，通常不进行窥器和盆腔检查，除非是作为麻醉下进行检查的一部分。应该始终记住，粗略或痛苦的检查很少能产生有用的信息，这可能导致患者将来拒绝检查，甚至在某些情况下（如输卵管异位妊娠）是危险的。

In a child or in a woman with an intact hymen, speculum and pelvic examination is usually not performed unless as part of an examination under anaesthesia. It should always be remembered that a rough or painful examination rarely produces any useful information and might result in future refusal to be examined, as well as in certain situations, such as tubal ectopic pregnancy, being dangerous.

在整个检查过程中，应警惕来自患者的言语和非言语的痛苦症状。任何要求停止检查的请求都应得到尊重。由于这些原因和前面提到的那些原因，在进行任何盆腔或妇科检查时，都应该有一个陪伴者在场（框 15-1）。

Throughout the examination, remain alert to verbal and non-verbal indications of distress from the patient. Any request that the examination be discontinued should be respected. For these reasons and those noted earlier, it is prudent to always have a chaperone present during any pelvic or gynaecological examination (Box 15.1).

（五）特殊情况（Special circumstances）

除非在紧急情况下，不讲英语的患者在没有翻译的情况下不应进行盆腔检查。你应该注意，而且对有特定文化或宗教期望的女性要敏感，这些因素可能会使检查更加困难。此外，一些女性接受了女性生殖器切割或女性割礼，这可能会限制阴道开口，使窥器检查和双合诊困难和痛苦。

Except in an emergency situation, pelvic examination should not be carried out for non-English-speaking patients without an interpreter. You should be aware of, and sensitive to, factors that may make the examination more difficult for the woman with particular cultural or religious expectations. Furthermore some women have undergone female genital mutilation or female circumcision, which can limit the opening of the vaginal introitus, making speculum and bimanual examinations difficult and painful.

对阴道检查有困难的女性，应给予一切机会，协助她们披露任何潜在的儿童期性虐待、强奸或目前的性和（或）婚姻困难。然而，不能假定所有盆腔检查困难的女性都有性虐待、家庭暴力或性生活欠佳的背景历史。

Women who experience difficulty with vaginal examination should be given every opportunity to facilitate disclosure of any underlying previous childhood sexual abuse, sexual abuse such as rape or current sexual and/or marital difficulties. However, it must not be assumed that all women who experience difficulty with pelvic examination have a background history of sexual abuse, domestic violence or sexual difficulties.

适用于对一般人群进行妇科检查的尊重、隐私、解释和同意等基本原则同样适用于对有暂时性或永久性学习障碍或精神疾病的女性进行此类检查。

The basic principles of respect, privacy, explanation and consent that apply to the conduct of gynaecological examinations in general apply equally to the conduct of such examinations in women who have temporary or permanent learning disabilities or mentalillness.

在检查麻醉患者时，所有工作人员都应像对待醒着的女性一样，以同样程度的敏感和尊重对待她。

When examining anaesthetized patients, all staff should treat the woman with the same degree of sensitivity and respect as if she were awake.

在检查所谓的性侵犯受害者时，应表现出特别温和的态度。应该让女性选择医生的性别，允许她们控制检查的节奏和位置。在进行指控性侵犯后的

框 15-1　GMC 指南：私密检查与陪伴	BOX 15.1　GMC Guidelines: intimate examination and chaperones

私密检查

私密检查可能会让患者感到尴尬或痛苦。当给患者做检查时，你应该对他们认为是私密的东西很敏感。这可能包括乳房、生殖器和直肠的检查，但也可能包括任何需要触摸，甚至接近患者的检查。

在本指南中，我们强调了进行私密检查所涉及的一些问题，但这并不能阻止你在必要时进行私密检查。你必须遵循此指导，并在检查时或检查后尽快做出详细和准确的记录。在进行私密检查之前，你应该：
①向患者解释为什么检查是必要的，给患者一个机会问问题。
②以患者可以理解的方式解释检查将包括什么内容，让患者清楚地知道会发生什么，包括任何疼痛或不适。
③检查前征得患者同意，并记录。
④为患者提供陪伴（见下述 8-13）。
⑤如果是儿童或年轻人 †
• 你必须评估他们是否有能力同意检查 ‡。
• 如果他们没有能力同意，您应该寻求他们父母的同意 **。
⑥给患者脱衣服和穿衣服提供隐私保护，并尽可能多地遮盖他们，以维护他们的尊严；不要帮助患者脱衣服，除非他们要求你这样做，或者你已经与他们确认他们需要你的帮助。

在检查过程中，你必须遵循医嘱：患者和医生共同做出决定。特别是你应该：
①解释前你要做什么，如果这不同于你以前告诉患者的情况，解释为什么，寻求患者的许可。
②停止检查，如果患者要求你停止的话。
③继续讨论相关的问题，不做不必要的个人评论。

对麻醉患者的私密检查

在你对一个被麻醉的患者进行私密检查之前，或者指导一个学生准备去检查，你必须先确保患者事先同意，通常是书面同意。

行为监督人

当你进行私密检查时，你应该给患者一个选择，让他们有一个公正的观察者（行为监督人）在场。无论你是否与患者性别相同，这都适用。

行为监督人通常应该是健康专业人士，你必须确信她会：
①敏感和尊重患者的尊严并保密。
②如果患者表现出痛苦或不适的迹象，则安抚患者。
③熟悉常规私密检查的程序。
④如果可行，检查全程在场，能看到医生正在做什么。
⑤如果他们担心医生的行为或动作，做好提出问题的准备。

Intimate examinations

Intimate examinations can be embarrassing or distressing for patients and whenever you examine a patient you should be sensitive to what they may think of as intimate. This is likely to include examinations of breasts, genitalia and rectum, but could also include any examination where it is necessary to touch or even be close to the patient.

In this guidance, we highlight some of the issues involved in carrying out intimate examinations. This must not deter you from carrying out intimate examinations when necessary. You must follow this guidance and make detailed and accurate records at the time of the examination, or as soon as possible afterwards. Before conducting an intimate examination, you should:
a. explain to the patient why an examination is necessary and give the patient an opportunity to ask questions
b. explain what the examination will involve, in a way the patient can understand, so that the patient has a clear idea of what to expect, including any pain or discomfort
c. get the patient's permission before the examination and record that the patient has given it
d. offer the patient a chaperone (see paragraphs 8-13 below)
e. if dealing with a child or young person[†]
• you must assess their capacity to consent to the examination[‡]
• if they lack the capacity to consent, you should seek their parent's consent[**]
f. give the patient privacy to undress and dress, and keep them covered as much as possible to maintain their dignity; do not help the patient to remove clothing unless they have asked you to, or you have checked with them that they want you to help.

During the examination, you must follow the guidance in consent: patients and doctors making decisions together. In particular you should:
a. explain what you are going to do before you do it and, if this differs from what you have told the patient before, explain why and seek the patient's permission
b. stop the examination if the patient asks you to
c. keep discussion relevant and don't make unnecessary personal comments.

Intimate examinations of anaesthetised patients

Before you carry out an intimate examination on an anaesthetised patient, or supervise a student who intends to carry one out, you must make sure that the patient has given consent in advance, usually in writing.

Chaperones

When you carry out an intimate examination, you should offer the patient the option of having an impartial observer (a chaperone) present wherever possible. This applies whether or not you are the same gender as the patient.

A chaperone should usually be a health professional and you must be satisfied that the chaperone will:
a. be sensitive and respect the patient's dignity and confidentiality
b. reassure the patient if they show signs of distress or discomfort
c. be familiar with the procedures involved in a routine intimate examination
d. stay for the whole examination and be able to see what the doctor is doing, if practical
e. be prepared to raise concerns if they are concerned about the doctor's behaviour or actions.

（续框）

框 15–1　GMC 指南：私密检查与陪伴	BOX 15.1　GMC Guidelines: intimate examination and chaperones
患者的亲戚或朋友不是公正的观察者，所以通常不适合作为行为监督人，但你应该遵守除行为监督人外让这样的人也在场的合理的要求。	A relative or friend of the patient is not an impartial observer and so would not usually be a suitable chaperone, but you should comply with a reasonable request to have such a person present as well as a chaperone.
如果你或者患者不希望在没有行为监督人在场的情况下进行检查，或者你或患者对监护人的选择不舒服，只要延迟检查不会影响患者的健康，你可以延迟检查，直到一个合适的行为监督人出现。	If either you or the patient does not want the examination to go ahead without a chaperone present, or if either of you is uncomfortable with the choice of chaperone, you may offer to delay the examination to a later date when a suitable chaperone will be available, as long as the delay would not adversely affect the patient's health.
如果你不想在没有行为监督人在场的情况下进行检查，但是患者拒绝有行为监督人在场，你必须清楚地解释为什么需要行为监督人在场。当然，必须优先考虑患者的临床需要。	If you don't want to go ahead without a chaperone present but the patient has said no to having one, you must explain clearly why you want a chaperone present. Ultimately the patient's clinical needs must take precedence.
你可以考虑将患者转给一位愿意在没有行为监督人的情况下为他们检查的同事，只要延迟不会对患者的健康造成不利影响。	You may wish to consider referring the patient to a colleague who would be willing to examine them without a chaperone, as long as a delay would not adversely affect the patient's health.
你应该在患者的病历中记录任何关于行为监督人的讨论和结果。如果有行为监督人在场，你应该把事实记录下来，并记下他们的身份。如果患者不想要，你应该记录下自己提出了建议及被拒绝的过程。	You should record any discussion about chaperones and the outcome in the patient's medical record. If a chaperone is present, you should record that fact and make a note of their identity. If the patient does not want a chaperone, you should record that the offer was made and declined.

†. 你们必须遵循 *Protecting Children and Young People: The Responsibilities of All Doctors*. General Medical Council (2012), London, GMC.

‡. 在评估年轻人的同意能力时，你应该记住：一个 16 岁的年轻人可被推定有同意的能力；一个 16 岁以下的年轻人可以被推定有同意的能力，这取决于他们的成熟程度和理解所涉及内容的能力。具体参见 General Medical Council (2007) *0–18 Years: Guidance for all Doctors*. London, GMC, paragraphs 24-26.

**. 参见 General Medical Council (2007) *0–18 Years: Guidance for All Doctors*, London, GMC, paragraphs 27-28.

引自 General Medical Council March 2013 Available at: https://www.gmc-uk.org/ethical-guidance/ethical-guidance-for-doctors/intimate-examinations-and-chaperones [accessed 7 May 2019]

†. You must also follow our guidance on *Protecting Children and Young People: The Responsibilities of All Doctors*. General Medical Council (2012), London, GMC.

‡. When assessing a young person's capacity to consent, you should bear in mind that:

at 16 a young person can be presumed to have the capacity to consent

a young person under 16 may have the capacity to consent, depending on their maturity and ability to understand what is involved.

General Medical Council (2007) *0–18 Years: Guidance for all Doctors*. London, GMC, paragraphs 24-26.

**. General Medical Council (2007) *0–18 Years: Guidance for All Doctors*, London, GMC, paragraphs 27-28.

General Medical Council March 2013 Available at: https://www.gmc-uk.org/ethical-guidance/ethical-guidance-for-doctors/intimate-examinations-and-chaperones [accessed 7 May 2019]

检查时，与附近的强奸和性侵犯中心进行讨论至关重要，以避免破坏和污染法医证据。

Exceptional gentleness should be displayed in the examination of victims of alleged sexual assault. The woman should be given a choice about the gender of the doctor and be allowed to control the pace of, and her position for, the examination. In the event of post-alleged sexual assault examination, a discussion with the nearby rape and sexual assault centre is crucial to avoid the disruption and contamination of forensic evidence.

另外，可以收集早期的样本，如首次尿液、穿的内衣和口腔冲洗液，以帮助保存法医证据，直到受过适当培训的卫生专业人员能够参加。在一些地区，有接受过这类检查培训的随叫随到的法医。

Furthermore, it may be that early samples can be collected, such as first urinary voids, underwear worn and oral rinses, to help preserve forensic evidence until an appropriately trained health professional can attend. In some areas, there are on-call forensic doctors trained in this type of examination.

（六）直肠检查（Rectal examination）

如果出现如排便习惯改变或直肠出血等症状，可能提示有肠道疾病或严重的子宫内膜异位症并伴有直肠疾病，则应进行直肠检查。偶尔，直肠检查联合阴道检查被用于评估盆腔肿块，并可以提供直肠阴道隔疾病的额外信息。

Rectal examination may be indicated if there are symptoms such as change of bowel habit or rectal bleeding, which may suggest bowel disease or severe endometriosis with associated rectal disease. It is occasionally used as a means of assessing a pelvic mass and, in conjunction with a vaginal examination, can provide additional information about disease in the rectovaginal septum.

三、描述你的发现（Presenting your findings）

先介绍患者的姓名和年龄，并给出主要的病因和入院情况。如果有多个问题，可依次处理。如果病史包含了一长串的事件，试着总结这些事件，而不是重述每一个事件。以一种逻辑结构的方式呈现病史的其余部分，而不是在不同项目之间来回跳转。最后，用一两句话总结一下。

Start by introducing the patient by name and age, and give the main reason for presentation and in turn admission. If there are several problems, deal with each in turn. If the history consists of a long narrative of events, try to summarize these rather than recap each event. Present the remainder of the history in a logical structured way, not skipping back and forward between items. At the end of your history give a summary in no more than one or two sentences.

除非患者要求你只讨论查体的某一部分，否则你应该从患者的总体情况开始，其中包括脉搏和血压。腹部检查应先列出视诊结果，然后是触诊和叩诊（如有腹胀或肿块）。

Unless you are asked only to discuss one particular part of the examination, always start by commenting on the patient's general condition, including pulse and blood pressure. For abdominal examinations, list the findings on inspection first followed by those on palpation and percussion (if there is abdominal distension or a mass).

如果有来自盆腔的肿块，可用妊娠子宫的大小来描述它（如一个肿块到达脐部将是一个相当于妊娠 20 周大的盆腔肿块）。如有压痛部位，应说明是否有腹膜炎（肌紧张和反跳痛）的迹象。

If there is a mass arising from the pelvis, describe it terms of a pregnant uterus (e.g. a mass reaching the umbilicus would be a 20-week-size pelvic mass). If there are areas of tenderness, specify whether they are associated with signs of peritonism (guarding and rebound).

在盆腔检查时，描述外阴视诊的结果，然后是子宫颈视诊结果（如果进行了窥器检查）。描述子宫的大小、位置、活动度和压痛。最后，请说明附件是否有可触及的肿块或压痛。

On pelvic examination, describe the findings on inspection of the vulva and then of the cervix (if a speculum examination was carried out). Describe the size, position and mobility of the uterus and any tenderness. Finally, say whether there were any palpable masses or tenderness in the adnexae.

病例分析：典型病史示例	Case study: Example of a typical history
Smith 女士，29 岁，孕 2 产 2，会计，因为出血和妊娠测试呈阳性，她的全科医生推荐她来诊所。Smith 女士在过去 3 天里有 3 次轻微无痛阴道出血。她的末次月经时间是 7 周前，在这之前她有一个规律的 28 天月经周期。	This is Ms Smith, a 29-year-old gravida 2 para 2 accountant who has been referred by her general practitioner to the clinic because of bleeding and a positive pregnancy test. Ms Smith has had three episodes of small painless vaginal bleeding over the last 3 days. Her LMP was 7 weeks ago, and prior to this she had a regular 28-day menstrual cycle.
她没有任何有记录的妇科病史，她唯一的子宫颈筛查是在 4 年前，结果为阴性。这是一次计划妊娠，在妊娠前她一直使用复方口服避孕药直到 3 个月前。她之前有过 2 次妊娠，都是无并发症的足月顺产。	She has no previous gynaecological history of note, and her only cervical screening test was 4 years ago and was negative. This is a planned pregnancy, and before conceiving she was using the combined oral contraceptive pill until 3 months ago. She has had two previous pregnancies with uncomplicated normal vaginal deliveries at term.
她 14 岁时接受了阑尾切除术，当时全身麻醉没有问题。她目前正在服用叶酸，没有任何过敏症状。她与爱人和两个孩子住在一起。她不吸烟也不饮酒。	She underwent an appendectomy at the age of 14 and had no problems with the general anaesthetic at the time. She is currently taking folic acid and has no known allergies. She lives with her partner and two children. She does not smoke or drink.
总之，Smith 女士是一位 29 岁的女性，在第 3 次妊娠的第 7 周出现无痛阴道出血。	In summary, Ms Smith is a 29-year-old woman with a history of painless vaginal bleeding at 7 weeks in her third pregnancy.

病例分析：临床表现示例	Case study: Example of presentation of clinical findings
经过全面检查，Smith 女士看上去很健康。她没有临床贫血，BMI 为 31。她的血压是 110/70mmHg，脉搏 88 次 /min，规律。胸部和心脏检查无明显异常。	On general examination, Ms Smith looked well. She was not clinically anaemic, and her BMI was 31. Her blood pressure was 110/70, and her pulse 88 and regular. Examination of the chest and heart was unremarkable.
在腹部检查时，在右下腹部有一个瘢痕，这与之前的开腹阑尾切除术的描述是一致的。触诊：腹部柔软，无压痛，无触痛肿块，没有器官肿大。	On abdominal examination, there was a scar in the right lower quadrant consistent with a previous open appendectomy. On palpation, the abdomen was soft and non-tender with no palpable masses and no organomegaly.
在盆腔检查中，除了会阴上有与以前撕裂或会阴切开术一致的旧伤疤外，外生殖器正常。经窥器检查，宫颈闭合，阴道内有少量游离血迹。子宫如孕 8 周大小，可移动，子宫前倾，没有可触及的附件肿块。	On pelvic examination, the external genitalia were normal, apart from an old scar on the perineum consistent with a previous tear or episiotomy. On speculum examination, the cervix was closed and there was a small amount of free blood in the vagina. She had a an 8-week-size, mobile, anteverted uterus, and there were no palpable adnexal masses.

本章概览	Essential information
病史 　**主诉** 　　• 主诉症状的发生和持续时间 　　• 与月经周期有关的相关症状 　　• 既往治疗和反应 　　• 特定的封闭式问题	**History** 　**Presenting complaint** 　　• Onset and duration of main complaint 　　• Associated symptoms, relationship to menstrual cycle 　　• Previous treatment and response 　　• Specific closed questions
既往妇科病史 　• 先前的调查或治疗 　• 避孕史 　• 性生活史 　• 子宫颈涂片检查 　• 月经史	**Previous gynaecological history** 　• Previous investigations or treatment 　• Contraceptive history 　• Sexual history 　• Cervical smear 　• Menstrual history
妊娠分娩史 　• 多少次 (妊娠孕次) 　• 结局 (产次) 　• 外科分娩，其中包括产钳 / 胎头吸引器分娩和任何会阴创伤	**Previous pregnancies** 　• How many (gravidity) 　• Outcome (parity) 　• Surgical deliveries, including forceps/vacuum delivery and any perineal trauma
既往手术和病史 　• 既往腹部手术 　• 主要心血管 / 呼吸系统疾病 　• 内分泌疾病 　• 血栓栓塞疾病 　• 乳房疾病 　• 药物史和过敏史	**Past surgical and medical history** 　• Previous abdominal surgery 　• Major cardiovascular/respiratory disease 　• Endocrine disease 　• Thromboembolic disease 　• Breast disease 　• Drug history and allergies
社会心理和家族史的细节 　• 家庭和生活环境 　• 支持 　• 心理健康史 　• 吸烟 　• 家族史	**Psychosocial and family history details** 　• Home and living circumstances 　• Support 　• Mental health history 　• Smoking 　• Family history

（续表）

本章概览	Essential information
检查 　**一般检查** 　　• 一般情况、体重、身高 　　• 脉搏、血压 　　• 贫血 　　• 甲状腺肿 　　• 乳房检查（如有需要） 　　• 第二性别特征、体毛 **腹部检查** 　• 视诊：膨胀、瘢痕 　• 触诊：肿块，器官肿大，压痛，腹膜炎，淋巴结，疝孔 　• 叩诊：腹水 **盆腔检查** 　• 解释、安慰、隐私、陪伴 　• 外生殖器检查 　• 窥器检查，宫颈筛查，拭子 　• 双合诊 　• 直肠检查（如有需要）	**Examination** 　**General examination** 　　• General condition, weight, height 　　• Pulse, blood pressure 　　• Anaemia 　　• Goitre 　　• Breast examination (if indicated) 　　• Secondary sex characteristics, body hair **Abdominal examination** 　• Inspection-distension, scars 　• Palpation-masses, organomegaly, tenderness, peritonism, nodes, hernial orifices 　• Percussion-ascites **Pelvic examination** 　• Explanation, comfort, privacy, chaperone 　• Inspection of external genitalia 　• Speculum examination, cervical screening, swabs 　• Bimanual examination 　• Rectal examination if indicated

第 16 章　妇科疾病

Gynaecological disorders

Ian S. Fraser　著　　杨　欣　译　　颜　磊　校

学习目标	LEARNING OUTCOMES
学习本章后，你应该能够：	After studying this chapter you should be able to:
知识标准	**Knowledge criteria**
• 描述月经失调的原因、意义和处理，其中包括经间、性交后和绝经后出血、月经不规律、月经过多、痛经和继发性闭经。	• Describe the causes, significance and management of disorders of menstruation, including intermenstrual, postcoital and postmenopausal bleeding, menstrual irregularity, heavy menstrual bleeding, dysmenorrhoea and secondary amenorrhoea.
• 描述 PALM COEIN 的概念，评估及分类异常子宫出血的原因。	• Describe the PALM COEIN concept of assessment and classification of causes of abnormal uterine bleeding.
• 描述青春期的问题，其中包括性早熟和青春期延迟。要认识到子宫内膜异位症通常始于青春期。	• Describe the problems of puberty, including precocious puberty and delayed puberty. Recognize that endometriosis is a condition that often starts in adolescence.
• 描述围绝经期的问题，其中包括异常出血、血管舒缩和其他症状、骨质疏松症和激素补充疗法。	• Describe problems of the perimenopause, including abnormal bleeding, vasomotor and other symptoms, osteoporosis and hormone-replacement therapy.
• 描述下生殖道的良性情况，其中包括外阴瘙痒、阴道分泌物和盆腔疼痛。	• Describe benign conditions of the lower genital tract, including vulval pruritus, vaginal discharge and pelvic pain.
• 描述 Bartholin 腺脓肿 / 囊肿、原因不明腹痛和急性非预期阴道出血的原因、意义和处理。	• Describe the causes, significance and management of Bartholin's abscess/cyst, abdominal pain of uncertain origin and acute unscheduled vaginal bleeding.
临床能力	**Clinical competencies**
• 对出现异常子宫出血、盆腔疼痛、阴道分泌物和闭经的患者进行初步评估和制订诊疗计划。	• Assess and plan the initial investigation of a patient presenting with abnormal uterine bleeding, pelvic pain, vaginal discharge and amenorrhoea.
• 解释良性妇科疾病的常见检查结果。	• Interpret the results of the common investigations in benign gynaecological disorders.
• 向患者解释关于妇科常见手术的指征、禁忌证、治疗原则和并发症。	• Counsel a patient about indications, contraindications, principles and complications of the common surgical procedures in gynaecology.

一、概述（Introduction）

社会和卫生系统常难以发现良性妇科疾病对女性生活的影响。女性常忍受良性疾病的许多方面，如月经过多（heavy menstrual bleeding，HMB）和使人衰弱的盆腔疼痛，这些有时也被卫生保健专业人员视为正常。其中，许多情况确实对女性的健康、福祉、家庭和社会关系、女性的工作生活及其妊娠能力产生重大影响。

Benign gynaecological conditions affect women's lives in ways that often remain hidden from society and from health systems. Many aspects of benign conditions such as heavy menstrual bleeding (HMB) and debilitating pelvic pain are often tolerated by women and sometimes dismissed as normal by health care professionals. Many of these conditions do have significant implications for women's health and wellbeing, family and social relationships, the working lives of women and their ability to conceive.

要确认良性妇科疾病，就需要教导女性哪些症状可视为正常育龄期的一部分，哪些症状可能需要检查和治疗。要充分了解妇科良性疾病，还需要保健专业人员对管理育龄期健康问题和确认潜在病理情况有更深入的了解。

The recognition of benign gynaecological conditions requires education of women about what symptoms can be considered part of normal reproductive life and what symptoms may require investigation and treatment. Full appreciation of benign gynaecological conditions also requires that health care professionals develop a deeper understanding of managing reproductive health issues and of identifying potential pathological conditions.

二、上生殖道的良性疾病（Benign conditions of the upper genital tract）

（一）子宫（The uterus）

子宫的形成是两个 Müllerian 管融合的结果；这种融合形成了阴道上 2/3、子宫颈和子宫体。先天性异常是由于融合失败，或者 1 个或 2 个 Müllerian 管缺失或部分发育而引起的。因此，这些异常可以从子宫底部轻微的凹陷到每个子宫角与子宫颈完全分离（图 16-1）。这些情况也通常伴随着阴道纵隔形成。

The formation of the uterus results from the fusion of the two Müllerian ducts; this fusion gives rise to the upper twothirds of the vagina, the cervix and the body of the uterus.

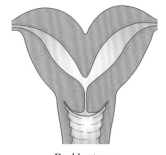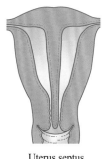

Double uterus
双子宫

Uterus septus
纵隔子宫

▲ 图 16-1　常见的子宫先天性畸形包括单宫颈双角子宫（双子宫，一个子宫颈，左）和纵隔子宫（纵隔子宫，右）

Fig. 16.1　Common congenital abnormalities of the uterus include uterus bicornis unicollis (double uterus, one cervix, *left*) and the subseptate uterus (uterus septus, *right*).

Congenital anomalies arise from the failure of fusion, or the absence or partial development of one or both ducts. Thus, the anomalies may range from a minor indentation of the uterine fundus to a full separation of each uterine horn and cervix (Fig. 16.1). These conditions are also commonly associated with vaginal septa.

1. 症状与体征（Symptoms and signs）

大多数子宫畸形是无症状的，通常因为妊娠并发症而得以诊断。然而，阴道隔的存在可能导致性交困难和性交后出血（pastcoital bleeding，PCB）。

The majority of uterine anomalies are asymptomatic and are usually diagnosed in relation to complications of pregnancy. However, the presence of a vaginal septum may result in dyspareunia and postcoital bleeding (PCB).

在常规阴道检查时，如果可以看到双宫颈，可能也可以确定双子宫的存在。双合诊阴道检查有时可触及子宫角分离，但多数情况下感觉子宫正常，只有一个子宫颈。当只有一个宫角的时候，可以触摸到子宫斜卧在骨盆内。两个子宫角和一个子宫颈的异常称为单宫颈双角子宫（图 16-2）。

The presence of a double uterus may also be established at routine vaginal examination, when a double cervix may be seen. The separation of the uterine horns is sometimes palpable on bimanual vaginal examination, but in most cases the uterus feels normal and there is a single cervix. When only one horn is present, the uterus may be palpable as lying obliquely in the pelvis. The abnormality of two uterine horns and one cervix is known as *uterus bicornis unicollis* (Fig. 16.2).

单角子宫部分闭锁或阴道隔阻塞从单角子宫流出的月经，可导致单侧阴道积血和宫腔积血并伴有经血逆流。在这种情况下，患者可能表现出痛经的

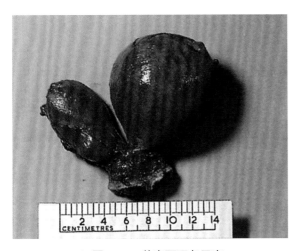

▲ 图 16-2　单宫颈双角子宫

Fig. 16.2　Uterus bicornis unicollis.

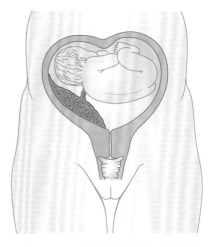

▲ 图 16-3　先露异常和不全子宫纵隔

Fig. 16.3　Malpresentation and a subseptate uterus.

症状，并有一个可触及的盆腔肿块。

Partial atresia of one horn of the uterus or a septate vagina resulting in obstruction to menstrual outflow from one horn of the uterus may result in a unilateral haematocolpos and haematometra with retrograde spill of menstrual fluid. In this case, the patient may present with symptoms of dysmenorrhoea and will have a palpable mass arising from the pelvis.

有子宫畸形的女性妊娠并发症包括以下几种情况。

- 复发性流产：先天性畸形在早期妊娠丢失中的作用尚不清楚。例如，在有正常生育史的女性中，纵隔子宫的发生率是相同的。然而，它与子宫颈功能不全有关，这可能导致妊娠中期流产。该问题通常与不全纵隔子宫有关，而在单角或双宫颈双角子宫中并不常见。

- 早产。

- 胎先露异常（图 16-3）。

- 胎盘残留。

The complications of pregnancy in women with these uterine anomalies include:

- Recurrent miscarriage: the role of congenital abnormalities in early pregnancy loss is unclear. For example, the incidence of uterine septa is the same in women with normal reproductive histories. However, there is an association with cervical incompetence, which may lead to mid-trimester miscarriage. This problem is usually associated with the subseptate uterus and is not common in unicornuate uterus or uterus bicornis bicollis.
- Pre-mature labour.

- Malpresentation of the fetus (Fig. 16.3).
- Retained placenta.

2. 诊断与处理（Diagnosis and management）

由于许多病例是无症状的，诊断可能只是偶然发现，不需要治疗或干预。如果病史提示诊断，应进一步检查子宫造影和宫腔镜。

As many cases are asymptomatic, the diagnosis may arise only as a coincidental finding and requires no treatment or intervention. Where the diagnosis is suggested by the history, further investigation should include hysterography and hysteroscopy.

3. 手术治疗（Surgical treatment）

由于没有对照研究证明手术重建对妊娠结局的好处，因此难以评估手术重建对双子宫不孕女性的作用。只有存在反复流产史，且为单宫颈双角子宫或有纵隔子宫的女性才应考虑。

The role of surgical reconstruction of a double uterus in women with infertility is difficult to assess, as there are no controlled studies demonstrating the benefits in pregnancy outcome. Consideration should be confined to women who have a history of recurrent miscarriage and where the abnormality is one of uterus bicornis unicollis or there is a uterine septum.

使两侧宫角融合或切除子宫纵隔的子宫重建术称为子宫成形术（图 16-4）。在子宫输卵管连接处之间的子宫底部作切口，注意不要触及输卵管的壁内部。然后，通过在前后平面将表面缝合在一起来重新接合空腔。如果有纵隔，只需用电能量器械将其分开，然后在前后平面缝合横切口闭合宫腔。这种类型的手术在某些情况下与术后不孕有关，并有后

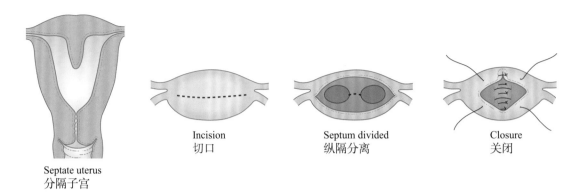

Septate uterus
分隔子宫

Incision
切口

Septum divided
纵隔分离

Closure
关闭

▲ 图 16-4   子宫成形术（右）用于双角子宫的子宫融合或纵隔子宫的分离（左）

Fig. 16.4   Metroplasty (*right*) for the reunification of a bicornate uterus or the division of a uterine septum (*left*).

续妊娠子宫破裂的风险。

The operation of plastic reconstruction of the uterus with unification of two uterine horns or excision of the uterine septum is known as metroplasty (Fig. 16.4). An incision is made across the fundus of the uterus between the uterotubal junctions, taking care not to involve the intramural portion of the tube. The cavities are then reunited by suturing the surfaces together in the anteroposterior plane. If there is a septum, it is simply divided by diathermy, and the cavity is then closed by suturing the transverse incision in the anteroposterior plane. Surgery of this type is associated with postoperative infertility in some cases and with a risk of uterine rupture in subsequent pregnancy.

另一种手术治疗方法是通过经子宫颈的宫腔镜使用电能量器械切开子宫纵隔。

An alternative surgical management is to divide the septum by diathermy through a hysteroscope inserted through the cervix.

（二）子宫内膜息肉（Endometrial polyps）

子宫内膜息肉（endometrial polyp，EP）是子宫内膜表面的局部性增生。从生育早期到绝经后的任何年龄都可能出现。EP 通常为良性病变，但常与不孕不育有关，因为去除这些病变可提高妊娠率和（或）减少妊娠丢失。不同的息肉在形态、功能和症状上存在差异，目前正在尝试开发一个详细的亚分类系统，作为 FIGO PALM-COEIN 系统的组成部分（见后述），这将有助于澄清和提高对不同类型的息肉的了解。

Endometrial polyps (EPs) are localized outgrowths from the surface of the endometrium. They appear at any age from the early reproductive years through to the postmenopausal period. EPs are usually benign lesions but have been implicated in subfertility, as removal of these lesions may improve rates of pregnancy and/or reduce pregnancy loss. There are differences in morphology, function and symptoms between different polyps, and attempts are now being made to develop a detailed subclassification system, as a component of the FIGO PALM-COEIN system (see later), which will allow clarification and improved understanding of the different types of polyps.

1. 症状（Symptoms）

子宫内膜息肉通常是无症状的疾病，但他们可能导致异常子宫出血（abnormal uterine bleeding，AUB）表现为经间出血（intermenstrual bleeding，IMB）、HMB 或绝经后出血。偶尔，通过子宫颈突出的息肉可能导致 PCB。子宫试图排出息肉时可能会引起腹部绞痛、痛经样疼痛。

EPs are usually asymptomatic lesions, but they may contribute to abnormal uterine bleeding (AUB) manifesting as either intermenstrual bleeding (IMB), HMB or postmenopausal bleeding. Occasionally, protrusion of the polyp through the cervix may result in PCB. Attempts by the uterus to expel the polyp may cause colicky, dysmenorrhoeic pain.

2. 体征（Signs）

通常在 AUB 和不孕症的检查中发现子宫内膜息肉。如果息肉从子宫颈突出，它可能难与宫颈息肉区分（图 16-5）。经阴道超声可以看到子宫内膜息肉，在月经周期的分泌期最容易发现，此时息肉中的非孕型腺体与周围正常的分泌型子宫内膜形成鲜明对比。如果临床上或经阴道超声检查怀疑 EP，可以通过经阴道超声宫腔造影检查（图 16-6）和（或）门诊或住院宫腔镜检查（伴或不伴直接切除活检）来进一步确定。

EPs are usually detected during the investigation for AUB and infertility. If the polyp protrudes through the cervix, it may be difficult to distinguish from an endocervical polyp (Fig. 16.5). EPs can be visualized on transvaginal ultrasound.

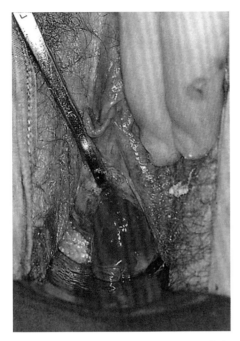

▲ 图 16-5 子宫内膜息肉通过宫颈口突出

Fig. 16.5 **Endometrial polyp protruding through the cervical os.**

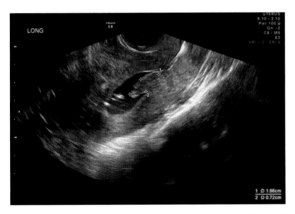

▲ 图 16-6 超声宫腔造影显示子宫内膜息肉（勾勒标记处）延伸至充满液体的腔内

Fig. 16.6 **Sonohysterogram demonstrating the endometrial polyp (outlined by the markers) extending into the fluid-filled cavity.**

They are most easily detected in the secretory phase of the menstrual cycle when the non-progestational type of glands in the polyp stand out in contrast to the normal surrounding secretory endometrium. If their presence is suspected either clinically or on transvaginal ultrasound, further clarification can be undertaken by performing a transvaginal sonohysterography (Fig. 16.6) and/or office or inpatient hysteroscopy, with or without directed excisional biopsy.

3. 病理（Pathology）

子宫内膜息肉是子宫内膜表层局部性的过度生

长。粗略来说，它们是光滑的圆柱形结构，切除后呈棕褐色至黄色。显微镜下，它们是由柱状上皮腺体覆盖的细纤维组织核心组成。包住息肉的子宫内膜可能是正常子宫内膜，也可能是对周期性激素影响无反应的子宫内膜。偶尔子宫内膜表面出现单纯型或复杂型增生，很少发生恶性改变。

EPs are localized overgrowths of the surface endometrium. Grossly, they are smooth, cylindrical structures, tan to yellow in colour after removal. Microscopically, they consist of a fine fibrous tissue core covered by columnar epithelium glands. The endometrium encasing the polyps varies from normal endometrium to endometrium that is unresponsive to cyclical hormonal influences. Occasionally the endometrial surface develops simple or complex hyperplasia and, rarely, malignant change occurs.

4. 治疗（Treatment）

小的（≤1cm）无症状的息肉可能自行消退，在这些病例中可选择观察性治疗。然而，有出血症状或不孕症的女性则需要切除息肉基底部。传统上，在全身麻醉下通过刮宫术（dilatation and curettage，D&C）来去除子宫内膜息肉，但盲刮在 50%～85% 的病例中会有遗漏，最好在宫腔镜引导下或进行刮术后再引入宫腔镜以确保所有病灶都已切除。使用现代设备，通常可以在没有麻醉或在宫颈局部注射麻醉药的情况下完成。

Small (1 cm or less) asymptomatic polyps may resolve spontaneously, and in these cases watchful waiting can be the treatment of choice. However, in women suffering from bleeding symptoms or infertility, surgical excision with removal of the polyp base is required. Traditionally, EPs were removed by dilatation and curettage (D&C) under general anaesthesia, but because blind curettage may miss EPs in 50–85% of cases, removal is best performed under hysteroscopic guidance or by performing curettage followed by reintroducing the hysteroscope to ensure that all the lesions have been removed. Using modern equipment, this can often be done without anaesthesia or with injection of local anaesthetic into the cervix.

（三）子宫肌层的良性肿瘤（Benign tumours of the myometrium）

1. 子宫平滑肌瘤（"子宫肌瘤"）[Uterine leiomyomas ('fibroids')]

子宫肌瘤（或者更准确地说，平滑肌瘤）是女性生殖道最常见的良性肿瘤，约 25% 的女性有明显的临床症状。它们是平滑肌肿瘤，大小差别很大，从显微镜下的生长到可能重量为 30～40kg 的大肿块。

子宫肌瘤可单发或多发，可发生在子宫颈或子宫体。

Uterine fibroids (or, more accurately, leiomyomas) are the most common benign tumour of the female genital tract and are clinically apparent in around 25% of women. They are smooth muscle tumours that vary enormously in size from microscopic growths to large masses that may weigh as much as 30–40 kg. Fibroids may be single or multiple and may occur in the cervix or in the body of the uterus.

根据解剖部位的不同，肌瘤主要有三种类型。其中最常见的位于子宫肌层内（壁间肌瘤）。位于浆膜或其外表面并向外伸展并使子宫正常轮廓变形的是浆膜下肌瘤。它们也可能是有蒂的，仅通过一个小茎与浆膜表面相连（图 16–7）。子宫肌瘤生长于子宫内膜内表面，使子宫内膜膨胀并延伸至子宫内膜腔内，引起腔内变形；如果有蒂，可能会填满宫腔，则为黏膜下肌瘤。宫颈肌瘤与子宫的其他部位相似。它们通常有蒂，但也可能无蒂，会长到足以填充阴道并扭曲盆腔器官的大小。

There are three main types of fibroids according to their anatomical location. The most common of these lie within the myometrium (intramural fibroids). Those located on the serosal or outer surface that extend outwards and deform the normal contour of the uterus are subserosal fibroids. These may also be pedunculated and only connected by a small stalk to the serosal surface (Fig. 16.7). Fibroids that develop near the inner surface of the endometrium distend the endometrium and extend into the endometrial cavity, either causing a distortion of the cavity or filling the cavity if they are pedunculated are submucous fibroids. Cervical fibroids are similar to other sites in the uterus. They are commonly pedunculated but may be sessile and grow to a size that will fill the vagina and distort the pelvic organs.

肿瘤的大小和位置对症状有相当大的影响。浆膜下肌瘤可压迫邻近器官，引起肠道和膀胱症状。黏膜下肌瘤可导致 HMB 和不孕。有黏膜下肌瘤时 HMB 可能非常严重。宫颈肌瘤的症状与其他宫颈息肉相似，此外，在试图排出宫颈肌瘤时，以及当有肌瘤发生变性或有蒂肌瘤扭转时可发生急性局部疼痛。现在强烈推荐使用 FIGO 的 PALM-COEIN 分类系统（见后述）来描述单个肌瘤的位置，并将这些特征与症状联系起来。

The size and site of the tumour have a considerable effect on the symptoms. Subserosal fibroids can put pressure on adjacent organs and cause bowel and bladder symptoms. Submucosal fibroids can lead to HMB and infertility. This HMB can be exceedingly heavy with submucous lesions. Cervical fibroids have symptoms similar to other cervical polyps, and in addition, during attempted extrusion, acute local pain can

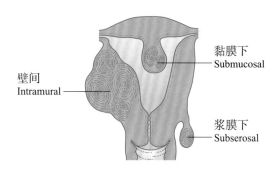

黏膜下 Submucosal

壁间 Intramural

浆膜下 Subserosal

▲ 图 16-7　子宫肌瘤产生的症状取决于其部位

Fig. 16.7 Uterine fibroids produce symptoms that are determined by their site.

occur, as well as when there is degeneration of a fibroid or torsion of a pedunculated fibroid. Nowadays there is a strong recommendation to use the FIGO PALM-COEIN classification system (see later) to describe the location of individual fibroids and link these characteristics with symptoms.

虽然遗传因素很重要，但肌瘤的病因目前还不是很清楚。非洲 – 加勒比民族、超重、未产妇、多囊卵巢综合征（PCOS）、糖尿病、高血压和肌瘤家族史的女性多见。妊娠导致肌瘤体积增大，而绝经则与肌瘤体积缩小有关。

The aetiology of fibroids is not well understood, although there is a significant genetic contribution. They are more common in women who are of Afro-Caribbean ethnicity, are overweight, are nulliparous, have polycystic ovary syndrome (PCOS), have diabetes, have hypertension and have a family history of fibroids. Pregnancy causes enlargement, and menopause is associated with some shrinkage.

2. 组织病理学（Histopathology）

肌瘤由呈漩涡状排列的平滑肌细胞、数量不等的纤维组织及伴随的结缔组织构成。肌瘤的主要血液供应位于肌瘤外面的假包膜内，正是这些薄壁小静脉导致了 HMB。

Myomas consist of whorled masses of unstriated muscle cells, varying amounts of fibrous tissue and accompanying connective tissue. The main blood supply of a fibroid is localized within the pseudo-capsule around the outside of the main muscle mass, and it is these thin-walled venules which contribute to HMB.

3. 病理改变（Pathological changes）

肌瘤可以发生一系列的病理改变，包括玻璃样变性、囊性变、钙化、感染和脓肿形成及坏死。后者，称为红色变性，可发生在妊娠或栓塞治疗后。极少发生肉瘤样变，其发生率为 0.13%～1%。

Fibroids can undergo a range of pathological changes, including hyaline degeneration, cystic degeneration, calcification, infection and abscess formation and necrobiosis. The latter, known as red *degeneration*, can occur in pregnancy or after treatment with embolization. Rarely, with an incidence of between 0.13% and 1%, sarcomatous change can occur.

4. 症状与体征（Symptoms and signs）

约 50% 患有肌瘤的女性没有症状，可能仅在常规的盆腔检查（宫颈细胞学检查或妊娠期管理）时发现。当症状确实发生时，往往与肌瘤的部位有关。常见症状如下。

Some 50% of women with fibroids are asymptomatic, and the condition may only be discovered during routine pelvic examination: either at the time of cervical cytology or in the management of a pregnancy. Where symptoms do occur, they are often related to the site of the fibroids. The common presenting symptoms are as follows:

- 异常子宫出血：黏膜下和壁间肌瘤常引起 HMB。黏膜下肌瘤可引起不规则阴道出血，特别是伴有子宫内膜炎或肌瘤表面坏死及溃烂时。黏膜下肌瘤可能会脱垂到宫颈，导致大量出血，虽然这种情况很少见。

- *Abnormal uterine bleeding*: Submucous and intramural fibroids commonly cause HMB. Submucous fibroids may cause irregular vaginal bleeding, particularly if associated with overlying endometritis or if the surface of the fibroid becomes necrotic or ulcerated. Although a rare occurrence, submucous fibroids may prolapse through the cervix, resulting in profuse bleeding.

- 疼痛：骨盆疼痛是一种相当常见的症状，可能与 HMB 有关。急性疼痛通常与带蒂肌瘤蒂扭转、黏膜下肌瘤脱垂至宫颈或妊娠时子宫平滑肌瘤内出血引起急性疼痛的“红色变性”有关。

- *Pain*: Pelvic pain is a fairly common symptom that may occur in association with HMB. Acute pain is usually associated with torsion of the pedicle of a pedunculated fibroid, prolapse of a submucous fibroid through the cervix or the 'red degeneration' associated with pregnancy where haemorrhage occurs within the leiomyoma, causing an acute onset of pain.

- 压迫症状：由于可触及腹部增大或膀胱或直肠受到压迫，大的肌瘤包块可能变得明显。女性可描述膀胱容量减少，伴随尿频和夜尿。后壁肌瘤对乙状结肠施加压力可导致便秘或里急后重。

- *Pressure symptoms*: A large mass of fibroids may become apparent because of palpable enlargement of the abdomen or because of pressure on the bladder or rectum. Women may describe reduced bladder capacity with urinary frequency and nocturia. A posterior-wall fibroid exerting pressure on the rectosigmoid can cause constipation or tenesmus.

- 妊娠并发症：复发性流产常见于黏膜下肌瘤女性。子宫肌瘤在妊娠期往往增大，更有可能发生红色变性。骨盆内大的子宫肌瘤可能阻碍分娩或使剖宫产更困难。产后出血的概率增加，子宫肌瘤增加了先兆早产和围产期并发症的危险。

- *Complications of pregnancy*: Recurrent miscarriage is more common in women with submucous fibroids. Fibroids tend to enlarge in pregnancy and are more likely to undergo red degeneration. A large fibroid in the pelvis may obstruct labour or make caesarean section more difficult. There is an increased chance of postpartum haemorrhage, and the presence of fibroids increases the risk of threatened pre-term labour and perinatal morbidity.

- 不孕症：在 3% 的不孕症女性中发现明显的肌瘤，但超声扫描显示出更高的比例。这一比例随着年龄的增长而大大增加（到更年期时达到 50%）。高达 30% 的患有子宫肌瘤的女性会有受孕困难。黏膜下和壁间肌瘤比浆液下肌瘤更容易影响受孕。其机制可能受到机械性、激素和局部分子调控因子的影响。

- *Infertility*: Obvious fibroids are found in 3% of women with infertility, but ultrasound scanning demonstrates a substantially higher number. The proportion increases greatly with age (up to 50% by the age of menopause). Up to 30% of women with uterine fibroids will have difficulty conceiving. Submucous and intramural fibroids are more likely to impair infertility than subserous ones. The mechanism may be mediated by mechanical, hormonal and local molecular regulatory factor effects.

通常可以通过经阴道超声扫描骨盆来确诊。然而，实性卵巢肿瘤有时会被误认为浆液下肌瘤，而肌瘤经囊性变后可能与卵巢囊肿相似。

The diagnosis can usually be confirmed by transvaginal ultrasound scans of the pelvis. However, a solid ovarian tumour may occasionally be mistaken for a subserous fibroid, and a fibroid undergoing cystic degeneration may mimic an ovarian cyst.

5. 子宫肌瘤的管理（Management）

大多数肌瘤是无症状的，不需要治疗。在有症状的女性中，治疗方法的选择可能取决于患者对未来生育能力的渴望、保留子宫的重要性、症状的严重程度和肿瘤特征等因素。

Most fibroids are asymptomatic and do not require treatment. In symptomatic women the choice of approach may be dictated by factors such as the patient's desire for future fertility, the importance of uterine preservation, symptom severity and tumour characteristics.

(1) 药物治疗（Medical treatment）：

口服避孕药、孕激素和非甾体抗炎药（nonsteroidal anti-inflammatory drug，NSAID）对肌瘤大小没有影响，但在控制月经量方面可能有价值。使用促性腺激素释放激素（GnRH）类似物，可使肌瘤大小缩小45%。然而，这些药物的长期使用受到其对骨密度影响的限制，并且当治疗停止时肌瘤会恢复到原来的大小。

The oral contraceptive pill, progestogens and nonsteroidal anti-inflammatory drugs (NSAIDs) have no effect on the size of fibroids but may be of value in controlling menstrual loss. A reduction of up to 45% in size can be achieved using gonadotrophin-releasing hormone (GnRH) analogues. However, the long-term use of these drugs is limited by their effect on bone density, and the fibroids return to their original size when treatment is stopped.

已发现使用孕激素受体调节剂米非司酮超过6个月可以有效地减少月经量和肌瘤大小，但仍缺乏长期数据支持其使用。其他选择性孕激素受体调节药，如乌利司他，也可能发挥作用，但它们的效用还有待临床试验、正式上市和潜在不良反应和罕见肝毒性的说明。

The progesterone receptor modulator mifepristone has been found to be effective in reducing blood loss and fibroid size over a 6-month period, but there is still a lack of long-term data to support its use. Other selective progesterone receptor modulators, such as ulipristal, may also have a role, but their utility awaits the outcome of clinical trials, formal marketing and the clarification of potential side effects and rare hepatotoxicity.

(2) 子宫动脉栓塞（Uterine artery embolization）：

子宫动脉栓塞（uterine artery embolization，UAE）包括经股动脉导管插入子宫动脉，并注射聚乙烯醇颗粒以减少对子宫和肌瘤的血液供应。肌瘤因缺血而萎缩。这项技术的优点是它避免了大手术的风险，并使患者保留生育能力，尽管有证据表明生育能力会受损，而且在妊娠的女性中，有可能增加不良妊娠结果的概率。生育力下降可能与栓塞引起小风险的卵巢损害有关。UAE的不良反应包括子宫缺血引起的疼痛以及变性肌瘤的败血症风险。目前，只在选定的情况下推荐使用它。

Uterine artery embolization (UAE) involves the catheterization of the uterine arteries via the femoral artery and the injection of polyvinyl particles to reduce the blood supply to the uterus and to the fibroids. The fibroid shrinks because of ischaemia. The advantages of this technique are that it avoids the risks of major surgery and allows the preservation of fertility, although there is evidence that fertility can be impaired and that in those women who do conceive, there may be an increased chance of an adverse pregnancy outcome. Impairment of fertility may be associated with a small risk of ovarian damage from the embolization. The side effects of UAE include pain from uterine ischaemia and risk of sepsis in the degenerating fibroid. At present its use is recommended only in selected cases.

(3) 手术治疗（Surgical treatment）：

如果保留生殖功能不重要，可选择的手术治疗是子宫切除术。事实上，在英国，子宫肌瘤占所有子宫切除术的1/3。在年轻女性或保留生殖功能很重要的女性，适合手术切除肌瘤或子宫肌瘤切除术。这个手术包括切开肌瘤的假包膜、剔除瘤体、用可吸收的缝合线间断缝合关闭瘤腔。

Where the preservation of reproductive function is not important, the surgical treatment of choice is hysterectomy. Indeed, fibroids account for about a third of all hysterectomies in the UK. In younger women or where the preservation of reproductive function is important, the removal of fibroids by surgical excision or myomectomy is indicated. This procedure involves incision of the pseudocapsule of the fibroid, enucleation of the bulk of the tumour and closure of the cavity by interrupted absorbable sutures.

子宫肌瘤切除术的并发症情况与子宫切除术的相似。如果不注意手术止血，在切除的肌瘤腔内可能会形成血肿。也不可能确定所有的肌瘤都被切除而不造成过多的子宫损伤；残留的幼小肌瘤有可能重新生长。

Myomectomy is associated with similar morbidity to hysterectomy. There may be haematoma formation in the cavity of the excised fibroid if care is not taken with surgical haemostasis. It is also impossible to be certain that all fibroids are removed without causing excessive uterine damage; there is always a possibility that residual seedling fibroids may regrow.

许多黏膜下肌瘤的内镜切除可以使用宫腔镜进行，而浆膜下和壁间肌瘤的切除通常可以使用腹腔镜技术完成。在熟练的操作人员中，与开腹手术相比，腹腔镜手术的并发症和复发率更低。如果肌瘤直径超过 3cm，术前或围术期使用 GnRH 类似物可以在术前减少肌瘤的大小。

Endoscopic resection of many submucous fibroids can be performed using the hysteroresectoscope, and resection of subserous and intramural myomas can often be accomplished using laparoscopic techniques. In skilled hands, these procedures tend to be associated with lower morbidity and recurrence rate compared to open procedures. If the fibroid is more than 3 cm in diameter, pre- or perioperative measures such as the use of GnRH analogues can used to reduce the size of the fibroid prior to surgery.

(4) 治疗进展（Treatments in development）：

临床试验表明，磁共振成像（MRI）引导的聚焦超声（仅在少数中心可用）利用定向能量加热并破坏肌瘤，是一种潜在的侵入性较小的治疗选择。该方法需要一次治疗一个肌瘤，不能用于有蒂肌瘤的治疗。此手术后不建议妊娠，且缺乏长期数据。

Clinical trials have shown that magnetic resonance imaging (MRI)-guided, focused ultrasound (that is only available in a few centres), which utilizes directed energy to heat and destroy the fibroid, is a potentially less invasive treatment option. The method requires treatment of one fibroid at a time and cannot be used for the management of pedunculated fibroids. Pregnancy is not recommended after the procedure, and long-term data are lacking.

（四）子宫腺肌症（Adenomyosis）

子宫腺肌症是一种以子宫内膜腺体和间质侵犯子宫肌层并周围有平滑肌增生为特征的疾病。它可能影响 5%～10% 的女性，直到最近，最常用的诊断仅是在子宫切除术后切除组织的组织学评估后做出的。随着 B 超医生通过使用现代超声设备，以及对腺肌症特征识别的技巧提高，或者使用 MRI，目前的使用影像学进行诊断越来越频繁。

Adenomyosis is a condition characterized by the invasion of endometrial glands and stroma into myometrium with surrounding smooth muscle hyperplasia. It probably affects around 5–10% of women and until recently the diagnosis was most commonly made only after histological assessment of tissue removed at hysterectomy. Diagnosis is now being made increasingly frequently with modern ultrasound equipment, increasing skills of the operators in recognizing the features or using MRI.

1. 症状和体征（Symptoms and signs）

与子宫内膜异位症不同，子宫腺肌症通常发生在经产妇中，通常在 40 岁时被诊断出来。它与 HMB 和日益严重的痛经有关。临床检查发现，子宫呈对称增大和压痛。症状在绝经后会减轻。

This condition, unlike endometriosis, typically occurs in parous women and is usually diagnosed in the fourth decade. It is associated with HMB and dysmenorrhoea of increasing severity. On clinical examination, the uterus is symmetrically enlarged and tender. The condition regresses after menopause.

2. 病理（Pathology）

子宫的肉眼表现为弥漫性增大。子宫腺肌症和肌瘤通常共存，尽管子宫很少扩大到肌瘤出现时的大小。子宫的后壁通常比前壁厚。子宫切面呈典型的螺旋状、小梁样外观，但偶见子宫肌层内边界分明的伴黑色出血点的结节。

The macroscopic appearances of the uterus are those of diffuse enlargement. Adenomyosis and myomas often co-exist, although the uterus is rarely enlarged to the size seen in the presence of myomas. The posterior wall of the uterus is usually thicker than the anterior wall. The cut surface of the uterus presents a characteristic, whorl-like, trabeculated appearance, but occasionally circumscribed nodules with dark haemorrhagic spots can be seen in the myometrium.

经阴道超声和 MRI 均显示对中度至重度子宫腺肌症的无创诊断具有较高的准确性，但 MRI 是最敏感的诊断技术（图 16-8）。显微镜下的诊断是基于子宫内膜腺体和间质侵犯子宫肌层的平滑肌层而形成的边界不清的区域。国际妇产科联合会（FIGO）和其他组织正在开发不同程度和特点的分类，以改进管理。

Both transvaginal ultrasound and MRI show high levels of accuracy for the non-invasive diagnosis of moderate to severe adenomyosis, but MRI is the most sensitive technique (Fig. 16.8). The microscopic diagnosis is based on the presence of a poorly circumscribed area of endometrial glands and stroma invading the smooth muscle layers of the myometrium. The International Federation of Gynecology and Obstetrics (FIGO) and others are developing improved

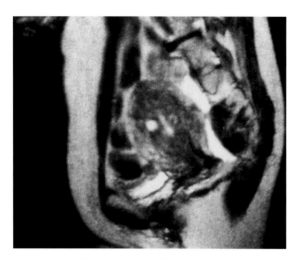

▲ 图 16-8 矢状面，磁共振成像显示子宫腺肌症增大的子宫

Fig. 16.8 Sagittal view using magnetic resonance imaging of a uterus enlarged by adenomyosis.

classifications of different degrees and characteristics for improved management.

3. 治疗（Treatment）

子宫腺肌病可以采用保守的药物治疗、UAE 治疗或手术治疗。药物和手术治疗方法都有争议。对于子宫内膜异位症，药物治疗在某些情况下是有效的，放置左炔诺孕酮宫内缓释系统能最大限度地缓解痛经和月经过多症状。有时前列腺素合成酶抑制药可能有帮助。

Adenomyosis can be managed conservatively with medical treatment, with UAE or surgically. Both medical and surgical approaches to treatment are controversial. Medical therapy, as for endometriosis, is effective in some cases, and symptomatic relief of dysmenorrhoea and heavy bleeding can best be obtained with insertion of a levonorgestrel-releasing intrauterine system. Prostaglandin synthetase inhibitors may sometimes help.

UAE 通常是一个有效的选择。子宫切除术是手术的选择，在有经验的内镜外科医生的专业单位，可采用创伤较小的手术，即选择性切除病灶区域。其他可能获得信任的新技术包括高强度聚焦超声热消融腺肌病灶。

UAE is often an effective alternative. Hysterectomy is the surgical procedure of choice, although less invasive techniques whereby the area of adenomyosis is specifically excised can sometimes be undertaken in specialized units with experienced endoscopic surgeons. Other new techniques that may gain credence include high-intensity focused ultrasound to thermally ablate the adenomyotic foci.

三、卵巢病变（Lesions of the ovary）

卵巢肿大通常是无症状的，恶性卵巢肿瘤的无症状性是这种癌症晚期发现的主要原因。卵巢肿瘤可以是囊性的或实性的、功能性的、良性的或恶性的。卵巢肿瘤的表现和并发症有共同的因素，没有直接的病理检查通常很难确定肿瘤的性质。卵巢肿瘤的诊断和治疗将在第 20 章详细讨论。

Ovarian enlargement is commonly asymptomatic, and the silent nature of malignant ovarian tumours is the major reason for the advanced stage of presentation of this cancer. Ovarian tumours may be cystic or solid, functional, benign or malignant. There are common factors in the presentation and complications of ovarian tumours, and it is often difficult to establish the nature of a tumour without direct pathological examination. The diagnosis and management of ovarian neoplasms are discussed in more detail in Chapter 20.

（一）症状（Symptoms）

卵巢肿瘤直径＜10cm 时很少有症状。常见症状如下。

- 腹部增大：出现恶性变化时，也可能与腹水有关。

- 压迫周围结构（如膀胱和直肠）的症状。

Tumours of the ovary that are less than 10 cm in diameter rarely produce symptoms. The common presenting symptoms include:

- Abdominal enlargement: in the presence of malignant change, this may also be associated with ascites.

- Symptoms from pressure on surrounding structures such as the bladder and rectum.

- 与肿瘤并发症有关的症状（图 16-9）如下。

 - 扭转：卵巢蒂的急性扭转导致肿瘤坏死；当肿瘤坏死时，会出现急性疼痛和呕吐，随后疼痛缓解。

 - 破裂：囊肿内容物溢入腹膜腔，引起弥漫性腹痛。

 - 肿瘤出血是一种不常见的并发症，但如果出血严重，可能导致腹痛和休克。

- Symptoms relating to complications of the tumour (Fig. 16.9); these include:
 - Torsion: acute torsion of the ovarian pedicle results in necrosis of the tumour; there is acute pain and

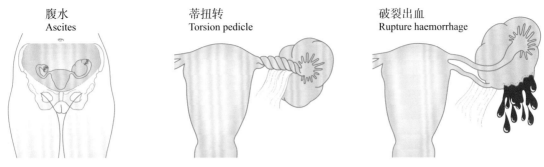

▲ 图 16-9 寻求医学咨询的卵巢肿瘤的常见并发症

Fig. 16.9 Common complications of ovarian tumours that precipitate a request for medical advice.

vomiting followed by remission of the pain when the tumour has become necrotic.

– Rupture: the contents of the cyst spill into the peritoneal cavity and result in generalized abdominal pain.

– Haemorrhage into the tumour is an unusual complication but may result in abdominal pain and shock if the blood loss is severe.

- 分泌激素的肿瘤可能出现月经周期紊乱。在分泌雄激素肿瘤中，患者可能表现出男性化的体征。虽然大部分的性索间质型肿瘤（见后述）是具有激素活性的，但临床实践中最常见的分泌型肿瘤是上皮型的。

– Hormone-secreting tumours may present with disturbances in the menstrual cycle. In androgen-secreting tumours, the patient may present with signs of virilization. Although a greater proportion of the sex-cord stromal type of tumour (see later) are hormonally active, the commonest type of secreting tumour found in clinical practice is the epithelial type.

（二）体征（Signs）

经查体，腹部可明显增大，在膨隆处叩诊可显示中央区浊音和侧方鼓音。大量的腹水可能掩盖这些体征。盆腔检查可发现小肿瘤，可在一个或两个穹隆内触诊发现。然而，随着肿瘤的长大，它会处于更中心的位置，如皮样囊肿通常位于子宫前方。大多数卵巢肿瘤触诊时没有触痛；如果疼痛，则应怀疑是否存在感染或扭转。良性卵巢肿瘤触摸时可与子宫体分开，通常活动度好。

On examination, the abdomen may be visibly enlarged. Percussion over the swelling will demonstrate central dullness and resonance in the flanks. These signs may be obscured by gross ascites. Small tumours can be detected on pelvic examination and will be found by palpation in one or both fornices. However, as the tumour enlarges, it assumes a more central position and, in the case of dermoid cysts, is often anterior to the uterus. Most ovarian tumours are not tender to palpation; if they are painful, the presence of infection or torsion should be suspected. Benign ovarian tumours are palpable separately from the uterine body and are usually freely mobile.

四、子宫内膜异位症（Endometriosis）

子宫内膜组织（腺体和间质）出现在子宫体外的部位时为子宫内膜异位症，通常被炎性反应浸润。有明显的炎症状态。5%～15% 的育龄女性患有此病。在出现盆腔疼痛或不孕症的女性，或者患有严重痛经或慢性盆腔疼痛的青少年中，患病率明显更高。

Endometriosis is a disease characterized by the presence of extrauterine endometrial-like tissue consisting of glands and stroma, often infiltrated by an inflammatory response. This is clearly an inflammatory condition. It affects between 5% and 15% of reproductive-age women. In women presenting with pelvic pain or infertility, or in adolescents with severe dysmenorrhoea or chronic pelvic pain, the prevalence is significantly higher.

患有子宫内膜异位症的女性通常会出现一系列使人衰弱的症状，其中包括盆腔疼痛、性交困难、排尿困难、排便困难和痛经。虽然子宫内膜异位症是良性疾病，但它对女性的健康造成了很大的负担，部分原因是从出现症状到确诊平均有 8～10 年的延迟。如果未确诊，病情会恶化，导致多年未得到治疗或无法有效治疗的盆腔疼痛。

Women suffering from endometriosis very often present with a complex of debilitating symptoms, including pelvic pain, dyspareunia, dysuria, dyschezia and dysmenorrhoea. Although benign, endometriosis causes a substantial burden to the woman's health, partly because of an average delay of 8–10 years between the onset of the symptoms and diagnosis. If undiagnosed, the condition can progress in severity and result in many years of untreated or ineffectively treated pelvic pain.

（一）病理生理学（Pathophysiology）

异常的子宫内膜病灶发生在许多不同的部位（图 16-10）。子宫内膜异位症通常发生在卵巢（图 16-11）、子宫骶韧带和直肠阴道隔。也可发生于覆盖子宫、输卵管、直肠、乙状结肠和膀胱的盆腔腹膜。在脐部、剖腹切口瘢痕（图 16-12）、疝瘢痕、阑尾、阴道、外阴、宫颈、淋巴结，以及极少数情况下在胸膜腔，也可发现远处的子宫内膜异位病灶。

Aberrant endometriotic deposits occur in many different sites (Fig. 16.10). Endometriosis commonly occurs in the ovaries (Fig. 16.11), the uterosacral ligaments and the rectovaginal septum. It may also occur in the pelvic peritoneum covering the uterus, tubes, rectum, sigmoid colon and bladder. Remote ectopic deposits of endometriotic tissue may occasionally be found in the umbilicus, laparotomy scars (Fig. 16.12), hernial scars, the appendix, vagina, vulva, cervix, lymph nodes and, on rare occasions, the pleural cavity.

目前，子宫内膜异位症通常表现为三种表型中的一种或多种：腹膜表面病变（浅表或深部），卵巢表面或深部囊性卵巢子宫内膜异位囊肿，或者深部盆腔病变，特别是在直肠阴道隔内。

Nowadays, endometriosis is usually recognized to present in one or more of three phenotypes, peritoneal surface lesions (superficial or deep), ovarian surface or deep cystic endometriomas, or as deep pelvic lesions, especially in the rectovaginal septum.

卵巢子宫内膜异位症表现为卵巢表面小的浅表病灶或较大的囊肿，即卵巢子宫内膜异位囊肿（图 16-13），可长到 10cm。这些囊肿有较厚的白色包膜层，内含血液呈巧克力样外观，因此被称为巧克力囊肿。卵巢子宫内膜异位囊肿通常与卵巢组织和周围其他结构紧密黏附。

Ovarian endometriosis occurs in the form of small superficial deposits on the surface of the ovary or as larger cysts known as *endometriomas* (Fig. 16.13), which may grow up to 10 cm in size. These cysts have a thick, whitish capsular layer and contain altered blood, which has a chocolatelike appearance. For this reason, they are known as *chocolate cysts.* Endometriomas are often densely adherent both to the ovarian tissue and to other surrounding structures.

这些囊肿可能漏出或偶尔破裂，8% 的子宫内膜异位症患者有急性腹膜刺激症状。

These cysts may leak or occasionally rupture, and in 8%

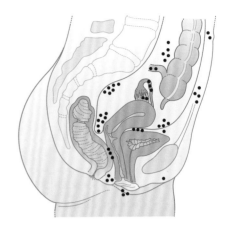

▲ 图 16-10　子宫内膜异位病灶的常见部位

Fig. 16.10　Common sites of endometriotic deposits.

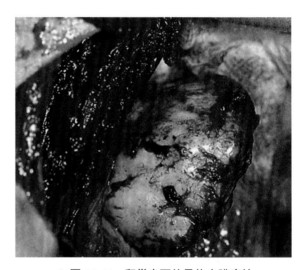

▲ 图 16-11　卵巢表面的异位内膜病灶

Fig. 16.11　Endometriotic patches on the surface of the ovary.

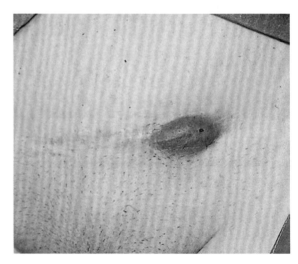

▲ 图 16-12　剖宫产术瘢痕子宫内膜异位症。在月经期间，伤口左侧的暗色有压痛的肿块变得压痛和增大

Fig. 16.12　Endometriosis in a caesarean section scar. The dark tender mass at the left of the wound becomes tender and enlarged during menstruation.

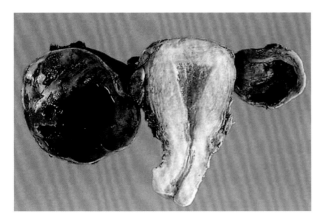

▲ 图 16-13　子宫切除术切除的双侧卵巢子宫内膜异位囊肿

Fig. 16.13　Bilateral endometriomas removed at hysterectomy.

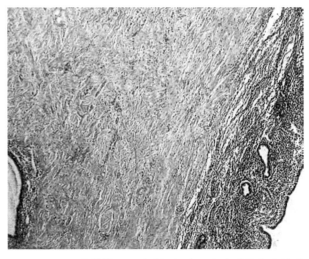

▲ 图 16-14　高倍镜显示瘢痕组织内子宫内膜异位病灶腔内活跃的上皮内膜

Fig. 16.14　High-powered magnification showing active epithelial lining of the cavity of an endometriotic deposit in scar tissue.

of cases, patients with endometriosis present with symptoms of acute peritoneal irritation

病变的显微特征可能是子宫内膜（图 16-14），其与子宫腔内的正常组织无法区分，但可发生广泛的变化，许多长期存在的病灶，因剥离和重复的月经出血可能导致子宫内膜所有的典型特征消失。

The microscopic features of the lesions may be of endometrium (Fig. 16.14) that cannot be distinguished from the normal tissue lining the uterine cavity, but there is wide variation, and in many long-standing cases, desquamation and repeated menstrual bleeding may result in the loss of all characteristic features of endometrium.

在囊肿的内层下面，通常有一个宽阔的区域，其内有包含含铁血黄素的吞噬细胞。也会存在包含玻璃样变的纤维组织的较宽区域。子宫内膜异位病变的特点之一是周围有强烈的纤维化反应，这也可能包含肌纤维。这种反应的强度往往导致在任何手术过程中解剖的巨大困难。尽管常发现与遗传因素有关，但子宫内膜异位症的发病机制尚不清楚。目前有大量研究正在进行，以提高诊断和疾病评估的准确性。

Underneath the lining of the cyst, there is often a broad zone containing phagocytic cells with haemosiderin. There is also a broad zone of hyalinized fibrous tissue. One of the characteristics of endometriotic lesions is the intense fibrotic reaction that surrounds them, and this may also contain muscle fibres. The intensity of this reaction often leads to great difficulty in dissection at the time of any operative procedure. The pathogenesis of endometriosis remains obscure, although a genetic component is frequently recognized. There is a great deal of ongoing research geared to improve the accuracy of diagnosis and assessment of this disease.

Sampson（1921）最初认为这种情况与月经期间

子宫内膜细胞逆行溢出有关，其中一些细胞会在适当的条件下植入腹膜腔和卵巢。这一假说不能解释腹膜腔外的子宫内膜异位病灶。另一种理论认为子宫内膜病变可能源于全身上皮表面的化生变化。

Sampson (1921) originally suggested that the condition was associated with retrograde spill of endometrial cells during menstruation and that some of these cells would implant under appropriate conditions in the peritoneal cavity and on the ovaries. This hypothesis does not account for endometriotic deposits outside the peritoneal cavity. An alternative theory suggests that endometrial lesions may arise from metaplastic changes in epithelium surfaces throughout the body.

（二）诊断（Diagnosis）

最初的评估包括详细记录盆腔疼痛的持续时间和性质，注意与月经周期的关系，是否存在排便和膀胱症状，是否存在性交困难以及姿势和运动对疼痛的影响。初步检查可能包括尿检、性传播感染筛查和经阴道超声扫描。

The initial assessment involves taking a detailed history of the duration and nature of pelvic pain with attention to the relationship to the menstrual cycle, the presence of bowel and bladder symptoms, the presence of dyspareunia and the impact of posture and movement on pain. Initial investigations may include urinalysis, screening for sexually transmitted infections and a transvaginal ultrasound scan.

如果由专家操作，超声对诊断卵巢子宫内膜异位囊肿和深部浸润性子宫内膜异位症有很高的敏感性和特异性，但在诊断常见的腹膜疾病类型时却很少使用。由于没有一贯可靠的无创伤性检查，由经验丰富的妇科内镜医师进行的诊断性腹腔镜检查仍然是确认或排除大多数类型子宫内膜异位症的最佳方法。

The ultrasound, if performed in expert hands, has a high degree of sensitivity and specificity for diagnosing ovarian endometriotic cysts and deep infiltrating bowel endometriosis but is of little use in identifying the commoner types of peritoneal disease. As there is no consistently reliable non-invasive test, diagnostic laparoscopy by an experienced gynaecological endoscopist remains the best way of confirming or excluding most types of endometriosis.

（三）管理（Management）

子宫内膜异位症是一种慢性疾病，通常需要终身治疗。药物治疗包括抑制排卵（和卵巢雌激素分泌）和创造稳定的激素环境。常用的药物包括口服孕激素、孕激素皮下埋植剂和（或）左炔诺孕酮宫内节育系统。

Endometriosis is a chronic disease that often requires lifelong management. Medical treatment involves suppression of ovulation (and ovarian oestrogen secretion) and creating a steady hormone environment. Commonly used medication includes oral progestogens, progestogen subdermal implants and/or the levonorgestrel intrauterine system.

雌孕激素联合的口服避孕药广泛用于子宫内膜异位症，但在患有雌激素敏感疾病的女性身上使用含有雌激素的制剂在逻辑上是不合理的。现代的避孕药为高效孕激素，可能效果很好。这些药物的耐受性都很好，并且在最初都比达那唑、GnRH 激动药和芳香化酶抑制药等替代品更好。药物治疗需要与手术治疗相结合。

Combined oral contraceptive pills are widely used, but it does not make logical sense to use an oestrogen-containing preparation in a woman with an oestrogen-sensitive disease. However, modern pills have a high progestogen balance and may work well. These medications are all generally well tolerated and are initially preferable to alternatives such as danazol, GnRH agonists and aromatase inhibitors. Medical therapy needs to be integrated with use of surgical therapies.

子宫内膜异位症的手术治疗通常包括完全切除可见病变。在 67%～80% 的手术患者中，这比尝试电凝消融病灶更可取，并减少疼痛和改善生活质量。为防止复发，手术后应始终考虑预防性药物治疗，除非有立即妊娠的愿望。

Surgical management of endometriosis usually involves complete excision of visible lesions. This is preferable to attempted diathermy ablation of the lesions and reduces pain and improves quality of life in 67–80% of operated patients. To prevent recurrences, preventive medical therapy after surgery should always be considered, unless pregnancy is immediately desired.

深部浸润性盆腔子宫内膜异位症累及乙状结肠或直肠需要结直肠外科医生进行多学科治疗。腹腔镜妇科专家越来越多地采用腹腔镜切除直肠阴道子宫内膜结节的"削片技术"，并进行重建，取代了肠切除和吻合。子宫内膜异位症的症状在妊娠期间通常会有所改善，有时妊娠后疼痛也会有长期的改善。然而，许多子宫内膜异位症患者在完成妊娠和母乳喂养后，症状会复发。

Deep infiltrating pelvic endometriosis that involves the sigmoid colon or rectum requires a multidisciplinary approach with a colorectal surgeon. Laparoscopic resection of the rectovaginal endometritic nodule by a 'shaving technique' with reconstruction by expert laparoscopic gynaecologists is increasingly practised instead of bowel resection and anastomosis. There is usually amelioration of endometriosis symptoms during pregnancy, and there may sometimes be longterm improvement in pain after pregnancy. However, many women with endometriosis will experience recurrence of symptoms as soon as pregnancy and breast-feeding have been completed.

五、异常子宫出血（Abnormal uterine bleeding）

AUB 是指发生在经期或经间期，或者月经过多、频发或经期延长的出血紊乱。这是一个概括的术语，用来描述各种原因的月经或月经周期的明显异常。FIGO 最近针对 AUB 的潜在原因设计了一个分类系统和精确的术语 –FIGO AUB 系统。这些建议可以使用首字母缩写 PALM-COEIN 将原因分类（表 16–1）。最常见的月经异常是经间期出血（常与 PCB 有关）和月经过多或不规则的月经出血。

AUB is any bleeding disturbance that occurs during or between menstrual periods, or that is excessive, frequent or prolonged. This is the overarching term to describe any significant disturbance of menstruation or the menstrual cycle. FIGO has recently designed a classification system and precise terminologies for underlying causes of AUB-The FIGO AUB Systems. These recommend that causes can be grouped under categories using the acronym PALM COEIN (Table 16.1). The most common menstrual abnormalities are intermenstrual (often associated with PCB) and heavy or irregular menstrual bleeding.

表 16–1　FIGO 对异常子宫出血的病因分类的建议

Table 16.1　FIGO recommendations on classification of causes underlying symptoms of abnormal uterine bleeding

分类 Examples		
结构性病变（"PALM"） Structural lesions ('PALM')		
息肉（子宫内膜息肉、宫颈息肉） Polyps (endometrial, endocervical)		
子宫腺肌症 Adenomyosis		
子宫平滑肌瘤（子宫肌瘤） Leiomyoma (uterine fibroids)		
子宫内膜恶变和增生 Malignancy and hyperplasia		
非结构性原因（"COEIN"） Non-structural causes ('COEIN')		
凝血功能障碍 Coagulopathies	血管性血友病 Von Willebrand disease 血小板功能障碍 Platelet dysfunctions 罕见的凝血因子缺乏 Rare clotting factor deficiencies 血小板减少症（低血小板） Thrombocytopenia (low platelets)	
排卵功能障碍 Ovulatory dysfunction	无排卵或排卵周期紊乱（雌激素正反馈或其他卵巢机制紊乱） Anovulatory or disturbed ovulatory cycles (disturbance of oestrogen positive feedback or other ovarian mechanisms) 多囊卵巢综合征 Polycystic ovary syndrome 甲状腺疾病 Thyroid disease	
子宫内膜局部异常 Endometrial primary causes	影响局部血管功能的子宫内膜分子途径的错误 Errors of endometrial molecular pathways affecting local vascular function	
医源性 Iatrogenic	这一类别包括源于治疗性或人为干预的所有病因。这包括医学治疗的不良反应，药物或设备的使用，如宫内节育器 A category including all causes from therapeutic or human interference. This includes AUB side effects of medicinal therapies, drugs or use of devices, e.g. IUCDs.	
未分类 Not yet classified	罕见的或新发的原因，目前不能归类为任何其他类型，可能会随着新的研究而改变分类。其中的 2 个例子一是子宫动静脉畸形，它可以引起严重的月经出血，二是新诊断的"剖宫产瘢痕憩室"（位于子宫下段"憩室"经常在剖宫产术后发现） Rare or novel causes which do not immediately or obviously fit into any of the other categories at this time. These may change with new research. Two examples of such conditions are uterine arteriovenous malformations, which can cause very heavy menstrual bleeding, or the novel diagnosis of 'isthmocoele' (the lower segment 'niche' frequently found following caesarean section).	

AUB. 异常子宫出血；FIGO. 国际妇产科联合会；IUCD. 宫内节育器

转载自 Munro MG, Critchley HO, Fraser IS, etal.（2011）FIGO 非妊娠育龄女性子宫异常出血原因分类系统（PALM-COEIN）。国际妇产科 113:3-13。

AUB, Abnormal uterine bleeding; FIGO, The International Federation of Gynecology and Obstetrics; IUCD, intrauterine contraceptive device.

Reproduced from Munro MG, Critchley HO, Fraser IS, etal. (2011) The FIGO classification system (PALM-COEIN) of causes of abnormal uterine bleeding in non-gravid women of reproductive age. Int J Gynecol Obstet 113:3-13

FIGO 分类是一个非常有用和灵活的系统，可以很容易地用于了解潜在病因的初始培训和应用于更加复杂专业的分类或研究性分类。

The FIGO classification is a very useful and flexible system, which can easily be used both for initial training in understanding underlying causes and for application to more complex specialized or research classifications.

（一）经间出血（Intermenstrual bleeding）

IMB 通常发生在明确的、周期性的、规律的月经期之间。

IMB generally occurs between clearly defined, cyclical, regular menses.

在每个周期中，出血可能在同一时间发生，也可能是随机的。这种症状通常与生殖道表面病变有关，这些女性也可能经历 PCB。未诊断的妊娠相关出血，包括异位妊娠和葡萄胎样疾病，可能导致类似 IMB 的不规则出血。在 1%～2% 的女性中，IMB 可能是生理性的，表现为在排卵期前后的点滴状出血。

The bleeding may occur at the same time in each cycle or may be random. This symptom is typically associated with surface lesions of the genital tract, and these women may also experience PCB. Undiagnosed pregnancy-related bleeding, including ectopic pregnancy and hydatidiform molar disease, may result in irregular bleeding mimicking IMB. In 1–2% of women, IMB may be physiological, with spotting occurring around the time of ovulation.

> **！注意**
>
> IMB 通常与激素避孕药的使用有关（当它被称为计划外或突破性出血），特别是复方口服避孕药、宫内避孕系统和使用单一孕激素方法，也包括药片和植入。
>
> IMB is commonly associated with the use of hormonal contraception (when it is known as unscheduled or breakthrough bleeding), particularly the combined oral contraceptive pill, intrauterine systems and use of progestogen-only methods, including the pills and implants.

在新发 IMB 的女性中，宫颈或阴道的性传播感染，特别是衣原体感染，应该被认为是一个可能的原因。较不常见的原因有阴道炎（非性传播）、宫颈外翻、子宫内膜或宫颈息肉、子宫内膜炎、子宫腺肌症、黏膜下肌瘤，有时还有宫颈癌或子宫内膜癌。

In women with new onset of IMB, sexually transmitted infection of the cervix or vagina should be considered as a possible cause, especially *Chlamydia*. Less common causes are vaginitis (non-sexually transmitted), cervical ectropion, endometrial or cervical polyps, endometritis, adenomyosis, submucous myomas and sometimes cervical or endometrial cancers.

在仔细检查下生殖道后，IMB 的检查应该始终要排除妊娠和感染。确保宫颈筛查是最新的，如果所有这些都是阴性的，盆腔超声或宫腔镜检查可能揭示宫内原因。

After a careful examination of the lower genital tract, the investigation of IMB should always exclude pregnancy and infection as a cause. Ensure that cervical screening is up to date, and if all these are negative, pelvic ultrasound or hysteroscopy may reveal an intrauterine cause.

（二）性交后出血（Postcoital bleeding）

PCB 是发生在性交过程中或之后的非月经性出血。每年约有 6% 的女性报告有这种症状。PCB 的病因包括生殖道表面病变，典型的是感染，宫颈或子宫内膜息肉，子宫颈、子宫内膜癌或阴道癌（很少），以及创伤。

PCB is non-menstrual bleeding that occurs during or after sexual intercourse. The symptom is reported by around 6% of women per year. Causes of PCB include surface lesions of the genital tract, typically infection; cervical or EPs; cervical, endometrial or (rarely) vaginal cancer; and trauma.

1%～39% 的宫颈癌女性会发生 PCB，如果有复发 PCB 的病史，无论是否伴有 IMB，即使巴氏涂片检查正常，也建议进行宫颈阴道镜检查。

PCB occurs in 1–39% of women with cervical cancer, and if there is a history of recurrent PCB, with or without IMB, colposcopy examination of the cervix is recommended even if the Pap smear is normal.

（三）绝经后出血（Postmenopausal bleeding）

阴道出血发生在最后一次自然月经后 1 年以上称为绝经后出血。虽然子宫内膜癌不是引起这种症状的最常见的原因，但也应考虑子宫体癌的可能性，并建议所有女性对子宫内膜进行评估，无论是用诊断性宫腔镜和子宫内膜活检，还是用高质量的经阴道超声测量子宫内膜的厚度和类型。当子宫内膜小于 3mm 时，子宫内膜病变的可能性很小。

Vaginal bleeding that occurs more than 1 year after the last natural menstrual period is known as *postmenopausal bleeding*. Although it is not the commonest cause of this symptom, the possibility of carcinoma of the body of the uterus should be considered, and an assessment of the endometrium is advised for all women, whether with diagnostic hysteroscopy and endometrial biopsy or with a high-quality transvaginal ultrasound measurement of the endometrial thickness and appearance. When the endometrium is measured at less than 3 mm, significant endometrial pathology is very unlikely.

绝经后出血的其他原因包括生殖道其他的良性和恶性肿瘤、外源性（或内源性）雌激素（如激素补充治疗 HRT 和来自卵巢肿瘤的雌激素）对子宫内膜的刺激、感染和绝经后萎缩性阴道炎。

Other causes of postmenopausal bleeding include other benign and malignant tumours of the genital tract, stimulation of the endometrium by exogenous (or endogenous) oestrogen (e.g. hormone replacement therapy [HRT] and oestrogens from ovarian tumours), infection and postmenopausal atrophic vaginitis.

六、月经过多（Heavy menstrual bleeding）

HMB 在研究中定义为每月月经量＞80ml，影响约 10% 的女性。推荐的"临床"HMB 定义（用于临床）是"过多的阴道出血导致干扰女性的身体、情感、社会和物质生活质量，并单独或与其他症状一起发生"。HMB 应该被认为对女性的生活质量有重大影响。尽管 HMB 通常是良性病变造成的，但它通常会导致铁缺乏或缺铁性贫血，可严重影响女性的社会、家庭和工作生活（通过处理失血过多的实际困难和不得不控制正常活动的负担）。

HMB, defined in research studies as more than 80 mL per month of loss, affects approximately 10% of women. The recommended 'clinical' definition of HMB (for use in the clinic) is 'excessive menstrual loss leading to interference with the physical, emotional, social and material quality of life of a woman, and which occurs alone or in combination with other symptoms'. HMB should be recognized as having a major impact on a woman's quality of life. Although HMB is usually caused by benign conditions, it commonly leads to iron deficiency or iron-deficiency anaemia, which can be part of the serious impact on a woman's social, family and working life (through the burden of managing the practical difficulties of excessive blood loss and having to curb normal activities).

HMB 通常是由子宫内膜局部水平的凝血和其他调节分子因子失衡引起的，不存在明显的结构性病变。然而，它也可能与一些良性妇科疾病有关，其中包括平滑肌瘤、EP、子宫腺肌症和子宫内膜增生，有时也与子宫内膜癌有关。HMB 的原因包括 AUB 的大部分整体原因。

HMB can commonly arise from an imbalance in the clotting and other regulatory molecular factors at a local endometrial level, without the presence of obvious structural pathology. However, it also can be associated with a number of benign gynaecological conditions, including leiomyomata, EPs, adenomyosis, endometrial hyperplasia and sometimes endometrial cancer. The causes of HMB include most of the overall causes of AUB.

（一）病因（Causes）

1. 结构性病变（FIGO 病因分类中的 PALM 成分）[Structural lesions (PALM component of the FIGO classification of causes)]

平滑肌瘤（稍后讨论）是最常见的结构性病变，导致规律性的月经过多，尽管大多数女性肌瘤月经量正常。子宫内膜癌在 40 岁以下罕见，最开始很可能引起不规则出血。子宫腺肌症通常与子宫均匀增大、触痛、HMB 和痛经有关。EP 是 HMB 的常见原因，但也常引起 IMB。子宫内膜增生是引起 HMB 的常见结构性病变，可能与月经不规则、无排卵周期有关。这可能是一种癌前病变。它可能与下面讨论的排卵紊乱相重叠。

Leiomyomata (discussed later) are the commonest structural lesions to cause heavy regular bleeding, although most women with fibroids do not experience abnormal loss. Endometrial carcinoma is rare under the age of 40 years and is more likely initially to cause irregular bleeding. Adenomyosis is usually associated with a uniformly enlarged tender uterus, HMB and dysmenorrhoea. EPs are a common cause of HMB but usually also cause IMB. Endometrial hyperplasia is a common structural lesion causing HMB and may be associated with irregular, anovulatory cycles. It may be a premalignant condition. It may overlap with the disturbed ovulation discussed in the next section.

2. 非结构性条件（FIGO 分类中的 COEIN 成分）[Non-structural conditions (COEIN component of the FIGO classification)]

排卵紊乱或不排卵会导致非常不规则，特别是稀发的月经周期，并伴有经期延长、月经过多和不规则的出血，有时甚至可能危及生命。在这种情况下，缺乏孕激素拮抗的雌激素往往导致子宫内膜极其增厚和增生。这种不稳定的子宫内膜最终会以一种不完整、不规则的方式脱落。大多数排卵障碍发生在绝经过渡期和青春期，或可追溯到内分泌疾病，如多囊卵巢综合征和甲状腺功能减退。

Disturbed ovulation or anovulation can result in very

irregular, especially infrequent, cycles with prolonged, heavy and irregular bleeding of such severity that it may occasionally be life threatening. In this situation, unopposed oestrogen often leads to the endometrium becoming greatly thickened and hyperplastic. This unstable endometrium eventually breaks down in a patchy and erratic fashion. Most ovulatory disorders occur in the menopause transition and in adolescence or can be traced to endocrinopathies, e.g. PCOS and hypothyroidism.

当有规律的大出血且没有潜在的结构性病变时，HMB 通常是原发性子宫内膜疾病的结果，调节局部子宫内膜"止血"的机制受到干扰。可能局部产生过多的纤溶因子（特别是组织型纤溶酶原激活物），局部产生不足的血管收缩物和局部产生增加的促进血管舒张的物质。大出血最常见的医源性原因是放置含铜宫内节育器（intrautering contraceptine device，IUCD）。

When there is regular heavy bleeding with no underlying structural lesion, HMB is usually the result of a primary endometrial disorder where the mechanisms regulating local endometrial 'haemostasis' are disturbed. There may be excessive local production of fibrinolytic factors (especially tissue plasminogen activator), deficiencies in local production of vasoconstrictors and increased local production of substances that promote vasodilation. The commonest iatrogenic cause of heavy bleeding is the presence of a copperbearing intrauterine contraceptive device (IUCD).

（二）病史和查体（History and examination）

一份准确的病史对于确定出血类型和症状持续时间至关重要。对失血量的临床评估是非常主观的，尽管血块的存在、夜间需要更换卫生防护措施和"血崩"（月经期间弄脏床单或内衣）更有可能表明明显出血过多。近期月经出血类型的改变和相关疼痛更有可能与结构性盆腔病变的发展有关。

An accurate history is essential to establish the pattern of bleeding and the duration of symptoms. Clinical estimation of the degree of blood loss is very subjective, although the presence of clots, the need to change sanitary protection at night and 'flooding' (the soiling of bedclothes or underwear during menstruation) are more likely to indicate significant bleeding. A recent change in the pattern of menstruation and associated pain are more likely to be associated with the development of structural pelvic pathology.

疼痛通常与子宫腺肌症和慢性盆腔炎（pelvic inflammatory disease，PID）有关。如果出血伴有疼痛，女性更有可能主诉 HMB。子宫内膜异位症有时会引起 HMB（及疼痛）。子宫和子宫颈的结构性表面病变更典型地引起 IMB 和 PCB。40 岁以下的子宫内膜恶性肿瘤很少见，但有糖尿病、高血压、多囊卵巢

综合征和肥胖病史的女性发生子宫内膜增生和子宫内膜癌的风险较高。

Pain is typically associated with adenomyosis and chronic pelvic inflammatory disease (PID). Women are more likely to complain of HMB if the bleeding is accompanied by pain. Endometriosis sometimes causes HMB (as well as pain). Structural surface lesions of the uterus and cervix more typically cause IMB and PCB. Endometrial malignancy is rare under the age of 40 years, but women with a history of diabetes, hypertension, PCOS and obesity are at increased risk of endometrial hyperplasia and carcinoma.

月经过多的女性应进行贫血和甲状腺疾病症状的全面检查，并进行盆腔检查（如有必要），其中包括宫颈检查。在盆腔检查中发现盆腔肿块最可能提示子宫平滑肌瘤（纤维瘤）的存在，但也可能提示子宫恶性肿瘤、子宫腺肌症或卵巢肿瘤。

Women with heavy periods should have a general examination for signs of anaemia and thyroid disease and a pelvic examination, including cervical screening test, if indicated. The finding of a pelvic mass on pelvic examination is most likely to indicate the presence of uterine leiomyomata (fibroids) but may indicate a uterine malignancy, adenomyosis or ovarian tumour.

（三）检查（Investigations）

在临床检查正常的情况下，开始治疗前只需要进行全血细胞计数包括血小板（有时血清铁蛋白和血清转铁蛋白受体饱和度以评估铁状态）。应该记住，铁缺乏是世界范围内最常见的缺铁性疾病。

A full blood count with platelets (and sometimes serum ferritin and serum transferrin receptor saturation to assess iron status) is the only investigation needed before starting treatment, provided that clinical examination is normal. It should be remembered that iron deficiency is the commonest deficiency disease worldwide.

如有下列情况，患者应转诊做进一步检查。

- 有反复或持续的不规则出血或 IMB 或子宫内膜癌高危因素的病史。

- 宫颈癌筛查异常。

- 盆腔检查异常。

- 有明显的盆腔疼痛，对单纯镇痛无反应。

- 6 个月的一线治疗无反应。

Patients should be referred for further investigation if:
- There is a history of repeated or persistent irregular or

IMB or of risk factors for endometrial carcinoma.

- The cervical screening test is abnormal.
- Pelvic examination is abnormal.
- There is significant pelvic pain unresponsive to simple analgesia.
- They do not respond to first-line treatment after 6 months.

额外的检查主要是确认或排除是否有盆腔的病变，特别是子宫内膜恶性肿瘤。主要检查方法有超声检查、子宫内膜活检、宫腔镜检查和经阴道超声检查（伴或不伴生理盐水子宫超声造影检查）。

Additional investigation is mainly to confirm or exclude the presence of pelvic pathology and in particular of endometrial malignancy. The main methods of investigation are ultrasound, endometrial biopsy, hysteroscopy and transvaginal ultrasound (with or without saline sonohysterography).

对月经异常的全身原因进行调查时，只有在有凝血病筛查史异常或年轻女性，才需要对止血障碍（凝血病）（其中轻度血管性血友病是与 HMB 相关的最常见的原因）进行部分凝血筛查。

Investigations for systemic causes of abnormal menstruation, such as a partial coagulation screen for the disorders of haemostasis-a coagulopathy-(of which mild von Willebrand disease is the commonest of these causes associated with HMB), are only indicated if a screening history for coagulopathies is suggestive or in young women.

甲状腺疾病是一种罕见的 HMB 病因，只有在检查中有其他特征或既往病史时才会进行调查。子宫内膜活检可作为门诊手术单独或与宫腔镜联合进行。

Thyroid disease is a rare cause of HMB, and investigation is only indicated if there are other features on examination or a previous history. Endometrial biopsy can be performed as an outpatient procedure either alone or in conjunction with hysteroscopy.

宫腔镜可通过宫颈插入 3mm 的内镜观察子宫腔，可以在全身麻醉或门诊局部麻醉下进行。宫腔镜和子宫内膜活检已经在很大程度上取代了传统且不可靠的盲法 D&C。

Hysteroscopy allows visualization of the uterine cavity using a 3-mm endoscope introduced through the cervix. It can be performed under general anaesthetic or as an outpatient investigation using local anaesthesia. Hysteroscopy with endometrial biopsy has largely replaced the traditional and unreliable blind D&C.

经阴道超声对鉴别生殖道的结构性病变有重要价值。在绝经前女性中，超声测量的子宫内膜厚度在月经周期的不同时间不同，但通常可以看到结构病变，如子宫内膜息肉。

Transvaginal ultrasound is of value in distinguishing the structural lesions of the genital tract. In premenopausal women, ultrasoundmeasured endometrial thickness will vary at different times of the menstrual cycle, but it is usually possible to visualize structural lesions such as polyps in the endometrial cavity.

（四）管理（Management）

1. 药物治疗（Medical treatment）

在没有恶性肿瘤的情况下，选择何种治疗取决于患者是否需要避孕、月经周期是否不规则，以及是否存在某些治疗的禁忌证。如果使用含铜节育器，可使用甲灭酸或氨甲环酸，或者使用左炔诺孕酮宫内系统（曼月乐）代替。

In the absence of malignancy, the treatment chosen will depend on whether contraception is required, whether irregularity of the cycle is a problem and the presence of contraindications to certain treatments. Where a copper IUD is in place, mefenamic or tranexamic acid can be used, or the device may be replaced by a levonorgestrel intrauterine system (Mirena).

2. 非激素治疗（Non-hormonal treatments）

NSAID，如甲灭酸或布洛芬，抑制前列腺素合成酶。它们可以减少 30% 左右的失血量，如果有相关的痛经，它们的镇痛特性可能是一个优势。主要的不良反应是轻微的胃肠道刺激。氨甲环酸是一种抗纤溶药，可减少约 50% 的失血。它是安全的，在许多国家不需要处方就可以买到。它不会引起静脉血栓形成，但在有血栓栓塞性疾病病史的患者中避免使用它是明智的。这两组药物的优点是只需要在月经期间服用。

NSAIDs, such as mefenamic acid or ibuprofen, inhibit prostaglandin synthetase enzymes. They reduce blood loss by around 30%, and their analgesic properties may be an advantage if there is associated dysmenorrhoea. The principal side effect is mild gastrointestinal irritation. Tranexamic acid is an anti-fibrinolytic agent that reduces blood loss by about 50%. It is safe and available over the counter without prescription in many countries. It does not cause venous thrombosis, but it is wise to avoid its use in patients with a previous history of thromboembolic disease. Both groups of drugs have the advantage of only needing to be taken during menstruation.

3. 激素治疗（Hormonal treatments）

采用复方口服避孕药或左炔诺孕酮宫内系统进行激素治疗，平均月失血量分别减少 30% 和 90%

（图 16-15）。左炔诺孕酮宫内释放系统被广泛推荐作为无禁忌证的 HMB 患者的首选药物。

Use of the combined oral contraceptive pill or the levonorgestrel intrauterine system is associated with around 30% and 90% reduction in average monthly blood loss, respectively (Fig. 16.15). The levonorgestrel-releasing intrauterine system is widely recommended as the first choice for medical therapy of HMB in those women who do not have contraindications to its use.

合成口服孕激素，如炔诺酮或醋酸甲羟孕酮，可以在 28 天中服用 21 天，以有效控制不规则的大出血，但往往有较高的不良反应发生率。它们也可以在急性情况下使用更高剂量来控制严重的 HMB（口服炔诺酮 5mg，或者醋酸甲羟孕酮 10mg，每日 3 次，共 21 天）。

Synthetic oral progestogens, such as norethisterone or medroxyprogesterone acetate, can be given for 21 days out of 28 over prolonged periods to effectively control irregular, heavy bleeding but do tend to be associated with a higher incidence of nuisance-value side effects. They can also be used in higher doses in an acute situation to control severe HMB (oral norethisterone 5 mg, or medroxyprogesterone acetate 10 mg, three times daily for 21 days).

达那唑是一种合成的、轻度受阻的雄激素衍生物，作用于下丘脑 - 垂体轴和子宫内膜，目前很少被使用。大剂量服用通常会导致闭经，但有 10% 的患者会有明显的不良反应。图 16-15 记录了各种药物治疗降低 HMB 的疗效。

Danazol is a synthetic, mild impeded androgen derivative that acts on the hypothalamic-pituitary axis and endometrium and is uncommonly used nowadays. Given at high doses, it will normally cause amenorrhoea but is associated with significant side effects in 10% of patients. The efficacy of various medical therapies in reducing HMB is documented in Figure 16.15.

（五）手术治疗（Surgical treatment）

1. 子宫内膜切除或消融术（Endometrial resection or ablation）

可以通过手术宫腔镜或第三代现代宫内加热或冷却装置来切除或破坏子宫内膜。第一代和第二代技术包括使用激光或行电切环切除，或者使用滚动球电凝或两者结合（图 16-16）。

The endometrium can be removed or destroyed using an operating hysteroscope or with a number of modern third-generation intrauterine heating or cooling devices that ablate the endometrium. The first- and second-generation techniques

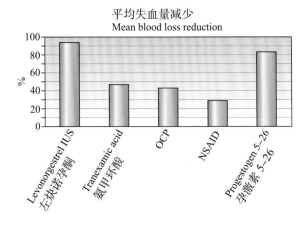

▲ 图 16-15　由于非结构性原因导致的月经过多的女性，不同治疗方法测量的出血量减少的平均百分比

IUS. 宫内节育器；OCP. 口服避孕药；NSAID. 非甾体抗炎药

Fig. 16.15　**Mean percentage reduction in measured blood loss with different therapies in women with heavy menstrual bleeding due to non-structural causes.**

IUS, Intrauterine system; OCP, Oral Contraceptive Pill ; NSAIDs, non-steroidal anti-inflammatory drugs.

involve using laser or diathermy resection with a wire loop or coagulation with a rollerball or a combination of the two (Fig. 16.16).

在术前使用达那唑或 GnRH 类似物治疗 4～8 周，子宫内膜可以变薄，以便更有效的消融。用灌洗液（如甘氨酸或生理盐水）使子宫腔膨胀。术中发生子宫穿孔和其他器官损伤需要开腹手术和修复的风险非常罕见。另一个潜在的并发症是由于过度吸收灌洗液而导致的液体潴留。

The endometrium can be thinned prior to treatment with danazol or GnRH analogues for 4–8 weeks before surgery, allowing for more effective ablation. The uterine cavity is distended with an irrigation fluid such as glycine or normal saline. There is a rare risk of intraoperative uterine perforation and possibly damage to other organs requiring laparotomy and repair. The other potential complication is fluid overload from excessive absorption of the irrigation fluid.

现在新的半自动技术已经在很大程度上取代宫腔镜手术，这种技术不需要同样的宫腔镜技术。球囊消融包括将充满液体的球囊插入子宫内膜腔，然后精确地加热，从而破坏整个子宫内膜。还有一系列其他的设备，它们都是基于使用不同的能量源对子宫内膜进行过度加热或冷却的原理，从而在不损害相邻结构的情况下精确地破坏子宫内膜。

Hysteroscopic procedures have now been largely replaced by newer semi-automatic techniques that do not require the same hysteroscopic skills. Balloon ablation involves inserting

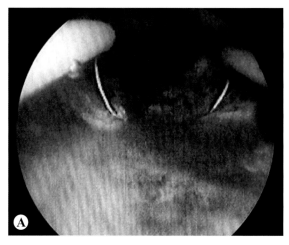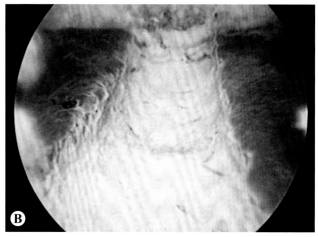

▲ 图 16-16　子宫内膜切除术。使用电切镜进行切除前 **(A)** 和切除后 **(B)** 的子宫腔视图

Fig. 16.16　Endometrial resection. View of the uterine cavity (A) before and (B) after excision using a resectoscope.

a fluidfilled balloon into the endometrial cavity, which is then very precisely heated so that it destroys the entire endometrium. A range of other devices are available, which are all based on the principle of excessively heating or cooling the endometrium using different energy sources so that it is very precisely destroyed without damaging adjacent structures.

有 30%～70% 的患者会闭经，还有 20%～30% 的患者 HMB 显著减少。少数患者最终需要进一步的手术和子宫切除术。

Around 30–70% of patients will become amenorrhoeic, with a further 20–30% achieving major reduction in HMB. A minority of patients will eventually need further surgery and hysterectomy.

2. 子宫切除术（Hysterectomy）

子宫切除术仍然是最终的治疗方法，与内科治疗或内镜手术相比，这更适合于有盆腔疾病的女性，如子宫腺肌症和子宫肌瘤。

This remains the definitive treatment and is more likely to be appropriate for those women with pelvic pathology, such as adenomyosis and fibroids, than medical treatment or endoscopic surgery.

子宫切除术的死亡率约为 1/2000，但患有良性妇科疾病的女性的死亡率应更低。明显的并发症发生在 25%～40% 的患者中，并且在接受经腹子宫切除术的患者中更常见。术中出血是主要的问题，术中应始终采取预防措施，尽量减少术后静脉血栓栓塞。

Hysterectomy is associated with a mortality of around 1 in 2000, although the mortality for women with benign gynaecological diseases should be less. Significant complications occur in 25–40% of patients and tend to be more common in patients undergoing abdominal hysterectomy. Intraoperative bleeding is the major concern, and intraoperative precautions should always be taken to minimize postoperative venous thromboembolism.

最常见的术后并发症是感染（尿路、呼吸系统或手术部位），但任何术后并发症也可能偶发在个体病例中。子宫切除术可以经腹部、经阴道或腹腔镜下进行。

The commonest postoperative complications are infections (urinary, respiratory or at the operation sites), but any postoperative complication may occasionally occur in individual cases. Hysterectomy can be undertaken abdominally, vaginally or laparoscopically.

经腹子宫切除术是通过腹下横切口或正中切口进行的。根据是否保留圆韧带、输卵管和卵巢血管，分别在卵巢内侧或远端切除并结扎（见后述）。打开子宫膀胱腹膜反折，将膀胱与子宫下段分离，使输尿管远离子宫血管，然后切断并结扎子宫血管。

Abdominal hysterectomy is carried out through a transverse lower abdominal or midline incision. The round ligaments, Fallopian tubes and ovarian vessels are cut and ligated on each side, either medial or distal to the ovaries, depending on whether these are to be conserved (see later). The uterovesical peritoneum is opened, and the bladder is reflected off the lower part of the uterus and cervix so as to displace the ureters away from the uterine vessels, which are then cut and ligated.

最后，切断子宫颈主韧带，打开宫颈周围的阴道壁，切除子宫。如果没有宫颈疾病史，可以在结扎子宫血管后，通过在子宫内口下方切除子宫体（子宫次全切除术）来保存宫颈。其指征为盆腔疾病使宫颈分离困难，以减少输尿管损害的风险，或者是患者的偏好。

Finally, the transverse cervical ligaments are cut and the vagina opened around the cervix, allowing removal of the uterus. If there has been no history of cervical disease, the cervix can be conserved by removing the uterine corpus just below the internal os after the uterine vessels have been ligated (*subtotal hysterectomy*). This may be indicated if other pelvic disease makes dissection of the cervix difficult in order to reduce the risk of ureteric damage or because of patient preference.

根治性经腹子宫切除术包括切除子宫、子宫颈、阴道上部和支持组织，在已知有子宫体癌或子宫颈癌时施行。

Radical abdominal hysterectomy involves removing the uterus, cervix, upper vagina and supporting tissues and is performed when there is known uterine or cervical cancer.

经阴道子宫切除术中（经阴道入口入路），在宫颈和膀胱周围切开阴道，向上分离膀胱进入盆腔。打开子宫膀胱和直肠阴道间隙上方的腹膜，钳夹、切断和结扎子宫颈部韧带。钳夹和结扎子宫和卵巢血管，摘除子宫，关闭腹膜和阴道壁。

In *vaginal hysterectomy* (with approach through the vaginal introitus), the vaginal skin is opened around the cervix and the bladder and reflected up into the pelvis. The peritoneum over the uterovesical and rectovaginal space is opened, and the cervical ligaments are clamped, cut and ligated. The uterine and ovarian vessels are clamped and ligated, the uterus is removed and the peritoneum and vaginal skin are closed.

可能摘除卵巢，但经阴道入路很少采用这种方法。由于没有腹部伤口，大大降低了术后的不良事件，因此这是大多数子宫切除术的首选方法。怀疑为恶性肿瘤者禁用。其他相对禁忌证包括子宫大小超过妊娠 14 周，存在子宫内膜异位症和需要同时切除病变卵巢的女性。

Removal of the ovaries is possible but is less commonly carried out by this route. The absence of an abdominal wound substantially reduces postoperative morbidity, making this the method of choice for most cases of hysterectomy. It is contraindicated where malignancy is suspected. Other relative contraindications include a uterine size of over 14 weeks, the presence of endometriosis and in women who require concurrent removal of the diseased ovaries.

腹腔镜子宫切除术是通过腹腔镜直视下，分离并夹闭或固定与子宫相连的组织，切除子宫，通过阴道拿出子宫，或者通过旋切器将子宫变成条状从

腹部切口拿出，由于子宫内膜异位症、粘连或需要切除卵巢等疾病而不能施行阴道子宫切除术时，熟练的内镜医师采用腹腔镜子宫切除术是最好的方法。

Laparoscopic hysterectomy involves dividing and occluding or fixing the attachments of the uterus under direct visualization through the laparoscope and then removing the uterus either vaginally or through the abdominal ports after reducing it to strips (morcellation). Laparoscopic hysterectomy by a skilled endoscopist is the best approach to hysterectomy when a vaginal hysterectomy cannot be performed because of the presence of diseases such as endometriosis, adhesions or when the ovaries need be removed.

在正常情况下，50 岁以下的女性接受子宫切除术治疗 HMB 通常建议保留卵巢，以避免手术引起的过早绝经。对于接近绝经期的女性，这一优势在概率上必须抵消后期可能发生卵巢恶性肿瘤的小风险，应该讨论是否选择切除卵巢。有卵巢癌家族史的患者通常考虑切除卵巢的决定。

Conservation of the ovaries, if normal, is usually recommended for women under the age of 50 years undergoing hysterectomy for HMB to avoid the onset of a surgically induced early menopause. For women near menopause, this advantage has to be offset against the small possible risk of later ovarian malignancy, and the option of oophorectomy should be discussed. Family history of ovarian cancer is usually considered in this decision.

七、继发性闭经和月经稀发（Secondary amenorrhoea and oligomenorrhoea）

继发性闭经的定义是既往有月经的女性，月经停止 6 个月或以上。月经稀发是指在 12 个月内月经≤ 5 次。在实践中，两者之间的区别可能有些武断，因为它们有许多相同的原因。

Secondary amenorrhoea is defined as the cessation of menses for 6 or more months in a woman who has previously menstruated. Oligomenorrhoea is the occurrence of five or fewer menstrual periods over 12 months. In practice, the distinction between the two can be somewhat arbitrary, as they share many of the same causes.

（一）病因学（Aetiology）

1. 生理性（Physiological）

生理原因（包括妊娠和哺乳）是生育年龄最常见的原因。母乳喂养会导致泌乳素的增加，从而抑制 GnRH 的释放，阻止正常的卵巢刺激。闭经的时

间长短取决于母乳喂养的程度、频率和时间长短。

Physiological causes, including pregnancy and lactation, account for most cases of amenorrhoea in the reproductive years. Breast-feeding causes a rise in prolactin, which inhibits GnRH release and prevents normal ovarian stimulation. The duration of amenorrhoea depends on the extent, frequency and length of time of breast-feeding.

2. 病理性（Pathological）

病理原因可分为下丘脑、垂体前叶、卵巢和生殖道疾病（图 16-17）。

Pathological causes can be divided into disorders of the hypothalamus, anterior pituitary, ovary and genital tract (Fig. 16.17).

3. 下丘脑疾病（Hypothalamic disorders）

功能性下丘脑闭经（functional hypothalamic amenorrhoea，FHA）是一种非器质性、可逆性的疾病，其中 GnRH 脉冲式分泌障碍起关键作用。FHA 有 3 种类型，即体重减轻相关的闭经、压力相关的闭经和运动相关的闭经。FHA 的特征是卵泡刺激素（FSH）和黄体生成素（LH）水平低或正常，泌乳素正常，垂体窝显像正常，雌激素分泌不足。

Functional hypothalamic amenorrhoea (FHA) is defined as a non-organic and reversible disorder in which the impairment of GnRH pulsatile secretion plays a key role. There are three types of FHA: weight loss-related amenorrhoea,

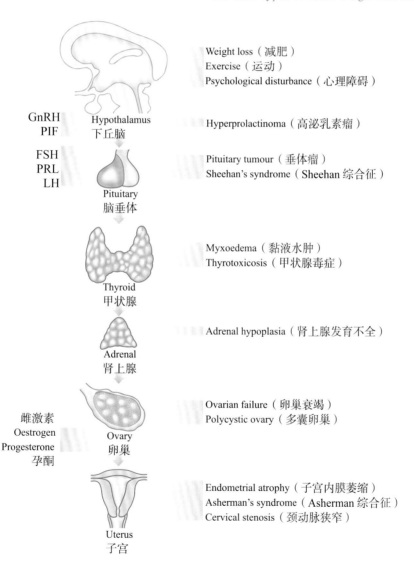

▲ 图 16-17　继发性闭经的原因

FSH. 卵泡刺激激素；GnRH. 促性腺激素释放激素；LH. 促黄体激素；PIF. 催乳素抑制因子；PRL. 泌乳素

Fig. 16.17　Causes of secondary amenorrhoea.

FSH, Folliclestimulating hormone; GnRH, gonadotrophin-releasing hormone; LH, luteinizing hormone; PIF, prolactin-inhibiting factor; PRL, prolactin.

stress-related amenorrhoea and exercise-related amenorrhoea. FHA is characterized by low or normal levels of follicle-stimulating hormone (FSH) and luteinizing hormone (LH), normal prolactin levels, normal imaging of the pituitary fossa and hypo-oestrogenism.

体重和月经之间有重要的关系。BMI 正常的体重减少 10%～15% 可能导致月经稀发或闭经。这可能是剧烈节食的结果，也可能是神经性厌食症的表现。这是一种精神疾病，其特征是对身体形象认知扭曲和对体重增加的强烈恐惧，即使是那些已经体重过轻的人。这些患者努力通过高强度运动、限制食物摄入或诱导餐后呕吐来减少体重。继发性闭经 3 个月是诊断的基本标准。

There is a critical relationship between body weight and menstruation. A loss of body weight of 10–15% of normal weight for height is likely to cause oligomenorrhoea or amenorrhoea. This may result from vigorous dieting, or it may be a manifestation of *anorexia nervosa*, a psychiatric condition characterized by disturbed body image and an intense fear of weight gain even in those already underweight. Those affected strive to reduce their body mass through intense exercising and limiting their food intake or inducing vomiting after meals. Secondary amenorrhoea of 3 months' duration forms part of the basic criteria for diagnosis of the condition in women.

参加大运动量训练的女性，如长跑、体操或芭蕾舞，可能会发展为继发性闭经（运动性闭经）。有几个因素共同促成了 FHA，其中包括低体脂、心理和生理压力及高能量消耗。

Women who participate in sports that require strenuous training, such as long-distance running or gymnastics, or ballet dancing, may develop secondary amenorrhoea (exercise-related amenorrhoea). Several factors combine to contribute to this FHA, including low body fat, psychological and physical stress and high energy expenditure.

来自工作、家庭、住房或关系状况变化的情绪压力也会导致 FHA。不善于应对压力的人似乎释放出更高的皮质醇水平，更容易发生 FHA。

Emotional stress from change in work, family, housing or relationship situations can also result in FHA. Individuals who cope less well with stress seem to release higher cortisol levels and are more prone to FHA.

 经验 虽然复方口服避孕药引起下丘脑 - 垂体 - 卵巢轴的抑制，但没有证据表明当停止服用避孕药时这种抑制会持续。

Although the combined oral contraceptive pill causes suppression of the hypothalamic-pituitary-ovarian axis, there is no evidence that this persists when the pill is discontinued.

4. 垂体性疾病（Pituitary disorders）

继发性闭经的垂体原因通常是高催乳素水平的结果。约 40% 的病例与垂体前叶泌乳素分泌肿瘤（微腺瘤或大腺瘤）有关，约 1/3 的患者发生泌乳（乳溢）。

The pituitary causes of secondary amenorrhoea are most commonly the result of high prolactin levels. Around 40% of cases are associated with a prolactin-secreting tumour of the anterior pituitary (microadenoma or macroadenoma), and secretion of breast milk (*galactorrhoea*) occurs in about one-third of patients.

所有继发性闭经的患者都应该评估泌乳素水平，如果水平异常升高，可以用计算机断层扫描（CT）或 MRI 检查垂体窝。垂体微腺瘤很常见，但大腺瘤很少见，因为相关的内分泌影响，患者通常就诊于内分泌专家。大腺瘤的生长可能由于压迫视交叉而引起双眼视野颞侧偏盲，但这种情况和其他脑神经压迫均不常见。

All patients with secondary amenorrhoea should have a prolactin estimation and, if the levels are abnormally raised, imaging of the pituitary fossa with computed tomography (CT) or MRI. Pituitary microadenomas are common, but macroadenomas are rare and usually present to an endocrinologist because of associated endocrine effects. Growth of a macroadenoma may cause bitemporal hemianopia as a result of compression of the optic chiasma, but this and other cranial nerve compressions are unusual findings.

垂体前叶泌乳素的释放受到神经递质多巴胺的抑制。具有抗多巴胺能作用的药物（框 16-1）会导致医源性催乳素水平升高和闭经。

The release of prolactin from the anterior pituitary is inhibited by the neurotransmitter dopamine. Drugs with anti-dopaminergic effects (Box 16.1) will result in iatrogenically elevated prolactin levels and amenorrhoea.

专框 16-1　可能引起高催乳素血症的药物	Box 16.1　Drugs that may cause hyperprolactinaemia
• 吩噻嗪类	• Phenothiazines
• 抗组胺药	• Antihistamines
• 丁酰苯类	• Butyrophenones
• 甲氧氯普胺	• Metoclopramide
• 西咪替丁	• Cimetidine
• 甲基多巴	• Methyldopa

在发达国家，由于严重的产科出血和低血压引起产后垂体前叶坏死可导致垂体闭经（Sheehan 综合征），但极少发生。

Rarely (in high-resource countries), pituitary amenorrhoea

may result from postpartum necrosis of the anterior pituitary from severe obstetric haemorrhage and hypotension (Sheehan's syndrome).

5. 卵巢疾病（Ovarian disorders）

(1) 卵巢衰竭（Ovarian failure）：

卵巢早衰（premature ovarian failure，POF）通常定义为卵巢功能在 40 岁前停止，以闭经和促性腺激素水平升高为特征。它影响 1% 的女性，而且通常是不可逆转的。遗传因素起着重要作用，20%～30% 患有 POF 的女性都有家族史。

Premature ovarian failure (POF) is usually defined as the cessation of ovarian function before the age of 40 and is characterized by amenorrhoea and raised gonadotrophin levels. It affects 1% of women and is most often nonreversible. Genetic factors play an important role, and 20–30% of women with POF have an affected relative.

一系列的遗传综合征导致了 POF，其中 Turner 综合征是最明显的。自发性 POF 中，有约 4% 的女性出现自身免疫性卵巢炎。这种情况通常与多个内分泌和其他器官的自身抗体有关，但也见于女性系统性红斑狼疮和重症肌无力。

A range of genetic syndromes lead to POF, of which Turner's syndrome is the most obvious. Autoimmune oophoritis is found in around 4% of women who present with spontaneous POF. This condition is most often associated with autoantibodies to multiple endocrine and other organs but has also been seen in women with systemic lupus erythematosus and myasthenia gravis.

手术切除卵巢、辐射破坏或感染会不可避免地导致继发性闭经。所有这些情况的特点是高水平的促性腺激素和低雌激素（高促性腺激素性性腺机能减退）。罕见的卵巢肿瘤，特别是与过量、异常的雌激素或睾酮分泌有关的肿瘤，可能导致闭经，但在已知的病因中只占很小的比例。

Surgical removal of the ovaries or destruction by radiation or infection inevitably results in secondary amenorrhoea. All these conditions are characterized by high levels of gonadotrophins and hypo-oestrogenism (*hypergonadotropic hypogonadism*). Rare ovarian neoplasms, particularly those associated with excessive, abnormal production of oestrogen or testosterone, may cause amenorrhoea but constitute only a very small percentage of known causes.

(2) 多囊卵巢综合征（Polycystic ovary syndrome）：

PCOS 影响 5%～10% 的育龄期女性，与 75% 的无排卵性不孕疾病和 90% 的月经稀发女性有关（框 16-2）。多囊卵巢综合征见于有雄激素过多症状的女性，90% 的女性有多毛和 80% 的女性有痤疮。约 50% 患有这种疾病的女性超重或肥胖。

PCOS affects 5–10% of reproductive-age women and is associated with 75% of all anovulatory disorders causing infertility and with 90% of women with oligomenorrhoea (Box

框 16–2　多囊卵巢综合征的特点	Box 16.2　Features of polycystic ovarian syndrome
月经稀发 / 闭经 Oligomenorrhoea/amenorrhoea	
多毛 / 痤疮 Hirsutism/acne	雄激素产生异常 Abnormal androgen production
肥胖 Obesity	
不孕 Infertility	
超声 – 卵巢 Ultrasound-ovaries	>8cm Size >8cm
多囊卵巢；卵巢内有 12 个或 12 个以上卵泡，直径 2～9mm，卵巢体积增大（>10ml） Polycystic ovaries; the presence of 12 or more follicles in either ovary measuring 2–9 mm in diameter and/or increased ovarian volume (>10 mL)	8 个直径<8mm 的液囊 8 ovarian cysts <8mm in diameter 卵巢间质回声 Echogenic ovarian stroma

16.2). PCOS is found in women with symptoms of androgen excess: in 90% of women with hirsutism and 80% of women with acne. Approximately 50% of women with the condition are overweight or obese.

多囊卵巢综合征最早是由美国妇科医生 Irving Stein 和 Michael Leventhal 于 1935 年描述的，他们注意到多囊卵巢、闭经和多毛症之间的联系。多囊卵巢症患者的卵巢明显增大，并含有多个（10～12 个及以上）、小的（<10mm）充满液体的结构，位于卵巢包膜下。

PCOS was first described by American gynaecologists Irving Stein and Michael Leventhal in 1935, who noticed the association between polycystic ovaries, amenorrhoea and hirsutism. The ovaries in PCOS appear enlarged and contain multiple (more than 10–12), small (less than 10 mm) fluid-filled structures just under the ovarian capsule.

这些是正常的小的窦性和闭锁性卵泡，不是真正的"囊肿"。与正常卵巢相比，它们的数量要多得多，但功能正常（图 16–18）。多囊的卵巢也有大量的卵巢间质增加，这可能导致内分泌功能异常。

These are small, normal antral and atretic follicles and are not true 'cysts'. They are present in much greater numbers than are present in the normal ovary, but they have the same functions as normal (Fig. 16.18). The polycystic ovary also has a greatly increased ovarian stroma, which may have abnormal endocrine properties.

超声检查发现多囊卵巢是很常见的，人群中约 25% 的女性会有这样的表现。这些女性中只有一小部分会患上多囊卵巢综合征（包括超声上的多囊卵巢外观，至少有高雄激素或排卵异常这两项中的一项）。

The presence of polycystic ovaries on ultrasound is very common, and around 25% of women in the population may have such appearances. Only a small proportion of these women will have the polycystic ovary syndrome (which comprises polycystic ovary appearances on ultrasound, associated with at least one of the androgenic or ovulation symptoms).

生化检查（图 16–19）表明 LH 水平异常升高，没有出现 LH 高峰。雌激素和 FSH 水平正常，因此 LH/FSH 比例升高。卵巢分泌睾酮、雄烯二酮和脱氢表雄酮可能增加。15% 的病例泌乳素水平增加。

Biochemical investigations (Fig. 16.19) indicate abnormally raised LH levels and absence of the LH surge. Oestrogen and FSH levels are normal and, as a result, there is an increase in the LH:FSH ratio. There may be increased ovarian secretion of testosterone, androstenedione and dehydroepiandrosterone. Prolactin levels are increased in 15% of cases.

①发病机制：PCOS 的确切病因尚不清楚，但有很强的遗传成分。主要障碍可能是雄激素生物合成异常和胰岛素抵抗。由于胰岛素抵抗和高脂血症，多囊卵巢综合征的女性很容易发展为非胰岛素依赖型糖尿病，而且患代谢综合征的风险更高。

Pathogenesis. The exact aetiology of PCOS is unknown, but there is a strong genetic component. The primary disorder may be abnormalities in androgen biosynthesis and insulin resistance. As a result of insulin resistance and hyperlipidaemia, women with PCOS are prone to developing non-insulin-dependent diabetes and are at greater risk of metabolic

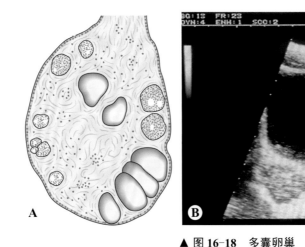

▲ 图 16-18　多囊卵巢

A. 卵巢包膜增厚，卵巢皮质内有许多小囊肿；B. 超声显示双侧卵巢呈斑点状，以多发小囊肿为特征

Fig. 16.18　Polycystic ovaries.

(A) The capsule of the ovary is thickened and there are numerous small cysts in the ovarian cortex. (B) Ultrasound showing mottled appearance of both ovaries characteristic of multiple small cysts.

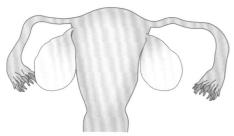

LH↑	LH ↑
LH surge absent	LH 极度缺乏
Δ^4-androstenedione↑	雄烯二酮 ↑
Dehydroepiandrosterone↑	脱氢表雄酮 ↑
Normal oestradiol levels	正常雌二醇水平
Normal FSH levels	正常 FSH 水平

▲ 图 16-19　Stein-Leventhal 综合征的生化特征

FSH. 促卵泡激素；LH. 促黄体激素

Fig. 16.19　Biochemical features of Stein-Leventhal syndrome.

FSH, Follicle-stimulating hormone; LH, luteinizing hormone.

syndrome.

许多患有 PCOS 的女性都有严重的肥胖。过量的雄激素中会抑制 FSH 的释放，并可能导致卵巢的"多囊"变化。雄激素的主要来源可能是卵巢和（或）肾上腺。一种来源于肾上腺的类固醇——硫酸脱氢表雄酮，在高达 50% 的 PCOS 患者中升高。

Many women with PCOS have substantial obesity. Inappropriate exposure of antral follicles to excessive concentrations of androgens results in inhibition of FSH release and may result in the 'polycystic' changes in the ovaries. The primary source of androgens may be both the ovary and/or the adrenals. The excretion of dehydroepiandrosterone sulphate-an exclusively adrenal steroid-is elevated in up to 50% of all women with PCOS.

PCOS 中由卵巢产生的主要雄激素包括睾酮和雄烯二酮。胰岛素和胰岛素样生长因子会显著增加它们的产量。它们不会被肾上腺激素抑制，但可以被 GnRH 激动剂抑制。在 PCOS 的女性中，有 10% 患者有 2 型糖尿病，30% 患者有糖耐量受损。

The principal androgens raised in PCOS and produced by the ovary include testosterone and androstenedione. Their production is significantly increased by insulin and insulinlike growth factors. They will not be suppressed by adrenal steroids but can be suppressed by GnRH agonists. About 10% of women with PCOS have type 2 diabetes, and 30% have impaired glucose tolerance.

②诊断：诊断（和定义标准）还存在争议。在鹿特丹国际共识会议提出的 PCOS 的定义如下，并被广泛采用。

符合以下三项中任意两项均可确诊。

a. 排卵稀发或停止排卵。

b. 高雄激素症（生化或临床）。

c. 超声检查多囊卵巢。

Diagnosis. Diagnosis (and criteria for the definition) is controversial. An international consensus meeting in Rotterdam proposed the following definition of PCOS, which has been widely adopted.

Any two of the following there are sufficion of contirm the diagnosis:

1. Oligoovulation or anovulation

2. Hyperandrogenism (biochemical or clinical)

3. Polycystic ovaries on ultrasound examination

6. 子宫的原因（Uterine causes）

手术切除子宫会导致继发性闭经。其他造成子宫内膜瘢痕并导致宫腔粘连和月经中断的情况包括肺结核和 Asherman 综合征。后一种情况大多发生在胎盘部分残留、粘连引起产后出血而行刮宫术；锐器刮宫已经破坏了子宫内膜的全层；并伴有低级别子宫内膜感染。

Surgical removal of the uterus will result in secondary amenorrhoea. Other conditions that scar the endometrium and cause intrauterine adhesions and loss of menses include infection from tuberculosis and Asherman's syndrome. The latter occurs mostly following dilatation and sharp curettage procedures for postpartum haemorrhage with retained, adherent placental fragments; where there has been damage to the full depth of endometrium by the sharp curettage; and where there is concurrent low-grade endometrial infection.

7. 隐经（字面意思为"隐藏的月经"）[Crypto-menorrhoea (literally 'hidden menstruation')]

外科手术或感染引起的宫颈狭窄引起经血流出受阻。

Cervical stenosis from surgical procedures or infection can cause blockage of menses through obstruction of outflow.

（二）闭经或月经稀发女性的检查（Investigations in women with amenorrhoea or oligomenorrhoea）

应该一直考虑妊娠的可能性，如果有必要，通过妊娠试验排除。病史应包括近期情绪压力、体重变化、更年期症状和目前药物治疗的细节。虽然体重指数（BMI）小于 $19kg/m^2$ 可能与体重相关的闭经有关，但大多数病例在临床检查中未发现异常。在缺乏甲状腺或肾上腺疾病的临床证据情况下，很难发现生化证据。

The possibility of pregnancy should always be considered and, if necessary, excluded by pregnancy test. The history should include details of recent emotional stress, changes in weight, menopausal symptoms and current medication. In the majority of cases, nothing abnormal is found on clinical examination, although a body mass index (BMI) of less than 19kg/m² is likely to be associated with weight-related amenorrhoea. In the absence of clinical evidence of thyroid or adrenal diseases, it is unusual to find biochemical evidence.

鉴别诊断是通过测定 FSH、LH、催乳素、雌二醇和甲状腺功能测试（thyroid function test，TFT）。盆腔超声可提供多囊卵巢综合征、卵巢肿瘤和下生殖道异常的额外证据。现在，通常不做常规的垂体窝成像，除非有泌乳素升高或一些不寻常的病史特征提示其他颅内病变。如果需要这样的成像，现在通常推荐 MRI。

The differential diagnosis is established by the measurement of FSH and LH, prolactin, oestradiol and thyroid function tests (TFTs). A pelvic ultrasound can provide additional evidence of PCOS, ovarian tumours and abnormalities of the lower genital tract. Nowadays, it is not usual to do routine imaging of the pituitary fossa, unless there is an elevated prolactin or some unusual features in the history suggesting other intracranial pathology. If such imaging is needed, MRI is now usually recommended.

> **！注意**
> 所有性行为活跃女性，在月经延迟或没有月经，甚至月经淋漓不尽时，都应排除妊娠。
> Pregnancy should be excluded in all women who are sexually active and who present with delayed or absent menses, even of long-standing menses.

黄体酮撤退试验有时用于诊断，每天给予醋酸甲羟孕酮 10mg，连续 5 天，在完成疗程后 2～7 天会产生撤退性出血。这是雌激素存在的体内生物测定。阳性检测表明子宫功能正常，子宫内膜完整，宫颈通畅，且循环雌激素水平足够。现在，血清雌二醇水平的现代测量足以提供这一证据。

The progesterone challenge test, in which medroxyprogesterone acetate 10 mg daily for 5 days is administered, should produce withdrawal bleeding 2–7 days after completing the course and is sometimes used as a diagnostic tool. This is really an in vivo bioassay of oestrogen presence. A positive test indicates a functional uterus with an intact endometrium and a patent outflow tract where circulating levels of oestrogen are adequate. Modern measurement of serum oestradiol levels is now usually

sufficient to provide this evidence.

（三）治疗（Management）

治疗方法取决于病因。除生理性外，大多数病例起源于下丘脑或 PCOS。大多数的这些症状最终会自动消失，而减肥是主要的潜在因素，重点应该是恢复正常的体重。然而，雌二醇水平较低，在某些情况下给予周期性的雌激素 – 孕激素治疗是有用的。

The treatment depends on the cause. Outside the 'physiological' group, the majority of cases are hypothalamic or PCOS in origin. Most of these will eventually resolve spontaneously, and where weight loss is the main underlying factor, the emphasis should be on restoring normal body mass. However, oestradiol levels are low, and in some cases it is useful to administer cyclical oestrogen-progestogen therapy.

停止使用任何多巴胺抑制药物或使用多巴胺激动药（如卡麦角林、溴隐亭或喹高利特）治疗，高催乳素血症通常会有所缓解。PCOS 治疗取决于哪一种症状最突出。生活方式的改变，其中包括减肥和锻炼，是基础，只要体重减少 5%，就可以改善月经模式、内分泌状况和生育能力。

Hyperprolactinaemia will usually respond to stopping any dopamine-inhibiting drugs or to treatment with dopamine agonists such as cabergoline, bromocriptine or quinagolide. Treatment for PCOS depends on which of the presenting symptoms predominate. Lifestyle changes, including weight loss and exercise, are the cornerstone, and a loss of as little as 5% in weight can improve the menstrual pattern, endocrine profile and fertility.

多毛症可通过局部使用脱毛辅助设备和电解治疗，周期性使用醋酸环丙孕酮并联合一种雌激素（如炔雌醇）对多毛症、痤疮和脱发有效。如果问题主要是不孕不育，那么可以使用克罗米芬或尿促性素刺激排卵。15%～40% 的 PCOS 女性存在克罗米酚抵抗，这可能是由其对子宫内膜和宫颈黏液的抗雌激素作用引起。二线治疗以前包括腹腔镜卵巢打孔，即多次刺破卵巢表面，但早期证据表明芳香化酶抑制剂的使用可能比手术干预更有效。口服降糖药、胰岛素增敏药二甲双胍在某些情况下似乎也有效。PCOS 的长期后遗症需要考虑。长期的无对抗的雌激素作用可能导致子宫内膜增生，这可能很少发生恶变。在使用孕激素如炔诺酮或醋酸甲羟孕酮后，增生通常会消退。PCOS 与代谢紊乱有关，并定期检测晚发型（2 型）糖尿病和血脂异常的进展。

Hirsutism can be treated by the local use of depilatory

aids and electrolysis, but the presence of hirsutism, acne and alopecia may also respond to antiandrogens such as cyproterone acetate combined with an oestrogen such as ethinylestradiol given on a cyclical basis. If the problem is primarily one of subfertility, then clomiphene citrate or carefully monitored human menopausal gonadotrophin can be used to stimulate ovulation. Approximately 15–40% of women with PCOS have clomiphene resistance, which may result from its antioestrogenic effects on the endometrium and cervical mucus. Second-line treatment has previously involved laparoscopic ovarian drilling, whereby the ovarian surface is punctured multiple times, but early evidence suggests the use of aromatase inhibitors may be more effective than surgical intervention. Medical management with the oral hypoglycaemic, insulin-sensitizing agent metformin also appears to be effective in some cases. The long-term sequelae of PCOS need to be considered. Prolonged unopposed oestrogen action may result in the development of endometrial hyperplasia, which may rarely undergo malignant change. Hyperplasia will often regress following the administration of a progestational agent, such as norethisterone or medroxyprogesterone acetate. PCOS is associated with metabolic disturbances, and regular testing for the development of late-onset (type 2) diabetes and lipid abnormalities should occur.

八、痛经（Dysmenorrhoea）

痛经，或者月经疼痛，是所有妇科症状中最常见的。它的特征通常是腹痛，从出血开始，在月经的前 1～5 天最明显。

Dysmenorrhoea, or painful menstruation, is the commonest of all gynaecological symptoms. It is usually characterized as colicky pain that starts with the onset of bleeding and is maximal in the first 1–5 days of the period.

原发性痛经发生在没有任何显著的盆腔疾病的情况下，是由于子宫内膜局部前列腺素（特别是 PGF2α）释放，导致子宫肌收缩过度引起的子宫缺血。通常在月经初潮后 6 个月至 2 年有排卵的周期中发生，通常在初潮早的年轻女性中发作得更频繁或更严重。

Primary dysmenorrhoea occurs in the absence of any significant pelvic pathology and is caused by excessive myometrial contractions producing uterine ischaemia in response to local release of prostaglandins (especially $PGF_{2\alpha}$) from the endometrium. It often begins with the onset of ovulatory cycles between 6 months and 2 years after the menarche, and it may occur more frequently or be more severe in young women whose periods start at an early age.

家庭成员往往有痛经史，母亲自己的经历会影响女儿对自己病情的认知。一些女性的疼痛可能会

很严重，剧烈的痉挛可能与恶心、呕吐、腹泻和头晕有关，这可能使其丧失行为能力并对其社会活动造成重大干扰。

There is often a family history of painful periods, and the mother's own experience can impact on the daughter's perception of her condition. The pain may be severe in some women, and the intense cramping can be associated with nausea, vomiting, diarrhoea and dizziness, which can be incapacitating and cause a major disruption to social activities.

疼痛通常只发生在有排卵的周期，位于下腹部和盆腔，但有时放射到大腿前部。通常在第一个孩子出生后疼痛消失或改善。盆腔检查未见异常。

The pain usually only occurs in ovulatory cycles and is lower abdominal and pelvic in nature but sometimes radiates down the anterior aspect of the thighs. Commonly the pain disappears or improves after the birth of the first child. Pelvic examination reveals no abnormality.

继发性或获得性痛经与某些盆腔疾病有关，通常（但并非总是）在月经初潮后某时发病。痛觉通常在月经开始前几天出现，并可能持续整个月经期。它往往是沉重的，牵扯性（通常称为充血性），可能放射到背部，腰部和腿部。

Secondary or acquired dysmenorrhoea occurs in association with some form of pelvic pathology and usually, but not always, has its onset sometime after menarche. The pain typically precedes the start of the period by several days and may last throughout the period. It tends to be of a heavy, dragging nature (often called congestive) and may radiate to the back, loins and legs.

继发性痛经可由子宫内膜异位症、肌瘤、子宫腺肌症、盆腔感染、粘连和发育异常引起。子宫内膜异位症疼痛往往开始于青春期严重的痛经，不应忽视这一潜在的诊断。

Secondary dysmenorrhoea may occur as a result of endometriosis, fibroids, adenomyosis, pelvic infections, adhesions and developmental anomalies. Endometriosis pain often begins with severe dysmenorrhoea in adolescence, and this potential diagnosis should not be overlooked.

如果青春期的"痛经"症状不常见或初始治疗无效，应高度怀疑子宫内膜异位症的存在。由于缺乏对子宫内膜异位症的相关医学认识，在青春期发病的子宫内膜异位症患者通常会延迟诊断（超过 10～12 年）。

A high degree of suspicion of the presence of endometriosis should be entertained if the features of 'dysmenorrhoea' in adolescence are unusual or do not respond to initial therapies. There is commonly a major delay (of more than 10–12 years) in making a diagnosis of endometriosis in those women in whom the symptom onset is in adolescence because of lack of medical awareness of this association.

（一）检查（Investigations）

仔细询问病史很重要，要注意发作的时间、疼痛的特点和相关症状，如性交痛和排尿痛。对于那些从未有过性活动的原发性痛经女性，应避免进行盆腔检查。应该个体化评估是否要做阴道检查，考虑到性行为和需要进行子宫颈涂片检查。原发性痛经的女性，阴道检查通常无盆腔压痛或任何异常。

A careful history is important with attention to the timing of the onset and characteristics of pain and associated symptoms, such as dyspareunia and dysuria. Pelvic examination is to be avoided in those women with primary dysmenorrhoea who have never been sexually active. The decision to perform a vaginal examination should be individually assessed, taking into account sexual activity and the need for a Pap smear. In women with primary dysmenorrhoea, there is usually no pelvic tenderness or any abnormality on vaginal examination.

在继发性痛经中，盆腔检查对评估包括子宫和附件的压痛、肿块和子宫活动度，以及后穹隆和宫颈摇摆痛是必要的。盆腔感染时应使用棉签取样，并行盆腔超声检查。

In secondary dysmenorrhoea, a pelvic examination is essential to assess uterine and adnexal tenderness, masses and uterine mobility, as well as the posterior fornix and cervical movement pain. Swabs should be taken for pelvic infection and a pelvic ultrasound organized.

虽然经阴道超声对子宫肌瘤是一个很好的检查方法，但对子宫腺肌症则不太可靠，通常也不能发现子宫内膜异位症，除非有子宫内膜异位囊肿或深部病变形成。有持续性或进行性疼痛症状且对药物治疗不缓解的患者需要腹腔镜检查。

Although transvaginal ultrasound is a good investigation for fibroids, it is less reliable for adenomyosis and will not commonly detect endometriosis, unless an endometrioma or deep lesion is present. Laparoscopy is required for women with persistent or progressive pain symptoms that are unresponsive to medical therapies.

（二）治疗（Management）

解释月经疼痛的原因是有帮助的，在适当的情况下，确保没有引起疼痛的潜在疾病。临床医生应采取全面的方法，注意饮食和生活方式因素，以及药物治疗。

An explanation of the causes of menstrual pain is helpful and, where appropriate, reassurance that there is no underlying pathology. Clinicians should adopt a holistic approach with attention to diet and lifestyle factors, as well as to medical therapies.

有充分的证据表明吸烟会增加痛经，也有一些证据表明运动是有益的。在小腹上使用热敷可以缓解疼痛，一些膳食补充剂也被研究过，如维生素 B_1 被认为是一种有效的治疗方法。

There is good evidence that smoking increases dysmenorrhoea and some evidence that exercise can be beneficial. Using a heat pack on the lower abdomen anecdotally provides relief, and several dietary supplements have been investigated, with vitamin B_1 indicated to be a helpful treatment.

药物治疗（Pharmacological）

非甾体抗炎药（NSAID）是治疗痛经最常用的药物，因为它能抑制前列腺素的合成。这些药物包括阿司匹林、甲芬钠酸、萘普生或布洛芬。非甾体抗炎药治疗 3 个月经周期无效的青少年和年轻人应该在接下来的 3 个月经周期内加用复方口服避孕药（非甾体抗炎药治疗可以继续）。

NSAIDs are the most commonly used drugs for the treatment of dysmenorrhoea due to their inhibition of prostaglandin synthesis. These drugs include aspirin, mefenamic acid, naproxen or ibuprofen. Adolescents and young adults with symptoms that do not respond to treatment with NSAIDs within three menstrual periods should be offered a combined oral contraceptive pill for the next three menstrual cycles (the NSAID therapy can be continued).

复方口服避孕药除了抑制排卵外，还能减少子宫前列腺素的释放。它可以持续使用以减少症状发生的频率。也可采用单一孕激素治疗方法，如醋酸甲羟孕酮注射、皮下植入和左炔诺孕酮宫内节育系统。对这些治疗无效的青少年和年轻人应评估其潜在的结构原因或感染原因。

The combined oral contraceptive pill, in addition to suppressing ovulation, reduces uterine prostaglandin release. It can be used in a continuous manner to reduce symptom frequency. Progestogen-only methods such as depo-medroxyprogesterone acetate injections, subdermal implants and the levonorgestrel intrauterine system can also be used. Adolescents and young adults who do not respond to these treatments should be evaluated for an underlying structural or infective cause.

在继发性痛经的病例中，治疗取决于相关的疾病性质。强化药物治疗可能有帮助，但也可能需要与手术相结合。如果病情不能接受药物治疗，有时只能通过子宫切除和切除相关病灶（如子宫腺肌症或子宫内膜异位症）来缓解症状。

In cases of secondary dysmenorrhoea, the treatment is dependent on the nature of the associated pathology. Intensive medical therapies may assist, but may also need to be combined with surgery. If the condition is not amenable to medical therapy, occasionally the symptoms may only be relieved by hysterectomy and excision of the associated pathology (such as adenomyosis or endometriosis).

九、经前期综合征（Premenstrual syndrome）

经前期综合征（premenstrual syndrome，PMS）的定义是反复出现的中度心理和生理症状，发生在月经周期的黄体期，并随着月经出血开始消退。约 20% 的育龄女性患有此病。经前焦虑障碍（premenstrual dysphoric disorder，PMDD）是更严重的类型，女性会经历身体、心理和行为方面的症状，严重到足以扰乱其社会、家庭或职业生活。

Premenstrual syndrome (PMS) is defined as recurrent moderate psychological and physical symptoms that occur during the luteal phase of the menstrual cycle and resolve with the onset of bleeding. It affects around 20% of reproductive-age women. In the more severe form, premenstrual dysphoric disorder (PMDD), women experience somatic, psychological and behavioural symptoms severe enough to disrupt social, family or occupational life.

（一）症状和体征（Symptoms and signs）

表 16-2 列出了与经前期综合征和经前焦虑障碍相关的症状。

The symptoms associated with PMS and PMDD are listed in Table 16.2.

表 16-2　经前期综合征或经前焦虑障碍女性最常表现的生理和心理症状

Table 16.2　The most commonly expressed physical and psychological symptoms in women suffering from PMS or PMDD

身体的 Physical	精神的 Psychological
腹部肿胀 Abdominal bloating	愤怒、烦躁 Anger, irritability
身体疼痛 Body pains	焦虑 Anxiety
乳房压痛或胀痛 Breast tenderness or fullness	食欲的变化（食欲增加，对食物的渴望） Changes in appetite (increased appetite, food cravings)
腹部疼痛和痉挛 Abdominal pain and cramps	性欲的变化 Changes in libido
疲劳 Tiredness	注意力下降 Decreased concentration
头痛 Headaches	情绪抑郁 Depressed mood
恶心 Nausea	失去控制的感觉 Feelings of loss of control
外周水肿 Peripheral oedema	情绪波动 Mood swings
体重增加 Weight gain	睡眠不好 Poor sleep
	退出社会和工作活动 Withdrawal from social and work activities

PMDD. 经前焦虑障碍；PMS. 经前期综合征

PMDD, Premenstrual dysphoric disorder; *PMS,* premenstrual syndrome.

（二）发病机制（Pathogenesis）

PMS 和 PMDD 的病因尚不清楚，但女性似乎对循环中的雌激素和黄体酮水平的变化更加"生理上"的敏感，并可能改变了中枢神经递质功能，特别是血清素。

The aetiology of PMS and PMDD is not known, but women appear to be more 'physiologically' sensitive to changes in circulating levels of oestrogen and progesterone, and may have altered central neurotransmitter function, particularly for serotonin.

（三）治疗（Management）

临床病史是诊断的关键，正确的诊断最好是通过要求女性前瞻性地收集详细的月经日记，最好超过两个周期的症状。这将辨别是否有可能提示其他医学或心理障碍的非黄体症状。治疗的目标是缓解症状，其中包括非药物和药物选择。

Clinical history is the key to diagnosis, and the correct diagnosis is best established by asking women to prospectively collect a detailed menstrual diary of their symptoms ideally over two cycles. This will clarify whether there are non-luteal symptoms that may suggest other medical or psychological disorders. The goal of treatment is relief of symptoms and involves both non-pharmacological and pharmacological options.

通常推荐的非药物疗法是增加锻炼，减少咖啡因和精制糖类的摄入量，但几乎没有证据支持这些行为。已研究过一些膳食补充剂，大量摄入钙和维生素 D 的女性少见 PMS 症状。

Non-pharmacological options frequently recommended are increasing exercise and reducing caffeine and refined carbohydrate intake, but there is little evidence to support these. A number of dietary supplements have been studied, and women with high intakes of calcium and vitamin D are less likely to have PMS symptoms.

维生素 B_6 和月见草油是治疗经前期综合征的常用处方。维生素 B_6（吡哆醇）是神经递质合成的辅助因子。虽然没有证据表明在 PMS 中真正缺乏这些物质，但最大的对照研究显示相比安慰剂的有效率为 70%，维生素 B_6 的有效率为 82%。有报道在高剂量时存在周围神经病变，但 100mg 的剂量可能是安全的。

Vitamin B_6 and evening primrose oil are frequently self-prescribed for PMS. Vitamin B_6 (pyridoxine) is a co-factor in neurotransmitter synthesis. Although there is no evidence of any actual deficit of these substances in PMS, the largest controlled study showed an 82% response rate to vitamin B6 compared to 70% on placebo. Peripheral neuropathy has been reported at high doses, but a dose of 100 mg is probably safe.

月见草油含有前列腺素的不饱和脂肪酸前体。有一些证据表明可改善某些症状，但推荐剂量每天 8 粒胶囊是难以维持的。抗前列腺素镇痛药（如布洛芬）可能对乳房疼痛和头痛有用。

Evening primrose oil contains the unsaturated fatty acid precursors of prostaglandins. There is some evidence of improvement in selected symptoms, but the recommended dose of eight capsules a day is difficult to sustain. Anti-prostaglandin painkillers, such as ibuprofen, may be useful for breast pain and headaches.

利尿药（如螺内酯）可能对少数经历了真性水潴留的女性有益，但应该只用于有明显体重增加的腹胀症状。蓖麻果的干提取物（20mg/d）也可以有效缓解烦躁、情绪变化、头痛和乳房胀痛的症状。认知行为疗法，虽然对其他情感障碍有用，但没有证据支持其在 PMD 或 PMDD 中的应用。

Diuretics such as spironolactone may be of benefit in the small group of women who experience true water retention but should only be used for symptoms of bloating where there is measurable weight gain. The dry extract of the *Agnus castus* fruit (20 mg daily) may also be effective in reducing symptoms of irritability, mood change, headache and breast fullness. Cognitive behaviour therapy, although useful for other affective disorders, has no evidence to support its use in PMD or PMDD.

药理（Pharmacological）

治疗严重 PMS 和 PMDD 的一线药物是选择性 5-羟色胺再摄取抑制药（SSRI）或 5-羟色胺和去甲肾上腺素再摄取抑制剂（SNRI）。这些药物（如舍曲林、西酞普兰和氟西汀）每日服用或在周期的黄体期服用，与安慰剂相比，已发现能显著减轻 PMS 的生理和心理症状。

The first-line medications for severe PMS and PMDD are the selective serotonin reuptake inhibitors (SSRIs) or the serotonin-norepinephrine reuptake inhibitors (SNRIs). These medications, such as sertraline, citalopram and fluoxetine, taken either daily or during the luteal phase of the cycle, have been found to significantly reduce the physical and psychological symptoms of PMS compared to placebo.

在服用药物的几周内通常可见对 PMS 的积极影响，但如果有相关的抑郁症，情绪改善可能需要 1 个月。

The positive impact on PMS is often seen within a few weeks of taking the medication, but improvement in mood, if there is associated depression, may take up to a month to improve.

复方口服避孕药通常用于治疗 PMS，但没有数据支持其有效性，除了一些关于含有抗利尿特性的孕激素药物的研究。几项研究表明，含有屈螺酮（一种螺内酯衍生物）的药丸，24 天 1 包，在减少 PMS 症状方面比安慰剂效果更好。此外，连续服用这些药片（每天服用激素片，不间断服用）比常规服用 28 天、间断 7 天的方法更有益。

The combined oral contraceptive pill has been commonly used to treat PMS, but there are no data to support its effectiveness, with the exception of some studies of pills containing progestogens with antidiuretic properties. Several studies suggest that pills containing drospirenone, a spironolactone derivative, in a 24-day pack are better than placebo in reducing the symptoms of PMS. Further, taking the pills in a continuous manner (hormone tablets every day without a break) is beneficial compared with taking a conventional 28-day pill with 7-day break.

GnRH 激动药在治疗过程中抑制卵巢功能并缓解症状。然而，当治疗停止时，这些症状会复发。因为成本和不良反应（包括绝经症状和骨质疏松症）而不适合长期使用。

GnRH agonists suppress ovarian function and relieve symptoms during treatment. However, these recur when treatment is stopped. They are unsuitable for long-term use because of their cost and adverse side effects, including menopausal symptoms and osteoporosis.

十、青春期的异常（Disorders of puberty）

（一）青春期、月经初潮（Puberty and menarche）

青春期代表着显著的生长和深刻的激素改变，这将导致身体发育成成人，以及在大多数情况下具有生育能力。还需要注意的是，这些变化通常与教育、社会和身体挑战同时发生。

Puberty represents a period of significant growth and profound hormonal changes that will lead to the development of an adult body and in the majority of cases the ability to reproduce. It needs also to be noted that these changes are usually occurring contemporaneously with educational, social and physical challenges.

性早熟或青春期发育延迟可能给年轻女孩或女性及其家人带来额外的社会心理困难。临床医生需要对这些问题敏感，任何治疗干预的目标都是减轻痛苦，同时最大化生长、发育和未来生育的潜力。

Precocious or delayed puberty may present the young girl or woman and her family with added psychosocial difficulties. The clinician needs to be sensitive to these issues, with the goal of any therapeutic intervention being to alleviate distress while maximizing potentials for growth, development and future fertility.

正常的青春期发育发生在一个有序的过程，涉及第二性征的获得，与快速生长有关，最终获得生殖能力。这一过程是由下丘脑以脉冲式分泌的 GnRH 数量的增加开始的，但这一事件的确切触发机制尚不清楚。

Normal pubertal development occurs in an ordered sequence and involves acquisition of secondary sex characteristics associated with a rapid increase in growth that culminates in reproductive capability. The process is initiated by increased amounts of GnRH secreted in a pulsatile manner from the hypothalamus, but the exact trigger of this event is not known.

脉冲式 GnRH 的释放导致垂体激素的释放，即 LH 和 FSH。前者刺激卵巢中雄烯二酮的产生，后者刺激雌二醇的合成。这种脉冲最初是夜间的，最终变成白天的。

The release of pulsatile GnRH leads to release of the pituitary hormones, i.e. LH and FSH. The former stimulates androstenedione production in the ovary, and the latter stimulates oestradiol synthesis. The pulses are initially nocturnal, becoming eventually diurnal.

与此同时，脑垂体分泌的生长激素的幅度也增加了。雄激素和雌激素都可以调节这种幅度。已证明性类固醇激素可以直接刺激骨骼生长。

At the same time there is an increase in amplitude of growth hormone from the pituitary. Both androgens and oestrogens may regulate this amplification. Sex steroids have also been shown to stimulate skeletal growth directly.

女性青春期的特征是加速线性生长，乳房发育（乳房萌发）、腋毛和阴毛生长（肾上腺功能初现），以及最终月经开始来潮，即月经初潮（图 16-20 和图 16-21）。一般来说，这些阶段都是依次向前发展的。

Puberty in females is characterized by accelerated linear growth, development of breasts, thelarche, axillary and pubic hair, adrenarche and eventual onset of menses, i.e. menarche (Figs 16.20 and 16.21). Generally, there is a forward progression through these stages.

然而，也会发生一些变化，如过早乳房萌发或肾上腺功能早现。一旦雌激素达到对下丘脑形成正反馈并建立排卵周期的水平，青春期就结束了。整

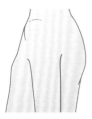 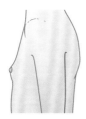 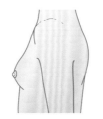 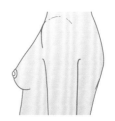 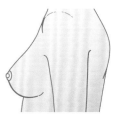

| Infantile breast 婴儿乳房 | Breast bud 乳芽 | Breast and areola enlarged 乳房和乳晕增大 | Nipple and areola enlarged 乳头和乳晕增大 | Adult breast 成人乳房 |

▲ 图 16-20　乳房萌发时期女性乳房的发育

Fig. 16.20　Development of the female breast during thelarche.

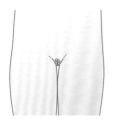 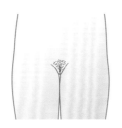 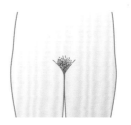 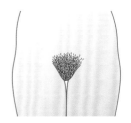

| Labia：sparse 阴唇：稀疏 | Symphysis pubis spread 耻骨联合展开 | Adult appearance：incomplete 成人外观：不完整 | Adult triangle distribution 成人三角分布 |

▲ 图 16-21　从肾上腺功能初现到完全性成熟期间的阴毛分布

Fig. 16.21　Pubic hair distribution leading up to full sexual maturation during adrenarche.

个过程的长度变化在 18 个月至 6 年。

However, several variations can occur such as premature thelarche or adrenarche. Puberty is complete once oestrogen rises to the level where positive feedback occurs on the hypothalamus and ovulatory cycles establish. The entire process is seen to vary in length considerably being between 18 months and 6 years.

Tanner 和 Davies 于 20 世纪 80 年代对北美女孩进行的纵向研究中记录了青春期的时间。他们发现，乳房萌芽发生在平均年龄 10.7 岁，标准偏差(standard deviation，SD) 为 1 岁，月经初潮发生在 12.7 岁（SD 1.3 岁）。乳房发育早于平均年龄 2.5SD，或在 8 岁以下发育定义为性早熟。

The timing of puberty was documented in longitudinal studies of North American girls performed by Tanner and Davies in the 1980s. Their studies found that breast budding occurred at the average age of 10.7 years with a standard deviation (SD) of 1 year and menarche at 12.7 (SD 1.3) years. The onset of breast development more than 2.5 SD from the mean or occurring in girls under the age of 8 is defined as precocious.

青春期发动的年龄受种族、家族史和营养的影响。有一段时间，Frisch 和 Revelle 在 20 世纪 70 年代提出了"临界体重"的假说，约 45kg 是刺激青春

期发育的必要条件。

The age at onset of puberty is seen to be influenced by race, family history and nutrition. It was felt for some time that a critical weight, as postulated in the 1970s by Frisch and Revelle, of approximately 45 kg was necessary to stimulate pubertal development.

这表明脂肪组织自身可能与青春期发动有关。然而，这一观点并没有得到后续研究的支持，身高、体重和青春期发育之间的关系明显更为复杂。尽管最近有更多的研究表明，青春期开始的平均年龄在下降，这可能是由肥胖率的上升引起的，但经典的青春期的定义并没有改变。

This suggested that fat tissue itself was responsible. However, this view has not been upheld by subsequent studies, and the relationship between height, weight and pubertal development is significantly more complex. Although more recent studies have suggested that the average age of onset of puberty is declining, possibly triggered by increasing rates of obesity, the definition of precious puberty has not changed.

(1) 乳房萌发（Thelarche）：

乳腺组织的发育始于乳晕下的乳腺芽，并在最初无对抗雌二醇的影响下发生。大约 80% 的女孩的青春期开始于乳房发育，其余的则首先经历肾上腺

功能初现。

Breast tissue development begins with a subareolar breast bud and occurs under the influence of initially unopposed oestradiol. Puberty begins with breast development in approximately 80% of girls, with the others experiencing adrenarche first.

(2) 肾上腺功能初现（Adrenarche）：

肾上腺雄激素的正常产生大约发生在阴毛初现，即青春期发动前 1~2 年。肾上腺功能初现不依赖于性腺功能初现、性腺成熟和性激素的分泌，但是先于性腺功能初现发生。

The normal onset of adrenal androgen production occurs approximately 1–2 years before pubarche, the onset of puberty. Adrenarche is independent of gonadarche, the maturation of the gonads and the secretion of sex steroids, but occurs prior.

(3) 月经初潮（Menarche）：

生殖成熟始于月经的开始。在英国，平均年龄为 12—13 岁。月经初潮通常发生在生长速度达到峰值之后。在最初的 6~18 个月里，月经周期通常不规律，因为排卵不频繁。

Reproductive maturity occurs with the onset of menstruation. In the UK, the average age is 12–13 years. Menarche usually occurs after the peak in growth velocity. The menstrual cycle is often irregular in the first 6–18 months as ovulation can initially be infrequent.

(4) 生长突增（Growth spurt）：

生长速度加快先于或与青春期发育同时发生。生长突增发生在 9.5—14.5 岁，依赖于生长激素和性腺类固醇。首先是腿部变长，其次是肩宽和躯干长度的增加。骨盆增大并改变形状。大多数女孩在乳房萌发后 2 年和月经初潮前 1 年左右达到最大生长速度。在 17—18 岁，股骨骨骺融合，身高达最大。

The acceleration in the rate of growth accompanies or precedes pubertal development. The onset of the growth spurt occurs between 9.5 and 14.5 years and is dependent on growth hormone as well as gonadal steroids. The first development is lengthening of legs followed by increase in shoulder breadth and trunk length. The pelvis enlarges and changes shape. Most girls reach maximum growth velocity approximately 2 years after thelarche and 1 year prior to menarche. Maximal height is reached between 17 and 18 years with fusion of the femoral epiphyses.

1. 性早熟（Precocious puberty）

对女孩来说，性早熟的定义是在 8 岁前出现青春期体征。因为乳腺组织对雌激素的反应比子宫内膜快，所以通常从过早乳房萌发发育到月经初潮。

In girls, precocious puberty is defined as the development of the physical signs of puberty before the age of 8 years. It usually progresses from premature thelarche to menarche because breast tissue responds faster to oestrogen than does the endometrium.

将可能性早熟的原因分为中枢原因，即 GnRH 依赖性，以及外周原因，即非 GnRH 依赖性。大多数病例没有病理基础。在 4 岁以上的女孩中，较少发现具体原因，大多数为特发性（80%）。年龄 4 岁以下以中枢神经系统（CNS）为主。

It is useful to categorize possible causes as central, i.e. dependent on GnRH secretion, and peripheral, i.e. GnRH independent. The majority of cases do not have a pathological basis. In girls older than 4 years old, specific causes are less likely to be found, with the majority being idiopathic (80%). Below this age, central nervous system (CNS) causes predominate.

中枢性（GnRH 依赖性）性早熟的原因，按发生频率排序如下。

Central (GnRH dependent) in order of frequency:

- 特发性。
- idiopathic
- 中枢神经系统肿瘤。
- CNS tumours
- 脑积水。
- hydrocephaly
- 继发于创伤或感染的中枢神经系统损伤，近期或过去。
- CNS injury secondary to trauma or infection, recent or past
- 中枢神经系统辐照。
- CNS irradiation
- 神经纤维瘤病。
- neurofibromatosis

患有中枢性性早熟的患者 GnRH 释放不受调节。FSH 和 LH 水平波动性大，因此需要更多样本，以了解夜间分泌的倾向。GnRH 刺激试验显示青春期 LH 水平升高 3 倍，FSH 也上涨但程度较轻。在中枢性早熟的青春期，其进展遵循通常的模式，尽管更早。

Patients with central precocious puberty have unregulated GnRH release. FSH and LH levels fluctuate, so multiple samples may be required, remembering a propensity to nocturnal secretion. A GnRH stimulation test will show a pubertal, threefold response in LH levels. FSH also rises but to a lesser degree. In central precocious puberty the progression follows the usual pattern, albeit earlier.

外周或非 GnRH 依赖性原因如下。

Peripheral or GnRH independent causes:

- 肾上腺或卵巢分泌激素的肿瘤。

  - hormonal secreting tumour of the adrenal gland or ovaries

- 产生促性腺激素肿瘤。

  - gonadotrophin-producing tumours

- 先天性肾上腺增生症（非经典）。

  - congenital adrenal hyperplasia (non-classical)

- McCune–Albright 综合征。

  - McCune-Albright syndrome

- 甲状腺功能减退。

  - hypothyroidism

- 外源性雌激素。

  - exogenous oestrogens

- 卵巢滤泡性囊肿

  - follicular cysts of the ovary

(1) 评估（Evaluation）：

评估性早熟女孩的第一步是获得完整的家族史，包括父母和兄弟姐妹青春期开始的年龄。应记录父母双方的身高，并计算出孩子的预期身高（图 16-22）。

The first step in evaluating a girl with precocious puberty is to obtain a complete family history, including the age of onset of puberty in parents and siblings. The heights of both parents should be recorded and the projected height of the child calculated (Fig. 16.22).

青春期发育的历史需要与其他症状一起记录，如头痛或视觉障碍。病史、创伤史、手术史和用药史也与此相关。体格检查应包括记录 Tanner 分期和其他提示外周性病因的体征检查，如皮肤损害或卵巢肿块。必须寻找男性化的迹象，其中包括痤疮、多毛和阴蒂肿大。

The history of pubertal development needs to be

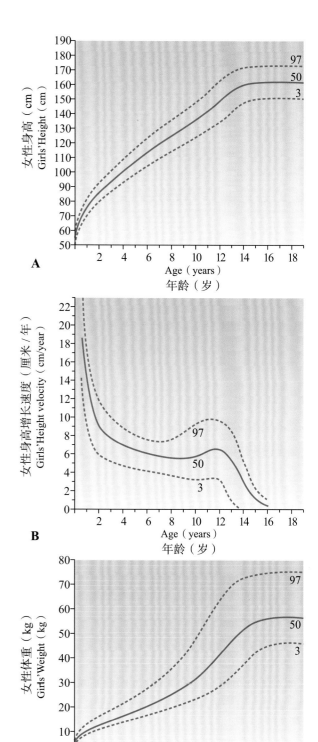

▲ 图 16-22　A. 女性身高的百分位数变化；B. 身高增长速度表明生长速度减缓，并在青春期前后出现二次加速；C. 体重的变化比身高的变化波动大

Fig. 16.22　(A) Centile change for height in the female. (B) Height velocity indicates the slowing down of the rate of growth with a secondary acceleration around the time of puberty. (C) Changes in weight show a wider scatter than with height.

documented along with other symptoms such as headache or visual disturbance. A history of illness, trauma, surgery and medications is also pertinent. Physical examination should include documentation of the Tanner stage and examination for other signs to indicate a peripheral cause, such as skin lesions or ovarian masses. Signs of virilization must be looked for, including acne, hirsutism and clitoromegaly.

(2) 检查（Investigations）：

确定性早熟的类型和缩小鉴别诊断范围是最重要的一步。血浆 FSH、LH 和雌二醇是必需的，TFT 也是。手部 X 线检查以确定骨龄很重要。体质性和脑性性早熟的骨龄提前，可能需要每隔 6 个月重复一次以确认成熟。

This is the most important step in determining which category of precocious puberty is responsible and narrowing the differential diagnosis. Plasma FSH, LH and oestradiol are essential, as is a TFT. X-ray of the hand to determine bone age is important. Bone age is advanced in the constitutional and cerebral forms and may need to be repeated at an interval of 6 months to confirm maturation.

应行腹部及骨盆超声检查，寻找肾上腺或卵巢肿瘤并建立正常解剖。卵巢在正常青春期、脑型和特发性性早熟表现为多囊卵巢。需要将滤泡囊肿与实性雌激素分泌性颗粒或卵泡膜细胞肿瘤区分开来。

Ultrasound of the abdomen and pelvis should be conducted, looking for adrenal or ovarian tumours and to establish normal anatomy. The ovary may show a multicystic appearance in normal puberty and in cerebral and idiopathic forms. Follicular cysts need to be distinguished from predominantly solid oestrogen-secreting granulosa or theca cell tumours.

长骨的放射学骨骼检查可能提示 McCune-Albright 综合征的溶骨性病变。如果结果与中枢性原因一致，则应安排头颅 CT 或 MRI，寻找蝶鞍异常、鞍上钙化等病变。

Radiological skeletal survey of the long bones may indicate osteolytic lesions of McCune-Albright syndrome. If results are consistent with a central cause, cranial CT or MRI should be arranged, looking for abnormalities of the sella turcica, suprasellar calcification and other lesions.

(3) 治疗（Management）：

治疗的关键目标是阻止甚至逆转青春期的体征，避免骨龄的快速发展，骨龄的快速发展可能导致最初的生长快于同龄人，但最终会导致过早的骨骺融合和比正常身材小。治疗中枢性进行性性早熟的主

要方法是 GnRH 激动剂，它使垂体脱敏，导致 LH 和 FSH 输出减少。这可能是每月注射 1 次或每 3 个月注射 1 次或鼻内制剂。一旦达到适当的年龄，药物就会停用，从而促进青春期的发育。

The key aims of treatment are to arrest and even reverse the physical signs of puberty and to avert the rapid development in bone age, which can result in initial growth advancement compared to peers but ultimately premature epiphyseal fusion and smaller-than-normal stature. The main treatment for central progressive precocious puberty is the GnRH agonist, which desensitizes the pituitary and leads to a reduction in LH and FSH output. This may be administered as monthly or trimonthly injections or as intranasal preparations. Once an appropriate chronological age is reached, the agent is withdrawn, allowing pubertal development to advance.

2. 正常青春期的变化（Variations on normal puberty）

(1) 肾上腺功能早现（Premature adrenarche）：

这是指 8 岁之前肾上腺雄激素的分泌。这通常是特发性和非进行性的。它通常表现为腋毛和（或）阴毛加上出现体味，有时痤疮和多毛症。重要的是要排除酶缺陷，如慢性肾上腺增生或雄激素分泌肿瘤，同时认识到大多数病例是自身限制性的。

This refers to the secretion of adrenal androgens before the age of 8 years. This frequently is idiopathic and nonprogressive. It presents usually with complaints of axillary hair and/or pubic hair plus the emergence of body odour, sometimes with acne and hirsutism. It is very important to exclude enzyme deficiencies, e.g. chronic adrenal hyperplasia or androgen-secreting tumours, while recognizing that the majority of cases will be self-limiting.

(2) 乳腺提前发育（Premature thelarche）：

该病的定义为 8 岁之前的乳房出芽，需要与性早熟区分开来，约有 10% 的患儿会发展为性早熟。它在婴儿中更常见，在这个群体中往往会自行消退。

Defined as breast budding prior to age 8 years, this condition needs to be differentiated from precocious puberty, as approximately 10% will progress. It is more common in infants and tends to resolve spontaneously in this group.

(3) 早熟的月经初潮（Precocious menarche）：

这是最不常见的变异，定义为无第二性征的周期性阴道出血。它可能是由于卵泡活动或子宫内膜敏感性升高引起的雌激素的短暂上升。仔细的病史是确定月经周期的必要条件，因为其他引起青春期前阴道出血的原因，包括感染、异物和肿瘤，都需

要排除。

This is the least common of the variants and is defined as cyclic vaginal bleeding without secondary sexual characteristics. It may be caused by a transitory rise in oestrogen as the result of follicular activity or a heightened endometrial sensitivity. A careful history is necessary to establish cyclicity, as other causes of prepubertal vaginal bleeding, including infection, foreign body and neoplasm, need exclusion.

3. 青春期延迟（Delayed puberty）

青春期延迟定义为女孩超过 13 岁乳腺没有发育。在 16 岁之前或青春期启动后 5 年内没有月经初潮也可作出诊断。大多数青春期延迟是体质性的，由下丘脑的 GnRH 分泌不足引起的。它也可能继发于慢性疾病，如神经性厌食症、哮喘、慢性肾脏疾病和炎症性肠病。需要排除解剖方面的病因，如流出道梗阻引起的阴道积血。以这种状态为特征的性腺机能减退可能与促性腺激素水平升高或降低同时发生。与性早熟一样，必须确定促性腺激素的状态以确定其原因（表 16-3）。

Delayed puberty is defined by the absence of breast development in girls beyond 13 years. The diagnosis is also made in the absence of menarche by age 16 or within 5 years after the onset of puberty. Mostly delayed puberty is constitutional, arising from inadequate GnRH from the hypothalamus. It may also be secondary to chronic illness such as anorexia nervosa, asthma, chronic renal disease and inflammatory bowel disease. Anatomical considerations such as outflow obstruction in haematocolpos need exclusion. The hypogonadism that characterizes this state may occur with both elevated and lowered levels of gonadotrophins. As with precocious puberty, it is essential to establish the status of the gonadotrophins to determine causation (Table 16.3).

（1）检查（Investigations）：

体格检查，注意身高、体重、BMI、Tanner 分期和生命体征，关注可能的病因，如 BMI 低和四肢寒冷，姿势下降提示可能的饮食失调。然而，实验室测试是辨别病因类别的关键。

Physical examination, noting height, weight, BMI, Tanner staging and vital signs, may draw attention to possible aetiologies such as low BMI and cold peripheries, with postural drop being suggestive of a possible eating disorder. However, once again laboratory tests hold the key to the category of causal agent.

FSH、LH、雌二醇、催乳素和 TFTs 将说明促性腺激素功能和卵巢反应以及可能与之有关的主要的

表 16-3 青春期某些方面发育迟缓的原因
Table 16.3 Causes of delay in some aspects of puberty

青春期延迟类型（% 频率） Delayed puberty types (% frequency)	原因 Causes
体质性性腺功能正常（25%） Constitutional eugonadism (25%)	
解剖性 Anatomical	处女膜闭锁 Imperforate hymen 阴道横隔 Transverse vaginal septum Müllerian 管发育不全：Rokitansky-Küster-Hauser 综合征及变异 Müllerian agenesis: Mayer-Rokitansky-Küster-Hauser syndrome and variant
持续性无排卵 Chronic anovulation	PCOS
高促性腺激素 Hypergonadotrophic 性腺功能亢进（45%） hypergonadism (45%)	

（续表）

青春期延迟类型（% 频率） Delayed puberty types (% frequency)	原因 Causes
染色体正常 Normal chromosomes	性腺发育不全 XY Gonadal dysgenesis XY 雄激素不敏感 Androgen insensitivity Swyer 综合征 Swyer's syndrome 新生或医源性 / 环境性卵巢早衰 Premature ovarian failure de novo or iatrogenic/environmental 卵巢抵抗综合征 Resistant ovary syndrome
异常染色体数组 Abnormal chromosomearray	特纳综合征 XO Turner's syndrome XO 混合性性腺发育不全 Mixed gonadal dysgenesis
性腺功能减退（30%） Hypogonadotrophic hypogonadism (30%)	体质性 Constitutional 先天或后天 Congenital or acquired 中枢神经系统肿瘤 CNS tumours 感染 Infection 创伤 Trauma
社会心理性 Psychosocial	药物摄入，鸦片和大麻吸入 Drug ingestion, opiates and marijuana inhalants 饮食失调 Eating disorders 锻炼 Exercise 压力 Stress
疾病（包括内分泌） Illness including endocrine	Kallman 综合征 Kallman's syndrome 孤立性 GnRH 缺乏 Isolated GnRH deficiency

（续表）

青春期延迟类型（% 频率） Delayed puberty types (% frequency)	原因 Causes
垂体破坏 Pituitary destruction	垂体破坏 Pituitary destruction
青春期延迟伴女性男性化 Delayed puberty with virilization	C-21 羟化酶缺乏症 C-21 hydroxylase deficiency 肿瘤 Neoplasm 部分型雄激素不敏感 Partial androgen insensitivity

GnRH. 促性腺激素释放激素；PCOS. 多囊卵巢综合征
GnRH, Gonadotrophin-releasing hormone; PCOS, polycystic ovary syndrome

内分泌疾病。盆腔超声将确定生殖道结构，记住经腹部 B 超可能很难看到青春期前的子宫。

FSH, LH, oestradiol, prolactin and TFTs will illustrate gonotrophin function and ovarian response together with the major endocrine disorders that may be responsible. Pelvic ultrasound will define genital tract architecture, bearing in mind that the prepubertal uterus may be very difficult to see on an abdominal pelvic ultrasound.

如果促性腺激素升高，首先检查患者的染色体核型，以确定是否存在特纳综合征，雄激素敏感性或 Swyer 综合征。如果核型正常，应寻找自身免疫性疾病。重要的是要确保核型分析至少探测 40 个细胞，以排除 Y 细胞系嵌合的可能性。

If the gonadotrophins are elevated, first check the patient's karyotype to determine whether Turner's syndrome, androgen sensitivity or Swyer's syndrome is present. If the karyotype is normal, explore for autoimmune disease. It is important to ensure that karyotyping explores at least 40 cells to exclude the possibility of a Y-cell line in mosaicism.

如果促性腺激素水平低或正常，调查饮食障碍、高强度训练和先天性或后天性脑损伤。性腺功能正常需要彻底排除解剖异常，这可能需要 MRI 来充分评估生殖道发育不全或发育不良。

If the gonadotrophins are low or normal, investigate for eating disorders, rigorous training and congenital or acquired cerebral lesions. Eugonadism requires a thorough exclusion of anatomical abnormalities, which may require MRI to adequately assess genital tract agenesis or dysgenesis.

(2) 治疗（Management）：

青春期延迟可以先用无对抗性的雌激素治疗，每天 0.3mg，然后慢慢增加，以促进乳房充分发育。一旦达到足够的生长水平，就应该周期性的添加孕激素来保护子宫内膜。

Delayed puberty can be treated initially with unopposed oestrogens beginning at 0.3 mg daily and slowly increasing to facilitate adequate breast development. Once adequate growth is achieved, progesterone should be added for endometrial protection and cyclicity.

其目标是治疗任何潜在的原因，以最大限度地提高生长和生育潜力。生育咨询和帮助 患者接受诊断是极其困难的，需要一定的敏感性。已证明同伴的支持对年轻女性面对不孕症和与这种差异做斗争很有价值。建议采用包括遗传学、内分泌学、心理学和妇科多学科方法联合治疗。

The goal is to treat any underlying cause to maximize growth and fertility potentials. Fertility counselling and help with accepting a diagnosis can be extremely difficult and require sensitivity. Peer support has been shown to be valuable for young women facing infertility and struggling with difference. A multidisciplinary approach, including genetics, endocrine, psychology and gynaecology, is suggested.

（二）绝经（Menopause）

绝经定义为是最后一次自然的月经周期，由于卵巢卵泡活性丧失而导致的月经永久停止，它标志着女性生殖功能的结束。该定义是在女性连续 12 个月没有月经时追溯得出的。

Menopause is the last natural menstrual period defined as the permanent cessation of menstruation resulting from the loss of ovarian follicular activity, and it marks the end of a woman's reproductive function. The definition is made retrospectively once a woman has had no periods for 12 consecutive months.

对大多数女性来说，绝经自然发生在 45—55 岁，平均年龄 51 岁左右。"过早绝经"可发生在 40 岁之前，因为自然卵巢功能停止或手术切除卵巢后或化疗或放疗后。

For most women, menopause occurs naturally between the ages of 45 and 55 years, with an average age of around 51 years. 'Premature menopause' may occur before the age of 40 due to either the cessation of natural ovarian function or after surgical removal of the ovaries or following chemotherapy or radiotherapy.

绝经过渡期（Menopause transition）

1. 世界卫生组织（WHO）将绝经过渡期或"围绝经期"定义为"紧接绝经前的内分泌、生物学和临床特征开始接近绝经的时期"。40 岁以上的女性月经周期缩短，周期长度的变化与卵泡期缩短有关。在月经周期的所有阶段，FSH 的水平都高于年轻女性的水平，而雌二醇水平可能会降低并伴随着不稳定的升高。在绝经过渡期的早期，FSH 和 LH 水平升高，月经周期经常不规律，周期可缩短、正常或延长。这些周期可能与卵泡发育延迟或间歇的"黄体失相"（LOOP）周期有关，并常常伴有不规律的重度月经。

The menopausal transition, or 'perimenopause', is defined by the World Health Organization (WHO) as 'that period of time immediately before menopause when the endocrinological, biological and clinical features of approaching menopause commence'. The menstrual cycle shortens in women over the age of 40 years, and the change in the cycle length is related to shortening of the follicular phase. FSH levels are higher at all stages of the cycle than levels seen in younger women, whilst oestradiol levels may be lower with erratic elevations. In the early part of the menopause transition, associated with rising FSH and LH levels, menstrual cycle irregularity often occurs with a predominance of short, normal-length or long cycles. These cycles may be associated with delayed follicle development, or intermittent 'luteal out-of-phase' (LOOP) cycles, and are often accompanied by erratically heavy periods.

在后面的阶段，FSH 和 LH 水平进一步升高，月经周期不规则以月经周期延长为主。虽然 AUB 在围绝经期很常见，但持续性不规则出血永远不能被认为是正常的，因为它可能与子宫肿瘤有关。

In the later stages where there are further elevations in FSH and LH, cycle irregularity occurs with a predominance of elongated menstrual cycles. Although AUB is common in perimenopause, persistent irregular bleeding should never be considered normal because it may be associated with uterine neoplasms.

2. 绝经后激素的变化（Hormone changes after menopause）

卵巢产生的雌激素，特别是雌二醇明显减少。有些雌激素产生于肾上腺，但雌二醇的主要来源是脂肪组织中雌酮和睾酮的外周转化。因此，高 BMI 的女性比苗条的女性有更高的循环雌激素水平。在绝经期，雌二醇的循环水平有相当大的差异，这可以解释更年期症状严重程度的差异。没有显著的雌激素产生导致过多的 FSH 和 LH 的释放，主要的增加发生在 FSH。促性腺激素的水平继续表现出类似于绝经前阶段的脉冲释放模式。卵巢和肾上腺产生的雄激素主要是雄烯二酮和睾酮，这些激素的水平在更年期女性下降。肾上腺雄激素分泌也减少，包括脱氢表雄酮（DHEA）和硫酸脱氢表雄酮。卵巢分泌的雌激素减少了，但睾酮的分泌却持续存在。

There is a marked reduction in ovarian production of oestrogen and, in particular, of oestradiol. Some oestrogen production occurs in the adrenal gland, but the major source of oestradiol arises from peripheral conversion of both oestrone and testosterone in fat tissue. Thus, women with a high BMI have higher circulating oestrogen levels than slender women. There is considerable variation in the circulating levels of oestradiol in menopause, and this may account for the variation in severity of menopausal symptoms. The absence of any significant oestrogen production results in excessive release of FSH and LH, with the major increases occurring in FSH. The levels of gonadotrophins continue to show pulsatile release similar to the pattern seen in the premenopausal phase. Androgens produced in the ovary and adrenal glands are mainly androstenedione and testosterone, and these levels fall in menopausal women. There is also a reduction in adrenal androgen secretion, including that of dehydroepiandrosterone (DHEA) and DHEA sulphate. Oestrogen production by the ovary is reduced, but the production of testosterone persists.

3. 绝经的症状和体征（Symptoms and signs of menopause）

与绝经有关的症状很多，但最显著的两个是潮热（通常与失眠有关）和阴道干燥。70% 的女性会出现这些症状，这是雌激素水平降低的结果。一系列其他症状无论是生理上还是心理上，都与绝经有关，其中包括心悸、头痛、骨骼和关节疼痛、虚弱、疲劳和乳房触痛。大多数女性的症状很少或只有轻微的症状。约 20% 的女性寻求帮助来控制她们的症状。

Numerous symptoms are described in relation to menopause, but the two that are the most significant are hot flushes (often associated with insomnia) and vaginal dryness. These symptoms are experienced by 70% of women and result from reduced oestrogen levels. A range of other symptoms, both physical and psychological, are associated with menopause, including palpitations, headaches, bone and joint pain, asthenia, tiredness and breast tenderness. Most women will have little or only mild symptoms. Around 20% of women seek help for management of their symptoms.

（1）躯体症状（Physical symptoms）：

①血管障碍：最常见的症状是潮热，约 75% 的女性会出现这种症状。这些症状通常持续 4-5 分钟，包括脸部、颈部和胸部的潮红和出汗。

Vascular disturbances. The commonest symptom, occurring in around 75% of women, is the development of hot flushes.

潮热通常发生在绝经后的第一年，最长可持续 5 年。虽然确切的病理生理学机制尚不清楚，但潮红与 LH 的脉动释放、皮肤温度急剧升高几度、心率短暂升高和心电图基线波动相一致。雌激素可以缓解这些症状，但其机制尚不清楚。夜间盗汗和失眠也会发生。

These episodes usually last for 4–5 minutes and consist of flushes and perspiration affecting the face, neck and chest. Hot flushes are typically experienced maximally in the first year after menopause and last up to 5 years. Although the exact pathophysiology remains elusive, the flushes coincide with pulsatile release of LH, an acute rise in the skin temperature of several degrees centigrade, a transient increase in heart rate and fluctuations in the electrocardiographic baseline. The administration of oestrogens relieves these symptoms, but the mechanism is unknown. Night sweats and insomnia also occur.

②尿道：子宫、阴道和膀胱的泌尿生殖组织含有雌激素和孕激素受体。雌激素缺失导致上皮细胞变薄，血管减少，肌肉体积减小和脂肪沉积增加。多达一半的女性在绝经后出现泌尿生殖系统症状，包括子宫阴道脱垂、阴道干燥和泌尿系统症状。

Urogenital tract. The urogenital tissues of the uterus, vagina and bladder contain oestrogen and progesterone receptors. Loss of oestrogen results in epithelial thinning, reduced vascularity, decreased muscle bulk and increased fat deposition. Up to half of women experience urogenital symptoms after menopause, including uterovaginal prolapse, dry vagina and urinary symptoms.

阴道壁失去了它们的皱褶，变得光滑和萎缩。

在严重的情况下，这也可能与慢性感染和萎缩性阴道炎有关。阴道和外阴干燥的主诉表现为性交时的不适或疼痛，以及性交后出血或点滴出血。宫颈变小，宫颈黏液分泌减少。子宫也会萎缩，子宫内膜也会萎缩。膀胱上皮也可能随着尿频、排尿困难和急迫性尿失禁的发展而萎缩。认识到这些症状是很重要的，因为它们可以通过雌激素替代疗法得到缓解。

The vaginal walls lose their rugosity and become smooth and atrophic. In severe cases, this may also be associated with chronic infection and atrophic vaginitis. The complaint of vaginal and vulval dryness can manifest as discomfort or pain during intercourse, as well as bleeding or spotting after sex. The cervix diminishes in size, and there is a reduction in cervical mucus production. The uterus also shrinks in size, and the endometrium becomes atrophic. The bladder epithelium may also become atrophic with the development of frequency, dysuria and urge incontinence. It is important to recognize these symptoms because they can be relieved by oestrogen replacement therapy.

③其他的躯体症状：身体上的皮肤变得更薄、更干燥，身体和面部的毛发变得更粗糙。卵巢雌激素的减少导致靶器官萎缩退化，其中包括乳房密度降低，体积缩小（图 16–23）。

Other physical symptoms. The skin over the body becomes thinner and drier, and body and facial hair become coarser. The reduction in ovarian oestrogen production results in involution and regression of target organs, including breasts that become less dense and reduce in size (Fig. 16.23).

（2）心理和情绪症状（Psychological and emotional symptoms）：

许多女性在绝经前后有心理症状，如焦虑、抑郁、记忆力减退、易怒、注意力不集中、疲倦和丧失信心。绝经的情绪障碍可能与女性对自身角色的不充分感和不确定感有关，如果她们是离家子女的主要照顾者。虽然没有证据表明这些症状与雌激素缺乏直接相关，但激素治疗（HT）/HRT 可能改善轻度抑郁症状；但是，中至重度抑郁症应采用抗抑郁药和其他疗法治疗。

Many women experience psychological symptoms around the time of menopause such as anxiety, depression, loss of memory, irritability, poor concentration, tiredness and loss of confidence. The emotional disturbances of menopause may be associated with feelings of inadequacy and uncertainty about the woman's role if they have been the primary caregiver of children who are leaving home. Although there is no evidence

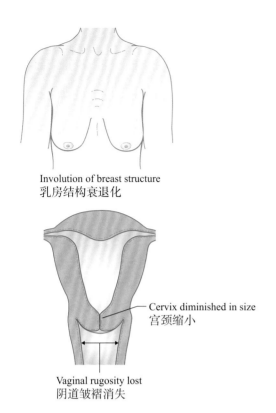

Involution of breast structure
乳房结构衰退化

Cervix diminished in size
宫颈缩小

Vaginal rugosity lost
阴道皱褶消失

▲ 图 16-23　绝经后乳房和生殖器的特征性变化

Fig. 16.23　**Characteristic changes in the breasts and genitalia following menopause.**

that these symptoms are directly related to oestrogen deficiency, hormone therapy (HT)/HRT may improve mild depressive symptoms; however, moderate to severe depression should be treated with antidepressant and other therapies.

(3) 其他症状（Other symptoms）：

雌二醇会影响心脏的电生理参数，女性通常会有心悸特别是在围绝经期，这影响生活质量。这种症状虽然常为良性，但也可由多种心脏疾病引起，如心肌病、心脏瓣膜病和冠状动脉疾病，虽然原发性心律失常是最常见的病因。

Oestradiol can affect the heart's electrophysiological parameters, and women commonly experience palpitations, especially in the perimenopausal period, that impact on quality of life. Although often benign, this symptom can also be brought on by a variety of cardiac disorders, such as cardiomyopathy, valvular heart disease and coronary artery disease, although primary cardiac arrhythmias is the most common cause.

①头痛：月经、妊娠和绝经影响女性头痛的频率和治疗。

Headaches. Menses, pregnancy and menopause affect the frequency and treatment of headaches in women.

在女性健康研究中，与不使用 HT 的患者相比，目前使用 HT 与偏头痛发生率高有关。

In the Women's Health Study, current use of HT was associated with higher reported rates of migraines than in non-users.

②骨和关节痛：许多女性在绝经前后都抱怨骨头和关节疼痛，骨关节炎可能在这个阶段表现出来。对所有女性来说，锻炼是管理这些症状的重要方式，而且，在一些女性中，激素替代疗法是有益的。

Bone and joint pain. Many women complain of bone and joint pain around the time of menopause, and osteoarthritis may manifest at this stage of life. For all women, exercise is an important way of managing these symptoms, and, in some women, HRT is beneficial.

4. 绝经的后果（Consequences of menopause）

(1) 骨的变化（Bone changes）：

骨质疏松症是一种以骨小梁丢失为特征的疾病。雌激素在维持骨骼强度方面起着重要作用，绝经后雌激素水平下降，前 4 年的骨质流失率约为每年 2.5%。骨折成为绝经女性发病的主要来源，60 岁以上的所有女性中至少有 50% 报告至少有一次因骨质疏松症而骨折。

Osteoporosis is a condition characterized by loss of trabecular bone. Oestrogen plays an important role in maintaining bone strength and, with a drop in oestrogen levels after menopause, bone loss occurs at a rate of about 2.5% per year for the first 4 years. Fractures become a major source of morbidity in the menopausal female, with at least half of all women over the age of 60 years reporting to have at least one fracture due to osteoporosis.

人工绝经的女性骨质流失最为严重。髋部骨折的发生率从 45 岁的 0.3‰ 增加到 85 岁的 20‰，Colles 骨折的发生率也增加了 10 倍。

Bone loss is most severe in women who have an artificial menopause. Hip fractures increase in incidence from 0.3/1000 at age 45 years to 20/1000 at age 85 years, and there is also a 10-fold increase in Colles' fractures.

骨质疏松症的诊断通常使用一种叫作双能 X 线吸收法（DXA 或 DEXA）的专门 X 线技术。DXA 测试结果以 T- 分值和 Z- 分值表示。T- 分值为与年轻女性（当骨密度达到峰值时）的骨密度进行比较。Z- 分值为与同龄女性的骨密度相比。T- 分值，而不是 Z- 分值，用于绝经前女性。

The diagnosis of osteoporosis is commonly made using a specialized X-ray technique called dual-energy X-ray absorption (DXA or DEXA). DXA test results are presented as a T-score and a Z-score. The T-score compares the bone density of the woman being scanned with that of a young woman (when peak bone mass is at its best). The Z-score compares the bone density of the woman being scanned with that of a woman of the same age as you. T-scores, not Z-scores, are used in premenopausal women:

- T– 分值＞–1 表示骨密度正常。

- T– 分值在 –1～–2.5 表示骨密度低，有时称为骨质减少。这意味着骨密度有一些流失，但还没有严重到被称为骨质疏松症。

- T– 分值≤–2.5 表示骨质疏松。当一个人发生影响轻微的骨折时，无论 T– 分值大小，也诊断骨质疏松症。

- T-score greater than −1 indicates <u>normal bone density</u>.

- T-score between −1 and −2.5 indicates <u>low bone density</u>, sometimes called osteopoenia. This means there is some loss of bone mineral density but not severe enough to be called osteoporosis.

- T-score of −2.5 or less indicates <u>osteoporosis</u>. When a person has a minimal impact fracture, regardless of the T-scores, osteoporosis is also diagnosed.

(2) 心血管并发症（Cardiovascular complications）：

与晚绝经女性相比，早绝经女性的心血管事件发生率和心血管事件死亡率更高。绝经后血清脂蛋白的变化包括胆固醇水平的升高和所有脂蛋白组分的升高，高密度与低密度脂蛋白比值降低。

The prevalence and incidence of cardiovascular events and death from cardiovascular events are higher in women who experience early mcnopausc compared to those having late menopause. The changes in serum lipoproteins that occur after menopause include a rise in cholesterol levels and an increase in all lipoprotein fractions, with a decrease in the ratio of the high- to low-density fractions.

这可以解释一些（但不是全部）心血管疾病发病率增加的原因，现在很明显，卵巢激素减少对心血管系统有广泛的影响，对血管壁生理有直接的有害影响。

This can explain some, but not all, of the increased cardiovascular morbidity, and it is now evident that ovarian hormone deprivation has a widespread impact on the cardiovascular system, with a direct harmful effect on vessel wall physiology.

5. 绝经治疗（Treatment of menopause）

许多女性绝经后没有任何症状，而且绝经后个体间的血清雌二醇水平差异很大。雌激素治疗是缓解症状的最有效的治疗方法，但可能与少数女性的显著不良反应有关。

Many women pass through menopause without any symptoms, and there is considerable variation in serum oestradiol levels between individuals after menopause. Oestrogen therapy is the most effective treatment for symptomatic relief but may be associated with significant adverse effects in a small minority of women.

使用 HRT 的决定是根据每个女性的病史、风险因素和个人偏好而做出的（表 16–4）。这应该以一种可以让患者理解的方式进行，以便每个女性都能做出知情的选择。

The decision to use HRT is made on an individual basis taking into account each woman's history, risk factors and personal preferences (Table 16.4). This should be done in a way that can be understood so that each woman can make an informed choice.

表 16–4 采用雌激素和孕激素联合替代疗法的女性相对风险及益处

Table 16.4 Relative risks and benefits seen in women taking combined oestrogen and progestogen hormone replacement therapy

	相对风险 vs. 安慰剂组（5 年） Relative risk vs. placebo group at 5 years
心脏病发作 Heart attacks	1.29
脑卒中 Stroke	1.41
乳腺癌 Breast cancer	1.26
静脉血栓形成 Venous thrombosis	2.11
股骨颈骨折 Fractured neck of femur	0.66
结直肠癌 Colorectal cancer	0.63

改编自 Rossouw JE, Anderson GL, Prentice RL, et al.（2002）Risks and benefits of estrogen plus progestin in healthy postmenopausal women: principal results from the Women's Health Initiative randomized controlled trial. JAMA 2002; 288:321-333.

Adapted from Rossouw JE, Anderson GL, Prentice RL, et al. (2002) Risks and benefits of estrogen plus progestin in healthy postmenopausal women: principal results from the Women's Health Initiative randomized controlled trial. JAMA 2002; 288:321-333.

(1) 激素补充治疗（Hormone replacement therapy）：

雌激素疗法可以单独或与孕激素联合或序贯治疗。建议的治疗类型取决于是否有子宫，以及治疗计划是短期或长期。任何女性长期 HRT 应该定期重新评估风险和收益。

Oestrogen therapy may be given on its own or as a combined or sequential therapy with a progestogen. The type of therapy recommended will depend on whether the uterus has been removed and whether the therapy planned is to be short or long term. There should be regular reappraisal of the risk and benefits on any woman taking long-term HRT.

①口服治疗：对于子宫完整的女性，持续给予微化雌二醇或孕马结合雌激素（倍美力），同时给予孕激素，以防止子宫内膜增生或恶性肿瘤的发展。孕激素通常每 4 周服用 10～14 天，以产生每月撤退性出血，但如果将其减少到每 12 周一次，也有保护作用。那些已绝经并希望避免进一步出血的女性可以使用包括连续使用雌孕激素的联合治疗。

Oral therapy. Micronized oestradiol or conjugated equine oestrogen (Premarin) is given continuously with concomitant administration of a progestogen in women with an intact uterus to prevent the development of endometrial hyperplasia or malignancy. Progestogens are commonly given for 10–14 days every 4 weeks to produce a monthly withdrawal bleed, but there is no loss of protective effect when this is reduced to 12-weekly intervals. Those women who have previously stopped their periods and wish to avoid further bleeds can be offered combination therapy that includes continuous progestogen administration with an oestrogen.

②胃肠道外治疗：雌激素也可以注射或皮下植入。将 100mg 的结晶雌二醇颗粒植入腹壁前方皮下组织，并与 50mg 的睾酮联合使用，这种植入方法具有温和的合成代谢作用和增强性欲的优势，通常可持续 6～12 个月，对手术绝经的女性有用。即使在正常或高雌二醇水平的情况下，埋植的间隔时间逐渐缩短的快速耐药性和症状复发有时也可能是一个问题。如果是子宫完整的女性进行皮下埋植，那么使用孕激素是很重要的，例如，在每个月的前 14 天使用醋酸炔诺酮 5mg。只要有活性的雌激素吸收，就会引起撤退性出血。

Parenteral therapy. Oestrogen can also be administered by injection or by subcutaneous implants. This can be achieved with crystalline oestradiol 100 mg in a pellet inserted in the subcutaneous tissue of the anterior abdominal wall. This is often combined with testosterone 50 mg, which has the advantage of a mild anabolic effect and of enhancing libido. The pellets usually last for 6–12 months and are useful in women who have experienced surgical menopause. Tachyphylaxis with progressively shorter intervals between implants and the return of symptoms even in the presence of normal or high oestradiol levels can occasionally be a problem. If the implants are given to a woman with an intact uterus, it is important to give a progestogen, such as norethisterone acetate 5 mg, for the first 14 days of each month. This will provoke withdrawal bleeding as long as active oestrogen absorption occurs.

③局部治疗：雌二醇可通过贴片或凝胶经皮给药。贴片应用于除脸部或乳房外的任何干净、干燥的皮肤区域，每周更换 2 次。这种凝胶每天涂在皮肤上一次。黄体酮既可以口服也可以经皮给药。这种方法的优点是绕过了肝脏代谢的"首过效应"，并且比植入剂提供了更稳定的血清激素水平。主要并发症之一是皮肤刺激。

Topical therapy. Oestradiol can be given percutaneously by self-adhesive patches or gel. Patches are applied to any area of clear, dry skin other than the face or breast and changed twice a week. The gel is rubbed into the skin once a day. A progestogen can be given either orally or transdermally. This route has the advantage of bypassing the 'first pass' liver metabolism and gives more stable serum hormone levels than with implants. The major complication is one of skin irritation.

④禁忌证：HRT 禁忌证有子宫内膜癌、乳腺癌、血栓栓塞性疾病（包括家族史）、急性肝病和缺血性心脏病。其他情况，如乳腺纤维囊性疾病、子宫肌瘤、家族性高脂血症、糖尿病和胆囊疾病都是相对禁忌证，但症状的缓解有时比其他考虑因素更重要。

Contraindications. HRT is contraindicated in the presence of endometrial and breast carcinoma, thromboembolic disease (including family history), acute liver disease and ischaemic heart disease. Other conditions such as fibrocystic disease of the breast, uterine fibroids, familial hyperlipidaemia, diabetes and gallbladder disease provide a relative contraindication, but relief of symptoms may sometimes be more important than other considerations.

⑤风险：HRT 的潜在并发症包括子宫内膜癌、乳腺癌和可能的卵巢癌的发病率升高。这些癌症的风险非常小，但可能会随着 HRT 的时间延长而增加。先前的观察性研究表明，它对心脏病和脑卒中有保护作用，但具有复杂和不确定性。静脉血栓形成的风险增加，但总体发生率很低。一些女性在雌激素治疗中发展成高血压，因此定期检查血压是很重要的。有胆囊病史的患者要小心。接受 HRT 治疗 6 个

月后出现不规则子宫出血是子宫内膜活检的适应证。

Risks. The potential complications of HRT include an increased incidence of carcinoma of the endometrium, breast and possibly ovary. The risk of these cancers is very small but may increase the longer that HRT is taken. Previous observational studies had suggested a protective effect against heart disease and stroke, but this is complex and uncertain. The risk of venous thrombosis is increased, but the overall incidence is very low. Some women develop hypertension on oestrogen therapy, and periodic checks on blood pressure are therefore important. Caution should be taken when there is a history of gallbladder disease. The development of irregular uterine bleeding after more than 6 months on HRT is an indication for endometrial biopsy.

> **！注意**
>
> HRT 不应再用于预防冠心病这一特定适应证。
>
> HRT should no longer be prescribed for the specific indication of prevention of coronary heart disease.

⑥益处：HRT 的主要益处是缓解绝经症状和预防骨质疏松症。HRT 的使用可以降低股骨颈骨折的风险和结直肠癌的发生率。

Benefits. The principal benefits of HRT use are in the relief of menopausal symptoms and the prevention of osteoporosis. HRT use is associated with a reduction in the risk of fracture of the neck of the femur and in the incidence of colorectal cancer.

(2) 对含雌激素 HRT 的替代选择（Alternatives to oestrogen-containing HRT）：

由于长期使用 HRT 的主要指征是预防骨质疏松症，患者需要认识到长期使用可能增加某些疾病的风险，以及预防骨质疏松症的可选治疗方案。

As the principal indication for long-term use of HRT is the prevention of osteoporosis, patients need to be aware of the possible increased risk of some conditions with longterm use and the alternative treatment options available to prevent osteoporosis.

替勃龙是一种合成的具有雌激素特性的弱雄激素。它不引起子宫内膜增生，所以没有撤退性出血，但只适合绝经一年以上的女性使用。它能有效减轻血管舒缩症状和骨质疏松症。

Tibolone is a synthetic weak androgen with oestrogenic properties. It does not cause endometrial proliferation, so there is no withdrawal bleed, but it is only advisable for women more than a year after menopause. It is effective at reducing vasomotor symptoms and osteoporosis.

选择性雌激素受体调节药（SERM）作用于骨中的雌激素受体而不影响乳房或子宫内膜。目前使用的药物在这方面是有效的，但不能缓解血管舒缩症状，并与传统的雌激素疗法一样，会增加血栓形成的风险。

Selective oestrogen receptor modulators (SERMs) act on oestrogen receptors in bone without affecting the breast or endometrium. Those currently available are effective at doing this but do not relieve vasomotor symptoms and are associated with the same increased risk of thrombosis as conventional oestrogen therapy.

可乐定是一种降压药，对血管舒缩症状有一定影响，但对其他症状或长期健康无影响。含 5- 羟色胺的抗抑郁药 SSRI 和 SNRI 似乎对潮热很有效，而且缓解症状的速度也很快。

Clonidine is an antihypertensive agent that has some effect on vasomotor symptoms but no effect on other symptoms or long-term health. The serotonergic antidepressants, the SSRIs and SNRIs, seem to be effective in hot flushes, and relief, if any, is rapid.

这些药物的长期使用，特别是对患有乳腺癌的女性来说，因为可能与他莫昔芬有相互作用，仍然存在争议。加巴喷丁是一种抗惊厥药物，在减少潮热的严重程度和频率方面比安慰剂更有效，而且在服用他莫昔芬的女性中可能是安全的。

The use of these medications in the long term, particularly in women who have had breast cancer as there may be an interaction with tamoxifen, remains in doubt. Gabapentin, an anticonvulsant drug, is more effective than placebo in reducing the severity and frequency of hot flushes and is likely to be safein women on tamoxifen.

草药疗法如黑升麻被广泛使用，但在随机对照试验中，缓解绝经症状的效果并不比安慰剂好。植物雌激素是一种非甾体植物化合物，由于其结构与雌二醇相似，具有轻微的雌激素作用。目前仍然缺乏使用这些化合物作为 HRT 替代治疗的控制良好的临床试验。它们可能对心血管疾病有微弱的积极影响，可能对乳腺癌有保护作用。它们还不能有效地防止骨质流失。

Herbal therapies such as black cohosh are widely used but in randomized controlled trials fare no better than placebo in relieving menopausal symptoms. Phyto-oestrogens are nonsteroidal plant compounds that, because of their structural similarity with oestradiol, have mild oestrogenic effects. There is still a lack of well-controlled clinical trials for the use of these compounds as alternatives to HRT. They probably have a weak positive impact on cardiovascular disease and may be protective against breast cancer. They are not potent enough to impact on bone loss.

十一、下生殖道的良性情况（Benign conditions of the lower genital tract）

（一）外阴瘙痒（Vulval pruritus）

瘙痒，是那些抱怨外阴不适最常见的症状。瘙痒常伴有抓挠和伴随的上皮损伤，通常是慢性的。结果，女性可能遭遇性方面的困难，经常报告在讨论她们的症状或寻求帮助时遇到问题。诊断和治疗对临床医生来说可能是困难的，因为症状和体征倾向于聚集，活检结果可能是模糊的，刺激或过敏反应可能会发展为需要各种药物和补救措施来治疗。

Pruritus, or itch, is the most commonly described symptom of those complaining of discomfort in the vulval area. The itch, so often accompanied by scratching with its attendant trauma to the epithelium, may often be chronic. Women may experience sexual difficulties as a consequence and often report problems in discussing their symptoms or seeking help. Diagnosis and management may be difficult for the clinician, as symptoms and signs tend to cluster, biopsy results can be equivocal and irritant or allergic reactions may develop to various medications and remedies tried.

幸运的是，大部分外阴瘙痒的原因是良性的（表 16–5）。然而，必须注意不要忽视或误诊罕见的恶性原因。外阴是皮肤，因此可以表现出身体其他部位的症状，如银屑病和皮炎。由于这一区域的性质，皮肤状况的外观可能会有很大的不同。外阴接近阴道，也可能表现为细菌性或病毒性阴道炎或宫颈炎伴对阴道分泌物过敏反应，如念珠菌病。因此，在评估一个外阴瘙痒症患者时，有一个非常广泛的病史是非常重要的，其中包括个人及家族皮肤病史、自身免疫性疾病，以及接触到可能的刺激物，如肥皂、香水、卫生产品等，并检查其他部位皮肤。特别要注意头皮、肘部、肘前窝和膝盖。对生殖器的检查一般不需要阴道镜检查，但重要的是，当有指征时，要从外阴病变和阴道或宫颈黏膜进行细菌和病毒培养。

Fortunately the majority of causes of vulval pruritus are benign (Table 16.5). However, care must be taken not to overlook or misdiagnose the rarer malignant causes. The vulva is skin and therefore may express conditions seen elsewhere on the body, e.g. psoriasis and dermatitis. Because of the nature of this area, the appearance of skin conditions may vary greatly. The vulva, in such proximity to the vagina, may also express features of bacterial or viral vaginitis or cervicitis with hypersensitivity reaction to productive discharge, as seen in candidiasis. It is therefore extremely important when assessing a patient with pruritus of the vulva to take a very wide-ranging history to include personal and family history of skin conditions; autoimmune disease; and exposures to possible irritants such as soaps, perfumes, sanitary products, etc. and to examine the rest of their skin. Particular attention should be paid to the scalp, elbows, anterior cubital fossae and knees. Inspection of the genitalia does not generally require colposcopic examination, but it is important to obtain bacterial and viral cultures both from vulval lesions and vaginal or cervical mucosa when indicated.

在成年女性中，进行穿刺活检的指征应该放宽。有血管增加的瘙痒、鳞状病变或治疗反应差应活检以排除恶性肿瘤。此外，由于一些皮肤病有类似的表现，活检可能是必要的，以确认诊断和确定治疗计划。

In adult women, the threshold to perform punch biopsy should be low. Itchy, scaly lesions with increased vascularity or poor treatment response should be biopsied to exclude malignancy. Further, as several dermatological conditions have similar presentations, biopsy may be necessary to confirm the diagnosis and ascertain treatment plans.

所有涉及外阴瘙痒的病例的治疗基础是确保消除刺激性或过敏刺激，保持该区域干燥和通风以促进愈合，处方中规定了防止重复损伤的屏障准备。肥皂、芳香卫生用品、滑石粉和带香味的润滑剂都应避免使用。使用纯水或油性低过敏性产品清洗；棉内衣；宽松的衣服；而经常使用山梨酚或类似的保湿剂是治疗的基本核心。

A cornerstone of treatment for all cases involving pruritus of the vulva is to ensure irritant or allergic stimuli are removed, that the area is kept dry and well ventilated to promote healing and that barrier preparations to prevent repeated insult are prescribed. Soap, perfumed hygiene products, talcum and flavoured lubricants should all be avoided. Washing with water alone or oil-based, hypoallergenic products; cotton underwear; loose clothing; and frequent moisturization with sorbolene or similar form an essential core of management.

（二）外阴肿瘤（Vulval neoplasia）

皮肤癌会发生在外阴，并伴有瘙痒，需要与良性皮肤病区分。应高度怀疑任何持续侵蚀性或鳞状病变和血管增生性病变，应放宽活检的指征（见第20章）。

表 16-5 外阴瘙痒的良性原因

Table 16.5 Benign causes of vulval pruritus

疾病 Condition	表现 Presentation	处理 Management
皮炎 Dermatitis	瘙痒，红斑性皮疹（内源性） Itchy, erythematous rash (endogenous) 特应性 / 脂溢性 Atopic/seborrhoeic 过敏或刺激（外源性） Allergic or irritant induced (exogenous)	轻至中效糖皮质激素随着症状减轻而减少用量（无论病因） Mild to moderate corticosteroid reducing as symptoms abate (regardless of the cause)
慢性单纯性苔藓 Lichen simplex chronicus	慢性刺激可导致皮肤增厚、肥大、红斑、脱皮 Chronic irritation results in thickening and hypertrophy of skin, erythema, excoriations 与黏膜无关 Mucosa not involved	孤立并消除诱发和加剧的因素 Isolate and remove provoking and exacerbating factors 强效局部类固醇 High-potency steroid locally 症状控制后减少用量 Reducing after symptom control
念珠菌病 Candidiasis	瘙痒不适，白色分泌物，排尿困难，性交痛 Itch discomfort, white discharge dyspareunia, dysuria 外阴过敏反应 Hypersensitivity reaction on vulva 确认诊断需要培养阳性 Requires positive culture to confirm diagnosis	轻度：克霉唑阴道栓 Mild: pessaries of clotrimazole 中度：长期治疗 ± 口服药物 Moderate: prolonged treatment ± oral drugs 严重 / 复发性：2~3 个月口服氟康唑。每周维持口服 150mg 或克霉唑阴道栓 500mg Severe/recurrent: 2–3 months oral fluconazole. Maintenance of oral 150 mg weekly or clotrimazole pessary 500 mg
外阴硬化性苔藓 Lichen sclerosis (LS)	增白羊皮纸般的斑块 Whitened parchment-like plaques 典型沙漏样外观，累及肛周皮肤 Classic hourglass appearance involving perianal skin 阴唇 / 阴蒂结构丧失，内腔狭窄 Loss of labial/clitoral architecture, introital narrowing 可能有撕裂或上皮下出血 / 瘀点与黏膜无关 May have tearing or subepithelial haemorrhage/petechiae 未涉及黏膜 Mucosa not involved	强效糖皮质激素 High-potency corticosteroids 每夜使用，直到临床症状好转（1~2 个月），然后减量 Nightly until clinical improvement (1–2 months) then reduce 每周维持治疗 1~2 次 Maintenance 1–2 per week 如症状复发，增加治疗强度至原强度，治疗 2 周 Increase treatment to original intensity for 2 weeks if symptoms recur
扁平苔藓 Lichen planus (LP)	慢性 LS 与 LP 难以鉴别 Chronic LS difficult to differentiate from LP 累及阴道口 Introits of vagina involved 粘连和糜烂可能对外科手术没有反应 Adhesions and erosions may occur not responsive to surgical division 口腔或牙龈可能受累 Oral/gingival involvement possible	强效糖皮质激素 High-potency corticosteroids 除了那些对治疗无效的轻度病例 Except in mild cases that are very resistant to treatment
银屑病 Psoriasis	瘙痒、鳞片、红色斑块不像皮肤上其他地方那么明显；检查头发 / 头皮、指甲 Itchy, scaly, red plaques not as well demarcated as elsewhere on the skin; examine hair/scalp, nails also	对于一般的牛皮癣，高效糖皮质激素加焦油产品 As for psoriasis in general; high-potency corticosteroid plus tar products 局部使用他克莫司 Local tacrolimus

Skin cancers will occur on the vulva and present with itchiness and need to be differentiated from benign dermatoses. Suspicion should be increased in any persistently eroded or scaly and hypervascular lesions with a very low threshold for biopsy (see Chapter 20).

（三）阴道分泌物（Vaginal discharge）

阴道分泌物是指任何液体通过阴道流出。而大部分分泌物是正常的，可以反映整个月经周期中的生理变化，一些分泌物可能由于感染或创伤而发生。白色分泌物通常在月经周期开始和结束时随激素的变化而产生，在月经中期，由于雌激素水平高，分泌物清亮。阴道分泌物异常的常见原因及处理方法见表 16-6。关于生殖道常见感染及其治疗的进一步细节见第 19 章。

Vaginal discharge describes any fluid loss through the vagina. While most discharge is normal and can reflect physiological changes throughout the menstrual cycle, some discharge can occur because of infection or trauma. White discharge usually occurs in response to hormonal changes at the beginning and the end of the cycle, whilst mid-cycle, with high oestrogen levels, the discharge is clear. The common causes and management of vaginal discharge are summarized in Table 16.6. Further details on the common infections of the genital tract and their treatment can be found in Chapter 19.

（四）宫颈息肉（Cervical polyps）

良性息肉起源于宫颈，有蒂，覆盖宫颈上皮和中央纤维组织核心。息肉呈鲜红色，血管增生，可

在常规检查中发现。目前的症状可能包括不规则的阴道出血或 PCB。

Benign polyps arise from the endocervix and are pedunculated, with a covering of endocervical epithelium and a central fibrous tissue core. The polyps present as bright red, vascular growths that may be identified on routine examination. The presenting symptoms may include irregular vaginal blood loss or PCB.

少见情况下，息肉起源于鳞状上皮，其外观类似于阴道上皮。小息肉可在门诊用息肉钳钳住，360°旋转撕脱。较大的息肉可能需要在全身麻醉下结扎蒂并切除息肉。

Less frequently, the polyps arise from the squamous epithelium, when the appearance will resemble the surface of the vaginal epithelium. Small polyps can be avulsed in the outpatient clinic by grasping them with polyp forceps and rotating through 360 degrees. Larger polyps may need ligation of the pedicle and excision of the polyp under general anaesthesia.

（五）外阴和阴道的良性肿瘤（Benign tumours of the vulva and vagina）

良性外阴囊肿包括皮脂腺囊肿、上皮包涵囊肿和 Wolffian 管囊肿（图 16-24），发生于小阴唇和尿道周围区域，以及 Bartholin 腺囊肿（见后述）。罕见的囊肿可起源于沿圆韧带的腹膜伸展，形成大阴唇积液。良性实体瘤包括纤维瘤、脂肪瘤和汗腺瘤。真性鳞状乳头状瘤表现为疣状生长，很少恶变。所

表 16-6 阴道分泌物：原因及治疗

Table 16.6 Vaginal discharge: Causes and treatment

分泌物特征及相关症状 Features of discharge and associated symptoms	可能原因 Possible causes	治疗 Treatment
黏稠、白、不痒 Thick, white, non-itchy	生理性 Physiological	
稠厚，白色，白干酪，外阴瘙痒，外阴疼痛和刺激，疼痛或不适 Thick, white cottage cheese, vulval itching, vulval soreness and initation, pain or discomfort	白色念珠菌 Candida albicans	局部或口服抗酵母菌药物 Topical or oral anti-yeast medication
黄绿色、发痒、泡沫状、恶臭（"鱼腥味"）的阴道分泌物 Yellow-green, itchy, frothy, foul-smelling ('fishy' smell) vaginal discharge	滴虫 Trichomonas	甲硝唑，性伴侣同治 Metronidazole and treatment of sexual partners
稀薄，灰色或绿色，鱼腥味 Thin, grey or green, fishy odour	细菌性阴道病 Bacterial vaginosis	甲硝唑 Metronidazole
黏稠白色分泌物，排尿困难，盆腔疼痛，宫颈脆弱 Thick, white discharge, dysuria and pelvic pain, friable cervix	淋病 Gonorrhoea	多变但以头孢菌素为基础 Variable but cephalosporins

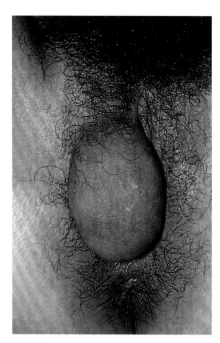

▲ 图 16-24　起源于残余 **Wolffian** 管的良性外阴囊肿

Fig. 16.24　Benign vulval cyst arising from remnant of the wolffian duct.

有这些病变均可通过简单的活检切除治疗。

Benign cysts of the vulva include sebaceous, epithelial inclusion and wolffian duct cysts (Fig. 16.24), which arise from the labia minora and the periurethral region, and Bartholin's cysts (see later). A rare cyst may arise from a peritoneal extension along the round ligament, forming a hydrocele in the labium major. Benign solid tumours include fibromas, lipomas and hidradenomas. True squamous papillomas appear as warty growths and rarely become malignant. All these lesions are treated by simple biopsy excision.

（六）阴道囊肿（Vaginal cysts）

1. 先天性（Congenital）

囊肿产生于阴道的胚胎残留；最常见的种类是来自 Gartner 管（Wolffian 管道残余）。阴道囊肿并不少见，发生在阴道前外侧壁，通常无症状，在常规检查中可以发现。

Cysts arise in the vagina from embryological remnants; the commonest varieties are those arising from Gartner's duct (wolffian duct remnants). These are not rare and occur in the anterolateral wall of the vagina. They are usually asymptomatic and are found on routine examination.

组织学上，囊肿内衬立方上皮，但有时可见扁平层状的复层鳞状上皮。

Histologically, the cysts are lined by cuboidal epithelium, but sometimes a flattened layer of stratified squamous

epithelium is seen.

囊肿的治疗方法是简单的手术切除，几乎不会引起任何困难。

The cysts are treated by simple surgical excision and rarely give rise to any difficulties.

2. 阴道包涵囊肿（Vaginal inclusion cysts）

包涵囊肿是由表皮下的小颗粒状或岛状阴道上皮形成的。囊肿常发生在会阴切开瘢痕处，内含淡黄色黏稠液体。治疗方法是简单的手术切除。

Inclusion cysts arise from inclusion of small particles or islands of vaginal epithelium under the surface. The cysts commonly arise in episiotomy scars and contain yellowish thick fluid. They are treated by simple surgical excision.

（七）子宫内膜异位症（Endometriosis）

子宫内膜异位病变可出现在阴道的任何部位，但最常见于后穹隆。病变可能表现为深褐色斑点或红色溃疡病变。诊断是通过切除组织活检来确定的，如果病变是多发的，则应与其他部位的病变一样进行药物治疗。

Endometriotic lesions may appear anywhere in the vagina but occur most commonly in the posterior fornix. The lesions may appear as dark brown spots or reddened ulcerated lesions. The diagnosis is established by excision biopsy. If the lesions are multiple, then medical therapy should be instituted as for lesions in other sites.

（八）实性良性肿瘤（Solid benign tumours）

阴道实性病变很少见，但可能来源于阴道内的任何组织。因此，息肉样肿瘤可能包括纤维肌瘤、肌瘤、纤维瘤、乳头状瘤和腺肌瘤。这些肿瘤可以通过简单的手术切除来治疗。

These lesions are rare but may represent any of the tissues that are found in the vagina. Thus, polypoid tumours may include fibromyomas, myomas, fibromas, papillomas and adenomyomas. These tumours are treated by simple surgical excision.

十二、阴道上皮的肿瘤性病变（Neoplastic lesions of the vaginal epithelium）

阴道上皮的肿瘤性病变见第 20 章。

Neoplastic lesions of the vaginal epithelium are covered in Chapter 20.

十三、妇科急症（Emergency gynaecology）

（一）盆腔感染（Pelvic infection）

PID 包括一系列女性上生殖道炎症性疾病，主要由宫颈或阴道上行感染引起。急性 PID 将在第 19 章详细介绍。

PID comprises a spectrum of inflammatory disorders of the upper female genital tract mainly caused by ascending infection from the cervix or vagina. Acute PID is covered in detail in Chapter 19.

（二）Bartholin 腺脓肿或囊肿（Bartholin's abscess/cyst）

Bartholin 腺位于阴道口的后壁，通过短导管分泌黏液样液体排入阴道。它们通常只有豌豆大小，但当导管被阻塞时，就会形成囊肿。这些囊肿可表现为在阴唇后方形成椭圆形肿块，有时长到高尔夫球大小或更大。它们通常是单侧的，会导致走路、坐着和性交时的不适。当腺体感染时，可发展成脓肿，最常见的是皮肤或泌尿生殖系统细菌，如葡萄球菌或大肠杆菌。巴氏脓肿比巴氏囊肿更急性发作，特别疼痛。

The Bartholin's glands lie in the posterior vaginal wall at the introitus and secrete mucus-like fluid via a short duct into the vagina. They are normally the size of a pea, but when the duct becomes blocked, a cyst can form. These cysts may present acutely as an oval-shaped lump in the posterior labia, sometimes growing to the size of a golf ball or larger. They are unusually unilateral and cause discomfort with walking, sitting and sexual intercourse. When the gland is infected, most commonly with skin or genitourinary bacteria, e.g. *Staphylococcus* or *Escherichia coli*, an abscess can develop. These arise more acutely than the Bartholin's cysts and are particularly painful.

小而无症状的囊肿可能不需要治疗，脓肿有时可以用抗生素治愈。然而，治疗大的囊肿和脓肿需要手术。该手术被称为"造口术"，通过切开囊肿壁，然后将其缝合到覆盖的皮肤上，形成一个通向腺体的囊状开口，以确保新的开口继续排出腺体中的液体（见第 19 章，图 19-13）。

Small asymptomatic cysts may not require treatment, and abscesses can sometimes resolve with antibiotics. However, treatment of large cysts and abscesses requires surgery. The procedure, called *marsupialization*, involves making a pouch-like opening to the gland by incising into the cyst wall and then suturing it to the overlying skin to ensure the new opening continues to drain the fluid from the glands (see Chapter 19, Fig. 19.13).

（三）外阴和阴道创伤（Vulval and vaginal trauma）

外阴和阴道的损伤可能导致严重的出血和血肿形成。外阴挫伤可能特别严重，因为在阴唇有丰富的静脉丛，通常是由跨摔伤造成的。阴道撕裂常与性交有关。外阴血肿经保守治疗后常消退，但有时需引流。重要的是要缝合阴道撕裂伤，并确定伤口没有穿透腹膜腔。

Injuries to the vulva and vagina may result in severe haemorrhage and haematoma formation. Vulval bruising may be particularly severe because of the rich venous plexus in the labia and commonly results from falling astride. Lacerations of the vagina are often associated with coitus. Vulval haematomas often subside with conservative management but sometimes need drainage. It is important to suture vaginal lacerations and be certain that the injury does not penetrate into the peritoneal cavity.

（四）原因不明的急性腹痛（Acute abdominal pain of uncertain origin）

对于出现急性腹痛的育龄女性，首先要了解疼痛的性质和有无相关症状。彻底的检查可以识别出最大的压痛、反跳痛和肌紧张的部位。排除妊娠，特别是异位妊娠至关重要。妊娠试验阴性和急性盆腔疼痛的妇科疾病包括 PID、功能性卵巢囊肿、卵巢或腹膜子宫内膜异位症和附件扭转。急性盆腔疼痛最常见的胃肠道原因包括阑尾炎、急性乙状结肠憩室炎和克罗恩病。

In a woman of reproductive age presenting with acute abdominal pain, it is first important to take a good history about the nature of the pain and the presence of associated symptoms. A thorough examination will identify the site of maximal tenderness, rebound tenderness and guarding. It is vital to always exclude pregnancy and particularly ectopic pregnancy. Gynaecological disorders in women with a negative pregnancy test and acute pelvic pain include PID, functional ovarian cysts, ovarian or peritoneal endometriosis and adnexal torsion. The most common gastrointestinal causes that can present with acute pelvic pain include appendicitis, acute sigmoid diverticulitis and Crohn's disease.

在评估患有急性盆腔疼痛的女性时，排除需要紧急干预的诊断如 PID、卵巢扭转和阑尾炎，是很重要的。前面讨论了 PID 的检查和诊断。卵巢扭转通常发生在卵巢增大时（见第 20 章）。卵巢扭转表现为突然发作的尖锐的单侧骨盆疼痛，常伴有恶心和呕吐。卵巢扭转的超声表现多种多样。卵巢增大，位置异常，位于子宫上方或后面。血流缺乏是重要的标志，多普勒超声缺乏静脉波形具有较高的阳性预测价值。然而，动静脉血流的存在并不排除扭转，任何临床怀疑扭转的病例都需要腹腔镜来观察附件。如果逆转早期扭转，卵巢可能得救。

It is important in the assessment of a woman with acute pelvic pain to exclude those diagnoses that require urgent intervention: PID, ovarian torsion and appendicitis. The investigation and diagnosis of PID were discussed earlier. Ovarian torsion usually occurs in the presence of an enlarged ovary (see Chapter 20). Women with torsion present with sudden onset of sharp unilateral pelvic pain that is often accompanied by nausea and vomiting. The sonographic findings in ovarian torsion are variable. The ovary is enlarged and can be seen in an abnormal location above or behind the uterus. The absence of blood flow is an important sign, and a lack of venous waveform on Doppler ultrasound has a high positive predictive value. However, the presence of arterial and venous flow does not exclude torsion, and any cases where it is suspected clinically require laparoscopy to visualize the adnexae. If the torsion is reversed early in the process, the ovary may be saved.

急性阑尾炎（Acute appendicitis）

典型的厌食和脐周疼痛，随后是恶心，右下腹（RLQ）疼痛和呕吐的病史只有 50% 的患者会出现。61%～92% 的患者有恶心症状；74～78% 的患者存在厌食症。

The classic history of anorexia and periumbilical pain followed by nausea, right lower quadrant (RLQ) pain and vomiting occurs in only 50% of cases. Nausea is present in 61–92% of patients; anorexia is present in 74–78% of patients.

（五）急性和严重的不定期阴道出血（Acute and excessively heavy unscheduled vaginal bleeding）

FIGO 最近将急性 HMB 定义为与妊娠无关的子宫大出血，需要紧急医疗干预。急性出血的女性通常有排卵障碍，但也可能有潜在的凝血系统疾病。急性 AUB/HMB 的处理可能需要 D&C，但通常可以非手术处理，给予性激素和（或）宫内填塞。以前，使用肠外结合雌激素，近期更多使用口服孕激素，有时双倍剂量的复方口服避孕药也证实能成功地控制出血。更安全的选择是高剂量的孕激素，有时与抗纤溶药氨甲环酸联合使用。静脉注射氨甲环酸被广泛用于治疗"急性"HMB，但还没有临床试验确认获益的程度。

The entity of acute HMB has recently been defined by FIGO as heavy uterine bleeding not associated with pregnancy that is of sufficient volume to require urgent or emergent medical intervention. Women presenting with acute bleeding most often have ovulatory dysfunction but may also have an underlying coagulopathy. The management of acute AUB/HMB can require D&C but can be usually managed non-surgically with the administration of gonadal hormones, and/or intrauterine tamponade. Previously, parenteral conjugated oestrogens were used, and more recently oral progestogens and sometimes double doses of the combined oral contraceptive pill have been shown to be successful. The safer option is high doses of progestogens, sometimes in combination with the anti-fibrinolytic agent, tranexamic acid. Intravenous tranexamic acid is widely used with benefit for 'acute' HMB, but there are no clinical trials to confirm the degree of this benefit.

炔诺酮 5mg，每日 2 次，可以用于止血。随访需要以确定出血的原因。对于非常严重的病例，在子宫腔内插入 Foley 导管球囊有助于实现子宫内膜填塞。

A regimen of norethisterone 5 mg tds can be used to settle the bleeding. Follow-up is required to establish the cause of the bleeding. For really severe cases, the insertion of a small inflated Foley catheter balloon into the uterine cavity can be useful to achieve endometrial tamponade.

本章概览	Essential information

青春期

- 正常顺序为乳房萌发、肾上腺功能初现、生长突增、月经初潮
- 月经初潮通常在 11—15 岁
- 早期无排卵
- 多数性早熟是体质性的
- 原发性闭经并不总是青春期延迟的同义词

继发性闭经

- 6 个月以上没有月经
- 生理原因：妊娠、哺乳
- 病理原因：下丘脑功能障碍、高催乳素血症、多囊卵巢综合征
- 询问：体重、压力，慢性病、药物、避孕
- 检查：妊娠检查、FSH、LH、PRL、超声

月经过多

- 长时间和（或）大出血
- 最常见的诊断是子宫内膜分子功能障碍和黏膜下子宫肌瘤
- 常规检查只需要全血细胞计数和血清铁蛋白
- 治疗的主体是药物

经前期综合征

- 周期性变化症状发生在月经周期的黄体期，并在月经开始时停止
- 最常见的症状：情绪变化、乳房压痛、腹胀和胃肠道症状
- 治疗方案有吡哆醇、月见草油、抑制排卵
- 安慰剂治疗反应高

绝经

- 更年期的一部分
- 开始于 50—51 岁
- 高促性腺激素性，性腺功能减退
- 与血管舒缩不稳定、生殖道和乳腺萎缩、心血管变化和骨质疏松有关
- HRT 对缓解症状和骨质疏松症有效

子宫先天畸形

- 由于 Müllerian 管融合或发育失败
- 通常无症状，除非经血阻塞
- 可能导致反复流产，畸形或胎盘滞留

子宫良性肿瘤

- 最常见的是 EP 和肌瘤
- 25% 的 30 岁以上女性患有肌瘤
- 症状取决于大小和部位，其中包括月经紊乱、压力症状和妊娠并发症
- 可能发生继发性改变，其中包括坏死或恶性改变 (0.13%～1%)

子宫内膜异位症和子宫腺肌症

- 异位的子宫内膜
- 最常见的部位是卵巢、子宫骶韧带和盆腔腹膜
- 可能由化生改变或种植引起
- 表现为生育力低下和（或）进行性加重的痛经

Puberty

- Normal sequence is thelarche, adrenarche, growth spurt, menarche
- Menarche normally between 11 and 15 years
- Early cycles anovulatory
- Most cases of precocious puberty are constitutional
- Primary amenorrhoea not always synonymous with delayed puberty

Secondary amenorrhoea

- Absence of menstruation for more than 6 months
- Physiological causes-pregnancy, breast–feeding
- Pathological causes-hypothalamic dysfunction, hyperprolactinaemia, polycystic ovarian syndrome
- Ask about-weight, stress, chronic illness, medication, contraception
- Investigations-pregnancy test, FSH, LH, prolactin, ultrasound

Heavy menstrual bleeding

- Prolonged and/or heavy bleeding
- Commonest diagnoses are disturbance of endometrial molecular function and submucous uterine fibroids
- Only routine investigations needed are full blood count and serum ferritin
- Mainstay of treatment is medical

Premenstrual syndrome

- Cyclical changes occurring in the luteal phase of the cycle and ceasing at the onset of menstruation
- Commonest symptoms-mood changes, breast tenderness, bloating and gastrointestinal symptoms
- Treatment options are pyridoxine, evening primrose oil, suppression of ovulation
- High placebo response rate

Menopause

- Part of climacteric
- Onset 50–51 years
- Hypergonadotrophic, hypogonadic
- Associated with vasomotor instability, atrophic changes in genital tract and breast, cardiovascular changes and osteoporosis
- HRT effective in symptom relief and osteoporosis

Congenital abnormalities of the uterus

- Due to failure of müllerian ducts to fuse or develop
- Usually asymptomatic unless menstrual flow obstructed
- May cause recurrent miscarriage, malpresentation or retained placenta

Benign uterine tumours

- Commonest are EPs and fibroids
- 25% of women over 30 years old have fibroids
- Symptoms depend on size and site and include menstrual disorders, pressure symptoms and complications of pregnancy
- May undergo secondary change, including necrosis or malignant change (0.13–1%)

Endometriosis and adenomyosis

- 'Ectopic' endometrium
- Commonest sites are ovaries, uterosacral ligaments and pelvic peritoneum
- May arise from metaplastic change or implantation
- Presents as subfertility and/or crescendic dysmenorrhoea

第 17 章　不孕症

Infertility

Eloïse Fraison　William Ledger　著　　管一春 译　颜 磊 校

学习本章后，你应当掌握：

知识标准
- 描述男性不育和女性不孕的常见原因
- 描述不孕夫妇评估中所使用的相关检查的适应证
- 讨论不孕症常用治疗方法的原则、适应证和并发症

临床能力
- 采集不孕夫妇的病史
- 制订不孕夫妇的初步检查计划

专业技能及态度
- 思考不孕症对夫妇双方的影响
- 思考不孕症管理相关的社会和伦理问题

LEARNING OUTCOMES

At the end of this chapter you should be able to:

Knowledge criteria
- Describe the common causes of male and female infertility
- Describe the indications for and interpretation of investigations used in the assessment of the infertile couple
- Discuss the principles of, indications for and complications of the common methods of treatment of infertility

Clinical competencies
- Take a history from a couple presenting with infertility
- Plan appropriate initial investigation of an infertile couple

Professional skills and attitudes
- Reflect on the impact of infertility on a couple
- Reflect on the social and ethical issues relevant to the management of infertility

在世界不同地区，不孕症患病率非常相似，其中，较发达国家的年患病率为 3.5%～16.7%，而欠发达国家为 6.9%～9.3%，预估总体中位患病率为 9%。例如，在英国，1/7 的夫妇由于受孕问题进行咨询。所有不孕夫妇中只有 50% 就医，较发达国家和欠发达国家的比例相似。根据这些预估数据和目前世界人口情况，有 7240 万女性患有不孕症，其中 4050 万女性正在寻求不孕症治疗。尽管很难找到确凿的证据，但在西方世界，不孕症的发病率似乎在上升，这是由于一系列因素造成的，其中包括患有性传播疾病的年轻人、肥胖人群及晚育女性人数的增加。

Estimates of the prevalence of infertility in different parts of the world give remarkably similar results, with a 12-month prevalence rate ranging from 3.5 to 16.7% in more developed nations and from 6.9 to 9.3% in less developed nations, with an estimated overall median prevalence of 9%. In the UK, for instance, one in seven couples consult due to problems in conceiving. Only half of all infertile couples seek medical help, with the proportion being similar in developed and less developed nations. Based on these estimates and on the current world population, 72.4 million women are currently infertile, and of these, 40.5 million are currently seeking infertility medical care. Although firm evidence is hard to find, it seems that the prevalence of infertility in the Western world is increasing due to a number of factors, including the increase in number of young people with sexually transmitted diseases, increase in obesity and increasing numbers of women deferring plans for childbearing until later in life.

原发不孕是指既往无妊娠或活产的不孕，继发不孕是指曾经有一次或多次妊娠后的不孕，无论曾经妊娠是正常妊娠、流产、宫外孕或自愿终止妊娠。不孕症检查方法的改进通常会暴露男女双方的问题，这就形成了相对低生育力的概念。较高生育力的女性通常会弥补其男性伴侣精子质量差的缺点，可以顺利受孕，反之亦然。

Primary infertility is defined as infertility without a previous pregnancy or live birth, and *secondary infertility* as failure to conceive after one or more pregnancies, whether successful or ending in miscarriage, ectopic pregnancy or voluntary termination. Improved methods for investigation of infertility frequently reveal a problem in both partners, leading to the concept of relative *subfertility*. A highly fertile female partner will often compensate for a male with poor sperm quality and conceive without difficulty, and vice versa.

在 25 岁时，每个周期的受孕率约为 25%，35 岁时是 12%，40 岁时，每周期仅为 6%。对于一对育龄夫妇，如果在正常性交 12 个月后没有受孕，这对夫妇应被视为潜在的不孕症患者，因为 80% 的夫妇通常在 1 年内受孕。因此，此时进行不孕症检查是合理的。然而，这一定义应该根据常识加以调整。例如，曾因宫外孕而切除双侧输卵管的女性或已知年轻时曾发生睾丸扭转情况的男性，都应尽早进行检查和治疗。

At the age of 25 years old, the conception rate per cycle is approximately 25%; at 35 years old, it is 12%; and at 40 years old, it is only 6% per cycle. For a couple of reproductive age, if conception does not occur after 12 months of regular sexual intercourse, the couple should be considered potentially infertile, as 80% of couples normally conceive within 1 year. It is therefore reasonable to proceed with investigations at this time. However, this definition should be tempered by common sense. For example, a woman who has lost both Fallopian tubes because of ectopic pregnancies or a man who is known to have had testicular torsion in his youth should not be denied early investigation and treatment.

不孕夫妇双方应一同就诊，因为不孕症可能是由男性或女性因素引起的，并且通常与两者混合因素密切相关。事实上，30% 的不孕症为男性因素，30% 为女性因素，女性和男性混合因素占 20%，另外 20% 为不明原因性不孕。

Both partners should be seen and investigated together, as infertility may result from male or female factors and is often associated with a combination of both. Indeed, in 30% the cause is due to male factor, 30% to female factor, 20% to both female and male factor and 20% cases of infertility are 'unexplained'.

针对不明原因性不孕症夫妇的长期随访研究表明，经不孕咨询后，30%～40% 的夫妇将在 7 年内受孕。许多不明原因性不孕症患者包括 35 岁以上的女性，进行体外受精（IVF）后会发现，可能存在卵巢刺激低反应和卵母细胞异常。年龄因素，尤其是女性年龄，无疑会影响生育力。IVF 成功率（由活产率定义）在 38 岁以后急剧下降（表 17-1）。年龄因素对男性生育力无显著影响，但高龄男性会出现异常精子和 DNA 碎片率的增加。

Long-term follow-up studies of couples with unexplained infertility have shown that 30–40% will conceive over a 7-year

表 17-1　2015 年英国女性各年龄段活产率（新鲜周期和冻融周期）

Table 17.1　Female age and live birth rate per embryo transfer (fresh and frozen) in the UK (2015).

	小于 35 岁 Under 35	35—37 岁	38—39 岁	40—42 岁	43—44 岁	大于 44 岁 Over 44
新鲜周期 Fresh	30	22	16	9	4	1
冻融周期 Frozen	25	23	18	14	9	6

数据引自 www.HFEA.gov.uk.

Data sourced from www.HFEA.gov.uk.

period after investigation. Many 'unexplained' cases involve women over age 35 years who may later be shown to have a poor response to ovarian stimulation and oocyte abnormalities if in vitro fertilization (IVF) is performed. Age, particularly female age, undoubtedly affects fertility. IVF success rates, defined by a live birth rate, fall sharply after age 38 (Table 17.1). The effect of age on the male is less pronounced, but older men exhibit more sperm abnormalities and DNA fragmentation.

致病因素的相对发生率因国家以及不孕症是原发性还是继发性而有所不同。此外，在许多夫妇中，不孕的原因是多方面的。表 17-2 展示了西方人群原发性不孕症的病因类型。

The relative incidence of causative factors will vary according to country and whether the problem is primary or secondary. Furthermore, in many couples there are multiple reasons for the infertility. Table 17.2 shows the pattern of causative factors of primary infertility in a Western population.

一、病史采集及体格检查（History and examination）

如前所述，初诊时应夫妇双方同时就诊。许多

医疗机构使用格式化调查问卷采集基础病史，从而合理利用初诊时间。基本检查，其中包括双方基本的血液检查和精液分析均可通过全科医师进行，并可在初诊时查看化验结果。

As mentioned, the initial consultation should involve both partners. Many clinics use a pro forma questionnaire to elicit basic information, allowing better use to be made of the time available in the consultation. Basic investigations, including baseline blood tests for both partners, and semen analysis can be organized through the general practice with results available at the initial meeting.

病史记录应包括以下内容。

The history should include the following:

- 双方的年龄、职业和教育背景。

- Age, occupation and educational background of both partners

- 不孕年限和避孕史。

- Number of years that conception has been attempted and the previous history of contraception

- 双方或其中一方的既往婚育史。

表 17–2　不孕原因

Table 17.2　Causes of infertility

诊断 * Diagnosis*	原发不孕组 Primary infertile group (n=167) N (%)	继发不孕组 Secondary infertile group (n = 151) N (%)	P 值 P-value
排卵问题 Ovulation problems	54（32.3）	35（23.2）	0.069
精子质量问题 Sperm quality problems	49（29.3）	36（23.8）	0.268
输卵管梗阻 Blocked Fallopian tubes	20（12）	21（13.9）	0.607
不明原因不孕 Unexplained infertility	49（29.3）	45（29.8）	0.928
子宫内膜异位症 Endometriosis	19（10.7）	15（10）	0.677
其他因素 Others	23（13.8）	32（21.2）	0.081

*. 每位女性不止一种诊断

数据引自一项苏格兰基于全科医学的研究 [Bhattacharya S, et al.（2010）The epidemiology of infertility in the North East of Scotland. Hum Reprod 24:3096–3107]. 苏格兰东北部被诊断不孕症女性自行上报了不孕原因，该数据包括试孕 12 个月或更长时间未成功和（或）已寻求医疗帮助的患者

*. Women have reported more than one diagnosis.

Data derived from a Scottish general practice-based survey (Bhattacharya S, et al. (2010) The epidemiology of infertility in the North East of Scotland. Hum Reprod 24:3096-3107). Self-reported cause of infertility amongst women who reported a diagnosis (northeast Scotland). The data reflect unsuccessful attempted conception for 12 months or longer and/or had sought medical help with conception.

- Previous conceptions of either partner in this or previous relationships

- 孕前、分娩和产后相关的并发症。

- Details of any complications associated with previous pregnancies, deliveries and postpartum

- 完整的妇科病史，其中包括月经的规律性、频率以及性质；宫颈涂片；经间期出血；阴道分泌物。

- Full gynaecological history, including regularity, frequency and nature of menses; cervical smears; intermenstrual bleeding; and vaginal discharge

- 性交史，其中包括性交频率、性交疼痛、性交后出血和勃起或射精功能障碍。

- Coital history, including frequency of intercourse, dyspareunia, postcoital bleeding and erectile or ejaculatory dysfunction

- 性传播疾病史及其治疗。

- History of sexually transmitted diseases and their treatment

- 一般病史，其中包括并发或既往严重疾病或

手术，尤其是与女性阑尾炎或男性疝修补术有关的病史；隐睾或睾丸固定术史。

- A general medical history to include concurrent or previous serious illness or surgery, particularly in relation to appendicitis in the female or herniorrhaphy in the male; a history of undescended testes or of orchidopexy

应考虑对双方进行检查，尽管在精液分析正常的情况下对男性的检查不大可能发现有意义的结果；如果高质量盆腔超声检查结果正常，对女性的检查可能同样不显著。无精子症男性应检查先天性双侧输精管缺如（congenital bilateral absence of the vas deferen，CBAVD），这与囊性纤维化突变有关。

Examination of both partners should be considered, although examination of the male is unlikely to reveal anything of significance in the presence of a normal semen analysis; that of the woman may well be equally unremarkable if there is a normal high-quality pelvic ultrasound. Azoospermic men should be examined for congenital bilateral absence of the vas deferens (CBAVD), which is associated with cystic fibrosis mutations.

病例分析	Case study
Y 女士和 Y 先生在尝试妊娠 5 年后仍未孕，被推荐至妇科门诊咨询。Y 女士 32 岁，她的母亲 38 岁时死于乳腺癌。她没有其他个人或家族病史。她的月经规律，无痛经，规律排卵。她最后一次宫颈涂片检查是 1 年前，结果正常。她的体重指数（BMI）为 23，临床检查正常。	Mrs and Mr Y were referred to the gynaecology clinic after trying to conceive for 5 years now without success. Mrs Y was 32 years old; her mother died of breast cancer at 38 years of age. She had no other personal or familial past history. Her menses were regular and painless, with regular ovulation. Her last cervical smear was 1 year previously and normal. Her body mass index (BMI) was 23 and clinical examination normal.
Y 先生 33 岁。没有既往病史。他有一个哥哥，未育。	Mr Y was 33 years old. He had no personal medical history. He had one brother older than him, with no children.
这对夫妇的初步检查结果显示，Y 女士的抗 Müllerian 管激素（AMH）为 30pmol/ml，卵泡刺激素（FSH）为 5U/L，黄体生成素（LH）为 3U/L，E2 为 130pmol/L。她排卵正常，第 21 天的孕酮水平为 53nmol/L。她的 B 超检查提示输卵管通畅。她咨询了遗传学家，未检测出 BRCA 突变。Y 先生是无精子和精液 pH 呈酸性。	The results of initial investigations for the couple showed that Mrs Y had an anti-müllerian hormone (AMH) of 30 pmol/mL, a follicle-stimulating hormone (FSH) of 5 IU/L, luteinizing hormone (LH) of 3 IU/L and E2 of 130 pMol/L. She was ovulating normally with a day-21 progesterone of 53 nMol/L. Her ultrasound was normal with evidence of tubal patency. She also saw a geneticist and did not have a detectable BRCA mutation. Mr Y was found to be azoospermia and with an acid seminal pH.
Y 先生咨询了一位男科专家。他做了临床检查和阴囊超声。临床检查提示 CBAVD，后经超声证实。他们进行了遗传咨询，并发现存在 CFTR 基因的杂合突变。他的妻子也接受了突变检测，结果呈阴性。	Mr Y was referred to an andrologist. He had a clinical examination and scrotal ultrasound. Clinical examination suggested CBAVD, which was confirmed by ultrasound. The patient was referred to a geneticist and was found to have a heterozygous mutation of the CFTR. His wife was also tested for the mutation and was negative.
在许多 CBAVD 病例中，可以通过手术从附睾或睾丸中穿刺取精。这可以用于卵胞质内单精子注射（intracytoplasmic sperm injection，ICSI）。在取精未成功的情况下，必要时需行供精。	In many cases of CBAVD it is possible to retrieve sperm from the epididymis or testis by surgical extraction. This can be used in an IVF cycle for intracytoplasmic sperm injection (ICSI). Use of donor sperm may be necessary in cases in which this is not possible.

二、女性不孕症（Female infertility）

年龄问题、严重的全身系统性疾病、营养不良、运动过度和情绪压力等一般因素都可能导致女性不孕。大多数女性不孕症是由于输卵管或子宫解剖或功能紊乱，或者卵巢功能障碍导致无排卵所引起的。较少见的疾病包括精子 - 宫颈黏液穿透困难、子宫内膜异位症和性交障碍。

General factors such as age, serious systemic illness, inadequate nutrition, excessive exercise and emotional stress may all contribute to female infertility. The majority of cases of female infertility follow from disorders of tubal or uterine anatomy or function, or ovarian dysfunction leading to anovulation. Less frequently observed disorders include cervical mucus 'hostility', endometriosis and dyspareunia.

（一）排卵障碍（Disorders of ovulation）

根据世界卫生组织（WHO）的定义，将排卵障碍分为四类。

Disorders of ovulation are divided into four categories, defined by the World Health Organization (WHO):

- Ⅰ型：低促性腺激素型性腺功能减退，为下丘脑 - 垂体衰竭所致。这种相对罕见的情况可能是先天性的（如 Kallman 综合征），也可能是后天获得性的，如继发于垂体腺瘤手术或放疗后。血清 LH、FSH 和雌二醇浓度异常低 / 检测不到，导致月经稀发或闭经。

- Type I-Hypogonadal hypogonadism resulting from failure of pulsatile gonadotrophin secretion from the pituitary. This relatively rare condition can be congenital (as in Kallman's syndrome) or acquired, for example, after surgery or radiotherapy for a pituitary tumour. Serum concentrations of LH and FSH and oestradiol are abnormally low/undetectable, and menses will be absent or very infrequent.

- Ⅱ型：促性腺激素正常型排卵障碍，最常见的原因是多囊卵巢综合征（PCOS；见第 16 章）。血清 FSH 正常，LH 正常或升高。血清 AMH 升高，血清睾酮或游离雄激素升高。

- Type II-Normogonadotropic anovulation, most commonly caused by polycystic ovary syndrome (PCOS; see Chapter 16). Serum concentrations of FSH will be normal and LH normal or raised. Serum AMH will be elevated, and there may also be elevation of serum testosterone or free androgen index.

- Ⅲ型：高促性腺激素型性腺功能减退，常为卵巢早衰所致，即 40 岁之前由于卵泡池耗尽而致不排卵。表现为血清促性腺激素水平增加，AMH 水平低或检测不到，且雌二醇浓度将至绝经后水平。

- Type III-Hypergonadotropic hypogonadism, frequently described as *premature ovarian failure*, describes cessation of ovulation due to depletion of the ovarian follicle pool before age 40 years. Serum gonadotrophin concentrations will be greatly raised and AMH low/undetectable, with postmenopausal (low) concentrations of oestradiol.

- Ⅳ型：高泌乳素血症，表现为血清泌乳素升高，血清 FSH 和 LH 低 / 正常。虽然通过垂体磁共振成像（MRI）或计算机断层扫描（CT）排除占位性的垂体大腺瘤是很重要的，但高催乳素血症通常由垂体微腺瘤所致。

- Type IV-Hyperprolactinaemia, with elevated serum prolactin and low/normal serum FSH and LH. Frequently due to a pituitary microadenoma, although it is important to rule out a space-occupying macroadenoma using pituitary magnetic resonance imaging (MRI) or computed tomography (CT).

- 无排卵通常可伴随闭经或月经过少的症状。月经周期的改变通常与压力、超重或肥胖有关，同时加剧了多囊卵巢综合征对于排卵的影响。或者，神经性厌食症或过度运动等极端情况将导致低促性腺激素型排卵障碍（Ⅰ型排卵障碍）。

- Anovulation is usually associated with amenorrhoea or oligomenorrhoea. Alterations in the menstrual cycle are commonly associated with periods of stress and with excessive weight gain or obesity, worsening the impact of PCOS on ovulation, or, at the other extreme, with anorexia nervosa or excessive exercise leading to hypogonadal (type I) anovulation.

（二）输卵管因素（Tubal factors）

输卵管必须首先从破裂的 Graafian 卵泡的排卵部位收集卵子，然后将卵子运输到输卵管壶腹部，壶腹部为受精部位。受精卵必须被运输到宫腔内，同时符合在月经周期中子宫内膜允许着床的正确时间点（"种植窗"）。输卵管因素占不孕症病例的 10%～30%：这因所涉及的人群而异。偶尔会存在先天性发育异常，但最常见的原因是输卵管炎。炎症可致输卵管伞端阻塞，在输卵管腔内聚集液体（输卵

病例分析	Case study
X 女士和 X 先生未避孕未孕 2 年。他们婚后性生活规律。	Mrs and Mr X presented with a 2-year history of trying to conceive without success. They were having regular intercourse.
X 女士，26 岁，家族史和既往史无异常。月经失调，曾服用罗可坦（异维 A 酸）治疗面部重度痤疮。体重指数为 28。体格检查，胸、腹部多毛体征。血压正常。	Mrs X was 26 years old and had no personal or familial past history. She had irregular menses and struggled with facial acne for which she took Roaccutane before her desire to become pregnant. Her BMI was 28. On clinical exam ination, she was found to have abnormal hirsutes on her breast and abdomen. Her blood pressure was normal.
X 先生 30 岁，无异常家族史、既往病史。	Mr X was 30 years old and had no personal or familial past history.
X 先生精液分析正常。X 女士盆腔超声检查提示子宫前位，输卵管通畅和卵巢多囊样改变。月经第 3 天内分泌检查显示 AMH 35 pmol/L，FSH 7 U/L，LH 9 U/L，E2 110 pmol/L，睾酮 3.2 nmol/L。	Mr X had a normal semen analysis. A pelvic ultrasound showed that Mrs X had an anteverted uterus, normal tubal patency and polycystic ovaries. Her blood test on day 3 showed an AMH of 35 pmol/L, FSH 7 IU/L, LH 9 IU/L, E2 at 110 pmol/L and testosterone at 3.2 nMol/L.
月经第 21 天孕酮 3.0 nmol/L。泌乳素、促甲状腺激素（TSH）与空腹血糖血脂均正常。宫颈涂片检查正常。风疹已免疫。	Progesterone on day 21 was 3.0 nMol/L. Her prolactin, thyroid-stimulating hormone (TSH) and fasting glucose lipid profiles were normal. Her cervical smear was normal, and she was rubella immune.
由于患者年龄在 30 岁以下，首先考虑改变其生活方式，帮助她进行至少 6 个月的健身和减重计划。减去 5% 的体重，可使 50% 的多囊卵巢综合征患者恢复正常排卵。可以使用 Clearblue 棒来追踪排卵。	As the patient is under 30 years old, the first consideration should be a lifestyle modification program to help her improve physical fitness and lose weight. This should continue for at least 6 months. Five percent weight loss can restore normal ovulation in 50% of women with PCOS. She can be advised to track her ovulation with a Clearblue stick.
如果她 6 个月后还未妊娠，考虑使用克罗米芬或来曲唑，可使约 70% 无排卵的 PCOS 患者恢复排卵，用药 6 周期后的妊娠率约为 60%。三线治疗可以是腹腔镜卵巢电打孔术（laparoscopic ovarian diathermy，LOD）或低剂量 FSH 卵巢刺激，但后者多胎妊娠的风险显著增加。	If she has not conceived after 6 months, consider use of clomiphene citrate or letrozole, which can restore ovulation in approximately 70% of women with anovular PCOS, with a pregnancy rate of approximately 60% after six cycles.
	Third-line treatment may be either laparoscopic ovarian diathermy (LOD) or low-dose FSH ovarian stimulation, although there is a significant risk of multiple pregnancy with the latter approach.
如果没有成功地诱导排卵，则最终的治疗方法将是在拮抗药控制的周期内进行低剂量 FSH 刺激的 IVF，采用激动药触发和全胚胎冷冻以避免卵巢过度刺激综合征（OHSS）的风险。	The ultimate approach to treatment if there is no success with ovulation induction would be an IVF with a low-dose FSH stimulation in an antagonist-controlled cycle, with an agonist trigger and 'freeze all' embryos to avoid risk of ovarian hyperstimulation syndrome (OHSS).

管积水）或脓液（输卵管积脓）（图 17–1）。

The Fallopian tube must first collect the ovum from its site of ovulation from the ruptured Graafian follicle and then transport the ovum to the ampullary segment, where fertilization occurs. The fertilized ovum must then be transported to the uterine cavity to arrive at the correct point in the menstrual cycle at which the endometrium becomes receptive to implantation (the 'implantation window'). Tubal factors account for about 10–30% of cases of infertility: this figure varies considerably according to the population involved. Occasionally, congenital anomalies occur, but the commonest cause of tubal damage is infection. Infection may cause occlusion of the fimbrial end of the tube, with the collection of fluid (hydrosalpinx) or pus (pyosalpinx) within the tubal lumen (Fig. 17.1).

! 注意

即使输卵管腔通畅，由于纤毛消失和输卵管蠕动障碍等对内部结构的损害也可能导致输卵管功能丧失。

Even in the presence of a patent tube, damage to the internal structure with depletion of cilia and impairment of tubal peristalsis may result in loss of tubal function.

在英国，急性输卵管炎最常见的病因是沙眼衣原体感染，但也可能是感染淋病奈瑟菌、大肠杆菌、厌氧菌和溶血性链球菌、葡萄球菌和梭状芽孢杆菌等其他微生物所致。输卵管损伤的发生率在盆腔炎初次发作后约为 8%，二次发作后为 16%，三次发作后为 40%。在英国，移民人口或其亲属中输卵管结核或子宫结核的发病率越来越高。

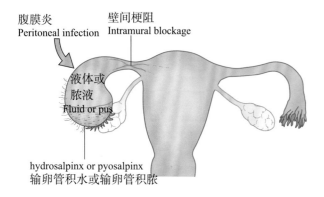

腹膜炎 Peritoneal infection
壁间梗阻 Intramural blockage
液体或脓液 Fluid or pus
hydrosalpinx or pyosalpinx
输卵管积水或输卵管积脓

▲ 图 17-1　输卵管梗阻与不孕症的发病机制，宫腔感染引起的输卵管壁间梗阻

Fig. 17.1　The pathogenesis of tubal occlusion and subfertility; intramural tubal obstruction results from intrauterine infection.

The commonest cause of acute salpingitis in the UK is infection with *Chlamydia trachomatis*, but it may also result from infection with other organisms such as Neisseria gonorrhoeae, Escherichia coli, anaerobic and haemolytic streptococci, staphylococci and *Clostridium welchii*. The incidence of tubal damage is approximately 8% after the first episode of pelvic infection, 16% after two and 40% after three episodes. Tubal or uterine tuberculosis has begun to be seen more frequently in the UK in the immigrant population or their relatives.

与腹膜炎相关的阑尾炎或包括克罗恩病或溃疡性结肠炎在内的炎症性疾病可能导致输卵管和卵巢周围粘连，而输卵管内部结构相对不受影响。

Disorders such as appendicitis associated with peritonitis or inflammatory conditions, including Crohn's disease or ulcerative colitis, can result in peritubal and peri-ovarian adhesions, leaving the internal structure of the Fallopian tube relatively unaffected.

（三）子宫因素（Uterine factors）

如果存在黏膜下肌瘤或先天性子宫畸形（如子宫纵隔等），受精卵着床的可能性较小。这些疾病常可通过手术矫正。浆膜下或完全的子宫肌壁间肌瘤似乎不影响受精卵着床。子宫腺肌病对着床的影响尚不明确，尽管发现其与胚胎反复种植失败和复发性流产有关。过度诊刮或术后感染（Asherman 综合征）所致的宫腔粘连会导致子宫内膜发育不良，闭经或月经过少，以及反复种植失败。

Implantation is less likely to occur if there is distortion of the uterine cavity due to submucous fibroids or congenital abnormalities such as an intrauterine septum. These disorders are often amenable to surgical correction. Subserous or entirely

intramural fibroids do not appear to affect implantation. The effect of adenomyosis on implantation is unclear, although the disorder has been linked to recurrent implantation failure and miscarriage. Intrauterine adhesions or synechiae following over-vigorous curettage or infection (Asherman's syndrome) result in inadequate endometrial development, absent or light periods and recurrent implantation failure.

子宫内膜异位症（Endometriosis）

子宫内膜异位症是一种病因不明的疾病，其病因学理论繁多，引起不孕的原因尚不明确。伴有大的卵巢囊肿和广泛粘连的重度内膜异位症会使输卵管解剖结构扭曲变形，干扰输卵管伞接近成熟卵泡，可能由于排卵障碍和输卵管"拾卵"功能受阻导致生育能力降低。然而，轻度的子宫内膜异位症也与不孕有关，一项大型随机对照试验表明，Ⅰ期和Ⅱ期子宫内膜异位症的手术治疗显著改善了自然妊娠率和活产率。

Endometriosis is an enigmatic condition with numerous theories related to aetiology and poorly defined links to infertility. Severe disease with large ovarian cysts and extensive adhesions distorting tubal anatomy and potentially interfering with approximation of the fimbriae to the mature follicle are likely to lead to subfertility due to impairment of ovulation and entrapment of the oocyte by the Fallopian tube. However, milder forms of the disorder have also been linked to problems of subfertility, and surgical treatment of grade I and II endometriosis led to a significant improvement in spontaneous pregnancy and live birth rates in a large randomized trial.

（四）宫颈因素（Cervical factors）

排卵时，宫颈黏膜细胞分泌丰富、透明、水样的宫颈黏液，其有高含水量和细长的糖蛋白分子，内含通道，有利于精子穿透进入宫腔。精子穿透发生在附着后的 2～3min。有 10 万～20 万个精子存在于宫颈黏液中，并在性交后保持这个水平约 24h。最终约有 200 个精子到达输卵管。排卵后，在孕酮的作用下，宫颈黏液不利于精子穿透。宫颈炎症或宫颈黏液或精浆中的抗精子抗体可抑制精子穿透力，从而导致不孕。

At the time of ovulation, endocervical cells secrete copious, clear, watery mucus, with high water content and elongated glycoprotein molecules containing channels that facilitate passage of spermatozoa into the uterine cavity. Sperm penetration occurs within 2–3 minutes of deposition. Between 100,000 and 200,000 sperm colonize the cervical mucus and remain at this level for approximately 24 hours after coitus. Approximately 200 sperm eventually reach the Fallopian

病例分析	Case study
30 岁的 Z 女士主诉为痛经和月经量过多。为了妊娠，她已于 3 个月前停止服用避孕药。她没有相关的既往史，她的丈夫也同样健康。她有一个姐姐，22 岁第一次分娩，24 岁第二次分娩。她的母亲也很健康，52 岁绝经。	A 30-year-old woman, Mrs Z, presented complaining of painful and heavy periods. She had stopped using the contraceptive pill 3 months earlier in order to conceive. She had no relevant general medical history, and her husband was equally healthy. She had one sister who had her first child at 22 years old and her second at 24. Her mother was healthy, having reached menopause at age 52.
Z 女士描述了 1 年前的手术，她被诊断为 IV 期子宫内膜异位症伴双侧子宫内膜异位囊肿，并被完全切除。术后，医生就给她开了口服避孕药。她的月经周期很规律。月经来的第一天，她每小时换一次卫生巾。她有中度性交疼痛，但无直肠或膀胱等相关症状。	Mrs Z described surgery 1 year previously at which she was diagnosed with stage 4 endometriosis with bilateral endometriomata, which were completely excised. She was prescribed the combined oral contraceptive pill from the time of surgery. Her cycles were regular. She changed her sanitary protection every hour on the first day of her period. She had moderate dyspareunia but no symptoms relating to bowel or bladder function. Her preoperative AMH was 15 pMol/L.
术前 AMH 15pmol/L。盆腔超声提示卵巢正常，但窦卵泡计数 (AFC) 为 3，右侧输卵管显示不清。AMH 2 pmol/L，FSH 10U/L，LH 5U/L，E2 130pmol/L。没有证据表明她的子宫内膜异位症存在复发现象。子宫体积增大，怀疑有早期弥漫性子宫腺肌病。精液分析结果正常。	Pelvic ultrasound showed normal ovaries, but the antral follicle count (AFC) was 3, and her right tube was not patent to contrast. Her AMH was 2 pmol/L, FSH 10 IU/L, LH 5 IU/L and E2 130 pMol/L. There was no evidence of recurrence of her endometriosis. The uterus was bulky with suspicion of early diffuse adenomyosis. Semen analysis was normal.
检查显示患者的卵巢储备功能下降，右侧输卵管损伤，这可能是由于子宫内膜异位症和卵巢手术造成的。可建议患者使用长效激动药方案进行 IVF 助孕，该方案包括至少 6 周采用促性腺激素释放激素（GnRH）激动药进行垂体下调调节。	The investigations indicated that she has a decreased ovarian reserve, and her right tube had probably been damaged, both probably due to consequences of endometriosis and ovarian surgery. She was advised to commence IVF treatment with a long agonist protocol involving at least 6 weeks of pituitary downregulation with a gonadotropin-releasing hormone (GnRH) agonist.

tube. After ovulation, mucus produced by the cervix under the influence of progesterone is hostile to sperm penetration. Cervical infection or antisperm antibodies in cervical mucus or seminal plasma can inhibit sperm penetration and result in subfertility.

三、男性不育症（Male infertility）

男性不育症可分为三类，即梗阻性无精症、非梗阻性无精症和混合性（梗阻性和非梗阻性无精症共存）。

Male infertility can be divided into three categories: obstructive azoospermia, non-obstructive azoospermia and mixed (association of obstructive and non-obstructive azoospermia).

（一）梗阻性无精症（Obstructive azoospermia）

梗阻性无精症可能是由于炎症、外伤或手术的副作用（如疝修补术）引起，导致生殖道阻塞，也可能是由于 CBAVD 或射精管狭窄所致。

Obstructive azoospermia may result from infection, trauma or side effects of surgery such as herniorrhaphy, leading

to an obstruction of the genital tract. It can also be due to CBAVD or a stenosis of the ejaculatory duct.

> **！注意**
> 如果发现了 CBAVD，则应该对患者进行遗传咨询，并寻找使患者成为囊性纤维化病携带者的基因突变位点，因为这对后代有明显的影响。
>
> If a CBAVD is found, the patient should have a genetic consultation and mutations in genes causing the patient to be a carrier for cystic fibrosis should be sought, since this has obvious implications for the potential offspring.

（二）非梗阻性无精症（Non-obstructive azoospermia）

非梗阻性无精症可能是因原发性睾丸疾病或继发于中枢性腺发育不良的一种性腺功能减退症。

Non-obstructive azoospermia can be due to primary testicular disorders or be secondary to central hypogonadal hypogonadism.

睾丸疾病包括雄激素不敏感综合征、染色体异常（如先天性曲细精管发育不全综合征）、隐睾病史、接受过性腺毒性化疗或其他一些药物治疗、先天性双侧无睾症、睾丸肿瘤或精索静脉曲张。男性性腺功能减退症可因先天性畸形（Kallman 综合征）、遗传异常（Prader-Willi 综合征或血色素沉着症等），也可因垂体肿瘤手术或放疗治疗所致。微腺瘤或大腺瘤或药物治疗（常用于治疗男性脱发或健美）引起的高泌乳素血症也可能是性腺功能减退症的原因。

Testicular causes include androgen insensitivity, chromosomal abnormalities such as Klinefelter's syndrome, past history of cryptorchidism, treatment with gonadotoxic chemotherapy or a number of other medications, bilateral anorchia, testicular tumour or varicocele. Hypogonadal hypogonadism in the male can result from congenital abnormalities including Kallman's syndrome, genetic abnormalities such as Prader-Willi syndrome or haemocromatosis or may follow surgery or radiotherapy to a pituitary tumour. Hypogonadal hypogonadism may also result from hyperprolactinaemia as a result of micro or macro adenoma or use of medications, including those commonly used to treat male alopecia or in bodybuilding.

四、不孕症检查（Investigation of infertility）

（一）女方检查（Investigation of the female partner）

所有不孕症女性患者均应进行风疹免疫学检查，如果血清学阴性，应在进一步治疗不孕症之前接种疫苗。还应建议他们从检查和治疗生育问题开始就补充叶酸，以降低后代患脊柱裂的风险。

All women presenting with infertility should have their rubella immunity checked and, if seronegative, be offered vaccination before undertaking further treatment for their infertility. They should also be advised to take folic acid supplementation from the outset of investigation and treatment of their fertility problem to reduce chances of spina bifida in their child.

1. 排卵监测（Detection of ovulation）

排卵评估取决于月经史。在月经周期规律的情况下，监测排卵可以通过基础体温（basal body temperature，BBT）测定，宫颈黏液或激素水平的变化，子宫内膜活检或 B 超检查。然而，对许多女性来说，BBT 需要每天测量体温并绘制图表，易给不孕症患者造成一定的精神压力。因此不推荐使用 BBT 测量。许多女性患者同样表明评估宫颈黏液性状变化十分困难，所以也不推荐使用这种方法。可以通过检测血液或尿液中的 LH 峰推断是否排卵，峰值约出现在排卵前 24h。使用现代商用 LH 检测试剂盒可以预测排卵情况，从而保证不延误性交时机。可以通过测量黄体期的血清孕酮来证明黄体生成，

其在黄体中期浓度超过 25nmol/L 通常被认为是排卵的证据，不同实验室的数值标准可能不尽相同。

The assessment of ovulation depends on the menstrual history. In the presence of a regular menstrual cycle, ovulatory status can be investigated by changes in basal body temperature (BBT), cervical mucus or hormone levels; by endometrial biopsy; or by ultrasound. However, measurement of BBT is difficult for many women to achieve and requires daily charting, increasing stress with a daily reminder of failure to conceive. Hence measurement of BBT is no longer recommended. Similarly, many women find assessment of cervical mucus changes difficult and challenging, and this method is also not recommended. Ovulation can be inferred by detection of the LH surge in blood or urine, with a peak that occurs approximately 24 hours before ovulation. Modern commercially available LH surge detection kits can provide reassurance and allow timing of intercourse. Formation of the corpus luteum can be demonstrated by measurement of serum progesterone in the luteal phase of the cycle. A mid-luteal concentration above 25 nmol/L is usually accepted as evidence of ovulation, although values vary from laboratory to laboratory.

> **！注意**
>
> 月经周期规律的女性无须测量甲状腺功能或泌乳素水平，除非她们有泌乳症状或甲状腺疾病的相关症状。
>
> There is no need to measure thyroid function or prolactin levels in women with regular menstrual cycles unless they have symptoms of galactorrhoea or thyroid disease.

(1) 超声检查（Ultrasonography）：

经阴道超声检查可用于监测卵巢内卵泡发育情况。卵泡直径可由排卵前 5 天的 11.5mm 增大至排卵前一天的 20mm，排卵后第 1 天卵泡直径减半，内部出现浑浊，最终生成黄体。这是最实用但是耗时的监测排卵的方法。超声检查对 PCOS 或卵巢型子宫内膜异位囊肿也具有诊断价值。

Transvaginal ultrasound examination of the ovaries can be used to track follicle growth. Follicular diameter increases from 11.5 mm 5 days before ovulation to 20 mm on the day before ovulation and decreases to approximately half this size on the day after ovulation, with opacification of the follicular remnant as the corpus luteum forms. This is a helpful, although time-consuming, way of monitoring the time of ovulation. Ultrasound may also be of value in the diagnosis of PCOS or ovarian endometrioma.

(2) 无排卵的检查（Investigation of anovulation）：

如果存在无排卵的证据，进一步的检查应包括以下方面。

If there is evidence of anovulation, further investigation should include measurement of:

- 在自然或人工月经周期的第 2 或第 3 天，测定血清 FSH、LH 和雌二醇，以及 AMH。

  - Serum FSH, LH and oestradiol on day 2 or 3 of a natural or induced menstruation, along with measurement of AMH

- 测定血清泌乳素和甲状腺功能。

  - Serum prolactin and thyroid function

- 如果泌乳素水平过高，进行蝶鞍 MRI 或 CT 检查。

  - MRI or CT of the sella turcica if prolactin levels are raised

(3) 卵巢储备功能评估（Assessment of ovarian reserve）：

女性高龄是决定体外受精治疗成功与否的最重要的预后因素之一。可通过测定血清中 AMH 和（或）经阴道行超声检查 AFC 估计个体的卵巢储备功能。与年龄相关的低 AMH 或低 AFC 水平预示着 IVF 助孕时卵母细胞数量可能较少及妊娠机会低于平均值，而其高于平均水平则预示着卵巢对促性腺激素的刺激反应良好。然而，尽管这些标记物有助于预测卵巢刺激后可获得的卵母细胞数量，但它们不能用以评价卵母细胞质量。卵子质量（受精、种植以及最终健康活产的潜力）似乎与女性年龄更紧密相关，年轻的卵巢低反应患者妊娠概率高，高龄的卵巢刺激反应良好的患者获卵数更多，但妊娠率仍然降低。

Advancing female age is one of the strongest prognostic factors that determines the success or otherwise of IVF treatment. Ovarian reserve testing using measurement of AMH in serum and/or AFC with transvaginal ultrasound allows an individual estimate of 'ovarian reserve' to be made. An age-related low AMH or low AFC predicts poor oocyte yield at IVF and a lower-than-average chance of pregnancy, whereas higher-than-average values predict a better ovarian response to gonadotrophin stimulation. However, although these markers are helpful in identifying predicted oocyte *quantity* after stimulation, they do not identify oocyte *quality* with the same precision. Quality (potential for fertilization and implantation leading to healthy live birth) seems to be more closely related to female age, such that a young 'poor responder' to stimulation has a good chance of pregnancy, whereas an older 'good responder' may obtain a larger-than-usual number of oocytes but there is still a reduced chance of pregnancy.

2. 输卵管通畅性检查（Investigation of tubal patency）

在进行诱导排卵或宫腔内人工授精之前，必须保证输卵管通畅。如果一对夫妇要直接进行 IVF 助孕，比如有严重的男性因素所致不育症，就无须进行输卵管通畅性检查。但应使用高分辨率经阴道超声检查或子宫输卵管造影术（hysterosalpingography，HSG）检查子宫的解剖结构。

It is essential to establish tubal patency before beginning ovulation induction or intrauterine insemination. Tubal patency need not be established if the couple are to proceed directly to IVF if, for example, there is a severe male factor. However, uterine anatomy should then be checked with high-resolution transvaginal ultrasound or hysterosalpingography (HSG).

(1) 子宫输卵管造影（Hysterosalpingography）：

对比剂注入宫腔和输卵管。不必进行全身麻醉。通过对比剂弥散勾勒出子宫腔的轮廓，并显示充盈缺损。其将提示是否存在输卵管阻塞及阻塞的部位（图 17-2）。输卵管造影应该在月经周期的前 10 天内进行，以避免意外辐射新受精的胚胎。女性应在行 HSG 前筛查沙眼衣原体或适当应用抗生素预防，以降低再次感染导致盆腔脓肿形成的风险。

A radio-opaque contrast medium is injected into the uterine cavity and Fallopian tubes. General anaesthesia is unnecessary. The contrast medium outlines the uterine cavity and will demonstrate any filling defects. It will also show whether there is evidence of tubal obstruction and the site of the obstruction (Fig. 17.2). HSG should be performed within the first 10 days of the menstrual cycle to avoid inadvertent irradiation of a newly fertilized embryo. Women should be screened for C. *trachomatis* infection or given appropriate antibiotic prophylaxis before HSG in order to reduce the risk of reactivation of infection leading to pelvic abscess formation.

(2) 子宫输卵管超声造影（Hysterosonocontrast sonography）：

子宫输卵管超声造影（Hysterosonocontrast sonography，HyCoSy）使用经阴道超声观察宫腔和输卵管的充盈缺损情况，最近已作为输卵管造影的替代检查。HyCoSy 避免暴露于电离辐射，并可以实时观察子宫和输卵管的解剖结构。高质量的超声设备和过硬的专业技术对于获得良好成像图是必不可少的因素。

Hysterosonocontrast sonography (HyCoSy) using transvaginal ultrasound to observe filling of the uterine cavity and Fallopian tubes has recently been introduced as an alternative to HSG. HyCoSy avoids exposure to ionizing radiation and allows real-time observation of uterine and tubal

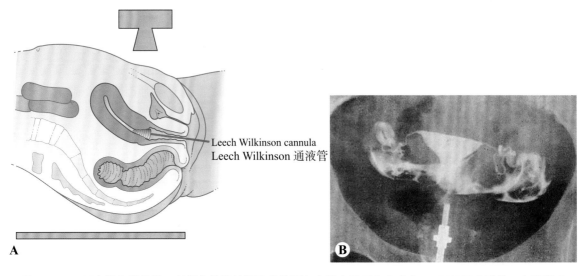

▲ 图 17-2　A. 子宫输卵管造影可以评估输卵管梗阻的位置和宫腔内是否存在病变；B. 可见子宫腔的三角形轮廓，对比剂从两侧输卵管伞端流出并扩散至邻近的肠管

Fig. 17.2　(A) Hysterosalpingography enables assessment of the site of tubal obstruction and the presence of pathology in the uterine cavity. (B) The triangular outline of the uterine cavity can be seen and the spill of dye on both sides from the fimbrial ends of the Fallopian tubes. The dye spreads over the adjacent bowel.

anatomy. High-quality ultrasound equipment and a degree of technical expertise are necessary to obtain good images.

(3) 腹腔镜下输卵管通液（Laparoscopy and dye insufflation）：

腹腔镜检查可以直接观察盆腔器官，并可以评估盆腔病变，如子宫内膜异位症或盆腔粘连。经宫颈口注入亚甲蓝溶液以评估输卵管的通畅性。腹腔镜检查可联合宫腔镜检查以评估宫腔情况。尽管手术可能导致盆腔结构受损，最好留给另一种场合让患者及其伴侣充分讨论手术的内涵，但"即看即治"可快速的经手术治疗轻度的子宫内膜异位症或粘连。腹腔镜检查几乎均需全身麻醉，腹腔镜检查对盆腔结构（包括肠、膀胱和输尿管）存在极小但严重的损伤风险，因此，除非有明确适应证，如盆腔炎或阑尾炎合并腹膜炎病史，临床一线应首选侵入性小的检查方法（图 17-3）。

Laparoscopy enables direct visualization of the pelvic organs and allows assessment of pelvic pathologies such as endometriosis or adhesions. Methylene blue is injected through the cervix in order to test tubal patency. Laparoscopy can be combined with hysteroscopy to assess the uterine cavity. A 'see-and-treat' policy allows for rapid surgical treatment of minor degrees of endometriosis or adhesions, although surgery that may result in damage to pelvic structures is better left to another occasion to allow full discussion of the implications of surgery to take place with the patient and her partner. Laparoscopy almost invariably requires general anaesthesia, and there

are small but significant risks of damage to pelvic structures, including bowel, bladder and ureter at laparoscopy, so less invasive methods are preferred as first-line investigations unless there is a specific indication, such as a history of pelvic inflammatory disease or appendicitis with peritonitis (Fig. 17.3).

3. 宫颈因素的不孕症检查（Investigation of cervical factor infertility）

宫颈因素不孕症检查，如性交后试验，因为缺乏既定的规范标准且与生育力之间的低相关性，因此不推荐不孕症夫妇进行例行检查。现代治疗不孕

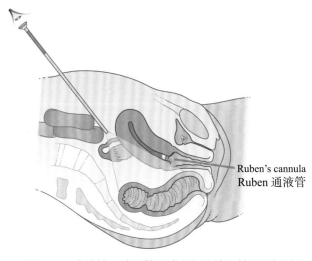

▲ 图 17-3　腹腔镜下输卵管通液术评估输卵管的通畅情况

Fig. 17.3　Dye laparoscopy for evaluation of tubal patency.

症的方法，如宫腔内人工授精（IUI）或体外受精（IVF），将避开宫颈黏液的影响，避免任何导致不孕症的潜在宫颈因素。

'Cervical factor' infertility tests, such as postcoital tests, are not recommended in the routine investigation of the infertile couple because of the lack of established normal criteria and poor correlation between findings and fertility. Modern treatments for infertility, such as intrauterine insemination (IUI) or IVF, will bypass cervical mucus and circumvent any possible cervical causes for infertility.

（二）男方检查（Investigation of the male partner）

精液分析是评价男性生育力最实用的检查方法。精液应在禁欲 3 天后用手淫法采集至无菌容器中，并于收集后 2h 内进行检查。最好在男科实验室附近的私密场所收集精液样本，以避免在运输过程中冷却并允许能准确识别男方信息。

The most useful investigation of the male partner is by semen analysis. Semen should be collected by masturbation into a sterile container after 3 days abstinence and examined within 2 hours of collection. The sample is best collected in a private facility adjacent to the andrology laboratory to avoid cooling during transportation and allow accurate identification of the male partner.

表 17-3 列出了精子参数（WHO 2010）的参考下限和 95%CI。

The lower reference limits and 95% confidence intervals for sperm parameters (WHO 2010) are given in Table 17.3.

精液特征的主要指标如下。

The major features of the semen analysis are:

- 体积：80% 的可生育男性一次射精 1～4ml。量少可能提示雄激素缺乏，量大则提示附属腺体功能异常

- Volume: 80% of fertile males ejaculate between 1 mL and 4 mL of semen. Low volumes may indicate androgen deficiency, and high volumes abnormal accessory gland function.

- 精子浓度：尽管可以通过经皮附睾穿刺精子抽吸术（PESA）或经睾丸穿刺取精术（TESA）或睾丸活检来获取患者的精子，但全部精子缺失（无精子症）仍表明其是不育症。精子的正常值下限在 1500 万～2000 万 /ml，因为精子浓度每天均有显著的波动性，所以不能仅凭单次取样结果进行判读。浓度异常过高，超过 2 亿 /ml，可能提示与生育力低下有关。

- Sperm concentration: The absence of all sperm (azoospermia) indicates sterility, although sperm may well be recoverable by percutaneous epididymal aspiration (PESA) or testicular aspiration (TESA) or testicular biopsy. The lower limit of normal is between 15 million and 20 million sperm/mL, but the findings should not be accepted on a single sample, as there is significant fluctuation from day to day. Abnormally high values, in excess of 200 million sperm/mL, may be associated with subfertility.

- 经正常分析后显示在采样后 1h 内 60% 的精子活力良好。向前运动力与其同等重要。WHO 根据以下标准对精子活力进行分级：

- A normal analysis should show good motility in 60% of sperm within 1 hour of collection. The characteristic of forward progression is equally important. The WHO grades sperm motility according to the following criteria:

- 等级 1：快速直线前向运动。

- Grade 1-rapid and linear progressive motility

- 等级 2：慢速或缓慢的线性或非线性运动。

- Grade 2-slow or sluggish linear or non-linear motility

- 等级 3：非前向运动。

- Grade 3-non-progressive motility

- 等级 4：不动。

- Grade 4-immotile

- 即使在生育力正常男性中，精子形态学也具有显著差异性，其对生育力的预测性远低于精子数或精子活力。白细胞是检查中一个重要的指标，因为它们的存在可能提示感染。如果存在脓液细胞，应将精液进行细菌培养。

- Sperm morphology shows great variability even in normal fertile males and is less predictive of subfertility than count or motility. It is important to look for leukocytes, as they may indicate the presence of infection. If pus cells are present, the semen should be cultured for bacteriological growth.

精子形成和精子功能可被多种毒素和药物影响。各种毒素和药物可能作用于曲细精管和附睾以抑制精子形成。化学药物，尤其是烷化剂，能抑制精子功能，而经常用于治疗克罗恩病的柳氮磺吡啶会降低精子活力和密度。患者在接受化疗或盆腔放疗前应该进行精子冷冻保存，这样一旦他们的疾病成功治愈后，他们就可以立即组建家庭（图 17-4）。此外，降压药可引起勃起功能障碍，用于健身的合成类固

表 17-3　精液各项参数的参考值下限（第 5 百分位数及 95% 的置信区间）

Table 17.3　Lower reference limits (5th centiles and their 95% confidence intervals) for semen characteristics

参数 Parameter	参考值下限 Lower reference limit
精液体积 (ml) Semen volume (mL)	1.5（1.4~1.7）
精子总数 (10^6 个 / 一次射精) Total sperm number (10^6 per ejaculate)	39（33~46）
精子浓度 (10^6/ml) Sperm concentration (10^6/mL)	15（12~16）
总活动率 (PR + NP, %) Total motility (PR + NP, %)	40（38~42）
前向运动精子 (PR, %) Progressive motility (PR, %)	32（31~34）
存活率（活精子，%) Vitality (live spermatozoa, %)	58（55~63）
精子形态 (正常形态，%) Sperm morphology (normal forms, %)	4（3.0~4.0）
其他公认阈值 Other consensus threshold values	
酸碱度 pH	≥7.2
过氧化物酶阳性白细胞（10^6/ml） Peroxidase-positive leukocytes (10^6/mL)	<1.0
混合抗球蛋白反应试验（与颗粒结合的活动精子，%） MAR test (motile spermatozoa with bound particles, %)	<50
免疫珠试验（与免疫珠结合的活动精子，%） Immunobead test (motile spermatozoa with bound beads, %)	<50
精浆果糖检测（μmol/ 一次射精量) Seminal fructose (μmol/ejaculate)	≥13
精浆中性葡萄糖苷酶检测 (mU/ 一次射精量) Seminal neutral glucosidase (mU/ejaculate)	≥20

数据引自 Cooper TG, Noonan E, von Eckardstein S, et al. (2010) World Health Organization reference values for human semen characteristics. Hum Reprod Update 16:231-245.

Data from Cooper TG, Noonan E, von Eckardstein S, et al. (2010) World Health Organization reference values for human semen characteristics. Hum Reprod Update 16:231-245.

醇可引起严重的生精障碍。

Spermatogenesis and sperm function may be affected by a wide range of toxins and therapeutic agents. Various toxins and drugs may act on the seminiferous tubules and the epididymis to inhibit spermatogenesis. Chemotherapeutic agents, particularly alkylating agents, depress sperm function, and sulfasalazine frequently used to treat Crohn's disease, reduces sperm motility and density. Patients who are prescribed chemotherapy or pelvic radiotherapy should be offered sperm cryopreservation before treatment to allow them to start a family later in life once their disease has been successfully treated (Fig. 17.4). Additionally, antihypertensive agents can cause erectile dysfunction, and anabolic steroids used for bodybuilding may produce profound hypospermatogenesis.

1. 精子 DNA 分析（Analysis of sperm DNA）

对精子浓度、精子活力和精子形态的标准化检测很难推断一对夫妇的受孕能力。精子染色体 DNA 的完整性对于正常受精和父系遗传信息的传递是必

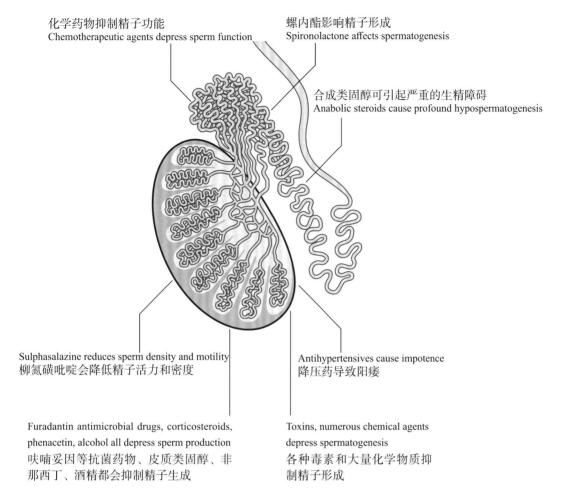

化学药物抑制精子功能
Chemotherapeutic agents depress sperm function

螺内酯影响精子形成
Spironolactone affects spermatogenesis

合成类固醇可引起严重的生精障碍
Anabolic steroids cause profound hypospermatogenesis

Sulphasalazine reduces sperm density and motility
柳氮磺吡啶会降低精子活力和密度

Antihypertensives cause impotence
降压药导致阳痿

Furadantin antimicrobial drugs, corticosteroids, phenacetin, alcohol all depress sperm production
呋喃妥因等抗菌药物、皮质类固醇、非那西丁、酒精都会抑制精子生成

Toxins, numerous chemical agents depress spermatogenesis
各种毒素和大量化学物质抑制精子形成

▲ 图 17-4　化学药物对精子形成的影响

Fig. 17.4　Influence of chemical agents on spermatogenesis.

不可少的，精子 DNA 完整性检测通常与常规精液检测项目相关，其中包括精子浓度或活力下降。当精子在男性和女性生殖道运输时，精子 DNA 受到保护避免损伤，精子 DNA 损伤可能导致生育力下降。

Standard tests of sperm concentration, motility and morphology are poorly predictive of the ability of a couple to conceive. The integrity of sperm chromosomal DNA is essential for normal fertilization and transmission of paternal genetic information, and tests of sperm DNA integrity generally correlate with routine semen variables, including impaired sperm concentration or motility. Sperm DNA is protected from damage while the sperm is transported through the male and female reproductive tracts, and damage to sperm DNA may lead to impaired fertility.

最常用的测量精子 DNA 损伤的方法是精子染色质结构分析（SCSA），它可测试精子染色质在吖啶橙酸性介质中的稳定性。当荧光剂与完整的 DNA 结合时发出绿色荧光，与碎片 DNA 结合时发出红色荧光；用流式细胞术测定发生 DNA 碎裂的精子比例，

用 DNA 碎片率（DNA fragmentation index，DFI）表示。其他常用的检测包括：①原位末端转移酶标记技术（TUNEL），进行流式细胞术对荧光激活的细胞进行分类；②单细胞电泳试验（Comet），使用电泳技术测量单链和双链 DNA 断裂；③光环试验（SCD），该试验可识别发生 DNA 碎裂的精子，因为它们在酸 / 盐处理后与琼脂糖混合时不能产生特征光环。每一种测定法都有其优缺点，不同试验之间不总是出现一致的正常或异常的结果。

The most frequently used measure of sperm DNA damage is the sperm chromatin structure assay (SCSA) that measures the stability of sperm chromatin in acid media with acridine orange. The dye gives rise to green fluorescence when bound to intact DNA and red when bound to fragmented DNA; the proportion of sperm with fragmented DNA is determined by flow cytometry and expressed as the DNA fragmentation index (DFI). Other commonly used tests include the deoxynucleotidyl transferase-mediated dUTP nick end labelling (TUNEL) assay in which fluorescence-activated cells are sorted by flow cytometry, the single cell electrophoresis assay (Comet) that measures single-strand and double-strand DNA breaks using electrophoresis and the Halo (SCD) test that identifies sperm with fragmented DNA because they fail to produce the characteristic halo when mixed with aqueous agarose following acid/salt treatment. Each assay has its strengths and weaknesses, and results imputing normality or abnormality do not always concur between assays.

在临床研究中，不育男性与正常生育力的男性相比，精子 DNA 完整性受损且精子质量较差。对中止避孕时具有正常生育能力的夫妇进行的妊娠时间的研究表明，SCSA 检测结果与妊娠率显著相关。然而，在 IVF 和 ICSI 研究中，精子 DNA 完整性结果与受精率或妊娠率的相关性并不明确。目前，对精子 DNA 完整性的评估仍应作为一种研究工具，而将其作为诊断性检查来常规应用则需要等待进一步的证据来区分那些愿意或不愿意受孕的夫妇。

In clinical studies, sperm DNA integrity is impaired among infertile compared with fertile men and with poor semen quality. Time-to-pregnancy studies with apparently normally fertile couples at the time of stopping contraception showed that results of the SCSA test were significantly associated with the probability of pregnancy. However, IVF and ICSI studies have been less conclusive in relating sperm DNA integrity results to fertilization or pregnancy rates. At present, assessment of sperm DNA damage should remain as a research tool, and routine use as a diagnostic test should await further evidence of ability to discriminate between those couples who will or will not conceive.

2. 男性内分泌激素测定（Endocrine assessment of the male）

血清高 FSH 和低 AMH 值提示睾丸可能受损，而正常水平提示梗阻性疾病。男性血清 FSH 和 LH 浓度低或检测不到提示垂体功能减退症，可以采用 FSH/LH 激素替代疗法。高 FSH、低 AMH 和无精子症需要进一步检查，它们均提示可能存在生精障碍。然而，即使 FSH 过高和 AMH 过低，睾丸活检仍可揭示精子发生过程中睾丸内病灶的位置，同时可取出精子用于 ICSI 助孕。

High serum concentrations of FSH and low AMH indicate testicular damage, whereas normal levels may indicate obstructive disease. Low or undetectable serum concentrations of FSH and LH are found in males with hypopituitarism, which may be treated with FSH/LH replacement therapy. The presence of high FSH, low AMH and azoospermia obviates the need for further investigation, as these findings indicate spermatogenic failure. However, testicular biopsy may reveal intratesticular foci of spermatogenesis, allowing retrieval of sperm for use in

ICSI, even if FSH is raised and AMH suppressed.

高泌乳素血症可继发于男性垂体腺瘤，可导致阳痿或少精症。

Hyperprolactinaemia may occur in the male in association with a pituitary adenoma and may cause impotence or oligospermia.

3. 细胞遗传学研究（Cytogenetic studies）

男性无精症患者的染色体分析可能提示 XXY 或 XYY 核型，偶尔在少精症患者中存在常染色体易位。少精症男性（活动精子少于 500 万）应进行囊性纤维化基因突变筛查。此类突变基因的携带者可能是健康的，但如果其伴侣也是该突变的携带者，则他们可能行 IVF 助孕后生育患有囊性纤维化病的子代。

Chromosome analysis in males with azoospermia may indicate the presence of a karyotype of XXY or XYY and, occasionally, autosomal translocation in the presence of oligospermia. Oligospermic men (fewer than 5 million motile sperm) should be screened for cystic fibrosis gene mutations. Carriers for such mutations may be healthy but could conceive a child with cystic fibrosis after IVF if their partner is also a carrier for the mutation.

4. 睾丸 / 附睾活检（Testicular/epididymal biopsy）

即使促性腺激素浓度升高，睾丸活检也能证明精子发生的存在。精子可以被抽吸并冷冻保存以备将来用于 ICSI。输精管梗阻的男性，如输精管切除术后，可进行 PESA，很大概率可获得合适的可行 ICSI 助孕的精子。

Testicular biopsy may demonstrate the presence of spermatogenesis even if there are elevated concentrations of gonadotrophins. Sperm may be aspirated and cryopreserved for later use in ICSI. Men with obstruction of the vas deferens, e.g. postvasectomy, may undergo PESA with a high chance of obtaining sperm that are suitable for ICSI.

5. 逆行射精（Retrograde ejaculation）

逆行射精是不孕的罕见原因，多继发于经尿道前列腺电切术后。通过检测高潮后尿液中的精子来进行诊断。可从患者高潮后的碱性尿液样本中提取精子，以用于 ICSI 助孕。

Retrograde ejaculation is a rare cause of infertility. It should be suspected following a transurethral resection of the prostate. The diagnosis is made by detecting spermatozoa in the urine following orgasm. Sperm can be retrieved from an alkalinized postorgasm urine sample for use in ICSI.

6. 男性不育的免疫学检查（Immunological tests for male infertility）

男性可能也会对精子产生免疫作用，对精子抗原的自身免疫作用可能与不育有关。抗原 - 抗体反应可通过阻断精子获能或卵母细胞透明带上的精子受体而导致自身免疫性不育。可以通过混合抗球蛋白反应试验（MAR）检测精浆中抗精子抗体是否与 IgG 和 IgA 相结合（IgG 和 IgA 是不同种类的免疫球蛋白）。当结合率超过 50% 时，抗精子抗体会对生育力产生重大的不利影响。

Immunity to sperm may occur in the male: autoimmunity to sperm antigens can be related to infertility. Antigen-antibody reactions may lead to autoimmune infertility by neutralizing sperm capacitation or by blocking sperm receptors on the oocyte zona pellucida. Sperm antibodies in seminal plasma appear in the IgG and IgA class (IgG and IgA are different kinds of immunoglobins) and can be detected using the mixed agglutination reaction (MAR). Sperm-bound antibodies appear to have a significant negative effect on fertility when there is more than 50% binding.

五、女性不孕症的治疗（Treatment of female subfertility）

如果双方的病史，体格检查和系统检查均正常，并且不孕年限少于 18 个月，应宽慰夫妇心理并建议其改变性生活的频率和生活方式，以提高妊娠机会。应建议双方停止吸烟并限制饮酒。应该鼓励 BMI 超过 30 的女性或男性参与具备专人监督的减肥计划。

If the history, examination and systematic investigation in both partners are normal and the duration of infertility is less than 18 months, the couple should be reassured and advised regarding coital frequency and simple lifestyle changes that may improve chances of conception. Both partners should be advised to stop smoking and limit their intake of alcohol. Women or men with a BMI of more than 30 should be encouraged to join a supervised programme of weight loss.

但是，如果女性超过 30 岁，则这种"观望"政策是不明智的，因为时机延误将对其 IVF 助孕的成功率产生显著的负面影响。应尽快将不孕症夫妇转诊至可行多种辅助生殖技术（assisted reproductive technology，ART）的生殖专科门诊进行后续治疗，其包括 IVF、ICSI、IUI 及供精和供卵治疗。

However, if the woman is over 30 years of age, this 'wait and see' policy is unwise, since delay will have a significant

adverse impact on her lifetime chance of conception using IVF. The couple should be referred rapidly to a specialist infertility clinic that has access to the full range of assisted reproductive technologies (ARTs), including IVF and ICSI, IUI and donor sperm and oocyte treatments.

（一）无排卵（Anovulation）

以 PCOS 为代表的 WHO Ⅱ 型无排卵，卵泡刺激素和泌乳素水平正常的情况下，首选用药仍是克罗米芬。应用克罗米芬后，80% 的受试者会排卵，其中约有 50% 的排卵者妊娠。从周期的第 2～6 天应用克罗米芬，初始剂量为 50mg/d，必要时增加到 100mg/d 和 150mg/d。排卵可以通过测量第 21 天的孕酮水平来监测，尽管正常的月经周期恢复后，随着排卵的恢复，通常会出现妊娠。据报道，双胎妊娠率为 6%～10%，三胎及以上妊娠发生风险约为万分之一。推荐用超声监测卵泡生长情况，如果有两个以上的成熟卵泡时应避免性交，以减少多胎妊娠的发生率。最近，芳香化酶抑制药来曲唑已被用作克罗米芬的口服替代药，现已被推荐作为一线治疗用药，提高了女性的排卵概率，可能获得更高的妊娠率。然而，来曲唑仍未获准用于治疗不孕症。

In the presence of WHO group II anovulation with stigmata of PCOS, normal FSH and prolactin levels, the drug of choice remains clomiphene citrate. Clomiphene will produce ovulation in 80% of subjects, leading to pregnancy in about one-half of those who ovulate. Clomiphene is administered from day 2 to 6 of the cycle with an initial dosage of 50 mg/day, increased to 100 and 150 mg/day where necessary. Ovulation can be monitored by measurement of day-21 progesterone levels, although restoration of a regular menstrual cycle is frequently followed by pregnancy as ovulation resumes. Rates of twin pregnancy of 6–10% have been reported, with higher-order pregnancies being reported in approximately 1:1000 patients. Ultrasound monitoring of follicle growth is recommended, with abstention from intercourse if there are more than two mature follicles to reduce the incidence of multiple pregnancy. More recently, the aromatase inhibitor letrozole has been used as an oral alternative to clomiphene and is now recommended as the first-line therapy, with an increase in the percentage of women who ovulate and possibly better pregnancy rates. However, letrozole remains unlicensed for treatment of infertility.

无排卵的二线治疗可能涉及 LOD，超过 70% 的 PCOS 患者会因 LOD 而排卵。LOD 的优势是诱导自然单卵 - 排卵，多胎妊娠的风险较前降低，一旦成功时，允许不使用药物和更多自然受孕的机会。另外，可以通过每日注射重组或尿源性 FSH 诱导排卵，尽管这可能花费昂贵，但由于反应过度和多胎妊娠的风险，需要进行超声和血液检查。谨慎使用低剂量，逐步递增的方案可以降低多胎妊娠率，同时妊娠率在可接受范围。

Second-line management of anovulation may involve LOD, which induces ovulation in over 70% of PCOS patients. LOD has the advantage of inducing natural monoovulation with a risk of multiple pregnancy no higher than background and, when successful, allowing a drug-free and more natural conception. Alternatively, ovulation may be induced with daily injection of recombinant or urinaryderived FSH, although this may be costly, and monitoring with ultrasound and blood tests is required due to the possibility of over-response and risk of multiple pregnancy. Careful management using a low-dose, step-up regimen can produce acceptable pregnancy rates with a low multiple pregnancy rate.

伴有垂体大腺瘤的高泌乳素血症无排卵可使用多巴胺受体激动药如卡麦角林治疗。卡麦角林优于溴隐亭，因为它易于给药且不良反应少。

Anovulation associated with hyperprolactinaemia in the absence of macroadenoma can be treated with a dopamine receptor agonist such as cabergoline. Cabergoline is preferred to bromocriptine due to its ease of administration and reduced incidence of side effects.

（二）输卵管病变（Tubal pathology）

在输卵管不孕症的治疗中，IVF 已几乎完全替代了输卵管显微外科手术。当患者存在输卵管积水的情况下，仍有必要在 IVF 前行腹腔镜下双侧输卵管切除术或双侧输卵管结扎术，以减少"有毒的"输卵管水样分泌物污染宫腔内子宫内膜的机会，或者进行初步的卵巢囊肿切除术或子宫肌瘤切除术。

Tubal microsurgery has been almost completely supplanted by IVF in the management of tubal infertility. Laparoscopic surgery may still be necessary to perform salpingectomy or tubal clipping prior to IVF in the presence of hydrosalpynx to reduce chances of contamination of the endometrial cavity with 'toxic' hydrosalpyngeal secretions, or for preliminary ovarian cystectomy or myomectomy.

输卵管粘连分离术用于分离输卵管周围粘连，若术后伞端良好，输卵管仍可具有一定的功能。一旦女性超过 30 岁，不要在此浪费过多时间，这是十分重要的。有时可以疏通梗阻的输卵管末端，即输卵管造口术（图 17-5）。进行任何输卵管手术均会增加异位妊娠的风险。

Salpingolysis to release peritubal adhesions still has a place if the fimbrial ends of the tubes are well preserved.

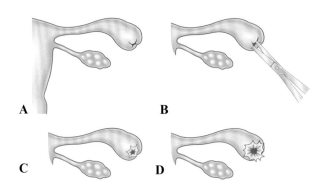

▲ 图 17-5　输卵管造口术治疗伞部纤毛闭锁及输卵管积水
A. 未经治疗的输卵管积水；B 和 C. 打开输卵管伞部纤毛；D. 缝合开放的输卵管积水部位

Fig. 17.5　Salpingostomy for fimbrial occlusions and hydrosalpynx. (A) Intact hydrosalpynx. (B, C) Opening of the fimbriae. (D) Suturing the opened hydrosalpinx.

However, it is important not to lose too much time if the woman is over 30 years of age. At times the blocked tubal end can be opened, i.e. salpingostomy (Fig. 17.5). There is an increased risk of ectopic pregnancy after all forms of tubal surgery.

（三）宫腔内人工授精（Intrauterine insemination）

使用柔性导管将精子注入宫腔这一技术已有多年的应用历史。通过清洗和分离活动精子制备精液样本及使用低剂量促性腺激素刺激排卵，使这项技术得以进一步发展。IUI 可被视为针对性交功能障碍和宫颈黏液异常的一种特殊治疗方法，但也经常用于治疗不明原因性不孕症和轻度男性因素不育症。进行 IUI 需要输卵管具有良好的通畅性。在高质量的生殖中心中，每个 IUI 周期活产率为 15%～20%。因其低剂量的促性腺激素、低水平监测和简化的实验室技术要求，IUI 仍然是 IVF 的一种经济有效的替代方法。

Placement of a sample of sperm into the uterine cavity using a soft, flexible catheter has been performed for many years. The technique has been enhanced by preparation of the semen sample by washing and isolation of motile sperm and by stimulation of ovulation using low-dose gonadotrophins. IUI can be seen as a specific treatment for coital dysfunction and for abnormalities of cervical mucus but is also used frequently to treat unexplained infertility and mild male factor infertility. IUI requires healthy, patent Fallopian tubes. Live birth rates in high-quality centres are between 15% and 20% per cycle, although IUI remains a cost-effective alternative to IVF because of the lower doses of gonadotrophins, reduced level of monitoring and simplified laboratory requirements.

（四）体外受精与胚胎移植（In vitro fertilization and embryo transfer）

自 1978 年 Louise Brown 出生以来，IVF 及其衍生技术发展而来的多种助孕技术已经使不孕不育的治疗发生了革命性的变化。40 年来，已经有超过 700 万儿童通过 IVF 出生，欧洲人类生殖与胚胎学会和美国生殖医学学会汇编了关于 IVF、ICSI 和胚胎冻存安全性的可靠数据。从本质上讲，体外受精包括使用重组或尿源性促性腺激素刺激多个卵泡发育，同时使用 GnRH 激动药或拮抗药，以预防 LH 峰过早出现和在取卵前排卵的情况。在经阴道超声引导下，使用穿刺针行卵泡抽吸法收集卵母细胞，将卵母细胞从卵泡液中分离出来，并与男方经处理后的精子共培养。受精卵（胚胎）可以被培养 5 天，当分裂至囊胚期阶段，可以对其形态学质量进行详细的评估。然后，使用移植管将"最优的"1～2 个囊胚移植至宫腔内，如果新鲜胚胎移植后未孕，剩余的囊胚将被冷冻保存以备后用（图 17–6）。

IVF and its many variants have revolutionized the management of infertility since the birth of Louise Brown in 1978. Forty years on, more than 7 million children have been born following IVF, and generally reassuring data on safety of IVF, ICSI and embryo cryopreservation have been compiled by the European Society for Human Reproduction and Embryology and the American Society for Reproductive Medicine. Essentially, IVF involves stimulation of multiple ovarian follicle development using recombinant or urinary-derived gonadotrophins, with concurrent use of a GnRH agonist or antagonist to prevent a premature LH surge and ovulation before oocytes are harvested. Oocytes are collected using transvaginal ultrasound-guided needle follicle aspiration, with the oocytes being isolated from the follicular fluid and cultured in the presence of a washed sample of the partner's sperm. Fertilized oocytes (embryos) can be cultured for up to 5 days, at which point they reach the blastocyst stage of division and it becomes possible to make a detailed assessment of their morphological quality. The 'best' one or two blastocysts are then transferred to the uterine cavity using a simple catheter, with remaining blastocysts being cryopreserved for use later if conception does not follow the fresh embryo transfer (Fig. 17.6).

这个主题具有灵活多变性，可以移植培养第 2 天或第 3 天的胚胎，而不移植囊胚，或者如果存在 OHSS 的风险，可以进行全胚胎冷冻而不进行新鲜移植。也可以对胚胎进行活检，行胚胎植入前遗传学诊断（PGD）或进行染色体或遗传疾病的筛查（PGS），

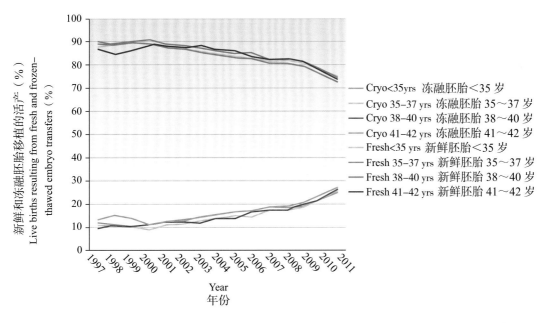

▲ 图 17–6　新鲜和冻融的胚胎移植的总活产率。数据源自一项美国的研究得出的数据显示，在不同年龄段接受辅助生殖技术助孕的人群中，冻融胚胎移植的活产率在总活产率中的占比越来越高

Cryo. 低温保存

经美国生殖医学学会许可转载 [Fertility and Sterility 2014; 102(1): 19-26]

Fig. 17.6　The contribution of fresh and frozen-thawed embryo transfers to the number of total live birth rate. Data derived from a U.S. study showing the increasing contribution of frozen embryo transfer in total live birth rate after assisted reproductive technology per age. Cryo, Cryopreserved.

Reprinted by permission from the American Society for Reproductive Medicine (Fertility and Sterility 2014;102(1):19-26).

仅移植筛选后正常的囊胚。ICSI 被广泛用于中至重度男性不育症，将单个精子直接注入卵母细胞的细胞质中，其受精率和妊娠率与 IVF 相似。女性年龄仍然是助孕结局的主要决定因素，越来越多的女性因自身的卵巢储备水平过低，无法获得正常妊娠和活产，她们寻求接受供卵作为一种助孕方式。虽然采用供卵助孕治疗健康活产的概率很高，但是孩子不具有其亲生母亲的 DNA，且由于无偿供卵者的短缺导致有偿供卵的国际市场环境逐步发展。在英国，有偿供精或供卵仍然是违法的，尽管在撰写本文时，人类受精与胚胎学管理局（HFEA）正在进行磋商讨论，以评估社会对这一伦理困境的态度。

There are many variations on this theme-embryos can be transferred on day 2 or 3 of development rather than as blastocysts, or all embryos may be cryopreserved without a fresh transfer if there is risk of OHSS. Embryos can also be biopsied for preimplantation genetic diagnosis (PGD) or screening (PGS) of chromosomal or genetic disorders with transfer only of those screened as normal. ICSI is widely used in cases of moderate to severe male factor infertility to inject a single spermatozoon directly into the cytoplasm of the oocyte, giving similar fertilization and pregnancy rates to IVF. Female age remains the main determinant of outcome, and an increasing number of women are resorting to treatment with donated oocytes from younger women as a means of achieving pregnancy at a time of life when their own ovarian reserve is too low to allow them the opportunity of healthy pregnancy and live birth. Whilst treatment with donor oocytes has a high chance of a healthy live birth, the child does not have the DNA of his or her birth mother, and the shortage of altruistic donors has led to development of an international market in oocytes from paid donors. Payment to oocyte or sperm donors remains illegal in the UK, although at time of writing a Human Fertilisation and Embryology Authority (HFEA) consultation is underway to assess societal attitudes to this ethical dilemma.

在英国，ART 由 HFEA 管理，其监督 IVF 治疗的各个方面。事实证明，HFEA 联接公众和政府之间以及 IVF 机构，允许其进行伦理辩论，并在临床和实验室安全领域实行"最佳实践"。HFEA 还整合了英国所有诊所的治疗结果，以简要介绍 ART 的成功率。IVF 受精率在 60%～80%，这在很大程度上取决于女性的年龄，大多数接受体外受精的患者都会进行胚胎移植。但是，着床率仍然相对较低，导致大多数中心每个周期活产率为 30%～40%。

In the UK, ART is regulated by the HFEA that oversees all aspects of IVF treatment. The HFEA has proven a useful interface between the public and government, on one hand, and IVF clinics, on the other, allowing for ethical debate and imposition of 'best practice' in areas of clinical and laboratory safety. HFEA also collates treatment results from all clinics in the UK, providing a snapshot of what can be achieved by ART. Fertilization rates after IVF are between 60% and 80%, depending largely on the age of the woman, and most patients who undertake IVF will have an embryo transfer. However, implantation rates remain relatively low, leading to a live birth in 30–40% of cycles in most centres.

IVF 助孕后发生产科和子代儿科问题的最常见原因是多胎妊娠导致的早产。在 ART 早期，在单个 IVF 周期中移植两个、三个或更多的胚胎是很普遍的，但是在以斯堪的纳维亚半岛国家为引领的许多国家中，大多数 IVF 周期都采取了单胚胎移植（SET）策略。在英国，多胎妊娠率仍约为 15%，但仍在稳步下降中（图 17-7）。SET 使用玻璃化冷冻技术后，冻融胚胎移植周期成功率的提高，使助孕夫妇倾向选择单胚胎移植（SET），因为在序贯移植一个新鲜胚胎后再移植一个冻融胚胎，与移植两个新鲜胚胎相比，活产率相似但无多胎妊娠的风险。在高龄助孕患者中，多胎妊娠的比例较高，但总体妊娠率偏低，导致患者和医生为了提高妊娠率不得不采取这一"亡命之计"。

The most frequent cause of obstetric and paediatric problems in offspring from IVF is the result of multiple pregnancy leading to premature birth. Transfer of two, three or more embryos in a single IVF cycle was commonplace in the early days of ART, but many countries, led by those in Scandinavia, have adopted a policy of single embryo transfer (SET) in the majority of IVF cycles. Multiple pregnancy rates remain at approximately 15% in the UK but are falling steadily (Fig. 17.7). Improved success rates from transfer of frozen embryos after cryopreservation using vitrification have made SET a more attractive option to couples, since their chances of a live birth after sequential transfer of one fresh then one frozen embryo are equivalent to those seen after transfer of two fresh embryos but without the risk of multiple pregnancy. The higher percentage of multiple pregnancies seen in the older patient groups reflects the lower overall chances of pregnancy, leading patients and practitioners to resort to desperate measures in order to try and achieve a pregnancy.

（五）植入前遗传学诊断或植入前遗传学筛查（Preimplantation genetic diagnosis or preimplantation genetic screening）

1990 年进行了首次植入前遗传学检测。早期研究使用荧光原位杂交技术（FISH），但是由于这种方法只能检查有限数量的染色体，因此结果常不尽如人意。现在更多时候采用新技术，如从最初的比较基因

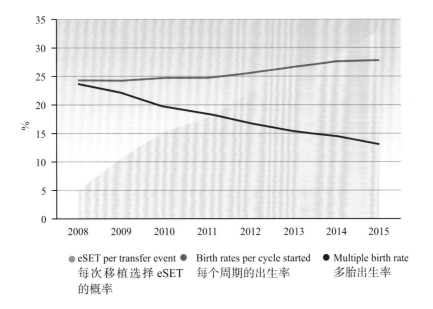

- eSET per transfer event ● Birth rates per cycle started ● Multiple birth rate
  每次移植选择 eSET　每个周期的出生率　多胎出生率
  的概率

▲ 图 17-7　2008-2015 年，英国的鲜胚和冻胚的活产率（每周期）和多胎妊娠率（每个活产）

eSET. 选择性单胚胎移植（数据源自 www.HFEA.gov.uk）

Fig. 17.7　UK live birth rate (per cycle started) and multiple birth rate (per live birth), fresh and frozen: 2008-2015.

eSET, Elective single embryo transfers. (Data sourced from www.HFEA.gov.uk.)

组杂交技术（CGH），至最近应用的高通量测序技术（NGS）。现在通常进行胚胎活检，从滋养外胚层收集细胞，以避免损伤内细胞团（图 17-8 和图 17-9）。

The first preimplantation genetic testing was performed in the 1990s. Early studies used fluorescent in situ hybridization (FISH), but as this only probed a limited number of chromosomes, results were often disappointing. New technologies, first comparative genomic hybridization (CGH) and, more recently, next-generation sequencing (NGS), are now used. Biopsy of the embryo is now usually done, collecting cells from the trophectoderm to avoid damage to the inner cell mass (Figs 17.8 and 17.9).

PGD 用于检测已经证实存在于父母一方或双方的特定单基因异常，如父母双方都是携带者的常染色体隐性疾病（如囊性纤维化病），常染色体显性疾病（如 Huntington 病），X 连锁遗传病（如 A 型血友病）或染色体平衡易位或倒位。计划妊娠的夫妇了解这一诊断结果多因存在先证者或于复发性流产筛查中被发现。这样做的目的是植入正常胚胎，避免纯合子导致隐性遗传疾病婴儿出生。PGS 的目的是筛查胚胎中的非整倍性，尽管父母双方均未发现遗传疾病。PGS 已应用于复发性流产、高龄孕妇、多次IVF 助孕失败或严重男性因素不育症的病例。目的是使用 PGS 选择最佳胚胎进行移植。在所有 IVF 病例中均提倡使用 PGS 进行非整倍体筛查，但任意应用

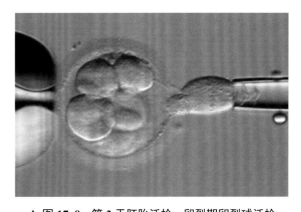

▲ 图 17-8　第 3 天胚胎活检，卵裂期卵裂球活检

Fig. 17.8　Embryo biopsy day 3, cleavage-stage blastomere biopsy.

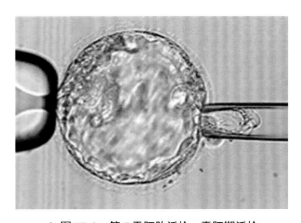

▲ 图 17-9　第 5 天胚胎活检，囊胚期活检

Fig. 17.9　Embryo biopsy day 5, blastocyst-stage biopsy.

PGS 是否有助于提高成功率仍有待证实。

PGD is used to detect specific single gene abnormalities that have been shown to exist in one or both parents, such as autosomal-recessive diseases in which both parents are carriers (e.g. cystic fibrosis), autosomal-dominant diseases (e.g. Huntington's disease), X-linked diseases (e.g. haemophilia A) or balanced chromosomal translocations or inversions. The diagnosis may be known by the potential parents due to the presence of an affected family member or found during a recurrent miscarriage screen. The aim is to avoid the birth of an affected child, preferably replacing a homozygous normal embryo. The purpose of PGS is to screen for aneuploidy in embryos, although both parents have no identified genetic abnormality. PGS has been used in cases of recurrent pregnancy loss, advanced maternal age, repeated unsuccessful IVF cycles or severe male factor infertility. The aim is to use PGS to select the best embryo for transfer. The use of PGS for aneuploidy screening in all cases of IVF has been advocated, but the contribution to improve success rates when used indiscriminately remains to be proven.

六、卵巢过度刺激综合征（Ovarian hyperstimulation syndrome）

OHSS 是促性腺激素过量使用的结果，导致卵泡过度发育及雌激素和血管内皮生长因子（VEGF）浓度过高。OHSS 具有潜在致命性，如果使用保守的促排卵方法，几乎可以完全避免。严重时，该病会导致卵巢明显肿大，液体从血管内腔转移到第三间隙，导致腹水、胸腔积液、钠潴留和少尿。患者可能会出现低血容量和低血压，并可能进展为肾衰竭、血栓栓塞和成人呼吸窘迫综合征。其主要病理生理特征与毛细血管通透性增加有关。

OHSS is the consequence of over-dosing with gonadotrophins, leading to excessive follicle development and high circulating concentrations of oestrogens and vascular endothelial growth factor (VEGF). OHSS is potentially lethal and is almost completely avoidable if a conservative approach to ovarian stimulation is used. In its severe form, the condition results in marked ovarian enlargement with fluid shift from the intravascular compartment into the third space, leading to ascites, pleural effusion, sodium retention and oliguria. Patients may become hypovolaemic and hypotensive and may develop renal failure, as well as thromboembolic phenomena and adult respiratory distress syndrome. The pathophysiology of this condition appears to be associated with an increase in capillary vascular permeability.

（一）治疗方法（Treatment）

如果血细胞比容低于 45%，并且体征和症状较

轻，患者可以在家接受治疗，但如果经超声检查提示有明显腹水，则应住院治疗。应测定基线电解质值和肝肾功能。可以使用人白蛋白或补充晶体液扩容治疗，如果伴随严重的腹水或胸腔积液症状，应穿刺引流以减少液体负荷。吲哚美辛和血管紧张素转化酶抑制药等药物可用于减轻病情的严重程度。最终，卵巢液囊自行吸收，卵巢将恢复至正常大小。接下来的促排卵剂量应考虑伴随 OHSS 时使用的原剂量方案。

If the haematocrit is below 45% and the signs and symptoms are mild, the patient can be managed at home, but where there is significant ascites as judged by ultrasound examination, she should be hospitalized. Baseline electrolyte values and liver and kidney function should be assessed. Volume expansion can be performed using human albumin, sometimes with crystalloid, and if there is severe ascites or pleural effusion, fluid should be drained to reduce the fluid load. Drugs such as indomethacin and angiotensin-converting enzyme inhibitors may be useful in reducing the severity of the episode. Eventually, the cysts will undergo resorption, and the ovaries will return to their normal size. Further attempts at ovarian stimulation should take into account the dosage regimens used during the episode of OHSS.

（二）预防措施（Avoidance of OHSS）

最近，已经发现了新的方案，几乎可以完全避免 OHSS 的风险（Devroey 等，2011）。

More recently, new strategies have been developed that allow almost total avoidance of risk of OHSS (Devroey et al. 2011).

该过程涉及 IVF 周期的"分割"，将促排卵与胚胎移植，黄体支持和妊娠阶段分开，并使用 GnRH 激动药"扳机"。卵巢刺激阶段由 GnRH 拮抗药调节。一旦达到了最终卵母细胞成熟的标准（通常，如果至少 3 个卵泡的直径超过 17mm），就给予单剂量的 GnRH 激动药。与自然周期一样，这会导致内源性 LH 峰。LH 激增最终诱导卵母细胞成熟和黄体化。然而，与传统的 hCG 扳机相比，这种效应的持续时间较短，持续时间少于 36h，而不是 4～5 天。通常使用经阴道超声引导的方法收集卵母细胞，使其受精并培养成囊胚。然后将所有高质量的囊胚冷冻，避免新鲜胚胎移植。由于天然黄体生成素的半衰期较短，以及避免在妊娠后暴露于人绒毛膜促性腺激素（hCG），因此避免了 OHSS 的风险。囊胚可在后续自然或人工周期中移植。

The process involves 'segmentation' of the IVF cycle, separating the stimulation phase from embryo transfer, luteal support and pregnancy, along with use of a GnRH agonist 'trigger'. The ovarian stimulation phase is regulated with a GnRH antagonist. Once the criteria for final oocyte maturation are reached (usually if at least three follicles exceed 17 mm in diameter), a single dose of a GnRH agonist is administered. This elicits an endogenous LH surge as in the natural cycle. The LH surge induces final oocyte maturation and luteinization. However, the duration of the effect is considerably less than seen with the traditional hCG 'trigger', lasting less than 36 hours compared with 4–5 days. Oocytes are collected using a transvaginal ultrasoundguided approach as usual, fertilized and cultured to blastocyst. All high-quality blastocysts are then frozen, avoiding fresh embryo transfer. The risk of OHSS is therefore avoided due both to the short half-life of the natural LH trigger and avoidance of exposure to human chorionic gonadotropin (hCG) following pregnancy. A blastocyst is then transferred later in a natural or medicated cycle.

七、男性不育症的治疗（Treatment of male infertility）

只有一小部分不育症男性可以进行特定的治疗。睾丸大小很重要，当存在小睾丸、无精子症、高卵泡刺激素和低 AMH 水平时，任何治疗都不太可能对其有所帮助。

Specific treatment is possible in only a small proportion of infertile males. Testicular size is important, and with the finding of small testes, azoospermia, high FSH and low AMH levels, it is unlikely that any therapy will help.

如果 FSH 水平正常且睾丸大小正常，则应怀疑输精管梗阻并进行睾丸活检。如果证实精子发生正常，则有必要进行输精管造影术和阴囊探查。外科吻合术可以重建生育能力。促性腺激素对罕见的低促性腺激素性性腺机能减退症男性有效，多巴胺激动药用于治疗高泌乳素血症的男性。未经证实但广泛应用于治疗男性不育的方法包括精索静脉曲张结扎术，应用抗氧化剂和补充剂以降低精子 DNA 碎片率。

Where FSH levels are normal and testicular size is normal, ductal obstruction should be suspected and testicular biopsy performed. If normal spermatogenesis is demonstrated, it is necessary to proceed to vasography and exploration of the scrotum. Surgical anastomosis may re-establish fertility. Gonadotrophins are effective in the rare cases of men with hypogonadotropic hypogonadism, and dopamine agonists are used in men with hyperprolactinaemia. Unproven but widely practised treatments for male infertility include ligation of a varicocele and antioxidants and supplements to reduce sperm DNA fragmentation.

男性不育症最成功的治疗方法是 ICSI。ICSI 是将单一固定的精子直接注射到卵母细胞的细胞质中。该技术与 IVF 具有相似的妊娠率。人们仍然担心，ICSI 后分娩儿童畸形率略高。畸形主要见于生殖道的发育过程（尿道下裂、睾丸下降不良），尽管遗传印记混乱的疾病（如 Angelman 综合征和 Beckwiths-Widemann 综合征）也在 ICSI 后更常见。

The most successful treatment for male infertility is ICSI. ICSI involves the direct injection of a single immobilized sperm into the cytoplasm of the oocyte. This technique produces pregnancy rates similar to those of in vitro fertilization. Anxieties remain concerning the slightly higher rate of abnormality in children conceived after ICSI. Abnormalities are mainly observed in the development of the genital tract (hypospadias, testicular maldescent), although cases of imprinting disorders such as Angelman and Beckwith-Widemann syndromes may also be seen more commonly after ICSI.

供精人工授精（Donor insemination）

如果无法获得可行 ICSI 的精子，或者男方是遗传病携带者，而这对夫妇希望避免遗传给孩子，则应与夫妇探讨供精人工授精问题。

If sperm cannot be obtained for ICSI or if the man is a carrier of a genetic disorder that the couple wish to avoid transmitting to their child, donor insemination should be discussed with the couple.

应从法律和个人的角度深入讨论这一助孕措施的潜在影响，并为双方提供独立咨询。2004 年，英国取消了匿名供精，由此导致供精短缺，许多夫妇从丹麦、美国等国外地区寻找精源并行助孕。根据法律规定，2004 年后行供精或供卵助孕治疗出生的儿童，在年满 18 岁时，可以在被监督的情况下与其遗传学父母相见。他们还可以参考 HFEA 数据库，检查潜在伴侣是否由同一名捐献者供精或供卵助孕后分娩，但如果在匿名法修改之前进行助孕治疗，捐献者的姓名不会被公布。

The implications of the procedure from both a legal and a personal point of view should be discussed in depth, with independent counselling for both partners. Anonymity for sperm donors was removed in the UK in 2004, and the resultant shortage of donor sperm has led many couples to seek treatment overseas or to import sperm from Denmark, the United States and elsewhere. Children conceived using donor oocyte or sperm collected after 2004 are legally allowed to meet their genetic parent under supervised conditions when they reach the age of 18. They can also check whether a potential partner was conceived using the same donor by referring to the HFEA database, although the name of the donor will not be released if the treatment preceded the change in the law regarding anonymity.

在英国，许多患者正在排队等待治疗，这为他们提供了充足的考虑时间。

Waiting lists for treatment in the UK are lengthy, although this does at least give adequate time for reflection.

本章概览	Essential information

不孕症
- 西欧患病率约为 9%
- 如果夫妻 12 个月后未孕可能是潜在不孕症患者
- 25 岁后生育力逐步下降
- 原因（原发 / 继发）：
  – 排卵障碍：32%/23%
  – 输卵管因素：12%/14%
  – 子宫内膜异位症：10%
  – 男性因素：29%/24%
  – 不明原因：30%
- PCOS 是无排卵的最常见原因
- 垂体肿瘤可引起继发性闭经
- 炎症（通常是衣原体感染）是输卵管损伤的最常见原因
- 宫内节育器（IUD）、流产和产褥期的感染通常会引起宫角阻塞
- 精子难以穿透子宫颈可能是由炎症、抗精子抗体或宫颈黏液异常所致

不孕症检查
- 黄体期孕酮值是预测排卵最重要指标之一
- 无排卵时激素水平
- HSG / 腹腔镜 / 超声检查输卵管通畅性
- 精液分析
  – 精子总数＞5000 万 / 一次射精
  – 60% 活动率
  – 形态学
- 不育症男性的激素水平
- 核型异常的无精症男性的染色体分析

不孕症治疗
- 无排卵
  – 克罗米芬或他莫昔芬
  – 如不成功，人类绝经期促性腺激素（hMG）（警惕 OHSS）
- 低促性腺素性功能减退症，给予 GnRH
- 输卵管病变
  – 手术
  – IVF
- 男性不育症的治疗只可能在少数患者中进行

Infertility
- Incidence about 9% in Western Europe
- Couple potentially infertile if no conception after 12 months
- Fertility declines progressively from the age of 25 years
- Causes (primary/secondary):
  – Disorders of ovulation: 32%/23%
  – Tubal: 12%/14%
  – Endometriosis: 10%
  – Male: 29%/24%
  – Unexplained: 30%
- PCOS most common cause of anovulation
- Pituitary tumours can cause secondary amenorrhoea
- Infection (often chlamydial) commonest cause of tubal damage
- Infections associated with intrauterine devices (IUDs), abortion and the puerperium commonly cause cornual blockage
- Poor cervical penetration by sperm may be caused by infection, antisperm antibodies or abnormal mucus

Investigation of infertility
- Luteal-phase progesterone is the most useful method of detecting ovulation
- Hormone levels in anovulation
- HSG/laparoscopy/ultrasound to investigate tubal patency
- Semen analysis:
  – Total sperm count >50 million per ejaculate
  – 60% motile
  – Morphology
- Hormone levels in infertile males
- Chromosome analysis in males with azoospermia-abnormal karyotype

Treatment of infertility
- Anovulation:
  – Clomiphene or tamoxifen
  – If unsuccessful, human menopausal gonadotropin (hMG) (beware OHSS)
- Hypogonadotropic hypogonadism-GnRH
- Tubal pathology:
  – Surgery
  – IVF
- Treatment of male infertility only possible in a small proportion of cases

第 18 章 早期妊娠护理
Early pregnancy care

Ian Symonds **著**　　李妍秋　谷牧青　阮祥燕　**译**　　石玉华　**校**

LEARNING OUTCOMES

学习目标	LEARNING OUTCOMES

学习本章后，你应当能够：

After studying this chapter you should be able to:

知识标准

- 列出早期妊娠出血、腹痛的原因
- 描述以下疾病的流行病学、病因学和临床特征
  - 流产
  - 异位妊娠
  - 葡萄胎妊娠
- 探讨超声和内分泌评估手段在早期妊娠疾病中的应用
- 描述早期妊娠常见疾病和并发症的处理，其中包括保守治疗、药物治疗和手术治疗
  - 流产（包括宫颈休克）
  - 复发性流产
  - 异位妊娠
  - 葡萄胎妊娠
  - 妊娠剧吐

临床能力

- 对于早期妊娠主诉阴道流血和（或）腹痛的女性，获取相关的妇科病史
- 进行尿妊娠试验并解释结果
- 对有早期妊娠疾病的女性进行循环评估和腹部检查，并确定需要立即干预的女性
- 对妊娠早期出现心血管功能衰竭的女性启动合理的复苏救治
- 能够与患者及亲属进行有效、谨慎的沟通

专业技能及态度

- 思考对一个能够给予帮助的环境的需求来解决与早期妊娠丢失有关的宗教和文化问题

Knowledge criteria

- List the causes of bleeding and/or pain in early pregnancy.
- Describe the epidemiology, aetiology and clinical features of:
  - Miscarriage
  - Ectopic pregnancy
  - Molar pregnancy
- Discuss the use of ultrasound and endocrine assessments in early pregnancy problems
- Describe the management of the common problems and complications of early pregnancy, ncluding the conservative, medical and surgical management of:
  - Miscarriage (including cervical shock)
  - Recurrent miscarriage
  - Ectopic pregnancy
  - Molar pregnancy
  - Hyperemesis gravidarum

Clinical competencies

- Take a relevant gynaecological history in a woman complaining of vaginal bleeding and/or abdominal pain in early pregnancy
- Perform a urinary pregnancy test and interpret the result
- Perform a circulatory assessment and abdominal examination of a woman with an early pregnancy problem, and identify those requiring immediate intervention
- Initiate appropriate resuscitation of a woman presenting in early pregnancy with cardiovascular collapse
- Be able to communicate effectively and sensitively with patients and relatives

Professional skills and attitudes

- Consider the need for a supportive environment that addresses religious and cultural issues around early pregnancy loss

一、早期妊娠出血（Bleeding in early pregnancy）

25% 的孕 20 周前的女性会发生阴道流血。这是所有女性，尤其是那些经历过流产的女性焦虑的主要原因，并且可能是异位妊娠等危及生命的疾病的表现症状。孕期出血应视为异常，并应进行适当的检查。

Vaginal bleeding occurs in up to 25% of pregnancies prior to 20 weeks. It is a major cause of anxiety for all women, especially those who have experienced previous pregnancy loss, and may be the presenting symptom of life-threatening conditions such as ectopic pregnancy. Bleeding should always be considered abnormal in pregnancy and investigated appropriately.

受精后 5～7 天囊泡植入子宫内膜时，可能会出现少量出血（植入出血）。如果这种出血发生在预期的月经期内，它可能会与经期混淆，从而影响以末次月经为依据来计算的孕周。

A small amount of bleeding may occur as the blastocyst implants in the endometrium 5–7 days after fertilization (implantation bleed). If this occurs at the time of expected menstruation, it may be confused with a period and so affect calculations of gestational age based the last menstrual period.

早期妊娠出血的常见原因有流产、异位妊娠和下生殖道良性病变。不太常见的原因可能是葡萄胎或宫颈恶性肿瘤的表现。

The common causes for bleeding in early pregnancy are miscarriage, ectopic pregnancy and benign lesions in the lower genital tract. Less commonly it may be the presenting symptom of hydatidiform mole or cervical malignancy.

二、流产（Miscarriage）

对于 24 周以下的妊娠丢失，推荐的医学术语是流产。在一些国家，如美国，这一术语用于描述胎儿存活前或胎儿体重小于 500g 的妊娠丢失。在澳大利亚的一些州，该术语用于描述任何小于 20 周的妊娠丢失。大多数流产发生于妊娠第二个或第三个月，并且 10%～20% 的临床妊娠会发生流产。有研究表明，如果诊断是基于血浆中 β- 人绒毛膜促性腺激素（hCG）的显著水平，那么妊娠早期流产的比例要高得多。

The recommended medical term for pregnancy loss

under 24 weeks is *miscarriage*. In some countries, such as the United States, this term is used to describe pregnancy loss before fetal viability or a fetal weight of less than 500 g. In some states in Australia, the term is used for any pregnancy loss under 20 weeks. Most miscarriages occur in the second or third month and occur in 10–20% of clinical pregnancies. It has been suggested that a much higher proportion of pregnancies miscarry at an early stage if the diagnosis is based on the presence of a significant plasma level of beta-subunit human chorionic gonadotrophin (hCG).

（一）流产的病因（The aetiology of miscarriage）

在许多情况下并不能找到流产的确切原因。确定病因尤为重要，因为其可对未来妊娠的预后将普遍高于平均水平。

In many cases no definite cause can be found for miscarriage. It is important to identify this group, as the prognosis for future pregnancy is generally better than average.

1. 流行病学因素（Epidemiological factors）

母亲年龄和流产次数是预测流产的独立危险因素。流产的风险从 20—24 岁女性的 11% 增加到 45 岁以上妊娠女性的 50% 以上。这一部分与胚胎中染色体异常（见后述）的风险增加有关，一部分与女性剩余卵母细胞数量和质量下降有关。当夫妇中男性年龄超过 40 岁时，流产的风险也更高。

Maternal age and the number of previous miscarriages are independent risk factors for further miscarriage. The risk of miscarriage increases from 11% in women aged 20–24 to more than 50% in women conceiving over the age of 45. This is in part related to the increased risk of chromosome abnormalities (see later) in the conceptus and in part a decline in the number and quality of the woman's remaining oocytes. The risk of miscarriage is also higher in couples where the man is over the age of 40.

(1) 遗传异常（Genetic abnormalities）:

染色体异常是早期流产的常见原因，可能导致胚胎发育失败、形成一个无胚胎发育的认识囊，或者随后排出异常胎儿。在任何形式的流产中，高达 57% 的妊娠物会出现异常核型。最常见的染色体缺陷是常染色体三体，占异常的 50%，而多倍体和单倍体 X 染色体各占 20%。尽管染色体异常在散发性流产中很常见，但父母染色体异常只出现在 2%～5% 的复发性流产中。这些异常通常是平衡倒位或 Robertsonian 易位或嵌合体。

Chromosomal abnormalities are a common cause of early miscarriage and may result in failure of development of the embryo, with formation of a gestation sac without the development of an embryo or with later expulsion of an abnormal fetus. In any form of miscarriage up to 57% of products of conception will have an abnormal karyotype. The most common chromosomal defects are autosomal trisomies, which account for half the abnormalities, while polyploidy and monosomy X account for a further 20% each. Although chromosome abnormalities are common in sporadic miscarriage, parental chromosomal abnormalities are present in only 2–5% of partners presenting with recurrent pregnancy loss. These are most commonly balance reciprocal or Robertsonian translocations or mosaicisms.

(2) 内分泌因素（Endocrine factors）：

孕酮的产生，在孕 8 周前主要依赖于黄体，而之后这一功能则由胎盘承担。黄体酮对维持妊娠至关重要，黄体的早期退化可能导致流产。然而，很难确定何时的血浆孕酮水平下降成为流产的主要原因，以及何时其为妊娠失败的指标。多囊卵巢综合征（PCOS）在复发性流产女性中的患病率明显高于一般人群。糖尿病控制不佳和甲状腺疾病未经治疗的女性流产和胎儿畸形的风险更高。

Progesterone production is predominately dependent on the corpus luteum for the first 8 weeks of pregnancy, and this function is then assumed by the placenta. Progesterone is essential for the maintenance of a pregnancy, and early failure of the corpus luteum may lead to miscarriage. However, it is difficult to be certain when falling plasma progesterone levels represent a primary cause of miscarriage and when they are the index of a failing pregnancy. The prevalence of polycystic ovarian syndrome (PCOS) is significantly higher in women with recurrent miscarriage than in the general population. Women with poorly controlled diabetes and untreated thyroid disease are at higher risk of miscarriage and fetal malformation.

(3) 母体疾病和感染（Maternal illness and infection）：

任何与感染有关的可引起发热的严重母体疾病，如流感、肾盂肾炎和疟疾，都容易导致流产。梅毒、单核细胞增生李斯特菌、支原体和弓形虫等特异性感染也可能与偶发性流产有关，但没有证据表明这些微生物会导致复发性流产，尤其是在中期妊娠。据报道，细菌性阴道病是早产和中期妊娠流产的危险因素，而不是早期妊娠流产的危险因素。其他涉及心血管、肝脏和肾脏系统的严重疾病也可能导致流产。

Any severe maternal febrile illnesses associated with infections, such as influenza, pyelitis and malaria, predispose to miscarriage. Specific infections such as syphilis, *Listeria monocytogenes*, mycoplasma and *Toxoplasma gondii* may also be associated with sporadic miscarriage, but there is no evidence that these organisms cause recurrent miscarriage, particularly in the second trimester. The presence of bacterial vaginosis has been reported as a risk factor for pre-term delivery and second-trimester, but not firsttrimester, miscarriage. Other severe illnesses involving the cardiovascular, hepatic and renal systems may also result in miscarriage.

2. 母体生活方式和用药史（Maternal lifestyle and drug history）

围孕期使用抗抑郁药和非甾体抗炎药与流产有关。吸烟、饮酒（每周超过 5 个标准饮酒单位）、咖啡（每天超过 3 杯）、可卡因和大麻与流产风险增加相关，尽管目前的证据不足以证实因果关系。有证据表明超重也与妊娠丢失相关。

Antidepressant use and periconceptual non-steroidal antiinflammatory drugs have been associated with miscarriage. Smoking, alcohol (more than 5 units a week), caffeine (more than 3 cups per day), cocaine and cannabis have been associated with an increase in the risk of miscarriage, although current evidence is insufficient to confirm a causal link. There is some evidence that obesity may also be associated with pregnancy loss.

(1) 子宫畸形（Abnormalities of the uterus）：

子宫的先天性畸形，如双角子宫或不完全纵隔子宫，在流产中发挥的具体作用仍有争议。据报道，复发性流产女性子宫畸形的发生率为 2%～38%。子宫畸形对妊娠的影响取决于畸形的性质，并且中期妊娠流产的女性子宫畸形的患病率似乎更高。胎儿存活率在纵隔子宫中最高，在单角子宫中最低。还必须牢记的是，超过 20% 的先天性子宫畸形的女性也同时有伴肾脏泌尿道畸形。子宫内膜和子宫壁损伤后，宫腔表面可能会粘连，从而部分闭塞子宫宫腔（Asherman 综合征）。这些粘连的存在可能导致复发性流产。

The exact contribution that congenital abnormalities of the uterine cavity, such as a bicornuate uterus or subseptate uterus, make to miscarriage remains controversial. The reported incidence of uterine anomalies in women with recurrent miscarriage varies from less than 2% to up to 38%. The impact of the abnormality depends on the nature of the anomaly, and the prevalence appears to be higher in women with second-trimester miscarriage. The fetal survival rate is best where the uterus is septate and worst where the uterus is unicornuate. It must also be remembered that over 20% of all women with congenital uterine anomalies also have renal tract anomalies. Following damage to the endometrium and inner uterine walls, the surfaces may become adherent, thus partly obliterating the uterine cavity (Asherman's syndrome). The presence of these synechiae may lead to recurrent miscarriage.

（2）宫颈功能不全（Cervical incompetence）：

宫颈功能不全通常会导致中期妊娠流产或早产。流产往往发生迅速、无痛，阴道流血少。诊断依据为非孕期宫颈口无困难通过 8 号 Hegar 扩宫棒或经超声或经前行子宫造影确诊。宫颈功能不全可能是先天性的，并与其他先天性子宫畸形有关，但最常见的原因是由于机械扩张、子宫颈手术或分娩时创伤造成的物理损伤所致。

Cervical incompetence typically results in second-trimester miscarriage or early pre-term delivery. The miscarriage tends to be rapid, painless and bloodless. The diagnosis is established by the passage of a Hegar 8 dilator without difficulty in the non-pregnant woman or by ultrasound examination or by a premenstrual hysterogram. Cervical incompetence may be congenital and associated with other congenital uterine malformations but most commonly results from physical damage caused by mechanical dilatation or surgery of the cervix or by damage inflicted during childbirth.

（3）自身免疫因素（Autoimmune factors）：

抗磷脂抗体——狼疮抗凝物（LA）和抗心磷脂抗体（aCL）存在于 15% 的复发性流产女性中，但只存在于 2% 的正常生育史女性中。未经治疗，原发性抗磷脂综合征女性的活产率可能低至 10%。妊娠丢失被认为是由于子宫胎盘血管系统血栓形成和滋养细胞功能受损。除外流产，宫内生长受限、先兆子痫和静脉血栓形成的风险也增加。

Antiphospholipid antibodies-lupus anticoagulant (LA) and anticardiolipin antibodies (aCL)-are present in 15% of women with recurrent miscarriage but only 2% of women with normal reproductive histories. Without treatment, the live birth rate in women with primary antiphospholipid syndrome may be as low as 10%. Pregnancy loss is thought to be due to thrombosis of the uteroplacental vasculature and impaired trophoblast function. In addition to miscarriage there is an increased risk of intrauterine growth restriction, pre-eclampsia and venous thrombosis.

（4）血栓形成缺陷（Thrombophilic defects）：

天然凝血抑制剂抗凝血酶Ⅲ、蛋白 C 和蛋白 S 的缺陷在复发性流产的女性中更为常见。活化蛋白 C 缺乏症的大多数病例继发于因子 V（Leiden）基因突变。

Defects in the natural inhibitors of coagulation-antithrombin III, protein C and protein S-are more common in women with recurrent miscarriage. The majority of cases of activated protein C deficiency are secondary to a mutation in the factor V (Leiden) gene.

（5）同种免疫因素（Alloimmune factors）：

对复发性流产的免疫学基础可能性研究广泛地探讨了正常保护性免疫反应障碍的可能性，或者是否由细胞滋养层表达得相对非免疫原性抗原导致了胎儿同种异体移植排斥。有证据表明，不明原因的自然流产与夫妇的人类白细胞抗原（HLA）位点 A、B、C 和 DR 相容数量异常的有关。父系淋巴细胞和免疫球蛋白治疗已被证明是无效的，并有潜在的危险。

Research into the possibility of an immunological basis of recurrent miscarriage has generally explored the possibility of a failure to mount the normal protective immune response or if the expression of relatively nonimmunogenic antigens by the cytotrophoblast may result in rejection of the fetal allograft. There is evidence that unexplained spontaneous miscarriage is associated with couples who share an abnormal number of human leukocyte antigen (HLA) antigens of the A, B, C and DR loci. Treatment with paternal lymphocytes and immunoglobulins has been shown not to be effective and is potentially dangerous.

（二）流产的临床类型（Clinical types of miscarriage）

1. 先兆流产（Threatened miscarriage）

即将流产的第一个迹象是妊娠早期阴道流血（图 18-1）。子宫增大，宫颈口闭合。下腹部疼痛轻微或无。大多数有先兆流产的女性会继续妊娠，无论采取何种治疗方法。

The first sign of an impending miscarriage is the development of vaginal bleeding in early pregnancy (Fig. 18.1). The uterus is found to be enlarged, and the cervical os is closed. Lower abdominal pain is either minimal or absent. Most women presenting with a threatened miscarriage will continue with the pregnancy irrespective of the method of management.

2. 难免流产 / 不全流产（Inevitable/incomplete miscarriage）

患者出现腹痛，通常伴有阴道流血增多，宫颈扩张，最终妊娠物排入阴道。如果出现部分妊娠物残留，则称为不全流产（图 18-2）。

The patient develops abdominal pain usually associated with increasing vaginal bleeding. The cervix opens, and eventually products of conception are passed into the vagina. However, if some of the products of conception are retained, the miscarriage remains incomplete (Fig. 18.2).

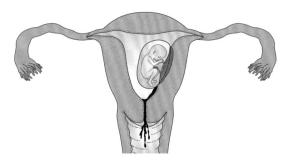

▲ 图 18-1　先兆流产：早期妊娠失血

Fig. 18.1　Threatened miscarriage: blood loss in early pregnancy.

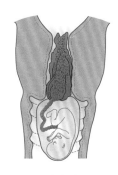

▲ 图 18-2　不全流产：伴随疼痛和出血的部分胎儿组织排出过程

Fig. 18.2　Incomplete miscarriage: progression to expulsion of part of the conceptus is accompanied by pain and bleeding.

> **！注意**
>
> 妊娠产物扩张宫颈管可导致低血压和心动过缓（宫颈性休克）。
>
> Distension of the cervical canal by products of conception can cause hypotension and bradycardia (cervical shock).

3. 完全流产（Complete miscarriage）

不全流产可自行演变成完全流产，此时腹痛会逐渐消失，阴道流血会随着子宫复旧而消退。孕 8～16 周胎盘组织残留很常见，孕 16 周后发生完全自然流产可能更大。

An incomplete miscarriage may proceed to completion spontaneously, when the pain will cease and vaginal bleeding will subside with involution of the uterus. Spontaneous completion of a miscarriage is more likely in miscarriages over 16 weeks' gestation than in those between 8 and 16 weeks' gestation, when retention of placental fragments is common.

4. 流产合并感染（败血症）[Miscarriage with infection (sepsis)]

在流产过程中或治疗性终止妊娠后，可能引起宫腔感染。败血症性流产的临床表现与不全流产相似，并伴有子宫和附件压痛。阴道流出物可能会化脓，患者会发热。在严重败血症的情况下，内毒素休克可能发展为严重且致命的低血压。其他临床表现包括肾衰竭、弥散性血管内凝血和多发性瘀点出血。通常侵入子宫腔的微生物有大肠埃希菌、粪链球菌、白色葡萄球菌和金黄色葡萄球菌、克雷伯菌和魏氏梭菌及产气荚膜梭菌。

During the process of miscarriage-or after therapeutic termination of a pregnancy-infection may be introduced into the uterine cavity. The clinical findings of septic miscarriage are similar to those of incomplete miscarriage with the addition of uterine and adnexal tenderness. The vaginal loss may become purulent and the patient pyrexial. In cases of severe overwhelming sepsis, endotoxic shock may develop with profound and sometimes fatal hypotension. Other manifestations include renal failure, disseminated intravascular coagulopathy and multiple petechial haemorrhages. Organisms which commonly invade the uterine cavity are *Escherichia coli*, *Streptococcus faecalis*, *Staphylococcus albus* and *aureus*, *Klebsiella* and *Clostridium welchii* and *perfringens*.

稽留流产（空孕囊、胚胎丢失、早期和晚期胎儿丢失）[Missed miscarriage (empty gestation sac, embryonic loss, early and late fetal loss)]:

在空孕囊（无胚妊娠或萎缩性胚囊）中，超声检查可见≥25mm 的妊娠囊（图 18-3），但 7 天后再

病例分析：不全流产	Case study: Incomplete miscarriage
一位 32 岁的亚洲女性，闭经 12 周，阴道流血伴严重下腹疼痛。入院时出汗，脸色苍白，血压低。脉搏 68/min。主诉广泛下腹痛。起初，由于疼痛和休克，怀疑输卵管妊娠破裂，直到阴道检查发现大量妊娠物从扩张的宫颈口突出。取出妊娠物在很大程度上减轻了疼痛，使子宫收缩，从而减少了失血。经过适当的复苏救治和准备，随后清除残余的妊娠物。	A 32-year-old Asian woman presented with a history of 12 weeks amenorrhoea and vaginal bleeding followed by severe lower abdominal pain. On admission to hospital, she was sweating, pale and hypotensive. Her pulse rate was 68 beats/minute. She complained of generalized lower abdominal pain. Initially, a ruptured tubal pregnancy was suspected because of the pain and shock, until vaginal examination revealed copious products of conception protruding from an open cervical os. Removal of these products largely relieved the pain and allowed the uterus to contract, thus reducing the blood loss. Subsequent evacuation of retained products of conception was performed after appropriate resuscitation and preparation.

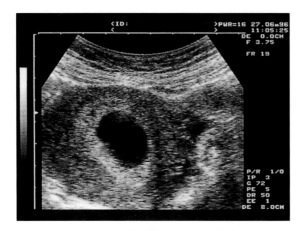

▲ 图 18-3　超声扫描显示无胚胎的空孕囊

Fig. 18.3　The empty gestation sac of anembryonic pregnancy seen on ultrasound scan.

次检测时，没有证据显示有胚胎极或卵黄囊或囊大小的变化。如果胎芽大小≥7mm 且无胎心搏动，或者超声检查 7 天后胚芽大小无变化，则诊断为胚胎丢失。早期胚胎停育是指超声已确认宫内妊娠且大小与 8～12 周一致，但未见胎心搏动。这些情况可能伴有出血和腹痛，或者是无症状的，仅在超声检查中被诊断出来。临床的流产类型可能提示了潜在的病因，如抗磷脂综合征，往往表现为复发性胎儿丢失。

In empty gestation sac (anembryonic pregnancy or blighted ovum), a gestational sac of ≥25 mm is seen on ultrasound (Fig. 18.3), but there is no evidence of an embryonic pole or yolk sac or change in size of the sac on rescan 7 days later. Embryonic loss is diagnosed where there is an embryo ≥7 mm in size without cardiac activity or where there is no change in the size of the embryo after 7 days on scan. Early fetal demise occurs when a pregnancy is identified within the uterus on ultrasound consistent with 8–12 weeks size but no fetal heartbeat is seen. These may be associated with some bleeding and abdominal pain or be asymptomatic and diagnosed on ultrasound scan. The pattern of clinical loss may indicate the underlying aetiology; for example, antiphospholipid syndrome tends to present with recurrent fetal loss.

5. 中期妊娠自然流产（Spontaneous second-trimester loss）

孕 12～24 周的流产与自发性胎膜破裂或宫颈扩张有关，尽管存在胎心搏动。

Pregnancy loss occurs between 12 and 24 weeks associated with spontaneous rupture of membranes or cervical dilation despite the presence of fetal heart activity

6. 复发性流产（Recurrent miscarriage）

复发性流产是指连续 3 次或 3 次以上的流产。

这一问题会影响 1% 的女性，这个数目大约是偶发性流产的 3 倍。大多数连续 2 次或 2 次以上流产的女性都急于寻找病因，并被证实不存在根本病因。不过，重要的是，在连续 3 次流产后，仍然有 55%～75% 的妊娠成功率。这意味着复发性流产不太可能是随机事件，有必要寻找原因。

Recurrent miscarriage is defined as three or more successive pregnancy losses prior to viability. The problem affects 1% of all women, approximately three times the number that would be expected by chance alone. Most women who have had two or more consecutive miscarriages are anxious to be investigated and reassured that there is no underlying cause. However, it is important to remember that after three consecutive miscarriages, there is still a 55–75% chance of success. This implies that recurrent miscarriage is unlikely to be a random event and that it is necessary to seek a cause.

（三）处理（Management）

对患者的检查应包括轻柔的阴道和窥器检查，以确定宫颈扩张。如果有发热症状，应采取阴道拭子细菌培养。有些女性可能不愿意接受检查，因为担心检查可能会促进流产，她们的意愿应该得到尊重。在专门的早孕评估单位（EPAU）进行管理可以减少住院和住院时间。超声检查对判断胎儿是否存活和正常很有价值。在早期妊娠常规应用超声检查可在没有任何迹象表明妊娠异常之前，就确定流产的诊断。有时最好在 1 周后重复检查，以使母亲接受诊断结果，而不是立即进行药物或人工清宫。

Examination of the patient should include gentle vaginal and speculum examination to ascertain cervical dilatation. If there is pyrexia, a high vaginal swab should be taken for bacteriological culture. Some women may prefer not to be examined because of apprehension that the examination may promote miscarriage, and their wishes should be respected. Management in dedicated early pregnancy assessment units (EPAUs) reduces the need for hospital admission and length of stay. An ultrasound scan is valuable in deciding if the fetus is alive and normal. One effect of the routine use of scans in early pregnancy is that the diagnosis of miscarriage may be established before there is any indication that the pregnancy is abnormal. It is sometimes preferable to repeat the scan a week later than proceed to immediate medical or surgical uterine evacuation, to enable the mother to come to terms with the diagnosis.

非致敏恒河猴血型（Rh）阴性女性在所有流产和异位妊娠的手术管理中应接受抗 D 免疫球蛋白治疗。

Non-sensitized Rhesus (Rh)-negative women should

receive anti-D immunoglobulin for all miscarriages and ectopic pregnancies managed surgically.

对于只接受药物治疗或期待治疗的流产或异位妊娠女性、先兆流产或不明部位妊娠的女性，无须给予抗 D 免疫球蛋白。

Anti-D immunoglobulin does not need to be given for women who have had only medical or expectant management for miscarriage or ectopic pregnancy, who have a threatened miscarriage or who have a pregnancy of unknown locations.

1. 先兆流产（Threatened miscarriage）

如果早期妊娠出现阴道流血，且确诊宫内妊娠伴有胎心搏动，应继续进行常规产前护理，如出血症状加重或症状持续 14 天以上时则建议就医治疗。

Women with bleeding in early pregnancy and a confirmed intrauterine pregnancy with a fetal heartbeat should be advised to return if bleeding gets worse or persists for more than 14 days but otherwise to continue with routine antenatal care.

2. *稽留流产和不全流产*（Missed or incomplete miscarriage）

流产可并发出血和剧烈疼痛，可能需要输血和使用阿片类镇痛药。如果有感染证据，应立即开始抗生素治疗，如果细菌培养鉴定对所用抗生素不敏感，则随后进行调整用药。

Miscarriage may be complicated by haemorrhage and severe pain, and may necessitate blood transfusion and relief of pain with opiates. If there is evidence of infection, antibiotic therapy should be started immediately and adjusted subsequently if the organism identified in culture is not sensitive to the prescribed antibiotic.

> **！ 注意**
>
> 败血症性流产并发内毒素休克常见的治疗方法是通过大量的抗生素治疗和足量的、谨慎的补液治疗。
>
> Septic miscarriage complicated by endotoxic shock is treated by massive antibiotic therapy and adequate, carefully controlled fluid replacement.

> **！ 注意**
>
> 如果有"宫颈休克"的征象，任何突出于宫颈口的妊娠物应使用组织钳抓住取出。
>
> If there is evidence of 'cervical shock' any products of conception protruding through the cervical os should be removed by grasping them with tissue–holding forceps.

>  **经验**
>
> 没有证据表明卧床休息可以改善先兆流产的预后，尽管对中期妊娠流产的高危女性或因宫颈功能不全导致胎膜脱垂进入宫颈管的女性来说，卧床休息可能有助于延长妊娠时间。
>
> There is no evidence that bed rest improves the prognosis in cases of threatened miscarriage, although it may be beneficial in prolonging pregnancy in women at high risk of second-trimester loss or where there is prolapse of membranes into the cervical canal as a result of cervical weakness.

3. 期待治疗（Expectant management）

对于确诊流产的女性来说，期待治疗是确诊流产后最初 7～14 天的最佳选择，除非该女性出血风险增加（如早孕晚期）、出血的影响风险增加、有感染证据。对一些女性来说，药物或外科治疗可能是一种更可接受的选择，应该被提供。治疗成功率取决于与临床处理能力等类似因素，但应提醒患者，完全流产可能需要 1～2 周。如果疼痛和出血在 7～14 天内消失，应建议女性重复进行尿妊娠试验，如果仍然阳性，应返院复查。如果期待治疗 14 天后还未开始出血或持续性出血，应进行复查。

This is the favoured option for the first 7–14 days for women with confirmed miscarriages unless the woman is at increased risk of bleeding (e.g. late first trimester) or she is at an increased risk of the effects of bleeding or there is evidence of infection. Medical or surgical management may be a more acceptable option for some women and should be offered as an alternative. Success rates depend on similar factors to those for medical management, but patients should be warned that it may take 1–2 weeks for complete miscarriage to occur. If pain and bleeding resolve within 7–14 days the woman should be advised to take a repeat urinary pregnancy test and return for review if this remains positive. A repeat scan should be organized if bleeding has not started or persists after 14 days of expectant management.

4. 药物治疗（Medical management）

当子宫内妊娠物还没有开始自然排出时，可以通过使用前列腺素类似物（如米索前列醇）来加速这个过程。妊娠物排出通常在 48～72h 内完成，但出血可能持续 3 周。药物治疗的成功率为 13%～96%，这取决于流产的类型、妊娠囊的大小和前列腺素的剂量。经阴道给予大剂量前列腺素治疗不完全流产成功率较高。药物治疗的优点是避免了全身麻醉，以及清宫的潜在并发症。接受药物治疗的患者应在 24h

内直接到医院咨询或入院，并应建议在治疗 3 周后进行尿妊娠试验，如果尿妊娠试验仍然阳性，则应返院复查，排除葡萄胎或异位妊娠。

When the uterine contents have not begun to be expelled naturally, the process can be expedited by the use of a prostaglandin analogue such as misoprostol. Passage of the products will normally be accomplished in approximately 48–72 hours, but bleeding may continue for up to 3 weeks. Success rates of medical treatment vary between 13% and 96% depending on the type of miscarriage, sac size and dose of prostaglandin. Higher success rates occur in incomplete miscarriage treated with high-dose prostaglandins given vaginally. The advantages of medical management are that a general anaesthetic is avoided, as are the potential complications of evacuation. Patients undergoing medical management should have 24-hour direct access to hospital services for advice or admission and should be advised to take a urinary pregnancy test 3 weeks after treatment and return for review if this remains positive to exclude molar or ectopic pregnancy.

5. 手术治疗（Surgical management）

妊娠残余物的手术清除手段包括宫颈扩张和抽吸刮除以清除妊娠残余物（图 18-4）。这是大出血或持续出血时，如果生命体征不稳定或存在受感染的残留妊娠组织时的选择方式。2% 手术治疗病例发生严重并发症，其中包括子宫穿孔、宫颈撕裂、腹腔损伤、宫腔粘连和大出血。宫内感染可导致输卵管感染和输卵管阻塞并继发不孕。应考虑进行包括沙眼衣原体在内的感染筛查，如有临床指征，应给予抗生素预防。如果怀疑子宫穿孔，并有证据表明腹腔内出血或肠损伤，应进行腹腔镜或开腹手术。无论选择哪种方法，如果可能的话，妊娠物都应该送去做组织学检查，因为一小部分病例会被证明是妊娠滋养细胞疾病（GTD）。

Surgical evacuation of retained products of conception involves dilatation of the cervix and suction curettage to remove the products (Fig. 18.4). This is the modality of choice when there is heavy bleeding or persistent bleeding, if the vital signs are unstable or in the presence of infected retained tissue. Serious complications of surgical treatment occur in 2% of cases and include perforation of the uterus, cervical tears, intra-abdominal trauma, intrauterine adhesions and haemorrhage. Intrauterine infection may result in tubal infection and tubal obstruction with subsequent infertility. Screening for infection, including *Chlamydia trachomatis*, should be considered and antibiotic prophylaxis given if clinically indicated. If uterine perforation is suspected and there is evidence of intraperitoneal haemorrhage or damage to the bowel, a laparoscopy or laparotomy should be performed.Whichever method is chosen,

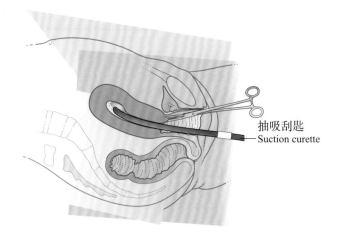

抽吸刮匙
Suction curette

▲ 图 18-4　妊娠残余物的清除
Fig. 18.4　Evacuation of retained products of conception.

products should be sent for histological examination if possible, as a small number will prove to be gestational trophoblastic disease (GTD).

6. 胎儿组织的妥善处理（Sensitive disposal of fetal tissues）

应该让女性或夫妇知道，如果他们希望就可以获得获取处理胎儿组织方式的信息。《火葬条例》不适用于孕 24 周以下的胎儿，但火葬机构可自行决定火葬。殡葬法规定没有法律义务埋葬（或火葬）孕 24 周前出生的死亡婴儿，但没有任何法律义务阻止任何一种埋葬选择。胎儿组织允许集体埋葬。

A woman or couple should be made aware that information on disposal options is available if they wish to have access to it. The cremation regulations do not apply to fetuses under 24 weeks' gestation, but cremation authorities may cremate them at their discretion. There is no legal duty under burial legislation to bury (or cremate) babies born dead before 24 weeks' gestation, but nothing to prevent either option. Communal burial is permitted for fetal tissue.

如果符合特定标准，女性或夫妇也可以选择在家安葬。

There is also the option for women or couples to bury at home, provided that certain criteria have been fulfilled.

任何婴儿，不论胎龄如何，出生时是活的，随后立即死亡，即为活产和新生儿死亡，在登记和处理方面应视为活产和新生儿死亡。

Any baby, irrespective of gestational age, who is born alive and then dies immediately afterwards is a live birth and neonatal death and should be treated as such in terms of registration and disposal.

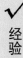

对于确诊的流产，药物和期待治疗是一种可替代手术治疗流产的有效方法。

Medical and expectant management is an effective alternative to surgical treatment in confirmed miscarriage.

7. 反复性流产（Recurrent miscarriage）

有复发性流产史的女性应转诊到专科诊所。如果可能的话，父母双方的染色体核型以及任何胎儿组织都应该进行检测。每隔 12 周至少两次检查孕妇血 LA 和 aCL。中期妊娠复发性流产的女性应进行血栓形成倾向筛查，其中包括 V-Leiden 因子、凝血因子Ⅱ基因突变和蛋白 S。应安排超声检查以评估多囊卵巢综合征的卵巢形态和宫腔。疑似子宫畸形（图 18-5）可能需要进一步检查，如宫腔镜或腹腔镜检查。患有持续性 LA 和 aCL 的女性应考虑在随后的孕期使用小剂量阿司匹林和肝素进行治疗。低剂量肝素治疗也可改善遗传性血栓性形成倾向女性的妊娠结局，而这与中期妊娠流产有关。有核型异常的夫妇应咨询临床遗传学家。宫颈功能不全患者孕 14～16 周行宫颈环扎术可降低早产的发生率，但尚未证明能提高胎儿存活率。采取预防性环扎术的另一替代选择是连续超声测量宫颈管长度，只有当宫颈长度缩短至 25mm 以下时才进行治疗。越来越多的证据表明孕酮（具有抗炎特性）能有效延长高危妊娠。细菌性阴道病与中期妊娠流产和早产有关。应用克林霉素（而不是甲硝唑）治疗细菌性阴道病似乎可以降低早产的风险，但没有证据支持经验性使用抗生素治疗中期妊娠丢失或其他感染。重要的是记住在相当一部分复发性流产的女性中并不能发现任何病因。在这些女性中仅给予支持性治疗通常可以获得好的预后，没有证据表明激素、阿司匹林、肝素或免疫治疗的经验性治疗可以改善结局。

Women with a history of recurrent miscarriage should be offered referral to a specialist clinic. The karyotype of both parents and, if possible, any fetal products should be tested. Maternal blood should be examined for LA and aCL on at least two occasions 12 weeks apart. Women with recurrent second-trimester miscarriage should be screened for thrombophilias, including factor V Leiden, factor II gene mutation and protein S. An ultrasound scan should be arranged to assess ovarian morphology for PCOS and the uterine cavity. Suspected uterine anomalies (Fig. 18.5) may require further investigation such as hysteroscopy or laparoscopy. Women with persistent LA and aCL should be considered for treatment with low-dose aspirin and heparin during subsequent pregnancies. Treatment with low-dose heparin may also improve pregnancy outcomes in women with inherited thrombophilias where these are associated with second-trimester miscarriage. Couples with karyotypic abnormalities should be referred to a clinical geneticist. Cervical cerclage carried out at 14–16 weeks in cases of cervical incompetence reduces the incidence of pre-term delivery but has not been shown to improve fetal survival. An alternative approach to the use of prophylactic cerclage is serial ultrasound measurement of the length of the cervical canal with treatment only if this drops below 25 mm. There is increasing evidence that progesterone (which has anti-inflammatory properties) is effective in prolonging high-risk pregnancies. Bacterial vaginosis has been associated with second-trimester losses and pre-term delivery. Treatment of this condition with clindamycin (not metronidazole) does appear to reduce the risk of pre-term delivery, but there is no evidence to support empirical antibiotic use in women with second-trimester loss or for other infections. It is important to remember that no cause will be identified in a significant proportion of women with recurrent miscarriage. The prognosis with supportive care alone in these women is generally good, and there is no evidence to suggest that empirical treatment with hormonal, aspirin, heparin or immunotherapy treatment improves the outcome.

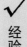

遗传异常是导致偶发性流产的最常见原因，但也是导致复发性流产的相对少见的原因。

Genetic abnormalities are the commonest cause of isolated miscarriage but a relatively uncommon cause of recurrent pregnancy loss.

三、异位妊娠（Ectopic pregnancy）

异位妊娠是指任何发生在子宫腔外的妊娠。

The term *ectopic pregnancy* refers to any pregnancy occurring outside the uterine cavity.

异位妊娠最常见的部位是输卵管，但也可能发生为卵巢妊娠、腹腔妊娠、宫颈妊娠或剖宫产瘢痕妊娠（CSP）（图 18-6）。

The most common site of extrauterine implantation is the Fallopian tube, but it may occur in the ovary as an ovarian pregnancy, in the abdominal cavity as an abdominal pregnancy, in the cervical canal as a cervical pregnancy or at the site of a previous caesarean section as a caesarean scar pregnancy (CSP) (Fig. 18.6).

在英国，每 1000 例妊娠中就有 11 例发生输卵管妊娠，尽管这一发病率在不同人群中有很大差异。异位妊娠仍然是妊娠最初三个月孕产妇死亡的一个重要原因（每 1000 例中有 0.2 例），在英国，每 3 年

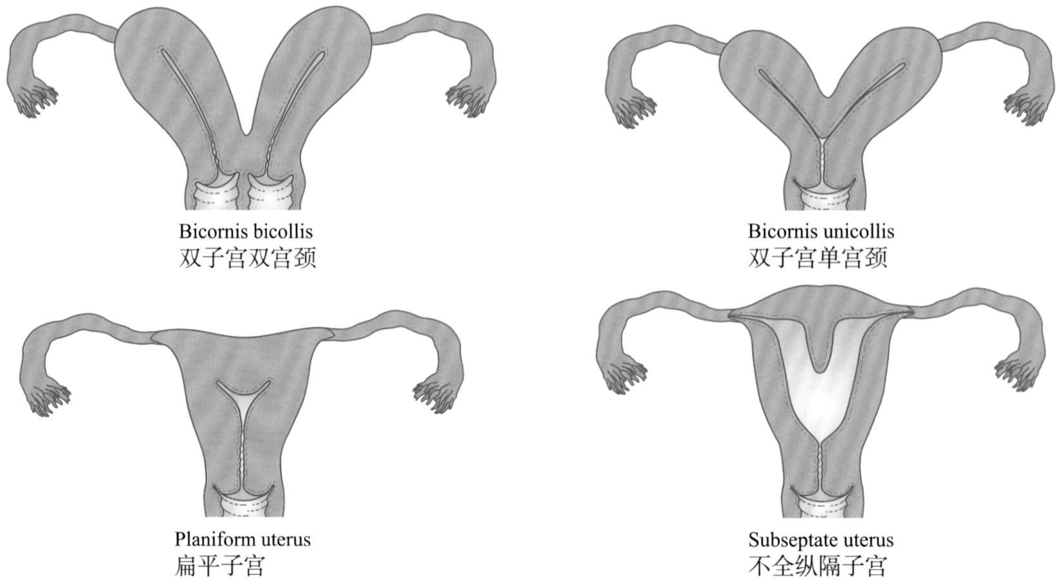

Bicornis bicollis
双子宫双宫颈

Bicornis unicollis
双子宫单宫颈

Planiform uterus
扁平子宫

Subseptate uterus
不全纵隔子宫

▲ 图 18-5 生殖道畸形

Fig. 18.5 Anomalies of the genital tract.

！注意

流产的心理因素

在西欧大多数女性确诊妊娠的时间比前几代人早得多。自然流产通常在医学上被认为并不严重，并且在第一次发生时很少被进一步探究原因。随访往往停留在初级护理阶段，很少有女性会到妇科了解及听取她们流产的原因。虽然没有证据表明流产与精神疾病发病风险的总体增加有关，但几乎 50% 的女性在流产后 6 周感到相当痛苦，并且经常感到愤怒、孤独和内疚。有过流产史且没有存活子女的女性、有过终止妊娠史的女性和有过精神病史的女性在流产后的几个月内最有可能患抑郁症。曾多次流产的女性尤其脆弱，应当得到妇科相关支持和咨询。

Psychological aspects of miscarriage

In Western Europe most women confirm their pregnancies considerably earlier than in previous generations. A spontaneous miscarriage is often regarded medically as not serious and is rarely investigated when it occurs for the first time. Follow-up is often left in primary care,and few women receive gynaecological attention or an explanation of their loss. Although there is no evidence to associate miscarriage with an overall increased risk of psychiatric morbidity, almost half of all women are considerably distressed at 6 weeks following miscarriage and often feel angry, alone and guilty. Women who have had a previous miscarriage and no live child, women who have had a previous termination of pregnancy and those with a previous psychiatric history are most at risk of becoming depressed in the months that follow miscarriage. Women who have had many miscarriages are particularly vulnerable and should probably receive gynaecological support and counselling.

就有 10～12 名女性死于异位妊娠。可悲的是，有证据表明其中有 2/3 病例的护理水平并不合格。输卵管妊娠可能发生在输卵管壶腹部、峡部和间质部，其结局取决于植入部位。

Tubal pregnancy occurs in 11 in 1000 pregnancies in the UK, although this incidence varies substantially in different populations. Ectopic pregnancy remains an important cause of maternal mortality (0.2 per 1000 cases) in the first trimester, with 10–12 women dying every 3 years from the condition in the UK. Sadly, there is evidence of substandard care in two-thirds of these cases. Tubal pregnancy may occur in the ampulla, the isthmus and the interstitial portion of the tube, and the outcome will depend on the site of implantation.

（一）诱发因素 [Predisposing factors (Table 18.1)]

大多数异位妊娠病例没有可识别的易感因素，但既往有异位妊娠、绝育、盆腔炎、生育能力低下的病史会增加异位妊娠的可能性（表 18–1）。宫内节育器（IUD）导致异位妊娠风险的增加只适用于带器妊娠。由于其作为避孕工具的有效性，放置宫内节育器的女性每年异位妊娠率低于不采取避孕措施女性。

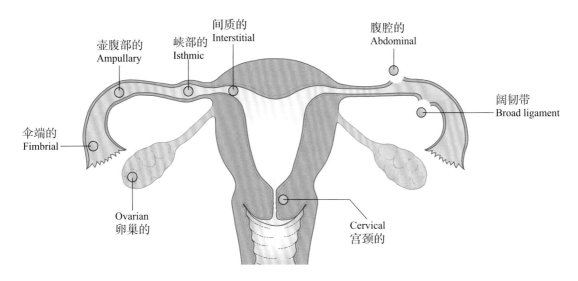

▲ 图 18-6　异位妊娠的植入部位

Fig. 18.6　Sites of implantation of ectopic pregnancies.

表 18-1　异位妊娠的危险因素

Table 18.1　Risk factors for ectopic pregnancy

	相对风险 Relative risk
既往有 PID Previous history of PID	4
既往输卵管手术 Previous tubal surgery	4.5
绝育失败 Failed sterilization	9
放置 IUD IUD in situ	10
既往异位妊娠 Previous ectopic pregnancy	10～15

IUD. 宫内节育器；PID. 盆腔炎性疾病

IUD, Intrauterine device; PID, pelvic inflammatory disease.

The majority of cases of ectopic pregnancy have no identifiable predisposing factor, but a previous history of ectopic pregnancy, sterilization, pelvic inflammatory disease and/or subfertility increases the likelihood of an ectopic pregnancy. The increased risk for an intrauterine device (IUD) applies only to pregnancies that occur despite the presence of the IUD. Because of their effectiveness as contraceptives, ectopic rates per year in IUD users are lower than in women not using contraception.

（二）临床表现（Clinical presentation）

1. 急性表现（Acute presentation）

典型的症状包括闭经、下腹痛和子宫出血。腹痛通常先于阴道流血，可从下腹一侧开始，但随着出血扩展至腹膜腔，腹痛范围迅速扩大。出血导致的膈下刺激会引起肩顶疼痛，并可能发生晕厥发作。

The classical pattern of symptoms includes amenorrhoea, lower abdominal pain and uterine bleeding. The abdominal pain usually precedes the onset of vaginal bleeding and may start on one side of the lower abdomen but rapidly becomes generalized as blood loss extends into the peritoneal cavity. Subdiaphragmatic irritation by blood produces referred shoulder tip pain, and syncopal episodes may occur.

停经时间一般为 6～8 周，但如果发生在输卵管间质部或腹腔妊娠，则可能更长。临床上常观察到休克，伴随低血压、心动过速和腹膜炎的迹象，其中包括腹胀、腹肌紧张和反弹压痛。由于急性疼痛不适，骨盆检查通常并不重要且应谨慎进行。不超过 25% 病例出现这种急性表现。

The period of amenorrhoea is usually 6–8 weeks but may be longer if implantation occurs in the interstitial portion of the tube or in abdominal pregnancy. Clinical examination reveals a shocked woman with hypotension, tachycardia and signs of peritonism, including abdominal distension, guarding and rebound tenderness. Pelvic examination is usually unimportant because of the acute pain and discomfort and should be undertaken with caution. This type of acute presentation occurs in no more than 25% of cases.

2. 亚急性表现（Subacute presentation）

短暂停经后，患者反复出现阴道流血和腹痛。患者可能出现的非妇科症状，如乳房压痛、胃肠道症状（排便疼痛）、泌尿系统症状、头晕或晕厥。任

病例分析：亚急性表现	Case study: Subacute presentation
一名 22 岁，孕 0 的女性，停经 8 周后因阴道流血入院。她用妊娠试剂盒测试阳性，并描述经阴道排出一些组织。超声检查显示子宫内无异常物质，但血清 β-hCG 仍呈阳性。疑似诊断为不全流产，并顺利进行了清宫术。她于术后第二天出院，但当晚因下腹疼痛再次入院；剖腹探查时发现输卵管壶腹异位妊娠破裂。几天后，最初清宫的组织学病理报告为 "A-S 反应蜕膜改变，未见绒毛"。	A 22-year-old woman, para 0, was admitted with vaginal bleeding after 8 weeks of amenorrhoea. She had had a positive home pregnancy kit test and described passing some tissue per vaginam. Ultrasound scan showed an empty uterus, although serum b-hCG was still positive. A presumptive diagnosis of incomplete miscarriage was made, and evacuation of the uterus carried out uneventfully. She was discharged the following day but readmitted that night with lower abdominal pain; a ruptured ampullary ectopic pregnancy was found at laparotomy. Some days later, histology of the original curettage was reported as 'decidua with Arias-Stella type reaction, no chorionic villi seen'.

何女性在闭经一段时间后出现下腹疼痛，都应被视为疑似异位妊娠。在亚急性期，可能引起压痛或感觉到阴道穹隆处有包块。

After a short period of amenorrhoea, the patient experiences recurrent attacks of vaginal bleeding and abdominal pain. Patients may present with non-gynaecological symptoms such as breast tenderness, gastrointestinal symptoms (pain of defecation), urinary symptoms, dizziness or syncope. Any woman who develops lower abdominal pain following an interval of amenorrhoea should be considered as a possible ectopic pregnancy. In its subacute phase, it may be possible to elicit tenderness or feel a mass in one fornix

其他检查结果可包括子宫增大伴宫颈举痛、皮肤黏膜苍白及下腹压痛。

Other findings on examination may include an enlarged uterus with cervical motion tenderness, pallor or lower abdominal tenderness.

（三）病理（Pathology）

胚胎着床可能发生在不同的部位，妊娠的结局取决于着床部位。腹腔妊娠可由胚胎直接植入腹腔或卵巢引起，在这种情况下称为原发性腹腔妊娠，也可由输卵管妊娠挤压并再次植入腹腔引起，称为继发性腹腔妊娠。胚胎着床可能发生在既往接受过子宫手术的部位，最常见的是之前的剖腹产瘢痕处，或发生在输卵管间质部分成为宫角妊娠。胚胎着床于子宫外仍会产生类似正常妊娠的激素变化。子宫增大，子宫内膜发生蜕膜改变。胚胎在输卵管伞端或壶腹内着床，包块在破裂发生前快速增大，而在输卵管间质部或峡部植入则出现出血或疼痛等的早期症状（图 18-7）。

Implantation may occur in a variety of sites, and the outcome of the pregnancy will depend on the site of implantation. Abdominal pregnancy may result from direct implantation of the conceptus in the abdominal cavity or on the ovary, in which case it is known as *primary abdominal pregnancy*, or it may result from extrusion of a tubal pregnancy with secondary implantation in the peritoneal cavity, which is known as *secondary abdominal pregnancy*. Implantation may occur at the site of previous uterine surgery, most commonly previous caesarean section, or in the interstitial portion of the Fallopian tube as a cornual pregnancy. Implantation of the conceptus outside of the uterus still results in hormonal changes that mimic normal pregnancy. The uterus enlarges, and the endometrium undergoes decidual change. Implantation within the fimbrial end or ampulla of the tube allows greater expansion before rupture occurs, whereas implantation in the interstitial portion or the isthmic part of the tube presents with early signs of haemorrhage or pain (Fig. 18.7).

滋养层细胞侵入管壁并侵蚀血管。这一过程将一直持续到妊娠物破入腹腔或阔韧带或胚胎死亡，

病例分析：急性表现	Case study: Acute presentation
一名 18 岁，孕 0 的女性，因下腹疼痛晕倒而送入急诊室。入院时，她出现休克，血压 80/40mmHg，脉搏 120 次/分钟，按压腹肌僵硬。阴道检查显示有轻微的血性分泌物，子宫增大，明显的宫颈举痛，右侧阴道穹隆可及一个质地柔软的包块。剖腹探查时，从腹腔取出 800ml 新鲜血液，发现右侧输卵管异位妊娠破裂。随后，反复盆腔感染和月经不规律史被发现。	An 18-year-old woman, para 0, was brought into casualty collapsed with lower abdominal pain. On admission, she was shocked with a blood pressure of 80/40, a pulse of 120 beats/min and a tender, rigid abdomen. Vaginal examination revealed a slight red loss, bulky uterus and marked cervical excitation with a tender mass in the right fornix. At laparotomy, 800 mL of fresh blood was removed from the peritoneal cavity and a ruptured right tubal ectopic pregnancy was found. Subsequently, a history of recurrent pelvic infections and irregular periods was elicited.

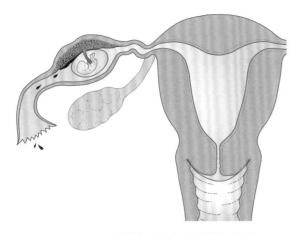

▲ 图 18-7　滋养细胞组织穿透输卵管壁

Fig. 18.7　**Penetration of the tubal wall by trophoblastic tissue.**

从而导致输卵管妊娠包块。在这种情况下，可能发生胚胎组织吸收或输卵管妊娠流产。胚胎排出到腹腔或不全流产时也可能发生持续的输卵管出血。

Trophoblastic cells invade the wall of the tube and erode into blood vessels. This process will continue until the pregnancy bursts into the abdominal cavity or into the broad ligament or the embryo dies, thus resulting in a tubal mole. Under these circumstances, absorption or tubal miscarriage may occur. Expulsion of the embryo into the peritoneal cavity or partial miscarriage may also occur with continuing episodes of bleeding from the tube.

（四）诊断（Diagnosis）

> **！注意**
>
> 如果早期妊娠伴有疼痛和出血，应始终怀疑异位妊娠。
>
> Ectopic pregnancy should always be suspected where early pregnancy is complicated by pain and bleeding.

虽然急性表现的异位妊娠诊断很少出现问题，但亚急性期的诊断可能要困难得多，可能被误认为是先兆流产或不完全流产，也可与急性输卵管炎或阑尾炎伴盆腔腹膜炎相混淆，有时可能与卵巢囊肿破裂或出血混淆。

Whilst the diagnosis of the acute ectopic pregnancy rarely presents a problem, diagnosis in the subacute phase may be much more difficult. It may be mistaken for a threatened or incomplete miscarriage. It may also be confused with acute salpingitis or appendicitis with pelvic peritonitis. It may sometimes be confused with rupture or haemorrhage of an ovarian cyst.

如果血液大量流失并进入腹腔，血红蛋白水平会降低，白细胞计数通常正常或略有升高。血清

hCG 检测阴性可以特异性高于 99% 地排除异位妊娠；尿 hCG 检测试剂盒可用于住院患者，可检测 97% 的妊娠。如果存在宫内活胎妊娠，85% 的病例在 48h 内血清 hCG 会翻倍（相比之下，异位妊娠为 15%）。正常宫内妊娠通常在血清 hCG 水平超过 1000U/L（识别区）时经超声扫描可见。在多达 85% 的病例中，通过连续测量血清 hCG 水平并结合超声诊断可以区分早期宫内妊娠与流产或异位妊娠。2% 的病例（图 18-8）的盆腔超声扫描可显示输卵管妊娠，或通过其他特征（如腹腔内游离液体）提示输卵管妊娠，但主要有助于排除宫内妊娠（表 18-2）。宫内妊娠通常可以在孕 6 周时通过经腹超声确诊，而在孕 5～6 周时通过经阴道超声可以更快地确诊。偶然有一些异位妊娠没有临床症状，但如果刮宫取出的组织病理学检查显示有蜕膜反应和 A-S 现象，则建议考虑腹腔镜探查。

If sufficient blood loss has occurred into the peritoneal cavity, the haemoglobin level will be low and the white cell count will be usually normal or slightly raised. Serum hCG measurement will exclude ectopic pregnancy if negative with a specificity of greater than 99%, and urinary hCG with modern kits that can be used on the ward will detect 97% of pregnancies. In the presence of a viable intrauterine pregnancy, the serum hCG will double over a 48-hour period in 85% of cases (compared to 15% of ectopic pregnancies). A normal intrauterine pregnancy will usually be visualized on scan where the serum hCG level is more than 1000 IU/L (the discriminatory zone). Serial measurements of serum hCG levels in conjunction with ultrasound diagnosis can distinguish early intrauterine pregnancy from miscarriage or ectopics in up to 85% of cases. Ultrasound scan of the pelvis may

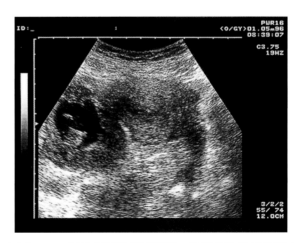

▲ 图 18-8　异位妊娠的超声图像，子宫体和宫腔位于中央，在子宫左侧的腔中可以看到一个胎芽

Fig. 18.8　**Ultrasound image of an ectopic pregnancy. The uterus and endometrial cavity can be seen centrally. A fetal pole can be seen in the cavity to the left of the uterus.**

表 18-2　经阴道超声诊断宫内妊娠及异位妊娠的特点

Table 18.2　Features of intrauterine and ectopicpregnancy on transvaginal scan

宫内妊娠 Intrauterine pregnancy	异位妊娠 Ectopic pregnancy
宫内妊娠囊（4～5 周） Intrauterine gestation sac (4–5 weeks)	空子宫 Empty uterus
卵黄囊（5～6 周） Yolk sac (5–6 weeks)	界限不清的输卵管环状包块伴随道格拉斯窝积液 Poorly defined tubal ring with fluid in pouch of Douglas
双蜕膜征（5 周） Double decidual sign (5 weeks)	宫内假性囊腔 Pseudo-sac in uterus
胎心搏动（7 周） Fetal heartbeat (7 weeks)	输卵管环状包块伴随宫外胎心搏动 Tubal ring with extrauterine heartbeat

demonstrate tubal pregnancy in 2% of cases (Fig. 18.8) or suggest it by other features, such as free fluid in the peritoneal cavity, but is mainly of help in excluding intrauterine pregnancy (Table 18.2). Intrauterine pregnancy can usually be identified by transabdominal scan at 6 weeks' gestation and somewhat sooner by transvaginal scan at 5–6 weeks gestation. Occasionally, there may be no clinical signs of an ectopic pregnancy, but if curettings submitted for histopathology show evidence of decidual reaction and the Arias-Stella phenomenon, then it is advisable to consider laparoscopy.

（五）治疗（Management）

对血流动力学稳定的疑似异位妊娠患者的理想治疗应在专用的 EPAU 同等设备或床旁超声基础上进行。血流动力学异常的患者应紧急转诊至急诊室，并抽取血液进行紧急交叉配血和输血。手术应尽快进行，并切除受损的输卵管。

Ideally management of haemodynamically stable patients with suspected ectopic pregnancy should take place in a dedicated EPAU or equivalent with access to point-of-care ultrasound. Patients who are haemodynamically compromised should be referred urgently to an emergency department and blood taken for urgent cross-matching and transfusion. Surgery should be performed as soon as possible with removal of the damaged tube.

未致敏的 Rh 阴性血女性任何一次异位妊娠，无论采用何种治疗方式，都应接受抗 D 免疫球蛋白治疗。

Non-sensitized Rh-negative women should receive anti-D immunoglobulin in any ectopic pregnancy, regardless of the mode of treatment.

1. 手术治疗（Surgical management）

一旦确诊，可采用以下治疗方案。

Once the diagnosis is confirmed, the options for treatment are:

（1）输卵管切除术：如果输卵管严重受损或对侧输卵管健康，正确的治疗方法是切除患侧输卵管。如果着床于输卵管间质部，除切除输卵管外，可能还需要切除部分宫角。

1. *Salpingectomy*-If the tube is badly damaged or the contralateral tube appears healthy, the correct treatment is removal of the affected tube. If implantation has occurred in the interstitial portion of the tube, it may be necessary to resect part of the uterine horn in addition to removing the tube.

（2）输卵管切开术：如果异位妊娠组织在输卵管内，则可以通过取出妊娠物和重建输卵管来保护输卵管。这种治疗方法在对侧输卵管缺如的情况下尤为重要。缺点是滋养层组织持续存在，需要进一步手术或药物治疗的病例高达 6%。

2. *Salpingotomy*-Where the ectopic pregnancy is contained within the tube, it may be possible to conserve the tube by removing the pregnancy and reconstituting the tube. This is particularly important where the contralateral tube has been lost. The disadvantage is the persistence of trophoblastic tissue requiring further surgery or medical treatment in up to 6% of cases.

尽管输卵管切开术后复发性异位妊娠的风险更大，但两种治疗后的宫内妊娠率相似。两者都可以通过开腹手术或腹腔镜手术进行。腹腔镜手术具有更快的恢复时间、更短的住院时间和更少的粘连形成，如果患者病情稳定并且护理标准符合预期，腹腔镜手术是首选方法。

Subsequent intrauterine pregnancy rates are similar after

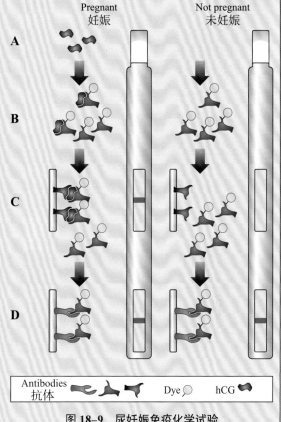

进行尿妊娠试验
Performing a urinary pregnancy test

虽然各种家庭式检测试剂的具体配置各不相同，但主要步骤如下（图 18–9）。

A. 将患者尿液样本放置在样本区域上。

B. 尿液通过毛细作用沿着试剂盒流向含有小鼠免疫球蛋白的区域，如果 hCG 存在于尿液中，则与 hCG 分子结合。这些抗体也与催化颜色变化的酶结合。

C. 结合和未结合的小鼠抗体通过毛细作用被提取到含有针对 hCG 和染料的固定多克隆抗体的第二区域。任何与 hCG 结合的小鼠抗体都会被捕获在这里，与之结合的酶会引起颜色变化（阳性结果）。

D. 任何剩余的未结合抗体将通过该区域携带到控制条带，在那里它们将被抗鼠抗体捕获并催化颜色变化（无论尿液中是否含有 hCG，这都将发生，有助于表明检测工作正常，并且第一个区域的阴性结果是由于缺乏 hCG 所致）。

Although the exact configuration of the various home kits varies, the principal steps are as follows: (Fig. 18.9)

A. A sample of the patient's urine is placed on the sample area (a).

B. The urine is drawn along the kit by capillary action towards an area containing mouse immunoglobulin, which binds to the hCG molecule if present in the urine. These antibodies are also conjugated to an enzyme that catalyzes a colour change.

C. Bound and unbound mouse antibodies are drawn up the kit by capillary action to a second area containing fixed polyclonal antibodies to hCG and dye (b). Any mouse antibodies bound to hCG will be trapped here, and the enzyme conjugated to them will cause a colour change (a positive result).

D. Any remaining unbound antibodies will carry on past this area to the control strip zone (c), where they will be trapped by anti–mouse antibodies and catalyze a colour change (this will occur whether the urine contains hCG or not but helps to show that the test is working properly and that a negative result in the first area is due to an absence of hCG).

图 18–9　尿妊娠免疫化学试验

（改编自 commons.wikimedia.org.）

Fig. 18.9　Immunochemistry of urinary pregnancy test
Figure adapted from commons.wikimedia.org.

---

both types of treatment, although the risk of recurrent ectopic pregnancy is greater after salpingotomy. Both can be carried out as an open procedure or laparoscopically. The laparoscopic approach is associated with quicker recovery time, shorter stay in hospital and less adhesion formation, and is the method of choice if the patient is stable and is now the expected standard of care.

2. 药物治疗（Medical management）

异位妊娠的药物治疗包括将甲氨蝶呤注射至全身或通过腹腔镜探查或超声引导注射至异位妊娠部位。并非所有类型异位妊娠都适合药物治疗。当疼痛不明显、异位妊娠包块大小<35mm，没有明显的胎心搏动，没有明确证据表明宫内活胎妊娠，药物治疗可以作为一线治疗。药物治疗的理想情况是 hCG 水平低于 1500U/L，但当 hCG 水平高达 5000U/L 时，在满足其他条件的前提下药物治疗可作为手术的替代方案，并且患者要理解需进一步接受干预的

可能性会增加，如果病情恶化需要紧急返院。药物治疗后，血清 hCG 检测应在 4 天和 7 天后复查，即之每周复查直到获得阴性结果。20% 的病例发生全身副作用，75% 发生腹痛。5%～10% 的病例发生输卵管破裂需手术治疗。异位妊娠经任何方法治疗后，85%～90% 的后续妊娠将是宫内妊娠，但只有 60% 的女性能够自然受孕，这反映了全球性的输卵管疾病的现状。

Medical treatment of an ectopic pregnancy involves the administration of methotrexate, either systemically or by injection into the ectopic pregnancy by laparoscopic visualization or by ultrasound guidance. Medical treatment is not suitable for all cases of ectopic pregnancy. It can be offered as first-line treatment where there is no significant pain, the ectopic is less than 35 mm in size with no visible heartbeat and there is no evidence of viable intrauterine pregnancy. Ideally the hCG level should be less than 1500 IU/L, although treatment can be offered as an alternative to surgery for levels up to 5000 IU/L, provided the other conditions are met and the woman understands that the chance of requiring further intervention is increased and there is a need to return urgently if her condition deteriorates. Following treatment the serum hCG should be repeated 4 and 7 days later and then weekly until a negative result is obtained. Systemic side effects occur in 20% of cases and abdominal pain in 75%. Tubal rupture requiring surgery occurs in 5–10% of cases. After an ectopic pregnancy treated by any method, 85–90% of subsequent pregnancies will be intrauterine, but only 60% of women will manage to conceive spontaneously, reflecting global tubal disease.

（六）不明部位妊娠（Pregnancy of unknown location）

这被定义为一种妊娠试验阳性并在超声检查中没有发现宫内宫外妊娠或妊娠残留物的迹象的情况，10% 的妊娠会出现这种情况。这可能表示宫内妊娠组织太小以至于在超声上无法看到，但需要随访以排除异位妊娠。连续测量 hCG 值和重复超声检查等保守治疗手段对无症状的女性是安全的。血清孕酮水平低于 20nmol/L 可预测妊娠失败，但无助于预测妊娠部位。

This is defined as a positive pregnancy test where there are no signs on ultrasound of either an intrauterine or ectopic pregnancy or retained products of conception, and it occurs in 10% of pregnancies. This may represent an intrauterine pregnancy that is too small to see on ultrasound but requires follow-up to exclude ectopic pregnancy. Conservative management with serial hCG measurement and repeat ultrasound is safe for asymptomatic women. A serum progesterone level of less than 20 nmol/L is predictive of pregnancy failure but does not help in predicting pregnancy location.

（七）其他类型的宫外妊娠（Management of other forms of extrauterine pregnancy）

1. 腹腔妊娠（Abdominal pregnancy）

腹腔妊娠对母体有生命危险。胎盘在子宫外植入，穿过肠组织和盆腔腹膜。任何试图去除妊娠组织的尝试都会导致极难控制的大出血。应通过开腹手术取出胎儿，胎盘留在原位等待再吸收或自然排出。

Abdominal pregnancy presents a life-threatening hazard to the mother. The placenta implants outside the uterus and across the bowel and pelvic peritoneum. Any attempt to remove it will result in massive haemorrhage, which is extremely difficult to control. The fetus should be removed by laparotomy and the placenta left in situ to reabsorb or extrude

spontaneously.

2. 宫颈妊娠（Cervical pregnancy）

宫颈妊娠通常表现为位于宫颈部位的自然流产。偶尔可以通过刮宫术清除妊娠组织，但出血可能很严重，50% 的病例需要进行子宫切除术以达到足够的止血效果。

Cervical pregnancy often presents as the cervical stage of a spontaneous miscarriage. Occasionally, it is possible to remove the conceptus by curettage, but haemorrhage can be severe, and in 50% of cases it is necessary to proceed to hysterectomy to obtain adequate haemostasis.

3. 宫角（间质）妊娠 [Cornual (interstitial) pregnancy]

这种情况发生在胚胎植入于输卵管间质部。既往输卵管切除术、残角子宫和近端宫腔内操作是诱发因素。妊娠组织包块破裂可伴有明显出血，诊断可能很困难，但如果在破裂发生前被发现，可选择用甲氨蝶呤治疗。对于包块破裂或直径大于 5cm，传统的治疗方法是经腹楔形切除宫角部，甚至行子宫切除术。但现在更多采用腹腔镜下宫角吻合术。

This occurs when implantation occurs in the interstitial portion of the tube. Previous salpingectomy, rudimentary horns and proximal intraluminal admissions are predisposing factors. Rupture can be associated with significant bleeding, and diagnosis can be difficult, but if recognized before rupture occurs, medical treatment with methotrexate is an option. For pregnancies that have ruptured or are >5 cm in size, the traditional treatment has been wedge resection of the cornua via laparotomy or even hysterectomy, but laparoscopic cornuostomy has been increasingly used.

4. 剖宫产瘢痕部位妊娠（Caesarean scar pregnancy）

当胚胎植入于既往剖宫产部位的纤维瘢痕组织内时，就会发生这种情况。这是一种罕见但可能危及生命的疾病，占所有异位妊娠的 6%，影响 0.15% 有剖宫产史女性。诊断通常是通过超声检查发现剖宫产瘢痕增大并伴有妊娠囊或混合性肿块。如果病情稳定，可进行药物治疗，局部或全身应用甲氨蝶呤，或者手术楔形切除妊娠组织包块。

This occurs when implantation takes place within the fibrous scar tissue at the site of a previous caesarean section. It is a rare but potentially life-threatening condition accounting for 6% of all ectopic pregnancies and affecting 0.15% of women with previous caesarean section. Diagnosis is usually made on ultrasound detection of enlargement of the caesarean section scar with an attached gestational sac or mixed mass.

Treatment can be medical if the patient is stable with local or systemic methotrexate, or surgical with wedge resection of the gestational mass.

四、妊娠滋养细胞疾病（Gestational trophoblast disease）

早期滋养层的异常可由胎盘组织发育异常引起，导致大量绒毛水肿，形成无血管绒毛组织。胎盘被称为葡萄胎的大量葡萄状囊泡所取代（图 18-10）。葡萄胎可分为完全性葡萄胎和部分性葡萄胎。后者通常含有胚胎或胎儿的物质。

Abnormality of the early trophoblast may arise as a developmental anomaly of placental tissue and results in the formation of a mass of oedematous and avascular villi. The placenta is replaced by a mass of grape-like vesicles known as a hydatidiform mole (Fig. 18.10). Hydatidiform moles can be classified as complete or partial. The latter usually contain embryonic or fetal material.

在 0.5%～4% 的部分性葡萄胎和 15%～25% 的完全性葡萄胎可发生恶变，被称为绒毛膜癌。

Malignant change occurs in 0.5–4% of partial moles and 15–25% of complete moles and is known as choriocarcinoma.

其他类型的 GTD 包括持续性 GTD、胎盘部位滋养细胞肿瘤和上皮样滋养细胞肿瘤。

Other types of GTD include persistent GTD, placenta site trophoblastic tumours and epithelioid trophoblast tumour.

（一）发病率（Incidence）

在英国，该病总患病率约为 1.5/1000，但在亚洲和东南亚要高得多。在生育的极限年龄更为常见。

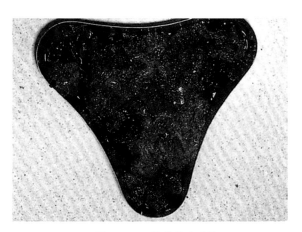

▲ 图 18-10　葡萄胎小囊泡

Fig. 18.10　Vesicles of a hydatidiform mole.

The overall prevalence of this condition is about 1.5 in 1000 pregnancies in the UK but is much higher in Asia and Southeast Asia. It is more common at the extremes of reproductive age.

（二）病理（Pathology）

葡萄胎妊娠被认为是由 2 个精子受精引起的，可以是无女性遗传物质的二倍体（完全葡萄胎），也可以是三倍体（部分葡萄胎）。良性葡萄胎仍局限于宫腔和蜕膜。组织病理学表现为绒毛样改变（图 18-11）。绒毛膜癌由柱状滋养细胞组成，无绒毛组织。广泛的血行转移是这种疾病的一个特点，直到最近，它的死亡率还是很高。转移可能发生在阴道局部，但最常见于肺部。1/3 的病例发生卵泡黄素化囊肿，这是由于血液循环中 hCG 水平过高所致。随着葡萄胎组织的清除，这些囊肿会自发地退化。50% 的绒毛膜癌病例与葡萄胎妊娠无关。

Molar pregnancy is thought to arise from fertilization by two sperm and can be diploid with no female genetic material (complete mole) or may exhibit triploidy (partial mole). Benign mole remains confined to the uterine cavity and decidua. The histopathology exhibits a villous pattern (see Fig. 18.11). Choriocarcinoma comprises plexiform columns of trophoblastic cells without villous patterns. Widespread blood-borne metastases are a feature of this disease, which, until recently, carried a very high mortality rate. Metastases may occur locally in the vagina but most commonly appear in the lungs. Theca lutein cysts occur in about one-third of all cases as a result of high circulating levels of hCG. These regress spontaneously with removal of the molar tissue. Fifty percent of cases of choriocarcinoma are not associated with molar pregnancy.

（三）临床表现（Clinical presentation）

葡萄胎妊娠最常见的表现为妊娠前半期出血，自然流产通常发生在孕 20 周左右。葡萄状绒毛有时预示着葡萄胎的存在。约有 50% 的病例子宫大于孕周，但这不是一个可靠指标，因为子宫有时可能小于孕周。妊娠剧吐，先兆子痫和不明原因的贫血都是提示这种疾病的因素。诊断可以通过超声扫描和血液、尿液中存在非常高水平的 hCG 来证实。

Molar pregnancy most commonly presents as bleeding in the first half of pregnancy, and spontaneous miscarriage often occurs at about 20 weeks' gestation. Occasionally, the passage of a grape-like villus heralds the presence of a mole. The uterus is larger than dates in about half the cases, but this is not a reliable sign, as it may sometimes be small for dates. Severe hyperemesis, pre-eclampsia and unexplained anaemia are all factors suggestive of this disorder. The diagnosis can be confirmed by ultrasound scan and by the presence of very high levels of hCG in the blood or urine.

（四）治疗（Management）

一旦确诊则抽吸刮宫终止妊娠。必须充分补充失血。虽然失血的风险增高，但关于常规使用催产素存在一个理论上的忧虑，即滋养层组织通过静脉系统传播的可能性。如有可能，这些工作应在清宫完成后开始。如果持续出血或血清 hCG 升高，有时可能需要重复清宫，但常规二次清宫并无效果。英国所有的葡萄胎妊娠病例都应该在其中一个滋养细胞疾病筛查中心登记，由该中心安排随访。对所有患者进行了至少 6 个月的连续 hCG 测量随诊（各国的具体细节各不相同）。

Once the diagnosis is established, the pregnancy is terminated by suction curettage. Adequate replacement of blood loss is essential. Although there is an increased risk of blood loss, there is a theoretical concern over the routine use of oxytocic agents because of the potential to disseminate trophoblastic tissue through the venous system. If possible, these should be commenced once the evacuation has been completed. Occasionally repeat evacuation may be required if there is persistent bleeding or a raised serum hCG, but routine second evacuation is not helpful. All cases of molar pregnancy in the UK should be registered with one of the trophoblastic disease screening centres, who will arrange follow-up. All patients are followed up with serial hCG measurements (details vary between countries) for at least 6 months.

如果组织学证据显示恶性改变，则采用甲氨蝶呤和放线菌素 D 化疗，可产生良好效果。在英国，这些病例由专门中心进行管理。澳大利亚和新西兰的一些州也有专门登记部门。

If the histological evidence shows malignant change, chemotherapy with methotrexate and actinomycin D is employed and produces good results. In the UK, management of these cases is concentrated in specialized centres. Some states in Australia and New Zealand have registries.

> **！注意**　值得注意，绒毛膜癌有时可能发生在流产或正常足月宫内妊娠之后。
>
> It must be remembered that choriocarcinoma sometimes can occur following a miscarriage or a normal-term intrauterine pregnancy.

直到血清 hCG 水平下降至正常的 6 个月后才可再次妊娠。含雌激素的口服避孕药和激素替代疗法（HRT）可在 hCG 水平一旦正常时即可使用。在随后

的妊娠中滋养细胞疾病复发的风险是 1/70，并且在随后任何一次妊娠的 6 周后应检查血清 hCG 水平。

Pregnancy is contraindicated until 6 months after the serum hCG levels fall to normal. Oestrogen-containing oral contraceptives and hormone replacement therapy (HRT) can be used as soon as hCG levels are normal. The risk recurrence in subsequent pregnancies is 1 in 70, and serum hCG levels should be checked 6 weeks after any subsequent pregnancy.

五、早期妊娠呕吐（Vomiting in early pregnancy）

恶心和呕吐是早期妊娠的常见症状（分别影响 80% 和 50% 的女性），通常从孕 4~10 周开始，孕 20 周前消失。13% 的病例症状持续至孕 20 周之后，但孕 12 周后出现的新症状不应归于剧吐。妊娠剧吐是指妊娠相关的持续性呕吐，伴有体重减轻 5% 以上和酮症。影响 0.3%~3% 的孕妇，该病与脱水、电解质失衡和维生素 B_1 缺乏有关。

Nausea and vomiting are common symptoms in early pregnancy (affecting 80% and 50% of women, respectively), usually starting between 4 and 10 weeks' gestation and resolving before 20 weeks. Symptoms persist beyond 20 weeks in 13% of cases, but new symptoms appearing after the twelfth week should not be attributed to hyperemesis. *Hyperemesis gravidarum* is defined as persistent pregnancy-related vomiting associated with weight loss of more than 5% of body mass and ketosis. Affecting 0.3–3% of all pregnant women, this is associated with dehydration, electrolyte imbalance and thiamine deficiency.

（一）病原学（Aetiology）

呕吐的病因是不确定的，多因素导致的，如内分泌、胃肠道和心理因素。多胎妊娠和葡萄胎时更常出现呕吐，提示与 hCG 水平有关。虽然短暂的甲状腺功能异常是常见的，但无其他甲状腺功能亢进的临床特征时并不需要治疗。感染幽门螺杆菌，这种与胃溃疡有关的微生物，也可能是病因之一。有过剧吐史的女性在随后的妊娠中很可能会再次经历剧吐。

The aetiology of hyperemesis is uncertain, with multifactorial causes such as endocrine, gastrointestinal and psychological factors proposed. Hyperemesis occurs more often in multiple pregnancy and hydatidiform mole, suggesting an association with the level of hCG. Although transient abnormalities of thyroid function are common, this does not require treatment in the absence of other clinical features

病例分析：滋养细胞疾病	Case study: Trophoblastic disease
一名 27 岁初产妇，因停经 12 周就诊，主诉阴道流血和下腹不适。腹部查体显示宫底大小为如孕 16 周。阴道流出新鲜血液，宫颈口闭合。尿 hCG 的滴度很高，超声扫描显示有暴风雪样图像，宫腔充满回声，但未显示胎儿（图 18-11）。第二天进行葡萄胎组织抽吸清除，并且恢复良好。	A 27-year-old primigravid woman attended the clinic with a history of 12 weeks of amenorrhoea, complaining of bright vaginal blood loss and lower abdominal discomfort. Abdominal examination revealed that the uterine fundus was 16 weeks in size. There was fresh blood in the vagina, and the cervical os was closed. There was a high titre of hCG in the urine, and an ultrasound scan showed a snowstorm appearance with the uterine cavity filled with echoes but no evidence of fetal parts (Fig. 18.11). Suction evacuation of molar tissue was performed the following day, and recovery was uneventful.

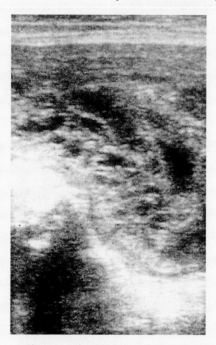

▲ 图 18-11　葡萄胎。葡萄胎组织的典型暴风雪外观很明显

Fig. 18.11　**Hydatidiform mole. The typical snowstorm appearance of molar tissue is apparent.**

of hyperthyroidism. Infection with *Helicobacter pylori*, the organism implicated in gastric ulcers, may also contribute. Women with a previous history of hyperemesis are likely to experience it in subsequent pregnancies.

（二）诊断（Diagnosis）

重要的是询问呕吐的频率、诱因及是否有其他家庭成员受到过影响。应询问既往孕期呕吐或非孕期呕吐史。吸烟和酗酒都会加重症状，应加以询问。若存在辅助生殖治疗或有双胞胎的密切家族史，多胎妊娠的可能性更大。早期妊娠出血或既往有滋养细胞疾病史可能提示葡萄胎。

It is important to ask about the frequency of vomiting, trigger factors and whether any other members of the family have been affected. A history of vomiting in a previous pregnancy or outside pregnancy should be sought. Smoking and alcohol can both exacerbate symptoms and should be

enquired of. If this pregnancy resulted from fertility treatment or there is a close family history of twins, a multiple pregnancy is more likely. Early pregnancy bleeding or a past history of trophoblastic disease may point to a hydatidiform mole.

脱水的临床特征包括心动过速、低血压和皮肤肿胀消失。需要排除非妊娠引起呕吐的病因，如甲状腺问题、尿路感染或肠胃炎等，因此应通过触诊腹部了解有压痛的部位，尤其是右上腹、下腹部和肾角。应进行尿液酮体、血细胞和蛋白质检测。

The clinical features of dehydration include tachycardia, hypotension and loss of skin turgor. Causes of vomiting not due to pregnancy, such as thyroid problems, urinary tract infection or gastroenteritis, need to be excluded, so the abdomen should be palpated for areas of tenderness, especially in the right upper quadrant, hypogastrium and renal angles. A dipstick analysis of the urine for ketones, blood or protein should be performed.

常规检查应包括全血计数、电解质、肝功和甲状腺功能检查。血细胞比容升高、电解质水平改变及酮尿症与脱水有关。因进行尿培养以排除感染，并安排超声波检查以检测多胎妊娠或 GTD。

Routine investigations should include full blood count, electrolytes and liver and thyroid function tests. Elevated haematocrit, alterations in electrolyte levels and ketonuria are associated with dehydration. Urine should be sent for culture to exclude infection and an ultrasound arranged to look for multiple pregnancy or GTD.

（三）治疗（Management）

如果呕吐是轻度到中度的，并且没有引起脱水的征象，通常需要的只是安慰和建议。

简单的措施如下。

- 少吃糖类食物，避免吃高脂肪食物。
- 姜根粉和吡哆醇（维生素 B_6）。
- 避免饮用大量的饮料，尤其是牛奶和碳酸饮料。
- 如果食管反流有问题，就抬高床头。

有持续严重呕吐史并有脱水迹象的患者需要入院进行症状评估和处理。

低血容量和电解质失衡应通过静脉补液纠正，应补充电解质平衡溶液或生理盐水。

If the vomiting is mild to moderate and not causing signs of dehydration, usually reassurance and advice will be all that is necessary.

Simple measures include:

- Taking small carbohydrate meals and avoiding fatty foods
- Powdered ginger root or pyridoxine (vitamin B_6)
- Avoiding large-volume drinks, especially milk and carbonated drinks
- Raising the head of the bed if reflux is a problem

A history of persistent, severe vomiting with evidence of dehydration requires admission to hospital for assessment and management of symptoms.

Hypovolaemia and electrolyte imbalance should be corrected by intravenous fluids. These should be balanced electrolyte solutions or normal saline.

> **！注意**
> 用 5% 葡萄糖快速补液可导致水中毒或脑桥中央髓鞘溶解。
> Overly rapid rehydration with 5% dextrose can result in water intoxication or central pontine myelinolysis.

应考虑使用加压袜和低分子肝素预防血栓形成。在这些支持措施下大多数女性会在 24～48h 安定下来。一旦呕吐停止，可摄入少量液体，最终重新摄入食物。

Thromboprophylaxis with compression stockings and low-molecular-weight heparin should be considered. Most women will settle in 24–48 hours with these supportive measures. Once the vomiting has ceased, small amounts of fluid, and eventually food, can be reintroduced.

镇吐疗法是保留给那些经支持措施后仍未稳定或持续复发的女性。当人们发现沙利度胺与因剧吐而服用该药的母亲所生孩子的严重畸形有关时，孕期抗呕吐药的使用得到了广泛的注意。目前抗组胺药如环己嗪是治疗恶心和呕吐的首选药物，而没有止呕药获准用于治疗。多巴胺拮抗药（甲氧氯普胺）和吩噻嗪类药物（丙氯拉嗪）在人身上尚未显示出致畸作用（尽管甲氧氯普胺在动物身上有致畸作用）。虽然患者的安全数据有限，选择性 5- 羟色胺拮抗药（如昂丹司琼）已被应用，因为它可以作为薄片给药，为不能耐受其他口服治疗的患者提供一种替代静脉注射的方法。

Anti-emetic therapy is reserved for those women who do not settle on supportive measures or who persistently relapse. The use of anti-emetics in pregnancy received widespread publicity when links were found between thalidomide and severe malformations of children born to mothers who had taken the drug for morning sickness. Currently antihistamines such as cyclizine are the recommended pharmacological first-line treatment for nausea and vomiting, with no anti-emetic being approved for treatment. Dopamine antagonists (metoclopramide) and phenothiazines (prochlorperazine) have not been shown to be teratogenic in man (though metoclopramide is in animals). 5HT-selective serotonin antagonists, such as ondansetron, have been used, although patient safety data are limited, because it can be given as a wafer and provides an alternative to parenteral administration in patients unable to tolerate other oral therapy.

尤其对于呕吐时间长的患者，应给予维生素补充剂，包括维生素 B_1。如果呕吐持续并且病史提示有严重食管反流或溃疡病，内窥镜检查是非常有价值的。这项技术在孕期是安全的。如果证实有严重的食道炎，可以给予适当的海藻酸钠和甲氧氯普胺治疗。溃疡病需应用 H_2 受体拮抗药治疗（雷尼替丁），如果病情非常严重需用奥美拉唑，尽管孕期治疗该病的经验有限。

Vitamin supplements, including thiamine, should be

given, particularly where hyperemesis has been prolonged. If vomiting continues and the history is suggestive of severe reflux or ulcer disease, endoscopy can be very valuable. It is a safe technique in pregnancy. If severe oesophagitis is confirmed, appropriate treatment with alginates and metoclopramide can be given. Ulcer disease will require H2 antagonist treatment (ranitidine) or, if very severe, omeprazole, though there is limited experience of this in pregnancy.

极少数情况下，有些女性经过这些综合措施仍未稳定。虽然药物试验仍在进行中，其中一些女性可能会通过类固醇治疗改善症状。这对于有肝功能异常的女性尤其受益。H₂ 受体拮抗药必须与类固醇治疗结合使用。对于严重蛋白质热量不足营养不良患者肠外营养很必要。特定的营养元素在这方面很有帮助。

Very occasionally, women do not settle with a combination of these measures. Some of these women may improve with steroid therapy, though trials are still ongoing. Women in whom there is liver function derangement may benefit particularly. H2 antagonists must be given in conjunction with the steroid treatment. Parenteral nutrition is necessary for some who develop severe protein-calorie malnutrition. Specialized nutrition units can be very helpful in this setting.

如果剧吐得不到治疗，母体的病情就会恶化。Wernicke 脑病是一种与缺乏维生素 B₁（硫胺素）相关的并发症。由于肝脏和肾脏受累，有昏迷和死亡的报道。终止妊娠可扭转这种情况，并在预防孕产妇死亡方面发挥作用。持续到晚期妊娠的呕吐需进一步检查，因为它可能是妊娠期急性脂肪肝等严重疾病的症状。

If hyperemesis is left untreated, the mother's condition worsens. Wernicke's encephalopathy is a complication associated with a lack of vitamin B_1 (thiamine). Coma and death have been reported because of hepatic and renal involvement. Termination of pregnancy may reverse the condition and has a place in preventing maternal mortality. Hyperemesis persisting into the third trimester should be further investigated, as it may be symptomatic of serious illness such as acute fatty liver of pregnancy.

本章概览 / Essential information

流产
- 孕 24 周前妊娠丢失
- 发生于 10%~20% 妊娠
- 通常与染色体异常相关
- 并不总是需要手术治疗

Miscarriage
- Pregnancy loss before 24 weeks
- Complicates 10–20% of pregnancies
- Commonly associated with chromosome abnormalities
- Does not always require surgical treatment

反复性流产
- 定义为连续 3 次以上流产
- 检查应包括抗磷脂抗体、染色体异常和多囊卵巢综合征的筛查
- 未经任何治疗，下一次成功妊娠的概率超过 60%
- 抗磷脂抗体阳性女性治疗异位妊娠时应给予小剂量阿司匹林和肝素

Recurrent miscarriage
- Defined as three consecutive pregnancy losses
- Investigations should include screening for antiphospholipid antibodies, chromosome abnormalities and PCOS
- Chances of a successful subsequent pregnancy more than 60% without any treatment
- Women with antiphospholipid antibodies should be offered treatment with low-dose aspirin and heparin

异位妊娠
- 1% 的妊娠出现异位妊娠
- 早期妊娠女性死亡的最重要原因
- 不典型症状很常见
- 异位妊娠最常见的部位是输卵管壶腹部
- 结合超声和 hCG 测量能精确诊断
- 腹腔镜治疗可降低发病率

Ectopic pregnancy
- 1% of pregnancies are ectopic
- Most important cause of maternal death in early pregnancy
- Atypical presentations are common
- Commonest site for ectopic pregnancy is the ampullary region of the Fallopian tube
- Can be accurately diagnosed by a combination of ultrasound and hCG measurement
- Laparoscopic treatment is associated with lower morbidity

滋养细胞疾病
- 在英国，每 650 例妊娠中就有 1 例患病
- 部分性葡萄胎是三倍体，完全性葡萄胎是二倍体
- 初始治疗是清宫术
- 50% 的绒毛膜癌发病无葡萄胎妊娠史
- 需要连续检测 hCG 进行随访

Trophoblastic disease
- Affects 1 in 650 pregnancies in the UK
- Partial moles are triploid, complete moles diploid
- Treated initially by surgical evacuation of the uterus
- 50% of choriocarcinomas occur without a history of molar pregnancy
- Requires follow-up with serial hCG measurement

（续表）

本章概览	Essential information
妊娠剧吐 • 孕 20 周前开始的持续呕吐伴有体重减轻和酮症相关 • 通常于中期妊娠症状消失 • 可能导致脑病、肾衰竭和肝衰竭 • 如果有脱水或电解质紊乱的症状，则应住院	**Hyperemesis gravidarum** • Persistent vomiting starting before 20 weeks in pregnancy associated with weight loss and ketosis • Usually resolves in second trimester • May lead to encephalopathy, renal and hepatic failure • Hospital admission is indicated where there is evidence of dehydration or electrolyte imbalance

（续表）

第 19 章　性和生殖健康

Sexual and reproductive health

Roger Pepperell　著　　王志坤　阮祥燕　译

学习目标

学习目标

学习本章后，你应当能够：

知识标准

- 描述避孕方法的有效率、收益、风险和不良反应
- 描述终止妊娠的手术和药物选择
- 讨论与节育有关的伦理和法律问题
- 描述常见性传播感染（包括 HIV）的病因、诊断、预防和治疗
- 描述男性和女性性功能障碍常见疾病的病因、检查和治疗

临床能力

- 采集与避孕和性卫生需求相关的病史
- 解释不同避孕方式的益处、风险和不良反应
- 就使用复方口服避孕药为女性提供咨询
- 就永久避孕为女性及其伴侣提供咨询
- 就紧急避孕为女性提供咨询
- 对有生殖道感染的男女进行适当的检查
- 就安全性行为为患者提供咨询

专业技能及态度

- 思考弱势群体的性卫生需求，如年轻人、性工作者和吸毒者
- 思考性传播感染和非意愿妊娠的心理影响
- 认识到必须尊重文化、宗教信仰和性的多样性

LEARNING OUTCOMES

After studying this chapter you should be able to:

Knowledge criteria

- Describe the methods of contraception in terms of efficiency, benefits, risks and side effects.
- Describe the surgical and medical options for termination of pregnancy.
- Discuss the ethical and legal issues relating to fertility control.
- Describe the aetiology, diagnosis, prevention and management of the common sexually transmitted infections, including HIV.
- Describe the aetiology, investigation and management of the common disorders of male and female sexual dysfunction.

Clinical competencies

- Take a history in relation to contraceptive and sexual health needs.
- Explain the benefits, risks and side effects of different forms of contraception.
- Counsel a woman about using the combined oral contraceptive pill.
- Counsel a woman and her partner about permanent contraception.
- Counsel a woman about emergency contraception.
- Plan appropriate investigation of men and women presenting with genital tract infections.
- Counsel a client about safe sexual behaviour.

Professional skills and attitudes

- Reflect on the sexual health care needs of vulnerable groups, e.g. the young, commercial sex workers and drug abusers.
- Reflect on the psychosocial impact of sexually transmitted infections and unplanned pregnancy.
- Recognize the need to respect cultural and religious beliefs as well as sexual diversity.

一、避孕和终止妊娠（Contraception and termination of pregnancy）

人为控制生育的能力，改变了人类生殖的流行病学和社会方面，家庭规模取决于很多因素，其中包括社会和宗教习俗、经济因素、避孕知识，以及是否有可靠的节育方法。

The ability to control fertility by reliable artificial methods has transformed both social and epidemiological aspects of human reproduction. Family size is determined by a number of factors, including social and religious customs, economic aspirations, knowledge of contraception and the availability of reliable methods to regulate fertility.

人工避孕方法主要通过以下途径起作用。

- 抑制排卵。

- 防止受精卵植入。

- 屏障避孕法，即防止精子进入子宫颈。

Artificial methods of contraception act predominantly by the following pathways:

- inhibition of ovulation
- prevention of implantation of the fertilized ovum
- barrier methods of contraception, whereby the spermatozoa are physically prevented from gaining access to the cervix

避孕方式的有效率，通过 1 年内使用此避孕方法的 100 个有生育能力且规律同房的女性，发生非意愿妊娠的次数来衡量，即 Pearl 指数（表 19-1）。

The effectiveness of any method of contraception is measured by the number of unwanted pregnancies that occur during 100 women-years of exposure, i.e. during 1 year in 100 women who are normally fertile and are having regular coitus. This is known as the *Pearl index* (Table 19.1).

（一）屏障避孕法（Barrier methods of contraception）

这些方法通过物理屏障减少精子到达女性上生殖道的概率。屏障避孕法还可以预防很多性传播感染（sexually transmitted infection，STI），使用这些避孕方法的女性，STI 相关盆腔炎性疾病（pelvic inflammatory disease，PID）的风险是 0.6。通常建议使用其他避孕方法的女性，同时使用避孕套，以降低原本可能增加的 STI 风险。

These techniques involve a physical barrier that reduces the likelihood of spermatozoa reaching the female upper genital tract. Barrier methods also offer protection against sexually transmitted infections (STIs). The relative risk of an STIinduced pelvic inflammatory disease (PID) is 0.6 for women using these methods. Women who use another method of contraception to prevent pregnancy are often advised to use a condom as well to reduce an otherwise-increased risk of STI.

1. 男用避孕套（Male condoms）

避孕套由一层可拉伸的薄乳胶套组成，它被模制成护套，润滑后包装在铝箔纸中。避孕套末端有一个储精囊用来收集精液。避孕套的缺点是必须在性交之前使用，以及会降低男性伴侣的快感。它的优点是易得、对女性没有不良反应，以及能防止性传播感染。尽管失败率有时高达"每年 100 名女性发生 15 次非意愿妊娠"，但是只要正确使用，避孕成功率高达 97%～98%。常见的失败原因有拔出阴茎时精液泄漏、生殖器接触后才戴上避孕套、使用润滑剂导致乳胶破裂和机械性破损。避孕套应该在生殖器接触之前完全展开套在阴茎上，当阴茎抽出时握住避孕套以避免精液泄漏。阴茎必须在疲软之前从阴道抽出，否则精液就会泄漏。

The basic condom consists of a thin, stretchable latex film, which is moulded into a sheath, lubricated and packed in a foil wrapper. The sheath has a teat end to collect the ejaculate. The disadvantages of sheaths are that they need to be applied before intercourse and they reduce the level of sensation for the male partner. The advantages are that they are readily available, are without side effects for the female partner and provide a degree of protection against infection. They have an efficiency of 97–98% with careful use, although typical failure rates can be as high as 15 pregnancies per 100 women-years. Common reasons for failure are leakage of sperm when the penis is withdrawn, putting the condom on after genital contact, use of lubricants that cause the latex to break and mechanical damage. Condoms should be unrolled completely on to the penis before genital contact occurs and held when the penis is withdrawn to avoid leakage. The penis needs to be withdrawn from the vagina before the erection is lost, or sperm will inevitably be lost from it.

2. 女用避孕套（Female condoms）

女用避孕套的使用不如男性避孕套广泛，但两者失败率和防止性传播感染的作用相似。它们都由聚氨酯制成，都是一次性的。

Female condoms are less widely used than the male equivalent but have a similar failure rate and give similar protection against infection. They are made of polyurethane and, like the male condom, are suitable for a single episode of intercourse only.

表 19-1　不同避孕方法的失败率（每百名女性）

Table 19.1　Failure rates per 100 women for different methods of contraception

	世卫组织使用的美国数据：使用后第一年内意外怀孕的女性百分比 a U.S. DATA USED BY WHO: % OF WOMEN HAVING AN UNINTENDED PREGNANCY WITHIN THE FIRST YEAR OF USE a		牛津/FPA 研究（所有已婚和 25 岁以上的女性）b OXFORD/FPA STUDY (ALL WOMEN MARRIED AND AGED ABOVE 25) b		
	一般使用 * Typical use *	正确使用 † Perfect use †	总体（任何使用时长） Overall (any duration)	25—34 岁（使用时长不超过 2 年） Age 25–34 (≤2 years use)	35 岁以上（使用时长不超过 2 年） Age 35+ (≤2 years use)
绝育（Sterilization）					
男性（无精后）[Male (after azoospermia)]	0.15	0.1	0.02	0.08	0.08
女性（Filshie 夹）[Female (Filshie clip)]	0.5	0.5	0.13	0.45	0.08
皮下植入（Subcutaneous implant Nexplanon）	0.05	0.05	–	–	–
注射（DMPA）[Injectable (DMPA)]	3	0.3	–	–	–
复方避孕药（Combined pills）					
50μg 雌激素（50μg oestrogen）	8	0.3	0.16	0.25	0.17
<50μg 雌激素（<50μg oestrogen）	8	0.3	0.27	0.38	0.23
避孕帖（Evra patch）	8	0.3	–	–	–
阴道环（NuvaRing）	8	0.3	–	–	–
Cerazette 单孕激素避孕药 Cerazette progestogen-only pill（POP）		0.17‡	–	–	–
旧款 POP（Old-type POP）	8	0.3	1.2	2.5	0.5
IUD[Intrauterine device (IUD)]					
左炔诺孕酮释放子宫内系统（LNG-IUS） Levonorgestrel-releasing intrauterine system (LNG-IUS)	0.2	0.2	–	–	–

（续表）

| | 世卫组织使用的美国数据：使用后第一年内意外怀孕的女性百分比 [a] U.S. DATA USED BY WHO: % OF WOMEN HAVING AN UNINTENDED PREGNANCY WITHIN THE FIRST YEAR OF USE [a] | | 牛津 /FPA 研究（所有已婚和 25 岁以上的女性）[b] OXFORD/FPA STUDY (ALL WOMEN MARRIED AND AGED ABOVE 25) [b] | | |
	一般使用 [*] Typical use [*]	正确使用 [†] Perfect use [†]	总体（任何使用时长） Overall (any duration)	25~34 岁（使用时长不超过 2 年） Age 25-34 (≤2 years use)	35 岁以上（使用时长不超过 2 年） Age 35+ (≤2 years use)
铜 T 形 380 IUD（T-Safe Cu 380 A）	0.8	0.6	—	—	—
其他 >300mm 铜线 Other >300 mm copper-wire IUDs（Nova-T 380, Multiload 375, Flexi-T 300）	≈1‡	≈1‡	—	—	—
男用避孕套（Male condom）	15	2	3.6	6.0	2.9
女用避孕套（Female condom）	21	5	—	—	—
阴道隔膜 [Diaphragm (all caps believed similar, not all tested)]	16	6	1.9	5.5	2.8
体外避孕法（Withdrawal）	27	4	6.7	—	—
仅用杀精剂（Spermicides alone）	29	18	11.9	—	—
节律法（Fertility awareness）	25	5	15.5	—	—
标准日法（Standard days method）	—	3~4	—	—	—
宫颈黏液观察法 [Ovulation (mucus) method]	—		—	—	—
Persona（排卵期检测）（Persona）	6‡		—	—	—
不避孕的年轻女性（No method, young women）	80~90		—	—	—
不避孕的 40 岁女性（No method at age 40）	40~50		—	—	—
不避孕的 45 岁女性（No method at age 45）	10~20		—	—	—
不避孕未绝经的 50 岁女性 [No method at age 50 (if still having menses)]	0~5		—	—	—

a. 引自 Trussell J (2007) Contraceptive efficacy. In: Hatcher RA, Trussell J, Nelson AL, et al. (eds). Contraceptive Technology: nineteenth revised edition. Ardent Media, New York.

其他注释 ① 年龄的影响：第五栏的概率均低于第四栏，而且预计 45 岁以上的概率更低。② 在其他相对不孕的状态下，如哺乳期，也可以获得更好的结果。③ Oxford/FPA 的样本在入组时已是确定的使用者，大大改善了屏障法的结果（Qs 1.19, 4.9）。④ Nexplanon、Ceracete 和 Persona 的结果来自制造商的售前研究，其给出 Pearl 指数的估计

b. 引自 Vessey M, Lawless M, Yeates D (1982) Efficacy of different contraceptive methods. Lancet 1(8276):841-842.

*. 一般使用：在刚开始使用这种避孕方法（不一定是第一次）的夫妇中，如果他们没有因为任何其他原因停止使用该方法，在第一年内非意愿妊娠的百分比

†. 正确使用：开始使用该避孕方法（不一定是第一次），然后能够正确使用该方法（始终如一且正确）的典型夫妇中，如果他们没有因任何其他原因停止使用该方法，则在第一年内意外妊娠的百分比

‡. Trussell 未提供数据，因此给出了最佳替代数据，例如来自制造商研究的数据

[此表引自 Guillebaud J, MacGregor A (2013) Contraception, 6th edn. ©Elsevier. 引自 Trussell J, Wyn LL (2008) Reducing unintended pregnancy in the United States. Contraception 77(1): 1-5.]

From ªTrussell J (2007) Contraceptive efficacy. In: Hatcher RA, Trussell J, Nelson AL, et al. (eds). Contraceptive Technology: nineteenth revised edition. Ardent Media, New York.

Other Notes (1) Note influence of age: all the rates in the fifth column being lower than those in the fourth column. Lower rates still may be expected above age 45. (2) Much better results also obtainable in other states of relative infertility, such as lactation. (3) Oxford/FPA users were established users at recruitment - greatly improving results for barrier methods (*Qs 1.19, 4.9*). (4) The Nexplanon, Cerazette and Persona results come from pre–marketing studies by the manufacturer, giving an estimate of the Pearl 'method–failure' rate.

b. Vessey M, Lawless M, Yeates D (1982) Efficacy of different contraceptive methods. Lancet 1(8276):841-842.

*. Typical use: Among typical couples who initiate use of the method (not necessarily for the first time), the percentage who experience an accidental pregnancy during the first year if they do not stop use for any other reason.

†. Perfect use: Among typical couples who initiate use of the method (not necessarily for the first time) and who then use it *perfectly* (both consistently and correctly), the percentage who experience an accidental pregnancy during the first year if they do not stop use for any other reason.

‡. Data not available from Trussell, so best alternative data given, e.g. from manufacturer's studies.

(This table was published in Guillebaud J, MacGregor A (2013) Contraception, 6th edn. ©Elsevier. Reproduced from Trussell J, Wyn LL (2008) Reducing unintended pregnancy in the United States. Contraception 77(1): 1-5, with permission.)

3. 阴道隔膜和宫颈帽（Diaphragms and cervical caps）

现代的阴道隔膜由一个乳胶薄膜和边缘的金属弹簧圈组成。这些隔膜的直径为 45～100mm，需要进行妇科检查来确定所需隔膜的大小。通过阴道检查确定子宫的大小和位置，并记录阴道后穹隆到耻骨联合的距离。置入适当的测量环，通常在 70～80mm。当置于正确的位置时，环或隔膜的前缘应位于耻骨联合后面，下后缘应位于后穹隆（图 19-1）。

The modern vaginal diaphragm consists of a thin latex rubber dome attached to a circular metal spring. These diaphragms vary in size from 45 to 100 mm in diameter. The size of the diaphragm required is ascertained by examination of the woman. The size and position of the uterus are determined by vaginal examination, and the distance from the posterior vaginal fornix to the pubic symphysis is noted. The appropriate measuring ring, usually between 70 mm and 80 mm, is inserted. When in the correct position, the anterior edge of the ring or diaphragm should lie behind the pubic symphysis and the lower posterior edge should lie comfortably in the posterior fornix (Fig. 19.1).

女性应采用仰卧位或跪撑位（kneeling position），向前弯曲时将阴道隔膜放入。只需从下方用示指钩住帽的边缘并将其拉出，即可将阴道隔膜取出。阴道隔膜两侧应涂上避孕药剂，通常建议圆顶朝下放入阴道隔膜。然而有些女性更喜欢圆顶朝上。

The woman should be advised to insert the diaphragm either in the dorsal position or in the kneeling position while bending forwards. The diaphragm can be removed by simply hooking an index finger under the rim from below and pulling it out. The diaphragm should be smeared on both sides with a contraceptive cream, and it is usually advised that it be inserted dome down. However, some women prefer to insert the diaphragm with the dome upwards.

阴道隔膜必须在性交之前置入，并且至少要等到 6h 后才能取下。这种方法的主要优点是除了偶尔对避孕乳膏产生反应外，它对女性没有不良反应。主要缺点是必须在性交前放入隔膜，失败率一般是"每年 100 名女性发生 6～16 次非意愿妊娠"。避孕失败的主要原因是隔膜尺寸太小、女性性高潮时阴道尺寸明显变化导致隔膜大小不再合适。

The diaphragm must be inserted prior to intercourse and should not be removed until at least 6 hours later. The main advantage of this technique is that it is free of side effects to the woman, apart from an occasional reaction to the contraceptive cream. The main disadvantages are that the diaphragm must be inserted before intercourse and typical failure rates are between 6 and 16 pregnancies per 100 women-years. The main reason for failure is probably that the diaphragm size chosen is actually too small and when orgasm occurs in the woman,

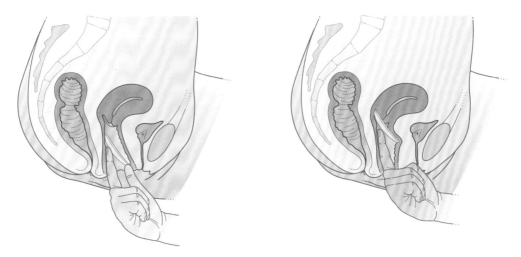

▲ 图 19-1　置入阴道横膈膜，覆盖宫颈和阴道前壁

Fig. 19.1　Insertion of a vaginal diaphragm to cover the cervix and anterior vaginal wall.

when the vaginal size can increase dramatically, the diaphragm no longer fits adequately.

有各种各样的宫颈帽，它们的直径比阴道隔膜小得多。适合宫颈较长或有一定程度脱垂的女性，但在其他方面比起阴道隔膜没有特别的优势。

There are a variety of vault and cervical caps, which are of much smaller diameter than the diaphragm. These are suitable for women with a long cervix or with some degree of prolapse but otherwise have no particular advantage over the diaphragm.

4. 杀精剂和避孕海绵（Spermicides and sponges）

一般来说，杀精剂通常只有与屏障避孕法结合使用时才有效。含有杀精剂的栓子或栓剂是水溶性或蜡基的。它们必须在性交前大约 15min 置入。常见的杀精剂是壬苯醇醚 –9 和苯扎氯铵。药剂中有乳化脂肪基，不易扩散，置入时必须小心地使杀精剂覆盖宫颈。

Spermicides are only effective, in general, if used in conjunction with a mechanical barrier. Pessaries or suppositories have a water-soluble or wax base and contain a spermicide. They must be inserted approximately 15 minutes befor intercourse. Common spermicides are nonoxynol-9 and benzalkonium. Creams consist of an emulsified fat base and tend not to spread. Care in insertion is essential so that the spermicide covers the cervix.

凝胶或糊状物具有水溶性，在体温下迅速扩散。因此，它们比乳霜更具优势，因为它们能布满阴道。

Jellies or pastes have a water-soluble base that spreads rapidly at body temperature. They therefore have an advantage over creams, as they spread throughout the vagina.

泡沫片和泡沫气溶胶含有碳酸氢钠，因此与水接触时会释放二氧化碳，泡沫将杀精剂扩散到整个阴道。妊娠率因药物不同而不同，但平均"每年 100 名女性中有 9～10 次非意愿妊娠"。

Foam tablets and foam aerosols contain bicarbonate of soda so that carbon dioxide is released on contact with water. The foam spreads the spermicide throughout the vagina. Pregnancy rates vary with different agents but average around 9–10 per 100 women-years.

避孕海绵由浸渍有壬苯醇醚 –9 的聚氨酯泡沫组成。避孕失败率为 9%～32%，因此不建议单独使用它们。在性交前至少 15min 置入，最多可以放置 12h。

Sponges consist of polyurethane foam impregnated with nonoxynol-9. The failure rate is between 9% and 32%, and their use in isolation is therefore not recommended. They are inserted at least 15 minutes before intercourse and can be left in for a maximum of 12 hours.

（二）宫内节育器（Intrauterine contraceptive devices）

在英国，有 6%～8% 的女性使用 IUD(intrauterine device，IUD)。已设计了各种各样的 IUD（图 19–2）。这些节育器的优点是，一旦置入，便可以保留，而无须采取其他避孕措施。它们似乎主要通过降低卵子活力、减少到达输卵管的精子数量来防止受精，从而起到避孕作用。

Intrauterine contraception is used by 6–8% of women in the UK. A wide variety of intrauterine devices (IUDs) have been designed for insertion into the uterine cavity (Fig. 19.2). These devices have the advantage that, once inserted, they are retained without the need to take alternative contraceptive precautions. It seems likely that they act mainly by preventing

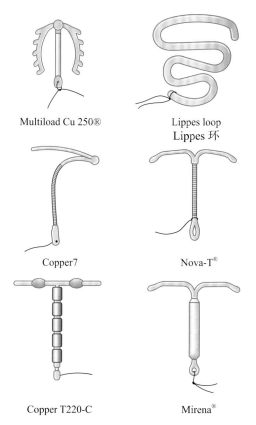

Multiload Cu 250®

Lippes loop
Lippes 环

Copper7

Nova-T®

Copper T220-C

Mirena®

▲ 图 19-2 一些宫内节育器；右列是左炔诺孕酮宫内节育系统

Fig. 19.2　Some intrauterine contraceptive devices; on the right, the levonorgestrel intrauterine system.

fertilization. This is a result of a reduction in the viability of ova and the number of viable sperm reaching the tube.

第一个被广泛使用的装置是 Grafenberg 环，它是由银铜合金制成的。从 20 世纪 30 年代开始使用，使用它时会出现出血、感染、流产和子宫穿孔等相当大的困难。后来，惰性塑料装置（如 Lippes 环）与使用者的月经量显著增加有关。含铜宫内节育器的发展提高了避孕效果，缓解了月经过量。

The first device to be widely used was the Grafenberg ring, which was made of a silver-copper alloy. Introduced in the 1930s, it ran into considerable difficulties with haemorrhage, infection, miscarriages and uterine perforation. Later, inert plastic devices such as the Lippes loop were associated with a significant increase in menstrual blood flow in many users. The development of copper IUDs has been associated with improved contraceptive efficacy and a lessening of excess menstrual blood loss.

1. IUD 的种类（Types of devices）

这些节育器是惰性或药物活性的。

The devices are either inert or pharmacologically active.

(1) 惰性 IUD（Inert devices）：

Lippes 节育环、纤维圈 T 形环和马古利斯螺旋环是塑料或者塑料涂层的器具，它们有一个从宫颈突出的长长的尾丝，用来让女性检查它的位置是否仍正常。惰性节育器往往比较大，它们现在已经不再使用了，但是一些使用过它的女性子宫内可能还有这种装置。

Lippes loops, Saf-T-coils and Margulis spirals are plastic or plastic-coated devices. They have a thread attached that protrudes through the cervix and allows the woman to check that the device is still in place. Inert devices tend to be relatively large. They are not now available but may still be found in situ in some older users.

(2) 药物活性 IUD（Pharmacologically active devices）：

将铜添加到避孕装置中，通过干扰子宫内膜雌激素结合位点和抑制胸腺嘧啶脱氧核苷进入 DNA，对子宫内膜产生直接影响，它还会损害子宫内膜中糖原的储存。比如铜 7 字形 IUD 和铜 T 形 IUD（第一代）、多载铜 250 IUD（第二代）和铜 T 形 380 IUD（第三代）。

The addition of copper to a contraceptive device produces a direct effect on the endometrium by interfering with endometrial oestrogen-binding sites and depressing uptake of thymidine into DNA. It also impairs glycogen storage in the endometrium. Examples of such devices are the Copper-T or Copper-7 (first generation), the Multiload Copper-250 (second generation) and the Copper-T 380 (third generation).

(3) 含孕激素节育器（Devices containing progestogen）：

曼月乐是释放左炔诺孕酮的宫内节育系统，含有 52mg 的左炔诺孕酮（图 19-2），它能抑制子宫内膜的正常增生，因此与大多数宫内节育器不同，它能减少月经出血。然而，在植入曼月乐的前 3 个月内，不规则少量的子宫出血的发生率很高。与之前的含孕激素节育器不同，它不会升高异位妊娠的风险。第三代含铜宫内节育器和左炔诺孕酮释放系统的优越功效，意味着它们现在是首选的节育器。

The levonorgestrel-releasing intrauterine system, or Mirena, contains 52 mg of levonorgestrel (see Fig. 19.2) which suppresses the normal buildup of the endometrium so that, unlike most IUDs, it causes a reduction in menstrual blood loss. However, there is a high incidence of irregular scanty bleeding in the first 3 months after insertion of the device. Unlike previous progestogen-containing devices, it does not appear to be associated with a higher risk of ectopic pregnancy. The superior efficacy of third-generation copper IUDs and the levonorgestrel-releasing system means that these are now considered the devices of choice.

2. 使用年限（Lifespan of devices）

铜 T 形 380 宫内节育器在英国和澳大利亚的有效期为 8 年（美国为 13 年）。其他含铜节育器和曼月乐的有效期为 5 年。然而，40 岁以上的女性不需要更换宫内节育器。50 岁之前绝经的女性，节育器需要保留到绝经后 2 年，50 岁以后绝经的女性，节育器需要保留 1 年。

The Copper-T 380 is licensed for 8 years in the UK and Australia (and 13 in the United States). Other copper devices and the Mirena are licensed for 5 years. However, IUDs do not need to be replaced in women over the age of 40 years. They should be left in place until 2 years after menopause if this occurs under age 50 and for 1 year otherwise.

3. 节育器的置入（Insertion of devices）

置入节育器的最佳时间是在月经周期的前半段，对于产后女性，最佳时间是产后 4～6 周。在治疗性流产时置入宫内节育器是安全的，如果有强烈意愿，可以在此时置入节育器。流产后置入宫内节育器是不明智的，因为有感染的危险。宫内节育器可以在分娩后几天内置入，但排出率很高。

The optimal time for insertion of the device is in the first half of the menstrual cycle. With postpartum women, the optimal time is 4–6 weeks after delivery. Insertion at the time of therapeutic abortion is safe and can be performed when motivation is strong. It is unwise to insert IUDs following a miscarriage because of the risk of infection. Devices may be inserted within a few days of delivery, but there is a high expulsion rate.

理想情况下，女性应处于截石位。如果有任何感染迹象，应进行子宫颈人乳头瘤病毒（human papilloma virus，HPV）检测或宫颈巴氏涂片检查，并取拭子进行培养。双合诊确定子宫大小、形状和位置。用消毒液擦拭子宫颈，双爪钳可以用在宫颈的前唇，尽管这是可能引起不适的非必需操作。

Ideally, the woman should be placed in the lithotomy position. A cervical human papilloma virus (HPV) assessment test or cervical Pap smear should be taken and a swab taken for culture if there is any sign of infection. The uterus is examined bimanually, and its size, shape and position are ascertained. The cervix is swabbed with an antiseptic solution, and a vulsellum can be applied to the anterior lip of the cervix, although this is not essential and may cause discomfort.

宫腔探针将显示子宫腔的深度和方向，宫腔的

尺寸（长度和宽度）可以通过空腔计（cavimeters）来评估。许多宫内节育器有不同的尺寸，空腔计有助于选择合适的宫内节育器。

The passage of a uterine sound will indicate the depth and direction of the uterine cavity, and the dimensions of the cavity may be assessed by devices known as cavimeters, which measure its length and breadth. Many IUDs are available in different sizes, and cavimeters help in choosing the appropriate IUD.

置入的宫内节育器的结构不尽相同，但通常由一个带有塞子的塑料管组成，塑料管中含有一个柱塞，用于挤压装置，可以是线性的，也可以是折叠的。将装置置入子宫腔平面，必须小心以免将其推过子宫底。

Insertion devices vary in construction but generally consist of a stoppered plastic tube containing a plunger to extrude the device, which may be linear or folded. The device is inserted in the plane of the lumen of the uterus, and care must be taken not to push it through the uterine fundus.

试图在宫颈管狭窄的地方置入宫内节育器，可能导致迷走神经性晕厥。置入后的急性疼痛可能表明子宫穿孔。应教导女性定期检查尾丝，如果无法触及尾丝，应立即通知医生。

Attempts at insertion of a device where the cervical canal is tight may result in vagal syncope. Acute pain following insertion may indicate perforation of the uterus. The woman should be instructed to check the loop strings regularly and to notify her doctor immediately if the strings are not palpable.

4. 并发症（Complications）

IUD 的并发症如图 19-3 所示。

The complications of IUDs are summarized in Figure 19.3.

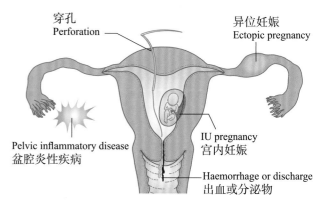

穿孔 Perforation
异位妊娠 Ectopic pregnancy
Pelvic inflammatory disease 盆腔炎性疾病
IU pregnancy 宫内妊娠
Haemorrhage or discharge 出血或分泌物

▲ 图 19-3　宫内节育器并发症
IU. 宫内
Fig. 19.3　Complications of intrauterine devices.
IU, Intrauterine.

(1) 妊娠率（Pregnancy rates）：

妊娠率因使用的 IUD 类型而异，使用非药物 IUD 的妊娠率为"每年 100 名女性 2～6 次非意愿妊娠"，使用早期含铜 IUD 的妊娠率为"每年 100 名女性 0.5～2 次非意愿妊娠"，使用第三代含铜和左炔诺孕酮 IUD 的妊娠率低于"每年 100 名女性 0.3 次非意愿妊娠"。带器妊娠的女性，流产发生率很高，如果尾丝容易触及，则应该将其取出以降低败血症流产的发生率，如果尾丝不易触及，尽管这会增加流产或胎膜早破的风险，还是应该先保留 IUD，在分娩时再将其取出。放置 IUD 后，避孕失败的风险逐年降低。

Pregnancy rates vary according to the type of device used, from 2 to 6/100 women-years for non-medicated IUDs and 0.5 to 2/100 for early-generation copper devices to less than 0.3/100 women-years for third-generation copper and levonorgestrel IUDs. If pregnancy does occur with an IUD in situ and its strings are easily grasped, it is sensible to remove it to reduce the incidence of a septic miscarriage, there being a high incidence of miscarriage in such pregnancies. If the strings are not accessible, the IUD should be left and removed at the time of delivery, although the risk of a miscarriage or premature rupture of the membranes would be increased. The risk of failure of the IUD diminishes with each year after insertion.

(2) 子宫穿孔（Perforation of the uterus）：

IUD 导致子宫穿孔的风险为 0.1%～1%。有时在置入 IUD 时发生部分穿孔，然后它移动导致完全穿孔。如果女性注意到 IUD 的尾丝消失，则可能是下面某种情况。

- IUD 已被排出。

- IUD 已在子宫腔内转动并拉起了尾丝。

- IUD 已穿透子宫，部分或全部位于腹腔内。

About 0.1–1% of devices perforate the uterus. In many cases, partial perforation occurs at the time of insertion and later migration completes the perforation. If the woman notices that the tail of the device is missing, it must be assumed that one of the following has occurred:

- The device has been expelled.
- The device has turned in the uterine cavity and drawn up the strings.
- The device has perforated the uterus and lies either partly or completely in the peritoneal cavity.

如果没有妊娠的证据，应对子宫行超声检查。如果 IUD 位于子宫腔内（图 19-4A），除非尾丝的一

部分可见，一般要在全身或局部麻醉下，扩张宫颈将其取出。如果在子宫内找不到该装置，可行腹部 X 线检查以显示其在腹腔内的位置（图 19-4B）。建议通过腹腔镜或剖腹手术取出宫外 IUD。惰性装置或可留下，但含铜 IUD 强烈刺激腹膜，必须要取出。

If there is no evidence of pregnancy, an ultrasound examination of the uterus should be performed. If the device is located within the uterine cavity (Fig. 19.4A), unless part of the loop or strings is visible, it will generally be necessary to remove the device with formal dilatation of the cervix under general or local anaesthesia. If the device is not found in the uterus, a radiograph of the abdomen will reveal the site in the peritoneal cavity (Fig. 19.4B). It is advisable to remove all extrauterine devices by either laparoscopy or laparotomy. Inert devices can probably be left with impunity, but copper devices promote considerable peritoneal irritation and should certainly be removed.

(3) 盆腔炎性疾病（Pelvic inflammatory disease，PID）：预先存在的 PID 是这种避孕方法的禁忌证。IUD 使用者发生急性 PID 的风险略有增加，但这主要发生在放置 IUD 的 3 周内。如果发现 PID，就开始抗生素治疗，如果治疗效果差，应移除 IUD，如果感染严重，最好在取出 IUD 前进行 24h 的抗生素治疗。无症状的放置 IUD 的女性，定期进行巴氏涂片，有时会发现放线菌，对于阳性，应该怎么处理还没有绝对的共识，有人会取出 IUD，3 个月后复查，如果涂片结果阴性，再置入另一个 IUD，而有些人会保留 IUD，并给予 2 周的青霉素治疗。

Pre-existing PID is a contraindication to this method of contraception. There is a small increase in the risk of acute PID in IUD users, but this is largely confined to the first 3 weeks after insertion. If PID does occur, antibiotic therapy is commenced, and if the response is poor, the device should be removed. If the infection is severe, it is preferable to complete 24 hours of antibiotic therapy before removing the device. It is not uncommon to find evidence of *Actinomyces* organisms in the Pap smear routinely collected in an asymptomatic woman who has an IUD in place. This is generally not due to an actinomycotic pelvic infection, but due to the presence of these organisms on the surface of the IUD. There is no absolute consensus of what should be done if such organisms are found in the Pap smear. Some would remove the IUD, repeat the smear in 3 months and reinsert another IUD if the smear is clear, whereas others would leave the IUD in place but give a 2-week course of penicillin therapy.

(4) 异常子宫出血（Abnormal uterine bleeding）：

很多使用惰性或含铜 IUD 的女性会出现月经过量的情况，但多数人可以耐受。然而，这些女性中，

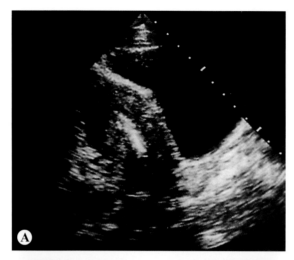

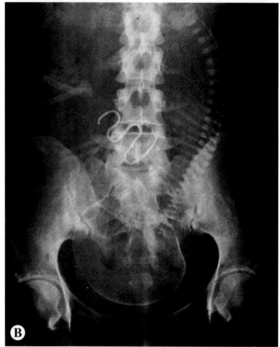

▲ 图 19-4　**A.** 塑料 **IUD** 的宫内超声诊断；**B.** 腹部 **X** 线片显示宫内节育器和足月妊娠

Fig. 19.4　**(A) Ultrasound diagnosis of a plastic intrauterine device (IUD). (B) Radiography of the abdomen showing an IUD and a full-term pregnancy.**

约有 15% 的患者病情严重到需要取出 IUD。可以通过药物如氨甲环酸或甲芬那酸来控制。经间出血也可能发生，但如果出血量少，不用取出 IUD。使用曼月乐的女性，至少有 20% 出现闭经，平均经期出血量减少了 90%。

Increased menstrual loss occurs in most women with an inert or copper IUD, but this can be tolerated by the majority. However, in 15% of such women, it is sufficiently severe to necessitate removal of the device. It can be controlled by drugs such as tranexamic acid or mefenamic acid. Intermenstrual

bleeding may also occur, but if the loss is slight, it does not constitute a reason for IUD removal. Amenorrhoea occurs in at least 20% of women using the Mirena, and average menstrual blood loss is reduced by 90%.

（5）盆腔疼痛（Pelvic pain）：

疼痛有时是慢性轻微疼痛的形式，有时是严重痛经。发病率变化很大，遭受疼痛的女性高达 50%。然而，不严重的疼痛是可以接受的，应该由患者综合考虑便利性和疼痛来决定是否使用此方法。

Pain occurs either in a chronic low-grade form or as severe dysmenorrhoea. The incidence is widely variable, with up to 50% of women suffering some pain. However, the pain may be acceptable if it is not severe, and this is a decision that has to be made by the patient in relation to the convenience of the method.

（6）阴道分泌物（Vaginal discharge）：

阴道分泌物可能是由感染引起的，但大多数使用 IUD 的女性会有轻微的水样或黏液性分泌物。

Vaginal discharge may be due to infection, but most women with an IUD develop a slight watery or mucoid discharge.

（7）异位妊娠（Ectopic pregnancy）：

与无保护性交的女性相比，使用 IUD 的女性的妊娠率较低（每年 100 名女性 1.2 次非意愿妊娠）。然而一旦妊娠，异位妊娠的风险更高（10%）。因此，使用 IUD 的女性，如果有腹痛和阴道不规则出血，必须考虑异位妊娠可能。

Compared with women having unprotected intercourse, the incidence of pregnancy is lower in women with an IUD in situ (1.2/100 women years). However, should pregnancy occur, there is a higher risk (10%) of the pregnancy being extrauterine. It is therefore essential to think of this diagnosis in any woman presenting with abdominal pain and irregular vaginal bleeding who has an IUD in situ.

> **！**
> **注意**
>
> 任何 IUD 在原位的妊娠女性都应该排除异位妊娠。
>
> Ectopic pregnancy should be excluded in any woman who conceives with an IUD in situ.

（三）激素避孕（Hormonal contraception）

口服避孕药（oral contraception pill，OCP）是雌激素和孕激素联合的，或者单孕激素的。

Oral contraception is given as a combined oestrogen and progestogen pill (OCP) or as progestogen only.

1. 复方避孕药（Combined pill）

目前大多数复方避孕药含有 20～30μg 的炔雌醇和 150～4000μg 的孕激素。使用的孕激素来自 17-羟孕酮或 19- 去甲睾酮（框 19–1）。

Most of the current combined pills contain 20–30 μg of ethinyl oestradiol and 150–4000 μg of progestogen. The progestogens used are derived from 17-hydroxyprogesterone or 19-norsteroids (Box 19.1).

框 19–1　避孕药的成分	Box 19.1　Progestogen content of contraceptive pills
复方避孕药 • 炔诺酮 • 炔诺孕酮 • 左炔诺孕酮 • 去氧孕烯 • 孕二烯酮 • 醋酸环丙孕酮 • 屈螺酮 • 地诺孕素	**Combined** • Norethisterone • Norgestrel • Levonorgestrel • Desogestrel • Gestodene • Cyproterone • Drospirenone • Dienogest
单孕激素避孕药 • 炔诺酮 • 左炔诺孕酮	**Progestogen only** • Norethisterone • Levonorgestrel

这种药片通常服用 21 天，然后是 7 天的无药片间隔期，在此期间出现撤药性出血，可用 7 片安慰剂片代替停服药片 1 周。激素的浓度在 21 天内可能相同（单相片），或者在整个周期内变化（双相片和三相片），以减少突破性出血。

The pill is usually taken for 21 days, followed by a 7-day pill-free interval during which there is a withdrawal bleed. Everyday (ED) preparations include seven placebo pills that are taken instead of a pill-free week. The concentration of the hormones may be the same throughout the 21 days (monophasic preparations) or vary across the cycle (biphasic and triphasic preparations) in order to reduce breakthrough bleeding.

如果女性希望完全避免经期，可以建议她每天服用复方避孕药，而不是每个月有 7 天服用没有激素的空白片，这意味着她可以连续 6 个月每天服用激素片。这经常会导致闭经，尽管有些不规则出血的女性通常只进行 3～4 个月的持续治疗。

If the woman concerned is keen to avoid having periods altogether, she could be advised to take the combined hormone preparation every day, rather than having 7 hormone-free days each month, meaning that she will take the hormone tablets every day for up to 6 continuous months. This will often result in amenorrhoea during that time, although some women do have irregular bleeding and are then usually advised to have

only 3–4 months of continuous therapy thereafter.

2. 单孕激素避孕药（Progestogen-only pill）

只含孕激素的药片含有炔诺酮或左炔诺孕酮，每天 1 片，连续服用。由于剂量较低，因此应每天同一时刻服用。

Progestogen-only pills contain either norethisterone or levonorgestrel and are taken continuously on the basis of one tablet daily. Because of the low dose, they should be taken at the same time every day.

3. 避孕药的作用方式（Mode of action of the contraceptive pills）

复方三相片通过抑制促性腺激素释放激素（gonadotrophin-releasing hormone, GnRH）和促性腺激素分泌，特别是抑制黄体生成激素峰值，从而抑制排卵。子宫内膜也变得不适合着床，宫颈黏液变得不利于精子通过。尽管单孕激素避孕药也会改变子宫内膜的成熟度，但是它们的主要作用是减少宫颈黏液的量和改变宫颈黏液的性质。只有 40% 的女性会被完全抑制排卵。

Combined and triphasic pills act by suppressing gonadotrophin-releasing hormone (GnRH) and gonadotrophin secretion and, in particular, suppressing the luteinizing hormone peak, thus inhibiting ovulation. The endometrium also becomes less suitable for nidation, and the cervical mucus becomes hostile. Progesterone-only pills act predominantly to reduce the amount and character of the cervical mucus, although they do alter the endometrial maturation as well. Ovulation is completely suppressed in only 40% of women.

4. 禁忌证（Contraindications）

避孕药有各种各样的禁忌证，有些是绝对禁忌证。

There are various contraindications to the pill, with some being more absolute than others.

绝对禁忌证包括妊娠、既往肺栓塞或深静脉血栓形成、镰状红细胞病、卟啉症、既往活动性肝病或既往胆汁淤积症（尤其是与既往妊娠有关的疾病）、先兆偏头痛或乳腺癌。有必要高度警惕静脉曲张、糖尿病、高血压、肾病和慢性心力衰竭的女性，但这些情况都不构成绝对禁忌证，在某些情况下，妊娠的不良影响可能大大超过避孕药的危害。吸烟和 35 岁以上的女性患冠状动脉和血栓栓塞疾病的风险显著增加。

The absolute contraindications include pregnancy, previous pulmonary embolism or deep vein thrombosis, sickle cell disease, porphyria, current active liver disease or previous cholestasis (particularly where it is associated with a previous pregnancy), migraine associated with an aura or carcinoma of the breast. It is necessary to maintain a high level of vigilance in women with varicose veins, diabetes, hypertension, renal disease and chronic heart failure, but none of these conditions constitute an absolute contraindication, and in some cases, the adverse effects of a pregnancy may substantially outweigh any hazard from the pill. Women who smoke and are also over the age of 35 years have a significantly increased risk of coronary artery and thromboembolic disease.

首次出现偏头痛、严重头痛、视觉障碍或短暂的神经系统改变是立即停药的指征。一些轻微的不良反应有时可以被利用，或者通过使用不同甾体激素复方药来抵消（表 19-2）。

The occurrence of migraine for the first time, severe headaches or visual disturbances or transient neurological changes are indications for immediate cessation of the pill. A series of minor side effects may sometimes be used to advantage or may be offset by using a pill with a different combination of steroids (Table 19.2).

5. 复方口服避孕药的其他治疗用途（Other therapeutic uses of the combined oral contraceptive pill）

避孕以外的治疗用途包括治疗月经过多、经前期综合征、子宫内膜异位症和痛经。

Therapeutic uses other than contraception include the treatment of menorrhagia, premenstrual syndrome, endometriosis and dysmenorrhoea.

6. 主要不良反应（Major side effects）

静脉血栓形成的风险从每年 5/10 万增加到每年 15/10 万，对于吸烟和既往静脉血栓形成的女性，此风险进一步增加。妊娠和产褥期女性静脉血栓形成的风险是 60/10 万。有几项研究提示尽管在这些研究中静脉血栓形成的风险比既往报道的要低，但是与含有其他孕激素的避孕药相比，含有去氧孕烯、孕二烯或屈螺内酯的所谓第三代和第四代复方避孕药，导致静脉血栓形成的风险要高出 2 倍。

The risk of venous thrombosis is increased from 5/100,000 to 15/100,000 women per year and is further increased in smokers and women with a previous history of venous thrombosis. This compares to a risk of venous thrombosis in pregnancy and the puerperium of 60/100,000 women. Several studies have suggested that so-called *third- and fourth-generation* combined pills containing desogestrel, gestodene or drospirenone are associated with a twofold greater risk of venous thrombosis than those containing other progestogens, although the risk of venous thrombosis was lower in these studies than had previously been reported.

动脉疾病风险增加，脑卒中增加 1.6～5.4 倍，心肌梗死增加 3～5 倍（尽管 25 岁以下女性或不吸烟者没有明显增加）。然而，这两种情况在 35 岁以下的女性中都很少见，因此总体风险仍然很低，服用复方避孕药导致的静脉血栓死亡不超过每年 1～2/100 万。

There is an increase in arterial disease, with a 1.6- to 5.4-fold increase in stroke and 3- to 5-fold increase in myocardial infarction (although there is no significant increase in women

表 19-2 复方口服避孕药的轻微不良反应

Table 19.2 Minor side effects of combined oral contraception

雌激素效应 Oestrogenic effects	孕激素效应 Progestogenic effects
液体潴留和水肿（Fluid retention and oedema）	经前期抑郁（Premenstrual depression）
经前紧张和易怒（Premenstrual tension and irritability）	阴道干燥（Dry vagina）
体重增加（Increase in weight）	粉刺，油发（Acne, greasy hair）
恶心呕吐（Nausea and vomiting）	食欲增加，体重增加（Increased appetite with weight gain）
头痛（Headache）	乳房不适（Breast discomfort）
黏液外流、宫颈柱状上皮外移（Mucorrhoea, cervical erosion）	腿和腹部抽筋（Cramps of the legs and abdomen）
月经过多（Menorrhagia）	性欲下降（Decreased libido）
过度疲劳（Excessive tiredness）	
静脉疾病（Vein complaints）	
突破性出血（Breakthrough bleeding）	

under 25 or in non-smokers). However, both these conditions are rare in women under the age of 35 years so the overall risk remains low, with deaths from venous thrombosis attributable to the combined pill of no more than 1–2/million women-years.

尽管一些报告表明，服用避孕药的人患乳腺癌（相对风险 1.24）和宫颈癌（相对风险 1.5～2）的相对风险略有增加，尤其是在首次妊娠前开始服用避孕药的人，但乳腺癌风险增加尚未得到明确证实，宫颈癌的发病率可能与 HPV 感染有关，而与口服避孕药无关。

Although some reports have suggested there is a small increase in the relative risk of breast cancer (relative risk 1.24) and cervical cancer (relative risk 1.5–2) in pill users, especially if it is commenced before a first pregnancy, the increased risk breast cancer is not definitely proven, and the cervical cancer risk is probably due to the incidence of HPV infection and not the taking of the OCP.

胆石形成和胆囊炎风险增加，糖耐量损害风险增加。

There is an increase in gallstone formation and cholecystitis and an increase in glucose intolerance.

服用单孕激素避孕药的失败率较高，而且可能导致不规则出血。如果避孕失败，异位妊娠风险更高。

The progestogen-only pill has a higher failure rate and is more likely to be associated with irregular bleeding. If it fails, there is also a higher risk of ectopic pregnancy.

7. 益处（Beneficial effects）

除了预防非意愿妊娠外，使用复方避孕药还可以减少 30% 的月经量、降低异位妊娠的发生率（0.4/1000）、对 PID 和良性卵巢囊肿有一定的保护

要求使用复方 OCP 的患者的临床实践
Practical care of a patient requesting to use the combined OCP

知识链接 ABC

重要的是，在开处方之前，要获得完整病史和检查，并每年体检，进行宫颈细胞学或 HPV 评估。一些药物在市场上可以买到，虽然是由不同的公司销售，但是成分相似。必须排除前面详述的禁忌证，检查应包括乳房检查、血压评估，除从未有过性行为的女性外，还应包括窥阴器检查、巴氏涂片或 HPV 检测和 PV 评估。应为特定患者选择合适的药物，然后按照以下思路进行咨询。

It is important to obtain a complete general history and examination before prescribing the pill and to perform annual check-ups and cervical cytology or HPV assessment. A large number of compounds are commercially available, and some pills are marketed by different companies but contain the same compounds at the same concentrations. The history taken must exclude the contraindications detailed earlier. Examination should include breast examination, blood pressure assessment and, except in women who have never been sexually active, speculum examination, Pap smear or HPV testing and PV assessment. An appropriate pill for that particular patient should then be chosen, and counselling then given along the following lines.

选择哪种药物？

Which pill should you choose?

一般来说，由于有效性和低成本，含 30μg 炔雌醇的避孕药通常是首选。含 20μg 的制剂价格更高，但许多女性更喜欢，而且不良反应较少，只是在治疗的前几个月更容易出现突破性出血。如果女性有雄激素过量、多毛症或临床多囊卵巢综合征（PCOS）的证据，应给予 OCP 达英 35，因为它的孕激素是酮醋环丙孕酮，能够拮抗雄激素。如果女性有液体潴留，建议选择包含屈螺酮的 OCP。

In general a 30-μg ethinyl oestradiol-containing pill is usually chosen first because of its effectiveness and low cost. The 20-μg-containing preparations are much more expensive but preferred by many women, and the side effects are usually less, except that breakthrough bleeding during the first few months of treatment is more common. If the woman had evidence of androgen excess, hirsutism or clinical polycystic ovarian syndrome (PCOS), the OCP Diane 35 should be given because its progestogen is cyproterone acetate, an anti-androgen. If the woman has fluid retention problems, an OCP containing drospirenone is usually advisable.

如果女性既往服用过 OCP 并且有突破性出血、在正确服用避孕药时妊娠，或者正在接受抗癫痫药物治疗，服用含有 50μg 炔雌醇的 OCP 更安全。

If the woman has used the OCP previously and had major problems with breakthrough bleeding, has conceived when taking the pill correctly or is on treatment with an anti-epileptic medication, it is safer to advise them to take an OCP containing50 μg of ethinyl oestradiol.

应该什么时候开始服药？

When should it be commenced?

最好在下一个月经周期的第 2～3 天开始，但可以随时开始。许多复方避孕药包括 7 天的安慰剂（"糖片"），以便用户每天服药，从而降低在 7 天不服药后忘记何时重新开始服药的风险（有时标记为 "ED" 或日常准备）。每个药片，包括安慰剂，都被标记上日历中的某周某天，安慰剂的颜色不同（图 19-5）。使用这些药片，女性应该在下一个月经周期的第一天开始服药，从对应当天的安慰剂药片开始。当从较高剂量的药片制备改为较低剂量的药片时，应建议女性在完成之前药片的最后一片后，立即开始服用新药丸的活性片，省略正常的 7 天间隙。

（续框）

It is best commenced on day 2–3 of the next period but can be commenced at any time. Many combined pills include 7 days of placebo ('sugar') tablets so that the user takes a pill every day of the month and so reduces the risk of forgetting when to restart the pill after the normal 7 'pill-free' days each cycle (sometimes labelled 'ED' or everyday preparations). Each tablet, including the placebos, is labelled with a day of the week in these calendar packs, with the placebos being a different colour (Fig. 19.5). With these pills a woman should start taking the pill on the first day of her next period starting with the inactive tablet corresponding to the current day of the week. When changing from a higher- to a lower-dose pill preparation women should be advised to start taking the active tablets of the new pill immediately on completing the last tablet of her previous pill, omitting the normal 7-day gap.

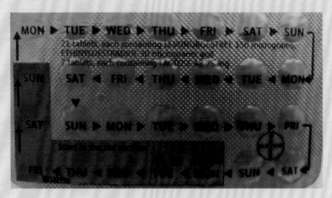

▲ 图 19-5　ED 复方口服避孕药

Fig. 19.5　The ED combined oral contraceptive pill.

什么时候达到避孕效果？

When will it achieve its contraceptive effect?

在连续 7 天每天服用活性片后。

When seven active hormone tablets have been taken on successive days.

如果漏服药片或恶心呕吐、腹泻怎么办？

What to do if a pill is missed or nausea, vomiting or diarrhoea occurs?

如果漏服时间大于 12h，这枚药片不再服用，但原始疗程仍在继续，并且在接下来的 7 天内使用其他避孕措施。如果漏服时间小于 12h，立即服用该药片，之后照常服用药片。当漏服药片的时间接近激素片停止和给予糖片的时间时，可以停止原始疗程，并在约 5~6 天后用一包新的药片，在这种情况下不需要额外的避孕措施。

If the missed pill is not discovered until more than 12 hours after it was meant to be taken, that pill should not be taken, but the original course continued and alternative contraception used for the next 7 days. If discovered <12 hours after the time it was meant to have been taken, take that pill now, and continue the cycle taking the next one at the appropriate time. When the missed pill is close to the time the hormone tablets were due to be ceased and sugar tablets given, the original course can be stopped and a new pack commenced about 5–6 days later. There is no need for additional contraception under such circumstances.

有哪些潜在的不良反应，如常见的突破性出血，如果发生这种出血怎么办？

What are the potential side effects, including the common ones of breakthrough bleeding, and what to do if such bleeding occurs?

主要的不良反应是突破性出血，尽管仍在服用激素片，但通常会出现轻微出血。这通常在服用 OCP 后 3 个月内自发消退，但如果持续存在，应给予更高剂量的药片。

The main nuisance side effect is breakthrough bleeding where generally light bleeding occurs despite the hormone tablets still being taken. This usually settles spontaneously within 3 months of starting the OCP, but if it persists a higher-dose pill should be given.

什么时候需要进一步评估，为什么？

When is further review needed and why?

应在 2~3 个月内对患者进行检查，以评估是否发生任何问题，并检查血压是否未升高。进一步评估，其中包括血压、乳房检查和妇科评估（包括巴氏涂片或 HPV 检测），通常每年都要进行。

She should be reviewed in 2–3 months to check if any problems have occurred and to check that blood pressure has not become elevated. Further reviews, when blood pressure, breast examination and gynaecological assessment including Pap smear or HPV testing should be done, are generally done annually.

作用。服用避孕药的人患子宫内膜癌和卵巢癌的风险也降低了 50%，这取决于服药的时间长短，停用 OCP 后，这种益处可以持续 10 年。

In addition to the prevention of unwanted pregnancy, the use of the combined pill is associated with a 30% reduction in blood loss at menstruation, a lower incidence of ectopic pregnancy (0.4/1000) and some protection against PID and benign ovarian cysts. Pill users also have a reduced risk of both endometrial and ovarian cancer of up to 50%, depending on the length of use, with this benefit lasting for up to 10 years after the OCP therapy has been ceased.

8. 甾体避孕药的药物相互作用（Interaction between drugs and contraceptive steroids）

许多药物影响避孕药的避孕效果，因此应采取其他预防措施（表 19-3）。呕吐和腹泻还会导致避孕

药流失，从而导致生育力恢复，特别是目前广泛使用的小剂量避孕药。为了保证单孕激素避孕药有效，必须每天服用。

Many drugs affect the contraceptive efficacy of the pill, and therefore additional precautions should be taken (Table 19.3). Vomiting and diarrhoea also result in loss of the pill and hence the return of fertility-particularly with the low-dose pills now widely in use. Progestogen-only pills must be taken every day if they are to be effective.

9. 失败率（Failure rates）

复方避孕药的失败率为"每年 100 名女性发生 0.27～5 次非意愿妊娠"，一般认为，失败率较高是因为女性未能正确服用避孕药、胃肠道疾病影响其吸收，或者正在接受的抗生素治疗减少其吸收。单孕

表 19-3　口服避孕药与其他药物的相互作用

Table 19.3　Interaction of various drugs with oral contraceptives

药物 Interacting drug	影响 Effects of interaction
镇痛药 Analgesics	可能增加对哌替啶的敏感性 Possible increased sensitivity to pethidine
抗凝药 Anticoagulants	可能减少抗凝药的作用，可能需要增加抗凝药的剂量 Possible reduction of effect of anticoagulant-increased dosage of anticoagulant may be necessary
抗惊厥药 Anticonvulsants	避孕可靠性下降 Possible decrease in contraceptive reliability
三环类抗抑郁药 Tricyclic antidepressants	抗抑郁药的反应减少；抗抑郁药毒性增加 Reduced antidepressant response; increase in antidepressant toxicity
抗组胺药 Antihistamines	避孕可靠性下降 Possible decrease in contraceptive reliability
抗生素 Antibiotics	避孕可靠性下降 Possible decrease in contraceptive reliability 可能突破性出血（利福平最有可能） Possibility of breakthrough bleeding (this is most likely with rifampicin)
降血糖药 Hypoglycaemic agents	糖尿病控制作用可能会降低 Control of diabetes may be reduced
抗哮喘药 Anti-asthmatics	同时口服避孕药可能会加重哮喘状况 Asthmatic condition may be exacerbated by concomitant oral contraceptive
全身皮质类固醇 Systemic corticosteroids	需要增加类固醇的剂量 Increased dosage of steroids may be necessary

激素制剂的失败率较高，约为"每年 100 名女性发生 0.3～8 次非意愿妊娠"。

The failure rate of combined pills is 0.27–5/100 women-years, with the higher end of this rate generally believed to be due to a failure of the woman to take the pill correctly, having a gastrointestinal disorder affecting its absorption or being on antibiotic therapy reducing its absorption. The failure rate for progestogen-only preparations is higher and varies between 0.3 and 8/100 women-years.

10. 避孕药与手术（The pill and surgery）

服用避孕药会增加深静脉血栓形成的风险，因此应在大手术前至少 6 周停用。在小手术前，尤其是在腹腔镜绝育手术前，不应停止。入院前非意愿妊娠的风险远大于血栓栓塞的风险。

The pill increases the risk of deep vein thrombosis and should therefore be stopped at least 6 weeks before major surgery. It should not be stopped before minor procedures-particularly before laparoscopic sterilization procedures. The risk of an unwanted pregnancy occurring before admission is substantially greater than the risk of thromboembolism.

11. 避孕药与哺乳（The pill and lactation）

复方制剂往往会抑制泌乳，因此最好避免服用，此时可以选择只含孕激素的避孕药，因为它对泌乳的影响很小，而且也许会促进泌乳。

Combined preparations tend to inhibit lactation and are therefore best avoided. The pill of choice at this time is the progestogen-only pill, as it has minimal effect on lactation and may indeed promote it.

12. 注射剂（Injectable compounds）

目前有主要两种类型：醋酸甲羟孕酮和依伴依。醋酸甲羟孕酮含有 150mg 醋酸甲羟孕酮，每 3 个月肌内注射一次。依伴依是一种含有依托孕烯的硅橡胶棒，皮下植入上臂，有效期长达 3 年。早期类型的植入物，释放左炔诺孕酮的诺普兰已经停止使用，但有些女性体内可能还保留着这些植入物。这些注射制剂都通过使宫颈黏液不利于精子通过，使子宫内膜不利于着床，以及抑制排卵发挥作用的。

There are currently two main types: Depo-Provera and Implanon. Depo-Provera contains 150 mg of medroxyprogesterone acetate and is given as a 3-monthly intramuscular injection. Implanon is a single Silastic rod containing etonogestrel that is inserted subdermally in the upper arm and is effective for up to 3 years. An earlier type of implant, the levonorgestrel-releasing Norplant Silastic rod, has been discontinued, but some women may still have this in place. Each of these injectable

preparations works by making the cervical mucus hostile and the endometrium hypotrophic and by suppressing ovulation.

失败率很低，第一年不到"每年 100 名女性发生 0.1 次非意愿妊娠"，5 年后上升到"每年 100 名女性发生 3.9 次非意愿妊娠"。失败的主要是在注射醋酸甲羟孕酮或植入依伴依时已经妊娠的女性，因此这些方法必须在终止妊娠时或在月经的前 5 天内开始，如果末次月经不正常，则通过血 β-hCG 检查来排除妊娠。

Failure rates are low, at less than 0.1/100 women-years in the first year rising to 3.9/100 over 5 years. Failures mostly relate to women already pregnant at the time of injection of the Depo-Provera or insertion of the Implanon device, so it is essential that these methods are commenced at the time of a pregnancy termination or within the first 5 days of menstruation, with pregnancy excluded by a plasma beta human chorionic gonadotropin (β-hCG) pregnancy test if the last menstrual period was not entirely normal.

肠胃外单独孕激素避孕药，长效、可逆、有效，避免首过效应，依从性要求低，并避免与雌激素有关的不良反应。但是，它们可能会导致不规则出血或闭经，这也许会引起怀疑妊娠的焦虑。去除植入物很困难，并且只能由经过相关程序培训的医生操作。一些女性会出现全身性的孕激素作用，如情绪变化和体重增加，或者出现雌激素缺乏症状。

Parenteral progestogen-only contraceptives are long-acting but easily reversible, are effective, avoid first-pass-effect liver metabolism, require minimal compliance and avoid the side effects associated with oestrogens. However, they may cause irregular bleeding or amenorrhoea, which can be a source of anxiety because of the possibility of pregnancy. Removal of the implants may be difficult and should only be carried out by a doctor trained in the procedure. Some women will experience systemic progestogenic effects such as mood changes and weight gain or develop symptoms of oestrogenic deficiency.

13. 激素避孕的新方法（Newer methods of hormonal contraception）

在过去的几年中，已引入激素透皮贴片和阴道避孕环的组合。其中每一种都与 OCP 一样有效，而且有很好的证据表明，与 OCP 相比，它们的实际激素水平变化较小，总量也较低。连续 3 周每周更换一次经皮避孕药贴片，第四周不使用贴片。对于阴道避孕环，将其留在阴道内 3 周，然后取出 1 周，然后置入新的阴道环。这些方法都与 OCP 一样，经期发生在未给激素的 1 周。

In the last few years combined hormone transdermal patches and a vaginal contraceptive ring have been introduced. Each of these is as effective as the combined OCP, and there is good evidence that the actual hormone levels achieved with either of these is less variable than that seen with oral therapy, and lower overall. The transdermal contraceptive patches are changed weekly for 3 weeks, and the fourth week is then patch free. For the NuvaRing, the device is left in the vagina for 3 weeks, then removed for 1 week, then a new vaginal ring inserted. With each of these methods, as with the OCP, the period occurs during the hormone-free week.

（四）紧急避孕（Emergency contraception）

在无保护性交、漏服复方避孕药或避孕套破裂后，性交 72h 内服用 1 片 750mg 左炔诺孕酮片，12h 后再服用 1 片。纯左炔诺孕酮的方法比以前使用的复方 OCP 方法不良反应少，在一些国家，16 岁以上的女性可以直接从药剂师那里获得此药。不良反应包括轻度恶心、呕吐（如果第一次给药后 2～3h 内呕吐，应再服用 1 片）和出血。应告知女性以下事宜。

After unprotected intercourse, a missed combined pill or a burst condom, a single 750-mg levonorgestrel tablet is taken within 72 hours of intercourse, followed by a second dose exactly 12 hours later. The levonorgestrel-only method has fewer side effects than the previously used combined OCP method and, in some countries, is available to women over the age of 16 years directly from pharmacists. Side effects include mild nausea, vomiting (an additional pill should be taken if vomiting occurs within 2–3 hours of the first dose) and bleeding. The woman should be advised that:

- 她的下一次月经可能推迟或提前。

- 在此之前，她需要使用屏障避孕法。

- 她如果有任何腹痛或者下一次月经不来或异常，需要复诊。

- Her next period might be early or late.
- She needs to use barrier contraception until then.
- She needs to return if she has any abdominal pain or if the next period is absent or abnormal.

如果下次月经期推迟 5 天以上，应考虑妊娠可能。紧急避孕措施可防止 85% 的预期妊娠。性行为后采取紧急避孕的时间间隔越长，功效越低。

If the next period is more than 5 days overdue, pregnancy should be excluded. Emergency contraception prevents 85% of expected pregnancies. Efficacy decreases with time from intercourse.

左炔诺孕酮在性行为后 72h 以上无效，但是如果仍在胚胎植入之前，可以置入 IUD。

If the woman concerned does not attend until more than 72 hours after the sexual activity occurred, levonorgestrel therapy is ineffective; however, an IUD can be inserted if it is still before the time implantation of any embryo produced would have occurred.

（五）非药物避孕的方法（Non-medical methods of contraception）

月经周期中生育能力最强的是排卵期。如果月经周期是 28 天，排卵是在第 13 或 14 天。生育期与宫颈黏液的变化有关，女性可以自我检查来识别，而激素的变化可以通过家用尿检试剂盒来检测。对于积极性很高的夫妇，避开生育期可能是一个非常有效的方法。

The most fertile phase of the menstrual cycle occurs at the time of ovulation. In a 28-day cycle, this occurs on day 13 or 14 of the cycle. The fertile phase is associated with changes in cervical mucus that a woman can learn to recognize by selfexamination and hormone changes that can be measured by home urine testing kits. Avoidance of the fertile period can be an extremely effective method in well-motivated couples.

计划生育的自然方法如下。

Natural methods of family planning include the following:

- 安全期避孕法：排卵前 6 天和排卵后 2 天避免性行为。这种方法的有效性取决于能否预测排卵时间。如果月经周期规律为 28 天，排卵预计在第 14 天，应该在第 8～16 天避免性行为。如果周期变化很大，在 24～32 天，排卵最早在第 10 天，最晚在第 18 天，因此在第 4～20 天需要避免性行为。

- *The rhythm method*: Avoiding intercourse mid-cycle and for 6 days before ovulation and 2 days after it. The efficacy of this method depends on being able to predict the time of ovulation. If a regular 28-day cycle occurs, ovulation is predicted for day 14, and abstinence should be from days 8 to 16. If the cycles are highly variable, varying between 24 and 32 days, the earliest ovulation would be on day 10 and the latest on day 18, so abstinence would be required between days 4 and 20.

- 宫颈黏液观察法：排卵前阶段由于宫颈黏液分泌导致阴道湿度增加，该避孕方法需要女性有识别这种阴道湿度增加的能力，并在此期间以及观察到湿度峰值后的 2 天内避免性行为。这种方法比安全期避孕法好得多，但许多女性在排卵之前 4 天才能识别出阴道湿度的增加，因此这之前 2 天的性行为可能导致妊娠。

- *The ovulation method*: This method takes into account the ability of a woman to recognize the increase in vaginal wetness due to cervical mucus production in the phase before ovulation and abstaining from sex during that time and for 2 days after the peak wetness has been observed. This method is much better than the rhythm method, but many women only get 4 days advanced warning of the time of ovulation, so intercourse on the preceding 2 days can result in a pregnancy.

- 体外射精法：一种传统的、仍然广泛使用的避孕方法，依赖于射精前抽出阴茎。这种避孕方法并不可靠，因为最好的精子往往在男性即将射精之前到达阴茎顶端，或者在激动的时候忘记抽出阴茎。

- *Coitus interruptus (withdrawal):* A traditional and still widely used method of contraception that relies on withdrawal of the penis before ejaculation. It is not a particularly reliable method of contraception, because the best sperm often reach the tip of the penis before the male experiences the imminent ejaculation, or he forgets in the 'heat' of the moment.

- 哺乳期无月经避孕法：母乳喂养历来是家庭"间隔"的最重要手段。母乳喂养的女性平均 4～6 个月后会恢复排卵。在孩子出生后的前 6 个月内，这是一种有效的避孕方法，母亲是完全母乳喂养，不给婴儿任何非母乳或其他食物，并保持闭经，如果所有这些特征都存在，失败率低至 1%。

- *Lactational amenorrhoea method:* Breast-feeding has historically been the most important means of family 'spacing'. Ovulation resumes, on average, 4–6 months later in women who continue to breast-feed. During the first 6 months after birth, this is an effective method of contraception in mothers providing they are fully breast-feeding, not giving the baby any non-breast milk or other food AND have remained amenorrhoeic, with failure rates as low as 1/100 women being seen if all of these features exist.

（六）绝育（Sterilization）

避孕技术的主要优点是易逆转，失败率低。缺点是在性行为之前，他们需要有意识地自主采取避孕措施。当家庭规模合适而不再有生育需求，或者有生育的禁忌证，可以考虑选择绝育。约有 30% 的夫妇选择绝育，而 40 岁以上的夫妇的绝育比例增加到 50%。

Contraceptive techniques have the major advantage that they are easily reversible and provide a high level of protection against pregnancy. They have the disadvantage that they require a conscious act on behalf of the individual before intercourse. When family size is complete or there is a specific medical contraindication to continuing fertility, sterilization becomes the contraceptive method of choice. Around 30% of couples use sterilization for contraception, and this increases to 50% in those over the age of 40 years.

1. 咨询（Counselling）

有必要就手术的性质及其影响向双方提供咨询，并讨论应该对男性还是女性伴侣进行绝育，在多数情况下，只有一个伴侣会要求绝育。然而重要的是要确保对替代方案进行充分讨论。

It is essential to counsel both partners about the nature of the procedures and their implications and to discuss whether it is better for the male or female partner to be sterilized. In many cases, only one partner will be seeking sterilization, in which case only one point of view needs to be considered. It is important, however, to ensure that there is a full discussion of the alternatives.

咨询应包括提及拟实施的方法及其风险和失败率（女性绝育为 1/200，男性绝育为 1/2000）。女性应该被告知，一旦绝育失败，她们患异位妊娠的风险就会增加。

Counselling should include reference to the intended method and its risks and failure rates (1/200 for female sterilization, 1/2000 for male sterilization). Women should be warned of the increased risk of ectopic pregnancy in the event of failure.

2. 绝育时机（Timing of sterilization）

绝育手术可以在月经周期的任何时候进行，但最好在卵泡期进行。如果女性月经推迟、月经未来潮或者她觉得可能妊娠了，应该在术前进行妊娠试验。

The operation can be performed at any time in the menstrual cycle but is best done in the follicular phase of the cycle. A pregnancy test should be performed preoperatively if a woman has a late or missed period or thinks she may be pregnant.

3. 绝育技术（Techniques）

(1) 女性绝育（Female sterilization）：

绝育手术的方式主要是输卵管的阻断，也有输

请记住，据报道第三代 / 左炔诺孕酮 IUD 的失败率与绝育相当，但男性绝育的失败率明显较低。

随着显微外科手术带来的改进，绝育不再是不可逆转的，应该根据采取的技术为患者提供咨询。哪个伴侣绝育是选择和动机的问题。如果某个伴侣因慢性病而预期寿命被缩短，那么该伴侣应绝育。

建议在绝育手术后月经期出现之前，女性继续使用其他避孕方法，直到绝育手术结束。男性绝育后，至少射精 10 次才能进行精液分析，在 2~4 周的连续两次精液分析显示无精子之前，男性应采取替代避孕方法。

Remember that the reported failure rate for third-generation/levonorgestrel IUDs is comparable to that of sterilization, but male sterilization has a significantly lower failure rate.

With the improvements brought about by microsurgery, it is no longer acceptable to say that sterilization is irreversible, and the patient should be counselled according to the technique to be used. The partner to be sterilized will be a matter of choice and motivation. If one partner has a reduced life expectancy from chronic illness, then that partner should be sterilized.

Women should be advised to continue to use other contraception until the period occurs following the sterilization procedure. Men should be advised to use alternative contraception until they have had two consecutive semen analyses showing azoospermia 2–4 weeks apart, with these analyses not done until at least 10 ejaculations have occurred.

卵管夹、全子宫切除术等方式。一般来说，手术越激进，绝育失败的可能性就越小。然而，现在应该选择避孕失败率低，并且可逆性强的绝育方法。

The majority of procedures involves interruption of the Fallopian tubes but may vary from the application of clips on the tubes to total hysterectomy. In general terms, the more radical the procedure, the less likely there is to be a failure. However, very low failure rates can now be achieved using methods with high reversibility prospects and these should be the methods of choice.

①腹腔镜绝育术：腹腔镜绝育手术大大缩短了住院时间。这是大多数发达国家的首选绝育方法，但在内镜设备或培训有限的国家，小型开腹手术更合适。

Laparoscopic sterilization. The use of the laparoscope for sterilization procedures has substantially reduced the duration of hospital stay. This is the method of choice in most developed countries, but an open approach through a mini-laparotomy may be more appropriate in countries where endoscopic facilities or training is limited.

- 输卵管夹：这是英国和澳大利亚使用最多的方法。输卵管夹由塑料和惰性金属制成，固定在输卵管上（图 19-6）。优点是对输卵管损坏小，但缺点是失败率较高。失败的原因可能是误夹了其他结构而不是输卵管、输卵管从输卵管夹中挤出、输卵管再通或输卵管夹破裂使其从输卵管上脱落。Filshie 夹的钛框架内衬硅橡胶，失败率最低（0.5%），更容易使用。Yoon 或 Fallope 环应用于管环上，类似于 Madlener 手术（见后述）。这种技术与较强的术后腹痛有关，失败率 0.3%~4%。此环不适用于产褥期肿胀和水肿的输卵管。

- Tubal clips. This is the most widely used method of sterilization in the UK and Australia. The clips are made of plastic and inert metals and are locked on to the tube (Fig. 19.6). They have the advantage of causing minimal damage to the tube, but their disadvantage is a higher failure rate. Failures may be due to application on the wrong structure, extrusion of the tube from the clip and recanalization or fracture of the clip so that it falls off the tube. The *Filshie clip*, which has a titanium frame lined by silicone rubber, has the lowest failure rate (0.5%) and is easier to apply. *Yoon or Fallope rings* are applied over a loop of tube and are similar to a Madlener procedure (see later). This technique is associated with considerably greater abdominal pain postoperatively, and the failure rates vary between 0.3% and 4%. The rings are not suitable for application to the tubes in the puerperium when the tube is swollen and oedematous.

- 输卵管电凝和分离：通过单极或双极电凝灼烧输卵管峡部 1~2cm 长来绝育。用这种技术可以破坏一定长度的输卵管。据说电凝后分离可以降低异位妊娠的风险。失败率取决于输卵管被破坏的长度。由于可能会引起热性肠损伤及渗漏和粪便性腹膜炎，所以除非机械方法在技术上有困难或在手术时失败，否则电凝法不应作为主要的绝育方法。

- Tubal coagulation and division. Sterilization is effected by either unipolar or bipolar diathermy of the tubes in two sites 1–2 cm from the uterotubal junction. A considerable amount of tube can be destroyed with this technique. Division of the diathermied tube is said to reduce the risk of ectopic pregnancy. The failure rate depends on the length of tube destroyed. Because

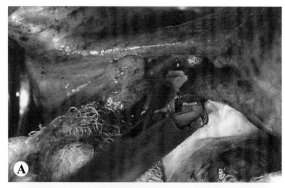

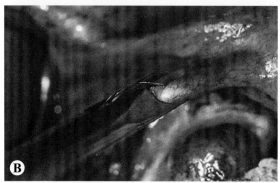

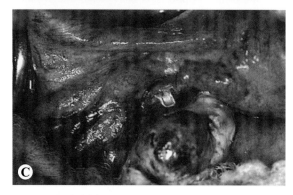

▲ 图 19-6　夹闭绝育（A）夹住右侧输卵管（B）夹闭，输卵管被破坏（C）Filshie 夹夹闭并锁定在输卵管上

Fig. 19.6　Sterilization by clip occlusion. (A) The right Fallopian tube is grasped with the clip. (B) The clip is closed and the tube is crushed. (C) The Filshie clip is closed and locked across the Fallopian tube.

of the risk of thermal bowel injury with subsequent leakage and faecal peritonitis, diathermy should not be used as the primary method of sterilization unless mechanical methods of tubal occlusion are technically difficult or fail at the time of the procedure.

②输卵管结扎术（图 19-7）：这些手术通常通过小切口剖腹术或在剖宫产时进行。随着腹腔镜手术的增加，它们的应用越来越少。现在更常见的是，即使由于某些原因不能做腹腔镜手术，也是使用夹子来阻塞输卵管。

Tubal ligation (Fig. 19.7). These procedures are usually performed through a small abdominal incision (minilaparotomy) or at the time of caesarean section. They are less widely used with the increase in laparoscopic procedures. Even when laparoscopy is contraindicated for some reason, it is still more common now to use clips to occlude the tubes.

结扎输卵管的最基本方法是 Madlener 手术，但失败率可能高达 3.7%。双折结扎切断法（Pomeroy 手术）是相同的，但管环被切除，并使用可吸收缝合材料进行结扎。该技术有几种变体，包括在分离阔韧带对侧输卵管的切端。切除的节段应进行组织学检查，以确认输卵管已被切除。

The most basic form of the procedure involving simple ligation of the tube is known as the *Madlener procedure*, but the failure rate may be up to 3.7%. The *Pomeroy technique* is the same, but the loop of tube is excised and absorbable suture material is used for the ligation. There are several variations of this technique, including the separation of the cut ends of the tubes on contralateral sides of the broad ligament. The excised segments should be examined histologically to confirm that the tube has been excised.

③ Essure 法：在宫腔镜检查时将一个小装置置入两侧输卵管，会导致双侧输卵管的纤维化，最终会阻塞。这种置入通常不需要麻醉，也不需要腹腔

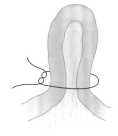

Madlener
Madlener 手术

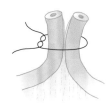

Pomeroy
Pomeroy 手术

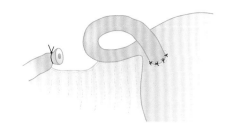

burial of tubal stumps
输卵管残端包埋

▲ 图 19-7　输卵管结扎术绝育

Fig. 19.7　Sterilization by tubal ligation.

镜。它的不锈钢线圈可以将其固定在输卵管的近端部分，内部的聚对苯二甲酸乙二酯纤维，在随后的 3 个月内会诱发良性纤维化反应。通过子宫输卵管造影检查输卵管是否完全阻塞。最近有报道称这种绝育法失败率在增加，因此在不久的将来它可能就会退出历史舞台。

The Essure procedure. This procedure consists of insertion of a small device into each tube at the time of a hysteroscopic examination, with this device resulting in fibrosis and ultimate occlusion of the tube on each side. This insertion can often be done without anaesthesia and does not require a laparoscopy. The device has a stainless steel coil, which holds the device in position in the proximal portion of the tube, and inner polyethylene terephthalate fibres, which induce the benign fibrotic reaction over the succeeding 3 months. Adequacy of tubal blockage is often checked by the performance of a hysterosalpingogram. Recent reports had detailed an increased failure rate with this technique of sterilization so it may be withdrawn from use in the near future.

④并发症：除了腹腔镜手术的并发症外，如果进行了绝育手术，那么输卵管绝育的长期并发症是输卵管再通和妊娠、异位妊娠、月经不调和性欲减退。

Complications. Apart from the complications of laparoscopy, if it was performed to enable sterilization, the longer-term complications of any tubal sterilization are tubal recanalization and pregnancy, ectopic pregnancy, menstrual irregularity and loss of libido.

(2) 输精管切除术（Vasectomy）：

这种手术通常在局部麻醉下进行。在精索上做两个小切口，切除 3～4cm 的输精管（图 19-8）。此法的优点是简单，缺点为不适立即有效，在精液不含精子之前不是不育的。平均来说，至少需要 10 次射精，在恢复无保护性交之前，应该通过精液分析来确认绝育的有效性。

This procedure is generally performed under local anaesthesia. Two small incisions are made over the spermatic cord and 3–4 cm of the vas deferens is excised (Fig. 19.8). The advantage of the technique is its simplicity. The disadvantages are that sterility is not immediate and should not be assumed until all spermatozoa have disappeared from the ejaculate. On average, this takes at least 10 ejaculations, and its effectiveness should be confirmed by a semen analysis before any unprotected intercourse is resumed.

输精管切除术比大多数形式的女性绝育更难以逆转，即使实现了令人满意的再吻合，由于精子制动抗体和精子凝集抗体的不利影响，只有约 50% 的

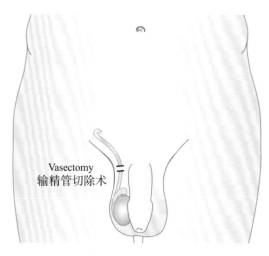

▲ 图 19-8　输精管切除术涉及一段输精管的切除
Fig. 19.8　Vasectomy involves excision of a segment of the vas deferens.

患者能恢复生育能力。失败率约为 1/2000。

The procedure is more difficult to reverse than most forms of female sterilization, and even when satisfactory re-anastomosis is achieved, only about 50% of patients will sire children, because of the adverse effect of the production of sperm-immobilizing and sperm-agglutinating antibodies. The failure rate is about 1/2000.

失败可能是由于输精管自发再通，或者切除的输精管长度不足。切除的节段应始终进行组织学检查，以确认输精管已被切除。手术并发症包括血肿形成、伤口感染和附睾炎。由于精子引起的异物反应，在输精管的切割端也可能形成疼痛的肉芽肿。

Failures may follow spontaneous recanalization and excision of an inadequate length of vas deferens. The excised segments should always be examined histologically to confirm that the vas has been excised. Complications of the operation include haematoma formation, wound infection and epididymitis. Also a painful granuloma may form at the cut end of the vas as a result of a foreign body reaction induced by spermatozoa.

4. 绝育对心理的影响（Psychological implications of sterilization）

有人认为女性绝育导致精神问题和性功能恶化。现代研究并未证实这一点。除了现代研究倾向于使用前瞻性标准化方法之外，21 世纪的绝育人群也与 40 年前的非常不同。以前绝育主要针对孩子很多、处于社会困境中和妇科健康状况差的老年女性。它是根据医学建议进行的，通常在分娩、堕胎或者在其他妇科手术后不久进行。而如今，绝育是所有年

龄段和社会阶层女性使用的一种广泛接受的避孕方法，因此在整个人口中更有代表性。绝育通常是由女性要求的，与分娩或流产无关。接受绝育的女性的孩子更少，总体健康状况比以前好。

Sterilization in women has acquired the reputation of leading to psychiatric problems and a deterioration in sexual function. Modern studies do not confirm this reputation. Apart from the fact that modern studies tend to use prospective standardized methodologies, the population being sterilized in the 21st century is very different to that of 40 years ago. Sterilization used to be performed predominantly on older women in poor gynaecological health, with large numbers of children and living in conditions of social adversity. It was carried out on medical recommendation, frequently shortly after childbirth, abortion or some other gynaecological procedure. Nowadays, sterilization is a widely accepted form of contraception used by women of all ages and social classes. They are therefore more representative of the population as a whole. Sterilization usually takes place at the request of the woman as an interval procedure unrelated to either childbirth or abortion. Women being sterilized have fewer children and are in better general health than previously.

绝育后精神疾病的发生率一般不高于一般女性人群。然而，分娩后立即进行绝育的女性，患产后抑郁症的风险增加。既往精神病史和对绝育的矛盾心理或不确定性是精神疾病的危险因素。产后状况、既往精神病史、矛盾心理和婚姻不和谐也是导致性心理功能下降和后悔的危险因素。一些学者还建议，在女性特质与生育能力密切相关的文化中，以及对避孕有罪恶感和羞耻感的文化中，应格外小心，以确保患者做好绝育准备。通常通过患者要求再通手术来判断患者后悔，而婚姻破裂和再婚似乎是有力的预测因素。

The rate of psychiatric disorder following sterilization is, in general, no higher than that in the general female population. However, for women who are sterilized immediately following childbirth, there is an increased risk of suffering from postnatal depression. A previous psychiatric history and ambivalence or uncertainty about sterilization are risk factors for psychiatric

disorders. Postpartum status, previous psychiatric history, ambivalence and marital discord are also risk factors for deterioration of psychosexual functioning and regret. Some authors have also suggested that in cultures where femininity is strongly associated with fertility and where there is guilt and shame about contraception, great care should be exercised to ensure that patients are properly prepared for sterilization. Regret, often measured by a request for reversal of sterilization, appears to be most strongly predicted by marital breakdown and subsequent remarriage.

（七）终止妊娠（Termination of pregnancy）

在英国，终止妊娠是根据 1967 年《堕胎法》的规定，在经批准的中心进行的。要求有 2 名医生同意，继续妊娠会对母亲或其他孩子的身体或精神健康产生危害，危害比终止妊娠更大，或者胎儿可能有严重致残性畸形（框 19-2）。该法案的最新修正案（1991 年）对第一个类别的终止妊娠做了 24 周内的限制，尽管实际上大多数是在 20 周之前进行的。

In the UK this is carried out in approved centres under the provisions of the Abortion Act 1967. This requires that two doctors agree that either continuation of the pregnancy would involve greater risk to the physical or mental health of the mother or her other children than termination or that the fetus is at risk of an abnormality likely to result in it being seriously handicapped (Box 19.2). The most recent amendment to the act (1991) set a limit for termination under the first of these categories at 24 weeks, although in practice the majority of terminations are carried out prior to 20 weeks.

在英国，所有的终止妊娠都要申报，年流产数在 1990 年最多，为 170 000，此后一直下降，直到 1996 年，"第三代"避孕药引发了对静脉血栓风险的恐慌。

All terminations carried out in the UK must be notified. Annual abortion numbers peaked in the UK in 1990 at 170,000 and declined after that until the scare over the risk of venous thrombosis with the 'third-generation' pills in 1996.

框 19-2　终止妊娠的适应证	Box 19.2　Indications for termination
A. 如果继续妊娠，孕妇的生命危险会更大	A. Risk to the life of the mother would be greater if the pregnancy continues
B. 防止对孕妇的精神或身体健康造成永久性伤害	B. To prevent permanent harm to mental or physical health of the mother
C. 如果继续妊娠，孕妇的健康风险更大	C. Risk to mother's health greater* if the pregnancy continues
D. 如果继续妊娠，对家庭其他孩子有风险	D. Risk to other children in the family* if the pregnancy continues
E. 儿童有严重残疾的危险	E. Risk of serious disability in the child

*. 仅妊娠小于 24 周

*. Only if less than 24 weeks.

在澳大利亚，各州终止妊娠的可得性和合法性各不相同，因此在执行任何此类操作前，必须仔细界定并遵守各州的规则。

The availability and legality of pregnancy termination in Australia vary from state to state, and the rules in each state must therefore be defined and followed carefully before any such procedure is performed.

1. 方法（Methods）

应该对所有终止妊娠的女性进行性传播感染（sexually transmitted infection，STI）的筛查和（或）给予抗生素预防感染。终止妊娠后，应对所有 Rh 阴性女性给予抗 D 免疫球蛋白治疗。应对所有患者随访一次，以检查是否有身体问题，以及是否采取了节育措施。

All women undergoing termination of pregnancy should be screened for STIs and/or offered antibiotic prophylaxis. Following termination, anti-D immunoglobulin should be given to all Rhesus-negative women. All women should be offered a follow-up appointment to check that there are no physical problems and that contraceptive measures are in place.

> **！注意**
>
> 在要求终止妊娠的女性中，衣原体感染率为 12%，如果手术流产时不给予适当的抗生素治疗，则有 30% 的风险患上 PID。
>
> The rate of infection with *Chlamydia* spp. is 12% of women requesting termination of pregnancy. In these women there is a 30% risk of PID if appropriate antibiotic treatment is not given at the time of a surgical termination.

(1) 手术流产（Surgical termination）：此法最常用于妊娠的最初 3 个月。结合妊娠周数，将子宫颈扩张，并用吸引器吸出妊娠物。一种变式是用卵圆钳零碎取出较大的胎儿部分（扩张和排空），可用于中期妊娠。在英国大多数流产手术都是在全身麻醉下进行的，但在许多国家中，很多 10 周前的流产手术采取了局部麻醉，从而减少患者在院时间。

This is the method most commonly used in the first trimester of pregnancy. The cervix is dilated by a number of millimetres equivalent to the gestation in weeks and the conceptus is removed using a suction curette. A variation involving piecemeal removal of the larger fetal parts with forceps (dilatation and evacuation) allows the method to be used for later second-trimester pregnancies. Although most procedures are carried out under general anaesthesia in the

UK, local anaesthesia is widely used in many countries for terminations before 10 weeks and reduces the time the patient needs to stay in the hospital or clinic.

> **经验**
>
> 术前应用前列腺素栓剂可使宫颈扩张更容易。
>
> Cervical dilation can be made easier by administration of prostaglandin pessaries before the operation.

(2) 药物流产（Medical termination）：药物流产常用于孕 14 周后，也越来越多地用于孕 9 周前，作为手术流产的替代方式。妊娠早期的标准用药方案是口服孕酮受体阻滞药米非司酮（RU 486），36~48h 后用前列腺素的阴道栓。有几种不同的给药方案，但成功率均超过 95%。妊娠中期引产也可以使用给予阴道前列腺素，每 3 小时一次，或者用气囊导管通过子宫颈进行羊膜外输液。米非司酮预处理可显著缩短前列腺炎给药至流产的时间间隔。在引产后，可能需要在全麻下检查以取出胎盘。

This is the method most commonly used for pregnancies after 14 weeks and is increasingly being offered as an alternative to surgical termination in first-trimester pregnancies up to 9 weeks' gestation. The standard regimens for first-trimester termination use the progesterone antagonist mifepristone (RU 486) given orally, followed 36–48 hours later by prostaglandins administered as a vaginal pessary. There are several different regimens, but all have a success rate of greater than 95%. Second-trimester terminations can also be performed using vaginal prostaglandins given 3-hourly or as an extra-amniotic infusion through a balloon catheter passed through the cervix. Pretreatment with mifepristone significantly reduces the time interval from the administration of the prostaglandin preparation to abortion. After delivery of the fetus, an examination under general anaesthetic may be necessary to remove the placenta.

2. 并发症（Complications）

早期并发症包括出血、子宫穿孔（可能损害其他盆腔内脏）、宫颈裂伤、妊娠物残留和败血症。有一定的失败率（0.7/1000）。晚期并发症包括不孕症、宫颈功能不全、同种免疫反应和精神问题。充分的咨询（书面资料支持）、解释流产及其风险是非常重要的。

Early complications include bleeding, uterine perforation (with possible damage to other pelvic viscera), cervical laceration, retained products and sepsis. All the procedures also have a small failure rate (overall rate 0.7/1000). Late complications include infertility, cervical incompetence, isoimmunization and psychiatric morbidity. Adequate counselling (supported by written information) and explanation of the procedures and their risks are essential.

3. 流产后心理后遗症（Psychological sequelae of termination）

大多数发现非意愿妊娠的女性都非常烦恼，尽管如此，有证据表明大多数女性没有经历中长期的心理后遗症，也没有任何证据表明精神病发病率增加。现有证据表明，终止妊娠后精神病发病率低于允许妊娠进行的情况。

The majority of women who find themselves with an unwanted pregnancy are very distressed. Despite this, evidence shows that the majority of women do not experience medium-to long-term psychological sequelae, nor is there any evidence of an increase in the rate of psychiatric morbidity. The available evidence is that the rate of psychiatric morbidity following termination of pregnancy is less than if the pregnancy was allowed to proceed.

(1) 妊娠早期流产不良后遗症的危险因素（Risk factors for adverse sequelae of first-trimester abortion）：对于已经结婚生子的女性，流产会导致内疚和后悔。这种情况下的女性在进行流产之前需要仔细的咨询。矛盾心理、强迫、既往终止妊娠、既往精神病史及与绝育相关的终止妊娠是导致精神问题的危险因素。

Being married and having children prior to a termination can lead to problems of guilt and regret. Women in such circumstances need careful counselling before proceeding with the termination. Ambivalence, coercion, previous termination of pregnancy, past psychiatric history and termination associated with sterilization are risk factors for psychiatric morbidity.

(2) 中晚期终止妊娠（Later terminations of pregnancy）：孕 12 周后，由于心理社会原因终止妊娠的女性人数正在下降。现在孕中期的终止妊娠占所有治疗性终止妊娠的比例低于 8%。这些女性有少数是因心理社会原因进行治疗性流产，大多数是因为胎儿畸形。

The number of women having terminations of pregnancy after 12 weeks for psychosocial reasons is falling. Secondtrimester terminations now account for fewer than 8% of all therapeutic terminations of pregnancy. A minority of these women are having a therapeutic abortion for psychosocial reasons; the majority for fetal abnormality.

与妊娠早期流产不同，妊娠中晚期终止妊娠可能会导致明显的心理困扰，使精神疾病发生率增加。在因为胎儿畸形流产的女性中，约有 39% 在术后 3～9 个月时抑郁，这个比例在术后 1 年时降至正常。因心理社会原因而终止妊娠的女性，痛苦和消极情绪发生率增加的原因，可能是推迟了提出终止妊娠的时间。这个群体中可能有非常年轻的女性、智力障碍者、慢性精神病患者、对妊娠有明显矛盾心理的女性。

Unlike first-trimester abortions, later terminations of pregnancy are associated with both marked psychological distress and an increased rate of psychiatric disorder. Some 39% of women having an abortion for fetal abnormality are depressed at 3–9 months postoperatively, although the rates fall to normal at 1 year. For women undergoing this procedure for psychosocial reasons, the cause for the increased rate of distress and morbidity is likely to be found in the delay in presenting for termination. The very young, the mentally handicapped and the chronically mentally ill may be found in this group, as well as those who have experienced marked ambivalence about their pregnancies.

因胎儿异常而终止妊娠的女性的情况有所不同。她们通常是年龄较大的女性，有强烈的妊娠意愿，并且由于以前的经历或筛查而被诊断出问题。通常只有经过深思熟虑和万分痛苦，才能决定终止妊娠。因此，终止妊娠的后果非常像更晚期妊娠的自发流产，这让她们非常悲伤。可以通过给她们冠名和安葬的尊严，来帮助她们进行社会心理康复。大多数终止妊娠都涉及引产和产程延长。这是令人痛苦的经历，而医生和护理人员的敏感而富有同情心的处理，将帮助她们心理康复。

The situation for women having a termination of pregnancy because of fetal abnormality is different. These are often older women who have a much-wanted pregnancy and whose problem has been diagnosed either because of a previous experience or as the result of screening. The decision to terminate the pregnancy is usually reached only after much thought and anguish. The consequence of termination is therefore very much like the spontaneous loss of a more advanced pregnancy, that is to say, a grief reaction. Their psychosocial recovery may be assisted by granting them the dignity of a naming and burial. Most late terminations of pregnancy involve the induction of labour and a prolonged process of giving birth. This can be a distressing and traumatic experience, and psychological recovery will be improved by sensitive and compassionate handling by the doctor and nursing staff.

4. 终止妊娠后的避孕（Contraception following termination）

终止妊娠的推荐也是讨论以后避孕措施并为其做好准备的机会。终止妊娠可以与绝育一起进行，这样做的好处是，对于那些确定不会再要孩子的女性，可以防止再次终止妊娠。几乎没有证据表明这与并发症发生率或之后避孕失败有关。但是，由于绝育的"后悔率"增加，通常建议在终止妊娠和绝育之间有一定的时间间隔。置入 IUD 可以在终止妊娠的同时进行，并不会增加穿孔或失败的风险。如果使用口服避孕药，可以在当日或次日开始。

Referral for termination should also be an opportunity to discuss future contraception and to ensure that adequate provision is made for this after the termination. The procedure can be combined with sterilization. This has the advantage of preventing further terminations for the woman who is certain that she has completed her family. There is little evidence that this is associated with an increase in the rate of complications or later contraceptive failure. However, because of the increase in the 'regret rate' for the sterilization, an interval procedure is generally recommended. IUD insertion can be carried out at the same time as termination and is not associated with an increased risk of perforation or failure. If the oral contraceptive is being used, this can be started on the same or following day.

5. 非法流产（Criminal abortion）

在某些国家，尤其是在无法进行合法堕胎的欠发达国家中，各种操作引起的流产占流产的很大比例。如果法律中关于流产的适应证是宽松的，那么非法流产就少，但在许多国家，非法流产在自然流产中占比很大。世界卫生组织估计，全世界每年有25 万女性因流产而死亡，其中大多数是非法流产。自 1967 年以来，英国孕妇的流产死亡率从 37/100 万降至 1.4/100 万，自 1982 年以来，英国孕妇没有因非法流产而死亡。

Miscarriage induced by a variety of techniques makes up a substantial percentage of miscarriage in some countries, particularly in under-developed countries where legal abortion is not available. Where the indications for legal miscarriage are liberal, criminal abortion is infrequent, but in many countries, it contributes to a high percentage of apparently spontaneous miscarriages. The World Health Organization estimates that 250,000 women per year in the world die as a result of abortions, most of which are illegal. Mortality from abortion in the UK has fallen from a rate of 37/million maternities to 1.4/million since 1967. There have been no deaths from illegal abortion in the UK since 1982.

二、生殖道感染（Genital tract infections）

女性生殖道直接进入腹膜腔。感染可能扩散到生殖道的任何位置，一旦到达输卵管，感染通常是双侧的。

The female genital tract provides direct access to the peritoneal cavity. Infection may extend to any level of the tract and, once it reaches the Fallopian tubes, is usually bilateral.

生殖道有丰富的血液和淋巴管，能够抗感染，特别是在妊娠期间。

The genital tract has a rich anastomosis of blood and lymphatic vessels that serve to resist infection, particularly during pregnancy.

其他抗感染的自然屏障包括以下情况。

- 阴裂和阴道壁的自然合拢。

- 阴道酸性环境 – 性成熟女性阴道的低 pH，不适合大多数细菌生长，这种抵抗力在青春期前和绝经后女性中减弱。

- 宫颈黏液可作为预防感染上行的屏障。

- 子宫内膜周期性剥脱。

There are other natural barriers to infection:
- The physical apposition of the pudendal cleft and the vaginal walls.
- Vaginal acidity-the low pH of the vagina in the sexually mature female provides a hostile environment for most bacteria; this resistance is weakened in the prepubertal and postmenopausal female.
- Cervical mucus that acts as a barrier in preventing the ascent of infection.
- The regular monthly shedding of the endometrium.

（一）下生殖道感染（Lower genital tract infections）

生殖道感染中最常见的是外阴和阴道的感染，阴道感染也会引起急性和慢性宫颈炎。

The commonest infections of the genital tract are those that affect the vulva and vagina. Infections that affect the vagina also produce acute and chronic cervicitis.

1. 症状（Symptoms）

外阴皮肤红肿，伴有疼痛、瘙痒和性交困难。阴道炎的症状包括阴道分泌物、瘙痒、性交困难和排尿困难。宫颈炎的症状有化脓性阴道分泌物、腰骶部疼痛和下腹痛、性交困难和排尿困难。宫颈靠近膀胱，常导致膀胱三角炎和尿道炎并存，尤其是淋球菌感染。

Swelling and reddening of the vulval skin is accompanied by soreness, pruritus and dyspareunia. When the infection is predominantly one of vaginitis, the symptoms include vaginal discharge, pruritus, dyspareunia and often dysuria. Cervicitis

采集冶游史 **Taking a sexual history**	知识链接 **ABC**

掌握准确的冶游史对于处理生殖道感染至关重要，冶游史与一系列其他表现相关，其中包括生育能力低下、盆腔疼痛和性功能紊乱。简明扼要的冶游史将有助于以下情况的确认。

Taking an accurate sexual history is essential to the management of genital tract infections, and aspects of sexual history are relevant to a range of other presentations, including subfertility, pelvic pain and disorders of sexual function. A concise sexual history will help to:

- 识别特定的风险行为。
- 评估症状以指导检测。
- 根据风险确定需要检测的解剖部位。
- 评估其他相关的性健康问题，如妊娠风险和避孕需求。
- 告知咨询进展、所需健康教育和追访。

- identify specific risk behaviours
- assess symptoms to guide examination and testing
- identify anatomical sites for testing based on risk
- assess other related sexual health issues such as pregnancy risk and contraceptive needs
- inform the counselling process, health education required and contact tracing

患者（和学生）经常焦虑不安，所以创造一个轻松友好的环境，保持一种尊重、不评判的态度是很重要的。在询问冶游史时，自我介绍、保持眼神交流和适当的肢体语言是良好沟通的重要方面。应解释保密性质，要使用患者可以理解的语言，避免标签化或做出评判。先问一般的问题，开放式提问。然后继续探索病因，更多地封闭式提问（见后述）。解释为了评估危险，每个人都必须被问到一些"普遍性"问题，避免基于外表主观判断性取向。

Patients (and students!) are often anxious so it is important to create a relaxed and friendly environment and have a respectful and a non-judgemental attitude. Introducing self and role, maintaining eye contact and having appropriate body language are important aspects of good communication when obtaining a sexual history. The confidential nature of the consultation should be explained. It is important to use language that is understandable and does not use labels or make judgements. Ask general questions first, using open-ended questions. Move on to the exploration of reasons for presentation and more closed-ended questions (see later). Explain there are some 'universal' questions that are explicitly asked of everyone to assess risk, and avoid making assumptions about sexual orientation based on appearance.

具体问题
Specific questions

主诉，包括症状

有关症状的直接问题可能包括以下内容。

- 症状持续时间和严重程度。
- 尿道和阴道分泌物，如量、颜色、气味、特征。
- 阴道或直肠异常出血。
- 生殖器和生殖器外皮疹、肿块或溃疡。
- 会阴、肛周和阴部瘙痒和（或）不适。
- 下腹痛或性交困难。
- 排尿、排便或性交困难 / 疼痛。

Reason for attendance: the problem/issue, including symptoms

Direct questions about symptoms may include:

- duration and severity of symptoms
- urethral and vaginal discharge: amount, colour, odour, character
- abnormal vaginal or rectal bleeding
- genital and extra-genital rashes, lumps or sores
- itching and/or discomfort in the perineum, peri-anal and pubic region
- lower abdominal pain or dyspareunia
- difficulties/pain with micturition, defecation or during intercourse

性行为风险评估

- 末次性交。
- 无保护性交史。
- 过去 3~12 个月的性接触人数和性别（应询问所有男性是否曾经与其他男性发生过性关系）。
- 性活动的类型（口腔、肛门、阴道、玩具）。
- 性传播感染的预防措施，以及是否始终使用并保持完好（避孕套）。
- 与性接触者的关系（固定、不固定、认识、不认识）。
- 最近任何性接触者有任何症状或感染。

（续框）

Sexual behaviour risk assessment:

- last sexual intercourse (LSI)
- history of unprotected intercourse
- number and gender of sexual contacts in last 3–12 months (all men should be asked if they have ever had sex with another man in the past)
- type of sexual activity practised (oral, anal, vaginal, toys)
- STI prevention used and whether consistently used and remained intact (condoms)
- relationship with sexual contacts (regular, casual, known, unknown)
- have any recent sexual contacts who had any symptoms or infections

性传播感染和血液传播病毒的风险评估：评估检测时机和其他风险的附加问题

检测和治疗计划

- 先前性传播感染和血液传播病毒测试的日期和结果。
- 目前或过去的注射吸毒史、共用针头、注射器或身体穿刺和（或）文身史，其中包括国家、何时实施，以及是否使用无菌设备。
- 他们是否在国外发生过性行为（不是与同行的人）。
- 性工作者或与性工作者的性接触。
- 疫苗接种史，其中包括甲型肝炎、乙型肝炎和人乳头瘤病毒。

STI and blood-borne virus (BBV) risk assessment: additional questions to assess timing of tests and other risks to inform

testing and management planning:

- date and results of previous STI and BBV testing
- current or past history of injecting drug use, sharing of needles, syringes or of body piercing and/or tattoos, including country, when it was done and whether sterile equipment was used
- whether they have had sex overseas other than with the person they are traveling with
- sex industry worker or sexual contact with a sex worker
- vaccination history, including hepatitis A and B and HPV

其他相关信息：识别可能与患者治疗相关的问题

- 目前或最近的用药。
- 过敏史，尤其是对青霉素的不良反应。
- 避孕和生殖健康史，其中包括避孕药具的使用、依从性和末次正常月经（LNMP）。
- 宫颈细胞学史（或宫颈 HPV 评估），其中包括最后一次检查的日期和结果，过去的异常细胞学检查结果。
- 既往诊疗史和手术史（包括任何国外诊疗和输血）。
- 饮酒、吸烟和其他吸毒史。

Other relevant information: to identify issues that may be associated with or influence client management:

- current or recent medications
- history of allergies, especially adverse reaction to penicillin
- contraceptive and reproductive health history, including contraceptive use and compliance and last normal menstrual period (LNMP)
- cervical cytology history (or cervical HPV assessment), including date of last test and result, past abnormal cytology
- past medical and surgical history (including any overseas medical treatment and transfusions)
- alcohol, tobacco and other drug use

引自 NSW Sexually Transmissible Infections Programs Unit 2011. NSW Health Sexual Health Services Standard Operating Procedures Manual 2011.

Reproduced from NSW Sexually Transmissible Infections Programs Unit 2011. NSW Health Sexual Health Services Standard Operating Procedures Manual 2011.

is associated with purulent vaginal discharge, sacral backache, lower abdominal pain, dyspareunia and dysuria. The proximity of the cervix to the bladder often results in co-existent trigonitis and urethritis, particularly in the case of gonococcal infections.

50%～60% 的经产妇有慢性宫颈炎。症状有时很轻微，可能有轻度的脓性分泌物，这不足以让女性警戒，只会当作偶然的发现，而未去积极治疗。严重的症状有大量的阴道分泌物、慢性腰骶部疼痛、性交困难和偶尔性交后出血。对分泌物行细菌培养

通常是无菌的。由于宫颈黏液不利于精子通过，这种情况可能会导致不孕。

Chronic cervicitis is present in about 50–60% of all parous women. In many cases, the symptoms are minimal. There may be a slight mucopurulent discharge, which is not sufficient to trouble the woman and may simply present as an incidental finding that does not justify active treatment. In the more severe forms of the condition, there is profuse vaginal discharge, chronic sacral backache, dyspareunia and occasionally postcoital bleeding. Bacteriological culture of the discharge is usually sterile. The condition may cause subfertility because of hostility of the cervical mucus to sperm invasion.

2. 体征（Signs）

体征取决于病因。外阴皮肤外观变红，有时伴有溃疡和脱屑，性成熟女性的阴道壁可能溃烂，附着白色念珠菌分泌物斑。原虫感染时，分泌物多，呈绿白色泡沫状。

These will depend on the cause. The appearance of the vulval skin is reddened, sometimes with ulceration and excoriation. In the sexually mature female, the vaginal walls may become ulcerated, with plaques of white monilial discharge adherent to the skin or, in protozoal infections, the discharge may be copious with a greenish-white, frothy appearance.

前庭大腺位于小阴唇后部和阴道壁之间，性交时分泌黏液作为润滑剂。导管和腺体感染会导致导管闭合，并形成前庭大腺囊肿或脓肿。这种情况经常复发，引起外阴疼痛和肿胀。前庭炎很容易通过肿胀的部位和性质来识别。

Bartholin's glands are sited between the posterior part of the labia minora and the vaginal walls, and these two glands secrete mucus as a lubricant during coitus. Infection of the duct and gland results in closure of the duct and formation of a Bartholin's cyst or abscess. The condition is often recurrent and causes pain and swelling of the vulva. Bartholinitis is readily recognized by the site and nature of the swelling.

在宫颈炎中，宫颈出现发红和溃疡，如疱疹性感染一样，并且由于宫颈内膜受累而有黏液脓性分泌物，通过检查和取宫颈分泌物培养来诊断。

In cervicitis the cervix appears reddened and may be ulcerated, as with herpetic infections, and there is a mucopurulent discharge as the endocervix is invariably involved. The diagnosis is established by examination and taking cervical swabs for culture.

3. 常见下生殖道感染(Common organisms causing lower genital tract infections）

（1）阴道假丝酵母菌病（Vaginal candidiasis）：白假丝酵母菌是一种酵母菌病原体，天然存在于皮肤和肠道中。感染可能是无症状的，或者呈阴道分泌物增多或改变，伴有外阴疼痛和瘙痒。没有男女性传播的证据。阴道窥器检查可见阴道上皮附着白色凝乳样分泌物，但并非所有病例都有此特征。

Candida albicans is a yeast pathogen that occurs naturally on the skin and in the bowel. Infection may be asymptomatic or associated with an increased or changed vaginal discharge associated with soreness and itching in the vulva area. There is no evidence of male-to-female sexual transmission. White curd-like collections attached to the vaginal epithelium may be seen on speculum examination, although these are not present in all cases.

假丝酵母菌感染常见的诱因有妊娠、服用避孕药、免疫抑制状态（如 HIV 感染）、糖尿病和长期服用类固醇。在这些情况下，阴道的 pH 升高，细菌生长被抑制，导致酵母病原体大量生长，因为在 pH 允许的环境下它很容易生长繁殖。菌丝和孢子可以用湿片法检查，并可以培养。

Candidal infections are particularly common during pregnancy, in women taking the contraceptive pill and in underlying conditions involving immunosuppression, e.g. HIV infection, diabetes or long-term steroids. In each instance, vaginal acidity is increased above normal and bacterial growth in the vagina is inhibited in such a way as to allow free growth of yeast pathogens, which thrive well in a low-pH environment. Candida hyphae and spores can also be seen in a wet preparation and can be cultured.

（2）滴虫病（Trichomoniasis）：阴道毛滴虫是一种有鞭毛的单细胞原生动物，可感染宫颈、尿道和阴道。在男性中，该病原体可以被携带在尿道或前列腺中，通过性传播进行感染。巴氏涂片上也经常能看到这种微生物，患者甚至没有症状。最常见的症状是异常阴道出血，其他症状包括阴道疼痛和瘙痒。阴道 pH 通常高于 4.5。阴道分泌物的新鲜生理盐水涂片可以显示出活动的滴虫（图 19-9），很容易识别鞭毛的特征运动，并且可以对其进行培养。

Trichomonas vaginalis is a flagellated, single-celled protozoal organism that may infect the cervix, urethra and vagina. In the male the organism is carried in the urethra or prostate and infection is sexually transmitted. The organisms are often seen on the Pap smear even in the absence of symptoms. The commonest presentation is with abnormal vaginal bleeding, but other symptoms include vaginal soreness and pruritus. The vaginal pH is usually raised above 4.5. A fresh wet preparation in saline of vaginal discharge will show motile trichomonads (Fig. 19.9). The characteristic flagellate motion is easily recognized, and the organism can be cultured.

（3）生殖器疱疹（Genital herpes）：生殖器疱疹是由单纯疱疹病毒（herpes simplex virus，HSV）2 型引起的，不太常见的是 1 型。这是一种性传播疾病。原发性单纯疱疹病毒感染通常是全身感染，伴有发热、肌痛，偶尔伴有脑膜炎。局部症状包括阴道分泌物、

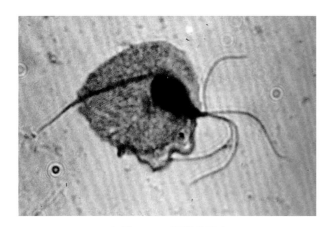

▲ 图 19-9　阴道毛滴虫

Fig. 19.9　*Trichomonas vaginalis.*

外阴疼痛、排尿困难和腹股沟淋巴结肿大。严重者可能有尿潴留。外阴病变包括生殖器周围出现水疱、糜烂或溃疡（图 19-10）。与宫颈发育不良的风险增加有关。伴侣可能无症状，潜伏期为 2～14 天。

The condition is caused by herpes simplex virus (HSV) type 2 and, less commonly, type 1. It is a sexually transmitted disease. Primary HSV infection is usually a systemic infection with fever, myalgia and occasionally meningism. The local symptoms include vaginal discharge, vulval pain, dysuria and inguinal lymphadenopathy. The discomfort may be severe enough to cause urinary retention. Vulval lesions include skin vesicles and multiple shallow skin ulcers (Fig. 19.10). The infection is also associated with an increased risk of cervical dysplasia. Partners may be asymptomatic, and the incubation period is 2–14 days.

诊断方法是从皮损处提取标本进行病毒培养或抗原检测。初次感染后病毒仍潜伏在骶神经节。复发可能由压力、月经或性交引起，但通常持续时间较短，比原发性发作轻。在已确定的皮损期血清抗体升高。

The diagnosis is made by sending fluid from vesicles for viral culture or antigen detection. After the initial infection the virus remains latent in the sacral ganglia. Recurrences may be triggered by stress, menstruation or intercourse but are normally of shorter duration and less severe than the primary episode. Serum antibodies are raised in well-established lesions.

(4) 细菌性阴道病（Bacterial vaginosis）：这是由于包括加德纳菌的厌氧微生物的过度生长，它不是性传播的。它可能是无症状的，或者有臭味的阴道分泌物和外阴刺激。它与 PID、尿路感染和产褥期感染的风险增加有关。下列 4 项中具备 3 项即可诊断。

This is due to an overgrowth of a number of anaerobic organisms, including *Gardnerella* spp. It is not sexually transmitted. It may be asymptomatic or cause a smelly vaginal

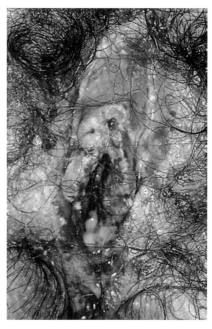

▲ 图 19-10　疱疹性外阴炎，病变也可发生在宫颈和外阴周围区域

Fig. 19.10　Herpetic vulvitis. Lesions can also occur in the cervix and in the perivulvar region.

discharge and vulval irritation. It is associated with an increased risk of PID, urinary tract infection and puerperal infection. Diagnosis is made by finding three of the following:

- 阴道分泌物 pH＞4.5。
- 典型匀质、稀薄、灰白色阴道分泌物。
- 在阴道分泌物里加入 10% 氢氧化钾溶液，产生烂鱼肉样的腥臭气味。
- 线索细胞阳性（图 19-11）。

- An increase in vaginal pH of more than 4.5
- A typical thin homogenous vaginal discharge
- A fishy odour produced when 10% potassium hydroxide is added to the discharge
- Clue cells on Gram-stained slide of vaginal fluid (Fig. 19.11)

(5) 淋球菌和衣原体性外阴阴道炎（Gonococcal and chlamydial vulvovaginitis）：这些微生物可导致盆腔炎性疾病（见后述），但也可能是无症状的，或仅仅表现为阴道分泌物和排尿困难。衣原体感染是目前最常见的 STI。

These organisms can result in extensive pelvic infection (see later) but may also be asymptomatic or indicated merely by vaginal discharge and dysuria. *Chlamydia* is the commonest STI seen today.

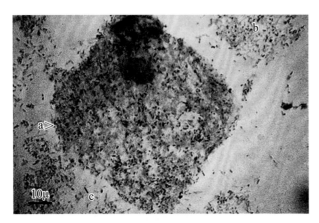

▲ 图 19-11　细菌性阴道病的线索细胞。它们是鳞状上皮细胞，表面附着多种细菌

a＞. 线索细胞；b. 正常上皮细胞；c. 细菌

Fig. 19.11　Clue cells in bacterial vaginosis. These are epithelial squamous cells with multiple bacteria adherent to their surface.

a＞, Clue Cell; b, Normal epithelial cell; c, bacteria.

（6）梅毒（Syphilis）：在感染梅毒螺旋体后 10～90 天左右开始出现症状。可出现原发性皮损，或者硬下疳，是一种硬丘疹，可形成溃疡，边缘隆起。这种病变最常发生在外阴，但也可能发生在阴道或宫颈。原发病灶可伴有腹股沟淋巴结肿大。硬下疳在 2～6 周内自行消退。

The initial lesion appears 10–90 days after contact with the spirochaete *Treponema pallidum*. The primary lesion or chancre is an indurated, firm papule, which may become ulcerated and has a raised firm edge. This lesion most commonly occurs on the vulva but may also occur in the vagina or cervix. The primary lesion may be accompanied by inguinal lymphadenopathy. The chancre heals spontaneously within 2–6 weeks.

硬下疳消失约 6 周后，出现二期梅毒的表现。皮疹发展为黄斑丘疹，常与脱发有关。出现丘疹，特别是在肛周、生殖器周围和口腔，并出现湿疣。

Some 6 weeks after the disappearance of the chancre, the manifestations of secondary syphilis appear. A rash develops which is maculopapular and is often associated with alopecia. Papules occur, particularly in the anogenital area and in the mouth, and give the typical appearance known as *condylomata lata*.

从原发性或继发性病变取拭子，暗视野下进行显微镜检查，可见螺旋体。血清学检测已在第 7 章中描述。

Swabs taken from either the primary or secondary lesions are examined microscopically under dark-ground illumination, and the spirochaetes can be seen. The serological tests have been described in Chapter 7.

然后，二期梅毒发展为三期梅毒。它可能影响身体的每一个系统，但最常见的长期病变是心血管系统和神经系统。

The disease then progresses from the secondary phase to a tertiary phase. It may mimic almost any disease process and affect every system in the body, but the common longterm lesions are cardiovascular and neurological.

（7）生殖器疣（尖锐湿疣）[Genital warts (condylomata acuminata)]：外阴和宫颈疣（图 19-12）是由 HPV 感染引起的。通常是通过性传播的，偶有其他传播方式。潜伏期长达 6 个月。在过去的 15 年中，发病率显著上升，尤其是在 16—25 岁的女性中，但是自从引入四价 HPV 疫苗，发病率已经显著下降。

Vulval and cervical warts (Fig. 19.12) are caused by HPV. The condition is commonly, although by no means invariably, transmitted by sexual contact. The incubation period is up to 6 months. The incidence had risen significantly over the last 15 years, particularly in women aged 16–25 years, but since the introduction of quadrivalent HPV vaccination the incidence has fallen considerably.

疣的外观与其他部位的相似，在外阴潮湿的环境中，尤其是在妊娠期间，疣通常会大量生长。经常伴有瘙痒和阴道分泌物，病变可扩散至肛周，有时合并继发感染。通常通过临床检查来诊断。

The warts have an appearance similar to those seen on the skin in other sites, and in the moist environment of the vulval skin are often prolific-particularly during pregnancy. There is frequently associated pruritus and vaginal discharge. The lesions may spread to the peri-anal region and in some cases become confluent and subject to secondary infection. Diagnosis is usually made by clinical examination.

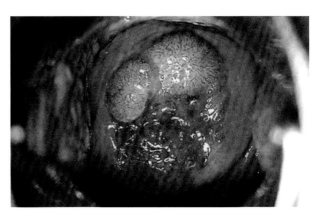

▲ 图 19-12　宫颈乳头状瘤病毒感染：尖锐湿疣

Fig. 19.12　Papilloma virus infection of the cervix: condylomata acuminata.

(8) 下生殖道感染的治疗（Treatment of lower genital tract infections）：通过检查和细菌学检测确定确诊后，即可采取适当的治疗措施。衣原体和淋病的治疗将在上生殖道感染讨论。只要诊断出性传播感染，就必须对患者（及其伴侣）进行其他感染筛查。

When the diagnosis has been established by examination and bacteriological tests, the appropriate treatment can be instituted. The treatment for *Chlamydia and gonorrhoea is* discussed later under infections of the upper genital tract. Whenever a diagnosis of STI is made, it is essential to screen patients (and their partners) for other infections.

外阴和阴道的假丝酵母菌感染可通过局部用药或口服制剂治疗，如单剂量的克霉唑栓剂或氟康唑口服。反复感染可通过口服酮康唑和氟康唑治疗。患者的伴侣应同时接受治疗。任何易感因素，如卫生条件差或糖尿病，都应予以纠正。

Vulval and vaginal monilial infections can be treated by topical or oral preparations. These include a single dose of clotrimazole given as a pessary or fluconazole taken orally. Recurrent infections can be treated by oral administration of ketoconazole and fluconazole. The patient's partner should be treated at the same time, and any predisposing factors such as poor hygiene or diabetes should be corrected.

滴虫感染和细菌性阴道病用甲硝唑 400mg 治疗，每天 2 次，连续 5 天，如果要避免感染复发，性伴侣双方都必须服用。甲硝唑可以 2g 的剂量单次给药，但孕期应避免大剂量给药。外用甲硝唑凝胶或克林霉素乳膏治疗细菌性阴道病也是有效的。

Trichomonas infections and bacterial vaginosis are treated with metronidazole 400 mg taken twice a day for 5 days, which must be taken by both sexual partners if recurrence of the infection is to be avoided. Metronidazole may be administered as a single dose of 2 g, but high-dose therapy should be avoided in pregnancy. Topical treatment with metronidazole gel or clindamycin cream is also effective for bacterial vaginosis.

如果患者常规巴氏涂片检查发现滴虫或念珠菌，但无症状，临床检查无阴道炎迹象，通常不需要对这些患者进行治疗。

If a patient is asymptomatic and there is no evidence of vaginitis on clinical examination but trichomonal or monilial organisms are identified in a routine Pap smear, treatment of these patients is usually not required.

非特异性阴道感染很常见，可使用阴道乳膏治疗，其中包括汞加芬、聚维酮碘、二碘羟基喹啉或磺胺乳膏。

Non-specific vaginal infections are common and are treated with vaginal creams, including hydrargaphen, povidone-iodine, di-iodohydroxyquinoline or sulphonamide creams.

梅毒首先用青霉素治疗，如果治疗失败，如合并感染耐青霉素的淋球菌，可使用盐酸多西环素或其他抗生素。

Syphilis is treated in the first instance with penicillin, and if this fails, for example in the case of co-infection with penicillin-resistant strains of the gonococcus, doxycycline hydrochloride or other antibiotics can be used.

萎缩性阴道炎可通过激素替代疗法进行治疗，即口服或阴道用雌激素制剂，如果有雌激素的禁忌证，可以使用乳酸栓子。对青少年外阴阴道炎也可采用同样的治疗方法，局部应用雌激素乳膏。

Infections of the vagina associated with menopausal atrophic changes are treated by the appropriate hormone replacement therapy using an oral or vaginal oestrogen preparation, or lactic acid pessaries when oestrogens are contraindicated. The same therapy may be used, with the local application of oestrogen creams, in juvenile vulvovaginitis.

前庭大腺的感染用抗相应菌的抗生素治疗。如果脓肿已经形成，应该椭圆形切开脓肿，并袋形缝合，从而使脓肿腔继续开放引流（图 19-13），这降低了脓肿复发的可能性。

Infections of Bartholin's gland are treated with the antibiotic appropriate to the organism. If abscess formation has occurred, the abscess should be 'marsupialized' by excising an ellipse of skin and sewing the skin edges to result in continued open drainage of the abscess cavity (Fig. 19.13). This reduces the likelihood of recurrence of the abscess.

外阴疣治疗或物理或化学透热疗法，使用鬼臼树脂直接用于表面的疣，还应治疗任何合并的阴道分泌物。

Vulval warts are treated with either physical or chemical diathermy using podophyllin applied directly to the surface of the warts. Any concurrent vaginal discharge should also receive the appropriate therapy.

众所周知，疱疹性感染对治疗有抵抗力，而且极易复发。最好的治疗方法是阿昔洛韦片剂，200mg，每日 5 次，连续 5 天，还局部使用 5% 的乳膏。

Herpetic infections are notoriously resistant to treatment and highly prone to recurrence. The best available treatment is acyclovir administered in tablet form 200 mg five times daily for 5 days or locally as a 5% cream.

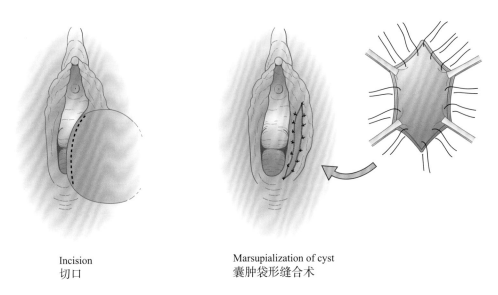

| Incision | Marsupialization of cyst |
| 切口 | 囊肿袋形缝合术 |

▲ 图 19-13　前庭大腺囊肿或脓肿的袋形缝合术，切口在囊肿的内侧（左），内层与皮肤缝合（右）

Fig. 19.13　Marsupialization of a Bartholin's cyst or abscess. The incision is made over the medial aspect of the cyst *(left)*, and the lining is sutured to the skin *(right)*.

急性宫颈炎通常与生殖道的广泛感染有关，根据微生物学诊断和治疗。对于慢性宫颈炎，因为很难识别出病原菌，抗生素也不能渗透宫颈腺的慢性微脓肿，所以药物治疗很少有效。如果宫颈拭子阴性，一个有效的治疗方法是在全身麻醉下对宫颈进行透热疗法。透热治疗后，应在阴道内放置抗菌乳膏，并应告知女性，2～3 周内分泌物会增加，但随后会减少。禁性生活 3 周，因为性生活可能导致继发性出血。

Acute cervicitis usually occurs in association with generalized infection of the genital tract and is diagnosed and treated according to the microbiology. Medical treatment is rarely effective in chronic cervicitis because it is difficult to identify an organism, and antibiotics do not penetrate the chronic microabscesses of the cervical glands. If the cervical swab is negative, the next most effective management is diathermy of the endocervix under general anaesthesia. Following diathermy, an antibacterial cream should be placed in the vagina, and the woman should be advised that the discharge may increase in amount for 2–3 weeks but will then diminish. She should also be advised to avoid intercourse for 3 weeks, as coitus may cause a secondary haemorrhage.

（二）上生殖道感染（Upper genital tract infections）

子宫内膜、子宫肌层、输卵管和卵巢的急性感染，通常是由下生殖道感染上行引起的。

Acute infection of the endometrium, myometrium, Fallopian tubes and ovaries are usually the result of ascending infections from the lower genital tract causing PID.

然而，阑尾炎或其他肠道感染可能会引起盆腔脓肿，从而引起上生殖道感染。阑尾穿孔合并盆腔脓毒症，仍然是输卵管阻塞和生育能力低下的常见原因。盆腔脓毒症也可能发生在产褥期、终止妊娠后或宫颈手术后。残留的胎盘组织和血液为来自肠道的微生物提供了极好的培养基，这些微生物包括大肠埃希菌、梭状芽孢杆菌、产气荚膜梭菌、金黄色葡萄球菌和粪链球菌。

However, infection may be secondary to appendicitis or other bowel infections, which sometimes give rise to a pelvic abscess. Perforation of the appendix with pelvic sepsis remains a common cause of tubal obstruction and subfertility. Pelvic sepsis may also occur during the puerperium and after pregnancy termination or after operative procedures on the cervix. Retained placental tissue and blood provide an excellent culture medium for organisms from the bowel, including *Escherichia coli*, *Clostridium welchii* or *C. perfringens*, *Staphylococcus aureus* and *Streptococcus faecalis*.

在发达国家，15—35 岁女性每年约有 1.7% 患有 PID。PID 患者中在 2 年内复发的比例高达 20%。PID 最常见于 15—24 岁女性，危险因素包括多个性伴侣、使用了经宫颈器械的手术。PID 是导致不孕的重要原因，在首发后，8% 的女性会输卵管不孕，复发导致的输卵管不孕的比例更是高达 2 倍。有 PID 病史的女性妊娠时，异位妊娠的可能性是正常人的 4 倍。

PID affects approximately 1.7% of women between 15 and 35 years of age per year in the developed world. Up to 20% of women with PID will have a further episode within 2 years. The disease is most common between the ages of 15 and 24 years, and particular risk factors include multiple sexual partners and procedures involving transcervical instrumentation. PID is an important cause of infertility. After a first episode, 8% of women will have evidence of tubal infertility; subsequent episodes approximately double this figure. Women with a past history of PID are four times more likely to have an ectopic pregnancy when they conceive.

 经验 有 3 次及以上 PID 发作的女性中，40% 有输卵管损伤。
Forty per cent of women who have had three or more episodes of PID have tubal damage.

1. 症状与体征（Symptoms and signs）

急性输卵管炎的症状包括几种情况。

The symptoms of acute salpingitis include:

- 急性双侧下腹痛：输卵管炎几乎都是双侧的；如果症状为单侧，则应考虑其他诊断。
- 严重性交疼痛。
- 异常月经出血。
- 白带脓性。
- Acute bilateral lower abdominal pain: Salpingitis is almost invariably bilateral; where the symptoms are unilateral, an alternative diagnosis should be considered
- Deep dyspareunia
- Abnormal menstrual bleeding
- Purulent vaginal discharge

然而，许多被确诊患有衣原体感染的女性根本没有任何症状。

However, many women shown to have chlamydial infection have no symptoms at all.

体征包括以下几种情况。

The signs include:

- 全身疾病伴发热和心动过速。
- 腹膜炎体征，肌紧张、反跳痛和腹壁局部强直（需要注意的是，如果腹腔内有出血，如异位妊娠，则很少出现肌紧张和腹壁强直，而即使没有腹膜炎，也会出现压痛和松反跳痛）。

- 盆腔检查时，宫颈刺激引起急性疼痛，阴道穹隆增厚，可能与输卵管内积脓引起的囊性输卵管肿胀有关，Douglas 腔内饱满表明存在盆腔脓肿（图 19-14）。
- 10%～25% 的患有衣原体性 PID 的女性会发生急性肝周围炎，这可能导致右上腹痛、肝功能紊乱以及肝表面和壁腹膜之间的多处粘连，被称为 Fitz-Hugh-Curtis 综合征。
- 38℃或以上的发热，有时伴寒战。

- Signs of systemic illness with pyrexia and tachycardia.
- Signs of peritonitis with guarding, rebound tenderness and often localized rigidity. (It should be noted that guarding and rigidity rarely are seen if blood is in the peritoneal cavity, such as due to an ectopic pregnancy, whereas tenderness and release tenderness are seen even in the absence of peritonitis.)
- On pelvic examination, acute pain on cervical excitation and thickening in the vaginal fornices, which may be associated with the presence of cystic tubal swellings due to pyosalpinges or pus-filled tubes; fullness in the pouch of Douglas suggests the presence of a pelvic abscess (Fig. 19.14).
- An acute perihepatitis occurs in 10–25% of women with chlamydial PID, which may cause right upper quadrant abdominal pain, deranged liver function tests and multiple filmy adhesions between the liver surface and the parietal peritoneum, and is known as the *Fitz-Hugh-Curtis syndrome*.
- A pyrexia of 38°C or more, sometimes associated with rigors.

2. 常见病原体（Common organisms）

PID 是主要由沙眼衣原体或淋病奈瑟菌（或两者）

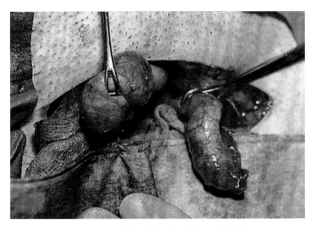

▲ 图 19-14 急性输卵管炎，输卵管肿胀、充血
Fig. 19.14 Acute salpingitis: the tubes are swollen and engorged.

感染引起的多种细菌感染，合并其他需氧菌和厌氧菌的机会性感染。

PID is thought to be the result of polymicrobial infection with primary infection by *Chlamydia trachomatis or Neisseria gonorrhoeae* (or both) allowing opportunistic infection with other aerobic bacteria and anaerobes.

(1) 衣原体（*Chlamydia*）：沙眼衣原体是专门的细胞内革兰阴性菌。在欧洲、澳大利亚和北美，它是最常见的细菌性的性传播感染，导致至少 60% 的 PID。在泌尿生殖诊所就诊的女性中，患病率为 11%～30%，在英国发病率最高的是 20—24 岁的女性。感染的主要部位是宫颈、尿道和直肠的柱状上皮，但许多女性无症状。宫颈感染女性中，约有 20% 发生上生殖道感染的上行。

C. trachomatis is an obligate, intracellular, Gram-negative bacterium. It is the commonest bacterial STI in Europe, Australia and North America and is thought to be the causative agent in at least 60% of cases of PID in those areas. Prevalence rates vary from 11% to 30% in women attending genitourinary medicine clinics, with the peak incidence in the UK in women aged 20–24 years. The main sites of infection are the columnar epithelium of the endocervix, urethra and rectum, but many women remain asymptomatic. Ascent of infection to the upper genital tract occurs in about 20% of women with cervical infection.

(2) 淋病奈瑟菌（*Gonorrhoea*）：淋病奈瑟菌是一种革兰阴性的胞内双球菌（图 19–15）。感染通常无症状，或有阴道分泌物。PID 的情况下，它会扩散到宫颈和子宫内膜表面，并在接触后 1～3 天内引起输卵管感染。它导致了 14% 的 PID，并与衣原体共同导致了另外 8% 的 PID。

N. gonorrhoeae is a Gram-negative, intracellular diplococcus (Fig. 19.15). Infection is commonly asymptomatic or associated with vaginal discharge. In cases of PID it spreads across the surface of the cervix and endometrium and causes tubal infection within 1–3 days of contact. It is the principal cause for 14% of cases of PID and occurs in combination with *Chlamydia* in a further 8%.

3. 鉴别诊断（Differential diagnosis）

急性盆腔感染通常很难确诊。与腹腔镜诊断相比，临床体征和症状的准确率为 65%～90%。鉴别诊断包括以下内容。

It is often difficult to establish the diagnosis of acute pelvic infection with any degree of certainty. The predictive value of clinical signs and symptoms when compared to laparoscopic diagnosis is 65–90%. The differential diagnosis

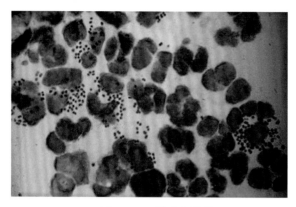

▲ 图 19-15　淋病奈瑟菌

Fig. 19.15　*Neisseria gonorrhoeae.*

includes the following:

- 输卵管异位妊娠：多数情况下初发疼痛是单侧的。可能有晕厥发作和膈肌刺激伴肩尖疼痛。白细胞计数正常或略有升高，但血红蛋白水平可能较低，具体取决于失血量，而在急性输卵管炎中，白细胞计数升高，血红蛋白浓度正常。

- Tubal ectopic pregnancy: Initially pain is unilateral in most cases. There may be syncopal episodes and signs of diaphragmatic irritation with shoulder tip pain. The white cell count is normal or slightly raised, but the haemoglobin level is likely to be low depending on the amount of blood lost, whereas in acute salpingitis, the white cell count is raised and the haemoglobin concentration is normal.

- 急性阑尾炎：疼痛是单侧的，盆腔检查通常不会显示出太多的疼痛和压痛，但必须记住，这两种情况有时是共存的，特别是感染的阑尾临近右输卵管。

- Acute appendicitis: The most important difference in the history lies in the unilateral nature of this condition. Pelvic examination does not usually reveal as much pain and tenderness, but it must be remembered that the two conditions sometimes co-exist, particularly where the infected appendix lies adjacent to the right fallopian tube.

- 急性尿路感染：可能产生类似症状，但很少产生腹膜炎症状，通常与尿路症状有关。

- Acute urinary tract infections: These may produce similar symptoms but rarely produce signs of peritonism and are commonly associated with urinary symptoms.

- 卵巢囊肿扭转或破裂。

- Torsion or rupture of an ovarian cyst.

4. 检查（Investigations）

当疑诊急性输卵管炎时，应住院治疗。完成病史和全身检查后，从阴道穹隆和宫颈管取拭子，送实验室进行培养和药敏试验。还应将中段尿样本送去进行培养，以排除可能的尿路感染。应另取一份尿样，通过聚合酶链反应（polymerase chain reaction，PCR）检测衣原体。尿道拭子可检测出宫颈拭子未发现的衣原体感染。与生殖道拭子相比，尿样的 PCR 检测具有相似或更好的灵敏度（90%），并为无症状女性的衣原体感染筛查提供了一种潜在手段。

When the diagnosis of acute salpingitis is suspected, the woman should be admitted to hospital. After completion of the history and general examination, swabs should be taken from the vaginal fornices and cervical canal and sent to the laboratory for culture and antibiotic sensitivity. A midstream specimen of urine should also be sent for culture to exclude a possible urinary tract infection. An additional endocervical swab urine sample should be taken for detection of *Chlamydia* by polymerase chain reaction (PCR). Urethral swabs may identify chlamydial infection not detected by endocervical swabs. PCR assays of urine samples have a similar or better sensitivity (90%) compared to genital tract swabs and offer a potential means for screening for chlamydial infection in asymptomatic women.

白细胞计数、血红蛋白测定和 C 反应蛋白的检测有助于确诊。如果发热明显，则需要进行血液培养。根据病史和检查结果对轻度至中度 PID 的诊断是不可靠的，如果不能确诊，需进行腹腔镜检查。

Examination of the blood for differential white cell count, haemoglobin estimation and C-reactive protein may help establish the diagnosis. Blood culture is indicated if there is a significant pyrexia. The diagnosis of mild to moderate degrees of PID on the basis of history and examination findings is unreliable and, where the diagnosis is in doubt, laparoscopy is indicated.

!
注
意
阴性拭子不排除 PID。

Negative swabs do not exclude the possibility of PID.

5. 治疗（Management）

当患者身体不适，出现腹膜炎、高热、呕吐或盆腔炎性包块时，应住院并按以下方式处理。

When the patient is unwell and exhibits peritonitis,

highgrade fever, vomiting or a pelvic inflammatory mass, she should be admitted to hospital and managed as follows:

- 静脉补液：呕吐和疼痛通常会导致脱水。

- 当临床怀疑 PID 时，应开始抗生素治疗。对于临床诊断的 PID，最初的抗生素治疗应该对沙眼衣原体、淋病奈瑟菌和以细菌性阴道病为特征的厌氧菌有效。如果女性出现急性不适，应静脉给予头孢呋辛和甲硝唑，同时口服多西环素等抗生素治疗，直至感染的急性期开始缓解。口服甲硝唑和多西环素应分别持续 7 天和 14 天。

- 使用非甾体抗炎症药物缓解疼痛。

- 如果子宫内有 IUD，开始抗生素治疗时立即取出。

- 卧床休息：在疼痛消退之前，必须制动。

- 避免性生活。

- Fluid replacement by intravenous therapy-vomiting and pain often result in dehydration.

- When PID is clinically suspected, antibiotic therapy should be commenced. Antibiotic therapy initially prescribed for clinically diagnosed PID should be effective against *C. trachomatis, N. gonorrhoeae* and the anaerobes characterizing bacterial vaginosis. If the woman is acutely unwell, treatment should be started with an antibiotic such as cefuroxime and metronidazole given intravenously with oral doxycycline until the acute phase of the infection begins to resolve. Treatment with oral metronidazole and doxycycline should then be continued for 7 and 14 days, respectively.

- Pain relief with non-steroidal anti-inflammatory drugs.

- If the uterus contains an IUD, it should be removed as soon as antibiotic therapy has been commenced.

- Bed rest-immobilization is essential until the pain subsides.

- Abstain from intercourse.

!
注
意
症状出现 3 天后就诊的女性，PID 后生殖力受损的风险，几乎是及时就诊女性风险的 3 倍。

Women who consulted after 3 days of symptoms had an almost threefold increased risk of impaired infertility after PID compared with those who consulted promptly.

全身情况良好的患者可以门诊治疗，使用单剂量阿奇霉素和 7 天疗程的多西环素，48h 后复查。

Patients who are systemically well can be treated as outpatients, with a single dose of azithromycin and a 7-day course of doxycycline, reviewed after 48 hours.

> **！注意**　在所有确诊的性传播感染病例中，性伴侣治疗非常重要，还要进行合适的性接触追溯。
>
> In all cases of confirmed STI, it is important to treat the partner and arrange appropriate contact tracing.

手术适应证（Indications for surgical intervention）：在大多数情况下，保守治疗能够完全缓解。开腹手术适于保守治疗不能缓解或盆腔有肿物。

In most cases, conservative management results in complete remission. Laparotomy is indicated where the condition does not resolve with conservative management and where there is a pelvic mass.

在大多数情况下，肿块是由输卵管积脓或输卵管卵巢脓肿引起的。可以引流，也可以行输卵管切除术。

In most cases, the mass will be due to a pyosalpinx or tubo-ovarian abscess. This can either be drained or a salpingectomy can be performed.

（三）慢性盆腔感染（Chronic pelvic infection）

急性盆腔感染可发展为慢性盆腔感染，并伴有输卵管扩张和阻塞，形成双侧输卵管积水和多发性盆腔粘连（图 19-16）。

Acute pelvic infections may progress to a chronic state with dilatation and obstruction of the tubes forming bilateral hydrosalpinges with multiple pelvic adhesions (Fig. 19.16).

1. 症状和体征（Symptoms and signs）

症状多种多样，其中包括以下情况。

- 慢性盆腔疼痛。

- 慢性的阴道脓性分泌物。

- 月经过多和痛经。

- 深部性交疼痛。

- 不孕。

Symptoms are varied but include:
- chronic pelvic pain
- chronic purulent vaginal discharge

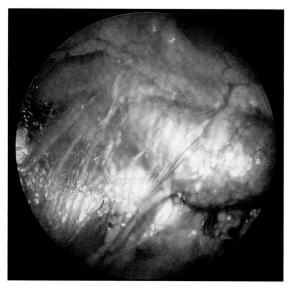

▲ 图 19-16　慢性盆腔炎性疾病，覆盖输卵管和卵巢的一层细粘连，埋入输卵管下方

Fig. 19.16　Chronic pelvic inflammatory disease: a sheet of fine adhesions covering the tubes and ovary, which is buried beneath the tube.

- epimenorrhagia and dysmenorrhoea
- deep-seated dyspareunia
- infertility.

慢性输卵管炎也与盆腔结缔组织感染有关，称为子宫旁炎。

Chronic salpingitis is also associated with infection in the connective tissue of the pelvis known as parametritis.

检查时，宫颈可能有脓性分泌物。子宫常后倾固定，穹隆增厚，双合诊疼痛。

On examination, there can be a purulent discharge from the cervix. The uterus is often fixed in retroversion, and there is thickening in the fornices and pain on bimanual examination.

> **经验**　有 PID 病史的女性中，25%～75% 会有慢性盆腔疼痛。
>
> Chronic pelvic pain occurs in 25–75% of women with a past history of PID.

2. 治疗（Management）

这种情况保守治疗很少有效，只有手术切除盆腔器官才能根治。有 PID 病史的女性行子宫切除术的可能性是普通人群的 8 倍。如果主要是由于输卵管疾病导致的不孕，最好的治疗方法是体外受精（in vitro fertilization，IVF）。如果存在输卵管积水，通常需要在 IVF 前切除输卵管，因为这样可以提高妊娠率。

Conservative management of this condition is rarely effective, and the problem is only eventually resolved by clearance of the pelvic organs. Women with a history of PID are eight times more likely to have a hysterectomy than the general population. If the problem is mainly infertility due to tubal disease, the best treatment is in vitro fertilization (IVF). Tubal removal prior to IVF is usually indicated if hydrosalpinges are present because this improves the pregnancy rate achieved.

（四）人类免疫缺陷病毒（Human immuno-deficiency virus，HIV）

HIV-1 和 HIV-2 是 RNA 反转录病毒，主要攻击人 CD4$^+$ T 淋巴细胞。最初被感染细胞比例很低，感染和临床症状之间有一个较长的潜伏期。可通过性交、受感染的血液制品、共用针头、母乳喂养和母婴传播。危险人群包括静脉注射吸毒者及其伴侣、双性恋男子的伴侣、血友病患者、性工作者和来自高危地区的移民。在发达国家，尽管 HIV 感染在男性中更为常见，但匿名检测显示，伦敦有 0.3% 的孕妇被感染，目前在 24—35 岁的非裔美国女性中，它是最常见的死亡原因。在撒哈拉沙漠以南的非洲地区，20%～30% 的孕妇携带 HIV。通过使用现代抗反转录病毒药物进行产前治疗、选择性剖腹产和避免母乳喂养，可将垂直传播率从 40% 降低到 1% 以下。尽管在过去，大多数 HIV 感染者会在几年内发展为艾滋病，像是无期徒刑，但通过现代的持续治疗，大多数感染都能够得到控制，而很少发展为艾滋病。

HIV-1 and HIV-2 are RNA retroviruses characterized by their tropism for the human CD4$^+$ (helper) T lymphocyte. The proportion of cells infected is initially low, and there is a prolonged latent phase between infection and clinical signs. Transmission occurs by sex, infected blood products, shared needles, breast-feeding and at the time of delivery. Risk groups include intravenous drug abusers and their partners, the partners of bisexual men, haemophiliacs, prostitutes and immigrants from high-risk areas. Although HIV infection is more common in men in the developed world, anonymous testing shows that 0.3% of pregnant women in London are infected, and it is now the most common cause of death in African American females aged 24–35 years in the United States. In parts of sub-Saharan Africa, 20–30% of all pregnant women are HIV positive. Vertical transmission rates can be reduced from 40% to less than 1% by antenatal treatment with the modern antiretroviral drugs, delivery by elective caesarean section and avoidance of breast-feeding. Although HIV infection was a life-ending

sentence for most people in the past, as most developed AIDS as an end result within a few years of becoming infected with HIV, with modern continuous therapy, most infections are able to be controlled and progression to AIDS is much less common.

主要临床特点如下。

- 感染后 3～6 个月出现流感样症状，与血清转化有关。

- 无症状免疫受损。

- 持续性全身淋巴结病。

- 艾滋病相关的特征性感染或肿瘤。

The main clinical states can be identified as:
- a 'flu-like' illness 3–6 months after infection, associated with seroconversion
- asymptomatic impaired immunity
- persistent generalized lymphadenopathy
- AIDS-related complex with pathognomonic infections or tumours.

常见的机会性感染包括念珠菌、单纯疱疹病毒、人乳头瘤病毒、分枝杆菌、隐孢子虫、卡氏支原体和巨细胞病毒。非感染性疾病包括体重减轻、腹泻、发热、痴呆、卡波西肉瘤和宫颈癌风险增加。

Common opportunistic infections include *Candida*, HSV, HPV, *Mycobacterium* spp., *Cryptosporidium* spp., *Pneumocystis carinii* and cytomegalovirus. Non-infective manifestations include weight loss, diarrhoea, fever, dementia, Kaposi's sarcoma and an increased risk of cervical cancer.

通过检测病毒抗体来诊断，但是这些抗体可能需要 3 个月才呈阳性。

The diagnosis is made by detecting antibodies to the virus, although these may take up to 3 months to appear.

三、女性性功能障碍（Disorders of female sexual function）

据报道多达 1/3 的女性有性功能障碍。有时，他们会意识到潜在的干扰因素，但往往，即使是对患者本人来说，这与其他情绪障碍之间的因果关系也是模糊的。因此，性功能障碍可能以精神或身体疾病，或者行为和关系障碍的形式出现，因此这不仅是医生的工作的一部分，而且是任何从事"护理"职业的人的工作的一部分。缺乏性知识和生殖道的解剖学知识的情况仍然很普遍，也是焦虑的根源。

Disorders of sexual function are reported by up to a third of women. Sometimes they are accompanied by awareness of the underlying disturbance, but often, as with other emotional difficulties, the link between cause and effect is obscure even to the sufferer. Sexual problems may therefore appear in the guise of mental or physical illness or disturbances of behaviour and relationships and thus form a part of the working experience not only of doctors but of anyone in the 'caring' professions. Lack of knowledge about sex and the anatomy of the genital tract remain common and a source of anxiety.

最常见的主诉包括以下几种情况。

- 性交疼痛。

- 阴道痉挛。

- 性欲丧失。

- 性高潮障碍。

The commonest complaints are:

- painful sex (dyspareunia)

- vaginismus

- loss of desire (libido)

- orgasmic dysfunction.

 经验 在问诊和检查过程中，应注意非语言交流。
Pay attention to the non-verbal communication during the consultation and examination.

（一）性交疼痛（Dyspareunia）

性交疼痛是指因疼痛而性交困难。这主要但不仅仅是女性的问题。根据疼痛是浅表的（阴道入口）还是深的（仅发生于阴茎深插入）来划分病因，因此获得简明扼要的病史尤为重要。

Dyspareunia is defined as painful intercourse. It is predominantly but not exclusively a female problem. The aetiology is divided on the basis of whether the problem is superficial (at the entrance to the vagina) or deep (only occurs with deep penile insertion), and it is therefore particularly important to obtain a concise history.

1. 浅表性交疼痛（Superficial dyspareunia）

浅表性交疼痛与外阴或阴道局部病变有关，病因如下。

Pain felt on penetration is generally associated with a local lesion of the vulva or vagina from one of the following causes:

- 感染：外阴和阴道的局部感染通常包括假丝

酵母菌性阴道炎和滴虫性阴道炎，前庭大腺的感染也会引起性交疼痛。

- Infection: Local infections of the vulva and vagina commonly include monilial and trichomonal vulvovaginitis. Infections involving Bartholin's glands also cause dyspareunia.

- 阴道口狭窄可能是先天性的，如处女膜狭窄或阴道狭窄。有时可能是阴道隔。导致阴道口狭窄的最常见原因是会阴切开伤口过度缝合、外阴裂伤或阴道脱垂修复。

- Narrowing of the introitus may be congenital, with a narrow hymenal ring or vaginal stenosis. It may sometimes be associated with a vaginal septum. The commonest cause of narrowing of the introitus is the over-vigorous suturing of an episiotomy wound or vulval laceration or following vaginal repair of a prolapse.

- 绝经期变化：由于雌激素缺乏引起的萎缩性阴道炎和阴道狭窄可能导致性交疼痛。萎缩性外阴疾病，如硬化性苔藓，也可引起行交疼痛。

- Menopausal changes: Atrophic vaginitis or the narrowing of the introitus and the vagina from the effects of oestrogen deprivation may cause dyspareunia. Atrophic vulval conditions such as lichen sclerosus can also caus pain.

- 外阴痛：病因不明，特点为外阴持续疼痛。

- Vulvodynia: This is a condition of unknown aetiology characterized by persisting pain over the vulva.

- 功能性改变：性刺激不充分导致润滑不足，以及情感问题、性交困难。

- Functional changes: Lack of lubrication associated with inadequate sexual stimulation and emotional problems will result in dyspareunia.

2. 深部性交疼痛（Deep dyspareunia）

深部插入疼痛常与盆腔病理学有关。任何在正常性生活后出现深度性交疼痛的女性，除非另有证据，否则都应考虑器质性原因。深部性交疼痛的常见原因包括以下情况。

Pain on deep penetration is often associated with pelvic pathology. Any woman who develops deep dyspareunia after enjoying a normal sexual life should be considered to have an organic cause for her pain until proved otherwise. The common causes of deep dyspareunia include:

- 急性或慢性 PID：其中包括宫颈炎、输卵管积脓和输卵管卵巢炎（图 19-16）。子宫可能会被固定，需要鉴别诊断异位妊娠。

- Acute or chronic pelvic inflammatory disease: including cervicitis, pyosalpinx and salpingo-oophoritis (see Fig. 19.16). The uterus may become fixed. Ectopic pregnancy must also be considered in the differential diagnosis in this group.

- 子宫后倾和卵巢脱垂：如果卵巢脱垂到 Douglas 腔中，并固定在该位置，则在性交插入较深时疼痛。

- Retroverted uterus and prolapsed ovaries: If the ovaries prolapse into the pouch of Douglas and become fixed in that position, intercourse is painful on deep penetration.

- 子宫内膜异位症：子宫内膜异位症的活动性病变和慢性瘢痕都可能引起疼痛。

- Endometriosis: Both the active lesions and the chronic scarring of endometriosis may cause pain.

- 宫颈和阴道肿瘤性疾病：这种情况下一部分疼痛与继发感染有关。

- Neoplastic disease of the cervix and vagina: At least part of the pain in this situation is related to secondary infection.

- 术后瘢痕：这可能导致阴道穹隆变窄和子宫失去活动性。狭窄通常发生在阴道修补术后，较少发生在阴道高位撕裂修补术后。阴道瘢痕也可能是由化学制剂引起的，如岩盐，在一些国家，岩盐被放入阴道以产生挛缩。

- Postoperative scarring: This may result in narrowing of the vaginal vault and loss of mobility of the uterus. The stenosis commonly occurs following vaginal repair and, less often, following repair of a high vaginal tear. Vaginal scarring may also be caused by chemical agents such as rock salt, which, in some countries, is put into the vagina in order to produce contracture

- 异物：有时阴道或子宫内的异物可能导致男性或女性伴侣疼痛。如折针的残余物，或者宫内节育器被挤出的部分，可能会导致男性伴侣剧烈疼痛。

- Foreign bodies: Occasionally, a foreign body in the vagina or uterus may cause pain in either the male or female partner. For example, the remnants of a broken needle or partial extrusion of an IUD may cause severe pain in the male partner.

3. 性交不能（Apareunia）

性交不能是指性交"缺失"或者无性交能力，

常见病因如下。

- 先天性无阴道。

- 处女膜闭锁。

Apareunia is defined as the 'absence' of intercourse or the inability to have intercourse at all. The common causes are:
- congenital absence of the vagina
- imperforate hymen.

4. 治疗（Treatment）

准确的诊断取决于详细询问病史和彻底的盆腔检查，治疗取决于病因。先天性无阴道可通过手术矫正（阴道成形术）治疗，处女膜闭锁可以进行切除术。

Accurate diagnosis is dependent on careful history taking and a thorough pelvic examination. The treatment will therefore be dependent on the cause. Congenital absence of the vagina can be successfully treated by surgical correction (vaginoplasty), and removal of the imperforate hymen is effective.

深部性交疼痛的药物治疗，其中包括使用抗生素和抗真菌药物治疗盆腔炎性疾病，以及使用局部或口服激素治疗绝经后萎缩性阴道炎。子宫内膜异位症的治疗见第 16 章。外科治疗包括矫正狭窄和切除疼痛瘢痕，对功能障碍患者进行安抚和性咨询是必要的。

Medical treatment for deep dyspareunia includes the use of antibiotics and antifungal agents for pelvic infection, and the use of local or oral hormone therapy for postmenopausal atrophic vaginitis. Treatment for endometriosis is discussed in Chapter 16. Surgical treatment includes correction of any stenosis and excision of painful scars where appropriate, and reassurance and sexual counselling are necessary in functional disorders.

（二）阴道痉挛（Vaginismus）

阴道痉挛是由于盆底肌肉和大腿内收肌痉挛而引起的症状，它会阻止阴茎插入，或者在尝试插入时导致强烈的疼痛。物理障碍可能存在，但不一定是病因，患者可能不允许任何人触摸外阴。原发性阴道痉挛通常是由于害怕插入性行为。继发性阴道痉挛更可能是感染、性侵、难产或手术后的性交疼痛的结果。即使在病情好转后，对再次疼痛的恐惧可能会导致阴道肌肉的非自主收缩，这本身就很疼痛，这是一个恶性循环。鼓励患者探索自己的阴道，自己感觉到没有异常或疼痛，有助于打破这种恶性

509

循环。诉诸手术很可能会加重患者的恐惧，而且无法改善症状。

Vaginismus is the symptom resulting from spasm of the pelvic floor muscles and adductor muscles of the thigh, which prevents or results in pain on attempted penile penetration. A physical barrier may be present but is not necessarily causative. The woman may be unable to allow anyone to touch the vulva. Primary vaginismus is usually due to fear of penetration. Secondary vaginismus is more likely to be the result of an experience of pain with intercourse after infection, sexual assault, a difficult delivery or surgery. Even after the condition has improved, fear of further pain may lead to involuntary contraction of the vaginal muscles, which is in itself painful, completing the vicious circle. Encouraging the patient to explore her own vagina and feel for herself that there is no abnormality or pain can help break this cycle. Resort to surgery is likely to confirm the patient's fears of abnormality and often leaves the presenting problem unchanged.

（三）性欲丧失（Loss of libido）

性欲丧失是女性性功能障碍最常见的症状。如果持续存在，可能是由于教育或宗教信仰而对性欲有羞耻感，从而压制性欲。这或许代表夫妻之间期望的差异。在曾有过令人满意的关系中，后来的性欲丧失可能是由于以下原因。

Loss of desire is the commonest symptom in women complaining of sexual dysfunction. If it has always been present, it may be a result of a repression of sexual thoughts as a result of upbringing or religious belief or a feeling that sex is dirty or unsuitable in some way. It may represent differences between the expectations of the couple. Loss of desire in a relationship that was previously satisfactory is more likely to be due to:

- 重大生活事件，如婚姻、妊娠。

- 生病、抑郁或悲伤。

- 内分泌或神经系统疾病。

- 性交疼痛。

- 药物（框 19–3）。

- 绝经期。

- 害怕妊娠或感染。

- 压力或慢性焦虑。

- major life events-marriage, pregnancy

- being ill, depressed or grieving

- endocrine or neurological disorders

- pain on intercourse

框 19–3　可能损害性欲的药物	Box 19.3　Drugs that may impair libido
• 抗雄激素，如环丙孕酮 • 抗雌激素，如三苯氧胺和一些避孕药 • 细胞毒性药物 • 镇静药 • 麻醉品 • 抗抑郁药 • 酒精和非法药物滥用	• Antiandrogens-cyproterone • Anti–oestrogens-tamoxifen and some contraceptives • Cytotoxic drugs • Sedatives • Narcotics • Antidepressants • Alcohol and illegal drug misuse

- medication (Box 19.3)

- menopause

- fear of pregnancy or infection

- stress or chronic anxiety.

1. 治疗（Treatment）

帮助夫妇寻找潜在的原因，有助于制订治疗方案。对于情感因素的夫妻，关系治疗可以作为一种选择。如果是绝经期的性欲减退，那么偶尔会对低剂量睾酮治疗和常规雌激素激素替代疗法产生反应。

Helping the couple to look at the underlying reasons involved helps to identify what they might do to correct the situation. Relationship therapy may be an option for suitably motivated couples. Where loss of libido is a feature of menopausal symptoms, this will occasionally respond to low-dose testosterone therapy, along with conventional oestrogen hormone replacement therapy.

（四）性高潮障碍（Orgasmic dysfunction）

到 40 岁时，有 5%～10% 的女性没有经历过性高潮。性高潮障碍通常与男性有责任给女性性高潮的观念有关。打破对自体刺激的抑制、鼓励在前戏和性交中进行良好沟通，对这个问题会有所帮助。

About 5–10% of women have not experienced orgasm by the age of 40 years. Orgasmic dysfunction is often linked to myths about it being the responsibility of the man to bring the woman to orgasm. The problem can be helped by breaking down inhibitions about self-stimulation and encouraging better communication during foreplay and intercourse.

四、男性性功能障碍（Disorders of male sexual function）

正常的男性性功能主要通过自主神经系统介导。勃起是副交感神经（胆碱能）兴奋引起血管充血的结果。高潮和射精主要是交感神经（肾上腺素能）支配。前列腺、输精管和精囊中的液体依次进入后尿道，膀胱颈的开放和闭合是由 α 肾上腺素能系统介导的，而外括约肌的开放（允许顺行射精）是通过阴部神经的躯体传输神经介导的。射精受到阴茎背神经的刺激，并涉及球海绵体、坐骨直肠肌和后尿道的收缩活动。皮质的影响、激素或神经或血管机制受损，容易抑制这些反应。

Normal male sexual function is largely mediated through the autonomic nervous system. Erection occurs as a result of parasympathetic (cholinergic) outflow causing vasocongestion. Orgasm and ejaculation are predominantly sympathetic (adrenergic). Emission occurs by the sequential expulsion of fluid from the prostate gland, vas deferens and seminal vesicles into the posterior urethra. Emission and closure of the vesical neck are mediated by alphaadrenergic systems, while opening of the external sphincter (to allow antegrade ejaculation) is mediated through the somatic efferent of the pudendal nerve. Ejaculation is stimulated by the dorsal nerve of the penis and involves contractile activity of the bulbocavernous and ischiorectal muscles as well as the posterior urethra. These responses are easily inhibited by cortical influences or by impaired hormonal, neural or vascular mechanisms.

男性性功能障碍的主要特征如下。

• 勃起不能。

• 射精问题。

• 性欲丧失。

The principal features of sexual dysfunction in men are:

• failure to achieve erection

• problems with ejaculation

• loss of libido.

这些症状的全部或任何一个，都可能从青春期开始出现，或者在有过健康性生活后的任何时间发病。性欲丧失的原因已在女性性功能障碍中描述过。

All or any of these may be present from adolescence or have their onset at any time of life after a period of healthy sexuality. The causes of loss of libido have been previously described under female sexual dysfunction.

（一）勃起功能障碍（Erectile dysfunction）

勃起功能障碍或阳痿，无法达到或维持完成性交所需的勃起状态，是最常见的问题。

Erectile dysfunction or impotence, the inability in the male to achieve erection for satisfactory penetration of the vagina, is the most common problem seen.

现在人们认识到，患有勃起功能障碍的男性中有很高比例（50%），有潜在的器质性病因，特别是40 岁以上的男性。其中，糖尿病最常见的原因，它引起大小血管损伤和神经病变。神经性阳痿也可能由脊髓、大脑和前列腺损伤及多发性硬化引起。高泌乳素血症与勃起功能障碍及性欲丧失有关。虽然雄激素对勃起不是必需的，但它们可以通过影响性欲和阴茎海绵体中氮氧化物的释放来影响勃起。酒精等娱乐性药物会导致勃起障碍，超过 200 种处方药会产生此不良反应。其中最常见的是降压药和利尿药，还包括抗抑郁药和镇静药。

Erectile dysfunction or impotence, the inability in the male to achieve erection for satisfactory penetration of the vagina, is the most common problem seen. It is now recognized that a high proportion (50%) of such men, especially those over the age of 40 years, have an underlying organic cause. Of these, diabetes is the commonest as a result of damage to the large and small blood vessels and neuropathy. Neurological impotence may also be caused by injuries to the spinal cord, brain and prostate and multiple sclerosis. Hyperprolactinaemia is associated with erectile dysfunction as well as with loss of libido. While androgens are not essential for erection, they influence it through their effects on libido and nitrogen oxide release in the cavernosum. Recreational drugs such as alcohol are known to cause erectile failure, and more than 200 prescription drugs are known to have it as a side effect. The most common of these are antihypertensive and diuretic agents. Others include antidepressant and sedative medications.

在年轻人中，原因更可能是心理因素。反应性或内源性的抑郁，是一个重要的病因或伴随条件。在不孕症的夫妇中，因迎合排卵而定时性交的压力可能导致勃起功能障碍。

In the younger age group, the cause is more likely to be psychogenic. Depression, reactive or endogenous, is an important aetiological or concomitant condition. The stress provoked by timing intercourse with ovulation may result in erectile dysfunction in couples undergoing treatment for infertility.

治疗（Treatment）

对于轻度的心因性患者，简单的治疗措施就会有效，如咨询、性治疗和感官集中训练。

Mild psychogenic cases will usually respond to simple measures such as counselling, sex therapy and sensate focusing exercises.

在催乳素水平升高的情况下，用溴隐亭治疗可以恢复性功能。

Treatment with bromocriptine may restore sexual function in cases where prolactin levels are raised.

虽然疼痛、对注射的恐惧会导致一些患者停止治疗，但是阴茎海绵体内注射前列腺素 E₁ 对精神性和器质性勃起功能障碍的患者都有效，西地那非是有效的口服替代药物，有 70% 的性交成功率，而安慰剂组只有 22%。它通过增强一氧化氮对血管平滑肌的作用，从而增加阴茎的血流量，达到促进勃起的作用。同时使用硝酸酯治疗心肌缺血性疾病的患者会出现显著的低血压。

Intracavernous injection of prostaglandin E_1 is effective in patients with both psychogenic and organic causes of erectile dysfunction, although pain and the fear of injection cause some patients to stop treatment. Sildenafil is an effective orally administered alternative, with up to 70% of attempts at intercourse being successful compared with 22% with placebo. It promotes erection by potentiating the effect of nitric oxide on vascular smooth muscle, thus increasing blood flow to the penis. Concurrent use in patients taking nitrate therapy for myocardial ischaemic disease causes significant hypotension.

（二）射精问题（Ejaculatory problems）

射精功能障碍包括早泄、射精迟缓、逆行射精和无射精。无射精和早泄多见于年轻患者。逆行射精通常是由器质性原因或手术引起的，如前列腺手术，此时通常根据病史作出诊断。

Ejaculatory dysfunction encompasses premature, retarded, retrograde and absent ejaculation. Anejaculation and premature ejaculation are more often seen in younger patients. Retrograde ejaculation is often a result of an organic cause or after surgery, e.g. prostate operations. The diagnosis is usually made on the presenting history.

治疗（Treatment）

对于早泄，使用 Masters 和 Johnson 描述的"挤捏法"，挤压龟头，这减少了射精的冲动，尽管成功率很低。替代方法包括使用局部麻醉剂和选择性 5-羟色胺再摄取抑制药。对于无射精和射精迟缓，可以通过教授手淫技术、夫妻咨询和感官集中练习来治疗。逆行射精主要是一个生育问题，治疗包括手术、α 肾上腺素受体激动药的药物治疗。

For premature ejaculation, the squeeze technique described by Masters and Johnson involves application of pressure to the top of the penis. This diminishes the urge to ejaculate, although the success rate is poor. Alternative approaches include the use of a local anaesthetic and selective serotonin-reuptake inhibitors. Anejaculation and retarded ejaculation can be treated by teaching masturbation techniques, couple counselling and sensate focus exercises. Retrograde ejaculation is regarded mainly as a fertility problem. Treatment may involve surgery or drug therapy with alpha-adrenoceptor agonists.

本章概览	Essential information
宫内节育器 • 防止受精和胚胎植入 • 惰性或药理活性 • 最适合高龄经产妇 • 可在分娩时置入 • 3～5 年后更换 • 失败率为每年 0.2～0.8 次 /100 名女性 • 并发症：穿孔、PID、异常出血、异位妊娠	**IUDs** • Prevent implantation and fertilization • Inert or pharmacologically active • Best for older multiparous women • Can be inserted at time of delivery • Replace after 3–5 years • Failure rate 0.2–0.8/100 women-years • Complications: perforation, PID, abnormal bleeding, ectopic pregnancy
复方避孕药 • 抑制促性腺激素，但也有其他作用 • 雌二醇和孕激素 • 妊娠、血栓栓塞和肝病禁忌 • 1.3/10 万的死亡率 • 失败率为每年 0.3 次 /100 名女性	**Combined OCP** • Suppress gonadotrophins, but have other effects as well • Oestradiol and progestogen • Pregnancy, thromboembolism and liver disease contraindicate • 1.3/100,000 mortality • Failure rate 0.3/100 women-years
绝育 • 1/200 失败率（女性） • 如果手术失败，异位妊娠风险增加 • 永久性 • 手术风险 • 替代方案	**Sterilization** • 1/200 failure rate (female) • Increased risk of ectopic pregnancy if procedure fails • Permanence • Risks of surgery • Alternatives

（续表）

本章概览	Essential information
终止妊娠 • 方法 　– 手术 　– 药物 • 并发症 　– 出血 　– 感染 　– 不孕 　– 组织残留 　– 反悔	**Termination of pregnancy** • Methods: 　– surgical 　– medical • Complications: 　– bleeding 　– infection 　– infertility 　– retained tissue 　– regret
外阴阴道炎 • 最常见的生殖道感染 • 表现为瘙痒、性交疼痛或阴道分泌物 • 常见原因是滴虫、细菌性阴道病和假丝酵母菌 • 易感因素包括妊娠、糖尿病、避孕药 • 可通过检查阴道分泌物的新鲜湿涂片进行诊断	**Vulvovaginitis** • Commonest infection of genital tract • Presents as pruritus, dyspareunia or discharge • Common causes are *Trichomonas*, bacterial vaginosis and *Candida* • Predisposing factors include pregnancy, diabetes, contraceptive pill • Can be diagnosed by examination of fresh wet preparation of vaginal discharge
生殖器疱疹 • 由 HSV 引起 • 阴道 / 外阴出现疼痛、出血、水疱或浅溃疡 • 与宫颈发育不良相关 • 易复发，但严重程度降低 • 如果活跃，在阴道分娩期间可传播给新生儿	**Herpes genitalis** • Caused by HSV • Presents with pain, bleeding and vesicles or shallow ulcers on the vagina/vulva • Associated with cervical dysplasia • Tends to be recurrent but with decreasing severity • Can be transmitted to the neonate during vaginal delivery if active
宫颈感染 • 急性（与全身感染相关）或慢性 • 阴道分泌物、性交疼痛、下腹痛或腰背痛、泌尿系统症状和产后出血 • 可能导致不育 • 慢性病时难以分离病原体 • 治疗包括适当的抗生素和烧灼术	**Infections of the cervix** • Acute (associated with generalized infection) or chronic • Discharge, dyspareunia, low abdominal pain or backache, urinary symptoms and postcoital bleeding • Can cause subfertility • Difficult to isolate an organism when chronic • Treatment includes appropriate antibiotics and cautery
上生殖道感染 • 通常来自下生殖道感染向上蔓延 • 可以发生于流产、正常分娩或子宫颈手术后 • 通常是由于沙眼衣原体或淋病奈瑟球菌的性传播引起 • 表现为疼痛、发热、阴道分泌物和月经周期不规则 • 刺激宫颈时双侧疼痛，白细胞计数升高 • 鉴别诊断包括异位妊娠、尿路感染和阑尾炎 • 治疗包括补液、抗生素、镇痛和休息 • 对于疑诊病例，手术（腹腔镜或开腹手术）可用于确诊、盆腔肿块引流和清理无反应性慢性患者的骨盆 • 全球不孕的主要原因，发作 3 次及以上后，导致 40% 的病例发生输卵管阻塞	**Upper genital tract infection** • Usually from ascending lower genital tract infection • Can follow abortion, normal delivery or an operative procedure on the cervix • Commonly due to *C. trachomatis or N. gonorrhoeae* when sexually transmitted • Presents as pain, fever, discharge and irregular periods • Bilateral pain on cervical excitation and raised white cell count • Differential diagnosis includes ectopic pregnancy, urinary tract infection and appendicitis • Management includes fluid replacement, antibiotics, analgesia and rest • Surgery (laparoscopy or laparotomy) is indicated to confirm diagnosis if in doubt, for drainage of pelvic mass and to clear pelvis in unresponsive chronic disease • Major cause of infertility worldwide, resulting in tubal obstruction in 40% of cases after three or more attacks

（续表）

本章概览	Essential information
HIV 感染 • 辅助性 T 淋巴细胞和中枢神经系统的反转录病毒感染 • 性、输血或垂直传播（分娩或母乳喂养） • 通过血清学、淋巴细胞计数或机会性感染进行诊断 • 可能无症状、引起全身不适和淋巴结病或艾滋病 • 药物治疗、选择性剖宫产和避免母乳喂养可降低垂直传播率 • 异性恋者发病率增加 • 进行反转录病毒治疗中，很少进展为艾滋病	**HIV infection** • Retrovirus infection of T-helper cells and central nervous system • Transmitted by sex, blood transfusion or to offspring (delivery or due to breast-feeding) • Diagnosis by serology, differential lymphocyte count or opportunistic infection • Can be asymptomatic, cause generalized malaise and lymphadenopathy or AIDS • Rates of vertical transmission can be reduced by drug treatment, elective caesarean section and avoiding breast-feeding • Incidence in heterosexuals increasing • With current retroviral therapy, progressing to AIDS is rare
性功能障碍 • 性交疼痛 　– 通常由感染、萎缩或缺乏润滑引起 　– 深部性交疼痛表明盆腔病变 • 阴道痉挛和性欲丧失通常是心理因素造成的 • 勃起障碍，如器质性（50%）或精神性	**Disorders of sexual function** • Dyspareunia: 　– often caused by infection, atrophic conditions or lack of lubrication 　– deep dyspareunia indicates pelvic pathology • Vaginismus and loss of libido are often psychogenic • Failure to achieve erection-organic (50%) or psychogenic

第 20 章　妇科肿瘤

Gynaecological oncology

Hextan Y. S. Ngan　　Karen K. L. Chan　著　　颜　磊　译　　石玉华　校

学习目标

学习本章后你应当能够：

知识标准
- 理解妇科肿瘤的流行病学、病因、诊断、处理和预后。
- 描述女性生殖道常见肿瘤的病因、流行病学和表现，其中包括：
  - 外阴和宫颈上皮内瘤变。
  - 外阴癌和阴道癌。
  - 宫颈癌。
  - 子宫内膜增生症。
  - 子宫内膜癌。
  - 卵巢恶性肿瘤。
- 讨论微创操作和影像诊断性操作在妇科肿瘤处理中的作用，其中包括：
  - 宫颈和内膜活检。
  - 超声。
  - 腹腔镜。
  - 宫腔镜。
  - MRI 和 CT。
- 列举妇科肿瘤药物和手术治疗的短期和长期并发症。
- 讨论筛查和预防接种在女性生殖道恶性疾病中的预防作用。

临床能力
- 为一名女性宫颈鳞癌临床前期筛查做咨询。
- 为具有生殖道恶性肿瘤症状的女性做初诊计划。
- 与女性及其家人就妇科肿瘤的诊断进行谨慎的沟通。

专业技能和态度
- 讨论妇科肿瘤姑息治疗原则。

LEARNING OUTCOMES

After studying this chapter you should be able to:

Knowledge criteria
- Understand the epidemiology, aetiology, diagnosis, management and prognosis of gynaecological cancer
- Describe the aetiology, epidemiology and presentation of the common neoplasms of the female genital tract, including:
  - Vulval and cervical intraepithelial neoplasia
  - Vulval and vaginal carcinoma
  - Cervical carcinoma
  - Endometrial hyperplasia
  - Endometrial carcinoma
  - Malignant ovarian tumours
- Discuss the role of minor procedures and diagnostic imaging procedures in the management of gynaecological cancers, including:
  - Cervical and endometrial sampling
  - Ultrasound
  - Laparoscopy
  - Hysteroscopy
  - Magnetic resonance imaging and computerized tomography
- List the short- and long-term complications of medical and surgical therapies for gynaecological cancer
- Discuss the role of screening and immunization in the prevention of female genital tract malignancy

Clinical competencies
- Counsel a woman about screening for the preclinical phase of squamous cell carcinoma of the cervix
- Plan initial investigation of women presenting with symptoms of genital tract malignancy
- Communicate sensitively with a woman and her family about the diagnosis of gynaecological cancer

Professional skills and attitudes
- Discuss the principles of palliative care in gynaecological cancers

一、外阴病变（Lesions of the vulva）

（一）外阴鳞状上皮内瘤变（Vulval intraepithelial neoplasia, VIN）

外阴鳞状上皮内瘤变（VIN）是一种以上皮结构失去极性和丧失为特征的疾病，可贯穿上皮全层。过去，世界卫生组织（WHO）根据异常发育不良细胞取代正常上皮的程度将 VIN 分为 VIN-1、VIN-2 和 VIN-3。然而，由于 VIN-1 主要对应的尖锐湿疣并不是癌前病变，VIN-1 这个术语已经被弃用，现在 VIN 在国际外阴疾病研究学会的最新分类中指的是之前的 VIN-2 和 VIN-3。

Vulval intraepithelial neoplasia (VIN) is a condition characterized by disorientation and loss of epithelial architecture extending through the full thickness of the epithelium. In the past, the World Health Organization classified VIN into VIN-1, 2 and 3 based on the extent to which normal epithelium is replaced by abnormal dysplastic cells. However, since VIN-1 mainly corresponds with condyloma that is not a precancerous lesion, the term VIN-1 has been abandoned, and VIN now refers to the previous VIN-2 and 3 in the latest classification of the International Society for the Study of Vulvar Disease.

根据不同的病理特征将 VIN 分为普通型 VIN（经典 VIN 或外阴鲍温病）和分化型 VIN（d-VIN）（框 20-1）。普通型 VIN 常见于 30—50 岁的年轻女性，与吸烟和人乳头瘤病毒（HPV）感染有关。患者可以无症状，也可以自诉瘙痒、疼痛、排尿困难和溃疡形成。病变可以是白色、粉红色或色素沉着的斑块或丘疹，最常见于阴唇和后阴唇系带。3%～4% 的普通型 VIN 可能进展为侵袭性疾病。

VIN is categorized into usual VIN (classic VIN or Bowen's disease) and differentiated VIN (d-VIN) based on the distinctive pathological features (Box 20.1). Usual VIN often occurs in young women between 30 and 50 years and is associated with cigarette smoking and human papilloma virus (HPV) infection. Patients can be asymptomatic, or they may complain of pruritus, pain, dysuria and ulceration. Lesions can be white, pink or pigmented in the forms of plaques or papules.

They are most frequently found in the labia and posterior fourchette; 3–4% of usual VIN may progress to invasive disease.

分化型 VIN 发生于绝经后女性，仅占所有 VIN 的 2%～10%。它与外阴鳞状上皮增生、硬化性苔藓和慢性单纯性苔藓有关，被认为是大多数 HPV 阴性的侵袭性角化鳞状细胞癌（squamous cell carcinomas, SCC）的前兆。患者的症状与硬化性苔藓相似。可见灰色、白色、红色结节、斑块或溃疡。它存在于高达 70%～80% 的癌旁组织，具有比普通型 VIN 更高的恶性潜能；因此，当发现分化型 VIN 时，排除恶性肿瘤是很重要的。

d-VIN occurs in postmenopausal women and accounts for only 2–10% of all VIN. It is associated with squamous hyperplasia, lichen sclerosus and lichen simplex chronicus and is considered the precursor of most HPV-negative invasive keratinizing squamous cell carcinomas (SCC). Patients have similar symptoms as with lichen sclerosus. Grey, white, red nodules, plaques or ulcers may be found. It is found in up to 70–80% of adjacent cancer and has a higher malignant potential than usual VIN. It is hence important to exclude malignancy when d-VIN is found.

与 VIN 发生于鳞状上皮不同，乳腺外的 Paget 病发生于顶浆分泌的腺上皮。病变的外观是可变的，它们呈丘疹样和隆起形，可能为白色、灰色、暗红色或不同深浅的棕色，可以局部分布或广泛分布（图 20-1）。这些情况很少见，该病的发病率为 0.53/10 万，常见于 50 岁以上的女性。在 20% 的病例中，Paget 病与其他部位的潜在腺癌或原发性恶性肿瘤相关，主要是乳腺和肠道。

Unlike VIN, which arises from squamous epithelium, extramammary Paget's disease arises from apocrine glandular epithelium. The appearance of the lesions is variable, but they are papular and raised; may be white, grey, dull red or various shades of brown; and may be localized or widespread (Fig. 20.1). These conditions are rare, with an incidence of 0.53/100,000, and commonly occur in women over the age of 50 years. Paget's disease is associated with underlying adenocarcinoma or primary malignancy elsewhere in 20% of cases, mainly breast and bowel.

框 20-1　外阴鳞状上皮内瘤变（VIN）	Box 20.1　Vulval intraepithelial neoplasia (VIN)
• 鳞状 VIN • 普通型 VIN（之前经典 VIN 或鲍温病） • 分化型 VIN（以前的"单纯"VIN） 　– 非鳞状 VIN • Paget 病	• Squamous VIN • Usual VIN (formerly classic VIN or Bowen's disease) • Differentiated VIN (formerly 'simplex' VIN) 　– Non-squamous VIN • Paget's disease

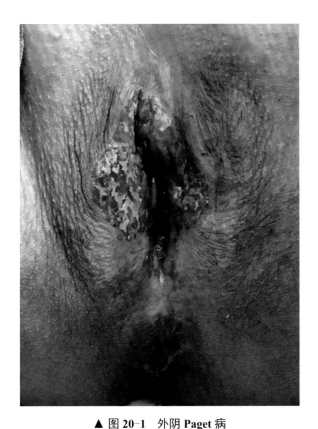

▲ 图 20-1　外阴 **Paget** 病

Fig. 20.1　Paget's disease of the vulva.

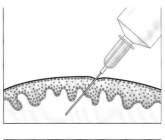

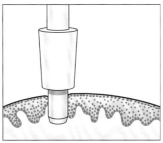

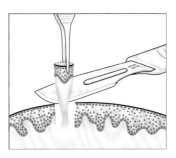

▲ 图 20-2　局部麻醉下 **Keye** 穿刺活检诊断外阴皮肤损伤

Fig. 20.2　Diagnosis of vulval skin lesions using Keye's punch biopsy under local anaesthetic.

治疗（Management）

重要的是通过活检确定诊断（图 20-2），并在其他部位（如宫颈和阴道）寻找上皮内瘤变，特别是当发现普通型 VIN 时。普通型 VIN 的治疗包括免疫调节剂咪喹莫特、激光治疗和皮肤病变的浅表切除。对于 d-VIN 药物治疗是无效的，进行手术切除会比普通型 VIN 手术切除更彻底。VIN 易复发且有恶性进展风险，尤其是分化型 VIN，因此需长期随访。

It is important to establish the diagnosis by biopsy (Fig. 20.2) and to search for intraepithelial neoplasia in other sites like the cervix and vagina, particularly when usual VIN is found. Treatment of usual VIN includes imiquimod, an immune modifier, laser therapy and superficial excision of the skin lesion. There is no role for medical treatment in d-VIN, and surgical excision tends to be more radical than that for usual VIN. Recurrence is common, and because there is a risk of malignant progression, especially in d-VIN, long-term follow-up is essential.

（二）外阴癌（Cancers of the vulva）

外阴癌占女性恶性肿瘤的 1%～4%；90% 的病变为鳞状细胞癌，5% 为腺癌，1% 为基底癌，0.5% 为恶性黑素瘤。外阴癌最常发生在 50—70 岁。

Carcinoma of the vulva accounts for 1-4% of female malignancies: 90% of the lesions are SCCs, 5% are adenocarcinomas, 1% are basal carcinomas and 0.5% are malignant melanomas. Carcinoma of the vulva most commonly occurs in the sixth and seventh decades.

外阴癌有两种不同的组织学类型，伴有两种不同的危险因素。基底细胞癌 / 疣状癌更常见，主要发生在年轻女性中，并与普通型 VIN 和 HPV 感染有关，有着与宫颈癌相似的危险因素。角化类型发生在老年女性，并与外阴硬化性苔藓有关。如前所述，在主体肿瘤附近可能有分化型 VIN 病灶。

Vulvar cancer has two distinct histological patterns with two different risk factors. The more common basoloid/warty types occur mainly in younger women and are associated with usual VIN and HPV infection, sharing similar risk factors as cervical cancer. The keratinizing types occur in older women and are associated with lichen sclerosus. As noted earlier, there may be foci of d-VIN adjacent to the main tumour.

1. 症状（Symptoms）

外阴癌患者会有瘙痒症状，并会发现外阴隆起的病变，可能伴有溃疡和出血（图 20-3）。恶性黑色素瘤通常为单发、有色素沉着和溃烂。外阴癌最常发生在大阴唇（50% 的病例），但也可能生长在阴蒂包皮、小阴唇、前庭大腺和阴道前庭。

The patient with vulval carcinoma experiences pruritus and notices a raised lesion on the vulva, which may ulcerate and bleed (Fig. 20.3). Malignant melanomas are usually single, hyperpigmented and ulcerated. Vulval carcinoma most frequently develops on the labia majora (50% of cases) but may also grow on the prepuce of the clitoris, the labia minora, Bartholin's glands and in the vestibule of the vagina.

2. 扩散方式（Mode of spread）

癌细胞可通过局部和淋巴系统发生扩散。受累淋巴结包括腹股沟浅、深淋巴结和股淋巴结（图 20-4）。除了累及阴蒂的原发病灶外，盆腔淋巴结通常只是继发性受累。血行播散出现较晚且罕见。该病通常进展缓慢，晚期伴有大面积溃疡、感染、出血和远处转移。在大约 30% 的病例中，两侧淋巴结受累。由国际妇产科联合会（FIGO）根据手术而不是临床结果来确定分期（表 20-1）。

Spread occurs both locally and through the lymphatic system. The lymph nodes involved are the superficial and deep inguinal nodes and the femoral nodes (Fig. 20.4). Pelvic lymph nodes, except in primary lesions involving the clitoris, have usually only secondary involvement. Vascular spread is late and rare. The disease usually progresses slowly, and the terminal stages are accompanied by extensive ulceration,

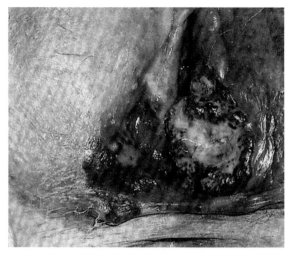

▲ 图 20-3 外阴鳞状细胞癌伴溃疡

Fig. 20.3 Ulcerative squamous cell carcinoma of the vulva.

infection, haemorrhage and remote metastatic disease. In some 30% of cases, lymph nodes are involved on both sides. Stages are defined by the International Federation of Obstetrics and Gynaecology (FIGO) on the basis of surgical rather than clinical findings (Table 20.1).

3. 治疗（Treatment）

ⅠA 期外阴癌可通过外阴局部扩大切除治疗。在中线外侧至少 2cm 的 ⅠB 期病变可采用局部扩大切除和单侧腹股沟淋巴结清扫术进行治疗。所有其他阶段的治疗采用广泛根治性局部切除或根治性外阴切除术和双侧腹股沟淋巴结清扫术。在经验丰富的

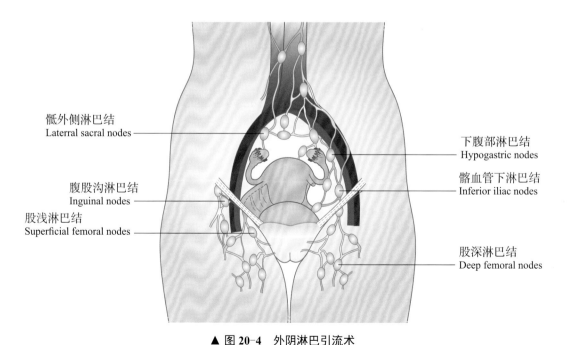

下腹部淋巴结
Hypogastric nodes

髂血管下淋巴结
Inferior iliac nodes

股深淋巴结
Deep femoral nodes

骶外侧淋巴结
Lateral sacral nodes

腹股沟淋巴结
Inguinal nodes

股浅淋巴结
Superficial femoral nodes

▲ 图 20-4 外阴淋巴引流术

Fig. 20.4 Lymphatic drainage of the vulva.

表 20-1　FIGO 卵巢癌分级（2009）

Table 20.1　FIGO staging of vulval cancer (2009)

I 期　肿瘤局限于外阴
　I A 期：病灶大小≤2cm，局限于外阴或会阴，间质浸润≤1.0mm*，无淋巴结转移
　I B 期：病灶大小＞2cm 或间质浸润＞1.0mm*，局限于外阴或会阴，阴性淋巴结

Stage I　Tumour confined to the vulva:
　Stage IA: Lesions ≤2 cm in size, confined to the vulva or perineum and with stromal invasion ≤1.0 mm*, no nodal metastasis
　Stage IB: Lesions >2 cm in size or with stromal invasion >1.0 mm*, confined to the vulva or perineum, with negative nodes

II 期　任何大小的肿瘤，侵犯邻近的会阴组织（尿道下 1/3，阴道下 1/3，肛门下），无淋巴结转移
Stage II　Tumour of any size with extension to adjacent perineal structures (lower third of urethra, lower third of vagina, anus) with negative nodes

III 期　任何大小的肿瘤，伴或不伴邻近会阴结构受侵（尿道下 1/3，阴道下 1/3，肛门），伴有腹股沟 - 股淋巴结转移
　III A 期：①1 个淋巴结转移（≥5mm）；②1～2 个淋巴结转移（＜5mm）
　III B 期：①≥2 个淋巴结转移（≥5mm）；②≥3 个淋巴结转移（＜5mm）
　III C 期：阳性淋巴结伴有淋巴结囊外扩散

Stage III　Tumour of any size with or without extension to adjacent perineal structures (lower third of urethra, lower third of vagina, anus) with positive inguinofemoral lymph nodes:
　Stage IIIA: (i) With 1 lymph node metastasis (≥5 mm) or (ii) 1–2 lymph node metastasis(es) (<5 mm)
　Stage IIIB: (i) With 2 or more lymph node metastases (≥5 mm) or (ii) 3 or more lymph node metastases (<5 mm)
　Stage IIIC: With positive nodes with extracapsular spread

IV 期　肿瘤侵犯其他区域（尿道上 2/3，阴道上 2/3）或远处结构
　IV A 期：肿瘤侵犯以下任何一种，①上尿道和（或）阴道黏膜、膀胱黏膜、直肠黏膜或固定于骨盆骨；②腹股沟 - 股淋巴结固定或溃疡
　IV B 期：包括盆腔淋巴结的任何部位远处转移

Stage IV　Tumour invades other regional (upper two-thirds of urethra, upper two-thirds of vagina) or distant structures:
　Stage IVA: Tumour invades any of the following: (i) upper urethral and/or vaginal mucosa, bladder mucosa, rectal mucosa or fixed to pelvic bone or (ii) fixed or ulcerated inguinofemoral lymph nodes
　Stage IVB: Any distant metastasis, including pelvic lymph nodes

*. 浸润深度的定义是肿瘤从邻近最浅表的真皮乳头的上皮间质交界处到浸润最深点

经许可，转载自 Pecorelli S & FIGO Committee on Gynecologic Oncology (2009). International Journal of Gynecology & Obstetrics, 105(2):103-104.

*. The depth of invasion is defined as the measurement of the tumour from the epithelial stromal junction of the adjacent most superficial dermal papilla to the deepest point of invasion.

Reproduced with permission from Pecorelli S & FIGO Committee on Gynecologic Oncology (2009). International Journal of Gynecology & Obstetrics, 105(2):103-104.

治疗中心，前哨淋巴结清扫术可以取代传统的淋巴结清扫术。术后放疗对于肿瘤延伸到接近切除边缘或累及腹股沟淋巴结的患者有作用。术前放疗，伴或不伴化疗，可用于病灶大的患者以减小肿瘤体积。根治性外阴切除术和腹股沟淋巴结清扫的并发症包括伤口破裂、淋巴囊肿和淋巴水肿（30%）、继发性出血、血栓栓塞、性功能障碍和心理疾病。对化疗的反应一般较差。术后每 3～6 个月随访一次，随访5 年。

　　Stage IA disease can be treated by wide local excision. Stage IB lesions that are at least 2 cm lateral to the midline are treated by wide local excision and unilateral groin node dissection. All other stages are treated by wide radical local excisions or radical vulvectomy and bilateral groin node dissection. Sentinel node dissection may replace conventional node dissection in centres with experience in the technique. Postoperative radiotherapy has a role in patients where the tumour extends close to the excision margin or there is involvement of the groin nodes. Preoperative radiotherapy, with or without chemotherapy, may be used in cases of extensive disease to reduce the tumour volume. Complications of radical vulvectomy and groin node dissection include wound breakdown, lymphocyst and lymphoedema (30%), secondary bleeding, thromboembolism, sexual dysfunction and psychological morbidity. Response to chemotherapy is generally poor. Patients are followed up at intervals of 3–6 months for 5 years.

4. 预后（Prognosis）

预后取决于肿瘤原发灶的大小和淋巴结受累情

况。可手术治疗的无淋巴结受累的患者的总生存率为90%，原发病灶小于 2cm 的患者总生存率高达 98%。如果有淋巴结受累，这个比例可降至 50%～60%，如果有双侧淋巴结受累，这个比例低于 30%。恶性黑色素瘤和腺癌预后差，5 年生存率为 5%。

Prognosis is determined by the size of the primary lesion and lymph node involvement. The overall survival rate in operable cases without lymph node involvement is 90% and is up to 98% where the primary lesion is less than 2 cm in size. This falls to 50–60% with node involvement and is less than 30% in patients with bilateral lymph node involvement. Malignant melanoma and adenocarcinoma have a poor prognosis, with a 5-year survival of 5%.

二、阴道上皮的肿瘤性病变（Neoplastic lesions of the vaginal epithelium）

（一）阴道上皮内瘤变（Vaginal intraepithelial neoplasia, VAIN）

阴道上皮内瘤变（VAIN）通常是多发的，倾向于多灶性，与类似的宫颈病变相关。2012 年，美国引入了两级而不是三级分级，其中包括低级别鳞状上皮内病变（low-grade squamous intraepithelial lesion, LSIL）和高级别鳞状上皮内病变（high-grade squamous intraepithelial lesion, HSIL），以取代 VAIN Ⅰ～Ⅲ级。阴道上皮内瘤变是无症状的，往往是由于涂片检查阳性或在阴道镜检查发现异常细胞时发现的，通常是在子宫切除术后被发现。该病变有进展为浸润性癌的风险，但在此之前疾病仍是浅表的，可以通过手术切除、激光消融或冷冻手术进行治疗。

Vaginal intraepithelial neoplasia (VAIN) is usually multicentric and tends to be multifocal and associated with similar lesions of the cervix. A two- instead of three-tiered grading classification comprising low-grade squamous intraepithelial lesion (LSIL) and high-grade squamous intraepithelial lesion (HSIL) replacing that of VAIN I-III was introduced in 2012 in the United States. The condition is asymptomatic and tends to be discovered because of a positive smear test or during colposcopy for abnormal cytology, often after hysterectomy. There is a risk of progression to invasive carcinoma, but the disease remains superficial until then and can be treated by surgical excision, laser ablation or cryosurgery.

（二）阴道腺病（Vaginal adenosis）

阴道腺病指阴道上皮出现柱状上皮，见于母亲妊娠期间接受己烯雌酚治疗的成年女性。通常情况

下可恢复为正常的鳞状上皮，但约 4% 的病例会发展为阴道腺癌；因此，通过连续的细胞学检查密切关注这些女性是很重要的。

This is the presence of columnar epithelium in the vaginal epithelium and has been found in adult females whose mothers received treatment with diethylstilboestrol during pregnancy. The condition commonly reverts to normal squamous epithelium, but in about 4% of cases the lesion progresses to vaginal adenocarcinoma. It is therefore important to follow these women carefully with serial cytology.

（三）阴道恶性肿瘤（Vaginal malignancy）

阴道浸润性癌可为鳞状细胞癌或偶尔也可为腺癌。原发性病变出现在 50—70 岁，但在英国是罕见的。阴道腺癌，通常是透明细胞癌，与在宫腔内己烯雌酚暴露有关，自从该药物在妊娠期禁用以来，其发病率已经下降。

Invasive carcinoma of the vagina may be a squamous carcinoma or, occasionally, an adenocarcinoma. Primary lesions arise in the sixth and seventh decades but are rare in the UK. The incidence of adenocarcinoma, typically clear cell, associated with in utero exposure of diethylstilboestrol has declined since this drug was withdrawn from use in pregnancy

宫颈癌和子宫内膜癌的继发病变常见于阴道的上 1/3，有时也可通过淋巴转移到阴道的下 1/3 处。

Secondary deposits from cervical carcinoma and endometrial carcinoma are relatively common in the upper third of the vagina and can sometimes occur in the lower vagina through lymphatic spread.

1. 症状（Symptoms）

其症状包括不规则阴道出血，以及当肿瘤坏死和随后发生感染时令人不适的阴道排液。局部扩散至直肠、膀胱或尿道，可导致瘘管形成。肿瘤可以表现为外生性病变，也可以表现为溃烂、固定的肿块。

The symptoms include irregular vaginal bleeding and offensive vaginal discharge when the tumour becomes necrotic and infection supervenes. Local spread into the rectum, bladder or urethra may result in fistula formation. The tumour may appear as an exophytic lesion or as an ulcerated, indurated mass.

2. 扩散方式（Method of spread）

如前所述，肿瘤的扩散是通过直接浸润或淋巴转移发生的。累及阴道上半部分的病变表现为类似

子宫颈癌的扩散模式。阴道下半部分的肿瘤与外阴癌的转移模式相似。

Tumour spread, as previously stated, occurs by direct infiltration or by lymphatic extension. Lesions involving the upper half of the vagina follow a pattern of spread similar to that of carcinoma of the cervix. Tumours of the lower half of the vagina follow a similar pattern of spread to that of carcinoma of the vulva.

3. 治疗（Treatment）

诊断是通过肿瘤活检来确定的。在开始治疗前进行分期（表 20-2）。

The diagnosis is established by biopsy of the tumour. Staging is made before commencing treatment (Table 20.2).

主要的治疗方法是放射治疗，其中包括外照射治疗和近距离放射治疗。

The primary method of treatment is by radiotherapy-both by external beam therapy and brachytherapy.

在特定的患者中也可以考虑手术治疗。例如，阴道上部病变的 I 期患者可采用根治性子宫切除术或阴道切除术加盆腔淋巴结清扫术。阴道下段病变的 I 期患者可能需要根治性外阴切除术。对于膀胱或直肠的局限性侵犯而无宫旁组织或淋巴结转移者，可考虑行盆腔廓清术。

Surgical treatment can also be considered in selected patients. For example, radical hysterectomy or vaginectomy and pelvic lymph node dissection can be considered in patients with stage I disease in the upper vagina, radical vulvectomy

may be needed in stage I disease in the lower vagina and pelvic exenteration may be considered in patients with localized invasion to the bladder or rectum without parametrial or lymph node metastasis.

4. 预后（Prognosis）

治疗的结果取决于最初的分期和治疗的方法。I 期和 II 期的 5 年生存率约为 60%，而 III 期和 IV 期的 5 年生存率则降至 30%～40%。阴道腺癌常发生在年轻女性，对放疗也有很好的反应。

Results of treatment depend on the initial staging and on the method of therapy. Stages I and II have a 5-year survival of around 60% but this figure falls to 30–40% for stages III and IV. Adenocarcinoma of the vagina, which often occurs in young females, also responds well to irradiation.

三、宫颈病变（Lesions of the cervix）

（一）宫颈癌（Cervical cancer）

宫颈癌是世界上第四大常见的女性癌症。全世界各地的发病率不同。在许多资源匮乏的国家，这是女性死于癌症的最常见原因。在英国，宫颈癌是第十四大常见的癌症，每年约有 3200 例新发病例，发病率最高的是在 2013—2015 年的 25—29 岁年龄组。宫颈癌有多种组织学类型，其中 SCC 占 70%～80%，腺癌占 10%～25%。其他亚型，如腺鳞癌、神经内分泌癌和未分化癌并不常见。宫颈癌最重要的危险因素是持续的 HPV 感染。导致持续 HPV 感染高危因素也是宫颈癌的危险因素，如初次性交年龄过早、伴侣数量、吸烟、社会经济地位低和免疫抑制治疗。

Cervical cancer is the fourth most common female cancer worldwide. Incidence varies across the world. In many lowresource countries, this is the most common cause of death from cancer in women. In the UK, cervical cancer is the fourteenth most common, with about 3200 new cases per year, with the highest incidence rates in the 25–29 age group between 2013 and 2015. Cervical cancer has several histological types, of which SCC accounts for about 70–80%, while adenocarcinoma accounts for about 10–25%. Other subtypes, such as adenosquamous, neuroendocrine and undifferentiated carcinomas, are uncommon. The most important risk factor for cervical cancer is persistent HPV infection. Factors leading to higher risk for persistent HPV infection are risk factors for cervical cancer, e.g. early age of first intercourse, number of partners, smoking, low socioeconomic status and immunosuppression.

表 20-2　阴道癌的临床分期

Table 20.2　Clinical staging of vaginal carcinoma

0 期　原位癌

Stage 0　Intraepithelial carcinoma

I 期　局限于阴道壁

Stage I　Limited to the vaginal walls

II 期　累及阴道壁下层组织，但未延伸至盆腔壁

Stage II　Involves the subvaginal tissue but has not extended to the pelvic wall

III 期　肿瘤已扩展到骨盆侧壁

Stage III　The tumour has extended to the lateral pelvic wall

IV 期　病变已扩展到邻近器官（IVA）或已扩散到远处器官（IVB）

Stage IV　The lesion has extended to involve adjacent organs (IVA) or has spread to distant organs (IVB)

人乳头瘤病毒感染及宫颈癌（HPV infection and cervical cancer）

几乎所有的宫颈癌病例（超过 99%）都是由高危 HPV 感染引起的。HPV 感染有 100 多种亚型。HPV 感染可感染生殖器和非生殖器部位。分为高危型和低危型。高危亚型与癌症有关，而低危亚型会导致疣。在 14 种高危亚型中，HPV16 和 HPV18 引起约 70% 的宫颈癌。HPV 感染主要通过皮肤 – 皮肤密切接触传播，如生殖器与生殖器的接触，以及肛交、阴道性交和口交。这是一种非常常见的感染，大多数性活跃的女性可能在她们一生中的某个时候被感染。然而，大多数感染是短暂的，并被人体的自然免疫系统清除。只有持续的感染才会导致癌变。除了宫颈癌，HPV 感染还会导致其他癌症，如外阴、阴道、肛门和口咽癌。

Almost all cases of cervical cancer (over 99%) are caused by high-risk HPV infection. There are more than 100 subtypes of HPV infection. HPV infection can infect genital and nongenital sites. The subtypes are classified as high risk or low risk. High-risk subtypes are associated with cancer, while the low-risk types cause warts. Amongst the 14 high-risk subtypes, HPV 16 and 18 cause about 70% of cervical cancer. HPV infection is mainly transmitted via close skin-to-skin contact, such as genital-to-genital contact and anal, vaginal and oral sex. It is a very common infection, where the majority of sexually active women would have been infected sometime during their lifetime. However, most infections are transient and are cleared by the body's natural immunity. Only persistent infections lead to cancer. Apart from cervical cancer, HPV infection also causes other cancers such as vulval, vaginal, anal and oropharyngeal cancers.

（二）病理生理学（Pathophysiology）

磷柱状交接部（squamocolumnar junction，SCJ）是子宫颈口外的鳞状上皮和子宫颈口内的柱状上皮之间的连接处。SCJ 的移动与解剖学宫颈外口相关。青春期、妊娠期或服用联合口服避孕药时雌激素的变化使 SCJ 向外移动，使柱状上皮暴露于阴道的较低 pH 环境。这使柱状上皮通过鳞状上皮化生过程转化为鳞状上皮。在当前的 SCJ 和向外移动到外子宫颈位置的 SCJ 之间的区域是转化区，这里是大多数癌前病变发生的地方。

The squamocolumnar junction (SCJ) is the junction between the squamous epithelium of the ectocervix and the columnar epithelium in the endocervix. The SCJ moves in relation to the anatomical external cervical os. Changes in oestrogen during puberty, pregnancy or while on the combined oral contraceptive pill move the SCJ outwards, exposing columnar epithelium to the lower pH of the vagina. This reacts by undergoing transformation back to squamous epithelium by a process of squamous metaplasia. The area that lies between the current SCJ and that is reached as it moves outwards across the ectocervix is the *transformation zone*, and it is here that most preinvasive lesions occur.

（三）宫颈癌预防（Cervical cancer prevention）

宫颈癌的自然史现在已经很清楚。HPV 感染子宫颈上皮。持续的 HPV 感染导致子宫颈上皮癌前病变，称为子宫颈上皮内瘤变（cervical intraepithelial neoplasia，CIN）。CIN 描述了鳞状上皮的变化，其特征是不同程度的分化和分层丧失以及核异型性（图 20–5）。它可以延伸到宫颈表面以下，但不超过基底膜。在英国，CIN 分为轻度（CIN-1）、中度（CIN-2）和重度（CIN-3），这取决于异常细胞替代的上皮细胞的比例。25% 的 CIN-1 在 2 年内发展为高级病变，30%～40% 的 CIN-3 在 20 年内发展为癌。约 40% 的低级病变（CIN-1）在不治疗的情况下可在 6 个月内恢复正常，尤其是在较轻的年龄组。在澳大利亚和新西兰，与 VAIN 类似，是用两级的低级鳞状上皮内病变（LSIL）和高级别鳞状上皮内病变（HSIL）来代替 CIN 1～3 级。从低级别到高级别病变的进展过程可以超过 3～10 年。由于从低级病变发展为浸润性癌需要 10～20 年的时间，这为我们筛选和治疗癌前病变提供了一个机会窗口，从而防止进展为浸润癌。

The natural history of cervical cancer is now well understood. HPV infects the cervical epithelium. Persistent HPV infection leads to premalignant changes in the cervical epithelium, known as *cervical intraepithelial neoplasia* (CIN). CIN describes the changes in the squamous epithelium characterized by varying degrees of loss of differentiation and stratification and nuclear atypia (Fig. 20.5). It may extend below the surface of the cervix but does not extend beyond the basement membrane. In the UK, CIN is graded as mild (CIN-1), moderate (CIN-2) or severe (CIN-3), depending on the proportion of the epithelium replaced by abnormal cells. Twenty-five per cent of CIN-1 will progress to higher-grade lesions over 2 years, and 30–40% of CIN-3 to carcinoma over 20 years. Around 40% of low-grade lesions (CIN-1) will regress to normal within 6 months without treatment, especially in the younger age group. Similar to VAIN, a two-tier instead of three-tier grading of LSIL and HSIL, replacing that of CIN 1–3, is used in Australia and New Zealand. The process of progression from lowgrade to high-grade lesions can be over 3–10 years. Since the progression from low-grade lesions to invasive cancer can take 10–20 years, this gives us a window

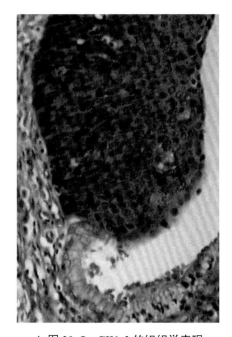

▲ 图 20-5 CIN-3 的组织学表现

Fig. 20.5 Histological appearance of CIN-3.

of opportunity to screen and treat the premalignant lesions, thus preventing the development of invasive cancers.

1. 一级预防：HPV 疫苗接种（Primary prevention-HPV vaccination）

既然我们现在知道宫颈癌的主要原因是 HPV 感染，预防 HPV 感染将是最好的主要预防宫颈癌的措施。已经研制出预防性的 HPV 疫苗。二价和四价疫苗在市场上已经有大约 10 年的时间。二价疫苗针对 2 种高危亚型 HPV16 和 HPV18，四价疫苗覆盖 HPV16、HPV18，以及 2 种会导致尖锐湿疣的低风险亚型 HPV6 和 HPV11。预防 HPV16 和 HPV18 感染理论上可以防止超过 70% 的宫颈癌病例。来自澳大利亚 10 年使用的确凿证据表明可减少 18—24 岁女性 77% 高危 HPV 血清型、30%～50% 的 HSIL 发生，以及减少 90% 的生殖器疣。这些疫苗在接触病毒之前，即初次性行为之前接种最有效。2007 年，澳大利亚开始为女孩接种四价疫苗。英国于 2008 年开始实施针对 HPV16 和 HPV18 感染的国家疫苗接种计划。自 2012 年以来，12—13 岁女孩定期接种四价疫苗，第一次 HPV 疫苗接种是在 8 年级时，第二次接种是在第一次接种后 6～12 个月。在其他一些国家，如澳大利亚，疫苗接种方案已扩展到男孩。虽然男孩不会得宫颈癌，但他们可以免受其他与 HPV 有关的癌症和生殖器疣的侵袭，而且他们的疫苗接种有

助于通过提高其未来伴侣对病毒的免疫力，降低传染给其未来伴侣的风险。HPV 疫苗已被证明能提供至少 10 年的保护，而且很可能是终身保护。最近有报道一种新的纳米疫苗。除了 HPV16 和 HPV18 之外，九价疫苗还可预防其他五种致癌类型（HPV31、HPV33、HPV45、HPV52、HPV58），它们与 HPV16 和 HPV18 一起占致宫颈癌类型的近 90%。

Since we now know that the main cause for cervical cancer is HPV infection, preventing HPV infections would be the best primary preventive measure. Prophylactic HPV vaccines have been developed. Bivalent and quadrivalent vaccines have been in the market for about a decade. The bivalent vaccine targets the two high-risk subtypes, HPV 16 and 18, while the quadrivalent vaccine covers HPV 16 and 18 as well as two low-risk subtypes, HPV 6 and 11, which cause genital warts. The prevention of HPV 16 and 18 infections could theoretically prevent more than 70% of cervical cancer cases, and indeed evidence from Australia after a decade of use has shown a 77% reduction in high-risk HPV serotypes in women aged 18–24 and 30–50% reaction in HSIL with a 90% reduction in genital warts. These vaccines are most effective when given before any exposure to the virus, i.e. before sexual debut. Vaccination using the quadrivalent vaccine was introduced for girls in Australia in 2007. In the UK, a national vaccination programme against HPV 16 and 18 infections was introduced in 2008. Since 2012, girls aged 12–13 years have been routinely offered the quadrivalent vaccine, with the first HPV vaccination given when they are in school year 8, and the second dose is offered 6–12 months after the first. In some other countries, e.g. Australia, the vaccination programme has extended to boys. Although boys do not get cervical cancer, they benefit from protection from other HPV-related cancers and genital warts, and their vaccination helps reduce the risk of transmission to their future partners by increasing her immunity to the virus. The HPV vaccine has been shown to offer protection for at least 10 years, and it is likely that the protection will be lifelong. Recently, a new nanovalent vaccine has been introduced. In addition to HPV 16 and 18, the nine-valent vaccine protects against five other oncogenic types (31, 33, 45, 52, 58) which, together with 16 and 18, account for nearly 90% of cervical cancers.

2. 二级预防：癌前病变的筛查（Secondary prevention-screening for premalignant lesions）

子宫颈普查计划的目的是在无症状人群中发现宫颈癌的非侵入性前期，即 CIN，以降低其死亡率和发病率。1988 年，英格兰和威尔士启动了国家保健服务全国子宫颈检查计划，到 1991 年，20—65 岁的所有女性中有 80% 每 5 年进行一次检查。从那时起，宫颈癌死亡率每年下降 7%。目前，所有年龄在 25—49 岁的女性每 3 年被邀请进行一次筛查，50—64 岁

的女性每 5 年被邀请进行一次筛查。通常，宫颈细胞学检查是从子宫颈取出的。这通常被称为宫颈涂片检查或巴氏涂片检查，以该检查的发明者 Georgios Papanicolaou 命名。传统的涂片是使用 Ayres 或 Aylesbury 压舌板 360° 从整个转化区的子宫颈上取细胞，并将细胞涂在玻璃载玻片上。近年来，液基细胞学（liquid-based cytology，LBC）在很大程度上取代了传统的涂片检查。LBC 是使用塑料颈刷从转化区取细胞。刷子以相同的方向旋转 5 圈，然后转移到一个有运输介质的容器中（见第 15 章）。LBC 允许对涂片进行自动化处理，并降低了不满意涂片的概率。该样本还可用于其他检测，如 HPV 检测。子宫颈细胞学检查（图 20-6 和图 20-7）主要用于筛查鳞状上皮病变，不能确切地排除宫颈管内病变。2017 年，澳大利亚的筛查改为以 HPV 为基础的检测，按巴氏涂片检查方法取样，只对被确定为多种高危型 HPV 阳性的女性进行 LBC 检测。与英国一样，筛查从 25 岁开始；如果结果为阴性，则每隔 5 年重复一次，直到 75 岁。

The aim of cervical screening programmes is to detect the non-invasive precursor of cervical cancer, CIN, in the asymptomatic population in order to reduce mortality and morbidity. The National Health Service (NHS) national cervical screening programme was introduced in England and Wales in 1988, and by 1991, 80% of all women between the ages of 20 and 65 were being tested on a 5-yearly basis. Since then mortality from cervical cancer has fallen by 7% a

year. Currently all women aged between 25 and 49 are invited for screening every 3 years, and those between 50 and 64 are invited every 5 years. Conventionally, cervical cytology is taken from the cervix. This is often referred to as a *cervical smear* or a *Pap smear*, named after the inventor of the test, Georgios Papanicolaou. Conventional smears involve taking cells from the cervix on the whole of the transformation zone with a 360-degree sweep using an Ayres or Aylesbury spatula and smeared onto a glass slide. In recent years, liquid-based cytology (LBC) has largely replaced the conventional smears. For LBC, the cells from the transformation zone are taken with a plastic cervical brush. The brush is rotated in the same direction for five turns and transferred into a container of transport medium (see Chapter 15). LBC allows automated processing of the smears, and it reduces the rate of unsatisfactory smears. The sample can also be used for additional tests such as HPV testing. Cervical cytology (Figs 20.6 and 20.7) is primarily for screening for squamous lesions and cannot reliably exclude endocervical disease. In 2017 screening in Australia was changed to an HPV-based test collected in the same way as the Pap smear support by LBC only in women identified as being positive for one of a number of high-risk HPV serotypes. As in the UK screening begins at age 25; if negative, it is repeated at 5-year intervals until age 75.

（四）宫颈细胞学分类（Classification of cervical cytology）

英国用于报道子宫颈涂片检查的术语由英国临床细胞学学会（British Society for Clinical Cytology）于 1986 年介绍，并于 2013 年更新。"核异质"一词用于描述位于正常鳞状细胞和恶性细胞之间的细胞，

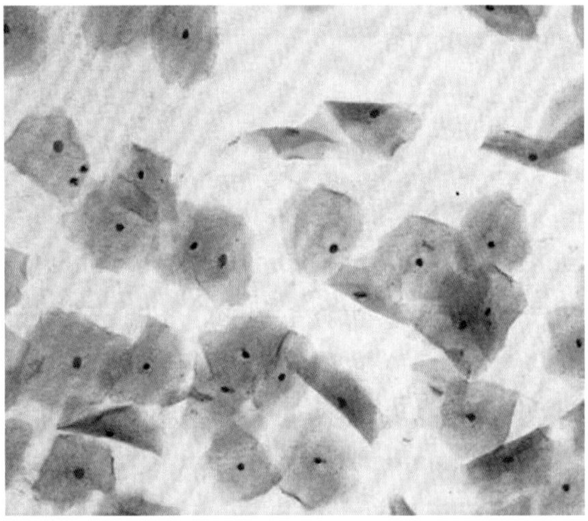

▲ 图 20-6　正常的子宫颈涂片显示浅层（粉红色）和中层（蓝色 / 绿色）脱落的子宫颈细胞（低倍放大）

Fig. 20.6　Normal cervical smear showing superficial (pink) and intermediate (blue/green) exfoliated cervical cells (low-power magnification)

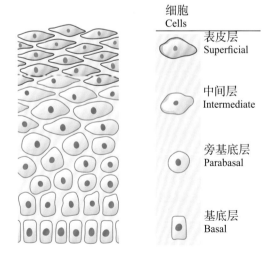

▲ 图 20-7　宫颈和阴道鳞状上皮细胞层

Fig. 20.7　Cell layers in the stratified squamous epithelium of the cervix and vagina.

并在恶变发生前表现出不同程度胞核改变（图 20-8）。达不到核异质异常程度的细胞称为交界性细胞。非典型腺细胞可能是宫颈管黏膜或子宫内膜癌前病变的表现。

The terminology used in the UK for reporting cervical smears was introduced by the British Society for Clinical Cytology in 1986 and updated in 2013. The term *dyskaryosis* is used to describe those cells that lie between normal squamous and frankly malignant cells and exhibit degrees of nuclear changes before malignancy (Fig. 20.8). Cells showing abnormalities that fall short of dyskaryosis are described as borderline. Atypical glandular cells may represent premalignant disease of the endocervix or endometrium.

恶性细胞显示核增大，而胞质变少（图 20-9）。细胞核呈分叶状轮廓。核染色强度增加，核分裂象数目增加。

Malignant cells show nuclear enlargement at the expense of cytoplasmic mass (Fig. 20.9). The nuclei may assume a lobulated outline. There is increased intensity of staining of the nucleus and an increase in the number of mitotic figures.

美国使用的 Bethesda 分类系统（表 20-3）的不同之处是，将中重度核异常合并为 HSIL，并使用意义不明的"非典型鳞状细胞"（ASCUS）一词而不是交界性。在当前版本的分类系统中，重点是尽量鉴别可能是高级别病变的疑似病例。这组疑似病变称为非典型鳞状细胞，不能排除高级别上皮内病变（ASC-H）。在澳大利亚和新西兰使用了 HSIL 和

LSIL 分类的改进版本，但使用的术语是可能的低级别鳞状上皮内病变（PLSIL）和可能的高级别鳞状上皮内病变（PHSIL），分别取代了 ASCUS 和 ASC-H。

The Bethesda system of classification used in the United States (Table 20.3) differs by combining moderate and severe dyskaryosis as HSIL and using the term *atypical squamous cells of undetermined significance (ASCUS)* instead of borderline. In the current edition of the classification system, the emphasis is to try and separate out borderline cases that may potentially be a high-grade lesion. This group of borderline lesions is called *atypical squamous cells, cannot exclude high-grade intraepithelial lesion (ASC-H)*. A modified version of this classification is used in Australia and New Zealand with HSIL and LSIL, but the terms *possible low-grade squamous intraepithelial lesions (PLSIL) and possible high-grade squamous intraepithelial lesions (PHSIL)* are being used instead of ASCUS and ASC-H, respectively.

高危型 HPV（HPV testing）检测对高级别 CIN 的敏感性约为 90%，比细胞学检查的敏感性高 25%。最常用的 HPV 检测方法之一是杂交捕获 Ⅱ（HC Ⅱ）检测，它检测 13 种高危 HPV 亚型。一些 HPV 检测不仅可以检测任何高危 HPV 亚型（类似于 HC Ⅱ），而且还可以检测 HPV16 和 HPV18，这两种类型的 HPV 高度病变的风险特别高。HPV 检测结合子宫颈细胞学检查（联合检测）或 HPV 单独检测作为一种初级筛查方法已得到评估。在美国，建议 30 岁以上的女性进行联合检测，而 25 岁以上的女性推荐单独进行 HPV 检测。高危 HPV 检测也有非常高的阴性预

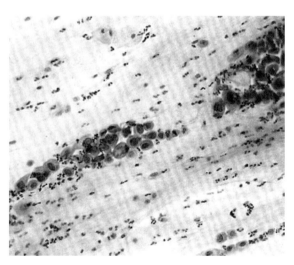

▲ 图 20-8　中度核异质。与正常细胞相比，细胞更小，核质比更高

Fig. 20.8　**Moderate dyskaryosis. The cells are smaller and the nuclear:cytoplasmic ratio is higher when compared with normal cells.**

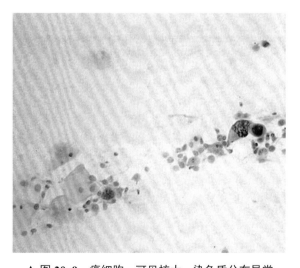

▲ 图 20-9　癌细胞。可见核大，染色质分布异常

Fig. 20.9　**Carcinoma cells. Note the large nuclei and abnormal distribution of chromatin.**

表 20-3 子宫颈细胞检验的分类

Table 20.3 Classification of cervical smears

英国系统（2013） UK system (2013)	美国 Bethesda 系统（2014） U.S. Bethesda system (2014)
阴性的 Negative	上皮内病变阴性 Negative for intraepithelial lesion
鳞状细胞边缘改变 Borderline change in squamous cells	非典型鳞状细胞（ASC-US）、ASC-H（不能排除 HSIL） Atypical squamous cells of undetermined significance (ASC-US), ASC-H (cannot exclude HSIL)
宫颈管细胞边界变化 Borderline change in endocervical cells	非典型宫颈内细胞、子宫内膜或腺细胞（NOS 或在注释中说明） Atypical endocervical, endometrial or glandular (NOS or specify in comments) 非典型宫颈内腔、子宫内膜或腺细胞，倾向于肿瘤 Atypical endocervical, endometrial or glandular cells, favour neoplastic
低级核异质 Low-grade dyskaryosis	低级 SIL Low-grade SIL
高级核异质（中度） High-grade dykaryosis (moderate)	高级 SIL High-grade SIL
高级核异质（严重） High-grade dyskaryosis (severe)	高级 SIL High-grade SIL
高级核异质 High-grade dyskaryosis 侵袭性鳞状细胞癌 invasive squamous cell carcinoma	鳞状细胞癌 Squamous cell carcinoma
宫颈内型腺瘤 Glandular neoplasia of endocervical type 腺瘤（非子宫颈的） Glandular neoplasia (non-cervical)	原位宫颈癌 Endocervical carcinoma in situ 腺癌：子宫颈内的、子宫外子宫内膜的、NOS Adenocarcinoma-endocervical, endometrial extrauterine, NOS

ASC-H. 非典型鳞状细胞（高度）；ASCUS. 意义不明的非典型鳞状细胞；NOS. 未另行指明；SIL. 鳞状上皮内病变

ASC-H, Atypical squamous cells (high-grade); ASCUS, atypical squamous cells of undetermined significance; NOS, not otherwise specified; SIL, squamous intraepithelial lesion.

测值，检测阴性的女性筛查间隔可以更长；而且对于接种疫苗的女性来说，这可能是一种更合适的初步筛查。然而，高危 HPV 检测的特异性较低，因为并非所有 HPV 感染都会导致癌前病变。如果对高危 HPV 阳性结果没有一个良好的分类系统，更多的女性将需要接受阴道镜检查（见后述章），从而导致更多不必要的干预。因此，英国部分地区已将 HPV 检测作为宫颈普查的主要方法，并将逐步在全国推广。对高危 HPV 检测呈阳性的女性将进行细胞学分诊（即做 LBC）。如果女性有高危 HPV 阳性和异常的细胞学结果（交界性或更差），将被转行阴道镜检查。在澳大利亚，HPV16 和 HPV18 型检测已经取代了子宫颈普查计划中的细胞学检查（见前述章）。

High-risk HPV testing has a sensitivity of about 90% for high-grade CIN, which is 25% more sensitive than cytology. One of the most commonly used HPV tests is the Hybrid Capture II (HCII) test, which tests for a pool of 13 high-risk HPV subtypes. Some HPV tests can not only test for the presence of any high-risk HPV subtypes (similar to the HC II) but also give individual results for HPV 16 and 18, which carry a particularly high risk for a high-grade lesion. HPV testing in conjunction with cervical cytology (co-test) or as a stand-alone test as a primary screening method has been evaluated. Co-testing is recommended in the United States for women over the age of 30, while HPV testing alone is recommended for women over age 25. High-risk HPV testing also has a very high negative predictive value, which allows a longer screening interval for women with a negative test, and it may be a more appropriate primary screening test for vaccinated women. However, high-risk HPV tests have lower specificity, since not all HPV infection would cause premalignant changes. Without a good triage system for high-risk HPV-positive results, more women would need to be referred for colposcopy (see later section) and result in more unnecessary interventions. Therefore, some areas in the UK have adopted the HPV test as the primary cervical screening method, and this would be gradually introduced across the country. Women testing positive for high-risk HPV would have cytology triage (i.e. have an LBC done). If the woman has a positive high-risk-positive test and an abnormal cytology result (borderline or worse), she would be referred for colposcopy. In Australia, the primary HPV test with genotyping for 16 and 18 has replaced cytology in its cervical screening programme (see earlier section).

（五）异常筛选结果的处理（Management of abnormal screening results）

异常的细胞学检查和 HPV 检测阳性是筛查试验。为了得到诊断，需要对异常区域进行活检。阴道镜检查有助于识别异常区域。阴道镜检查是用带有光源的低倍率双目显微镜（阴道镜）检查宫颈和下生殖道。这是一种门诊手术，使用窥器显露子宫颈。在不同的国家，异常筛选试验后进行阴道镜检查的详细方案各不相同。一般而言，如果一项筛查试验提示有重大病变的可能性很高，患者应接受阴道镜活检。在英国，有高级别核异质（中度或重度）或细胞学检查中怀疑为浸润性癌的女性应转行阴道镜检查。有交界性改变或低级别核异常的女性需要进行高危 HPV 检测。如果高危 HPV 阳性，应转行阴道镜检查；如果是阴性，他们就会恢复常规筛查。以 HPV 筛查代替子宫颈细胞学检验作为主要筛查手段的女性，转行阴道镜的标准会比较复杂。由于许多高危 HPV 感染会自行消退，不会引起任何癌前病变，将所有高危 HPV 结果转诊将导致许多不必要的阴道镜检查。因此，需要进行第二次检测来筛选那些确实存在高级别病变风险的患者。这种分诊检查可以是细胞学检查，也可以是 HPV16 和 HPV18 的基因分型，它们特别与高级别病变相关。例如，在澳大利亚，如果一名女性是高危 HPV 阳性，并且其子宫颈涂片显示 HSIL，或者无论细胞学检查结果如何，只要她的 HPV16 或 HPV18 检测呈特异性阳性，那么她将被转介进行阴道镜检查。

Abnormal cytology and positive HPV tests are screening tests. To get a diagnosis, a biopsy of the abnormal area is needed. A colposcopic examination helps identify the abnormal areas. Colposcopy is examination of the cervix and lower genital tract with a low-power binocular microscope with a light source (a colposcope). It is an outpatient procedure performed using a speculum to expose the cervix. Detailed protocols for referral to colposcopy after an abnormal screening test vary in different countries. In general, if a screening test is suggestive of a high possibility of a significant lesion, the patient should be referred to colposcopy for a biopsy. In the UK, women with highgrade dyskaryosis (moderate or severe) or suspicions for invasive carcinoma in her cytology should be referred for colposcopy. Women with borderline changes or low-grade dyskaryosis would have a reflex high-risk HPV test done. If high-risk HPV positive, they should be referred to colposcopy; if negative, they would return to routine recall. For women who undergo HPV testing instead of cervical smear as their primary screening methods, referral criteria would be more complicated. As many high-risk HPV infections would regress spontaneously and would not cause any premalignant changes, referring all high-risk HPV results would lead to many unnecessary colposcopies. Therefore a second test to triage those who are really at risk of a highgrade lesion is needed. This triage test can be a cytology test or can be genotyping for HPV 16 and 18, which are particularly associated with highgrade lesions. For example, in Australia the woman would be referred for colposcopy if she is high-risk HPV positive and her cervical smear shows HSIL or she tests positive specifically for HPV 16 or 18, regardless of the results of the cytology

1. 阴道镜原理（Principles of colposcopy）

在进行阴道镜检查时，阴道镜医师会涂抹醋酸，其次是卢戈碘液，以确定在最不正常的部位进行活组织检查。与正常鳞状上皮细胞相比，肿瘤细胞有较多与细胞质有关的核物质和较少的表面糖原。它们与底层脉管系统的过度生长程度相关。当暴露于 5% 的醋酸时，核蛋白会凝固，使得肿瘤细胞呈现出典型的白色外观（图 20-10）。上皮下的小血管由于毛细血管组织增加，可见点状（斑点状）或铺路石状（镶嵌状）。肿瘤细胞不会与卢戈碘（Schiller 试验）发生反应，不同于正常会染成深棕色的鳞状上皮（图 20-11）。早期侵袭性癌症的特征是，有异常血管、脆弱组织、明显镶嵌状粗糙斑点的隆起或溃烂区域。触诊宫颈质硬，并且触诊时常有接触性出血。在较晚期的疾病中，宫颈变得固定，或者被易碎的疣状肿块所取代（图 20-12）。

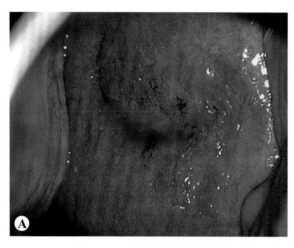
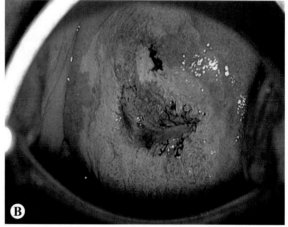

▲ 图 20-10　阴道镜下应用醋酸前（A）后（B）的高级别病变和。应用醋酸后外观为醋酸白

Fig. 20.10　Colposcopic appearance of a high-grade lesion before (A) and after (B) application of acetic acid. Note acetowhite appearance after the application of acetic acid.

At colposcopy, the colposcopist adds acetic acid, followed by Lugol's iodine, to identify the most abnormal areas to take biopsies. Neoplastic cells have an increased amount of nuclear material in relation to cytoplasm and less surface glycogen than normal squamous epithelium. They are associated with a degree of hypertrophy of the underlying vasculature. When exposed to 5% acetic acid, the nuclear protein will coagulate, giving the neoplastic cells a characteristic white appearance (Fig. 20.10). Small blood vessels beneath the epithelium may be seen as dots (punctation) or a crazy paving pattern (mosaicism) due to the increased capillary vasculature. The neoplastic cells do not react with Lugol's iodine (Schiller's test), unlike the normal squamous epithelium that will stain dark brown (Fig. 20.11). Early invasive cancer is characterized by a raised or ulcerated area with abnormal vessels, friable tissue and coarse punctation with marked mosaicism. It feels hard on palpation and often bleeds on contact. In more advanced disease, the cervix becomes fixed or replaced by a friable warty-looking mass (Fig. 20.12).

2. 高级别癌前病变的治疗（Treatment of high-grade preinvasive lesions）

如果经阴道镜活检显示为低级别病变，大多数情况下只需要定期检查。然而，如果活检显示高级别病变，则需要进行切除或破坏病变区域（通常是整个转化区）的治疗。

If the colposcopic-directed biopsy shows a low-grade lesion, only regular surveillance would be required in most cases. However, if the biopsy shows a high-grade lesion, treatment by excision or destruction of the affected area (usually the whole of the transformation zone) is required.

激光消融、冷冻术和凝固透热等破坏 / 消融方法只适用于能看到整个转化区，没有腺体异常或侵袭性疾病的证据，并且细胞学和组织学结果之间没

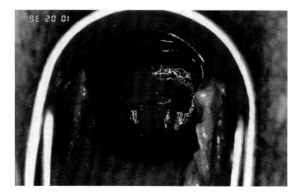

▲ 图 20-11　CIN-2 的阴道镜表现。异常的上皮无法被碘染色

Fig. 20.11　Colposcopic appearances of CIN-2. The abnormal epithelium fails to stain with iodine.

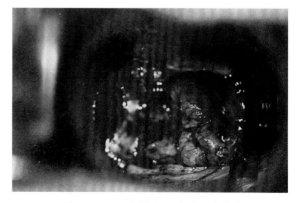

▲ 图 20-12　浸润性宫颈癌的阴道镜表现

Fig. 20.12　Colposcopic appearance of invasive carcinoma of the cervix.

有重大差异的情况。首选的治疗方法是切除而不是消融，因为切除的标本可以送去做组织学诊断，以确认活检结果。最常见的切除方法是转化区大环切除（LLETZ）（图 20-13），这是一种用电切环进行的切除，可以在门诊局部麻醉下完成。当无法看到 SCJ 或怀疑腺上皮病变时，我们需要进行更深的"锥形"活检，以确保对所有的宫颈内膜取样（图 20-14）。约 5% 的女性在治疗后会出现持续性或复发性疾病，因此随访很重要。不同国家的后续方案各不相同。例如，在英国，女性通常在 6 个月后被邀请再次进行细胞学 ± HPV 检测，作为治愈测试。如果细胞学检查和高危 HPV 均阴性，该女性可能在 3 年内复发；如果高危 HPV 呈阳性，她则需要再次进行阴道镜检查；如果 HPV 无法检测，那么她需要进行重复的细胞学检查。

Destructive/ablative methods such as laser ablation, cryocautery and coagulation diathermy are only suitable when the entire transformation zone can be visualized, there is no evidence of glandular abnormality or invasive disease and there is no major discrepancy between the cytology and histology results. Excision instead of ablation is the preferred treatment because the excised specimen can be sent for a histological diagnosis to confirm the biopsy result. The commonest excisional method is the large loop excision of the transformation zone (LLETZ) (Fig. 20.13), which is excision with a diathermy wire loop, which can be done under local anaesthetic in the outpatient clinic. When the SCJ cannot be seen or a lesion of the glandular epithelium is suspected, a deeper 'cone' biopsy is required to ensure that all of the endocervix is sampled (Fig. 20.14). About 5% of women will have persistent or recurrent disease following treatment; therefore, follow-up is important. Follow-up protocols vary in

For example, in the UK, women are usually invited to return for repeat cytology ± HPV test as a test of cure 6 months later. If both cytology and high-risk HPV are negative, the woman can return in 3 years. If high-risk HPV is positive, she will need to have colposcopy again. If HPV is not available, then she needs to have repeat cytology.

（六）宫颈癌（Cervical cancer）

1. 病理学（Pathology）

浸润性宫颈癌有两种类型，70%～80% 的病变为 SCC，20%～30% 为腺癌。组织学上，侵袭程度决定了疾病的分期（表 20-4）。

There are two types of invasive carcinoma of the cervix. Approximately 70–80% of lesions are SCC and 20–30% adenocarcinomas. Histologically, the degree of invasion determines the stage of the disease (Table 20.4).

2. 肿瘤的扩散（The spread of tumour）

宫颈癌通过直接浸润和通过淋巴管和血行转移。约 0.5% 的 IA_1 期女性发生淋巴转移，IA_2 期女性淋巴转移率上升至 5%，Ⅱ 期女性则为 40%。淋巴优先转移到髂外、髂内和闭孔淋巴结。次级水平也可转移到腹股沟、骶前和主动脉淋巴结。血源性转移发生在肺、肝、骨和肠。

Cervical carcinoma spreads by direct local invasion and via the lymphatics and blood vessels. Lymphatic spread occurs in approximately 0.5% of women with stage IA1 disease, rising to 5% for stage IA2 and 40% of women with stage II disease. Preferential spread occurs to the external iliac, internal iliac and obturator nodes. Secondary spread may also occur to inguinal, sacral and aortic nodes. Blood-borne metastases occur in the lungs, liver, bone and bowel.

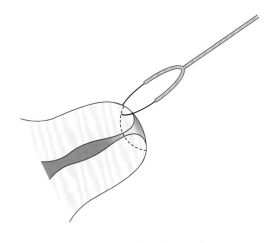

▲ 图 20-13　宫颈大环切除
Fig. 20.13　Large loop excision of the cervix.

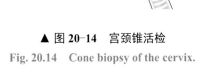

▲ 图 20-14　宫颈锥活检
Fig. 20.14　Cone biopsy of the cervix.

表 20-4 FIGO 宫颈癌的分类（2009 年）

Table 20.4 FIGO classification of cervical cancer (2009)

Ⅰ期 肿瘤严格局限于子宫颈（不考虑扩展到主体）
 Ⅰ A 期：仅依靠镜检即可诊断的浸润性癌，浸润最深≤5mm，最大延伸≤7mm
 Ⅰ A₁ 期：测定间质浸润深度≤3.0mm，浸润范围≤7.0mm
 Ⅰ A₂ 期：测得间质浸润>3.0mm，≤5.0mm，浸润范围≤7.0mm
 Ⅰ B 期：肉眼可见癌灶仅限于宫颈或镜下病灶大于Ⅰ A*
 Ⅰ B₁ 期：肉眼可见癌灶最大尺寸≤4.0cm
 Ⅰ B₂ 期：肉眼可见癌灶最大尺寸>4.0cm

Stage Ⅰ Carcinoma is strictly confined to the cervix (extension to the corpus would be disregarded):
Stage ⅠA: Invasive carcinoma that can be diagnosed only by microscopy, with deepest invasion ≤5 mm and largest extension ≤7 mm
Stage ⅠA₁: Measured stromal invasion of ≤3.0 mm in depth and extension of ≤7.0 mm
Stage ⅠA₂: Measured stromal invasion of >3.0 mm and not >5.0 mm with an extension of not >7.0 mm
Stage ⅠB: Clinically visible lesions limited to the cervix uteri or preclinical cancers greater than IA*
Stage ⅠB₁: Clinically visible lesion ≤4.0 cm in greatest dimension
Stage ⅠB₂: Clinically visible lesion >4.0 cm in greatest dimension

Ⅱ期 宫颈癌浸润子宫外，但浸润没有达到骨盆壁或未达阴道的下 1/3
 Ⅱ A 期：没有子宫旁组织的浸润
 Ⅱ A₁ 期：肉眼可见癌灶最大尺寸≤4.0cm
 Ⅱ A₂ 期：肉眼可见癌灶最大尺寸>4.0cm
 Ⅱ B 期：有明显的宫旁组织浸润

Stage Ⅱ Cervical carcinoma invades beyond the uterus but not to the pelvic wall or to the lower third of the vagina:
Stage ⅡA: Without parametrial invasion
Stage ⅡA₁: Clinically visible lesion ≤4.0 cm in greatest dimension
Stage ⅡA₂: Clinically visible lesion >4.0 cm in greatest dimension
Stage ⅡB: With obvious parametrial invasion

Ⅲ期 肿瘤延伸至盆腔壁和（或）累及阴道下 1/3，和（或）引起肾盂积水或肾功能不全**
 Ⅲ A 期：肿瘤累及阴道下 1/3，未延伸至骨盆壁
 Ⅲ B 期：扩展到骨盆壁和（或）肾积水或肾功能不全

Stage Ⅲ The tumour extends to the pelvic wall and/or involves lower third of the vagina and/or causes hydronephrosis or non-functioning kidney:**
Stage Ⅲ A: Tumour involves lower third of the vagina with no extension to the pelvic wall
Stage Ⅲ B: Extension to pelvic wall and/or hydronephrosis or non-functioning kidney

Ⅳ期 肿瘤已延伸至真骨盆以外或已侵犯膀胱或直肠黏膜（活检证实）。因此，大疱性水肿不属于Ⅳ期
 Ⅳ A 期：转移到邻近的器官
 Ⅳ B 期：转移到远处的器官

Stage Ⅳ The carcinoma has extended beyond the true pelvis or has involved (biopsy proven) the mucosa of the bladder or rectum. A bullous oedema, as such, does not permit a case to be allotted to stage IV:
Stage ⅣA: Spread of the growth to adjacent organs
Stage ⅣB: Spread to distant organs

经许可，转载自 Pecorelli S & FIGO Committee on Gynecologic Oncology (2009). International Journal of Gynecology & Obstetrics, 105(2):103-104.

*. 所有肉眼可见病变，即使有浅表浸润，均为Ⅰ B 期肿瘤。浸润仅限于间质浸润，最大深度 5.0mm，水平延伸不>7.0mm。取自原组织鳞状或腺上皮间质浸润深度不应>5.0mm。浸润深度应以毫米为单位报告，即使是"早期（最小）间质浸润"（≈1mm）的病例也应如此。血管 / 淋巴间隙的累及不应改变分期

**. 直肠检查时，肿瘤与骨盆壁之间没有无瘤间隙。所有肾盂积水或肾功能不全的病例均包括在内，除非已知有其他原因

Reproduced with permission from Pecorelli S & FIGO Committee on Gynecologic Oncology (2009). International Journal of Gynecology & Obstetrics, 105(2):103-104.

*. All macroscopically visible lesions-even with superficial invasion-are allotted to stage IB carcinomas. Invasion is limited to a measured stromal invasion with a maximal depth of 5.0 mm and a horizontal extension of not >7.0 mm. Depth of invasion should not be >5.0 mm taken from the base of the epithelium of the original tissue-squamous or glandular. The depth of invasion should always be reported in millimetres, even in those cases with 'early (minimal) stromal invasion' (≈1 mm). The involvement of vascular/lymphatic spaces should not change the stage allotment.

**. On rectal examination, there is no cancer-free space between the tumour and the pelvic wall. All cases with hydronephrosis or non-functioning kidney are included, unless they are known to be due to another cause.

3. 临床特征（Clinical features）

ⅠA 期在发病时通常无症状，并且在常规宫颈细胞学检查时发现。宫颈浸润癌的常见症状包括性交后出血，有时带血的恶臭稀水样分泌物，以及肿瘤坏死时的阴道不规则出血。宫旁组织横向浸润可累及输尿管，最终导致输尿管梗阻和肾衰竭。侵犯神经和骨骼会引起难以忍受和持续的疼痛，累及淋巴通道可能导致淋巴阻塞伴下肢顽固性水肿。

Stage IA disease is usually asymptomatic at the time of presentation and is detected at the time of routine cervical cytology. The common presenting symptoms from invasive carcinoma of the cervix include postcoital bleeding, foulsmelling discharge which is thin and watery and sometimes blood-stained, and irregular vaginal bleeding when the tumour becomes necrotic. Lateral invasion into the parametrium may involve the ureters, leading eventually to ureteric obstruction and renal failure. Invasion of nerves and bone causes excruciating and persistent pain, and involvement of lymphatic channels may result in lymphatic occlusion with intractable oedema of the lower limbs.

肿瘤也可向前或向后扩散，分别累及膀胱或直肠。累及膀胱可产生尿频、排尿困难和血尿等症状。如果累及肠道，可发生里急后重、腹泻和直肠出血。肿瘤最初可能在宫颈内生长，宫颈扩大如圆柱状、桶状，肿瘤的外在表现很少。

The tumour may also spread anteriorly or posteriorly to involve the bladder or rectum, respectively. Involvement of the bladder produces symptoms of frequency, dysuria and haematuria; if the bowel is involved, tenesmus, diarrhoea and rectal bleeding may occur. The neoplasm may initially grow within the endocervix, producing a cylindrical, barrelshaped enlargement of the cervix with little external manifestation of the tumour.

外生性肿瘤生长在子宫颈的阴道部分，呈菜花样肿瘤。肿瘤最终脱落并取代了正常的宫颈组织并延伸到阴道壁。

The exophytic tumour grows over the vaginal portion of the cervix and appears as a cauliflower-like tumour. The tumour eventually sloughs and replaces the normal cervical tissue and extends on to the vaginal walls.

4. 检查（Investigation）

我们通过对肿瘤进行活检来建立组织学诊断，活检深度应大于 5mm，以区分微小浸润癌和浸润性癌。诊断性 LLETZ 可能是必要的。除了ⅠA₁ 期，一般建议对紧张的患者在麻醉下进行阴道和直肠检查，加或不加用膀胱镜检查。腹部和盆腔的磁共振成像（MRI）用于评估宫旁和淋巴结状况。如果怀疑有肺转移，也需要胸部 CT。可考虑用 PET-CT 在晚期疾病中评估远处转移。

The diagnosis is established histologically by biopsy of the tumour, which should be greater than 5 mm in depth to distinguish between microinvasive and invasive disease. Diagnostic LLETZ may be necessary. Examination under anaesthesia in tense patients by vaginal and rectal examination, with or without cystoscopy is generally recommended except in stage IA1 disease. Magnetic resonance imaging (MRI) of the abdomen and pelvis is performed for assessment of the parametrium and lymph node status. Computed tomography (CT) of the thorax may also be needed if lung metastasis is suspected. Positron emission tomography (PET)-CT may be considered in advanced disease to assess for distant spread.

5. 浸润性癌的治疗（Treatment of invasive carcinoma）

我们通过手术、放疗 / 放化疗或两者的结合进行治疗。对于希望保留生育能力的ⅠA 期患者，局部锥切是一种选择。对于那些已经完成生育的ⅠA₁ 期患者，单纯子宫切除术即可。

Treatment is by surgery or radiotherapy/chemoradiation or a combination of both methods. Local excision by cone biopsy is an option for patients with stage IA lesions who wish to preserve fertility. Simple hysterectomy suffices for stage IA1 disease for those who have completed family.

广泛子宫切除术或放疗可用于治疗ⅠB～ⅡA 期患者。手术和放疗的治愈率相似，但前者通常阴道狭窄的长期发病率较低。手术还可以保护绝经前女性的卵巢功能。疾病Ⅱ～Ⅳ期通常采用放化疗，每周以铂类为基础的化疗、腔内放疗和外照射。

Extended hysterectomy or radiotherapy can be used to treat stage IB–IIA. The cure rate is similar for both surgery and radiotherapy, but the former is generally associated with less long-term morbidity from vaginal stenosis. Surgery can also preserve ovarian function for those premenopausal women. Stage II–IV disease is usually treated with chemoradiation with weekly platinum-based chemotherapy and intracavity and external beam radiotherapy.

(1) 手术：根治性子宫切除术和盆腔淋巴结清扫术（Surgery-radical hysterectomy and pelvic lymph node dissection）。子宫切除术（图 20-15）包括切除子宫、宫旁组织和阴道上 1/3。卵巢可被保留。这种治疗方法，配合髂内外及闭孔淋巴结清扫术，适合ⅠB₁ 期及早期ⅡA₁ 期患者。并发症包括出血、感染、盆腔血肿、淋巴囊肿 / 淋巴水肿、膀胱功能障碍和输尿管或膀胱损伤，这可能导致 2%～5% 病例瘘管形成。然而，手术治疗阴道狭窄的发生率低于放疗，因此性交功能得以更好地保留，这使其成为年轻女性患者的首选治疗方法。如果希望保留生育功能，可以考虑对体积小的 Ⅰ B₁ 期肿瘤（<2cm）行根治性子宫颈切除术并进行盆腔淋巴结清扫和预防性宫颈环扎术。

Radical hysterectomy (Fig. 20.15) includes removal of the uterus, parametrium and upper third of the vagina. The ovaries may be conserved. This method of treatment, together with internal and external iliac and obturator lymph node dissection, is appropriate for patients with stage IB1 and earlystage IIA1 diseases. Complications include haemorrhage, infection, pelvic haematomas, lymphocyst/lymphoedema, bladder dysfunction and damage to the ureters or bladder, which may result in fistula formation in 2–5% of cases. However, the incidence of vaginal stenosis is less than after radiotherapy, and so coital function is better preserved, making it the treatment of choice in the younger woman. Radical trachelectomy with pelvic lymph node dissection and prophylactic cervical cerclage can be considered in small-stage IB1 tumour (less than 2 cm) if preservation of fertility is desired.

(2) 放疗 / 放化疗（Radiotherapy/chemoradiation）：这种疗法适用于治疗其他分期的宫颈癌和那些肿瘤体积大的 Ⅰ B 期或不适合手术的患者。疾病早期的分期生存率与手术相似。辅助放化疗也用于那些在手术时发现有淋巴结受累的患者。

This is to treat other stages of cervical cancer and those patients with bulky stage IB disease or who are unfit for surgery. Survival stage-for-stage in early forms of the disease is similar to that for surgery. Adjuvant chemoradiotherapy is also used for those patients who have been found to have lymph node involvement at the time of surgery. Chemotherapy is platinum based and given weekly in conjunction with radiotherapy.

化疗以铂为基础，每周配合放疗。放射治疗的方法是将镭（Ra）、铯 –137（^{137}Cs）和铱 –192（^{192}Ir）局部放入宫腔和阴道穹窿，并对骨盆侧壁进行外照射。并发症包括过度辐射对正常组织的影响，并可能导致放射性膀胱炎或直肠炎，以及瘘管形成和阴道狭窄。

Radiotherapy is administered by local insertion of a source of radium, cesium-137 and iridium-192 into the uterine cavity and the vaginal vault and by external beam radiation to the pelvic side wall. Complications include the effects of excessive radiation on normal tissues and may lead to radiation cystitis or proctitis, as well as fistula formation and vaginal stenosis.

6. 预后（Prognosis）

预后主要取决于诊断时的分期和淋巴结状态。5 年生存率结果如下。

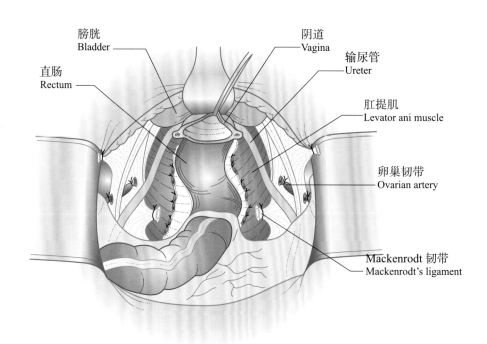

▲ 图 20-15 根治性子宫切除术包括切除子宫、子宫旁组织和阴道上 1/3

Fig. 20.15 **Radical hysterectomy involves excision of the uterus, parametrium and upper third of the vagina.**

- Ⅰ期：85%。

- Ⅱ期：60%。

- Ⅲ期：30%。

- Ⅳ期：10%。

This depends mainly on the stage at diagnosis and lymph node status. The results for 5-year survival are:

- stage I: 85%
- stage II: 60%
- stage III: 30%
- stage IV: 10%.

1/3 的病例出现复发性宫颈病变，预后较差。当局部复发累及膀胱或直肠，但未扩展到其他结构时，有时可通过根治性切除或脏器切除实现治疗切除，其中包括全膀胱切除术和直肠切除。

Recurrent cervical lesions occur in a third of cases and have a poor prognosis. Where local recurrence involves the bladder or rectum but does not extend to other structures, curative excision may occasionally be achieved by radical excision or exenteration, including total cystectomy and removal of the rectum.

四、子宫恶性疾病（Malignant disease of the uterus）

（一）子宫内膜癌（Endometrial carcinoma）

在发达国家，子宫内膜腺癌是最常见的女性肿瘤之一。在英国，它是第四大最常见的女性肿瘤，占所有女性肿瘤的 5%（2015 年）。在过去的 10 年里，它的发病率增加了 21%。它主要见于绝经后的女性。发病率在 65—69 岁的女性中最高。

In developed countries, endometrial adenocarcinoma is one of the commonest female cancers. In the UK, it is the fourth most common female cancer, accounting for 5% of all female cancers (2015). Over the last decade, the incidence has increased by 21%. It mainly affects postmenopausal women. The incidence peaks in women aged 65–69.

一些特定的因素与子宫体癌的风险增加相关，如未生育、绝经晚、糖尿病和高血压。它也可能是遗传的。患有遗传性非息肉性结直肠癌（HNPCC）综合征的女性患子宫内膜癌、卵巢癌及结直肠癌的风险增加。然而，最重要的危险因素是高雌激素状态。

Specific factors are associated with an increased risk of corpus carcinoma, such as nulliparity, late menopause, diabetes and hypertension. It can also be hereditary. Women with hereditary non-polyposis colorectal cancer (HNPCC) syndrome have increased risk of endometrial and ovarian cancers, as well as colorectal cancer. However, the most important risk factors are associated with a hyperoestrogenic state:

- 肥胖：绝经后卵巢间质继续产生雄激素，并在脂肪组织中转化为雌激素。在子宫内膜上起着无对抗的雌激素作用，导致子宫内膜增生和恶性肿瘤。

- Obesity: The ovarian stroma continues to produce androgens after menopause, which are converted to oestrone in adipose tissue. This acts as unopposed oestrogen on the endometrium, resulting in endometrial hyperplasia and malignancy.

- 外源性雌激素：无对抗的雌激素作用，如单独使用雌激素而不用孕激素抵抗，这与子宫内膜癌发病率的增加有关。每个月至少增加 10 天的孕激素可以降低这种风险，联合口服避孕药可以降低该病的发病率。

- Exogenous oestrogens: Unopposed oestrogen action, e.g. having oestrogen alone without progestogen for hormonal replacement, is associated with an increased incidence of endometrial carcinoma. The addition of a progestogen for at least 10 days of each month can reduce this risk, and the combined oral contraceptive pill reduces the incidence of the disease.

- 内源性雌激素：产生雌激素的卵巢肿瘤，如颗粒细胞肿瘤，与子宫内膜癌的风险增加有关。

- Endogenous oestrogens: Oestrogen-producing ovarian tumours, such as granulosa cell tumours, are associated with an increase in the risk of endometrial cancer.

- 他莫昔芬在乳腺癌中的作用：乳腺癌患者服用他莫昔芬后发生子宫内膜癌的风险略高，但多数早期发现，预后良好。

- Tamoxifen in breast cancer: Breast cancer patients on tamoxifen have a slightly increased risk of endometrial cancer, but most of these are detected in early stages nd have good prognosis.

- 子宫内膜增生症：用无对抗性的雌激素长期刺激子宫内膜可导致子宫内膜增生，出现闭经，随后出现大量或不规则的出血。子宫内膜增生可分为有异型性和无异型性。有不典型增生的女性并发癌的机会高达 50%，未来发展为癌的概率为30%。这些女性通常采用子宫切除术和双侧输卵管卵巢切除术（bilateral salpingo-oophorectomy，BSO）。无异型增生的患者患癌的风险要低得多（<5%）。这些女性中绝大多数可以通过孕激素保守治疗。

- Endometrial hyperplasia: Prolonged stimulation of the endometrium with unopposed oestrogen may lead to hyperplasia of the endometrium with periods of amenorrhoea followed by heavy or irregular bleeding. Endometrial hyperplasia can be classified into those with or without atypia. Women with atypical hyperplasia have an up to 50% chance of concurrent carcinoma and 30% chance of future progression to carcinoma. These women are usually treated by hysterectomy and bilateral salpingo-oophorectomy (BSO). The risk of carcinoma in those with hyperplasia without atypia is much lower (<5%). The majority of these women can be treated conservatively by progestogen therapy.

1. 症状（Symptoms）

最常见的症状是绝经后出血。然而，对于绝经前的女性，子宫内膜癌与不规则阴道出血和月经量逐渐增加有关。伴有子宫积脓的老年患者也应怀疑是子宫内膜癌。这些女性通常有带脓的阴道分泌物。

The commonest symptom is postmenopausal bleeding. However, in the premenopausal woman, endometrial carcinoma is associated with irregular vaginal bleeding and increasingly heavy menses. Endometrial cancer should also be suspected in elderly patients with pyometra. These women usually present with purulent vaginal discharge.

2. 病理学（Pathology）

子宫内膜癌可分为两种类型。Ⅰ型指子宫内膜样腺癌。这种类型与高雌激素状态有关，因此所有危险因素都与高雌激素相关，如肥胖、糖尿病、无对抗的雌激素等。Ⅱ型内膜癌代表其他组织学类型，如浆液性乳头状和透明细胞亚型。这些分型往往是恶性，预后较差。人们正在根据它们的分子图谱其进行更好的分类。

Endometrial carcinoma can be divided into two types. Type I refers to endometrioid adenocarcinoma. This type is related to the hyperoestrogenic state and hence all the risk factors associated with hyperoestrogenism, such as obesity, diabetes, unopposed oestrogen, etc. Type II represents other histological types, such as serous papillary and clear cell subtypes. These tend to be aggressive tumours with poorer prognosis. Work is underway to better classify them according to their molecular profiles

大多数子宫内膜癌是子宫内膜样腺癌（Ⅰ型）。显微镜下表现为细胞结构的改变，多面体样细胞密集，细胞核染色深，有大量的有丝分裂。

Most endometrial cancer is endometrioid (type I) cancer. The microscopic appearances include changes in the architecture with the development of closely packed polyhedral cells with dark-staining nuclei and considerable numbers of mitoses.

子宫内膜癌在局部生长（图20-16）。肿瘤通过直接侵犯子宫肌层，然后经阴道、经输卵管和癌物质外溢而扩散。肿瘤也可以通过淋巴转移到盆腔和

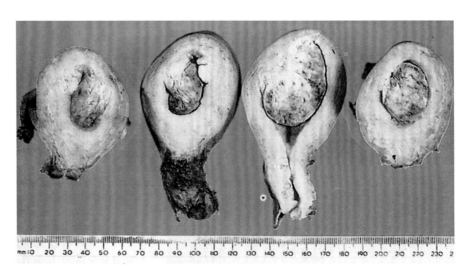

▲ 图 20-16　子宫内膜腺癌。多个切片显示子宫内膜癌浸润子宫肌层

Fig. 20.16　Endometrial adenocarcinoma. Multiple sections showing a large endometrial carcinoma invading the substance of the myometrium.

主动脉旁淋巴结。

Endometrial cancer grows locally (Fig. 20.16). The tumour spreads by direct invasion into the myometrium and then transcervically, transtubally and by spillage of carcinomatous material. There can also be lymphatic spread to the pelvic and para-aortic nodes

3. 检查（Investigations）

初步检查包括经阴道超声扫描以评估子宫内膜厚度，以及通过子宫内膜抽吸获得子宫内膜组织进行组织学评估。绝经后女性经阴道超声检查子宫内膜厚度＜5mm，表明患子宫内膜癌的风险非常低。然而，对绝经前或围绝经期女性使用子宫内膜厚度进行参考不太可靠，因为子宫内膜厚度随月经周期变化。对于 40 岁以上有异常阴道出血的女性，子宫内膜抽吸物应该是评估子宫内膜的一线检查。子宫内膜抽吸可使用各种子宫内膜取样器，如 Pipelle 取样器。Pipelle 取样器是一种直径非常小（如 3mm）的透明塑料套管，不用扩宫即可通过宫颈口，也无须麻醉可在诊室内进行取样。然而，如果子宫内膜抽吸不成功或不确定，或者症状持续，尽管子宫内膜抽吸结果阴性，诊断性宫腔镜检查和活检仍是必需的。这些手术可以在门诊进行，也可以在全身麻醉的情况下进行。宫腔镜是一种狭窄的、坚硬的镜子，在诊断性宫腔镜检查中，其可通过宫颈口进入子宫腔。将其用气体或液体扩张，可以直接显示子宫腔，并且可以对子宫内膜的任何病变进行定位活检。这种手术的风险很小，但可能会发生并发症，如子宫穿孔、宫颈撕裂、盆腔感染和对膨宫介质的反应。子宫内膜癌的诊断是通过组织学上子宫内膜活检结果确定的。

Initial investigations include a transvaginal ultrasound scan to assess the endometrial thickness and an endometrial aspirate to obtain endometrial tissue for histological assessment. An endometrial thickness of less than 5 mm on transvaginal ultrasound in a postmenopausal woman indicates a very low risk of endometrial cancer. However, using endometrial thickness is less reliable in premenopausal or perimenopausal women because the endometrial thickness varies with the menstrual cycle. In women over 40 years old who have abnormal vaginal bleeding, an endometrial aspirate should be the first-line investigation to assess the endometrium. Endometrial aspirate can be done with various endometrial samplers such as the Pipelle sampler. The Pipelle is a transparent plastic cannula with a very small diameter, e.g. 3 mm, that can be passed through the cervical os without dilation and can be done in the office without anaesthesia. However,

if the endometrial aspirate is unsuccessful or inconclusive or symptoms persist despite a negative endometrial aspirate result, a diagnostic hysteroscopy and biopsy are required. These can be carried out as outpatient procedures or under general anaesthesia. During a diagnostic hysteroscopy, a hysteroscope, which is a narrow, rigid telescope, is passed through the cervical os and the uterine cavity is distended by either gas or fluid. This allows direct visualization of the uterine cavity, and directed biopsies of any endometrial lesions can be taken. The risk of this procedure is small, but complications can occur, such as uterine perforation, cervical laceration, pelvic infection and reaction to distension media. The diagnosis of endometrial cancer is established histologically by the endometrial biopsy result.

4. 治疗（Treatment）

治疗的主要手段是全子宫切除和双附件切除。对所有患者常规行盆腔和主动脉旁淋巴结清扫术的治疗价值是有争议的。术前检查包括全血细胞计数、肾功能和肝功能检查和胸部 X 线检查，以及根据个人健康状况进行如心电图（ECG）、血糖水平等额外检查。肿瘤（或糖类）抗原 125（CA-125）可能在疾病晚期升高，其术前的基线值对后续疾病监测有用。宫外出现病变的危险因素包括高级别病变、不利的组织学亚型（如浆液或透明细胞组织学）、肿瘤大小和子宫肌层浸润深度。分级和组织学亚型可通过子宫内膜活检进行评估。肿瘤的大小和子宫肌层浸润可以通过术前影像学检查（如超声、CT 或 MRI）来评估。MRI 是目前应用最广泛的技术。它有助于评估子宫肌层浸润、宫颈浸润和淋巴结转移情况。尽管如此，MRI 的准确性也是有限的，并不是对所有患者都有好的成本效益。全子宫切除术可以通过开腹、腹腔镜或经阴道手术来完成。我们应对患者进行个体化评估，以确定最佳手术方式。

The mainstay of treatment is total hysterectomy and BSO. The value of routine pelvic and para-aortic lymphadenectomy for all patients is controversial. Preoperative investigations include full blood count, renal and liver function test and a chest X-ray, as well as any additional investigations depending on individual health status such as electrocardiogram (ECG), blood sugar levels, etc. Cancer (or carbohydrate) antigen 125 (CA-125) may be raised in advanced disease, and a preoperative baseline value can be useful for subsequent disease monitoring. Risk factors for extrauterine disease include high-grade lesions, unfavourable histological subtypes (e.g. serous or clear cell histology), tumour size and depth of myometrial invasion. The grading and histological subtypes can be assessed by endometrial biopsy. The tumour size and myometrial invasion can be assessed by preoperative imaging such as ultrasound, CT or MRI. Currently, MRI is the most widely used technique. It helps to assess myometrial invasion, cervical invasion and lymph node involvement. Nonetheless, MRI has limited accuracy and may not be cost-effective for all patients. Total hysterectomy can be done by open laparotomy, laparoscopically or vaginally. Patients should be individually assessed to determine the best route.

对于有复发高危因素的患者，我们常给予辅助放疗。阴道近距离放疗可减少穹窿局部复发。骨盆外束照射可用于有复发风险的患者。远处高复发风险患者，应该考虑化疗。肿瘤晚期患者的治疗方法是先行减瘤术，然后再进行化疗伴或不伴放疗。

Adjuvant radiotherapy is often given to patients with high risk of recurrence. Vaginal brachytherapy can reduce local vault recurrence. External beam pelvic irradiation can be given to those with risk of pelvic recurrence. Chemotherapy should be considered for patients with high risk of distal recurrence. Patients with advanced disease are treated by debulking the tumour followed by chemotherapy with or without radiotherapy.

5. 预后（Prognosis）

子宫内膜癌靠手术分期（表 20–5）。子宫内膜癌的预后很大程度上取决于疾病的分期及其他预后因素，包括年龄、组织学亚型和分级。对于 I 期 I 级，子宫肌层浅表浸润者 5 年生存率可达 90% 以上；而对于子宫肌层深部浸润和Ⅲ级病变患者，即使病变局限于子宫，5 年生存率也仅为 60% 左右。对于Ⅱ期、Ⅲ期和Ⅳ期患者，5 年生存率分别为 70%~80%、40%~50% 和 20%。浆液性乳头状癌和透明细胞癌预后较差，5 年生存率分别为 50% 和 35%。

Endometrial cancer is surgically staged (Table 20.5). Prognosis largely depends on the stage of the disease as well as other prognostic factors that include age, histological subtype and grading. For stage I grade I, the 5-year survival can be over 90% for those with superficial myometrial invasion, but for those with deep myometrial invasion and grade III disease, the 5-year survival is only about 60% even if the disease is still confined to the uterus. For stage II, III and IV diseases, the 5-year survival is about 70–80%, 40–50% and 20%, respectively. Serous papillary and clear cell carcinomas have poorer prognosis, with 5-year survival rates of 50% and 35%, respectively.

（二）子宫恶性间质肿瘤（Malignant mesenchymal tumours of the uterus）

非上皮肿瘤仅占子宫恶性肿瘤的 3%。一般来说，它们起源于子宫平滑肌（平滑肌肉瘤）或子宫内膜间质（间质肉瘤）。混合型米勒管或癌肉瘤包含来自子宫内膜上皮和间质的恶性成分，被认为是子宫内膜癌的变异。

Non-epithelial tumours account for only 3% of uterine malignancies. In general, they arise from either myometrial smooth muscle (leiomyosarcomas) or stroma of the endometrium (stromal sarcomas). Mixed müllerian duct or carcinosarcomas contain malignant elements from both the endometrial epithelium and stroma and are considered variants of endometrial cancer.

1. 子宫内膜间质肉瘤（Endometrial stromal sarcomas）

这些肿瘤起源于子宫内膜间质，占子宫肉瘤的不到 10%，约占所有子宫恶性肿瘤的 1%，可分为子宫内膜间质结节（ESN）、低级别子宫内膜间质肉瘤（LGESS）、高级别 ESS（HGESS）和未分化子宫肉瘤（UUS）。ESN 为良性，其余为恶性。HGESS 与 LGESS 相比更具侵袭性，高复发率和高死亡率，而 UUS 的预后最差。与其他伴有阴道排液和出血的子宫肿瘤相比，它们往往出现在较小的年龄组（45—50 岁）。子宫内膜间质肉瘤与子宫腺肌症和子宫内膜异位症有关。标准的治疗方法是全子宫切除术加双附件切除术。Ⅰ期年轻女性患者保留卵巢可能是一种选择。LGESS 的雌激素受体和孕激素受体通常呈阳性，因此激素治疗，如孕激素和芳香化酶抑制剂，通常用于疾病晚期。HGESS 和 UUS 复发风险高。尽管不清楚是否任何形式的辅助治疗可以提高生存率，但经常使用化疗。

These tumours, arising from the stroma of the endometrium, account for less than 10% of uterine sarcomas and about 1% of all uterine malignant tumours. They are classified as endometrial stromal nodule (ESN), low-grade endometrial stromal sarcoma (LGESS), high-grade ESS (HGESS) or undifferentiated uterine sarcoma (UUS). ESN is benign, while the others are malignant. HGESS is more aggressive and is associated with more recurrences and higher mortality than LGESS, and UUS has the worst prognosis. They tend to present in a younger age group (45–50 years) than other uterine tumours with vaginal discharge and bleeding. Endometrial stromal sarcoma is found in association with adenomyosis and endometriosis. The standard treatment is by total hysterectomy and BSO. Retention of the ovaries in young women with stage 1 disease may be an option. LGESS is usually positive for oestrogen and progesterone receptors, and hormonal treatment, such as progestins and aromatase inhibitors, is commonly given for advanced disease. HGESS and UUS have a high risk of recurrence. Chemotherapy is often

表 20-5　FIGO 分期子宫内膜癌（2009）

Table 20.5　FIGO staging for endometrial cancer (2009)

Ⅰ期 *　局限于子宫体的肿瘤：
　Ⅰ A 期：肿瘤浸润深度<1/2 肌层
　Ⅰ B 期：肿瘤浸润深度≥1/2 肌层

Stage I *　Tumour confined to the corpus uteri:
　Stage IA: No or less than half myometrial invasion
　Stage IB: Invasion equal to or more than half of the myometrium

Ⅱ期 *　肿瘤侵犯宫颈间质，但无宫体外蔓延 **

Stage Ⅱ *　Tumour invades cervical stroma but does not extend beyond the uterus **

Ⅲ期 *　肿瘤局部和（或）区域扩散
　Ⅲ A：肿瘤累及子宫浆膜和（或）附件 #
　Ⅲ B：肿瘤累及阴道和（或）宫旁组织 #
　Ⅲ C：盆腔淋巴结和（或）腹主动脉旁淋巴结转移 #
　Ⅲ C$_1$：盆腔淋巴结转移
　Ⅲ C$_2$：腹主动脉旁淋巴结转移伴（或不伴）盆腔淋巴结转移

Stage Ⅲ *　Local and/or regional spread of the tumour:
　Stage Ⅲ A: Tumour invades the serosa of the corpus uteri and/or adnexae #
　Stage Ⅲ B: Vaginal and/or parametrial involvement #
　Stage Ⅲ C: Metastases to pelvic and/or paraaortic lymph nodes #
　Stage Ⅲ C$_1$: Positive pelvic nodes
　Stage Ⅲ C$_2$: Positive para-aortic lymph nodes with or without positive pelvic lymph nodes

Ⅳ期 *　肿瘤侵犯膀胱和（或）直肠黏膜，和（或）远处转移
　Ⅳ A：肿侵及膀胱和（或）直肠黏膜
　Ⅳ B：远处转移，其中包括腹腔内和（或）腹股沟淋巴结转移

Stage Ⅳ *　Tumour invades bladder and/or bowel mucosa, and/or distant metastases:
　Stage Ⅳ A: Tumour invasion of bladder and/or bowel mucosa
　Ⅳ Stage Ⅳ B: Distant metastases, including intra-abdominal metastases and/or inguinal lymph nodes

*. G1、G2 或 G3

**. 宫颈腺受累应只视为Ⅰ期，而不再是Ⅱ期

#. 阳性细胞学必须单独报告，而不改变分期

经许可，转载自 Pecorelli S & FIGO Committee on Gynecologic Oncology (2009). International Journal of Gynecology & Obstetrics, 105(2):103-104.

*. Either G1, G2 or G3.

**. Endocervical glandular involvement only should be considered stage I and no longer stage II.

#Positive cytology has to be reported separately without changing the stage.

Reproduced with permission from Pecorelli S & FIGO Committee on Gynecologic Oncology (2009). International Journal of Gynecology & Obstetrics, 105(2):103-104.

given, although it is not clear if any form of adjuvant treatment would improve survival.

2. 平滑肌肉瘤（Leiomyosarcoma）

这些平滑肌肿瘤发生于子宫肌层，仅占子宫恶性肿瘤的 1.3%。这些疾病比较少见（0.7/10 万），52 岁为发病高峰，比肌瘤发病高峰约晚 10 年。虽然肌瘤发生恶性变化的风险很小（0.3%～0.8%），但平滑肌肿瘤在现有的肌瘤中有 5%～10% 的发生率。平滑肌肉瘤可根据分化程度进行分类。它们可能表现为疼痛、绝经后出血或快速生长的"肌瘤"，但通常无症状，并在子宫肌瘤切除术后确诊。治疗方法是子宫切除术。辅助放疗和（或）化疗有时被认为可以降低复发风险，但它们在提高生存率方面的作用尚不清楚。

These smooth muscle tumours arise in the myometrium of the uterus and account for only 1.3% of uterine malignancies. They are uncommon (0.7/100,000), with a peak incidence at the age of 52 years, about 10 years later than the peak incidence for fibroids. Between 5% and 10% arise in existing fibroids, although the risk of malignant change occurring in a fibroid is small (0.3–0.8%). Leiomyosarcomas are classified according to the degree of differentiation. They may present with pain, postmenopausal bleeding or a rapidly growing 'fibroid' but are often asymptomatic and diagnosed following hysterectomy for fibroids. Treatment is by hysterectomy. Adjuvant radiotherapy and/or chemotherapy are sometimes considered to reduce the risk of recurrence, but their role in improving survival is unknown.

3. 癌肉瘤（Carcinosarcoma）

癌肉瘤（图 20–17）由上皮细胞和间叶细胞组成。上皮细胞通常是子宫内膜样细胞，但也可以是鳞状细胞或混合型。其基质成分可以是异源的（成软骨细胞瘤、骨肉瘤、纤维肉瘤）或同源的（平滑肌肉瘤、前肉瘤）。它们的处理方法与高级别子宫内膜癌相似。癌肉瘤平均发病年龄为 65 岁。检查时常发现子宫不规则增大，并有肿瘤从宫颈口突出。子宫外转移发生较早，所以只有 25% 的患者在确诊时疾病仅限于子宫内膜。

These tumours (Fig. 20.17) consist of both epithelial and esenchymal elements. The epithelial elements are usually endometrioid but can be squamous or a mixture. The stromal elements are either heterologous (chondroblastoma, osteosarcoma, fibrosarcoma) or homologous (leiomyosarcoma, presarcoma). They are managed in a similar way to that of a high-grade endometrial cancer. The mean age at presentation is 65 years. An enlarged, irregular uterus with tumour protruding through the cervical os is a common finding at examination. Extrauterine spread occurs early, and only 25% of patients have disease limited to the endometrium at the time of diagnosis.

五、卵巢病变（Lesions of the ovary）

卵巢肿大通常是无症状的，卵巢恶性肿瘤的无症状性是导致疾病进展到晚期的主要原因。卵巢肿瘤可以是囊性的或实性的、功能性的、良性的或恶性的。卵巢肿瘤的表现和并发症有一些共同因素，如果没有直接检查通常很难确定肿瘤的性质。

Ovarian enlargement is commonly asymptomatic, and the silent nature of malignant ovarian tumours is the major reason for the advanced stage of presentation. Ovarian tumours may be cystic or solid, functional, benign or malignant. There are common factors in the presentation and complications of ovarian tumours, and it is often difficult to establish the nature of a tumour without direct examination.

（一）症状（Symptoms）

直径 <10cm 的卵巢肿瘤很少出现症状。常见症状如下。

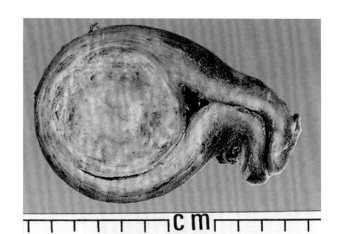

▲ 图 20-17　大的米勒管混合瘤
Fig. 20.17　Large mixed müllerian tumour.

- 腹部增大——出现恶变时，也可能与腹水有关。

- 压迫周围组织（如膀胱和直肠）的症状。

- 与肿瘤并发症有关的症状（图 20–18）如下。

  - 扭转：卵巢蒂的急性扭转导致肿瘤坏死；会出现急性疼痛和呕吐，肿瘤坏死后疼痛缓解。

  - 破裂：囊肿内容物溢入腹膜腔，引起泛发性腹痛。

  - 出血：肿瘤出血是一种不常见的并发症，但如果出血严重，可导致腹痛和休克。

  - 激素分泌肿瘤：可表现为月经周期紊乱。在雄激素分泌肿瘤中，患者可能表现出男性化的迹象。虽然大部分的性索间质型肿瘤（见后文）是激素活跃的，但临床实践中最常见的激素分泌肿瘤是上皮性的。

Tumours of the ovary that are less than 10 cm in diameter rarely produce symptoms. The common presenting symptoms include:

- Abdominal enlargement-in the presence of malignant change, this may also be associated with ascites.

- Symptoms from pressure on surrounding structures such as the bladder and rectum.

- Symptoms relating to complications of the tumour (Fig. 20.18). These include:

  - Torsion: Acute torsion of the ovarian pedicle results in necrosis of the tumour; there is acute pain and

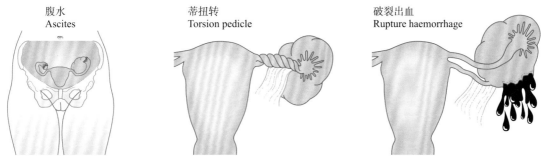

▲ 图 20-18　需要立即就医的卵巢肿瘤的常见并发症

Fig. 20.18　Common complications of ovarian tumours that precipitate a request for medical advice.

vomiting followed by remission of the pain when the tumour has become necrotic.

- Rupture: The contents of the cyst spill into the peritoneal cavity and result in generalized abdominal pain.
- Haemorrhage into the tumour is an unusual complication but may result in abdominal pain and shock if the blood loss is severe.
- Hormone-secreting tumours may present with disturbances in the menstrual cycle. In androgen-secreting tumours, the patient may present with signs of virilization. Although a greater proportion of the sex-cord stromal type of tumour (see later) are hormonally active, the commonest type of secreting tumour found in clinical practice is the epithelial type.

（二）体征（Signs）

体格检查时，腹部可明显增大。在膨胀处叩诊可显示中央性浊音和两侧共振。大量腹水可掩盖这些体征。虽然小于 5cm 的肿瘤通常无法触及，盆腔检查可发现小肿瘤，可在触诊时于一侧或两侧穹窿内发现。随着肿瘤的增大，它会处于更加正中的位置。大多数卵巢肿瘤触诊时无压痛；如果出现压痛，则应怀疑是否存在感染或扭转。良性卵巢肿瘤可与子宫体分开触到，通常可自由活动。

On examination, the abdomen may be visibly enlarged. Percussion over the swelling will demonstrate central dullness and resonance in the flanks. These signs may be obscured by gross ascites. Small tumours may be detected on pelvic examination and will be found by palpation in one or both fornices, although tumours smaller than 5 cm are often not palpable. As the tumour enlarges, it assumes a more central position. Most ovarian tumours are not tender on palpation; if they are painful, the presence of infection or torsion should be suspected. Benign ovarian tumours may be palpable separately from the uterine body and are usually freely mobile.

六、卵巢良性肿瘤（Benign ovarian tumours）

（一）功能性卵巢囊肿（Functional cysts of the ovary）

这些囊肿只发生在有月经的时期，直径很少超过 6cm。

These cysts occur only during menstrual life and rarely exceed more than 6 cm in diameter.

1. 滤泡囊肿（Follicular cysts）

滤泡囊肿（图 20-19）是卵巢最常见的功能性囊肿，可以是多发的和双侧的。囊肿直径很少超过 4cm，囊壁由几层颗粒细胞和富含性激素的透亮液体组成。囊肿大多数无症状，并在几个月内自行消退。这些囊肿可能发生在用克罗米酚或促性腺激素刺激卵巢时（图 20-20）。

Follicular cysts (Fig. 20.19) are the commonest functional cysts in the ovary and may be multiple and bilateral. The cysts rarely exceed 4 cm in diameter, with the walls consisting of layers of granulosa cells and the contents of clear fluid, which is rich in sex steroids. Most are asymptomatic and resolve spontaneously within a few months. These cysts may occur during ovarian stimulation with clomiphene or human menopausal gonadotrophin (Fig. 20.20).

2. 黄体囊肿（Lutein cysts）

黄素化卵巢囊肿有以下两种类型。

There are two types of luteinized ovarian cysts:

- 颗粒细胞黄体囊肿是黄体的功能性囊肿，直径可达 4~6cm，发生于月经周期的后半期。这种囊肿持续分泌黄体酮可能导致闭经或月经来潮延迟。该病常引起疼痛，由于病

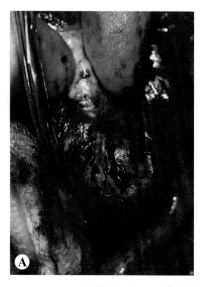

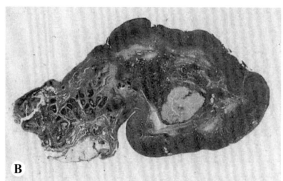

▲ 图 20-19　A. 接近月经周期中期的小卵泡囊肿；B. 组织学特性

Fig. 20.19　(A) Small follicular cyst near mid-cycle. (B) Histological features.

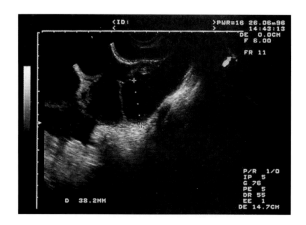

▲ 图 20-20　盆腔超声显示卵巢过度刺激并有多个卵泡

Fig. 20.20　Pelvic ultrasound showing ovarian hyperstimulation with multiple follicles.

史和检查结果与输卵管异位妊娠相似，故很难鉴别诊断。偶尔囊肿出血时，可伴随破裂并导致腹腔内积血。囊肿通常会自行消退，只有在出现腹腔内出血症状时才需要手术治疗。

- Granulosa lutein cysts, functional cysts of the corpus luteum, may be 4–6 cm in diameter and occur in the second half of the menstrual cycle. Persistent production of progesterone may result in amenorrhoea or delayed onset of menstruation. These cysts often give rise to pain and therefore present a problem in terms of differential diagnosis, as the history and examination findings mimic tubal ectopic pregnancy. Occasionally, haemorrhage occurs into the cyst, which may rupture and lead to a haemoperitoneum. The cysts usually regress spontaneously and require surgical intervention only when they give rise to symptoms of intra-abdominal haemorrhage.

- 卵泡膜黄体囊肿通常与高水平的人绒毛膜促性腺激素（hCG）有关，因此可见于葡萄胎患者。囊肿可以是双侧的，有时破裂可引起出血。一旦囊肿形成，就可以通过超声检测出来。它们通常会自发退化，但如果有卵巢大量出血，则可能需要手术治疗。

- Theca lutein cysts commonly arise in association with high levels of chorionic gonadotrophin and are therefore seen in cases of hydatidiform mole. The cysts may be bilateral and can on occasion give rise to haemorrhage if they rupture. Once the cysts have been formed, they can be detected by ultrasound. They usually undergo spontaneous involution, but surgical intervention may be necessary if there is significant haemorrhage from the ovaries.

（二）良性赘生性囊肿（Benign neoplastic cysts）

这些肿瘤起源于卵巢的特定细胞系，可以是囊性或实性的。世界卫生组织对卵巢肿瘤的完整分类说明了卵巢来源肿瘤的复杂性；在此只讨论比较常见的疾病。

These tumours may be cystic or solid and arise from specific cell lines in the ovary. The full World Health Organization classification of ovarian tumours illustrates the complexity of tumours arising from the ovary; only the commoner ones will be discussed in this section.

1. 良性上皮性肿瘤（Benign epithelial tumours）

（1）浆液性和黏液性囊腺瘤（Serous and mucinous cystadenomas）：浆液性和黏液性囊腺瘤是最常见的卵巢良性肿瘤。它们可以是单房的也可以是多房的，大小也可以不同。黏液性肿瘤往往是多房性的，并且体积可能很大，有时能充满腹腔（图 20-21）。切开囊腺瘤时可见浆液性肿瘤含有浆液，而黏液性肿瘤中可见黏稠的黏液。我们通过组织学进行诊断——浆液性囊腺瘤的内衬细胞类似于输卵管细胞，而黏液性囊腺瘤的内衬细胞类似于宫颈或胃肠道细胞。由于这些囊肿多发生在育龄女性且为良性，所以通过卵巢囊肿切除术切除囊肿即可。除非囊肿很大，腹腔镜是首选的治疗入路。

These cysts are the commonest benign ovarian tumours. They can be unilocular or multilocular, and the size can also vary. Mucinous tumours tend to be more likely to be multilocular and can become very large, sometimes filling the peritoneal cavity (Fig. 20.21). When cut open, serous tumours contain serous fluid, while thick mucinous fluid is seen in mucinous tumours. The diagnosis is made histologically-the cells lining a serous cystadenoma resemble those from the Fallopian tube, while those lining a mucinous cyst are similar to cells in the endocervix or the gastrointestinal tract. Since these cysts tend to occur in women of reproductive age and they are benign, removal of the cyst by ovarian cystectomy is usually sufficient. Laparoscopy is the preferred route unless the cyst is very large.

> **！注意**
>
> 应注意避免囊肿破裂，因为黏液上皮可种植入腹腔内，引起腹膜假性黏液瘤。大量的胶冻状物质可在腹膜腔积聚。
>
> Care should be taken to avoid rupture of the cysts because mucinous epithelium may implant in the peritoneal cavity, giving rise to a condition known as pseudomyxoma peritonei. Huge amounts of gelatinous material may accumulate in the peritoneal cavity.

（2）子宫内膜异位囊肿（Endometriotic cysts）：子宫内膜异位囊肿含有巧克力色液体，代表着改变的血液的积聚，并有厚的纤维包膜（图 16-13）。内衬细胞可能由子宫内膜细胞组成，但在陈旧性囊肿中这些细胞可能消失。治疗方法通常是卵巢囊肿切除术（见第 16 章子宫内膜异位症部分）。

Endometriomas contain chocolate-coloured fluid representing the accumulation of altered blood and have a thick fibrous capsule (see Fig. 16.13). The lining may consist of endometrial cells, but in old cysts these may disappear.

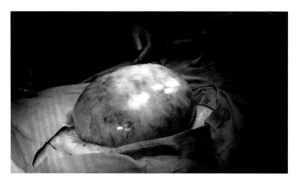

▲ 图 20-21　占据腹腔的巨大良性黏液囊腺瘤

Fig. 20.21　Large benign mucinous cystadenoma occupying the abdominal cavity.

Treatment is usually by ovarian cystectomy. (Also refer to section on endometriosis in Chapter 16.)

2. 性索间质肿瘤（Sex cord stromal tumours）

这是一种不常见的肿瘤，起源于卵母细胞周围的细胞。它们可以是良性的，也可以是恶性的。可以是纯性索肿瘤（如颗粒细胞瘤）、纯间质肿瘤（如纤维瘤和卵泡膜瘤），或者混合有性索和间质成分（如 Sertoli-Leydig 细胞肿瘤）。颗粒细胞肿瘤通常被认为是恶性的，而约 25% 的 Sertoli-Leydig 细胞肿瘤是恶性的，这些将在恶性肿瘤部分中讨论。

This is an uncommon group of tumours arising from the cells surrounding the oocytes. They can be benign or malignant. They can be pure sex cord tumours, such as granulosa cell tumours; pure stromal tumours, such as fibromas and thecomas; or they can have a mixed sex cord and stromal components, e.g. Sertoli-Leydig cell tumours. Granulosa cell tumours are generally considered malignant, while about 25% of Sertoli-Leydig cell tumours are malignant, and these would be discussed under the malignant section.

（1）纤维瘤（Fibroma）：这是最常见的性索间质瘤。纤维瘤是一种良性实性肿瘤，主要见于绝经后的女性。它们不具有激素活性。治疗方法是输卵管卵巢切除术。Meig 综合征指的是卵巢纤维瘤伴有腹水或胸腔积液的情况。通常，腹水和胸腔积液会随着肿块的切除而消失。

This is the commonest sex cord stromal tumour. Fibromas are benign solid tumours found mainly in postmenopausal women. They are not hormonally active. Treatment is by salpingo-oophorectomy. Meig's syndrome refers to the condition where the ovarian fibroma is associated with ascites or pleural effusion. Usually, the ascites and pleural effusion would resolve with removal of the mass.

（2）卵泡膜细胞瘤（Thecoma）：卵泡膜细胞瘤

起源于梭形的膜细胞，但常与颗粒细胞混合。它们通常是良性的实性肿瘤，主要见于绝经后的女性。它们可能产生雌激素，进而导致异常阴道出血或绝经后出血和子宫内膜增生。绝经后女性，可以考虑经腹全子宫切除术（total abdominal hysterectomy，TAH）和双附件切除术。对于年轻女性，单侧输卵管卵巢切除术（unilateral salpingo-oophorectomy，USO）加子宫内膜取样是治疗的首选。

Thecomas or theca cell tumours arise from the spindle-shaped thecal cells but are often mixed with granulosa cells. They are usually benign, solid tumours found mostly in postmenopausal women. They may produce oestrogen, which may in turn lead to abnormal vaginal bleeding or postmenopausal bleeding and endometrial hyperplasia. In postmenopausal women, total abdominal hysterectomy (TAH) BSO can be considered. In young women, unilateral salpingo-oophorectomy (USO) with endometrial sampling is the treatment of choice.

3. 生殖细胞肿瘤（Germ cell tumours）

起源于生殖细胞的肿瘤可以复制模拟早期胚胎的阶段。这些肿瘤可以是良性的也可以是恶性的。

Tumours of germ cell origin may replicate stages resembling the early embryo. These tumours can be benign or malignant.

成熟囊性畸胎瘤（皮样囊肿）[Mature cystic teratoma (dermoid cyst)]：良性囊性畸胎瘤占卵巢肿瘤的 12%～15%。它们含有大量的胚胎成分，如皮肤、毛发、脂肪、肌肉组织、骨骼、牙齿和软骨（图 20-22）。有些成分可以在影像学上识别出来。

Benign cystic teratomas account for 12–15% of ovarian

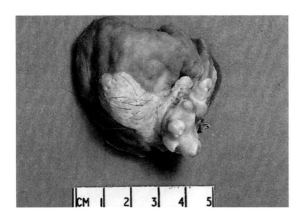

▲ 图 20-22　皮样囊肿（良性囊性畸胎瘤），内含牙齿和毛发

Fig. 20.22　Dermoid cyst (benign cystic teratoma) containing teeth and hair.

neoplasms. They contain a large number of embryonic elements such as skin, hair, adipose and muscle tissue, bone, teeth and cartilage (Fig. 20.22). Some of the components can be recognized on imaging.

这些肿瘤通常是偶然发现的，因为它们通常无症状，除非发生扭转或破裂。12% 的病例是双侧的。有时会有一种特殊的部分占主导地位，例如，在卵巢甲状腺肿中，甲状腺组织占主导地位。这有时可引起甲状腺功能亢进状态。治疗方法是卵巢囊肿切除术，同时注意不要在手术中使囊肿破裂。囊肿内容物如皮脂腺物质的溢出可引起化学性腹膜炎。

These tumours are often chance findings, as they are commonly asymptomatic unless they undergo torsion or rupture. They are bilateral in 12% of cases. Sometimes, one specialized element becomes predominant, e.g. in struma ovarii, thyroid tissue dominates. This may occasionally induce a state of hyperthyroidism. Treatment is by ovarian cystectomy while taking care not to rupture the cyst during the operation. Spillage of the cyst contents, such as the sebaceous material, may cause chemical peritonitis.

 经验　皮样囊肿是年轻女性最常见的实性卵巢肿瘤。

Dermoid cysts are the commonest solid ovarian neoplasm found in young women.

七、卵巢恶性肿瘤（Ovarian malignancy）

卵巢癌是英国女性第六大常见癌症，是英国女性因恶性疾病死亡的第十四大常见原因（2014 年）。虽然它是仅次于子宫内膜癌的第二常见妇科癌症，但它是导致妇科癌症死亡的最常见原因。在 2014 年，英国女性一生中罹患卵巢癌的风险约为 1/52。卵巢癌的发病率随年龄增长而增加，80% 的患者年龄在 50 岁以上。存活率低的一部分原因是卵巢癌确诊较晚，因为许多女性没有明显症状。

Ovarian cancer is the sixth most common cancer in females in the UK and is the fourteenth most common cause of death from malignant disease in women in the UK (2014). Although it is the second most common gynaecological cancer after endometrial cancer, it is the commonest cause of gynaecological cancer deaths. The lifetime risk of developing ovarian cancer was about 1 in 52 women in the UK in 2014. The incidence increases with age, with 80% being diagnosed in women over the age of 50 years. The poor survival is partly attributable to late diagnosis, as many women present late due to lack of obvious symptoms.

（一）病因学（Aetiology）

卵巢癌的确切病因仍在调查研究中。不同的组织学亚型可能有不同的病因。近年来，越来越多的证据表明高浆液型卵巢癌起源于输卵管内发现的前体细胞。

The exact aetiology of ovarian cancer is still under investigation. Different histological subtypes may have different aetiologies. In recent years, there is increasing evidence that the high-grade serous subtypes originate from precursors found in the Fallopian tube.

1. 遗传（Genetic）

10%～20% 的卵巢癌具有遗传性。BRCA1 和 BRCA2 基因的遗传突变是最常见的遗传原因。它是通过常染色体显性模式遗传的。携带 BRCA1 和 BRCA2 突变的女性患卵巢癌的平均累积风险分别为 45% 和 12%；此外，许多其他基因也被发现与卵巢癌风险的增加有关。

About 10–20% of ovarian cancers are hereditary. Germline mutation of the BRCA1 and BRCA2 genes is the commonest genetic cause. It is inherited via an autosomal-dominant pattern. Women carrying the BRCA1 and BRCA2 mutations will have an average cumulative risk of 45% and 12%, respectively, in the development of ovarian cancer. Many other genes have also been found to be associated with the increased risk of ovarian cancers.

2. 分娩和生育（Parity and fertility）

经产妇患卵巢癌的风险比未产妇低 40%，而不孕治疗失败的女性患卵巢癌的风险似乎更高。使用避孕药可使卵巢癌的发病率减少 60%。

Multiparous women are at 40% less risk than nulliparous women of developing ovarian cancer, whereas women who have had unsuccessful treatment for infertility seem to be at increased risk. The use of the contraceptive pill may produce up to a 60% reduction in the incidence of the disease.

（二）病理学（Pathology）

1. 原发性卵巢癌（Primary ovarian carcinoma）

卵巢癌的组织学类型分布如下。

The distribution of histological types of ovarian cancers is as follows.

(1) 上皮型（Epithelial type）：这占卵巢癌病例的 85%。上皮性肿瘤包括以下亚型。

• 浆液性囊腺癌：是卵巢癌最常见的组织学类型（40%），通常为单房性，可能为双侧。与良性肿瘤相比，这些肿瘤更有可能包含实性成分。

• 黏液囊腺癌：这些多囊性肿瘤（图 20-23）的特征是充满黏液的囊肿，囊内排列着柱状腺上皮细胞，并且可能与阑尾肿瘤有关。

• 子宫内膜样囊腺癌：类似于子宫内膜腺癌，20% 的病例与子宫癌相关。

• 透明细胞囊腺癌：这是最常见的与卵巢子宫内膜异位症相关的卵巢恶性肿瘤。单房薄壁囊内排列着具有典型靴钉样外观，胞质清晰的上皮细胞。

• Brenner 或移行细胞囊腺癌：常与黏液性肿瘤相关，但预后优于膀胱来源的类似肿瘤。

This makes up 85% of cases of ovarian malignancy. Epithelial tumours include the following subtypes:

• Serous cystadenocarcinoma is the most common histological type of ovarian carcinoma (40%) and is usually unilocular. They may be bilateral. These tumours are more likely to contain solid areas than their benign counterparts.

• Mucinous cystadenocarcinomas: These multicystic tumours (Fig. 20.23) are characterized by mucin-filled cysts lined by columnar glandular cells and may be associated with tumours of the appendix.

• Endometrioid cystadenocarcinomas resemble endometrial adenocarcinomas and are associated with uterine carcinomas in 20% of cases.

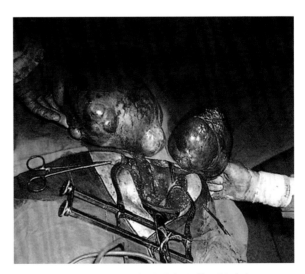

▲ 图 20-23　双侧多囊性卵巢恶性肿瘤

Fig. 20.23　Bilateral multicystic malignant ovarian tumours.

妇产科学（原书第 6 版） Essential Obstetrics and Gynaecology (6th Edition)

- Clear-cell cystadenocarcinoma is the most common ovarian malignancy found in association with ovarian endometriosis. The unilocular thin-walled cysts are lined by epithelium with a typical hobnail appearance and clear cytoplasm.
- Brenner's or transitional cell cystadenocarcinoma is often found in association with mucinous tumours but has a better prognosis than similar tumours arising from the bladder.

低度恶性或交界性潜在肿瘤占原发上皮癌的 10%～15%。它们通常是浆液性或黏液性肿瘤。具有恶性肿瘤细胞学改变，其中包括细胞异型性，有丝分裂增加，呈复层性，但没有侵袭性。它们的预后明显优于侵袭性疾病，Ⅰ期病变的 5 年生存率超过 95%，但晚期复发率为 10%～15%。

Tumours of low malignant or borderline potential account for 10–15% of primary epithelial carcinomas. They are commonly serous or mucinous tumours. There are cytological changes of malignancy, including cellular atypia, with increased mitosis and multilayering but without invasion. They have a significantly better prognosis than invasive disease, with a 5-year survival of more than 95% for stage I lesions, but there is a 10–15% incidence of late recurrence.

(2) 恶性性索间质肿瘤（ Malignant sex cord stromal tumours ）：这类肿瘤相对罕见，因为它们只占原发性卵巢恶性肿瘤的 6%。

These tumours are relatively rare, as they make up only 6% of primary ovarian malignancy.

(3) 颗粒细胞肿瘤（ Granulosa cell tumours ）：源于卵巢颗粒细胞的肿瘤（图 20–24 ）通常表现为单侧巨大实性肿块。从组织学上看，颗粒细胞具有"咖啡豆"形细胞核，这些肿瘤的特征是存在 Call-Exner 小体，其细胞在中央腔周围成小簇排列。这些肿瘤大多生长缓慢，但有些表现出侵犯性行为。大约 95% 的成年颗粒细胞肿瘤发生在中年女性身上，剩下的 5% 是幼年颗粒细胞肿瘤，这类肿瘤通常在青春期之前发生于年轻女孩，而且通常比成人类型更具侵犯性。卵巢颗粒细胞肿瘤是最常见的雌激素分泌肿瘤。由于颗粒细胞肿瘤可以在任何年龄发生，所以症状取决于肿瘤发生的年龄。青春期前出现的肿瘤会导致性早熟；对于育龄女性，长期的雌激素刺激会导致子宫内膜增生和长时间不规则阴道流血。约 50% 的病例发生在绝经期后并伴有绝经后阴道出血。卵巢颗粒细胞瘤的治疗方法是全子宫切除术和双附件切除术。对于局限于卵巢的年轻患者，保留生育功

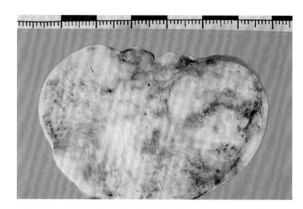

▲ 图 20-24 颗粒细胞 / 膜细胞瘤。这显示了切除肿瘤的白色固体表面上的出血区域

Fig. 20.24 Granulosa cell/theca cell tumour. This shows haemorrhagic areas in the solid white surface of the cut tumour.

能的单侧附件切除可能是可行的。然而，如果不做子宫切除术，那么就应该谨慎进行宫腔镜检查和子宫内膜取样，以排除子宫内膜增生症。

Arising from ovarian granulosa cells, these tumours (Fig. 20.24) usually present as a unilateral, large, solid mass. Histologically, granulosa cells have the 'coffee bean' grooved nuclei, and these tumours are characterized by the presence of Call-Exner bodies where cells are arranged in small clusters around a central cavity. The majority of these tumours are slow growing but some exhibit aggressive behaviour. About 95% of the adult granulosa cell tumours that occur in middle-aged women and the remaining 5% are juvenile granulosa cell tumours, which affect young girls, usually before puberty, and they are usually more aggressive than the adult type. These tumours are the commonest oestrogen-secreting tumours. As granulosa cell tumours can present at any age, the symptoms depend on the age of occurrence. Tumours arising before puberty produce precocious sexual development, and in women of reproductive age, prolonged oestrogen stimulation results in endometrial hyperplasia and irregular and prolonged vaginal bleeding. Around 50% of cases occur after menopause and present with postmenopausal bleeding. Treatment is by total hysterectomy and BSO. Fertility-sparing surgery with USO may be feasible in young patients with disease confined to the ovary. However, if hysterectomy is not done, it is prudent to proceed with a hysteroscopy and endometrial sampling to exclude endometrial hyperplasia.

(4) Sertoli Leydig 细胞肿瘤（ 雄母细胞瘤 ）[Sertoli-Leydig cell tumours（androblastomas）]：这类肿瘤是含有 Sertoli-Leydig 细胞的肿瘤，其中大约 25% 是恶性的。它是一种罕见的雄激素分泌肿瘤，通常发生在 20—30 岁。肿瘤的症状是雄激素过多，如面部和身体多毛，嗓音加粗和阴蒂增大。该疾病的诊断是通过在一个卵巢中发现肿瘤并排除男性化肾上腺肿

544

瘤来确定的。治疗方法是切除受累的卵巢。

These are tumours of Sertoli-Leydig cells. Approximately 25% of these tumours are malignant. They are rare androgensecreting tumours that occur most frequently between 20 and 30 years of age. They present with symptoms of androgen excess, such as increasing facial and body hirsutism, deepening of the voice and enlargement of the clitoris. The diagnosis is established by the exclusion of virilizing adrenal tumours and the identification of a tumour in one ovary. The condition is treated by excision of the affected ovary.

(5) 恶性生殖细胞瘤（Malignant germ cell tumours）

• 无性生殖细胞瘤：这些实体肿瘤可以很小，也可大到足以填满腹腔。肿瘤切面呈灰粉红色，显微镜下，肿瘤由大的多边形细胞组成，排列在瘤巢中，由纤维组织相隔。

• Dysgerminomas: These solid tumours may be small or large enough to fill the abdominal cavity. The cut surface of the tumour has a greyish-pink colour, and microscopically, the tumour consists of large polygonal cells arranged in alveoli or nests separated by septa of fibrous tissue.

• 未成熟畸胎瘤：恶性或未成熟的畸胎瘤最常见实性、单侧和异质性的多种组织成分。这类肿瘤可能产生人绒毛膜促性腺激素和甲胎蛋白。

• Immature teratomas: The malignant or immature form of teratoma is most commonly solid, unilateral and heterogenous with multiple tissue elements. These tumours may produce human chorionic gonadotrophin and alpha-fetoprotein.

• 内胚窦瘤或卵黄囊瘤：虽然这类肿瘤只占生殖细胞肿瘤的 10%～15%，但它们是儿童中最常见的生殖细胞肿瘤。它们是实性、包裹性肿瘤，排列着扁平的间皮细胞。这些肿瘤会产生甲胎蛋白。

• Endodermal sinus or yolk sac tumours: Although these tumours make up only 10–15% of germ cell tumours, they are the most common germ cell tumour in children. They are solid, encapsulated tumours containing microcysts lined by flat mesothelial cells. These tumours produce alpha-fetoprotein.

2. 继发性卵巢癌（Secondary ovarian carcinomas）

卵巢是乳腺、生殖道、消化系统和造血系统原发性恶性肿瘤的继发肿瘤的常见部位。

The ovaries are a common site for secondary deposits from primary malignancies in the breast, genital tract, gastrointestinal system and haematopoietic system.

Krukenberg 瘤是来自消化系统的转移性肿瘤。它们呈实性增长，且几乎总是双侧生长。间质常富含细胞，可呈肌瘤性。上皮细胞呈明显的腺泡簇状，细胞表现出黏液样改变，称为印戒细胞。

Krukenberg's tumours are metastatic deposits from the gastrointestinal system. They are solid growths that are almost always bilateral. The stroma is often richly cellular and may appear to be myomatous. The epithelial elements occur as clusters of well-marked acini, with cells exhibiting mucoid change, known as *signet ring cells*.

（三）卵巢癌的分期（Staging of ovarian carcinoma）

原发性卵巢肿瘤可以通过直接扩散、淋巴扩散或血液扩散。卵巢癌手术按照 FIGO 分期系统进行分期（表 20-6）。一个分期手术包括全子宫切除和双附件切除、大网膜切除术和对腹膜表面进行仔细检查和取样，以及腹膜后（盆腔和腹主动脉旁）淋巴结清扫。卵巢癌的分期对预后和治疗都很重要。

Spread of primary ovarian tumours can be by direct extension, lymphatics or via the bloodstream. Ovarian cancer is surgically staged according to the FIGO staging system (Table 20.6). A staging procedure includes total hysterectomy with BSO, omentectomy and careful inspection and sampling of peritoneal surfaces and retroperitoneal (pelvic and para-aortic) lymph node dissection. Staging of ovarian carcinoma is important in determining both prognosis and management.

（四）诊断（Diagnosis）

早期卵巢癌大多无症状。最常见的症状是腹部不适或腹胀。临床上可发现盆腔肿块，并有腹水。经阴道超声可排除其他原因的盆腔肿块，如肌瘤，它也有助于评估提示恶性肿瘤的特征，如双侧病变、多房囊肿、实性区域、乳头状突起、转移、腹水和血流增加（多普勒）。CA-125 是 85% 上皮肿瘤脱落的糖蛋白，可作为卵巢癌的肿瘤标志物。绝经后女性通常使用 35u/L 的临界值。单独使用 CA-125 缺乏敏感性和特异性。只有 50% 的早期卵巢癌会出现假阳性结果，而其他恶性肿瘤（肝脏、胰腺）和许多良性疾病，如子宫内膜异位症、盆腔炎和早期妊娠也会出现假阳性结果。恶性肿瘤风险指数（RMI）可根据绝经状态、超声特征和 CA-125 水平计算。RMI= U×M×CA-125，其中 U 代表超声评分，M 代表绝经期状态。超声结果为以下特征各 1 分：多房囊

表 20-6　2014 年 FIGO 卵巢癌分类

Table 20.6　FIGO classification of ovarian carcinoma 2014

分期特征 Stage Characteristics	
I	局限于卵巢的肿瘤 Tumour confined to ovaries
	I A　肿瘤局限于一个卵巢 I A　Tumour limited to one ovary
	I B　肿瘤局限于两个卵巢 I B　Tumour limited to both ovaries
	I C　肿瘤局限于一个或两个卵巢，具有下列任何一种 I C　Tumour limited to one or both ovaries, with any of the following:
	I C$_1$　手术导致肿瘤破裂 I C$_1$　Surgical spill
	I C$_2$　手术前包膜破裂或卵巢表面有肿瘤 I C$_2$　Capsule ruptured before surgery or tumour on ovarian surface
	I C$_3$　腹水或腹膜冲洗液中有恶性细胞 I C$_3$　Malignant cells in ascites or peritoneal washing
II	伴有盆腔扩散的肿瘤（骨盆边缘以下） Tumour with pelvic extension (below pelvic brim)
	II A　子宫、输卵管或卵巢的扩散 II A　Extension on uterus or Fallopian tubes or ovaries
	II B　蔓延到其他盆腔腹膜组织 II B　Extension to other pelvic intraperitoneal tissues
III	肿瘤扩散至骨盆外腹膜 ± 转移至腹膜后淋巴结 Tumour spread to peritoneum outside pelvis ± metastasis to retroperitoneal node
	III A$_1$　仅腹膜后淋巴结阳性 III A$_1$　Positive retroperitoneal node only
	III A$_2$　显微镜下盆腔外腹膜受累 III A$_2$　Microscopic extrapelvic peritoneal involvement
	III B　肉眼可见盆腔外腹膜转移≤2cm III B　Macroscopic peritoneal metastasis ≥2 cm
	III C　肉眼可见盆腔外腹膜转移>2cm III C　Macroscopic peritoneal metastasis >2 cm
IV	远处转移 Distant metastasis

引自 Prat J & FIGO Committee on Gynecologic Oncology (2015) FIGO's staging classification for cancer of the ovary, fallopian tube,and peritoneum: abridged republication. J Gynecol Oncol 26(2):87-89. 开放获取。

From Prat J & FIGO Committee on Gynecologic Oncology (2015) FIGO's staging classification for cancer of the ovary, fallopian tube, and peritoneum: abridged republication. J Gynecol Oncol 26(2): 87-89. Open access.

肿、实性区域、转移、腹水和双侧病变。超声评分 0 分时 U=0；1 分时 U=1；2～5 分时 U=3。绝经前女性的绝经状况评分为 M=1，绝经后女性的评分为 M=3。如果有盆腔肿块且 RMI＞200 的女性应转诊给妇科肿瘤医生做进一步的检查和治疗。其他评分系统如恶性肿瘤风险算法（ROMA）或国际卵巢肿瘤分析（IOTA）分类也可以使用。ROMA 是一种结合两个肿瘤标志水平：CA-125 和一种新的肿瘤标志物 HE4（人附睾蛋白 4）来判断囊肿是否可能为恶性的方法。IOTA 分类是基于超声表现。进一步的影像学检查，如腹部和盆腔的 CT、MRI 或 PET-CT 可以评估任何转移（图 20-25），胸部 X 线检查肺转移和胸腔积液。通过对手术标本的组织学评估来做出诊断。

Early ovarian carcinomas are mostly asymptomatic. The commonest symptoms are abdominal discomfort or distension. Clinically, a pelvic mass may be detected, and there may be ascites. A transvaginal ultrasound scan can exclude other causes of pelvic mass such as fibroids, and it is also useful in assessing features suggestive of malignancy, such as bilateral lesions, multilocular cysts, solid areas, papillary projections, metastases, ascites and increased blood flow (Doppler). CA-125 is a glycoprotein shed by 85% of epithelial tumours and can be used as a tumour marker for ovarian cancer. A cut-off level of 35 u/L is commonly used for postmenopausal women. CA-125 lacks sensitivity and specificity if used alone. It is only raised in 50% of early-stage ovarian cancers, and false-positive results occur in other malignancies (liver, pancreas) and many benign conditions such as endometriosis, pelvic inflammatory disease and early pregnancy. A risk of malignancy index (RMI) can be calculated based on the menopausal status, ultrasound features and CA 125 levels. RMI = U × M × CA125, where U represents the ultrasound score and M represents the menopausal status. The ultrasound result is scored 1 point for each of the following features: multilocular cysts, solid areas, metastases, ascites and bilateral lesions. U = 0 for ultrasound score of 0, U = 1 for score of 1 and U –3 for score of 2–5. Menopausal status is scored as M = 1 for premenopausal women and M = 3 for postmenopausal women. Women with a pelvic mass with an RMI more than 200 should be referred to gynaecological oncologists for further workup and management. Other scoring systems such as the Risk of Malignancy Algorithm (ROMA) or the International Ovarian Tumor Analysis (IOTA) classification can also be used. ROMA is a formula for classifying whether the cyst is likely to be malignant by combining the two tumour marker levels: CA 125 and a new tumour marker, HE4 (human epididymis protein 4). IOTA classification is based on ultrasound appearances. Further imaging such as CT or MRI of the abdomen and pelvis or PET-CT can be done to assess for any metastases (Fig. 20.25) and a chest X-ray to look for lung metastases and pleural effusions. The diagnosis is made by histological assessment of the surgical specimens.

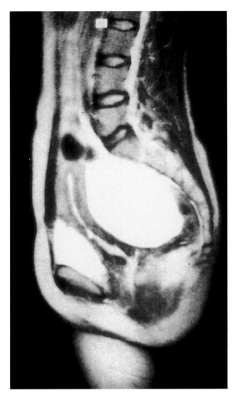

▲ 图 20-25 卵巢大囊肿磁共振成像。可见肿瘤使子宫扩展并拉长子宫内膜

Fig. 20.25 Magnetic resonance image of a large ovarian cyst. The tumour can be seen distending the uterus and elongating the endometrium.

（五）处理（Management）

手术是卵巢癌的主要治疗方法，其次是化疗。对于局限于卵巢的早期疾病，可行分期开腹手术（见前文）。在疾病晚期，目的是去除所有肉眼可见的病灶（完全减灭）。随后的预后与初次手术后残余的病灶量成正比。手术后通常是辅助化疗。在特定的晚期病例中，初次手术前的新辅助化疗可以降低手术并发症发病率，并有更高的概率实现最佳的肿瘤切除。生殖细胞肿瘤往往发生在年轻女性身上。即使是在转移性疾病存在时，保留生育功能的手术，如保留子宫和对侧卵巢的单侧附件切除，也应被考虑，因为肿瘤对化疗具有高度敏感性。

Surgery is the mainstay of treatment of ovarian cancer, followed by chemotherapy. For early disease confined to the ovary, a staging laparotomy (see earlier) is done. In advanced disease, the aim is to remove all macroscopic disease (complete debulking). Subsequent prognosis is proportional to the amount of disease remaining after primary surgery. Surgery is often followed by adjuvant chemotherapy. In selected advanced cases, neoadjuvant chemotherapy before primary surgery can decrease morbidity of surgery with higher chance of achieving optimal removal of tumour. Germ cell tumours tend to occur in young women. Fertility-sparing surgery, e.g. USO with preservation of the uterus and the other ovary, should be considered even in the presence of metastatic disease because the tumour is highly chemosensitive.

1. 化学疗法（Chemotherapy）

复发风险高的患者，如高分级、组织学亚型差、ⅠC 期及以上的患者，常接受辅助化疗。铂类药物顺铂和卡铂是目前主要的治疗药物。主要不良反应有骨髓抑制、神经毒性和肾毒性。目前，卡铂由于不良反应较小，已在很大程度上取代了顺铂，而且常与另一种对卵巢癌有效的药物紫杉醇联合使用。整体反应率高达 80%。

Patients with high risk for recurrence, e.g. those with highgrade, poor histological subtypes or stage IC or above, are often given adjuvant chemotherapy. The platinum-based drugs cisplatin and carboplatin are currently the mainstay of treatment. The main side effects are marrow suppression, neurotoxicity and renal toxicity. Carboplatin has now largely replaced cisplatin due to its better side effect profile, and it is often combined with paclitaxel, another active agent for ovarian cancer. The overall response rate is up to 80%

靶向治疗（Target therapy）：使用抗血管生成药物（如贝伐珠单抗）可以提高无进展生存期，但不能提高总生存期。在 BRCA 突变的卵巢癌中使用聚（ADP- 核糖）聚合酶（PARP）抑制药也可以延长无进展生存期。许多靶向疗法正在进行试验，如靶向免疫通路、PD1（程序性细胞死亡蛋白 1）和 PDL1（程序性细胞死亡配体 1）的疗法。

The use of an anti-angiogenetic agent such as bevacizumab improves the progression-free survival but not overall survival. The use of poly (ADP- ribose) polymerase (PARP) inhibitor in BRCA-mutated ovarian cancer can also prolong progression-free survival. Many target therapies were undergoing trials, such as those targeting immunopathway, PD1 (programmed cell death protein 1) and PDL1 (programmed cell death ligand 1).

2. 交界性肿瘤（Borderline tumours）

对于希望保留生育功能的年轻女性，可以通过单侧卵巢切除术进行治疗，但需要仔细、长期的随访。

These can be treated by unilateral oophorectomy in young women wishing to preserve their reproductive capacity, although careful, long-term follow-up is required.

3. 复发的随访和治疗（Follow-up and treatment of recurrence）

患者的随访内容包括任何症状，如腹部不适，肿瘤标志物和临床体格检查。如怀疑复发，可安排影像学检查。化疗是治疗复发的主要手段。如果肿瘤是局部的且复发间隔较长，则肿瘤的减瘤术是可行的。对于铂敏感患者，即那些在初始治疗结束后 6 个月（部分敏感）和 12 个月后复发的患者，建议重新接受一线化疗（以卡铂为基础的）。除此之外，还有各种二线化疗药物，如脂质体阿霉素、吉西他滨和拓扑替康，但它们的反应率只有 20%～30%。

Patients are followed up for any symptoms such as abdominal discomfort, tumour markers and clinical examination. Imaging can be arranged if there is suspicion of recurrence. Chemotherapy is the mainstay of treatment for recurrence. Debulking of the tumour may be feasible if it is localized and there is a long interval to recurrence. In platinum-sensitive patients, i.e. those that recur after 6 months (partially sensitive) and 12 months from completion of primary treatment, rechallenge with first-line chemotherapy (carboplatin based) is recommended. Otherwise, there are wide ranges of second-line chemotherapy agents such as liposomal doxorubicin, gemcitabine and topotecan, but their response rates are only about 20–30%.

（六）预后（Prognosis）

5 年生存率取决于肿瘤的分期以及肿瘤是否被完全切除（表 20-7）。

The 5-year survival figures depend on the stage and on whether the tumour has or has not been completelyremoved (Table 20.7).

表 20-7　卵巢癌的生存率

Table 20.7　Survival rates for ovarian cancer

分期 Stage	5 年生存率（%） 5-year survival (%)
I 期 Stage I	89
II 期 Stage II	66
III 期 Stage III	34
IV 期 Stage IV	18

（七）卵巢癌筛查（Screening for ovarian cancer）

由于早期疾病患者的预后好于晚期，如果无症状的女性能更早地诊断出疾病，总生存率可能会提高。然而，最好的筛查策略还不清楚。两种主要方法是超声和 CA-125 测定。

Because the prognosis for early-stage disease is better than that for advanced disease, overall survival might be improved if the disease could be diagnosed earlier in asymptomatic women. However, the best screening strategy is unclear. The two main methods proposed are ultrasound and CA-125 measurement.

经阴道超声对发现卵巢包块很敏感，但对区分卵巢癌和良性卵巢囊肿还不够准确。这会导致许多不必要的手术。

Transvaginal ultrasound is sensitive in picking up ovarian masses, but it is not accurate enough to differentiate between ovarian cancer and benign ovarian cysts. This leads to many unnecessary operations.

单独使用 CA-125 缺乏敏感性和特异性。

CA-125 lacks both sensitivity and specificity if used alone.

在大规模随机试验中研究了经阴道超声与连续 CA-125 测定联合，如英国卵巢癌筛查合作试验（UKCTOCS）。筛查是否能降低死亡率仍在研究中。可以考虑对卵巢癌高风险女性（如 BRCA 携带者）进行筛查，以在早期发现卵巢癌，但这是否会转化为总体生存率的提高仍不清楚。

Combining transvaginal ultrasound with serial CA-125 has been investigated in large-scale randomized trials, e.g. the UK Collaborative Trial of Ovarian Cancer Screening (UKCTOCS). Whether screening can reduce mortality is still under investigation. Screening may be considered in women at high risk for ovarian cancer, such as *BRCA* carriers, to detect ovarian cancer at an earlier stage, but whether this would translate into improved overall survival is still not known.

（八）降低卵巢癌风险的手术（Risk-reducing surgery for ovarian cancer）

预防 BRCA 携带者（见前述）卵巢癌最有效的方法是降低风险的输卵管切除术（RRSO），可降低 80% 的风险。推荐的 RRSO 年龄在 35—40 岁。BSO 通常可以通过腹腔镜进行。需要对手术标本进行细致的处理，以排除输卵管内隐匿的癌症。随着许多高级别浆液性癌的发现，BSO 已经被提出，但其确切的有效性仍在研究中。

The most effective way to prevent ovarian cancer in *BRCA* carriers (see earlier) is risk-reducing salpingo-ophrectomy (RRSO) with an 80% decreased risk. The recommended age of RRSO is around 35–40. BSO can usually be done laparoscopically. Meticulous processing of the surgical specimen is needed to rule out occult cancer in the tube. With the discovery that many high-grade serous carcinomas arise from the tube, BSO has been proposed, but its exact effectiveness is still under investigation.

八、妇科肿瘤姑息治疗原则（Principles of palliative care in gynaecological cancer）

尽管有最佳的初始治疗，对一定比例的妇科肿瘤患者，疾病的复发和进展是不可避免的。在许多这样的情况下，治疗已不再是一个现实的选择，但这决不意味着要撤回医疗专业人员的投入。在姑息治疗团队的大力支持下，通过多学科途径为患者提供支持性治疗是至关重要的。姑息治疗的目的是提供身体和精神上的支持，以及为死亡的最终来临做准备。在生命的最后阶段，生活质量、患者的自主性和尊严是最重要的。患者和她的照料者之间良好的沟通和信任关系是实现这些目标的关键。理想情况下，姑息治疗的概念应该在适当的时候引入，而不是在临床的关键时刻引入，以便患者和她的家人有时间去接受和做出切实的选择。决定是继续还是停止抗肿瘤治疗，需要考虑生活质量的综合效益，考虑治疗而不是疾病带来的额外压力和不良反应。

Despite optimal initial treatment, disease recurrence and progression are inevitable in a certain proportion of women with gynaecological cancer. In many of these situations, a cure is no longer a realistic option, but this by no means translates into withdrawal of the input from medical professionals. A multidisciplinary approach, with strong input from the palliative team to provide supportive care to the individual, is crucial. Palliative care aims to provide both physical and emotional support, as well as preparation for the eventual outcome of death. Quality of life and the patient's autonomy and dignity are the most important aspects in this final phase of life. Good communication and a trusting relationship between the patient and her carers are key to achieving these aims. Ideally, the concept of palliative care should be introduced in good time and not at a clinically critical moment so that the patient and her family can have time to develop acceptance and realistic expectations. The decision to either continue or stop anticancer treatment needs to take into account the overall benefit in quality of life, bearing in mind the additional stress and side effects arising from the treatment rather than the disease.

无法控制的症状可引起严重的痛苦，而控制症状是姑息治疗的主要范畴之一。患者几乎不可避免地会经历疼痛，这可能是疾病或治疗的结果。疼痛是一种主观感觉。因此，要达到良好控制，既要减少疼痛刺激，又要提高个人的疼痛阈值。减轻疼痛刺激需要通过良好的病史来仔细评估病因。治疗措施可以针对所涉及的机制，例如，非甾体抗炎药物适用于炎症引起的疼痛或抗痉挛药物适用于肠痉挛，而神经性疼痛可以通过三环抗抑郁药或抗惊厥药物（如加巴喷丁）来缓解。

Uncontrolled symptoms can cause severe distress, and symptom control is one of the main areas for palliative care. Patients almost inevitably experience pain, which can be a result of the disease or the treatment. Pain is a subjective sensation; therefore, to achieve good control, it is important both to reduce the pain stimulus and to increase the personal pain threshold. Reducing pain stimulus requires careful assessment of the cause by taking a good history. Therapeutic measures can then be targeted at the mechanisms involved, e.g. non-steroidal anti-inflammatory drugs would be appropriate for pain arising from inflammation or antispasmodic agents for bowel spasms, while neuropathic pain can be relieved by tricyclic antidepressants or anticonvulsant drugs such as gabapentin.

增加疼痛阈值需要良好的心理支持，可能需要抗抑郁药和抗焦虑药的帮助。世界卫生组织（WHO）已经研发出一种缓解肿瘤疼痛的"三阶梯"疗法。给药顺序如下：非阿片类药物（如对乙酰氨基酚和阿司匹林），弱阿片类药物（可待因），然后是强阿片类药物（如吗啡）。每一步都可以添加"佐剂"。佐剂的主要适应证并非缓解疼痛，但能帮助缓解某些情况下的疼痛，如抗惊厥药和抗抑郁药。阿片类药物非常有效，但需要在正确的时机给以正确的剂量。应该定期给药，并且可以根据突破性疼痛的需要开额外剂量的处方。常见的阿片类药物不良反应包括恶心、呕吐和便秘；因此，在开始使用阿片类药物时，还应开止吐药和常规通便药。应当让患者放心，说明适当使用阿片类药物不会导致成瘾。

Increasing the pain threshold involves good psychological support, possibly with the help of antidepressants and anxiolytics. The World Health Organization has developed a three-step 'ladder' for cancer pain relief. Administration of drugs should be in the following order: non-opioids (such as paracetamol and aspirin), mild opioids (codeine), then strong opioids such as morphine. At each step, 'adjuvant' agents can be added. Adjuvants are medications that have a primary indication other than pain control but can also help to relieve pain in certain situations, such as anticonvulsant and antidepressant agents. Opioids are very effective, but they need to be given at the right dose and at the right time. They should be given at regular intervals, and additional doses can be prescribed as required for breakthrough pain. Common opioid side effects include nausea, vomiting and constipation; therefore anti-emetics and regular laxatives should also be prescribed when starting opioids. Patients should be reassured that appropriate use of opioids would not cause addiction.

患有广泛腹腔内疾病的女性，如晚期卵巢癌，出现肠梗阻和腹水是常见的。肠梗阻的症状很难完全治愈。手术治疗可能有最好的姑息效果，但由于广泛疾病造成的多处梗阻往往不可行。保守治疗的目的是通过镇吐药 ± 鼻胃管或胃切开术减少恶心和呕吐，并通过静脉输液维持水化。偶尔，短期糖皮质激素药物减少肠道周围炎症性水肿的试验可能对缓解肠梗阻有效。腹膜疾病来源的腹水经穿刺可有效缓解，但腹水易再次积聚，需多次穿刺。利尿药（如螺内酯）可以尝试减少再积聚发生的速度。

In women with extensive intra-abdominal disease, such as those in advanced ovarian cancer, bowel obstruction and ascites are common. Symptoms from bowel obstructions are difficult to deal with entirely. Surgical intervention can potentially give the best palliative effect but is often not feasible due to multiple sites of obstruction from extensive disease. Conservative management aims to reduce nausea and vomiting with anti-emetic ± nasogastric tube or gastrotomy and maintaining hydration by intravenous fluid. Occasionally, a trial of shortcourse corticosteroid drugs to decrease inflammatory oedema around the bowels may be effective in relieving the obstruction. Ascites from peritoneal disease can be effectively relieved by paracentesis, but they tend to reaccumulate, and often repeated paracentesis is required. Diuretics such as spironolactone can be tried to reduce the rate of re-accumulation.

最后，当患者濒临死亡时，关怀计划应集中于为患者及其家人提供一个和平和有尊严的环境。应尽量减少无效的医疗干预，同时应充分控制痛苦症状。最后但也很重要的是，了解患者的文化和精神偏好很重要，这样患者和她的家人都能感到她已经有了一个"好的结局"。

Eventually, when the patient is very close to death, care plans should concentrate on providing a peaceful and dignified environment for the patient and her family. Futile medical interventions should be minimized, while distressing symptoms should be adequately controlled. Last but not least, it is important to be aware of the individual's cultural and spiritual preferences so that both the patient and her family can feel that she has come to a 'good end'.

本章概览	Essential information
恶性外阴的病变 • 在六十多岁最常见。 • 大多数是鳞癌（92%）或腺癌（5%）。 • 临床表现为皮肤瘙痒、病灶出血。 • 通过–局部浸润、腹股沟–股淋巴结转移。 • 首选治疗是外阴根治性切除和腹股沟淋巴结清扫，个体化。 • 局限于外阴者预后良好。	**Malignant vulval lesions** • Commonest in sixth decade • Majority are squamous (92%) or adenocarcinomas (5%) • Present with pruritus, bleeding lesions • Spreads by local invasion and via inguinal and femoral nodes • Primary treatment by radical vulvectomy and groin node dissection with individual modification • Good prognosis if confined to vulva at presentation
阴道恶性肿瘤 • 原发肿瘤少见，鳞癌起自于阴道上 1/3。 • 最常见的转移性肿瘤来自宫颈和子宫。 • 临床表现为疼痛、出血和瘘管形成。 • 局部浸润和淋巴转移。 • 通常采用放射治疗。	**Malignant vaginal tumours** • Primary malignancy rare, squamous carcinomas arising in upper third • Common site for spread from cervix and uterus • Presents as pain, bleeding and fistula formation • Spreads by local invasion and lymphatics • Usually treated by radiotherapy
子宫颈普查及疫苗注射 • 25—65 岁每 3～5 年宫颈细胞学检查。 • 25—74 岁每 5 年筛查 HPV。 • 异常的筛查结果需要进行阴道镜检查及活检。 • 12—13 岁女孩接种 HPV16、HPV18 或纳米疫苗。	**Cervical screening and vaccination** • Cytology 3-5-yearly intervals from 25 to 65 years of age • HPV testing in screening every 5 years from 25 to 74 • Abnormal screening tests results require colposcopy and biopsy • HPV 16 and 18 or nanovalent vaccination in girls (and in Australia boys) aged 12–13 years old

（续表）

本章概览	Essential information
宫颈癌 • 与 HPV 感染有关。 • 可以无症状，或者表现为阴道出血、疼痛和肠道或膀胱症状。 • 通过局部浸润和髂 / 闭孔淋巴结转移。 • 疾病早期治疗是根治性宫颈切除和盆腔淋巴结清扫，其他情况放疗。 • 5 年生存率依据分期为 10%～90%。	**Cervical cancer** • Associated with HPV infection • May be asymptomatic or present with vaginal bleeding, pain and bowel or bladder symptoms • Spreads by local invasion and iliac/obturator nodes • Treatment is radical hysterectomy and pelvic nodes dissection for early-stage disease, chemoradiotherapy otherwise • 5-year survival varies from 10% to 90% depending on stage
子宫内膜癌 • 危险因素包括肥胖、未产、晚绝经、糖尿病和无雌激素拮抗，遗传性非息肉性结肠癌或林奇综合征。 • 常表现为异常阴道流血或绝经后流血。 • 通过直接蔓延传播，最初倾向于在子宫内。 • 早期高分化者可手术治疗，晚期需要化疗和（或）放疗。 • 如果早期诊断，5 年生存率 90%。	**Endometrial carcinoma** • Risk factors include obesity, nulliparity, late menopause, diabetes and unopposed oestrogens, HNPCC or Lynch's syndrome • Commonly presents as abnormal vaginal bleeding or postmenopausal bleeding • Spreads by direct invasion but tends to remain localized within the uterus initially • Well-differentiated early-stage disease can be treated by surgery alone; more advanced lesions require chemotherapy and/or radiotherapy • Has 90% 5-year survival if diagnosed early
卵巢恶性肿瘤 • 75% 病例表现为晚期。 • 绝大多数为上皮性卵巢癌。 • 预后依赖于疾病的分期和初次手术后剩余病灶程度。 • 首选治疗是手术，其次是铂类基础的化疗。 • 5 年生存率为 35%～40%。	**Malignant ovarian tumours** • 75% of cases present with advanced disease • Most cases are epithelial in type • Prognosis depends on stage at diagnosis and extent of residual disease after initial surgery • The primary treatment is surgery, followed by platinumbased chemotherapy • 5-year survival 35–40%
姑息治疗的原则 • 多学科举措来控制和缓解症状，物理和情感支持。 • 加或不加佐剂的三阶梯疗法。 • 临终关怀和家庭支持。	**Principles of palliative care** • Multidisciplinary approach for symptom control and relief, physical and emotional support • Three-step ladder for pain relief with or without adjuvant • Care plan for terminal stage and support to family

第21章 泌尿系脱垂和功能失调

Prolapse and disorders of the urinary tract

Ajay Rane   Mugdha Kulkarni   Jay Iyer   著   颜 磊 译   石玉华 校

<table>
<tr><td>

学习目标

学习本章后你应当能够:

知识标准
- 描述子宫和阴道的正常支撑。
- 描述维持排尿控制的正常机制和正常排尿的生理学。
- 描述与尿失禁、尿频、泌尿道感染和泌尿生殖系统脱垂相关的流行病学、病因学和临床特征。
- 评估常见的用于治疗尿失禁和生殖器脱垂的手术和非手术治疗,其中包括导尿、膀胱再训练、盆底锻炼、药物治疗、伴或不伴子宫切除术后的阴道修复、吊带悬吊和阴道尿道悬吊术。

临床能力
- 为一名表现出肠道、膀胱和性生活症状的女性患者收集病史。
- 进行盆腔检查,以评估泌尿生殖系统脱垂和盆底张力。
- 解释用于评估尿失禁和脱垂的调查,其中包括微生物学、尿动力学、膀胱镜检查和成像。

专业技能和态度
- 考虑尿失禁对女性和社区的影响。

</td><td>

LEARNING OUTCOMES

After studying this chapter you should be able to:

Knowledge criteria
- Describe the normal supports of the uterus and vagina.
- Describe the normal mechanisms that maintain urinary continence and the physiology of normal micturition.
- Describe the epidemiology, aetiology and clinical features associated with urinary incontinence, urinary frequency, urinary tract infections and genitourinary prolapse.
- Evaluate the common surgical and non-surgical treatments used in the management of urinary incontinence and genital prolapse, including catheterization, bladder retraining, pelvic floor exercises, medical therapies, vaginal repair with or without hysterectomy, sling procedures and colposuspension.

Clinical competencies
- Take a history from a woman presenting with bowel, bladder and sexual symptoms.
- Perform a pelvic examination to assess genitourinary prolapse and pelvic floor tone.
- Explain the investigations employed in the assessment of incontinence and prolapse, including microbiology, urodynamics, cystoscopy and imaging.

Professional skills and attitudes
- Consider the impact of urinary incontinence on women and the community.

</td></tr>
</table>

一、子宫阴道脱垂（Uterovaginal prolapse）

阴道和子宫的位置取决于各种支持筋膜和韧带，后者是由特定区域增厚的支持筋膜形成的（图 21-1 至图 21-4）。我们对盆底支持的解剖学和盆腔脏器脱垂发展的病理生理学的理解已经有了范式的转变。盆腔器官支持的三个层次具有临床相关性，概念上更容易掌握。子宫骶韧带负责对阴道上段和子宫颈提供第一水平的支持（并延伸到子宫），它在第 2、第 3 和第 4 骶椎骨有广泛的附着，由子宫颈和阴道上段结合部出发，向后经直肠两侧附着于骶前。另一个重要的结构是盆筋膜腱弓（ATFP；图 21-3 和图 21-5），也称为白线——闭孔内肌骨盆侧蜂窝结缔组织缩聚而成。ATFP 从坐骨棘延伸至耻骨结节，其末端内侧端称为髂耻骨韧带（Cooper 韧带），为做腹股沟和股疝手术的普通外科医生熟知。从白线向中间延伸的是缩聚的盆腔结缔组织，悬吊着阴道前后壁以及它们下面的器官，即膀胱和直肠，提供第二水平的支撑。膀胱的前支撑以前被称为耻骨膀胱宫颈筋膜或膀胱支柱，而直肠的后支撑被称为直肠阴道筋膜。

The position of the vagina and uterus depends on various fascial supports and ligaments derived from specific thickening of areas of the fascial support (Figs 21.1–21.4). There has been a paradigm shift in our understanding of the anatomy of pelvic floor supports and with it the pathophysiology of development of pelvic organ prolapse. Three levels of pelvic organ support are clinically relevant and conceptually easier to grasp. The uterosacral ligaments responsible for providing level I support to the upper vagina and the cervix (and by extension to the uterus) have a broad attachment over the second, third and fourth sacral vertebrae arising posteriorly from the junction of the cervix and the upper vagina running on each side lateral to the rectum towards the sacral attachments. The other important structure is the arcus tendineus fasciae pelvis (ATFP; see Figs 21.3 and 21.5), also known as the *white line*-a condensation of pelvic cellular tissue on the pelvic aspect of the obturator internus muscle. The ATFP runs from the ischial spines to the pubic tubercle, and its terminal medial end is known as the *iliopectineal ligament* (Cooper's ligament), well known to general surgeons who operate on inguinal and femoral hernias. Extending medially from the white lines are condensed sheets of pelvic cellular tissue suspending the anterior and posterior vaginal walls and the organs underlying these, namely the urinary bladder and the rectum providing level II support. The anterior support to the bladder was previously referred to as the *pubovesicocervical fascia or bladder pillars*, whereas the posterior support to the rectum was termed the *rectovaginal fascia*.

第三水平支撑由会阴体后部和耻骨尿道韧带前部提供。会阴体是一个复杂的纤维肌块，有几种结构插入其中。头侧紧邻直肠阴道隔（Dennonviller 筋膜），尾侧紧邻会阴皮肤，前侧紧邻肛管直肠壁，外侧紧邻坐骨支。三维结构被比作红松（落叶松），它形成了盆底的基石，一个 4cm×4cm 的肌纤维结构不仅在前方为下 1/3 的阴道壁（生殖器裂隙的一部分）提供支持，后方还为肛门外括约肌提供支持。附着

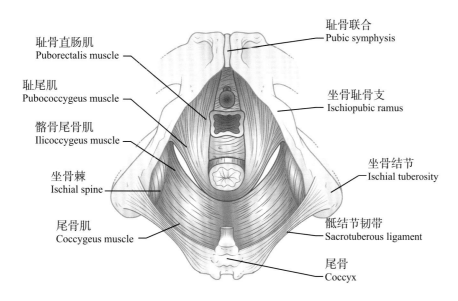

▲ 图 21-1　盆膈自下往上示意

Fig. 21.1　The pelvic diaphragm viewed from below.

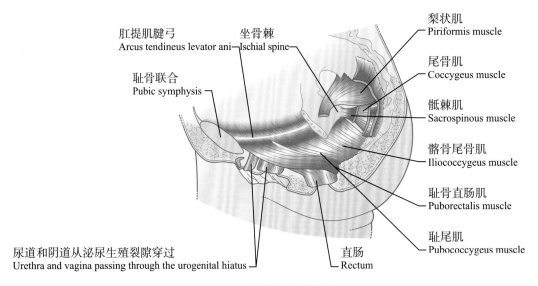

肛提肌腱弓
Arcus tendineus levator ani

坐骨棘
Ischial spine

梨状肌
Piriformis muscle

尾骨肌
Coccygeus muscle

骶棘肌
Sacrospinous muscle

髂骨尾骨肌
Iliococcygeus muscle

耻骨直肠肌
Puborectalis muscle

耻尾肌
Pubococcygeus muscle

耻骨联合
Pubic symphysis

尿道和阴道从泌尿生殖裂隙穿过
Urethra and vagina passing through the urogenital hiatus

直肠
Rectum

▲ 图 21-2　盆底肌肉（侧面观）

Fig. 21.2　Muscles of the pelvic floor, lateral view.

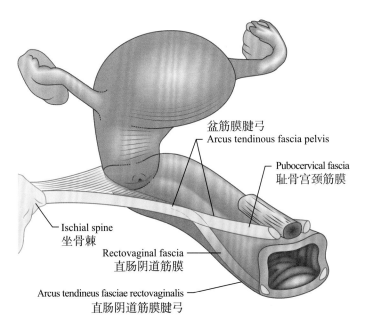

盆筋膜腱弓
Arcus tendinous fascia pelvis

Pubocervical fascia
耻骨宫颈筋膜

Ischial spine
坐骨棘

Rectovaginal fascia
直肠阴道筋膜

Arcus tendineus fasciae rectovaginalis
直肠阴道筋膜腱弓

▲ 图 21-3　耻骨宫颈筋膜（PCF）和直肠阴道筋膜（RVF）外侧附着到骨盆侧壁。图中还显示了盆筋膜腱弓（ATFP）、直肠阴道筋膜腱弓（ATFRV）和坐骨棘（IS）

Fig. 21.3　The lateral attachments of the pubocervical fascia (PCF) and the rectovaginal fascia (RVF) to the pelvic sidewall. Also shown are the arcus tendineus fascia pelvis (ATFP), arcus tendineus fasciae rectovaginalis (ATFRV) and ischial spine (IS).

在会阴体侧面的是会阴浅横肌和深横肌。

Level III support is provided by the perineal body posteriorly and the pubourethral ligaments anteriorly. The perineal body is a complex fibromuscular mass into which several structures insert. It is bordered cephalad by the rectovaginal septum (Dennonviller's fascia), caudal by the perineal skin, anteriorly by the wall of the anorectum and laterally by the ischial rami. The three-dimensional form has

been likened to the cone of the red pine (*Pinus resinosa*), and it forms the keystone of the pelvic floor, a 4 cm × 4 cm fibromuscular structure providing support not just to the lower third of the vaginal wall (part of the genital hiatus) anteriorly but also to the external anal sphincter posteriorly. Attaching laterally to the perineal body are the superficial and deep perineal muscles.

阴道前壁由耻骨膀胱宫颈筋膜支撑，后者是从

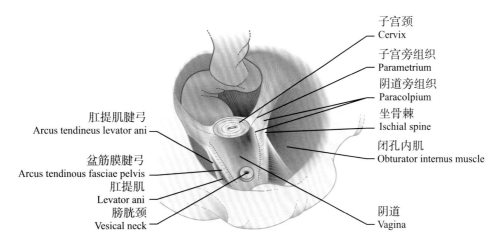

子宫颈
Cervix

子宫旁组织
Parametrium

阴道旁组织
Paracolpium

坐骨棘
Ischial spine

闭孔内肌
Obturator internus muscle

肛提肌腱弓
Arcus tendineus levator ani

盆筋膜腱弓
Arcus tendinous fasciae pelvis

肛提肌
Levator ani

膀胱颈
Vesical neck

阴道
Vagina

▲ 图 21-4　骨盆内筋膜的三维观。注意子宫颈的位置在阴道前段附近

Fig. 21.4　Three-dimensional view of the endopelvic fascia. Notice the location of the cervix in the proximal anterior vaginal segment.

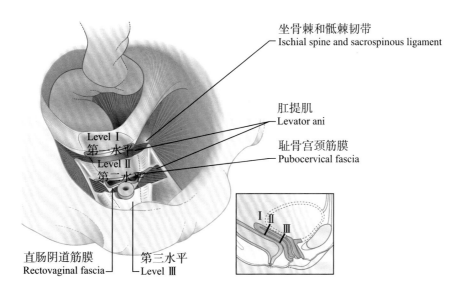

坐骨棘和骶棘韧带
Ischial spine and sacrospinous ligament

肛提肌
Levator ani

耻骨宫颈筋膜
Pubocervical fascia

Level I
第一水平

Level II
第二水平

直肠阴道筋膜
Rectovaginal fascia

第三水平
Level III

▲ 图 21-5　子宫切除术后患者的骨盆内筋膜按照 DeLancey 的生物力学水平分级：第一水平，近端悬吊；第二水平，侧向附着；第三水平，远端融合

经许可改编自 DeLancey JO (1992) Anatomic aspects of vaginal eversion after hysterectomy. Am J Obstet Gynecol 166:1717. ©Elsevier 版权所有

Fig. 21.5　The endopelvic fascia of a post-hysterectomy patient divided into DeLancey's biomechanical levels: level I, proximal suspension; level II, lateral attachment; level III, distal fusion.

Modified with permission from DeLancey JO (1992) Anatomic aspects of vaginal eversion after hysterectomy. Am J Obstet Gynecol 166:1717. © Elsevier.

一侧的 ATFP 延伸到另一侧的 ATFP，提供吊床状第二水平的支撑。阴道后壁由直肠阴道隔纤维组织支撑，该纤维组织仅在中线清晰可见；侧向上，吊床状支撑起自 ATFP。

The anterior vaginal wall is supported by the pubovesicocervical fascia, which extends from the ATFP on one side to the ATFP of the other, providing a hammock-like

level II support. The posterior vaginal wall is supported by the fibrous tissue of the rectovaginal septum that is well defined only in the midline; laterally the hammock-like supports arise from the ATFP.

子宫由阴道壁支撑组织提供间接支撑，但直接由子宫骶韧带支撑。圆韧带和阔韧带对阴道和子宫提供微弱的支撑。完整的肛提肌（骨盆底）间接地支撑着阴道和子宫的下 1/3。后者的作用尚不清楚，但肛提肌的耻骨直肠肌部分在妊娠和分娩过程中对生殖器裂隙的扩张起着重要作用，这使其非常容易受伤。这块肌肉的损伤被认为是晚年阴道脱垂的原因。

The uterus is supported indirectly by the supports of the vaginal walls but directly by the uterosacral ligaments. The round and broad ligaments provide weak, if any, support to the vagina and uterus. Indirect support of the lower third of the vagina and uterus is provided by the intact levator ani (pelvic floor). The role of the latter has always been in doubt, but the puborectalis portion of the levator ani plays a significant role in the distension of the genital hiatus in labour and delivery, making it very prone to injury. Injury to this muscle has been postulated to be the cause for vaginal prolapse later in life.

（一）定义（Definitions）

1. 阴道脱垂（Vaginal prolapse）

阴道前壁脱垂可影响尿道（尿道膨出）和膀胱（膀胱膨出，图 21-6）。查体可看到尿道和膀胱下降并膨出向阴道前壁，严重者膨出物在阴道口处或口外可见。尿道膨出是第三水平支撑（前部）损伤的结果，即耻骨尿道韧带。膀胱膨出通常是由于丧失第二水平支撑和耻骨膀胱宫颈筋膜中线缺损造成的。然而，近一半的前部脱垂也有顶部缺损。直肠膨出是由以下两个因素共同形成的：①直肠阴道筋膜缺损导致的直肠疝；②与 ATFP 提供的第二水平支撑的

侧向脱离。通常可以看到的是直肠通过阴道后壁可见的隆起。它常与会阴部缺陷和松弛有关。这是影响会阴体的典型的第三水平缺损（后部）。

Prolapse of the anterior vaginal wall may affect the urethra (*urethrocele*) and the bladder (*cystocele*, Fig. 21.6). On examination, the urethra and bladder can be seen to descend and bulge into the anterior vaginal wall and, in severe cases, will be visible at or beyond the introitus of the vagina. A urethrocele is the result of damage to level III (anterior) support, i.e. the pubourethral ligaments. Cystoceles usually result due to a loss of level II support and usually due to a midline defect in pubovesicocervical fascia. However, nearly half of anterior prolapses have apical defects as well. A *rectocele* is formed by a combination of factors: a herniation of the rectum through a defect in the rectovaginal fascia, as well as a lateral detachment of the level II support from the ATFP. This can usually be seen as a visible bulge of the rectum through the posterior vaginal wall. It is often associated with a deficiency and laxity of the perineum. This is the classical level III defect (posterior) affecting the perineal body.

肠膨出是小肠通过子宫直肠窝（即道格拉斯陷窝），通过阴道穹隆的上部脱垂形成的（图 21-6）。这种情况可以单独发生，但通常与子宫脱垂相关联。当阴道穹隆的支持不足时，子宫切除术后也可能发生肠膨出。这代表的是第一水平支撑的损伤。

An *enterocele* is formed by a prolapse of the small bowel through the rectouterine pouch, i.e. the pouch of Douglas, through the upper part of the vaginal vault (see Fig. 21.6). The condition may occur in isolation but usually occurs in association with uterine prolapse. An enterocele may also occur

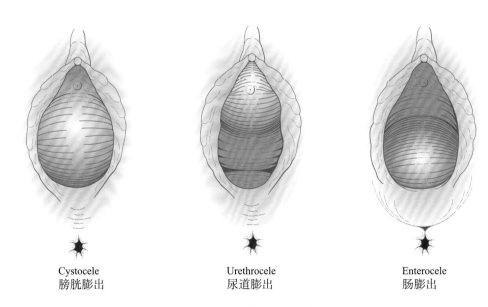

| Cystocele 膀胱膨出 | Urethrocele 尿道膨出 | Enterocele 肠膨出 |

▲ 图 21-6　阴道脱垂临床表现

Fig. 21.6　The clinical appearance of vaginal prolapse.

following hysterectomy when there is inadequate support of the vaginal vault. This represents damage to level I support.

2. 子宫脱垂（Uterine prolapse）

当第一水平支持不足时发生子宫下降，可能不伴阴道壁脱垂，但更常见的是与阴道脱垂同时发生。子宫 I 度脱垂常与子宫后位和子宫颈在阴道内下降有关。如果子宫颈下降到阴道口外，脱垂被定义为 II 度。III 度子宫脱垂是指子宫颈、子宫体和阴道壁完全突出于阴道口。Procidentia 这个词实际上的意思是"脱垂"或"下落"，但通常用于描述完全或 III 度脱垂（图 21-7）。

Descent of the uterus, which occurs when level I support is deficient, may occur in isolation from vaginal wall prolapse but more commonly occurs in conjunction with it. Firstdegree prolapse of the uterus often occurs in association with retroversion of the uterus and descent of the cervix within the vagina. If the cervix descends to the vaginal introitus, the prolapse is defined as second degree. The term *procidentia* is applied to where the cervix and the body of the uterus and the vagina walls protrude through the introitus. The word actually means 'prolapse' or 'falling' but is generally reserved for the description of total or third-degree prolapse (Fig. 21.7).

（二）症状和体征（Symptoms and signs）

症状通常取决于脱垂的严重程度和部位（表 21-1）。

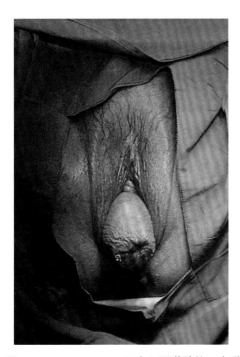

▲ 图 21-7　Procidentia：子宫和阴道壁的三度脱垂

Fig. 21.7　Procidentia: a third-degree prolapse of the uterus and vaginal walls.

Symptoms generally depend on the severity and site of the prolapse (Table 21.1).

> **！注意**
>
> 经产妇常有轻度脱垂，可能无症状。
>
> Mild degrees of prolapse are common in parous women and may be asymptomatic.

有些症状是所有形式脱垂的共同症状，其中包括以下症状。

- 与拖拽不适相关的阴道充盈感。

- 宫颈和阴道壁可见的突出。

- 骶背痛，通常在躺下时缓解。

症状往往是多重的，并与脱垂的性质有关。重要的是要注意，脱垂的症状（和体征）在一天结束时更严重。因此，对于那些有典型脱垂症状但无明显体征的患者，安排一天中稍晚一点的时间来检查是有一定价值的。

Some symptoms are common to all forms of prolapse; these include:

- A sense of fullness in the vagina associated with dragging discomfort

- Visible protrusion of the cervix and vaginal walls

- Lower backache is usually relieved on lying down

Symptoms are often multiple and related to the nature of prolapse. It is important to note that the symptoms (and signs) of prolapse are worse at the end of the day. It is therefore of some value to schedule examination of patients who have typical symptoms of prolapse without its obvious signs a little later in the day.

1 尿道膨出和膀胱膨出（Urethrocele and cystocele）

典型的患者主诉是，阴道"有东西掉下来"。有时膀胱有不完全排空感，这和重复排尿有关，即在明显排尿完成后想立即再次排尿。患者可能会有不得不手动将脱垂物复位到阴道以排尿的病史。有些患者可能由于膀胱排空不完全而反复发生尿路感染。有时患者可能会主诉隐匿性压力性尿失禁，即腹内压升高引起的不自觉漏尿，这种情况在咳嗽时并不容易表现出来，但可在脱垂程度减轻时出现。

Typically patients complain of 'something coming down' per vaginam. At times there may be incomplete emptying of the bladder, and this will be associated with double micturition, the desire to repeat micturition immediately after apparent completion of voiding. The patient may give a history of having

表 21-1　不同支撑水平的诊断和相关症状

Table 21.1　Levels of supports with diagnosis and co-relation with symptoms

盆腔脏器支撑水平 Level of pelvic organ support	受累器官 Organ affected	突出类型 Type of prolapse	症状 Symptoms
I 级：子宫骶韧带 Level I -uterosacral ligaments	子宫 / 阴道穹窿（子宫切除术后） Uterus/vaginal vault (post-hysterectomy)	子宫宫颈 / 穹窿 / 肠膨出 Uterocervical/vault prolapse/enterocele	阴道压迫，骶背痛，"有东西掉下来"，性交困难，阴道分泌物 Vaginal pressure, sacral backache, 'something coming down', dyspareunia, vaginal discharge
II 级：盆筋膜腱弓（ATFP） Level II -arcus tendineus fascia pelvis (ATFP)	膀胱 Urinary bladder	膀胱膨出 Cystocele	"有东西掉下来"，重复排尿，隐匿性压力性尿失禁，反复泌尿系感染 'Something coming down', double voiding, occult stress incontinence, recurrent urinary tract infection
	直肠 Rectum	直肠膨出 Rectocele	"有东西掉下来"，排便困难，用手指排便 'Something coming down', difficult defecation, manual digitation
III 级：前（耻骨尿道韧带） Level III -anterior (pubourethral ligaments)	尿道 Urethra	尿道膨出 Urethrocele	"有东西掉下来"，压力性尿失禁 'Something coming down', stress incontinence
III 级：后（会阴体） Level III -posterior (perineal body)	阴道下 1/3 或阴道口或肛管 Lower third of the vagina/vaginal introitus/anal canal	生殖道裂隙增宽 Enlarged genital hiatus	阴道松弛，性交障碍，阴道胀气，需要给会阴施压以协助排便 Vaginal looseness, sexual dysfunction, vaginal flatus, needing to apply pressure to the perineum to evacuate faeces

to manually replace the prolapse into the vagina to void. Some patients may get recurrent urinary tract infections as a result of incomplete emptying of the bladder. Occasionally the patient may complain of occult stress incontinence, i.e. the involuntary loss of urine following raised intra-abdominal pressure that is not readily demonstrable on coughing but appears on reducing the prolapse.

通过仰卧体位检查确定诊断。单叶 Sim 窥器可以用来观察阴道前壁。当患者被要求屏气用力时，可以看到阴道前壁的隆起，而且经常出现在阴道口处。对尿液标本进行培养以排除感染的存在是很重要的。鉴别诊断仅限于阴道前壁囊肿或肿瘤，以及尿道或膀胱憩室。

The diagnosis is established by examination in the dorsal position. A single-bladed Sims' speculum can be used to visualize the anterior vaginal wall. When the patient is asked to strain, the bulge in the anterior vaginal wall can be seen and often appears at the introitus. It is important to culture a specimen of urine to exclude the presence of infection. The differential diagnosis is limited to cysts or tumours of the anterior vaginal wall and diverticulum of the urethra or bladder.

2. 直肠膨出（Rectocele）

经阴道后壁的直肠膨出通常与会阴体的盆底缺陷和提肛肌分离有关。这主要是由分娩过程中过度扩张的阴道口和盆底导致的问题。

The prolapse of the rectum through the posterior vaginal wall is commonly associated with a deficient pelvic floor, disruption of the perineal body and separation of the levator ani. It is predominantly a problem that results from over-distension of the introitus and pelvic floor during parturition.

直肠膨出的症状包括排便困难，偶尔需要"用手指"。一般的主要症状是感觉到一个可还纳的肿块进入阴道或通过阴道口膨出。

The symptoms of a rectocele include difficulty with evacuation of faeces with an occasional need to 'manually digitate'. Needless to say, the awareness of a reducible mass bulging into the vagina and through the introitus is often the presenting symptom.

对外阴的检查通常发现会阴缺如（测量长度＜ 3cm），使后面的阴唇系带与前面的肛缘紧密贴合。

患者可能会抱怨由此导致阴道松弛和性功能障碍。在直接询问时可以发现阴道"胀气"的症状并不罕见。

Examination of the vulva usually shows a deficient perineum (measuring less than 3 cm in length) bringing the posterior fourchette in close apposition with the anterior anal verge. Patients can complain of vaginal looseness and sexual dysfunction as a result of this. Not uncommonly the symptom of vaginal 'flatus' can be uncovered on direct questioning.

3. 肠膨出（Enterocele）

如果子宫被切除，道格拉斯囊疝通常通过阴道穹窿发生。由于阴道压力感是相同的，通常很难区分高位直肠膨出和肠膨出。对于无明显脱垂体征但有盆腔拖曳感或骶背痛的女性，偶尔站姿检查或双指检查可发现肠膨出。罕见的肠膨出发生在阴道穹窿前部，可近似于膀胱膨出。

Herniation of the pouch of Douglas usually occurs through the vaginal vault if the uterus has been removed. It is often difficult to distinguish between a high rectocele and an enterocele, as the symptoms of vaginal pressure are identical. Occasionally an examination in the standing position or a bidigital examination may reveal an enterocele in a woman with no obvious signs of prolapse but complaints of a dragging sensation in the pelvis or a low backache. Uncommonly the enterocele occurs anterior to the vaginal vault and may mimic a cystocele.

大的肠膨出可包含肠管，并可合并肠嵌顿和肠梗阻。

A large enterocele may contain bowel and may be associated with incarceration and obstruction of the bowel.

4. 子宫脱垂（Uterine prolapse）

子宫的下降最初与子宫颈的延伸和子宫体的下降有关。通常受影响的宫颈部位是在阴道以上，即在阴道穹窿上方。症状是阴道受压，最终子宫通过阴道口完全突出。在这个阶段，子宫脱垂可产生坐时的不适，摩擦性溃疡可导致出血。有时有轻微脱垂或先天性脱垂的患者可能会有阴道下的宫颈延伸，这经常导致对脱垂的分度混淆，因为它可能看起来比实际上分级更高。

Descent of the uterus is initially associated with elongation of the cervix and descent of the body of the uterus. Mostly the affected portion of the cervix is supravaginal, i.e. above the level of the vaginal fornices. The symptoms are those of pressure in the vagina and, ultimately, complete protrusion of the uterus through the introitus. At this stage, the prolapsed uterus may produce discomfort on sitting, and decubitus ulceration may result in bleeding. Sometimes patients with minor degrees of prolapse or with congenital prolapse may have infravaginal cervical elongation that often leads to confusion in staging the degree of prolapse, as it may appear to be in a more advanced stage than it actually is.

尿路感染可发生于输尿管受压，以及由于膀胱不能完全排空导致的肾盂积水。患者经历性交困难并非罕见，但不太容易出现于此症状。

Urinary tract infection may occur because of compression of the ureters and consequent hydronephrosis due to incomplete emptying of the bladder. Not unusually, patients experience dyspareunia but are not very forthcoming with this symptom.

（三）脱垂的分期/分级（Staging/grading of prolapse）

Baden-Walker 半程系统（图 21-8 和表 21-2）

Baden-Walker halfway system (Fig. 21.8 and Table 21.2)

该系统的开发是为了引入更多的客观指标量化盆腔器官脱垂程度。例如，用厘米来代替主观分数。如图 21-9 所示，记录了 9 种具体的测量。

This system was developed in an effort to introduce more objectivity into the quantification of pelvic organ prolapse. For example, measurements in centimetres are used instead of subjective grades. Nine specific measurements are recorded, as indicated in Figure 21.9.

（四）发病机制（Pathogenesis）

脱垂可能是先天性或获得性的。

- 先天性：年轻或未产妇的子宫脱垂是由于支撑子宫和阴道穹隆的力量薄弱。有最低程度的阴道壁脱垂。

- 获得性：脱垂最常见的形式是在多种因素的影响下获得的。这种类型的脱垂包括子宫和阴道，但也必须记住阴道壁脱垂也可以在没有任何子宫下降的情况下发生。其诱发因素包括以下几种。

  - 多产次：子宫阴道脱垂是已产妇的一种情况。骨盆底对阴道壁提供直接或间接的支持，当这种支持被撕裂或过度扩张破坏时，就容易导致阴道壁脱垂。使用产钳/胎头吸引，特别是中腔产钳和旋转产钳，可能导致在以后的生活中发生尿失禁和脱垂。

  - 腹内压升高：肿瘤或腹水可能导致腹内压

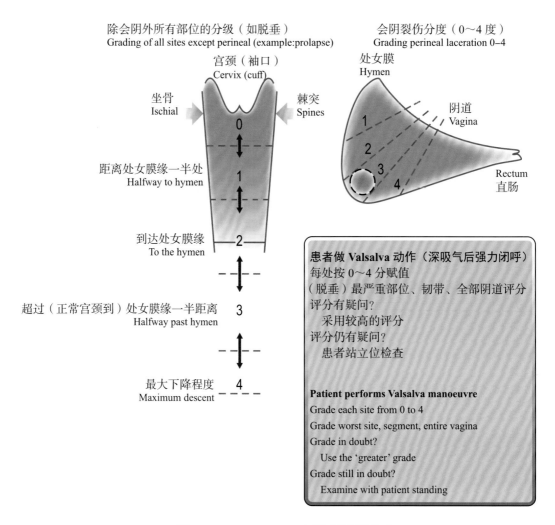

除会阴外所有部位的分级（如脱垂）
Grading of all sites except perineal (example:prolapse)

会阴裂伤分度（0～4 度）
Grading perineal laceration 0–4

宫颈（袖口）
Cervix (cuff)

处女膜
Hymen

坐骨
Ischial

棘突
Spines

阴道
Vagina

距离处女膜缘一半处
Halfway to hymen

直肠
Rectum

到达处女膜缘
To the hymen

超过（正常宫颈到）处女膜缘一半距离
Halfway past hymen

最大下降程度
Maximum descent

患者做 Valsalva 动作（深吸气后强力闭呼）
每处按 0～4 分赋值
（脱垂）最严重部位、韧带、全部阴道评分
评分有疑问？
　采用较高的评分
评分仍有疑问？
　　患者站立位检查

Patient performs Valsalva manoeuvre

Grade each site from 0 to 4

Grade worst site, segment, entire vagina

Grade in doubt?

　Use the 'greater' grade

Grade still in doubt?

　Examine with patient standing

▲ 图 21-8　Baden-Walker 半程系统评分指南

（经许可转载自 Baden WF, Walker T (1992) Surgical repair of vaginal defects. Lippincott, Williams & Wilkins, Philadelphia.）

Fig. 21.8　Guidelines on how to assign grades in the Baden-Walker halfway system.

(Reproduced with permission from Baden WF, Walker T (1992) Surgical repair of vaginal defects. Lippincott, Williams & Wilkins, Philadelphia.)

升高，但更常见的原因是慢性咳嗽和慢性便秘。

- 激素变化：脱垂的症状往往在绝经期迅速恶化。雌激素的缺少导致阴道壁和子宫的支撑组织变薄。虽然脱垂通常在绝经前出现，但绝经期症状变得明显，脱垂下降的程度明显恶化。初次阴道分娩的年龄影响以后生活中脱垂和尿失禁的发生率。据推测，分娩年龄增大易导致肛提肌损伤，使这些女性更容易发生盆底疾病。

Prolapse may be:

• Congenital: Uterine prolapse in young or nulliparous women is due to weakness of the supports of the uterus and vaginal vault. There is a minimal degree of vaginal wall prolapse.

• Acquired: The commonest form of prolapse is acquired under the influence of multiple factors. This type of prolapse is both uterine and vaginal, but it must also be remembered that vaginal wall prolapse can also occur without any uterine descent. Predisposing factors include:

– *High parity*: Uterovaginal prolapse is a condition of parous women. The pelvic floor provides direct and indirect support for the vaginal walls, and when this support is disrupted by laceration or over-distension, it predisposes to vaginal wall prolapse. Instrumental delivery employing forceps/ventouse, especially mid-cavity rotational forceps delivery, may play a contributory role in the causation of urinary incontinence and prolapse in later life.

表 21-2　在 Baden-Walker 半程系统中使用的每个部位的主要和次要症状

Table 21.2　Primary and secondary symptoms at each site used in the Baden-Walker halfway system

解剖部位 Anatomical site	主要症状 Primary symptoms	次要症状 Secondary symptoms
尿道 Urethral	尿失禁 Urinary incontinence	脱落 Falling out
膀胱 Vesical	排尿困难 Voiding difficulties	脱落 Falling out
子宫 Uterine	脱落、沉重等 Falling out, heaviness, etc.	
后穹隆 Cul-de-sac	骨盆压力（站） Pelvic pressure (standing)	脱落 Falling out
直肠 Rectal	真正的肠袋 True bowel pocket	脱落 Falling out
会阴 Perineal	肛门失禁 Anal incontinence	太松（气体 / 粪便） Too loose (gas/faeces)

经许可转载自 Baden WF, Walker T (1992) Surgical repair of vaginal defects. Lippincott, Williams & Wilkins, Philadelphia, p. 12.

Reproduced with permission from Baden WF, Walker T (1992) Surgical repair of vaginal defects. Lippincott, Williams & Wilkins, Philadelphia, p. 12.

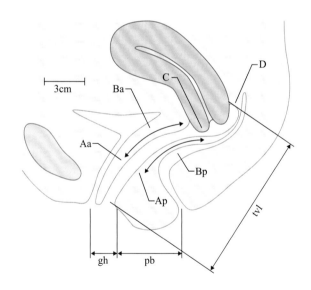

▲ 图 21-9　盆腔脏器脱垂量化评分系统（POP-Q）

Fig. 21.9　Pelvic organ prolapse quantification system (POP-Q).

- *Raised intra-abdominal pressure*: Tumours or ascites may result in raised intra-abdominal pressure, but a more common cause is a chronic cough and chronic constipation.
- *Hormonal changes:* The symptoms of prolapse often worsen rapidly at the time of menopause. Cessation of oestrogen production leads to thinning of the vaginal walls and the supports of the uterus. Although the prolapse is generally present before menopause, it is at this time that the symptoms

become noticeable and the degree of descent visibly worsens. The age at first vaginal childbirth affects the incidence of prolapse and urinary incontinence in later life. It has been postulated that increased maternal age predisposes to levator trauma, making these women more prone to developing pelvic floor disorders.

（五）处理（Management）

脱垂的处理包括保守治疗和手术治疗。

The management of prolapse can be conservative or surgical.

1. 预防（Prevention）

在子宫切除术时用良好的手术技巧来支撑阴道穹窿可以减少后期穹窿脱垂的发生率。避免分娩时第二产程延长和不适当或过早地向下用力，鼓励分娩后盆底功能锻炼，准确地使用器械分娩与适当的个体化会阴切开术，可能都有助于减少今后生活中脱垂的风险。

Good surgical technique in supporting the vaginal vault at the time of hysterectomy reduces the incidence of later vault prolapse. Avoiding a prolonged second stage of labour and inappropriate or premature bearing-down efforts, encouraging pelvic floor exercises after delivery and the judicious use of instrumental delivery with appropriately individualized episiotomies may all help reduce the risk of prolapse in later life.

561

2. 保守治疗（Conservative treatment）

> **！注意**
>
> 许多女性有轻微的无症状子宫阴道脱垂。如果偶然发现脱垂，那么应该建议女性不要接受任何手术治疗。
>
> Many women have minor degrees of uterovaginal prolapse, which are asymptomatic. If the recognition of the prolapse is a coincidental finding, the woman should be advised against any surgical treatment.

轻微程度的脱垂在分娩后是常见的，应该通过盆底锻炼或使用子宫托来治疗。手术干预至少推迟到分娩后 6 个月，因为组织血供丰富并可能发生进一步的自我修复。

Minor degrees of prolapse are common after childbirth and should be treated by pelvic floor exercises or the use of a pessary. Operative intervention is deferred for at least 6 months after delivery, as the tissues remain vascular and may undergo further spontaneous improvement.

激素替代疗法可用于术前的组织准备，但其本身在缓解症状方面的益处有限。

Hormone replacement therapy may be used preoperatively to prepare the tissues but by itself is of limited benefit in alleviating symptoms.

如果需要短期支持或女性的一般健康状况使得手术治疗具有潜在危险，则阴道壁和子宫脱垂都可以通过使用阴道内放子宫托进行治疗。然而如果要保留子宫托，必须有一些盆底支撑。

Where short-term support is required or the general health of the woman makes operative treatment potentially dangerous, both vaginal wall and uterine prolapse can be treated by using vaginal pessaries. It is, however, necessary to have some pelvic floor support if a pessary is to be retained.

最常用的子宫托（图 21-10）包括以下几种。

- **环形托：**此托由可塑塑料环组成，直径为 60～105mm。子宫托插于后穹窿和耻骨联合后面。阴道壁的扩张会对阴道壁脱垂起到支持作用。

- **Hodge 子宫托：**这是一个坚硬的、拉长、弯曲的卵圆形子宫托，以类似于环形托的方式插入，主要用于子宫后倾。

- **Gelhorn 子宫托：**这种子宫托形状像一个颈扣，用于治疗严重程度的脱垂。

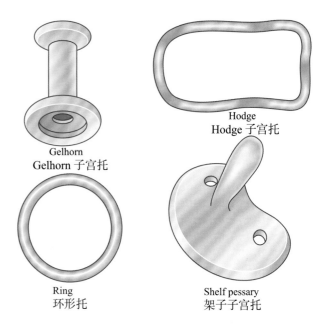

▲ 图 21-10　用于子宫阴道脱垂保守治疗的不同类型的子宫托

Fig. 21.10 Various types of vaginal pessaries used in the conservative management of uterovaginal prolapse.

- **架子子宫托：**形状像衣钩，主要用于治疗子宫或阴道穹窿脱垂。

The most widely used pessaries (Fig. 21.10) are:

- Ring pessary: This pessary consists of a malleable plastic ring, which may vary in diameter from 60 to 105 mm. The pessary is inserted in the posterior fornix and behind the pubic symphysis. Distension of the vaginal walls tends to support the vaginal wall prolapse.

- Hodge pessary: This is a rigid, elongated, curved ovoid which is inserted in a similar way to the ring pessary and is principally useful in uterine retroversion.

- Gelhorn pessary: This pessary is shaped like a collar stud and is used in the treatment of severe degrees of prolapse.

- Shelf pessary: This is shaped like a coat hook and is used mainly in the treatment of uterine or vaginal vault prolapse.

长期使用子宫托的主要问题是阴道穹窿的溃疡，如果子宫托被"忽视"或"遗忘"，通常在膀胱和阴道之间会形成罕见的瘘管。子宫托应每 4～6 个月更换一次，应检查阴道是否有溃疡的迹象。对绝经后的女性来说防止溃疡的做法是给予阴道雌激素乳膏 / 片。

The main problem with long-term use of pessaries is ulceration of the vaginal vault, and rarely a fistula may form, usually between the bladder and the vagina, if the pessary is 'neglected' or 'forgotten'. Pessaries should be replaced every 4–6 months, and the vagina should be examined for any signs of ulceration. In postmenopausal women it is considered good practice to prescribe vaginal oestrogen creams/tablets to prevent ulceration.

3. 盆底物理治疗（Pelvic floor physiotherapy）

见尿失禁部分。

See the section on urinary incontinence.

4. 手术治疗（Surgical treatment）

子宫阴道脱垂的手术治疗近年来有了许多变化。越来越多地使用移植材料和组织锚点来增加脱垂修复的耐久性，因此脱垂修复可分为筋膜修复和移植物增强修复。

The surgical management of uterovaginal prolapse has seen many changes in recent years. There was an increasing use of graft material and tissue anchors for increasing durability of the prolapse repair. Thus prolapse repairs can be classified into fascial repairs and graft-augmented repairs.

（1）筋膜修复（Fascial repairs）：膀胱突出的经典

手术治疗是阴道前壁修补术（图 21–11）。该手术包括从阴道皮瓣剥离脱垂的内脏（膀胱），用坚韧的延迟可吸收缝合线缝合耻骨膀胱宫颈筋膜，并缝合阴道壁。目前的做法不包括切除"多余的阴道皮肤"，因为预期阴道将重塑，并在 6～8 周内这种感觉上的松弛几乎会消失。

Classically surgical treatment of a cystocele is by anterior colporrhaphy (Fig. 21.11). The operation consists of dissection of the prolapsed viscus (the urinary bladder) off the vaginal flaps, buttressing the pubovesicocervical fascia with durable delayed absorbable sutures and closure of the vaginal skin. Current practice does not include excision of 'excess vaginal skin', as the vagina is expected to remodel and the perceived laxity all but disappears in 6–8 weeks' time.

直肠膨出的修复方法是再次将脱垂的内脏（在本例中是直肠）从覆盖的阴道皮肤上剥离，并通过用延迟可吸收缝合线缝贴直肠阴道筋膜撕裂的末端来实现强有力的修复。有时可以辨认出筋膜撕裂处，通常将撕裂端再缝接即可。直肠膨出常伴有会阴体缺损，会阴肌肉萎缩或向外侧收缩，患者主诉"阴道

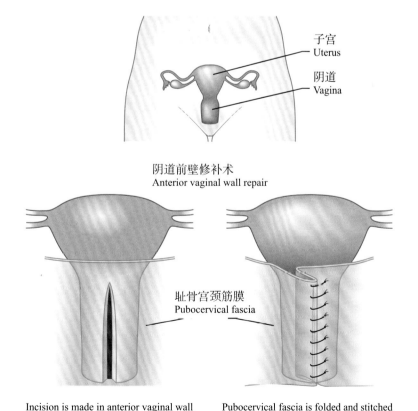

阴道前壁修补术
Anterior vaginal wall repair

子宫
Uterus

阴道
Vagina

耻骨宫颈筋膜
Pubocervical fascia

Incision is made in anterior vaginal wall
阴道前壁切开

Pubocervical fascia is folded and stitched
耻骨宫颈筋膜折叠并缝合

▲ 图 21-11　膀胱膨出的前部筋膜修补
Fig. 21.11　Anterior fascial repair of cystocele.

松弛"或性功能障碍。阴道内会阴成形术是一种旨在治疗这些症状的手术，其中包括侧壁剥离以识别会阴肌肉的末端，将两侧肌肉拉至中线并缝合肌肉到切口顶点。这一手术有助于重建会阴体，缩小生殖器裂隙的大小，从而改善阴道张力，并矫正阴道轴。该手术是会阴修复术的一种改进，后者会阴皮肤首先被切开然后被切除，但仍然不能达到前面所述的目标。

Rectocele is repaired by again dissecting the prolapsing viscus (in this case the rectum) off the overlying vaginal skin and effecting a robust repair by apposing the torn ends of the rectovaginal fascia together with delayed absorbable sutures. Sometimes it is possible to identify the tears in the fascia, and often a reattachment of the torn ends suffices. Not uncommonly a rectocele is accompanied by a deficient perineal body where the perineal muscles are attenuated or retracted laterally, with the patient complaining of 'vaginal laxity' or sexual dysfunction. Intravaginal perineoplasty is the operation designed to treat these symptoms and involves lateral dissection to identify the retracted ends of the perineal muscles, apposing these in the midline and suturing the apposed muscles to the apex of the incision. This procedure helps re-create the perineal body and reduces the size of the genital hiatus, thus improving vaginal tone, and also corrects the vaginal axis. This operation is an improvement on the perineorrhaphy where the perineal skin is first incised and later excised but still fails to achieve the objectives stated earlier.

如果有肠膨出，选择的手术是 McCall 穹窿成形术。这包括通过子宫骶韧带和中间腹膜的切口放置延迟可吸收缝合线，将这些缝合线依次固定到阴道穹窿。该手术的目的不仅是治疗肠膨出，而且要防止穹窿脱垂的发生。

Where there is an enterocele, the procedure of choice is a McCall's culdoplasty. This involves the placement of delayed absorbable sutures through the cut ends of the uterosacral ligaments and the intervening peritoneum, hitching these successively to the vaginal vault. The aim of this operation is not just to treat the enterocele but also to prevent occurrence of vault prolapse.

子宫脱垂的治疗选择取决于女性是否愿意保留其生育潜能。如果她的家庭完整，那么经阴子宫切除术同时修复脱垂的阴道壁是首选方法。如果需要保留生育功能，那么可以通过简单地切除延长的子宫颈到适当的长度，并将主韧带缝合在子宫颈残端前来保存子宫。这种手术被称为 Manchester 或 Fothergill 修复术。然后用环缝法将阴道皮肤缝合到宫颈残端。此外，手术医生可能会选择通过称为骶棘宫颈固定术 / 子宫固定术的骶棘韧带缝合来支撑宫颈。

The treatment of choice for uterine prolapse depends on the woman's preference for retaining her reproductive potential. If her family is complete, then a vaginal hysterectomy, usually with repair of the prolapsed vaginal walls, is the preferred approach. If preservation of reproductive function is required, then the uterus can be conserved by simply excising the elongated cervix that is fashioned to an appropriate length with suturing of the cardinal ligaments in front of the cervical stump. This procedure is known as a *Manchester or Fothergill repair*. The vaginal skin is then sutured into the cervical stump using circumferential sutures. Additionally the operating surgeon may elect to suspend the cervix by means of sutures taken through the sacrospinous ligament called *sacrospinous cervicopexy/ hysteropexy*.

类似的操作可用于治疗子宫切除术后发生的穹窿脱垂；这个过程被称为骶棘阴道固定术（colpos Gk: vagina）。

A similar procedure may be employed to treat vault prolapse occurring after hysterectomy; the procedure is then called *sacrospinous colpopexy* (*colpos* Gk: vagina).

(2) 移植物修复（Graft repairs）：最早使用补片的修补是治疗穹窿脱垂（图 21–12）。治疗阴道穹窿脱垂的方法是用合成网将阴道穹窿悬挂在骶骨前纵韧带上。这种手术被称为骶骨阴道固定术，可以通过腹腔镜、机器人或开腹手术进行。打捆针驱动的网片用于修复阴道脱垂。2008 年，美国食品药品管理局（FDA）发布了一份报道，将这些并发症归类为罕见的并发症。然而，随着阴道补片使用的增加，这种情况在 2011 年发生改变，并发症不再被认为是罕见的。目前的文献表明，大多数盆腔脏器脱垂的病例可以不用补片治疗，没有令人信服的证据表明补片更有效，特别是对于穹窿和后盆腔。

The earliest repairs using mesh have been to treat vault prolapse (Fig. 21.12). The prolapsed vaginal vault is treated by suspending the vaginal vault from the anterior longitudinal ligament of the sacrum using a synthetic mesh. This procedure is known as *sacrocolpopexy*-a procedure that can be performed laparoscopically, robotically or through a laparotomy. Needle-driven mesh kits were used for repair of vaginal prolapse. A Food and Drug Administration (FDA) report released in 2008 classified complications occurring from these to be rare. However, with increasing use of vaginal mesh, this was changed in 2011 where the complications were no longer considered to be rare. Current literature suggests that most cases of pelvic organ prolapse could be treated without mesh, and there is no compelling evidence of greater success with mesh, particularly for vault and posterior compartment.

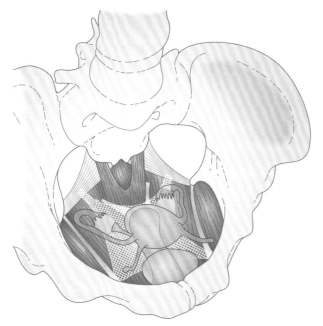

▲ 图 21-12　用于阴道脱垂（膀胱膨出）的移植物（网片）

Fig. 21.12　Graft (mesh) used for vaginal prolapse repair (cystocele).

这一证据主要针对较旧的补片，目前还没有关于较新、较轻补片的随机对照试验（RCT）。此证据不适用于腹部使用的网片。腹腔镜骶骨阴道固定术仍然被认为是治疗第一水平脱垂的好方法。

This evidence is mainly for older mesh, and there are no current randomized controlled trials (RCTs) about newer, lighter mesh. This does not apply to mesh used abdominally. Laparoscopic sacrocolpopexy is still considered a good option for level I prolapse.

（六）并发症（Complications）

无论是筋膜性还是非筋膜性的修复，都可能导致被治疗的内脏损伤，如膀胱、小肠、直肠或肛管。当进行 McCall 穹窿成形术时，乙状结肠或输尿管可能会受到额外的损伤。打捆针驱动的网片很少伴有骨盆深层血管的损伤，而阴道网片外露是相对更常见并发症。原发性、保守性和继发性出血以及感染均可在这些手术后发生。经阴子宫切除术的直接并发症包括出血、血肿形成、感染和较少发生的尿潴留。远期的并发症是性交困难和阴道容积减少，特别是如果阴道黏膜切除不当时。筋膜修补，特别是前筋膜室，可能在大约 1/3 的病例中复发。后筋膜室修补术的效果更好，只有 20% 的复发率。对阴道顶部的支持不足可能会导致阴道穹窿脱垂的复发。补片修补术的效果更强，复发率更低。

Repairs, whether fascial or otherwise, can result in injury to the viscus being treated, i.e. bladder, small intestines, rectum or anal canal. The sigmoid colon or the ureters may additionally be injured when a McCall's culdoplasty is performed. The needle-driven devices were known to be rarely associated with damage to the deeper vessels in the pelvis and with more common occurrence of vaginal mesh exposure. Primary, reactionary and secondary haemorrhage may all occur with these procedures, as may infection. The immediate complications of vaginal hysterectomy include haemorrhage, haematoma formation, infection and, less commonly, urinary retention. The long-term complications are dyspareunia and reduced vaginal capacity, especially if vaginal skin is inappropriately excised. Fascial repairs, especially of the anterior compartment, may recur in about a third of cases. Posterior compartment fascial repairs perform better with only 20% recurrence. Inadequate support to the vaginal apex may result in recurrence of the prolapse of the vaginal vault. Mesh repairs were found to be more robust with lower rates of recurrence.

二、尿道疾病（Urinary tract disorders）

（一）尿道的结构和生理（Structure and physiology of the urinary tract）

膀胱是一个中空肌性器官，有外膜层，以及称为逼尿肌的平滑肌层和内层的移行上皮。

The urinary bladder is a hollow muscular organ with an outer adventitial layer, a smooth muscle layer known as the *detrusor muscle* and an inner layer of transitional epithelium.

膀胱神经包含交感神经和副交感神经。交感神经纤维起源于脊髓的胸段下两段和腰段上两段，副交感神经纤维来自第 2、第 3 和第 4 骶关节段。

The innervation of the bladder contains both sympathetic and parasympathetic components. The sympathetic fibres arise from the lower two thoracic and upper two lumbar segments of the spinal cord, and the parasympathetic fibres from the second, third and fourth sacral segments.

尿道本身起始于膀胱外壁，在尿道的远 2/3 处，与阴道融合，它与阴道有共同的胚胎起源。尿道从膀胱颈到尿生殖膈下筋膜段，起自于膀胱中、远 2/3 的交界处，分有好几层。在外层，环形骨骼肌层（泌尿生殖器括约肌）与一些环形平滑肌纤维混合。在这一层内有纵行平滑肌层包围着血供丰富的黏膜下静脉丛，以及对雌激素刺激有反应的非角化的鳞状上皮。排尿控制机制由泌尿生殖括约肌维持，辅之以尿道上皮的黏膜接合和黏膜下静脉丛提供的"膨胀"效应。

The urethra itself begins outside the bladder wall. In its distal two-thirds, it is fused with the vagina, with which it shares a common embryological derivation. From the vesical neck to the perineal membrane, which starts at the junction of the middle and distal thirds of the bladder, the urethra has several layers. An outer, circularly oriented skeletal muscle layer (urogenital sphincter) mingles with some circularly oriented smooth muscle fibres. Inside this layer is a longitudinal layer of smooth muscle that surrounds a very vascular submucosal venous plexus and non-keratinized squamous epithelium that responds to estrogenic stimulation. The continence mechanism is maintained by the urogenital sphincter, aided by the mucosal co-aptation of urethral epithelium and the 'bulking-up' effect provided by the submucosal venous plexus.

排尿时，膀胱内压力上升，超过尿道内压力，尿道阻力下降。膀胱颈周围肌纤维的张力因骶神经丛运动神经元受中枢抑制而减弱。膀胱以 1~6ml/min 充盈。由于膀胱壁的顺应性和逼尿肌的反射性抑制，膀胱内压力仍然很低。同时，横纹肌括约肌的紧张性收缩和尿道黏膜的张力使尿道内口关闭。当腹腔内压力升高时，如咳嗽或打喷嚏，排尿控制是通过传递压力上升到近端尿道（通常位于腹腔内）和肛提肌张力的增加来维持。

During micturition, the pressure in the bladder rises to exceed the pressure within the urethral lumen, and there is a fall in urethral resistance. The tone of muscle fibres around the bladder neck is reduced by central inhibition of the motor neurons in the sacral plexus. The bladder fills at 1–6 mL/min. The intravesical pressure remains low because of compliance of the bladder wall as it stretches and reflex inhibition of the detrusor muscle. At the same time the internal urethral meatus is closed by tonic contraction of the rhabdosphincter and the tone of the urethral mucosa. During rises in intraabdominal pressure such as coughing or sneezing, continence is maintained by transmission of the pressure rise to the proximal urethra (which lies normally within the intraabdominal space) and an increase in the levator tone.

输尿管长 25~30cm。它沿着腰椎横突，在腰大肌前走形，与卵巢血管交叉，在髂总血管分叉进入骨盆。从这里，它在髂内血管前面走形，到坐骨棘，在此向内侧转到子宫颈。它再次转向前到阴道穹窿外侧 1.5cm 处，穿过子宫血管下方进入膀胱的后表面。

The ureter is 25–30 cm long. It runs along the transverse processes of the lumbar spine, anterior to the psoas muscle, is crossed by the ovarian vessels and enters the pelvis anterior to the bifurcation of the common iliac vessels. From there it runs anterior to the internal iliac vessels to the ischial spines, where it turns medially to the cervix. It turns again anteriorly 1.5 cm lateral to the vaginal fornix, crossing below the uterine vessels

to enter the posterior surface of the bladder.

！注意

输尿管在盆腔的两个部位特别容易受到手术损伤。一个是输尿管在卵巢悬韧带的外侧进入骨盆处。在切除一个大的卵巢肿瘤时，由于肿瘤被拉到内侧，输尿管可从骨盆侧壁提离，钳夹卵巢悬韧带时可能会夹住输尿管。第二，在子宫切除术时，在输尿管进入膀胱前流经子宫动脉下的位置，夹住或剥离子宫血管，可能会造成损伤。

The ureters are particularly vulnerable to surgical damage at two sites in the pelvis. One is the point at which the ureter enters the pelvis under the lateral origin of the suspensory ligament. At the time of removal of a large ovarian tumour, clamping of the ligament may incorporate the ureter as the tumour is pulled medially and the ureter is lifted off the lateral pelvic wall. Second, during a hysterectomy the ureter may be damaged by clamping or dissection at the point where it passes under the uterine artery before entering the bladder.

（二）常见的膀胱功能障碍（Common disorders of bladder function）

常见的膀胱功能障碍包括以下症状。

- 尿失禁。

- 尿频。

- 排尿困难。

- 尿潴留。

- 夜间遗尿。

The common symptoms of bladder dysfunction include:

- urinary incontinence
- frequency of micturition
- dysuria
- urinary retention
- nocturnal enuresis.

1. 尿失禁（Incontinence of urine）

非自主漏尿可能与膀胱或尿道功能障碍或瘘管形成有关。尿失禁的类型如下。

- 真性尿失禁是通过阴道持续流失尿液，它通常与瘘管形成有关，但偶尔也可能是尿潴留并溢尿的表现。

- 压力性尿失禁是在短时间内腹内压升高时发

生的不自觉小便丢失。它通常与前面描述的控制机制损伤和缺乏雌激素刺激有关，通常在绝经前后表现出来。检查发现咳嗽时不自觉的漏尿，通常伴有尿道过度蠕动和阴道前壁脱垂。

- 急迫性尿失禁是由突然的逼尿肌收缩与不受控制的失尿而产生。这种情况可能是由于特发性逼尿肌不稳定或与尿路感染、梗阻性尿路病变、糖尿病或神经系统疾病相关。排除尿路感染尤为重要。

- 混合失禁和压力性尿失禁在相当多女性中会出现。有急迫性尿失禁的女性也会有真正的压力性尿失禁，在纠正压力性尿失禁之前治疗逼尿肌不稳定是特别重要的。如果不这样做可能会导致情况恶化。

- 充盈性尿失禁发生于膀胱扩张或弛缓，而张力 / 功能很小或没有。这在阴道分娩后或脊髓麻醉后膀胱被"忽略"时并不罕见。膀胱扫描通常显示膀胱残留其容量的一半以上。膀胱会变得"懒惰"，当它充满的时候就会外排。

- 混合性尿失禁包括感染、药物治疗、长期制动和认知障碍，在某些情况下可能会导致尿失禁。

The involuntary loss of urine may be associated with bladder or urethral dysfunction or fistula formation. Types of incontinence are as follows:

- True incontinence is continuous loss of urine through the vagina; it is commonly associated with fistula formation but may occasionally be a manifestation of urinary retention with overflow.

- Stress incontinence is the involuntary loss of urine that occurs during a brief period of raised intraabdominal pressure. It is usually related to injury to the continence mechanism described earlier and lack of estrogenic stimulation and usually manifests around menopause. Examination reveals the involuntary loss of urine during coughing usually accompanied by hypermobility of the urethra and descent of the anterior vaginal wall.

- Urge incontinence is the problem of sudden detrusor contraction with uncontrolled loss of urine. The condition may be due to idiopathic detrusor instability or associated with urinary infection, obstructive uropathy, diabetes or neurological disease. It is particularly important to exclude urinary tract infection.

- Mixed urge and stress incontinence occurs in a substantial number of women. Women with urge incontinence also have true stress incontinence, and it is particularly important to treat the detrusor instability prior to correcting stress incontinence. Failure to do so may lead to a worsening of the condition.

- Overflow incontinence occurs when the bladder becomes dilated or flaccid with minimal or no tone/function. It is not uncommon after vaginal delivery or when the bladder is 'neglected' after a spinal anaesthetic. A bladder scan usually reveals the presence of a residual of more than half the bladder capacity. The bladder then becomes 'lazy' and empties when it becomes full.

- Miscellaneous types of incontinence include infections, medications, prolonged immobilization and cognitive impairment and in certain situations may precipitate incontinence.

2. 尿频（Urinary frequency）

尿频是一种无法抑制的排尿欲望，一天排尿超过 7 次或一晚超过 1 次。年龄在 30—64 岁的女性中有 20% 的人患有此病，可由妊娠、糖尿病、盆腔包块、肾衰竭、使用利尿药、过量液体摄入或习惯引起，但最常见的原因是尿路感染。尿频可发生在日间（白天）或夜间。

Urinary frequency is an insuppressible desire to void more than seven times a day or more than once a night. It affects 20% of women aged between 30 and 64 years and can be caused by pregnancy, diabetes, pelvic masses, renal failure, diuretics, excess fluid intake or habit, although the most common cause is urinary tract infection. The frequency may be diurnal (daytime) or nocturnal.

膀胱收缩性增强在没有感染时也可发生，膀胱容量减少也可导致尿频。

However, enhanced bladder contractility may occur without the presence of infection. Reduced bladder capacity may also result in frequency of micturition.

3. 排尿困难（Dysuria）

这种症状是由感染引起的。在排尿时局部尿道感染或外伤引起灼烧或烫伤感，但膀胱感染更容易在排尿完成后引起耻骨上疼痛。建议所有主诉排尿时灼热的女性都要进行阴道检查，因为尿道炎与阴道炎和阴道感染有关。

This symptom results from infection. Local urethral infection or trauma causes burning or scalding during micturition, but bladder infection is more likely to cause pain suprapubically after micturition has been completed. It is always advisable to perform a vaginal examination on any woman who complains of scalding on micturition because urethritis is associated with vaginitis and vaginal infection.

4. 尿潴留（Urinary retention）

急性尿潴留对女性来说是少见的问题，但是在下列情况时可发生。

- 阴道分娩和会阴侧切术后。

- 手术分娩。

- 阴道修复手术后，特别是涉及阴道后壁和会阴的手术。

- 绝经期：自发性梗阻性尿潴留更有可能发生于绝经期女性。

- 妊娠期：在妊娠早期的尾声，子宫后倾可能会在盆腔压迫膀胱。

- 当外阴有炎性病变时。

- 未经治疗的膀胱过度膨胀（如分娩后），神经病变或恶性肿瘤。

Acute urinary retention is less of a problem in women. However, it can be seen:

- after vaginal delivery and episiotomy
- following operative delivery
- after vaginal repair procedures, particularly those operations that involve the posterior vaginal wall and perineum
- in menopause-spontaneous obstructive uropathy is more likely to occur in menopausal women
- in pregnancy-a retroverted uterus may become impacted in the pelvis towards the end of the first trimester
- when inflammatory lesions of the vulva are present
- as a result of untreated over-distension of the bladder
- (such as following delivery), neuropathy or malignancy.

5. 夜间遗尿或尿床（Nocturnal enuresis or bed-wetting）

这是发生在睡眠中的尿失禁，可能自儿童时期有心理基础。

This is urinary incontinence occurring during sleep and may have a psychological basis to it from childhood.

（三）诊断（Diagnosis）

诊断最初是由病史来提示的。持续地漏尿表明

有瘘，但并非所有的瘘都持续漏尿。瘘管交通常发生于膀胱与阴道之间（膀胱阴道瘘）、输尿管与阴道之间（输尿管阴道瘘）。瘘管形成存在以下原因。

- 与难产有关的产科创伤。

- 手术创伤。

- 恶性疾病。

- 放疗。

The diagnosis is initially indicated by the history. Continuous loss of urine indicates a fistula, but not all fistulas leak urine continuously. The fistulous communication usually occurs between the bladder and vagina, *vesicovaginal fistula*, and the ureter and vagina, *ureterovaginal fistula*. Fistula formation results from:

- obstetric trauma associated with obstructed labour
- surgical trauma
- malignant disease
- radiotherapy.

还有其他类型存在于肠道和尿道之间、肠道和阴道之间的瘘管，但这些不常见。

There are other types of fistula with communications between bowel and urinary tract and between bowel and vagina, but these are less common.

直肠阴道瘘有类似的发病机制，附加因素为三度裂伤后的会阴破裂。

Rectovaginal fistulas have a similar pathogenesis, with the additional factor of perineal breakdown after a third-degree tear.

尿瘘定位依据以下检查。

- 膀胱镜检查。

- 静脉尿路造影。

- 经尿管膀胱灌注亚甲蓝，阴道出现染色提示存在膀胱阴道瘘。

Urinary fistulas are localized by:

- cystoscopy
- intravenous urogram
- instillation of methylene blue via a catheter into the bladder; the appearance of dye in the vagina indicates a vesicovaginal fistula.

压力性尿失禁和急迫性尿失禁的鉴别诊断比较困难，且往往不能令人满意。如果要进行正确的手术或避免手术，充分的术前评估是很重要的。用有

效的患者问卷（改良的 Bristol 女性下尿路症状问卷就是一个很好的例子）、3 天的排尿日记和尿垫试验来评估患者是很重要的。这些有助于临床医生深入了解尿失禁症状如何影响患者的日常基础生活。膀胱和尿道在实验室通过尿动力学进行评估。这个过程通常包括三个基本步骤。

The differential diagnosis between stress and urge incontinence is more difficult and is often unsatisfactory. Adequate preoperative assessment is important if the correct operation is to be employed or if surgery is to be avoided. It is important to assess patients with a validated patient questionnaire (the Modified Bristol Female Lower Urinary Tract Symptoms Questionnaire is a good example) with a 3-day urinary diary and a pad test. These help the clinician gain an insight into how the symptoms of urinary incontinence affect the patient on a day-to-day basis. The bladder and urethra are assessed in the laboratory by urodynamics. This procedure usually involves three basic steps:

1. 尿流率测定

要求患者将尿液排入专门设计的马桶，以测量排尿量、最大和平均尿流速率。流量＞15ml/s 被认为是可以接受的，正常的膀胱可以完全排空。流速＜15ml/s，提示排尿功能障碍，在女性通常提示"功能性梗阻"，而非解剖性梗阻。有时，强大的逼尿肌可能导致膀胱收缩来对抗关闭的内尿道，进而引起排尿功能障碍，这种情况称为逼尿肌 - 括约肌协同障碍。

1. Uroflowmetry: The patient is asked to pass urine into a specially designed toilet that measures voided volume, maximal and average urinary flow rates. Flow rates of >15 mL/sec are considered acceptable, and it is expected that a normal bladder will completely empty itself. Flow rates of <15 mL/sec are indicative of voiding dysfunction and in the female often indicate a 'functional obstruction' rather than an anatomical one. Occasionally a powerful detrusor may cause the bladder to contract against a closed internal urethral meatus resulting in dysfunctional voiding, a condition termed *detrusor-sphincter dyssynergia*

2. 膀胱内压测量图（图 21-13）

压力可通过膀胱内和阴道内测量，或者直肠内测量（较少），因为阴道内压力代表腹内压力，减去膀胱内压力即可测量逼尿肌压力。第一次排空时，膀胱内的液体容量通常约为 150ml。正常的膀胱容量达 400ml 时，出现强烈的排尿欲。低容量、高逼尿肌压力反映了慢性感染相关的膀胱异常敏感。充盈过程中不应出现逼尿肌收缩，在这种情况下出现的

任何收缩都表明逼尿肌不稳定。逼尿肌不活跃表现为膀胱完全充盈时无收缩，提示神经控制异常。膀胱平均容量为 250～550ml，但容量是评价膀胱功能的较差指标。因此，膀胱内压测量是评估逼尿肌功能或逼尿肌不稳定的有效方法，后者会导致急迫性尿失禁。在尿道功能不全的情况下会出现静息时尿道压力低，尿道压力无自发升高不能中止尿流，以及向尿道腹部段传递的压力减少，测量频率 / 容积时容积大。因为可能会有压力性尿失禁和急迫性尿失禁的混合存在，这两种尿失禁之间并没有明确的界限。然而，区分膀胱颈部无力、压力性尿失禁、逼尿肌不稳定和急迫性尿失禁的主要影响是很重要的。

2. The cystometrogram (Fig. 21.13): Pressure is measured intravesically and intravaginally or, less commonly, intrarectally because intravaginal pressure represents intra-abdominal pressure and is subtracted from the intravesical pressure to give a measure of detrusor pressure. The volume of fluid in the bladder at which the first desire to void occurs is usually about 150 mL. A strong desire to void occurs at 400 mL in the normal bladder. High detrusor pressure at a lower volume reflects an abnormally sensitive bladder associated with chronic infection. There should be no detrusor contraction during filling, and any contraction that occurs under these circumstances indicates *detrusor instability*. An underactive detrusor shows no contraction on complete filling and indicates an abnormality of neurological control. The average bladder has a capacity of 250–550 mL, but capacity is a poor index of bladder function. Thus, cystometry is a useful method for assessing detrusor muscle function or detrusor instability, which may result in urge incontinence.In the presence of urethral incompetence, there is low resting urethral pressure, no voluntary increase in urethral pressure, inability to stop midstream, decreased pressure transmission to the abdominal urethra and large volumes in the frequency/volume measurements. There is not always a clear-cut demarcation between the two conditions, as there may be a mixture of both stress and urge incontinence. Nevertheless, it is important to differentiate between the predominant influence of bladder neck weakness and stress incontinence and detrusor instability and urge incontinence.

3. 尿道压力图

这是在膀胱测压的最后阶段进行的，测量的是中尿道的压力，特别是最大尿道闭合压力（MUCP）。这对于预测治疗尿失禁手术后的成功率是有价值的。压力小于 20 厘米水柱预示着不良的结果。在一些机构，膀胱内镜检查和盆底超声扫描是评价女性尿失禁的额外流程。

3. Urethral pressure profile: This is performed at the very end of the cystometry and measures the pressure within

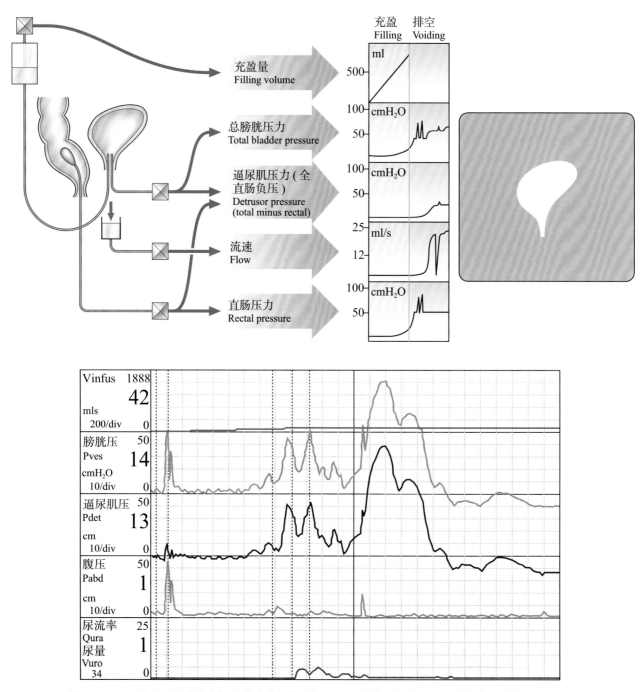

▲ 图 21-13　A. 检查下尿道综合征的膀胱动力学研究；B. 一位特发性逼尿肌不稳定患者的膀胱内压测量图
Fig. 21.13 (A) Bladder flow studies in the investigation of lower urinary tract symptoms. (B) Cystometrogram from a patient with idiopathic detrusor instability.

the mid-urethra, in particular, the maximum urethral closure pressure (MUCP). This is of value in predicting the likelihood of surgical success after an anti-incontinence procedure. Pressures <20 cm of H_2O are predictive of poorer outcomes.In some units an endoscopic view of the bladder called cystoscopy and an ultrasound scan of the pelvic floor are the additional procedures performed in the evaluation of the incontinent woman.

（四）处理（Management）

1. 尿道瘘（Urinary tract fistula）

在发达国家，大多数尿道瘘是由手术创伤造成的。最常见是膀胱阴道瘘或输尿管阴道瘘，是由子宫切除术时的手术创伤造成的，有时是在剖宫产术后。

In the developed world, most urinary tract fistulas result from surgical trauma. The commonest fistulas are vesicovaginal or ureterovaginal and result from surgical trauma at the time of hysterectomy, or sometimes following caesarean section.

膀胱阴道瘘通常会在术后第一周表现出来。如果瘘管很小，可能自行闭合。

A vesicovaginal fistula will usually become apparent in the first postoperative week. If the fistula is small, closure may be achieved spontaneously.

应给患者留置尿管并持续引流。如果 2～3 个月后瘘口仍未闭合，则瘘口不太可能自主闭合，建议手术闭合。做进一步手术的时机仍然是一个有争议的问题。直到不久前仍建议延迟 6 个月，但越来越多的证据表明，早期手术干预可以获得良好的结果，不过前提是瘘管部位无感染。

The patient should be treated by catheterization and continuous drainage. If closure has not occurred after 2–3 months, the fistula is unlikely to close spontaneously, and surgical closure is recommended. The timing of further surgery is still a subject of controversy. Until recently, a delay of 6 months was recommended, but there is increasing evidence that good results can be obtained with early surgical intervention. However, the fistulous site should be free of infection.

手术闭合可以通过经阴道精细地分离瘘管边缘、分层关闭膀胱和阴道来实现。术后护理包括持续留置尿管引流 1 周，以及抗生素全覆盖。腹部入路可用于瘘管修补，一些优势在于有大瘘管的情况下，可以插入大网膜填补。

Surgical closure may be achieved vaginally by meticulous separation of the edges of the fistula and closure in layers of the bladder and vagina. Postoperative care includes continuous catheter drainage for 1 week and antibiotic cover. An abdominal approach to the fistula can also be used and has some advantages, allowing the interposition of omentum in cases where there is a large fistula.

输尿管阴道瘘的治疗方法通常是将受损的输尿管重新植入膀胱。

Ureterovaginal fistulas are usually treated by reimplantation of the damaged ureter into the bladder.

2. 压力性尿失禁（Stress incontinence）

压力性尿失禁应首先通过盆底物理治疗来处理。保守治疗无效时，应行手术治疗。在阴道前壁脱垂时行阴道前壁修补加膀胱颈处进行支撑缝合，具有简单的优点。它肯定会缓解脱垂，但就压力性尿失禁而言结果是多样的，有 40%～50% 的病例得到缓解。在没有脱垂的情况下，手术是没有价值的。

Stress incontinence should be managed initially by pelvic floor physiotherapy. Surgical treatment is indicated where there is a failure to respond to conservative management. In the presence of anterior vaginal wall prolapse, *anterior repair*, with the placement of buttressing sutures at the bladder neck, has the virtue of simplicity. It will certainly relieve the prolapse, but the results are variable as far as the stress incontinence is concerned, with relief in about 40–50% of cases. It is of no value in the absence of evidence of prolapse.

以下是常用的手术方法。

- 中尿道悬吊（图 21-14）

    - 耻骨后悬吊：可以通过放置无张力阴道条索实现中尿道支持。聚丙烯带通过尿道下阴道切口插入，由针引导，经膀胱周围从耻骨联合后方穿出。这可以在局部麻醉、区域麻醉或全身麻醉的情况下进行，条索以无张力的方式放置在尿道中部。术中进行膀胱尿道镜检查以排除对膀胱和尿道的损伤。由于该手术的微创性，大多数女性能够在 1～2 周内恢复正常活动。手术的长期成功率在 80% 左右。

    - 经闭孔悬吊术：相比与耻骨后悬吊术，将针穿过闭孔创伤较小。

The following procedures are commonly used:
- Mid-urethral slings (Fig. 21.14):
    - Retropubic sling: Mid-urethral support can be achieved by placement of a tension-free vaginal tape. A polypropylene tape is inserted through a sub-urethral vaginal incision and guided via a needle paravesically to exit behind the symphysis pubis. This can be carried out under local, regional or general anaesthetic, and the tape is placed mid-urethrally in a tension-free manner. A cystourethroscopy is performed intraoperatively to rule out damage to the bladder and urethra. As this procedure is minimally invasive, most women are able to return to normal activity within 1–2 weeks. The long-term success rates are around 80%.
    - Trans-obturator sling: Less invasive compared to retropubic sling, performed by passing needles through the obturator foramina.

- 仍在流行的其他各式手术

    - 腹腔镜 Burch 阴道悬吊术：通过在腹腔镜

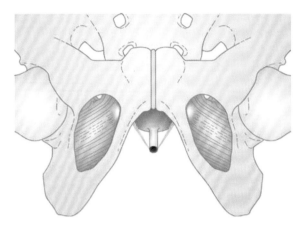

▲ 图 21-14　中尿道悬吊治疗压力性尿失禁

Fig. 21.14　Mid-urethral sling used in the treatment of stress incontinence.

下缝合阴道上侧壁与髂耻骨韧带，以抬高膀胱颈部。成功率约为 60%，该手术会导致绝大多数患者出现排尿功能障碍。由于更流行和更安全的中尿道悬吊，这种手术变得或多或少更加无效，但现在由于对网片的担忧，该手术重新流行起来。

- 经尿道注射：通过膀胱镜将可注射的膨胀剂注射到中尿道。步骤简单，围术期并发症很少，成功率为 40%～60%。这些都是对中尿道悬吊的有用的辅助，特别是对复发和多次手术失败的女性。最常用的试剂是胶原蛋白（戊二醛交联牛胶原蛋白）、硅（大的硅颗粒）、硬晶石（热解碳被覆珠）、丁香酰胺等。

- Miscellaneous procedures still in vogue:
  - Laparoscopic Burch colposuspension involves bladder neck elevation by suturing the upper lateral vaginal walls to the iliopectineal ligaments under laparoscopic control. The success rates are around 60%, and the procedure results in voiding dysfunction in a significant majority of patients. This procedure was more or less invalidated by the more popular and safer mid-urethral slings but now is resurging due to the concerns around mesh.
  - Transurethral injections: Injectable bulking agents can be injected via a cystoscope into the mid-urethra. These are simple procedures with very little perioperative morbidity and have success rates of about 40–60%. These are useful adjuncts to the mid-urethral slings, especially in recurrences and in women with multiple failed operations. The commonest agents employed are collagen

(glutaraldehyde cross-linked bovine collagen), silicon (macroparticulate silicon particles), Durasphere (pyrolytic carbon-coated beads), Bulkamid, etc.

（五）不稳定膀胱：膀胱过度活跃综合征（OAB）[The unstable bladder: overactive bladder syndrome (OAB)]

膀胱不稳定的特点是尿频、夜尿、尿急和急迫性失禁。当面临这一病史重要的是获得一些有关摄入液体量和出量频率的一些指标，因此患者需要记录一张图表来阐明这一方面。

The features of the unstable bladder are those of frequency of micturition and nocturia, urgency and urge incontinence. When confronted with this history, it is important to obtain some indication of the frequency as related to fluid intake and output. A chart should therefore be kept by the patient to clarify this aspect.

易感因素的评估包括尿培养、尿流速率和尿动力学研究。

The assessment of predisposing factors includes urine culture, urinary flow rates and urodynamic studies.

治疗显然要针对病因，因此存在泌尿道感染就需要适当的抗生素治疗。绝经后女性阴道上皮菱缩和尿急、尿频的症状往往对低剂量雌激素替代治疗有反应。

Treatment will obviously be directed at the cause, so the presence of urinary tract infection necessitates the administration of the appropriate antibiotic therapy. Postmenopausal women with atrophic vaginal epithelium and symptoms of urgency and frequency often respond to replacement therapy with low-dose oestrogens.

1. 病因不明的逼尿肌不稳定（Detrusor instability of unknown aetiology）

如果问题出现在大脑层面，就需要采取心理治疗措施。膀胱训练是按一定的记录模式逐渐增加排尿间隔的方法。短期有效，但复发率高。

If the problem arises at a cerebral level, psychotherapeutic measures are indicated. Bladder drill involves a regimen of gradually increasing the voiding interval on a recorded pattern. This is effective in the short term, but the relapse rate is high.

逼尿肌不稳定安慰剂治疗的反应率超过 40%，并出现自发缓解。

The placebo response rate in detrusor instability is more than 40%, and spontaneous remissions occur.

2. 药物治疗（Drug treatment）

另一种方法是使用作用于膀胱壁水平的抗胆碱能药物。它们作用于膀胱壁上的毒蕈碱受体，引起弛缓。其中一些药物更具有特异性，作用于M_3受体。药物的特异性越强，出现不良反应的情况的可能性就越小。表 21-3 所列药物是按特异性和更小的不良反应的顺序递增排列。

The alternative approach is to use anticholinergic drugs that act at the level of the bladder wall. These act on the muscarinic receptors on the bladder wall and cause relaxation. Some of these drugs are more specific and act on M_3 receptors. The more specific the drug, the less likely it is to cause side effects. The drugs listed in Table 21.3 are in increasing order of specificity and better side effect profile.

A 型肉毒杆菌毒素（Botox）：这种药物现在被有效地用于治疗 OAB 和神经源性膀胱。肉毒杆菌可

表 21-3　膀胱过度活跃的药物治疗

Table 21.3　Drug therapy of overactive bladder

药物名称 Drug name	药物类型 Drug type	用量 Dosage	可获得的规格 Available doses	不良反应 Side effects
奥昔布宁 Oxybutynin	抗毒蕈碱类 Antimuscarinic	2.5～5mg，口服，一日3 次 2.5–5 mg PO tid	5mg 片剂 5-mg tablet, 5mg/ml 糖浆 5-mg/mL syrup	口干，便秘，眩晕，心悸，厌食，恶心，弱视 Dry mouth, constipation, dizziness, palpitations, anorexia, nausea, amblyopia
奥昔布宁（贴皮剂） Oxybutynin (transdermal)	同上 See earlier	3.9mg/d，每2 周更换 3.9 mg/d; patch changed twice weekly	36mg 每贴 36-mg patch	
托特罗定（短效） Tolterodine (short-acting)	选择性抗毒蕈碱 M_3 受体类 M_3-selective antimuscarinic	1～2mg 口服，一日2 次 1–2 mg PO bid	1mg、2mg 片剂 1-, 2-mg tablet	
托特罗定（长效） Tolterodine (long-acting)	同上 See earlier	2～4mg 每日顿服 2–4 mg PO once daily	2mg、4mg 胶囊 2-, 4-mg capsule	
曲司氯胺 Trospium chloride	抗毒蕈碱季胺基类 Antimuscarinic quaternary amine	20mg，口服，一日2 次 20 mg PO bid	20mg 片剂 20-mg tablet	
达非那新 Darifenacin	选择性抗毒蕈碱 M_3 受体类 M_3-selective antimuscarinic	7.5～15 mg，口服，一日1 次 7.5–15 mg PO daily	7.5mg、15mg 片剂 7.5-, 15-mg tablet	
索利那新 Solifenacin	选择性抗毒蕈碱 M_3 受体类，口服 5～10mg/d M_3-selective antimuscarinic 5–10 mg PO once daily	5～10mg 每日顿服 5–10 mg PO once daily	5mg、15mg 片剂 5-, 10-mg tablets	
盐酸咪丙嗪 Imipramine hydrochloride	三环抗抑郁药、抗胆碱能药、肾上腺素类、抗组胺药 Tricyclic antidepressant, anticholinergic, adrenergic, antihistamine	10～25mg，口服，一日2～3 次 10–25 mg PO bid–tid	10mg、25mg、50mg 片剂 10-, 25-, 50-mg tablets	
米拉贝隆 Mirabegron	β_3 受体激动药 B_3 agonist	25～50mg，每日顿服 25–50 mg once daily	25mg、50mg 缓释片剂 25-, 50-mg tablet extended release	心悸，头痛 Palpitations, headache

以在局部麻醉、镇静或全身麻醉的情况下注射。每个开展这些治疗的机构都需要确保有一个严格的试验无效方案（TOV）和备用计划，以防出现排尿功能障碍。

Botulinum toxin A (Botox): This drug is now being used effectively to manage OAB and neurogenic bladder. Botox can be injected under local, sedation or general anaesthesia. Each unit performing these needs to ensure they have a strict trial of void (TOV) protocol and back-up plan in case of voiding dysfunction.

3. 盆底理疗：盆底肌肉训练（Pelvic floor physiotherapy: pelvic floormuscle training）

对于有轻到中度尿失禁症状的女性，盆底肌肉训练（PFMT）即使不能治愈，也可以改善症状。PFMT，也被称为凯格尔运动，需要提肛肌的自主收缩。这些需要每天重复几次最多 50 或 60 次，以达到一些临床受益。

In women who have mild to moderate symptoms of urinary incontinence, pelvic floor muscle training (PFMT) may allow improvement, if not cure. Also known as *Kegel exercises*, PFMT entails voluntary contraction of the levator ani muscles. These need to be repeated several times a day up to 50 or 60 times to be of any clinical benefit.

盆底肌训练具体细节是有些多变的，取决于临床医生个体化和临床环境。大多数患者发现单独训练提肛肌具有挑战性的，通常会代之以收缩腹肌；因此，这些练习必须由对盆底康复特别感兴趣的理疗师来示范说明。为了增强这些练习的效果，在做凯格尔运动时，可以在阴道内放置加重的阴道锥或闭孔器，这些器械为骨盆底肌肉的运动提供了阻力。

The specifics are a bit variable, being very clinician specific and dependent on the clinical setting. Most patients find isolating the levator ani muscles most challenging and often contract their abdominal muscles instead. Therefore it is imperative that these exercises be demonstrated by a physiotherapist with a special interest in pelvic floor rehabilitation. To augment efficacy of these exercises, weighted vaginal cones or obturators may be placed into the vagina during Kegel exercises. These provide resistance against which pelvic floor muscles can work.

4. 电刺激（干预疗法）[Electrical stimulation (interferential therapy)]

作为主动骨盆底收缩的替代或辅助手段，可用阴道探头对提肛肌进行低频电刺激。虽然机制尚不清楚，电刺激可用于改善压力性尿失禁（SUI）或急迫性尿失禁。对于急迫性尿失禁，传统上使用低频，而较高的频率用于 SUI。

As an alternative/adjunct to active pelvic floor contraction, a vaginal probe may be used to deliver low-frequency electrical stimulation to the levator ani muscles. Although the mechanism is unclear, electrical stimulation may be used to improve either stress urinary incontinence (SUI) or urge incontinence. With urge incontinence, traditionally a low frequency is applied, whereas higher frequencies are used for SUI.

5. 生物反馈疗法（Biofeedback therapy）

许多行为治疗技巧通常被认为是生物反馈疗法，可测量生理信号，如肌张力，然后实时显示给患者。一般来说，在这些疗程期间，视觉、听觉和（或）口头反馈线索都被传送至患者。这些线索为患者提供即时的表现评估。具体来说，在 PFMT 的生物反馈过程中的典型应用就是通常使用无菌阴道探头来测量提肛肌收缩期间阴道内的压力变化。读数反映的是对肌肉收缩力的估计。治疗疗程是个体化的，由潜在的功能障碍决定，并根据对治疗的反应进行修改。在许多情况下，在随后的不同时间间隔进行强化训练也显示是有益的。

Many behavioural techniques, often considered together as *biofeedback therapy*, measure physiological signals such as muscle tension and then display them to a patient in real time. In general, visual, auditory and/or verbal feedback cues are directed to the patient during these therapy sessions. These cues provide immediate performance evaluation to a patient. Specifically, during biofeedback for PFMT, a sterile vaginal probe that measures pressure changes within the vagina during levator ani muscle contraction is typically used. Readings reflect an estimate of muscle contraction strength. Treatment sessions are individualized, dictated by the underlying dysfunction and modified based on response to therapy. In many cases, reinforcing sessions at various subsequent intervals may also prove advantageous.

6. 改变饮食习惯（Dietary modifications）

鼓励患者避免饮用碳酸饮料和咖啡因，并开始服用蔓越莓片，因为这些通常有助于减轻尿急和尿频的症状。

Patients are encouraged to avoid carbonated drinks and caffeine and commence cranberry tablets because these often help with reducing symptoms of urgency and frequency.

7. 定时排尿（Timed voiding）

鼓励患者"按时间"排尿，以减少 OAB 患者经常的出现紧急症状。随着时间的推移，膀胱能够承受不断增加的容积，而不会导致漏尿。

Patients are encouraged to void 'by the clock' in an attempt to limit the waves of urgency that patients with OAB symptoms often experience. Over time the bladder is able to hold successively increasing volumes without resulting in leakage.

8. 阴道用雌激素（Vaginal oestrogen）

雌激素可以增加尿道血流量，增加肾上腺素 α 受体的敏感性，从而增加尿道适应力和尿道闭合压力。理论上，雌激素可能会增加胶原沉积，增加尿道周围毛细血管丛的血管密度。据说这些是为了改善尿道适应性。因此，对于阴道萎缩伴尿失禁的女性，使用外源性雌激素是合理的。

Oestrogen has been shown to increase urethral blood flow and increase alpha-adrenergic receptor sensitivity, thereby increasing urethral coaptation and urethral closure pressure. In theory, oestrogen may increase collagen deposition and increase vascularity of the periurethral capillary plexus. These are purported to improve urethral coaptation. Thus, for incontinent women who are atrophic, administration of exogenous oestrogen is reasonable.

（六）膀胱出口梗阻（Bladder outlet obstruction）

女性原发性膀胱颈梗阻可能是由于排尿时膀胱颈未能打开所致，可采用 α 肾上腺素受体拮抗药（如坦索罗辛）、尿道扩张术或尿道切开术等治疗。继发性出口梗阻通常与先前的尿失禁手术有关，可能对尿道扩张术有反应，但效果不是特别好。

Primary bladder neck obstruction in the female probably results from the failure of the vesical neck to open during voiding and can be treated either with α-adrenergic blocking agents like tamsulosin, urethral dilatation or urethrotomy. Secondary outlet obstruction is usually associated with previous surgery for incontinence and may respond to urethral dilatation, but the results are not particularly good.

（七）神经源性膀胱（The neuropathic bladder）

膀胱功能丧失可能与影响中枢神经系统的各种情况有关。这些情况也可能与肠功能改变、性功能障碍和下肢功能丧失有关。

Loss of bladder function may be associated with a variety of conditions that affect the central nervous system. These conditions may also be associated with alteration in bowel function, sexual dysfunction and loss of function of the lower limbs.

1. 表现（Presentation）

神经源性膀胱是逼尿肌和膀胱括约肌活动失调的反映。这导致了各种各样的障碍，从通过在高或低压力下潴留与溢出的"自动膀胱"到完全的压力性尿失禁。它也可能与肾衰竭有关。

The neuropathic bladder is a reflection of dyssynergy between the activity of the detrusor muscle and the bladder sphincter. This results in a variety of disorders ranging from the 'automatic bladder' through retention with overflow at high or low pressure to total stress incontinence. It may also be associated with renal failure.

2. 病因（Aetiology）

原因可能在脑桥上部，如脑血管意外、帕金森病或脑瘤。脑桥下症的病因包括脊髓损伤或压迫、多发性硬化和脊柱裂。影响膀胱功能的周围性自主神经病变可能是先天性的或糖尿病引起，偶尔继发于手术损伤。

The causation may be suprapontine, such as a cerebrovascular accident, Parkinson's disease or a cerebral tumour. Infrapontine causes include cord injuries or compression, multiple sclerosis and spina bifida. Peripheral autonomic neuropathies that affect bladder function may be idiopathic or diabetic and, occasionally, secondary to surgical injury.

3. 诊断（Diagnosis）

诊断是建立在包括膀胱内压测量、尿流率研究、神经系统筛查、脑部扫描、肾盂造影和肾脏同位素扫描等系统性检查来确定的。

The diagnosis is established by a systematic search for the cause involving cystometry, urinary flow rate studies, neurological screening, brain scan, pyelography and renal isotope scans.

4. 处理（Management）

治疗显然取决于确定病因，但从症状上看，治疗也包括非手术治疗，即使用吸收尿垫和清洁间歇性自我导尿。抗胆碱能药物也在一些患者中占有一席之地。手术治疗包括使用人工括约肌和骶神经刺激法。姑息疗法可以用耻骨上膀胱造瘘插管。

The management clearly depends on establishing the cause, but symptomatically it also involves non-surgical management using absorptive pads and clean intermittent self-catheterization. Anticholinergic drugs also have a place for some patients. Surgical treatment includes the use of artificial sphincters and sacral nerve stimulators. Palliative therapy can be in terms of suprapubic catheters.

（八）膀胱疼痛综合征（Painful bladder syndrome）

无明确病因的慢性膀胱疼痛称为间质性膀胱炎（interstitial cystitis，IC）。膀胱疼痛综合征与 IC 可互换使用。其发病机制尚不清楚，治疗的目的主要是缓解症状。它通常在 40 多岁时被诊断出来，但是注意到较年轻的人群中也出现症状。

Chronic bladder pain in the absence of a known aetiology was known as interstitial cystitis (IC). Painful bladder syndrome and IC can be used interchangeably. The pathogenesis is poorly understood, and the aim of treatment is mainly towards symptom relief. It is usually diagnosed in the fourth decade of life, but symptoms in younger populations have been noted.

诊断是根据病史的特定症状，并排除其他原因的疼痛。

Diagnosis is made on the basis of history of specific symptoms and excluding other causes for the pain.

处理（Management）

可考虑采用保守的药物治疗和（或）膀胱注射或灌注的系统性治疗。自我管理和行为修正扮演着重要的角色。避免某些会加剧症状的运动、食物和饮料会有所帮助。口服、经皮和膀胱灌注镇痛药也可以使用。

A systematic approach with conservative medical therapies and/or bladder injections or instillations is considered. Self-management and behaviour modification play an important role. Avoiding certain activities, foods and beverages that exacerbate symptoms can help. Analgesics in the form of oral, transdermal and bladder instillations can be done as well.

已经发现阿米替林、聚硫戊聚糖钠和抗组胺药有一定的效果。三线治疗包括膀胱扩张和黏膜下注射类固醇和局部麻醉。进一步的骶神经调节剂和环孢素的治疗正在研究中。

Amitriptyline, pentosan polysulphate sodium and antihistamines have been found to have a modest effect. Third-line therapy involves bladder distension and submucosal injection with steroids and local anaesthetic. Further management with sacral neuromodulation and cyclosporine is being studied.

本章概览	Essential information
脱垂 • 可包括阴道前壁或后壁脱垂伴随不同程度的子宫下降。 • 诱发因素包括多产、长期增高腹部压力和激素变化。 • 症状取决于脱垂的程度，以及是否包括肠或膀胱颈的脱垂。 • 产后 6 个月内可能自然改善。 • 治疗的选择是手术修复 ± 子宫切除术。 • 无症状的轻度脱垂不需要治疗。	**Prolapse** • May involve anterior or posterior vaginal wall with varying degrees of uterine descent • Predisposing factors include high parity, chronically raised intra-abdominal pressure and hormonal changes • Symptoms depend on degree of prolapse and whether bowel or bladder neck involved • May undergo spontaneous improvement up to 6 months postpartum • Treatment of choice is surgical repair ± hysterectomy • No treatment required for asymptomatic minor degrees of prolapse
压力性尿失禁 • 无意识性尿失禁导致的社会或卫生问题，在客观上是显而易见的。 • 常与盆腔前部脱垂相关。 • 达 30% 病例与逼尿肌不稳定相关。	**Stress incontinence** • Involuntary loss of urine causing social or hygienic problems and objectively demonstrable • Commonly associated with prolapse of the anterior compartment • Associated with detrusor instability in up to 30% of cases
逼尿肌不稳定 • 表现为尿频、尿急、夜尿和尿失禁。 • 通常为特发性，但需要与梗阻性尿路病、糖尿病、神经系统疾病和感染区分。 • 可能表现为压力性尿失禁。 • 治疗包括膀胱造瘘、抗胆碱能药物和抗感染治疗。	**Detrusor instability** • Presents as frequency, urgency, nocturia and incontinence • Usually idiopathic but needs to be distinguished from obstructive uropathy, diabetes, neurological disorders and infection • May present as stress incontinence • Management includes bladder drill, anticholinergics and treatment of infection

附录部分

附录 A　围术期管理原则
Principles of perioperative care

Stergios K. Doumouchtsis　**著**　　杨慧霞　**译**　　石玉华　**校**

<table>
<tr><td>

学习目标

学习本附录后你应当能够:

知识标准
- 列举感染控制原则。
- 描述血液和血液制品的合理使用方法。
- 讨论术后管理中的一般病理学原理。
- 描述伤口愈合和水电解质平衡的原理。
- 了解手术室中手术安全的各个方面。
- 描述术后加速恢复的原则。

临床技能
- 设计普通妇科手术患者的围术期管理方案。
- 认识正常的术后过程。
- 解释相关的术后检查。
- 识别常见术后并发症的症状和体征。
- 制订常见或严重的术后并发症的管理计划。

</td><td>

LEARNING OUTCOMES

After studying this appendix you should be able to:

Knowledge criteria
- List the principles of infection control.
- Describe the appropriate use of blood and blood products.
- Discuss the general pathological principles of postoperative care.
- Describe the principles of fluid-electrolyte balance and wound healing.
- Understand aspects of surgical safety in the operating theatre.
- Describe principles of enhanced recovery.

Clinical competencies
- Plan perioperative care for a patient undergoing the common gynaecological procedures.
- Recognize the normal postoperative course.
- Interpret relevant postoperative investigations.
- Recognize symptoms and signs of common postoperative complications.
- Initiate a management plan for common/serious postoperative complications.

</td></tr>
</table>

一、术前管理（Preoperative care）

（一）患者咨询和知情同意（另请参阅附录 C）[Patient counselling and consent (see also Appendix C)]

为患者选择适合的手术方案时，首先应对患者进行详细的咨询，签署知情同意书。应告知患者建议的手术术式及其风险和益处，相关不良事件，必要时会采取的其他手术操作，住院时间，麻醉相关事项，术后恢复情况，手术标本的存放、组织学检查和处置，使用多媒体记录，相关教学工作，以及其他可供选择的治疗方案，其中包括期待治疗。如果有患者明确表示不希望进行的手术操作，需要记录在案。

Selecting the appropriate procedure for the appropriate patient should include detailed counselling and informed consent. The patient should be informed about the proposed procedure and its risks and benefits, adverse events and other procedures that may become necessary; length of hospital stay; anaesthesia; recovery; tissue examination, storage and disposal; use of multimedia in records; teaching; and alternative therapies available, including no treatment. If there are any procedures that the patient would specifically not wish to be performed, this needs to be documented.

理想情况下，应根据各项危险因素计算不良事件发生率，并用频率或百分比的形式呈现给患者。应当由能够完成该手术或有该手术经验的医师提供知情同意的咨询，由手术医师或其上级医师进行确认。

Risks should ideally be presented as a frequency or percentage and estimated according to individual risk factors. Consent should be obtained by someone who is capable of performing the procedure or has experience of the procedure and confirmed by the operating or supervising surgeon.

（二）术前评估（Preoperative assessment）

1. 临床病史（Clinical history）

临床病史应包括内外科病史、药物治疗史和过敏史，以及拟手术治疗的疾病相关信息；合并症和并发症的危险因素；血栓栓塞的个人史、家族史或危险因素；麻醉并发症的个人史或家族史。

Clinical history should include medical and surgical history, medications and allergies, as well as information related to the medical condition for which the procedure is planned; co-morbidities and factors related to risks of complications; personal or family history or risk factors for thromboembolism; and personal or family history of anaesthetic complications.

术前评估还应包括以下方面：患者是否有胸痛或呼吸困难、心绞痛或心脏病史、脑卒中、癫痫、颈部或下颌问题、肝肾或甲状腺疾病、哮喘、糖尿病、支气管炎和其他呼吸道疾病等。

The preoperative medical assessment should also include questions on chest pain or breathlessness, history of angina or heart attack, stroke, epilepsy, neck or jaw problems, kidney liver or thyroid disease, asthma, diabetes, bronchitis and other respiratory conditions.

2. 临床检查（Clinical examination）

对疾病和危险因素进行术前评估后，行临床检查，其中包括心血管和呼吸方面的检查，以评估是

否适合行麻醉。术前应行全面的盆腔检查。麻醉后重复盆腔检查，以确认先前的发现。

Preoperative screening of medical conditions or risk factors should be followed by clinical examination, including cardiovascular and respiratory examination to evaluate fitness for anaesthesia. A complete pelvic examination should be performed preoperatively. A pelvic examination is often repeated under anaesthesia to confirm the previous findings.

3. 化验检查（Investigations）

术前血液检查包括全血细胞计数；高血压或糖尿病患者以及使用利尿剂的患者行尿素和电解质检查以筛查肾脏疾病；有酗酒或肝病病史的患者需行肝功能检查；如果有大出血风险或患者存在特殊血型抗体，术前应筛查并明确血型，并在手术前交叉配血。如果严重大出血的风险高，应考虑行自体血液回收。

Preoperative blood investigations include full blood count; urea and electrolytes for screening for renal disease in patients with hypertension or diabetes and in women on diuretics; liver function tests for patients with a history of alcohol abuse or liver disease; and group and screen prior to procedures with risk of bleeding and cross-match if heavy bleeding is anticipated or antibodies are present. The availability of a cell saver should be considered if significant bleeding is anticipated.

术前应检查血糖和 HbA1c 用于筛查糖尿病和评估血糖控制情况。除非患者患有出血性疾病或服用抗凝药物，否则无须常规行凝血功能检查。患有胸部疾病的患者应行胸部 X 线检查。所有育龄期女性患者均应行妊娠试验。心脏病、高血压患者和高龄患者术前必须行心电图检查。

Blood glucose tests and HbA1C are indicated to screen for diabetes and assess diabetic control. Routine coagulation screening is not necessary unless the patient has a known bleeding disorder or has been on medication that causes anticoagulation. A chest X-ray is indicated for patients with chest disease. A pregnancy test should be undertaken in all women of reproductive age. An electrocardiogram (ECG) is mandatory preoperatively in patients with cardiac disease, hypertension and advanced age.

4. 药物（Medications）

应在术前 7～10 天停用阿司匹林，因为阿司匹林会不可逆地抑制血小板环氧化酶，停药后血小板聚集试验可在长达 10 天里呈异常结果。非甾体类抗炎药（NSAID）也会抑制血小板环氧化酶，但其作

用是可逆的。

Aspirin should be discontinued 7–10 days before surgery, as it inhibits platelet cyclooxygenase irreversibly, so platelet aggregation studies can be abnormal for up to 10 days. Non-steroidal anti-inflammatory drugs (NSAIDs) cause inhibition of cyclooxygenase, which is reversible.

口服抗血小板药氯吡格雷对血小板聚集率的抑制作用呈剂量依赖性，停药 5 天后出血时间恢复正常。服用抗凝药的患者术前需要换用低分子量肝素（LMWH）进行桥接。应由血液科专家在内的多学科团队管理这类患者。

Clopidogrel bisulphate, an oral antiplatelet agent, causes a dose-dependent inhibition of platelet aggregation and takes about 5 days after discontinuation for bleeding time to return to normal. Patients on oral anticoagulants need to be converted to low-molecular-weight heparin (LMWH). Management of these patients should be undertaken by a multidisciplinary team involving haematologists.

有静脉血栓栓塞（VTE）危险因素的女性应使用 LMWH 预防血栓形成。应在大手术前 4~6 周停用复合口服避孕药，以将 VTE 的风险降至最低，并向患者提供其他避孕方法。单纯孕激素制剂是否增加 VTE 风险目前不详。尽管激素替代治疗是术后 VTE 的危险因素，但因风险较低无须术前停药。在手术当天，应告知患者需服用哪种药物。

Women with risk factors for venous thromboembolism (VTE) should receive LMWH thromboprophylaxis. The combined oral contraceptive pill should be stopped 4–6 weeks prior to major surgery to minimize the risk of VTE, and alternative contraception should be offered. The progesterone-only pill is not known to increase the risk of VTE. Although hormone replacement therapy is a risk factor for postoperative VTE, this risk is small and it is not necessary to stop prior to surgery. On the day of surgery, patients should be advised which of their medications they should take.

（三）术前准备（Preoperative preparation）

1. 贫血管理（Management of anaemia）

缺铁性贫血患者应在术前补铁治疗。重组促红细胞生成素（Epo）可用于提高血红蛋白浓度。为了增加治疗有效性，铁储备必须充足，应在使用 Epo 之前或同时补充铁剂。如果拒绝使用血液制品的患者术中大出血风险高，可在术前使用 Epo 来增加血红蛋白浓度。

Iron-deficiency anaemia should be treated with iron therapy before surgery. Recombinant erythropoietin (Epo)

can be used to increase haemoglobin concentrations. To be effective, iron stores must be adequate, and iron should be given before or concurrently with Epo. When significant blood loss is anticipated in women who will not accept blood products, Epo may be used to increase the haemoglobin concentration preoperatively.

异常子宫出血患者术前可使用促性腺激素释放激素激动药止血并增加血红蛋白浓度。

Gonadotropin-releasing hormone agonists may be used preoperatively to stop abnormal uterine bleeding and increase haemoglobin concentrations.

自体输血避免了感染 HIV、肝炎和出现输血反应的风险。

Autologous blood donation avoids the risks of HIV or hepatitis infection and transfusion reactions.

2. 预防性使用抗生素（Antibiotic prophylaxis）

在手术开始前应预防性静脉使用抗生素。在手术时间延长或术中出血较多时，应追加抗生素。常用抗生素包括复合阿莫西林 – 克拉维酸，或者头孢菌素联合甲硝唑。对有药物过敏的患者，可选用广谱药物包括克林霉素联用庆大霉素、环丙沙星或氨曲南、甲硝唑联用庆大霉素，或者甲硝唑联用环丙沙星。对于有耐甲氧西林金黄色葡萄球菌（MRSA）感染史或定植史的患者，建议加用万古霉素。对患有急性传染疾病风险的女性，建议行术前筛查，并使用能够治疗衣原体的多西环素或阿奇霉素。

Antibiotic prophylaxis should be administered intravenously before the start of the procedure. In prolonged procedures or where the estimated blood loss is excessive, additional doses should be administered. Co-amoxiclav or cephalosporins with metronidazole are the commonly used antibiotics. For patients with known hypersensitivity, alternative broad-spectrum agents include combinations of clindamycin with gentamicin, ciprofloxacin or aztreonam; metronidazole with gentamicin; or metronidazole with ciprofloxacin. In patients with a known history of methicillin-resistant *Staphylococcus aureus* (MRSA) infection or colonization, addition of vancomycin is recommended. Preoperative screening is recommended in women at risk for sexually transmitted infections, and antibiotic cover for *Chlamydia* with doxycycline or azithromycin should be given.

术前备皮和消毒皮肤可以降低感染的风险。小手术不需要预防性使用抗生素。

Skin preparation with an antiseptic and a sterile technique reduces the risks of infection. Minor procedures do not require antibiotic prophylaxis.

3. 糖尿病管理（Management of diabetes）

围术期良好的血糖控制对于预防糖尿病酮症酸中毒、伤口愈合并发症和感染并发症很重要。除了血糖控制较好的小手术患者，口服降糖药应在手术当天停止使用，换用滑尺胰岛素注射法。患有 1 型糖尿病的患者应在术日开始使用滑尺胰岛素注射法。

Good glucose control in the perioperative period is important for the prevention of diabetic ketoacidosis and healing and infectious complications. Oral hypoglycaemics should be stopped on the day of surgery and replaced by an insulin sliding scale, except for minor procedures in a well-controlled patient. People with type 1 diabetes should have a sliding scale commenced on the day of surgery.

4. 手术室的手术安全（Surgical safety in the operating theatre）

手术室中应设置标准系统以预防和识别可能导致不良事件的潜在错误和故障。降低风险的常用措施包括团队全体成员互相介绍，检查患者的知情同意书，使用核查表和手术前后内部信息通报。核查表必须包括如下信息：确保在正确的地点进行正确的操作；合理预防性应用抗生素；耐心地处理问题，确保仪器和其他设备的可用性，以及在需要时可使用成像系统。

Standard systems should be in place in the operating theatre to prevent and identify potential errors and failures that may lead to adverse events. Common measures to reduce risk include introduction of all team members, review of the patient's informed consent, checklists and team briefings before and after surgery. Ensuring the correct procedure on the correct site, administration of the appropriate antibiotic prophylaxis, patient handling issues, availability of instruments and other equipment and use of imaging when required are essential parts of a checklist.

手术开始前应完成一份标准化核查表，以确保所有安全措施得到落实，如世界卫生组织（WHO）外科手术安全核查表（图 A1-1），该核查表列举了在手术的三个阶段（麻醉诱导前、术前和手术结束）需要核查的项目。

A standardized checklist should be completed prior to the start of each procedure to ensure that all safety measures are followed. An example is the World Health Organization (WHO) surgical safety checklist (Fig. A1.1), which provides a set of checks to be done at three stages of a surgical procedure (sign in, time out and sign out).

世界卫生组织外科手术安全核查表的制订旨在增加手术中的团队合作和沟通，减少错误和不良事件发生。使用该核查表可以显著降低发病率和死亡率，减少术后并发症，目前已被全世界大多数手术机构采用。

The WHO Surgical Safety Checklist was developed with an aim to reduce errors and adverse events and increase teamwork and communication in surgery. The use of this checklist has been associated with significant reductions in both morbidity and mortality, as well as postoperative complications, and is now used by the majority of surgical settings worldwide.

手术前应进行术前内部信息通报或"术前讨论"。

Before surgery, a preoperative team briefing, or 'huddle', should be performed.

整个团队都需参加，其中包括外科医生、麻醉师、巡回护士和器械护士。术前内部信息通报应包括以下内容。

The entire team participates, including the surgeon(s), anaesthetist(s), circulating nurse(s) and scrub nurse. A preoperative briefing should include the following elements:

- 团队成员介绍，包括姓名和分工。
- Team introductions by names and roles
- 确认患者身份和知情同意书，拟行的手术，手术的部位、侧别或平面。
- Confirmation of patient identity and consent; the planned surgical procedure; and the site, side or level of surgery
- 研究患者的病情和检查结果，制订并发症管理方案。
- Identifying the patient's medical status and investigation results, with a management plan for medical comorbidities
- 讨论抗生素使用。
- Discussion of antibiotic administration
- 评估和预防静脉血栓栓塞（VTE）风险。
- Confirmation of VTE risk assessment and prophylaxis
- 确认血型和备血情况，或者血液制品的可用性。
- Ensuring blood group and save or blood product availability
- 确定对患者进行理想监控的设备及其可用性。
- Determining ideal patient status monitoring and availability of equipment
- 确认所有必要的手术设备和器械的可用性及

手术安全核查表
Surgical Safety Checklist

患者安全
Patient Safety
为了更安全的护理
A Wold Allance for Safer Heslth Care

诱导麻醉前 Before induction of anaesthesia	皮肤切开前 Before skin incision	患者离开手术室前 Before patient leaves operating room
（至少有护士与麻醉师共同完成） (with at least nurse and anaesthetist)	（由护士、麻醉师和外科医师共同完成） (with nurse, anaesthetist and surgeon)	（由护士、麻醉师和外科医师共同完成） (with nurse, anaesthetist and surgeon)

诱导麻醉前

患者是否确认了自己的身份，手术部位和手术名称，并已签署知情同意书？
Has the patient confirmed his/her identity,site, procedure, and consent?
□是的 Yes

是否标记了手术部位？
Is the site marked?
□是的 Yes
□不适用 Not applicable

是否完成了对麻醉机和麻醉药物的检查？
Is the anaesthesia machine and medication check complete?
□是的 Yes

患者是否佩戴了脉氧仪，脉氧仪是否正常工作？
Is the pulse oximeter on the patient and functioning?
□是的 Yes

患者是否有已知的过敏史？
Does the patient have a: Known allergy?
□没有 No
□有 Yes

是否为困难气道，或有误吸风险？
Difficult airway or aspiration risk?
□无 No
□是的，已安排好急救设备或人员
Yes, and equipment/assistance available

是否有出血超过 500ml 的风险？（儿童出血超过 7ml/kg）
Risk of > 500ml blood loss (7ml/kg in children)?
□无 No
□有，开放了两条静脉通道 / 中心静脉，已准备好静脉用液体
Yes, and two IVs/central access and fluids planned

皮肤切开前

□确认所有团队成员介绍了各自的姓名和角色
Confirm all team members have introduced themselves by name and role.

□确认患者的姓名、手术名称和切口位置
Confirm the patient's name, procedure, and where the incision will be made.

在术前 60min 内是否预防性使用了抗生素？
Has antibiotic prophylaxis been given within the last 60 minutes?
□是的 Yes
□不适用 Not applicable

预计发生的重要事件
Anticipated Critical Events
外科医生：
To Surgeon:
□本台手术中关键手术步骤或非常规手术步骤是什么？ What are the critical or non-routine steps?
□手术时间预计多久？ How long will the case take?
□估计术中出血多少？ What is the anticipated blood loss?
麻醉师：
To Anaesthetist:
□是否存在患者特有的问题？ Are there any patient-specific concerns?
护理团队：
To Nursing Team:
□是否确认了各项无菌指标（包括指标结果）？
Has sterility (including indicator results) been confirmed?
□手术设备是否有问题？ Are there equipment issues or any concerns?

图像显示屏是否摆放好？
Is essential imaging displayed?
□是的 Yes
□不适用 Not applicable

患者离开手术室前

护士口头确认：
Nurse Verbally Confirms:
□手术名称 The name of the procedure
□已清点手术器械、纱布和缝针计数 Completion of instrument, sponge and needle counts
□确认标本标签（大声读出标本的标签和患者姓名）Specimen labelling (read specimen labels aloud, including patient name)
□手术设备是否存在问题 Whether there are any equipment problems to be addressed

外科医师，麻醉师和护士：
To Surgeon, Anaesthetist and Nurse:
□该患者术后恢复与管理的关键因素？ What are the key concerns for recovery and management of this patient?

此核查表并不全面，建议增加或修改以符合当地医疗机构临床常规的项目。修订于 2009 年 1 月 © WHO, 2009

This checklist is not intended to be comprehensive. Additions and modifications to fit local practice are encouraged. Revised 1 / 2009 © WHO, 2009

图 A1-1　WHO 手术安全核查表（经世界卫生组织许可转载）

Fig. A1.1　The WHO Surgical Safety Checklist. (Reproduced with permission of the World Health Organization.)

能否正常运行，并发现可能的问题。

- Verifying availability and proper functioning of all necessary surgical equipment and instruments and identifying any concerns

- 讨论患者合适的体位，垫板放置位置和皮肤

准备。

- Discussion of appropriate patient positioning, padding and skin preparation

- 确保团队预期关键或非常规手术步骤。

- Ensuring team anticipation of critical or non-routine

steps

- 讨论术后管理计划（如去特护病房或重症监护室）。

- Discussion of postoperative plan (e.g. high-dependency or intensive care unit if appropriate)

- 请所有团队成员提出问题并就任何存在顾虑的地方发表意见。

- Invitation to all team members to ask questions and to speak up regarding any concerns

术后汇报以确保所有步骤完成，并发现存在的所有问题或危险，并提出改进建议。术后汇报核查表包括以下内容。

A debriefing postoperatively aims to establish that all steps have been completed, as well as to identify any problems or hazards and suggest improvements. A debriefing checklist includes:

- 已完成所有书面记录。

- Completion of all documentation

- 检查标本和标本状态以行病理学检查。

- Checking of specimens and specimen forms for pathology

- 讨论可能遇到的任何设备问题。

- Discussion of any equipment problems that may have been encountered

- 识别与安全或效率有关的任何错误和问题。

- Identification of any errors and issues on safety or efficiency

- 讨论术后的患者转运和对患者的指导。

- Discussion of patient transfer and patient instructions after surgery

- 信息通报中发现的错误和几乎发生的差错对于临床管理和质量改进是必不可少的。

- Errors and near-misses identified during debriefing are essential to be used in clinical governance and quality improvement processes.

二、术中并发症（Intraoperative complications）

（一）局部麻醉和全身麻醉（Regional and general anaesthesia）

与局部和全身麻醉有关的并发症包括液体过量、电解质紊乱和气体栓塞。

Complications related to regional and general anaesthesia include fluid overload, electrolyte disturbances and gas embolization.

（二）局部麻醉（Local anaesthesia）

严重的不良反应很少见，多由静注药品时出现疏忽、药物剂量过大和药物清除延迟导致。中枢神经系统的不良反应包括口腔刺痛、震颤、头晕、视物模糊、癫痫发作、呼吸抑制和呼吸暂停。心血管系统的不良反应是心肌抑制（心动过缓和心血管衰竭）。

Serious adverse reactions are uncommon, but they are secondary to inadvertent intravascular injection, excessive dose and delayed clearance. Central nervous system side effects include mouth tingling, tremor, dizziness, blurred vision, seizures, respiratory depression and apnoea. Cardiovascular side effects are those of myocardial depression (bradycardia and cardiovascular collapse).

注意药物总剂量并避免静脉给药错误，可减少与局部麻醉药相关的不良事件。

The adverse events associated with injectable local anaesthetic agents are reduced by attention to total dosage and avoidance of inadvertent intravascular administration.

局部用药全身吸收后也可能导致不良事件。

Topical agents can also be associated with adverse events secondary to systemic absorption.

（三）患者体位导致的并发症（Complications secondary to patient positioning）

1. 急性骨筋膜室综合征（Acute compartment syndrome）

膀胱截石位可导致患者腿部骨筋膜室内肌肉受压缺血，再灌注后出现毛细血管渗漏，导致神经肌肉组织进一步水肿和横纹肌溶解，从而导致骨筋膜室综合征。使用腿架或下肢循环驱动、患者体重指数高和手术时间延长均是危险因素。

Compartment syndrome in the legs may occur due to the lithotomy position when the pressure in the muscle of an osteofascial compartment is increased, causing ischaemia followed by reperfusion, capillary leakage from the ischaemic tissue and further increase in tissue oedema resulting in neuromuscular compromise and rhabdomyolysis. Leg holders, pneumatic compression stockings, high body mass index and prolonged surgical time are risk factors.

采用减压技术和早期理疗可减少远期后遗症。

Decompression techniques and early physiotherapy may reduce long-term sequelae.

2. 神经系统损伤（Neurological injury）

膀胱截石位和手术时间延长可导致腰骶神经丛的运动神经（股神经、闭孔神经和坐骨神经）和感觉神经（髂腹下神经、髂腹股沟神经、生殖股神经、阴部神经、股神经、坐骨神经和股外侧皮神经）损伤。

Injury to motor nerves arising from the lumbosacral plexus (femoral, obturator and sciatic nerves) and the sensory nerves (iliohypogastric, ilioinguinal, genitofemoral, pudendal, femoral, sciatic and lateral femoral cutaneous nerves) can occur with the lithotomy position and prolonged operative time.

股神经疾病可继发于髋关节过度屈曲、外展和外旋导致的神经压迫。坐骨神经和腓神经分别固定于坐骨切迹和腓骨颈，伸直膝关节后屈曲髋关节，同时大腿过度外旋会导致这些部位受到拉伸。坐骨神经会因髋关节过度屈曲而受到创伤。腓总神经也容易压迫损伤。

Femoral neuropathy may occur secondary to excessive hip flexion, abduction and external hip rotation, which contribute to nerve compression. The sciatic and peroneal nerves are fixed at the sciatic notch and neck of the fibula, respectively. Flexion of the hip with a straight knee and excessive external rotation of the thighs cause stretch at these points. The sciatic nerve can be traumatized with excessive hip flexion. The common peroneal nerve is also susceptible to compression injury.

理想的膀胱截石位要求膝关节和髋关节适度屈曲，限制其外展和外旋。外科医生和助手应避免倚靠在患者的大腿上。

Ideal lithotomy positioning requires moderate flexion of the knee and hip, with limited abduction and external rotation. The surgeons and assistants should avoid leaning on the thigh of the patient.

（四）出血（Haemorrhage）

术中大出血是指出血量超过 1000ml，或者出血过多需要输血。严重大出血是急性出血量超过患者血容量的 25%，或出血过多需要抢救。

Intraoperative haemorrhage is blood loss of more than 1000 mL or blood loss that requires blood transfusion. Massive haemorrhage is defined as acute loss of more than 25% of the patient's blood volume or a loss that requires a lifesaving intervention.

出血量超过血容量 30%～40% 时可导致循环系统不稳定。出血量超过血容量的 40% 会有生命危险。

严重大出血时，需要在 1h 内抢救，否则可导致多脏器功能衰竭甚至死亡。

A loss of 30–40% of the patient's blood volume may result in cardiovascular instability. More than 40% blood loss is life threatening. Severe haemorrhage can lead to multiple organ failure and death unless resuscitation takes place within an hour.

止血的第一步是压迫出血部位。在腹腔镜手术中，可使用止血钳加压止血，但大血管破裂出血时，常需中转开腹手术止血。

The first step is pressure applied to the bleeding area. In laparoscopic surgery, pressure can be applied with an atraumatic laparoscopic grasper. In large-vessel bleeding, a laparotomy is usually required.

电凝、缝合或钳夹止血可用于控制小血管出血。结扎血管前应将血管与周围组织分离，以免造成意外损伤。

Diathermy, suturing or surgical clips can be used to control small-vessel bleeding. Vessels should be separated from surrounding structures before ligation to avoid inadvertent injury.

如果上述措施止血失败，则应考虑结扎双侧髂内动脉，但只能由经验丰富的外科医生操作。

If initial attempts to arrest bleeding fail, bilateral internal iliac artery ligation should be considered but only performed by surgeons experienced with this procedure.

控制低容量静脉的弥漫性出血可使用局部止血药物，其中包括明胶海绵 / 凝血酶（辉瑞公司），这是一种可吸收的明胶基质；止血纱布（爱惜康公司），是由氧化的再生纤维素制成；止血凝胶（百特公司），是一种止血剂，由人的血浆，明胶和凝血酶混合制成；纤维蛋白胶（百特公司），是凝血酶和高度浓缩的人纤维蛋白原的混合物。

Topical haemostatic agents for control of diffuse, lowvolume venous bleeding include Gelfoam/thrombin (Pfizer), an absorbable gelatine matrix; Surgicel (Ethicon), made of oxidized regenerated cellulose; FloSeal (Baxter), a haemostatic agent made from human plasma and constituted by mixing gelatine and thrombin; and Tisseel (Baxter), a mixture of thrombin and highly concentrated human fibrinogen.

应持续监测患者的血流动力学状态。应考虑静脉输液和输血及血液制品。必要时需呼叫麻醉师、另一位高年资妇科医生、多名护士、手术室工作人员和血管外科专家进行协助。应交叉配血，并检测血红蛋白、血小板计数、部分凝血活酶时间（PTT）和活化的部分凝血活酶时间（aPTT）。如果 PTT 和

aPTT 超过正常上限的 1.5 倍，应输注新鲜冰冻血浆。相关研究表明，输注红细胞与新鲜冰冻血浆的比例为 1 ：1 至 1.5 ：1 时死亡率降低，故输注红细胞与新鲜冰冻血浆的比例应小于 2 ：1。如果纤维蛋白原水平低，应由血液科医生协助处理，应输注冷沉淀。

The patient's haemodynamic status should be continuously monitored. Fluid replacement and transfusion of blood and blood products should be considered. Assistance of a second senior gynaecologist and anaesthetist, additional nursing and theatre staff and an additional surgeon with expertise in vascular surgery may be necessary. Blood should be cross-matched. Haemoglobin, platelet count, partial thromboplastin time (PTT) and activated partial thromboplastin time (aPTT) should be checked. If the PTT and aPTT exceed 1.5 times the control value, fresh frozen plasma should also be given. The ratio of red blood cells (RBCs) to fresh frozen plasma should be <2:1, as studies on trauma suggest that ratios of 1–1.5:1 are associated with reduced mortality. If fibrinogen is low, cryoprecipitate should be given and a haematologist involved.

如果血小板计数低于 50 000/ml，需输注血小板。应监测酸碱平衡以及血浆钙和钾水平。

Platelet transfusion is indicated if the platelet count is less than 50,000/mL. Acid-base balance and plasma calcium and potassium levels should be monitored.

患者收缩压＜ 70mmHg，出现酸中毒和体温过低时体内凝血酶活性抑制，出现凝血功能障碍的风险增加。大量输液和输注红细胞会稀释凝血因子和血小板，也会导致凝血功能障碍。当有凝血功能障碍或微血管弥漫性出血时，应行成分输血。

A systolic blood pressure <70 mmHg, acidosis and hypothermia inhibit clotting enzymes and increase the risk of coagulopathy. Large volumes of fluids and transfusion of packed RBCs dilute the clotting factors and platelets and predispose to coagulopathy. Component therapy is used when there is clinical evidence of coagulopathy or microvascular diffuse bleeding.

如果其他措施未能止血，可在骨盆中持续放置压力包 48～72h。放置盆腔引流管有利于监测到持续的内出血。留置导尿管可监测尿量。

If other measures fail to control bleeding, a pressure pack may be left in the pelvis for 48–72 hours. A pelvic drain will enable monitoring of continued bleeding. An indwelling urinary catheter allows urine output monitoring.

（五）输尿管和膀胱损伤（Ureteric and bladder injury）

妇科大手术中输尿管和膀胱的损伤率分别为 2/1000～6/1000 和 3/1000～12/1000。

The incidence of ureteric and bladder injury during major gynaecological surgery is 2–6 per 1000 cases and 3–12 per 1000 cases, respectively.

膀胱损伤的危险因素包括子宫内膜异位症、感染、膀胱过度膨胀和粘连。在有粘连时，行子宫全切术时锐性分离膀胱很重要，因为钝性分离可能导致膀胱损伤。在腹腔镜手术中，应充分导尿避免膀胱充盈，以免行腹部套管针穿刺时损伤膀胱。与耻骨上穿刺相比，侧腹部套管针穿刺能减少膀胱损伤的风险。膀胱热损伤会延迟出现，在术后数天方有临床表现。

Risk factors for bladder injury include endometriosis, infection, bladder over-distension and adhesions. In cases with adhesions, it is important to use sharp dissection of the bladder during a hysterectomy, as blunt dissection may result in injury. During laparoscopic surgery, the bladder should be empty to avoid injury with the trocars. Lateral rather than suprapubic trocar insertion will reduce the risk of bladder injury. Bladder thermal injury may be delayed and clinically manifest several days postoperatively.

膀胱上小于 1cm 的破口可自愈，无须修复。较大的破口可使用可吸收缝线双层连续缝合。可用靛蓝胭脂红或亚甲基蓝液体充盈膀胱来评估膀胱的完整性。可通过放置输尿管支架或静脉输注靛蓝胭脂红后观察输尿管内染料通过情况，评估输尿管的通畅性。尿管应留置 7～14 天。

Small defects less than 1 cm heal spontaneously and do not need to be repaired. A larger injury is closed in two layers using a running absorbable suture. The integrity of the bladder can be assessed by filling the bladder with indigo carmine or methylene blue dye. Ureteric patency is assessed using indigo carmine intravenously to demonstrate dye efflux from both ureters or by ureteric stenting. An indwelling catheter should be inserted for 7–14 days.

输尿管外伤可能是由横断伤、挤压伤、去血管化或热损伤引起的。如果怀疑损伤了输尿管，可以术中使用染料结合膀胱镜检查或放置输尿管支架来评估其通畅性。如果怀疑输尿管发生损伤，应咨询泌尿科医师，确定输尿管损伤后，可以进行输尿管端端吻合术或输尿管再植入术。

Ureteric trauma may be caused by transection, crush injury, de-vascularization or thermal injury. If ureteric injury is suspected, patency can be evaluated by intraoperative cystoscopy with dye or ureteric stenting. If there is doubt, a urologist should be consulted and, in case of confirmed injury, an end-to-end anastomosis or re-implantation can be undertaken.

在所有脱垂或失禁手术中应尽可能行膀胱镜检查，以排除膀胱或输尿管损伤。漏诊输尿管损伤时，患者会出现腹痛、发热、血尿、侧腹部痛和腹膜炎的症状。

Cystoscopy should be performed intraoperatively where possible after all prolapse or incontinence surgery to rule out bladder or ureteric injury. In undiagnosed ureteric injuries, patients present with symptoms of abdominal pain, fever, haematuria, flank pain and peritonitis.

（六）胃肠道损伤（Gastrointestinal injury, GI）

妇科手术中的胃肠道（GI）损伤发生率为 0.05%～0.33%。术中胃肠道损伤的患者死亡率高达 3.6%。胃肠道损伤可发生于气腹针穿刺或放置套管针时，以及分离粘连、离断血管或使用能量器械时。既往有腹部手术史会增加粘连的风险。在这种情况下，腹腔镜检查应采用开放（Hassan）式入路或先行左上腹部穿刺（Palmer 点）。

Gastrointestinal injury (GI) during gynaecological surgery occurs in between 0.05% and 0.33% of cases. Intraoperative GI injury has a mortality rate as high as 3.6%. Injury may occur during Veress needle or trocars insertion, adhesiolysis, tissue dissection, devascularization and electrosurgery. Previous abdominal surgery increases the risk of adhesions. In these cases, laparoscopy should be undertaken using an open (Hassan) technique or entry through the left upper quadrant (Palmer's point).

如果怀疑损伤，应对肠管进行检查，如有不确定，应请外科医生台上会诊。若患者术后 2～4 天出现恶心、呕吐、腹痛和发热时，可疑出现胃肠道损伤。

If an injury is suspected, the bowel should be examined and a surgeon's opinion should be sought if in doubt. Unrecognized injuries present 2–4 days postoperatively with nausea, vomiting, abdominal pain and fever.

穿刺针损伤在没有出血或伤口撕裂时通常不需要修复。肠刺伤但没有撕裂时，由于肠内细菌载量高，应对腹腔进行细致的冲洗并予抗生素治疗，这一点十分重要。肠损伤时应双层缝合修复。对于肠管撕裂伤，建议行肠管节段性切除。肠管热损伤后存在组织坏死的风险，需要扩大肠管切除范围，否则临床上可能需要几天的时间才能出现相关症状。

Veress needle injuries do not usually need to be repaired in the absence of bleeding or a tear. For punctures of the large intestine without tearing, meticulous irrigation of the peritoneal cavity and antibiotic treatment are important, as the large intestine contents have a high bacterial load. Intestinal injury should be repaired in two layers. In extended lacerations, a segmental resection is recommended. Thermal injuries require wide resection due to the risk of tissue necrosis, which may take days to manifest clinically.

乙状结肠和直肠的损伤可以通过乙状结肠直肠镜来检查。

Injury to the rectosigmoid colon may be detected by proctosigmoidoscopy.

在广泛结肠损伤或肠系膜损伤时应行结肠造口术。

A diverting colostomy is indicated in extensive colon injuries or injuries involving the mesentery.

有上腹部手术史的患者可能在行腹腔镜手术时出现胃穿孔，麻醉诱导后因疏忽导致患者胃内气体膨胀后行穿刺针穿刺也可导致胃穿孔。气腹针造成的胃损伤若无出血，可仅进行冲洗。较大的损伤（如套管针穿刺损伤）需要由胃外科经验丰富的外科医生进行双层缝合修复。应冲洗腹腔以清除胃内容物。术后多行鼻胃管负压吸引，直到患者消化道功能恢复正常。

Gastric perforation during laparoscopy may occur in cases with prior upper abdominal surgery and an inadvertently gas-distended stomach following induction of anaesthesia. Small Veress needle punctures with no bleeding can be treated by irrigation. Larger defects such as trocar injuries require repair in two layers by a surgeon experienced in gastric surgery. The abdominal cavity should be irrigated to remove any gastric contents. Nasogastric suction usually is maintained postoperatively until normal bowel function returns.

三、术后管理（Postoperative care）

（一）镇痛（Analgesia）

术前应制订术后镇痛方案。较大的腹部手术多需要硬膜外镇痛或患者自控镇痛泵（PCA）。可逐渐过渡为使用对乙酰氨基酚和非甾体类消炎药，必要时加用阿片类药物来缓解疼痛。开具阿片类药物时，应同时开具止吐药和大便软化剂。

Analgesia should be planned preoperatively. Major abdominal surgery is likely to require an epidural or patientcontrolled analgesia (PCA). This can then be gradually converted to regular paracetamol and an NSAID, with or without opioids for breakthrough pain. Anti-emetics and stool softeners should be prescribed with opioids.

（二）水电解质平衡（Fluid and electrolyte balance）

对于静脉输液的患者，术后保持液体平衡和监测血浆电解质水平十分重要。正常人体每日液体摄入量约为 2.5L，由于术中出血和不显性失水，手术患者需补充丢失的液体。对于高钾血症患者，可行心电图评估心律，可予葡萄糖酸钙预防和控制心律不齐，可静滴胰岛素 – 葡萄糖液体降低血钾水平。低钾血症可通过在静脉输液中添加钾来纠正。低钠血症通常由于液体摄入过多导致，高钠血症则是由于脱水导致。尿量下降到 0.5ml/(kg·h) 以下可能表明液体摄入不足。液体摄入不足可通过补充胶体后观察尿量是否增加来判断。在老年患者或心脏病患者中，补充液体需要谨慎，可能会加重肺水肿。补充液体后如未观察到尿量增加，则需要评估心脏和肾脏功能。

In the immediate postoperative period, it is important to maintain fluid balance and monitor serum electrolyte levels whilst a patient is on intravenous fluids. The normal fluid intake of approximately 2.5 L/24 hours requires additional replacement of fluid deficit due to intraoperative blood loss and insensible water losses. In cases of hyperkalaemia, an ECG is indicated for the assessment of cardiac rhythm, as well as calcium gluconate for prevention and management of arrhythmia and an insulin-dextrose infusion for the reduction of potassium levels. Hypokalaemia is treated by adding potassium in the intravenous fluids. Hyponatraemia is usually caused by excessive fluid intake, and hypernatraemia by dehydration. A fall in the urine output below 0.5 mL/kg/hour may indicate insufficient replacement. This can be confirmed with a fluid challenge of a colloid. Fluid challenges should be given with caution in elderly patients or those with cardiac disease, as this may exacerbate pulmonary oedema. If no improvement in urine output is seen, an assessment of cardiac and renal function is required.

（三）循环系统稳定（Cardiovascular stability）

术后低血压的常见原因有硬膜外镇痛、脱水和出血，会导致组织灌注减少、伤口愈合减慢、脑梗死、肾功能衰竭和多器官功能衰竭。除非患者一般情况稳定，定向性好，心率在 50～100 次 / 分，远端肢体皮温正常，毛细血管再充盈速度 < 2s，且尿量较多，否则需要进一步查明术后低血压原因。

Epidural analgesia, dehydration and bleeding are common causes of postoperative hypotension. This in turn can result in reduced tissue perfusion and impaired healing, cerebral

infarction, renal failure and multiple organ failure. Unless the patient is stable, orientated, with pulse 50–100 beats/ min, warm peripheries, capillary refill <2 seconds and a good urine output, further investigations to identify the cause are required.

（四）膀胱护理（Bladder care）

术后留置导管可以精确监测尿量，预防继发于全身麻醉或疼痛的尿潴留发生。患者能够下床活动后，应取出导尿管。排尿试验包括监测排尿量，以及使用便携式膀胱超声估算残余尿量。若残余尿量＞150ml，则需再次留置导尿管 24～72h。若仍然排尿困难，患者需带导尿管回家，并在 7～10 天后返回，取出导尿管进行排尿试验；或者使患者学会自行间断导尿，直到膀胱功能恢复正常，能够自主控制排尿。

An indwelling catheter in the postoperative period allows for accurate measurement of urine output and prevents urinary retention secondary to the general anaesthetic or pain. The catheter should be removed when the patient is able to mobilize. The trial of void involves measurement of the voided volume and estimation of the post-void residual volume using a portable bladder ultrasound scan. If greater than 150 mL, re-catheterization for 24–72 hours is indicated. With persistent voiding difficulty, the patient may need to go home with an indwelling catheter and return after 7–10 days for a trial without catheter or be taught intermittent self-catheterization until bladder function is normal, i.e. she has control of micturition.

（五）进食（Oral intake）

术后尽早恢复饮食饮水可缩短患者的住院时间，不会增加肠梗阻。若患者呕吐，则应推迟进食。若患者持续呕吐，应排除肠梗阻。肠梗阻的其他症状包括腹痛和无排气排便，体征包括腹胀、腹痛和肠鸣音亢进。行腹部 X 线检查可显示肠管扩张。肠梗阻的处理包括禁食、静脉补液和插鼻胃管。如果没有改善，则需要行进一步的影像学检查识别梗阻部位，以行外科手术干预。如果发生麻痹性肠梗阻的风险很高（肠管扰动过多或肠损伤），则应插鼻胃管，并注意推迟进食。

Early postoperative oral hydration and feeding may reduce the length of patient stay without any increase in ileus. If there is vomiting, feeding should be delayed. With persistent vomiting, bowel obstruction should be excluded. Other symptoms include abdominal pain and an absence of passage of flatus or faeces. Signs include abdominal distension and tenderness with pronounced bowel sounds. An abdominal X-ray would show dilated loops of bowel. Management involves nil by mouth, intravenous fluids and insertion of a nasogastric tube.

If there is no improvement, further contrast imaging is required to identify the site of obstruction for surgical intervention. In cases at high risk of paralytic ileus (excessive bowel handling or bowel injury), a nasogastric tube should be inserted with slower introduction of diet.

四、术后并发症（Postoperative complications）

（一）术后出血（Postoperative haemorrhage）

腹腔内出血的表现包括心动过速、低血压、腹胀、少尿、意识模糊、出汗和腹痛。少量出血可以在严密监测下期待治疗，可动态监测血红蛋白水平，必要时输血。较小的腹膜后血肿可能自行吸收。休克患者和腹围持续增加的腹腔内出血患者需要立即手术探查。

Signs of intra-abdominal bleeding include tachycardia, hypotension, abdominal distension, oliguria, confusion, sweating and abdominal pain. Minimal bleeding can be managed expectantly with monitoring, serial haemoglobin measurements and transfusion if indicated. Small retroperitoneal hematomas may eventually be reabsorbed. Patients with shock and increasing abdominal girth require immediate surgical exploration.

对于血流动力学稳定并伴有活动性出血的女性，可以考虑盆腔动脉栓塞。

Pelvic arterial embolization can be considered for haemodynamically stable women with active arterial bleeding.

（二）发热（Pyrexia）

在术后第一个 24h 内，发热超过 38℃但无其他症状，保守治疗后通常可好转。但若术后持续发热或术后 24h 后出现发热，感染可能性较大，应查明感染来源、早期抗感染治疗，以降低并发症发生率。应对心脏、胸部、腹部、切口部位和下肢进行查体，并行血液检查，查全血细胞计数、C 反应蛋白、尿素、电解质和肝功能等。应行中段尿或尿管内取样行镜检、培养和药敏检查，并行血培养和痰培养。

An isolated episode of pyrexia >38°C within the first 24 hours will usually resolve with conservative measures, but persistent pyrexia or pyrexia after 24 hours is likely to represent infection. Identification of the source and early treatment aim to reduce morbidity. Examination of the chest, heart, abdomen, wound and legs should be followed by blood tests, including full blood count, C-reactive protein, urea and electrolytes and liver function tests. A mid-stream urine or catheter specimen should be sent for microscopy, culture and sensitivity along with blood and sputum cultures.

胸部 X 线检查可以检查是否患肺炎或肺不张。常规服用对乙酰氨基酚可减少发热，应做好液体管理，补充液体损失。

A chest X-ray enables investigation for pneumonia or atelectasis. Regular paracetamol will reduce pyrexia, and fluid administration is required to replace increased losses.

（三）手术部位感染（Surgical site infections, SSI）

手术部位感染（SSI）可由皮肤或阴道内的定植菌引起。腹部切口 SSI 的常见病原体包括金黄色葡萄球菌、凝固酶阴性葡萄球菌、肠球菌和大肠埃希菌。阴道手术 SSI 的病原体包括来自阴道和会阴的革兰阴性杆菌、肠球菌、B 族链球菌和厌氧菌。术后盆腔脓肿通常与厌氧菌有关。

Surgical site infections (SSIs) can be caused by endogenous flora of the skin or vagina. Common organisms in SSIs of abdominal incisions are S. *aureus*, coagulase-negative staphylococci, *Enterococcus* spp. and *Escherichia coli*. SSIs of vaginal procedures include Gram-negative bacilli, enterococci, group B streptococci and anaerobes from the vagina and perineum. Postoperative pelvic abscesses are commonly associated with anaerobes.

SSI 的危险因素包括糖尿病、吸烟、全身类固醇药物治疗、放疗、营养不良、肥胖、长期住院和输血治疗。与 SSI 相关的手术因素包括手术时间长、出血多、体温低、手术部位剃毛和外科引流。

Risk factors include diabetes, smoking, systemic steroid medication, radiotherapy, poor nutrition, obesity, prolonged hospitalization and blood transfusion. Surgical factors associated with SSIs include prolonged operating time, excessive blood loss, hypothermia, hair removal by shaving and surgical drains.

SSI 可发生在表浅切口、深切口，并可累及器官或体腔，如阴道顶端蜂窝组织炎和盆腔脓肿。

SSIs can be superficial incisional, deep incisional and involve organ or space, i.e. vaginal cuff cellulitis and pelvic abscess.

最严重的 SSI 是坏死性筋膜炎，通常由多种微生物感染引起，可迅速导致周围组织坏死、脓毒症和终末器官损伤。

The most serious form of SSI is necrotizing fasciitis, often caused by a poly-microbial infection that can rapidly lead to necrosis of the surrounding tissue, sepsis and endorgan damage.

实验室检查包括全血细胞计数和切口或脓肿部位分泌物培养。当怀疑器官或体腔 SSI 时，应行计算机断层扫描（CT）、磁共振成像（MRI）或超声检查以确定感染部位。

Laboratory investigations include a full blood count and culture from the incision or abscess discharge. When organ or space SSIs are suspected, computed tomography (CT) scan, magnetic resonance imaging (MRI) or ultrasonography is indicated to localize the site of infection.

治疗（Treatment）

伤口蜂窝织炎患者可以在门诊口服抗生素。但若出现发热、腹膜炎、腹腔或盆腔脓肿，无法耐受口服抗生素，或者有其他脓毒症迹象，应入院静脉注射抗生素治疗。局部伤口感染时，需切开引流。在没有脓肿的情况下，可以口服抗生素治疗阴道顶端蜂窝织炎。

Patients with wound cellulitis can be treated as outpatients with oral antibiotics. Admission and intravenous antibiotic treatment are indicated in cases of pyrexia, peritonitis, intra-abdominal or pelvic abscess; inability to tolerate oral antibiotics; or other signs of sepsis. In a localized wound infection, incision and drainage are indicated. In the absence of an abscess, cuff cellulitis can be treated with oral antibiotics.

如果发生深切口或器官/体腔感染，应静脉应用广谱抗生素直到患者无发热并且连续 24～48h 临床一般情况较好。如果静脉使用抗生素后患者一般情况没有改善，48h 内仍有发热，应请微生物感染科专家会诊后，重复影像学检查并更换抗生素。

In case of deep incisional or organ/space infections, intravenous broad-spectrum antibiotics should be continued until the patient is apyrexial and clinically well for at least 24–48 hours. If patients do not demonstrate systemic improvement and if there is no resolution of fever within 48 hours, repeat imaging and change of antibiotics following consultation with a microbiologist should be considered.

对于无脓肿或血肿，广谱抗生素治疗无效的患者，应排除脓毒性盆腔血栓性静脉炎。脓毒性盆腔血栓性静脉炎的治疗包括使用抗生素和静脉应用肝素。

Septic pelvic thrombophlebitis should be ruled out in patients who are not responding to broad-spectrum antibiotics in the absence of an abscess or haematoma. Treatment includes antibiotics and intravenous heparin.

浅表脓肿应切开引流。对坏死组织清创后，可通过包扎、负压吸引或待伤口肉芽化后闭合切口来促进愈合。深部切口和器官/体腔感染时，有时也需行清创和引流。

Superficial abscesses should be opened and drained. After debridement of necrotic tissue, wound healing may be facilitated with packing, wound vacuum or secondary closure after re-granulation. In deep incisional and organ/space infections, debridement and drainage are occasionally required.

坏死性筋膜炎危及生命，需要立即行局部扩大范围的清创和静脉应用广谱抗生素。

Necrotizing fasciitis is life threatening and requires immediate, wide, local debridement and broad-spectrum intravenous antibiotics.

（四）心血管和呼吸系统并发症（Cardiovascular and respiratory complications）

手术和全身麻醉会增加心肌梗死风险，尤其是有危险因素的患者。胸痛患者应行心电图和心肌酶检查。患者出现心律失常时，应与脓毒症、低血容量、电解质异常和药物中毒相鉴别。

Surgery and general anaesthesia increase the risk of myocardial infarction, especially in those with risk factors. An ECG and cardiac enzymes should be considered in a patient with chest pain. In cases of arrhythmia, differential diagnosis includes sepsis, hypovolaemia, electrolyte abnormalities and drug toxicity.

呼吸系统并发症包括呼吸道感染、肺不张、肺水肿和肺栓塞。需要非吸氧状态下行血气分析来确定严重程度并调整吸氧治疗。对于氧饱和度 < 90% 或 $PO_2 < 8.0kPa$ 的患者，应考虑行辅助通气以及入住重症监护病房。

Respiratory complications include respiratory tract infection, atelectasis, pulmonary oedema and pulmonary embolism. A blood gas on air is required to determine the severity and adjust oxygen therapy. Assisted ventilation and admission to intensive care unit should be considered for patients with oxygen saturations <90 % or a PO_2 <8.0 kPa.

（五）静脉血栓栓塞（Venous thromboembolism）

如果临床上怀疑有肺栓塞（pulmonary embolism，PE），需要行诊断性影像学检查。如果无法及时检查，应予治疗剂量的低分子肝素（LMWH）。

If there is clinical suspicion of pulmonary embolism (PE), diagnostic imaging is required. If there is a delay in obtaining imaging, a treatment dose of LMWH should be administered.

如果临床怀疑深静脉血栓形成（deep vein thrombosis，DVT），但腿部多普勒超声检查为阴性，应持续抗凝治疗并在 1 周后复查超声。

If there is high clinical probability of a deep vein

thrombosis (DVT) but a negative leg Doppler ultrasound, it may be appropriate to continue with treatment and repeat the scan after 1 week.

对于怀疑 PE 的患者，推荐在行胸部 X 线检查后，行计算机断层扫描肺血管造影（CTPA）和同位素肺扫描。对于确诊 PE 的患者，应予治疗剂量的 LMWH，并在患者稳定及出血风险降低后换为口服抗凝药。应将患者转诊至血液科医生和抗凝方面专家的门诊或病房接受治疗。

Computerized tomography pulmonary angiogram (CTPA) and isotope lung scanning after a chest X-ray are the recommended imaging investigations. In a positive diagnosis, a treatment dose of LMWH should be commenced and converted to oral anticoagulants once the patient is stable and the risk of bleeding is reduced. The patient should be referred to a haematologist and anticoagulation specialist.

五、出院（Discharge from hospital）

出院总结中应提供围术期事件的相关信息，并为患者提供足量的止痛药和其他药物，对于有并发症或有疑问的患者，提供医院联系方式。

A discharge summary should provide information of the perioperative events, and the patient should be supplied with adequate analgesia and medications, as well as contact information in case of complications or concerns.

六、加速恢复（Enhanced recovery）

加速恢复是术前、术中和术后基于循证医学证据的临床管理路径，可减轻生理应激和减少器官功能障碍发生，使患者更快恢复、尽早下床活动，最终缩短住院时间。加速恢复可减轻术后疼痛，减少患者护理需求，提高患者满意度和生活质量。加速恢复管理路径应个性化。

Enhanced recovery is a care pathway that combines evidence-based elements of care pre-, intra-, and postoperatively to reduce physiological stress and organ dysfunction and enable patients to recover and resume activity earlier and to have a shorter hospital stay. Enhanced recovery pathways have been associated with reduced pain and nursing requirements and improved patient satisfaction and quality of life. These pathways should be individualized as indicated.

行妇科择期手术且术后需留院观察的患者适合加速恢复管理路径。

Patients undergoing elective gynaecological surgery with an overnight stay are potential candidates for enhanced recovery.

加速恢复的目的是优化患者教育，实现患者对围术期体验的期望，缩短围术期禁食时间，维持患者的血流动力学稳定和体温正常，增加活动量，有效缓解疼痛，预防恶心和呕吐，并减少导管和引流的使用。

Enhanced recovery focuses on optimizing patient education and perioperative expectations, decreasing the perioperative fasting period, maintaining haemodynamic stability and normothermia, increasing mobilization, providing effective pain relief, nausea and vomiting prophylaxis and decreasing use of catheters and drains.

术前加速恢复要点是评估患者的身体情况和手术适应证，优化任何发现的问题，进行术前准备及患者教育（口头和书面指导）。

Preoperative enhanced recovery elements include assessment of the patient's health and fitness for a surgical procedure and optimization of any problems identified and preoperative patient preparation, as well as patient education (verbal and written instructions).

术中加速恢复的实施需要麻醉师和外科医生参与。手术当天为避免脱水，麻醉前禁水时间缩短至 2h。围术期予镇痛治疗。避免使用长效镇静类麻醉药以利于术后尽早下床活动。加速恢复路径的常用措施还包括使用短效麻醉药、通气措施，预防和避免术后恶心和呕吐，避免使用（或尽早取出）鼻胃管。强烈建议行微创手术。

Intraoperative elements of enhanced recovery involve both the anaesthetists and surgeons. On the day of the surgical procedure, the period of starvation is reduced to 2 hours for clear fluids prior to anaesthetic to avoid dehydration. Interventions aim at perioperative pain control. Avoidance of long-acting sedative pre-medication is associated with earlier postoperative mobilization. Short-acting anaesthetic agents, ventilation measures, prophylaxis for postoperative nausea and vomiting and avoidance (or early removal) of nasogastric tubes are intraoperative measures commonly applied in enhanced recovery pathways. The use of minimal access techniques is strongly encouraged.

术后加速恢复的重点是早进食，减少静脉输液，镇痛，促进肠道功能恢复和下床活动。妇科手术后患者常在 1~2 天内出院。

Postoperative enhanced recovery measures focus on early feeding, reducing intravenous fluid infusions, pain management, bowel function and mobilization. After gynaecological procedures, patients are usually discharged within 1–2 days.

出院标准包括可正常饮食饮水，可下床活动，以及口服镇痛药止痛。应为患者提供有关术后恢复的书面建议，以及急诊的联系方式。

Criteria for discharge include ability to eat and drink, ambulation and pain management with oral analgesia. Patients should be provided written advice on recovery and expected return to normal function, as well as emergency contact information.

附录 B　管理、审查与研究
Governance, audit and research

Tahir Mahmood　Sambit Mukhopadhyay　著　　杨惠茜　杨慧霞　译　　石玉华　校

学习目标	LEARNING OUTCOMES
学习本附录后你应当能够：	After studying this appendix you should be able to:

知识标准

- 理解数据存储、检索、分析和展示的原则。
- 讨论临床数据的使用范围、有效解读和保密问题。
- 列出《数据保护法》的基本原则。
- 描述适用于当地和全国妇产科的数据审查周期（特别是与母亲与胎儿死亡率相关的数据）。
- 讨论指南、临床管理路径和临床常规的作用，如英国国家卫生和临床卓越研究所和皇家妇产科学院指南。
- 描述临床有效性的要素，其中包括基于循证医学的临床实践、临床试验类型、证据分类和推荐等级。
- 描述风险管理（包括事件报告）的原则。
- 对比审查与研究之间的差异。

专业技能和态度

- 理解良好的研究设计和研究批判性分析（包括数据统计和伦理问题）的原则。

Knowledge criteria

- Understand the principles of storage, retrieval, analysis and presentation of data.
- Discuss the range of uses of clinical data, its effective interpretation and associated confidentiality issues.
- List the basic principles of the Data Protection Act.
- Describe the audit cycle as applied to obstetrics and gynaecology locally and nationally (specifically related to maternal and perinatal mortality).
- Discuss the role of guidelines, integrated care pathways and protocols, e.g. National Institute for Health and Clinical Excellence and the Royal College of Obstetricians and Gynaecologists guidelines.
- Describe the elements of clinical effectiveness, including evidence-based practice, types of clinical trial, evidence classification and grades of recommendation.
- Describe the principles of risk management, including incident reporting.
- Contrast the differences between audit and research.

Professional skills and attitudes

- Consider the principles behind good research design and critical analysis of research, including statistics and ethical issues.

一、国民医疗服务体系（NHS）的数据收集 [Data collection in the National Health Service (NHS)]

患者可以去社区医院或大医院就诊。首诊通常在社区医院，占就医的 80%。

Patients connect with their doctors either in the primary care or in the hospital setting. The first interface usually occurs in the primary care setting, and that accounts for 80% of contact between the patient and the health system.

在大医院，患者常在门诊就诊或通过紧急通道到急诊就诊。少数患者需收入院行进一步诊治，治疗包括手术治疗和药物治疗。在患者就医的每个环节，医生通过纸质形式的病历记录或电子数据系统（无纸质记录）收集信息。

In the hospital setting, patients are seen either in outpatient clinics or as an emergency through acute admission units. A small proportion of patients will eventually be admitted to inpatient beds, either for further diagnostic workup or requiring surgical or medical intervention. At each stage of the patient's journey, information is collected either in paper form (case notes) or entered into electronic data systems (paperless notes).

卫生保健规划人员面临的挑战是，首先要确保在各级医院收集的信息可以链接到国家数据库，以确定疾病模式、人群的需求和未来卫生服务计划的趋势。

The challenge for health care planners is first to ensure that the information collected at the primary and secondary interfaces can then be linked to national databases to define trends in disease patterns, population needs and future health service planning.

第二个挑战是要确保数据库的健全和"简练"，以易于数据分析。这些数据有助于开展流行病学研究，如统计孕产妇死亡率。这些数据可以在国际范围互相比较，例如，世界卫生组织（WHO）关于国际孕产妇死亡率的报告，以及英国不同地区剖宫产和子宫切除率的报道。

The second challenge is to assure that data sets are robust and 'clean' in such a format which can be easily analyzed. These data help in carrying out epidemiological studies such as maternal mortality rates. These data also allow international comparisons such as the World Health Organization (WHO) report on Maternal Mortality and regional comparisons in caesarean section and hysterectomy rates in England.

第三个挑战是，当地的质量改进项目和成本效益在很大程度上取决于这些数据的准确性。英国国民医疗服务体系的精准医疗部是一个分部，向改善医疗服务成本的专员提供数据。

Third, local quality improvement projects and cost efficiency heavily depend upon the accuracy of these data. NHS Right Care, a division of NHS England, provides data to commissioners for potential cost improvement in delivery of health care.

（一）收集数据的来源和计算系统（Sources of data collection and computing systems）

1. 全科医生咨询和登记（General practitioner consultations and registrations）

患者在社区医院就诊的所有情况都被记录了下来，以便了解患者就诊于全科医生（general practitioner, GP）的原因，如抑郁症、上呼吸道感染、关节炎、轻伤、阴道出血、有避孕需求等。此外，可通过设置警报线来敦促国家医疗质量目标的实现，例如以下目标。

All patient interfaces with primary care are captured so that a picture can evolve on why patients are making contact with their general practitioners (GPs), such as diagnosis of depression, upper respiratory tract infection, arthritis, minor injuries, vaginal bleeding, contraceptive requirements, etc. Furthermore these data can also be used to meet national quality targets by setting alert signals, for example:

- 超过 90% 应行宫颈细胞学检查的女性已进行了筛查。
- That >90% of women eligible for cervical cytology have been screened

2. 出生和死亡登记（Registration of births and deaths）

自 1838 年以来，英格兰和威尔士实行了强制性的出生和死亡登记制度。低年资医生需填写死亡证明。严格按照说明进行操作并正确输入信息十分重要。死亡证明分为以下两部分。

Since 1838 there has been an enforced system of registration of birth and deaths in England and Wales. As a junior doctor, you may be asked to complete a death certificate. It is important to follow the instructions carefully and make correct entries. A death certificate has two sections:

- 死亡的直接原因。
- A direct cause of death

- 导致死亡的影响因素。
- Contributory factors to the cause of death

不论出生地点在哪，法律规定需对所有出生进行登记。据此可准确地知道在家中或在产房中分娩的婴儿比例。

It is a legal requirement to register all births irrespective of the place of birth. Therefore, it is possible to accurately know what proportion of babies have been born at home or in obstetric units.

使用这些数据，还可以详细研究每千人口新生儿出生率和死亡率的变化。出生率减去死亡率可得出人口的年增长率。

Using these data, it is also possible to study in detail the changes in birth rates and death rates per 1000 population. Subtraction of the death rates from the birth rates gives the annual growth rate of a population.

3. 医院病情统计（Hospital Episode Statistics, HES）

医院病情统计（HES）收集了住院患者病历记录中的管理信息和临床数据。临床数据包括患者主要疾病和伴随疾病的情况，以及手术记录和日期。管理信息包括患者开始排队住院的日期、入院的方式和日期、所在科室、出院或死亡的日期，以及出院或转院的目的地。该数据提供了总体医疗活动的数据，如手术次数（如子宫切除术和剖宫产），可用于调整医院服务，例如根据当地对产床的需求进行相应调整。

Hospital Episode Statistics (HES) collects inpatient administrative and clinical data transcribed from patients' case notes. The clinical data include the principal condition causing admission, other relevant conditions and the description and date of any operation performed. The administrative data include the date the patient was put on the waiting list, the source and date of admission, the specialty, the date of discharge or death and the destination on discharge or transfer. The data provide overall activity data such as number of operations performed such as hysterectomies and caesarean sections, and this information can be used in the planning of hospital services such as local needs for maternity beds.

（1）死亡率统计（Mortality rates statistics）：以下是根据患者住院信息计算得出的。自 1952 年以来，英国的孕产妇死亡率数据每 3 年进行一次报告。该报告显示产后出血、妊娠期高血压疾病、感染和静脉栓塞病仍然是孕产妇死亡的主要原因。自 2012 年以来，孕产妇死亡率报告改为每年一次，每次有一个主题，该报告对于减少孕产妇死亡作出了更大的贡献。英国国家患者结局和死亡保密调查（NCEPOD）年度报告分析了围术期死亡的数据，称只有 22% 的

高危患者在重症监护病房得到护理，并指出没有为患者提供恰当的治疗导致了患者死亡。

These are calculated from hospital admissions. The maternal mortality data in the UK have been reported through a triennial report since 1952. These reports tell us that major postpartum haemorrhage, hypertensive disease of pregnancy, infection and venous embolic disease remain the major causes for maternal deaths. However, since 2012, the maternal mortality report is now published on an annual basis and addresses one particular theme making a bigger contribution towards maternal deaths. The *National Confidential Enquiry into Patient Outcome and Death* (NCEPOD) annual report analyzes data on perioperative deaths and has reported that only 22% of the high-risk group were cared for in a critical care unit, thus receiving suboptimal care leading to their deaths.

英国对每年的围产期死亡率（PNMR）数据进行了收集，其中包括妊娠期死产数和每 1000 例活产中新生儿生后一周死亡数。这些数据包括所有妊娠 20 周以上或胎儿体重 500g 以上的死亡。早产是围产期死亡的最常见原因，其次是先天缺陷和小于胎龄儿。PNMR 是用于比较一个国家内各产科机构的医疗服务质量的主要指标，并用于比较世界各国的医疗质量。英国皇家妇产科学院（RCOG）已获得资助对所有胎儿死亡进行深入的研究，以查明每个病历中胎儿死亡的根本原因，从而改变产前或产时处理策略以减少胎儿死亡率。RCOG 发布了《每个婴儿都很重要》的年度报告，具体可登录 www.rcog.org.uk 查看。

Data on perinatal mortality rates (PNMRs) are collected annually. They include the number of stillbirths during pregnancy and deaths in the first week of life per 1000 live births. These data include all fetuses after 20 weeks of gestation or 500 g. Pre-term births are the most common cause of perinatal death, followed by birth defects and small-for-gestation babies. PNMR is a major marker used to compare the quality of health care delivery among maternity units within a country and to compare quality of care worldwide. The Royal College of Obstetricians and Gynaecologists (RCOG) has been funded to study all stillbirths in depth to identify underlying cause(s) in each case to see if antenatal or intrapartum policy changes within obstetric units can reduce these losses. The RCOG publishes an annual report, Every Baby Counts, which is accessible at www.rcog.org.uk.

（2）发病率统计（Morbidity rates statistics）：英国利用患者的住院数据来查看特定疾病的发病率：如通过计算严重产后出血（失血量＞2.5L），产后转入重症监护室，孕期脑卒中、肺栓塞和深静脉血栓形成等的发病率来获取妊娠相关并发症发生率。在苏格兰，所有严重的母体并发症均报告给 NHS 苏格

兰国家医疗服务质量改进协会，该协会在年度报告（接近过失事件调查）中对比了所有产科机构的调查数据。

Hospital admissions data are utilized to look at the morbidity data related to specific diseases: for example, pregnancyrelated morbidity data are captured by calculating the incidence of major postpartum haemorrhage (blood loss >2.5 L), admission to intensive care unit following delivery, stroke during pregnancy, pulmonary embolism and deep vein thrombosis, etc. In Scotland all cases of severe maternal morbidity are reported to NHS Quality Improvement Scotland, and an annual report (near-miss survey) is published showing comparative data for all the obstetric units.

4. 研究与数据链（Research and data linkage）

数据库的相互关联为我们提供了疾病的全过程以及单一个体患不同疾病的情况。不同数据库之间的相互关联有助于进行质控，例如，了解患者术后因深静脉血栓再次入院率，或者二次手术率。

Linkage of records gives us a picture of the full course of illness and of the different illnesses occurring in the life of an individual. It is also possible to use record linkage between different databases to develop quality indicators such as patients' re-admission rates within 28 days with a diagnosis of deep vein thrombosis or the number of patients having a re-operation.

（二）数据保护法（Data Protection Act）

英国和澳大利亚的《数据保护法》力求在维护个人权利和合法使用个人信息（有时影响个人利益）之间取得平衡。保存或处理个人数据的员工必须遵守以下原则。

The Data Protection Acts in the UK and Australia seek to strike a balance between the rights of the individual and the sometimes-competing interests of those legitimate reasons for using personal information. Staff who hold or process personal data must abide by the following principles.

个人信息必须符合以下。

Personal information must be:

- 公平合法地处理。
- Fairly and lawfully processed
- 为有限的目的而处理。
- Processed for limited purposes
- 足够，相关且不过多。
- Adequate, relevant and not excessive
- 准确且最新。

- Accurate and up to date
- 保留信息的期限合理。
- Not kept longer than necessary
- 处理个人信息要保护其权利。
- Processed in accordance with the individual's rights
- 时刻保护信息的安全。
- Kept secure at all times
- 不得将信息转移到其他国家，除非该国对个人有足够的保护。
- Not transferred to other countries unless the country has adequate protection for individuals

1. 通用数据保护条例（GDPR），2018 年（General Data Protection Regulations, 2018）

旧数据保护法是在 20 世纪 90 年代制定的，未能跟上技术变革的步伐。《通用数据保护条例》（GDPR）于 2018 年 5 月 25 日出台，更新了个人数据使用规则。这是欧盟法律中针对欧盟和欧洲经济区（EEA）所有个人的数据保护和隐私保护的强制性法规。它还解决了将个人数据导出到 EEA 和欧盟以外的问题。因此，即使在欧洲经济区和欧盟之外注册，但在欧洲范围内运营的公司和组织也必须遵守该条例。

The previous data protection laws were put in place during the 1990s and have not been able to keep pace with the levels of technological change. The General Data Protection Regulations (GDPR) were introduced on 25 May 2018 to update personal data rules. It is a mandatory regulation in EU law on data protection and privacy for all individuals within the European Union and European Economic Area (EEA). It also addresses export of personal data outside the EEA and EU. Therefore even companies and organizations registered outside the EEA and EU but operating within Europe must comply with this regulation.

实际上 GDPR 为人们提供了访问公司和组织中他们自己信息的新权利，这些组织有义务更好地管理数据，否则有承担罚款的风险。

Essentially the GDPR offers new rights for people to access the information companies/organizations hold about them, and there are obligations for organizations for better management of data or to risk a new regimen of fines.

GDPR 中的两个关键术语是个人数据和敏感数据。个人数据是可以直接或间接识别出个体的信息。可能是名称、地址，甚至是 IP 地址。它包括自动生成的个人数据，以及可识别出个人的匿名数据。

The two key terms in the GDPR involve personal and sensitive data. Personal data can be anything that allows a *living* person to be identified directly or indirectly. This may be name, address or even an IP address. It includes automated personal data and anonymized data if a person can be identified.

敏感数据包括特殊类型的信息，涉及性取向、宗教信仰、政治见解和种族信息等。

Sensitive personal data include special categories of information. These involve sexual orientation, religious beliefs, political opinions, racial information, etc.

根据 GDPR，个人数据的使用必须符合以下原则。

Under GDPR, personal data use must be:

- 合理（用诚实善意的方式使用数据）。

  - Fair (defined as good-faith approach to data use)

- 合法（需要符合相关法律）。

  - Lawful (requires compliance with any applicable law)

- 透明（进行通知和必要的交流）。

  - Transparent (this includes the notification and related communication obligation)

- 法律依据——数据处理应符合以下条件之一：知情同意、合同、法律义务、重大利益、公共任务和合法利益。

  - Legal basis-data processing should have one of the following conditions: consent, contract, legal obligation, vital interests, public task and legitimate interest

此外，如果个人数据与健康有关，也必须符合其他相关法律。其中最相关的是以下内容。

In addition, where the personal data relate to health, another legal basis must apply. The most relevant of these will be:

- 卫生保健条款。

  - The provision of health care

- 明确的知情同意。

  - Explicit consent

- 对于无法进行知情同意的患者，保护他们的切身利益。

  - Protection of vital interests of an individual where they cannot consent

GDPR 还详细说明了数据主体的权利。患者对于他们的数据有新的权利。

The GDPR also specifies data subject rights. Patients have new rights over their data.

- 知情权，由隐私条款规定。

  - The right to be informed, usually covered by privacy notices

- 有权看自己的病历记录，无论是电子的还是纸质的。

  - The right of access to case notes, whether electronic or paper

- 修改权。

  - The right to rectification

- 删除权。

  - The right to erasure

- 限制处理权。

  - The right to restrict processing

- 数据携带权。

  - The right to data portability

- 反对权。

  - The right to object

- 自动决策和资料收集相关的权利。

  - Rights in relation to automated decision-making and profiling

GDPR 还建议使用可靠的方法传输数据。如果通过互联网传输数据，则应使用加密的通信协议。传真机应作为不得已的方式，只有具有合法权利的人才能使用传真机。

The GDPR also advises using reliable methods for transmitting data. If transmitting data over the Internet, an encrypted communication protocol should be used. Fax machines should be used as a last resort, and fax machines should only be accessible to people with legitimate rights.

良好的旧邮政系统被认为更为可靠。

The good old postal system is still considered to be more reliable.

2. Caldicott 原则（Caldicott principles）

在英国，《Caldicott 报告》（1997 年）建议在每个 NHS 组织中任命一名 Caldicott 管理员，负责处理患者信息，并确保信息传递时（即通过口头、书面、电子信息或其他方式）符合 Caldicott 原则。

In the UK the Caldicott Report (1997) recommended the

appointment of a Caldicott Guardian in each NHS organization and that staff who handle patient-identifiable information ensure that the Caldicott principles are met whenever information is transferred, i.e. by word of mouth, written, by electronic or any other means.

当进行临床审计，需要审查病历记录时，必须寻求医院的 Caldicott 管理员的允许。这样可确保遵守信息管理的原则，并且提取的数据是匿名的。不得将数据存储在私人计算机上。只能使用授权加密的 USB 驱动器。

When you consider undertaking a clinical audit which would require review of case notes, you must seek permission from the Caldicott Guardian of your hospital. This process ensures that you observe the principles of information governance and the data extracted are anonymized. You must not store data on your private computer. You can only use authorized encrypted USB drives.

（三）社交媒体（Social media）

社交媒体是当今社会生活的重要部分。大众最为熟悉的社交媒体网络是 Facebook、Twitter、Instagram 和 Snapchat。在每个平台中有一些主题性的网络，如 LinkedIn、Mumsnet、Patients Like Me、Metoo、博客、视频共享等。

Social media forms an important part in today's practice. The most familiar social media networks are Facebook, Twitter, Instagram and Snapchat. Within each platform there can be thematic networks like LinkedIn, Mumsnet, Patients Like Me, Metoo, blogs, video sharing, etc.

据估计，英国 60% 的成年人在使用某种形式的社交媒体。社交媒体对年轻人的吸引率更高。如果医生和卫生保健从业人员与社交媒体合作，可能会带来潜在的利益和风险。专业人员使用社交网络后可使大众获得健康相关信息，但在维护隐私性、专业性和个人界限方面存在困难。因此，所有医生都必须了解并遵守通用医学委员会对使用社交媒体的指导。

It is estimated that 60% of the UK adult population use some form of social media. The uptake amongst the younger population is higher. There are potential benefits and risks for doctors and health care professionals if they are engaging with social media. Whilst there are advantages of networking professionally and socially and the public accessing health-related information from professionals, challenges exist in maintaining confidentiality and professional and personal boundaries. It is therefore important that all doctors be aware of and adhere to the General Medical Council's guidance on the use of social media.

二、循证卫生保健（Evidence-based health care）

基于循证医学的临床实践是系统地查阅和使用同时期的研究结果作为临床决策的依据，并且是临床管理中不可分割的部分。为了促进循证医学的发展，需要进行以下步骤。

Evidence-based practice is the process of systematically finding and using contemporaneous research findings as a basis for clinical decision-making and is an integral part of a clinical governance framework. In order to facilitate the development of evidence-based practice, the following processes need to be applied:

- 确定可以提出明确的临床问题的领域。
- Identify areas in practice from which clear clinical questions can be formulated.
- 从可用的文献（如指南）中找出最相关的证据。
- Identify the best related evidence from available literature such as guidelines.
- 严格评估证据的有效性和临床实用性。
- Critically appraise the evidence for validity and clinical usefulness.
- 将相关发现应用于临床实践。
- Implement and incorporate relevant findings into practice.
- 记录后续临床结局，并与预期和同行进行比较。
- Subsequently measure performance against expected outcomes or against peers.
- 通过为循证实践、教育和培训提供充足的资源，确保医务人员得到支持和发展。
- Ensure staff are supported and developed through adequate resourcing of evidence-based practice, education and training programmes.

（一）临床审计（Clinical audit）

临床审计是对临床管理质量进行系统的和批判性的分析，包括疾病的诊治流程、相关资源的使用及患者结局。临床审计旨在通过临床医生根据最佳循证医学证据检查并改进其临床处理，以改善临床管理的质量和患者结局（框 B1-1）。

A clinical audit is the systematic and critical analysis of the quality of clinical care, including the procedures used for

框 B1–1　临床审计的关键因素	Box B1.1　Key facts about clinical audits
• 临床审计不是研究，而是专注于改善对患者的管理 • 临床审计需要花时间并需要多专业人员参与 • 临床审计应该有一个明确的问题，需要根据最佳循证证据进行解决 • 临床审计需要足够的时间来设计，需要与领导层沟通，收集可靠数据，进行数据分析并将结果呈现给团队 • 一个明确的、经过深思熟虑的策略对于传播、实施和监测最佳临床实践以及改进临床管理非常重要	• A clinical audit is not research but is focused on improving patient care. • A clinical audit takes time and requires multiprofessional involvement. • A clinical audit should have a clearly defined question which needs to be addressed derived from the best evidence-based practice. • A clinical audit requires adequate time for planning, engagement with stakeholders, collecting reliable data, analyzing and then presenting the results to the team. • A clearly thought-out strategy is important to disseminate the best practice, implement it, monitor and demonstrate improvement in clinical care.

diagnosis and treatment, the associated use of resources and the resulting outcome for the patient. A clinical audit should seek to improve the quality and outcome of patient care through clinicians examining and modifying their practice according to standards of what could be achieved based on the best available evidence (Box B1.1).

临床审计的四个步骤（Four steps of a clinical audit）

（1）明确问题（Defining best practice）：确定的问题必须有助于改善临床管理质量，如剖宫产后的高感染率。

The area identified must address important aspects of practice about quality of care, such as high infection rates following caesarean section.

接下来是将描述当前临床实践情况，说明问题，并确定需要改进的地方。这可以通过查看以下资源来完成，即 RCOG 指南、苏格兰学院间指南网络（SIGN）、英国国家卫生和临床卓越研究所（NICE）、RANZCOG 关于女性健康情况的声明和 NHS 证据网站。

The next stage is to describe current practice to illustrate the problem and identify areas for improvement. This can be done by looking at resources such as the RCOG Green Top Guidelines, Scottish Intercollegiate Guidelines Network (SIGN), National Institute of Health and Clinical Excellence (NICE), RANZCOG statements on women's health and the NHS evidence website.

最终，在指南中明确一个特定的领域，这有助于定义一个"标准"（基于最佳循证医学证据阐述的良好的临床管理），根据该标准可以衡量当前的临床管理（条件）。条件包括达到标准（结构）所需的资源，以及必须采取的行动（过程）和结果（结局）。

Finally a particular area of interest is identified in the guideline that would help to define a 'standard' (a broad statement of good practice based on the best possible evidence) against which current practice can be measured (this is termed *criteria*). The criteria refer to resources used for the successful achievement of the standard (structure), the actions that must be undertaken (process) and the results (outcomes).

（2）准备监测（Preparing to monitor）：条件应易于衡量和收集相关数据，并将收集的数据在临床上进行应用。首先收集基础数据，这提供了一个可以衡量进度的起点。该标准应通过简讯和部门会议广泛传播给病房和临床人员，以使他们了解审计情况。

The criteria should be easy to measure and to collect relevant data, and the collected data are useful clinically. Baseline data are collected first, which provides a starting point from which progress can be measured. The standard should be widely disseminated through newsletters and departmental meetings to the wards and the clinical staff to make them aware of the audit.

（3）监控进度（Monitoring your achievement）：与临床管理者商定样本数量和时间框架以完成审计周期非常重要。医院信息系统人员可提供有关特定临床情况的患者数量的信息，以便估计收集数据需花费的时间。接下来需明确谁负责在审计软件收集和记录数据，以便及时反馈。

It is important to agree on a sample size and time frame with your clinical supervisor to complete the audit cycle. The hospital information system manager may have information about the number of patients with particular clinical conditions so that you can estimate how long it might take to collect your data. The next step would be to agree who will be collecting data and who will be recording it on an audit software package in order to generate timely feedback.

（4）改善计划（Planning for improvement）：一旦

收集了审计数据，应完成审计情况总结并仔细检查结果，以便为临床团队提供建设性反馈。应与专业小组讨论结果，征求他们关于解释结果和制订行动计划的意见。临床管理较好的方面和需要改善的方面均需要明确记录。应指定专人实施和监控对于现有政策的适当更改。

Once the audit data have been collected, the audit summary should be completed and the results carefully looked at in order to provide constructive feedback to the clinical team. The results should be discussed with the professional groups to ask for their comments for the interpretation of results and action planning. Areas of good practice are clearly highlighted, and areas that need to be addressed are clearly documented. A named individual should be identified so that appropriate changes in the policy can be implemented and monitored.

重要的是要记住，临床审计是一个持续的过程，以及一次临床审计通常会导致第二次临床审计，以证明第一次审计的方面已经进行了重大改变，使得医院的政策得到更新或采用了新的管理方式，以达到国家标准。因此，进行临床审计的医生有责任撰写详细的报告，并就下一小组的医生继续完成相同的主题提出适当的建议，以确保第二或第三次审计完成。

It is important to remember that a clinical audit is a continuing process, and one clinical audit quite often leads to a second clinical audit to demonstrate that the first audit cycle has made measurable changes leading to redefining unit policy or adopting new ways of delivering care to meet national standards. Therefore it is the responsibility of the doctor undertaking a clinical audit to write a detailed report and to make appropriate recommendations on how the next group of foundation doctors could continue with the same theme in order to ensure that the second or third audit cycle is completed.

（二）英国国家临床审计（National clinical audits）

孕产妇死亡率和并发症发生率数据被用作全球各国和国际衡量妇产科质量的指标。若孕产妇死亡有产科原因，并且死亡发生在妊娠期或分娩后的 42 天内，产科原因被归类为直接原因。孕产妇死亡的直接原因最常见的是严重的产后出血、妊娠期高血压疾病、社区获得性感染和深静脉血栓形成。间接原因包括非产科原因，如在分娩后 1 年内发生自杀。专家小组对每例孕产妇死亡进行了深入分析。围产儿死亡率也进行了收集，对数据的分析可提供围产儿死亡原因的数据和趋势，围产儿死亡的主要原因是不明原因的胎儿死亡和与早产有关的死亡。

Maternal mortality and morbidity data are used as quality indicators for maternity services nationally and internationally. The maternal deaths are categorized as direct causes where there are obstetric causes and the death occurs during pregnancy or within the first 42 days following delivery. The commonest causes of direct maternal deaths are major postpartum haemorrhage, hypertensive disease of pregnancy, community-acquired infection and deep vein thrombosis. The indirect causes of death include non-obstetric causes such as suicide occurring within 1 year of childbirth. Every maternal death is analyzed in depth by a panel of experts. Similarly, perinatal mortality data are also collected. Their analyses provide data and trends on causes of perinatal deaths, and the main causes are unexplained stillbirths and deaths related to prematurity.

（三）临床指南（Clinical guidelines）

临床指南的定义为系统地制订的声明，以帮助医疗人员就特定临床情况作出适当的医疗管理和决策。RCOG 的 Green Top 指南是一个极好的资源。

Clinical guidelines have been defined as systematically developed statements to assist practitioners in patient management decisions about appropriate health care for specific clinical circumstances. The Green Top Guidelines of the RCOG are an excellent resource.

临床指南的制订是一个相当耗时的过程，从开始到完成可能需要 18～24 个月的时间。在早期阶段，先就拟制订指南中的临床问题达成一致，从而提供了框架便于对可用证据进行系统评价。通过使用"推荐等级、评价、发展和评估"（GRADE）工作组对文献进行综合，并对证据进行分级。对于许多治疗方案，没有随机对照试验或系统评价也是可以的，这种情况下观察性研究可能会提供更好的证据。

The development of clinical guidelines is a fairly timeconsuming procedure and it can take between 18 and 24 months to develop the guideline from inception to completion of the task. At an earlier stage the clinical questions within a guideline are agreed. They provide the framework for the systematic review of the available evidence. The literature is synthesized and evidence is graded by using the Grading of Recommendations, Assessment, Development and Evaluation (GRADE) working group. It is also accepted that for many therapies, randomized controlled trials or systematic reviews of randomized controlled trials may not be available. In those instances observational data may provide better evidence, as is generally the case for their outcomes.

GRADE 证据级别：从 1 级（对随机对照试验进行的系统评价）到 4 级（专家意见）：更多详细信息请访问 www.sign.ac.uk。一旦针对每个临床问题进行了证据整理，就需对证据进行评估和审查。

GRADE evidence levels: They are graded from level 1 (randomized controlled trials for a systematic review) to level 4 (expert opinion): more details are available at www.sign.ac.uk. Once the evidence has been collated for each clinical question, it is then appraised and reviewed.

根据证据水平，在临床指南中提出建议。

Based on the level of evidence, recommendations are made within a clinical guideline.

推荐等级：基于证据的指南推荐等级为 A 级（基于 Meta 分析、系统评价或随机对照试验），医生的临床常规作为推荐共识（www.rcog.org.uk）。

Grading of recommendation: The recommendations for guidelines based on evidence are graded as Grade A (based on meta-analysis, systematic reviews or randomized controlled trials) to Good Practice point where clinicians make a consensus recommendation (www.rcog.org.uk).

综合管理路径被描述为患者在医疗保健系统内诊治疾病的过程，其中包括患者从社区医院到二级和三级医院的所有过程。综合管理路径里的每个步骤都应有明确的诊疗核查表，以确保医务人员遵守了诊疗常规，并提供了恰当的处理。

Integrated care pathways have been described as the journey of a patient through all interfaces within the health care system and should take care of all the steps of patient journey from primary care to secondary and tertiary care. Each stage of an integrated care pathway should have a clearly defined checklist of recommended measures to ensure that the care providers have adhered to those recommendations and appropriate care has been provided.

临床指南中的诊疗原则可能需要改动，以适宜各医院具体应用（形成本地诊疗常规），这可促进开发和使用更为便捷的临床路径，更容易遵循常规对患者进行诊治，并能监测诊治过程。

The principles enshrined in a clinical guideline need to be adapted for local use (local protocol) so that a care pathway is developed for easy access to instructions on how to look after a patient within the local service provision and adherence to the local protocol can be monitored.

（四）研究（Research）

研究的主要目的是普及新知识，而审计的目的是监测临床管理是否标准。

The primary aim of research is to drive generalizable new knowledge, whereas the aim of an audit is to measure standards of care.

对于临床研究，需要经人员构成合理的研究伦理委员会批准申请，而临床审计常不需要此类批准。

For clinical research, application is made for approval from a suitably constituted research ethics committee, whereas no such approval is normally required for a clinical audit.

进行研究时要从法律和道义上最大限度地尊重参与者及其隐私，即使该研究与临床管理无关。获得明确的同意后才能将有个人信息的数据用于医学研究，尤其是在非临床工作人员可接触到数据的多中心研究或二次研究。管理和使用研究数据库人员的技能、态度和承诺对于保护数据主体的隐私很重要。

There is a legal and a moral impetus to ensure that research is conducted with maximum respect for participants and their privacy, even if the research is not linked to clinical care. It is generally believed that explicit consent should be obtained to use identifiable personal data for medical research, particularly for multi-centre or secondary research where people who are not part of the clinical team need access to data. The skills, attitude and commitment of the people who manage and use a research database are important to protect the privacy of its data subjects.

研究中普遍存在的不当行为得到了普遍关注。为职业晋升或获得经济报酬而发表错误研究的不诚实行为破坏了公众对医学研究的信心。

Concern has been expressed regarding widespread misconduct in research. This dishonesty in publishing erroneous findings in order to promote careers or to get financial rewards has undermined public confidence in medical research.

研究类型包括如下几种类型。

Types of research studies

（1）描述性研究（Descriptive studies）：此类研究可用于检验其他研究提出的病因学假说。例如，流行病学研究首先发现了烟草的慢性毒性作用及其与肺癌的关系。描述性研究也常用于证实其他来源的疑虑，例如，母体己烯雌酚治疗引起的儿童期阴道癌，母体孕期高血糖导致巨大儿，以及石棉暴露引起胸膜间皮瘤等。与此相似，有关多发性硬化症的数据显示此病在美国北部各州的非洲裔美国人和白种人中发生率相同，该观察性研究表明，环境对于疾病发生率的影响是至关重要。

Descriptive studies provide information that can be used to test an aetiological hypothesis generated by other research methods. For example, the long-term toxic effects of tobacco and the relationship to the development of lung cancer were first discovered by epidemiological studies.

Quite often descriptive studies have been used to substantiate suspicions arising from other sources, e.g. vaginal carcinoma in childhood resulting from maternal stilboestrol therapy, maternal hyperglycaemia during pregnancy associated with large-for-dates babies and pleural mesothelioma from asbestos exposure. Similarly, data on multiple sclerosis show that it occurs with the same degree of frequency in African Americans and Caucasians in the northern U.S. states. This observation suggests that environmental influences are critically important in determining whether the disease is common or rare.

（2）分析性研究（Analytical studies）：此类研究指的是在个体而不是人群中进行的两种流行病学观察后，提供证据表明特定事件可能是特定疾病的原因。其中，病例对照研究是比较患有疾病的人与未患疾病的人；队列研究是比较暴露于可疑原因与未暴露的人群。两种类型的研究回答了两个不同的问题。

Two kinds of epidemiological observations are made in groups of individuals rather than populations and provide evidence that a particular event may be a cause of a particular disease. Case *control studies* compare people with the disease and those without it. *Cohort studies* compare people exposed to the suspected cause and those not exposed. The two types of studies answer two different questions.

为了解释这一点，我们假设需要调查产钳助产对婴儿头部造成的创伤是否会导致脑损伤（可表现为儿童癫痫）。

To explain this, suppose that investigation is required to determine whether delivery by forceps and the accompanying trauma to the infant's head can result in brain damage, which can then manifest itself as childhood epilepsy.

病例对照研究将比较研究组癫痫儿童和对照组非癫痫儿童的产科史。如果发现研究组产钳助产的比例超过了对照组，则表明产钳助产可能是癫痫的原因。但是还有许多其他导致癫痫的因素，因此在癫痫人群中，只有一小部分病例可归因于产钳助产。该比例可以通过使用数学公式来计算。

A *case control study* would involve comparing the obstetric histories of a group of epileptic children with those of a control group of non-epileptic children. If it is found that the proportion of epileptic children with a history of forceps delivery exceeded the proportion of control children, this would suggest that forceps delivery may be a cause of epilepsy; but there are many other determinants of epilepsy so that among the group of epileptics only a small percentage of cases may be attributed to forceps delivery. This proportion can be calculated by using a mathematical formula.

针对同一问题的队列研究将比较产钳助产的儿童与正常分娩的儿童。如果发现产钳助产分娩的孩子发生癫痫的比例超过了未用产钳的孩子，则表明产钳助产与癫痫有关并且可能是癫痫的原因。产钳助产并不一定会导致癫痫，这种情况只发生在小部分的儿童中。通过使用数学计算，可以计算出超额或归因风险。

A *cohort study* of the same problem would compare a group of children delivered by forceps with a group of children delivered normally. If it is found that the proportion of forceps-delivered children who developed epilepsy exceeded the proportion of normally developed children, this would suggest that forceps delivery is associated with and may be a cause of epilepsy. Forceps delivery does not invariably lead to epilepsy, which occurs in only a small percentage of children delivered in this way. By using mathematical calculations, it is possible to calculate the excess or attributable risk.

（五）临床试验（Clinical trials）

临床试验用于在医学研究和药物开发中收集安全有效的数据以进行健康干预。临床试验设计的目的包括以下几个方面。

Clinical trials are carried out in medical research and drug development to allow safety and efficacy data to be collected for health interventions. A clinical trial may be designed to:

- 评估新药的安全性和有效性，如抗生素类。
  - Assess the safety and effectiveness of new medication, e.g. antibiotics
- 评估常用药物不同剂量的安全性和有效性，例如在第三产程中使用 5U 催产素代替 10U。
  - Assess the safety and effectiveness of a different dosage of medication than is commonly used, e.g. 5 IU of oxytocin instead of 10-IU dose for the third stage of labour
- 评估手术器械的安全性和有效性，如腹腔镜手术器械。
  - Assess the safety and effectiveness of a surgical device, e.g. laparoscopic surgical instruments
- 比较两个或多个已经批准的干预措施的有效性，如比较药物 1 和药物 2。
  - Compare the effectiveness of two or more already approved interventions, e.g. comparing medication 1 against medication 2

临床试验通常分为三个阶段。

Clinical trials are usually conducted in three phases:

- 第 1 阶段用于少数健康人，以检测药物是否安全。

- *Phase 1* to test the treatment in a few healthy people to learn whether it is safe to take.

- 第 2 阶段用于少数患者，以检测在短期内是否对这种疾病有效。

- *Phase 2* to test the treatment in a few patients to see if it is active against the disease in the short term.

- 第 3/4 期临床试验通常在不同的诊所或医院，对数百至数千名患者进行应用。试验过程中通常将新疗法与已使用的疗法进行比较，或者少数情况下也将新疗法与未使用的疗法进行比较。

- Phase 3/4 trials to test the treatment on several hundred to several thousand patients, often at many different clinics or hospitals. These trials usually compare the new treatment with either a treatment already in use or occasionally with no treatment.

随机临床试验可以是下列几种。

Randomized clinical trials can be:

(1) 双盲：参与研究的受试者和研究人员均不知道受试者接受了哪种治疗。这种双盲的目的是为了防止偏倚，以使医师不知道哪位患者正在接受治疗，哪位患者在使用安慰剂，或者在两药比较研究中，不知道该患者是使用了药物 A 还是药物 B。

- *Double blind*: The subjects and the researchers involved in the study do not know which study treatment they receive. This blinding is to prevent bias so that the physician should not know which patient was getting the study treatment and which patient was getting the placebo or, in a two-drug comparison study, whether it was drug A or drug B.

(2) 安慰剂对照：使用安慰剂（假治疗）可去除药物的治疗作用。假治疗与活性药物治疗紧密对照十分重要。对两组患者进行治疗效果和不良反应的密切监测。

- *Placebo controlled:* The use of a placebo (fake treatment) allows the researchers to isolate the effects of the study treatment. It is important that the dummy treatment is closely matched to the active drug treatment. The patients in both study groups are monitored very closely for the impact of treatment and the side effects experienced by patients in both groups.

所有临床试验均应获得伦理委员会批准并由专家小组监督。在招募患者参加临床试验之前必须签署知情同意书，这一点十分重要。在临床试验开始

之前患者应同意随机化处理。

All clinical trials should be approved by the ethics committee and overseen by a panel of experts. It is important that before recruiting a patient into a clinical trial, an informed consent has been signed. The process of randomization is agreed to before the start of a clinical trial.

临床研究人员有责任确保受试者的安全得到了密切监测，以发现任何不良结局。因此，药物的临床试验需要排除育龄期女性、孕妇和（或）在研究期间怀孕的女性。

It is the responsibility of the clinical researcher to ensure that the safety of the subjects is closely monitored for any adverse outcomes. Therefore clinical trials of drugs are designed to exclude women of childbearing age, pregnant women and/or women who become pregnant during the study.

药物试验的结果被发送到适当的国家许可机构。

The results of the drug trials are sent to the appropriate national licensing authority.

（六）临床管理（Clinical governance）

临床管理被定义为通过降低临床风险来持续改善患者管理的框架（框 B1-2）。

Clinical governance has been defined as a framework for the continual improvement of patient care by minimizing clinical risks (Box B1.2).

（七）风险管理（Risk management）

风险管理即"建立良好的临床规范，减少不良事件的发生"。临床风险定义为，与预期的治疗、护理、治疗或诊断结果有出入的临床错误，可能会导致不良结果。例如，如果产科患者在剖宫产后发生伤口感染，将导致患者住院时间延长、不适感增加，以及该部门工作人员的工作量和花费增加。重要的是要考虑围绕这一情况的更广泛的问题，例如，病房的清洁未遵守感染控制条例，未能遵循预防脓毒症的国家指南，以及解决员工的教育和培训需求。每个部门都应制订临床风险策略，并建立适当的系统来报告、监测和评估临床不良事件和接近过失事件。接近过失事件被描述为"可能对患者/医务人员造成不良后果的潜在有害事件"。同样，应该建立投诉报告、监测以及从这些投诉中学习的系统，以改善患者护理。

Risk management simply means 'to develop good practice and reduce the occurrence of harmful or adverse incidents'. Clinical risk is defined as 'a clinical error to be at variance from

框 B1-2 团队质量提升的关键点	Box B1.2 Key attributes associated with promotion of a quality organization
• 整个团队采用综合的质量改进方法。 • 根据专业和临床需求培养领导技能。 • 存在促进循证医学发展的基础设施。 • 重视创新，并在团队内外分享优秀的临床实践。 • 风险管理系统到位。 • 用一种主动的途径来报告和处理不良事件，并从中吸取教训。 • 认真对待投诉，并采取措施防止再次发生。 • 识别不良的临床实践，从而防止对患者或工作人员造成潜在伤害。 • 临床实践和专业进步与临床管理保持一致。	• There is an integrated approach to quality improvement throughout the whole organization. • Leadership skills are developed in line with professional and clinical needs. • Infrastructures exist that foster the development of evidence-based practices. • Innovations are valued and good practices are shared within and without the organization. • Risk management systems are in place. • There is a proactive approach to reporting, dealing with and learning from untoward incidents. • Complaints are taken seriously and actions taken to prevent any recurrence. • Poor clinical performance is recognized, thus preventing potential harm to patients or staff. • Practice and professional development are aligned and integral to the clinical governance framework.

高质量的临床数据可用于有效监测患者管理和临床结局（NHS 白皮书，DH 1997）

Clinical data are of the best quality and can be used effectively to monitor patient care and clinical outcomes [White Paper *The New NHS; Modern, Dependable* (DH 1997)].

intended treatment, care, therapeutic intervention or diagnostic result; there may be an untoward outcome or not'. For example, if patients in an obstetric unit develop wound infections following caesarean section, this results in an extended length of stay, increased patient discomfort and increased workload and cost for staff working in that unit. It is important to consider the broader issues surrounding this situation, such as ward cleanliness, lack of adherence to infection control policies, failure to follow national guidelines on sepsis prophylaxis and addressing education and training needs of the staff. Each unit should have a clinical risk strategy and a system in place for reporting, monitoring and evaluating clinical incidences and near-misses. Near-misses have been described as 'potentially harmful incident that could have adverse consequences for the patient/carer'. Similarly, there should be a system in place for *complaints reporting*, monitoring and learning from these complaints to improve patient care.

美国国家临床过失信托计划（CNST）成立于 1995 年。对于专门应用于妇科的 CNST，每个部门根据其规模和 CNST 标准认证的等级支付保险费，并获得临床风险管理的补助。CNST 认证分为三个等级，达到的等级越高，补助就越高。CNST 促进了风险管理的改进和临床风险的降低。

The National Clinical Negligence Scheme for Trusts (CNST) was established in 1995. With CNST specifically in obstetrics, each unit pays a premium based on the size of the unit and level achieved through CNST standards and receives a discount for managing clinical risks. There are three levels of CNST accreditation: the higher the level you achieve, the higher the discount. It has been recognized that the CNST

standards have done much to advance risk management and reduce clinical risks.

临床事件报告（Clinical incident reporting）

医务人员和患者需要临床事件报告，以发现个人或团队无法提供符合标准的临床服务的部分。事件报告提供了监测不良事件和接近过失事件的框架，使得能够尽快采取行动，汲取经验教训，对临床工作进行审查并共享信息，以防止再次发生。以监测三度和四度会阴裂伤为例，对其进行事件报告和信息整理后，每月的报告中将确定三度或四度会阴裂伤的病例数量是否随着器械助产增加而增加。该监测将评估这些医生是否具有适当的技能，以及是否受过训练和受到监督。

Clinical incident reporting is required for staff and patients in highlighting any areas where an individual or organization fails to deliver the appropriate standard of care. Incident reporting offers a framework for the detection of untoward incidents and near-misses, which enable actions to be taken and lessons to be learned, practices to be reviewed and information to be shared to prevent any recurrence. Let us take an example of monitoring third- and fourth-degree perineal tears in an obstetric unit. These incidents are reported, and information is collated. Monthly reports will identify if the number of third- or fourth-degree tears are increasing following instrumental deliveries. That observation would call into question whether the doctors undertaking those procedures are appropriately skilled, trained and supervised.

三、结论（Conclusion）

重要的是要意识到，临床管理是要确保持续不断的质量改进，这只有通过拥有适当团队支持，进行了最佳临床实践的，意志坚定并持续努力的临床和非临床工作人员才能实现。质量改进基于以下的系统和流程。

It is important to appreciate that clinical governance is about assuring sustained, continuous quality improvement that can only be achieved by determined and conscious efforts by the clinical and non-clinical staff who have the appropriate support of their organization to deliver best practice. Quality improvement is based around the following robust systems and processes:

- 临床风险管理和临床审计。

  - clinical risk management and clinical audit

- 持续的临床实践和专业发展。

  - continued practice and professional development

- 在 NHS 组织内实施和持续进行的专业发展。

  - implementing and continuing professional development within the NHS organization

- 研究与发展。

  - research and development

- 循证医学。

  - evidence-based health care.

603

附录 C 妇产科相关法律问题
Medicolegal aspects of obstetrics and gynaecology

Roger Pepperell 著   杨慧霞 译   石玉华 校

学习目标	LEARNING OUTCOMES
学习本附录后你应当能够：	After studying this appendix you should be able to:
知识标准	**Knowledge criteria**
• 讨论 16 岁以下孩子（Fraser 能力）和弱势成年人的隐私和知情同意问题。	• Discuss the issues of confidentiality and consent in under-16-year-olds (Fraser competency) and vulnerable adults.
• 列举流产、性侵和辅助生殖技术相关的法规，以及胎儿和孕妇的相对法律地位。	• Outline the legal regulation of abortion, sexual offenders and assisted reproduction and the relative legal status of the fetus and the mother.
• 描述儿童保护原则。	• Describe the principles of child protection.
• 描述知情同意的原则和相关法律问题。	• Describe the principles and legal issues surrounding informed consent.
临床能力	**Clinical competencies**
• 签署妇产科常见手术的知情同意书。	• Obtain informed consent for the common procedures in obstetrics and gynaecology.
专业技能和态度	**Professional skills and attitudes**
• 了解孕妇的合法权利和相关法规。	• Be aware of the legal rights of and provisions for pregnant women.

一、知情同意书的原则和法律问题
（ Principles and legal issues around informed consent ）

当患者同意接受外科手术或特定的治疗方案时，必须向患者解释其利益和风险的影响，或者获得对这种治疗的知情同意。医生必须获得患者对任何药物或外科手术治疗的知情同意，这是医学和法律的基本原则。在未获得患者的知情同意时，手术可能构成对患者的侵犯或侵害行为。

When a woman agrees to a surgical procedure or a specific method of treatment, it is essential that the implications of benefits and risks are explained to her or informed consent to such treatment is obtained. Indeed, it is a fundamental law of medical and legal practice that a doctor must obtain consent from the patient for any medical or surgical treatment and that without appropriate consent, a procedure may constitute an act of assault or trespass against the person.

然后，患者必须对任何建议的治疗方案都有足够的了解，才能做出有效的选择。同意书应提供患者同意进行该手术的证据，只有在患者确实已经了解该手术的本质和意义的情况下，该同意书才有意义。

Second, the patient must receive sufficient knowledge of any proposed treatment to make a valid choice about whether to consent. The consent form provides evidence that consent has been given for a procedure, but it only has meaning if it is evident that the patient did understand the nature and implications of the procedure.

在向任何患者解释手术的本质时，说明手术的目的和潜在的并发症十分重要。鉴于任何手术都可能存在一系列并发症，因此出现了一个问题，即对所有潜在并发症的解释程度，因为这可能会引起患者对一系列极低风险的事件产生过多的焦虑。

In explaining the nature of a procedure to any woman, it is important to explain the purpose of the operation and the potential complications. Given that there may be a range of complications for any operation, the question arises as to how far it is necessary to go in explaining all the potential complications, given that this may induce disproportionate anxiety about a series of very remote risks.

一般而言，应向患者解释发生率超过 1% 的不良事件，尽管这只是源于指南而非绝对数字。如果风险远低于 1% 但很严重，一旦发生就会影响生活质量，也需要详细解释，以便患者可以就是否希望手术进行决定。但是，2015 年蒙哥马利诉拉纳克郡案的案中，因没有向矮胖且患有糖尿病的母亲告知分娩时存在发生胎儿肩难产和缺氧性损伤的风险，引发了人们对如何解释风险和征得患者知情同意的新认识。法院裁定，应该向患者解释任何可能发生的重大风险，而不是仅医生认为应该告知的重大风险。这将使知情同意过程更费时，但会使患者更满意。可使用非手术方案代替手术方案时，也需要向患者进行解释。

In general terms, a risk of more than a 1% chance should be explained to the patient, although this is a guideline rather than an absolute figure. Where the risk is well under 1% but is serious and would influence the quality of life subsequently if it occurred, this also needs to be explained in detail so that an informed decision can be made by the patient as to whether she wishes to proceed. However, the 2015 ruling on *Montgomery v. Lanarkshire* where a shortstatured diabetic mother was not told about possible risk of shoulder dystocia and risk of hypoxic injury has brought in a new understanding of how risks should be explained and consent should be taken. The court ruled that whatever could be considered material risk to the patient should be explained to the patient rather than what the doctor thinks is the material risk that should be told. This would make counselling consent time consuming but more satisfying to the patient. Where non-surgical methods of treatment could be used instead of a surgical procedure, these also need to be explained to the patient.

一个常见的例子可以说明知情同意中的问题，就是行绝育术前告知患者避孕失败率。在 20 世纪 80 年代，大量的法律诉讼里患者未被告知常用绝育术式后存在较高避孕失败风险，可能造成后续妊娠。提出索赔的患者通常称没有告知避孕失败和意外妊娠的风险，如果进行了告知，则不会进行手术，或者将在术后继续服用避孕药。现今的标准做法是告知所有女性和男性患者绝育术后避孕失败风险，并记录已告知此信息。关于绝育术，应牢记月经周期的特点。如果月经量大或不规则的月经在使用口服避孕药（OCP）期间得到缓解，则在行绝育术后患者停止服用 OCP 后，月经异常复发的概率极高，如果告知患者这种可能，她很可能决定继续服用 OCP 而不是行绝育术。

A common example that addresses the issues of informed consent is the information given to patients before sterilization about potential failure rates. During the 1980s a substantial number of legal actions were based on alleged failure to inform patients that there was a significant risk of failure and that pregnancy could follow any of the commonly used sterilization procedures. The patient bringing a claim would generally allege that no advice was given about the risk of failure and subsequent pregnancy and that, had such advice been given, either the woman would not have had the operation or she would have continued to use contraception after the sterilization procedure. It is now standard practice to advise all patients, both female and male, that there is a risk of failure and to record a statement to the effect that such advice has been given. Regarding sterilization, the character of the menstrual cycle also needs to be borne in mind. Where the periods have been particularly heavy or irregular and have been controlled during treatment with the oral contraceptive pill (OCP), when the OCP is ccascd after the sterilization, the abnormal periods will almost certainly return. If the patient is made aware of this likelihood, she may well decide to just continue the OCP rather than having the sterilization performed.

男性或女性的绝育术都可能由于操作失败或再

通而失败。在女性患者体内，金属夹子可能夹错位置，放置过程中可能横切输卵管，或者未保持闭合状态。在这些情况下，怀孕通常在手术后的 6 个月内发生。避孕失败的第二个原因是输卵管或输精管再通。这可能会导致多年后妊娠，是手术不可避免的风险。尽管签署了告知手术失败风险的知情同意书，通常无法避免发生这种错误操作。

The failure of a sterilization procedure in either sex may result from a method failure or recanalization. In the female, a clip may be applied to the wrong structure, may transect the tube during application or may not remain closed. In each of these instances, pregnancy usually occurs within 6 months of the procedure. The second cause of failure is recanalization of the Fallopian tubes or, in men, the vas deferens. This may result in a pregnancy many years later and is an unavoidable risk of the procedure. Despite the signing of a consent form that records the risk of failure, errors of technique are generally indefensible.

> **！注意**
>
> 如果手术失误，知情同意书既不能保护患者，也不能保护外科医生。
>
> A consent form does not protect either the patient or the surgeon if performance of the procedure is faulty.

重要的是，必须由有资格的医生取得同意，并在解释手术的性质和潜在的并发症后与患者签署知情同意书。理想情况下，绝育手术应在卵泡期进行，或者在进行了避孕的月经周期中进行。

It is important that consent is obtained by a member of staff who is medically qualified and who signs the consent form with the patient after explaining both the nature of the procedure and the potential complications. Ideally the procedure should be performed in the follicular phase of the cycle or alternative contraception given in that cycle.

同样重要的是要确保患者姓名和手术细节信息准确无误。例如，当手术操作可能是电灼输卵管、钳夹输卵管或结扎输卵管时，仅写"绝育术"来描述手术是不够的。实际进行的术式必须写在知情同意书上。

It is also important to ensure that the details concerning the patient's name and the description of the procedure to be performed are correct. For example, it is not sufficient to write 'sterilization' to describe the operation when the procedure may be tubal cautery, clip sterilization or tubal ligation. The actual procedure to be performed must be written on the consent form.

知情同意书必须始终可见，必须在患者入院时

> **经验**
>
> 理想情况下，应由手术医生签署患者的知情同意书。鉴于知情同意书中的合理信息有限，通常的做法是在同意书中或患者病历中写上一般性声明，说明风险和手术预期的目的已向患者解释。在为医学法律案件辩护时，通常会发现这样的一般性陈述是不充分的，如果在签署知情同意书时将讨论的事项的标题记录在知情同意书上或病历中则更好。
>
> Ideally, consent should be obtained by the surgeon who is performing the procedure. There are limitations as to what can be reasonably included in a consent form, and it is common practice to include a general statement, either in the text of the consent form or in the patient's records, that the risks and the intended purpose of the procedure have been explained to the patient. Such a general statement is often found to be inadequate when defending a medicolegal case, and it is much better if headings of the matters discussed are recorded on the consent form or within the medical record at the time the consent form is signed.

和手术开始前检查知情同意书，然后才能开始手术。若手术是在术前评估 4 周后进行，应再次评估患者情况，其中包括最后一次月经的日期和情况，因为患者可能在此期间妊娠，可能希望改变以前建议的治疗方法。

The consent form must always be available and must be checked at the time of admission to hospital and in theatre before any operation is commenced. The condition of the patient at that time, including the date and normality of the last menstrual period, should also be checked, where the procedure is being done more than 4 weeks after the previous review. The patient may have conceived in the interim and wish a change in the treatment previously proposed.

二、妇产科诉讼（Litigation in obstetrics and gynaecology）

妇产科诉讼对孕产妇保健产生了深远影响。在英国和澳大利亚，该问题在一定程度上被英国国家赔偿及澳大利亚的类似赔偿所掩盖，政府为在公共卫生部门执业的所有医生和助产士提供了保险。但是，在诸如美国这样的国家，由于诉讼的风险以及为案件辩护或进行赔偿的成本较大，关闭产科部门和减少孕产妇保健工作是司空见惯的事。保险费用必须赔偿给母亲，否则产科保健工作将无法进行。现实情况是，不管出现的过错是什么，孕产妇保健

机构无法购买商业保险，除非赔偿是有上限的。美国的许多地区，妇产科医生因为他们的专业风险太大而无法购买保险。

Litigation in obstetrics and gynaecology has had a profound effect on the provision of maternity services. In the UK and Australia, the problem has been masked to some extent by Crown indemnity and its equivalent in Australia. The government provides insurance coverage for all doctors and midwives practising within the public health services. However, in countries such as the United States, closure of maternity units and the reduction of maternity services are common events because of the risk of litigation and the size of the costs to defend a case or settle the damages awarded. The costs of insurance must be passed on to the mothers, or the services cannot survive. The reality of the situation is that, regardless of the issues of fault, unless damages are capped, maternity services are often commercially uninsurable. Indeed, in many parts of the United States, obstetricians cannot purchase insurance coverage, as their specialty is too high risk.

当患者决定向其医生提出索赔时，她将联系她的律师。如果律师认为有正当理由，将通过发传票来推进诉讼，寻求有关的病历记录，然后提出听证申请。如果此案继续进行，在英格兰和威尔士将由皇后区高等法院的法官进行审理。如果费用低于某个水平，也可以在县法院审理案件。在英国，案件是由法官而非陪审团审理的。在澳大利亚，案件通常由法官和陪审团共同审理。原告的律师先概述他们认为存在的问题和接受的医疗服务。案件常在日报中进行报道，通常在报纸的第一页或第二页上以大号字体显示，常常对医生或医院造成严重的负面宣传。如果最终证明医生或医院没有过错，很少有媒体如此详尽地报道结果，评论也往往隐藏在出版物的小号字体中。

When a patient decides to make a claim against her doctor, she will approach her solicitor. If the solicitor considers there is justification, she or he will advance the action by issuing a summons, seek access to the relevant case note records and then lodge an application for a hearing. If the case is to proceed, in England and Wales it will be heard in the High Court by Masters of the Queen's Bench Division. Cases may also be heard in the County Court if the costs are below a certain figure. In the UK, cases are heard before a judge and not a jury. In Australia, cases are usually heard before a judge and jury. The case usually commences with the barrister for the plaintiff outlining their perceived problem and the care given. This is generally reported widely in the daily press, often in large type on the first or second pages of the paper and often resulting in severe adverse publicity for the doctor or hospital concerned. If it is ultimately proven that the doctor or hospital was not at fault, it is rare for the press to detail these findings

as widely, and the comments tend to be almost hidden in small type deep in the publication.

患者发现问题后可能立即提出医学诉讼，也可能会延迟数年。如果不涉及儿童，须在"不良事件"发生后的 7 年内将诉讼文件递交给相关法院。如果诉讼的原因涉及儿童，则应在儿童"成年"后的 7 年内将诉讼递交给法院；换句话说，"不良事件"发生后的 25 年内可能发生诉讼。因为没有人能确切记得 12 个月前发生的事情，更不用说 25 年前了，所以任何不良事件都必须详尽记录。在发出传票到听证会开始之间，以及在确定审判到实际审判日期之间，往往也会有很长的间隔。

Medical litigation may occur soon after a problem has been perceived to have occurred by a patient but may be delayed for some years. Where the problem does not involve a child, the litigation process must generally be submitted to the Court involved within 7 years of the 'adverse' event occurring. Where the condition of the child is the reason for the litigation, the case should reach the Court within 7 years of that child reaching 'maturity'-in other words, the case can reach the Court any time in the 25 years after the 'adverse' event occurred. Because no one can remember exactly what happened 12 months ago, let alone 25 years ago, the documentation about any adverse event must be extensive and detailed. There also tends to be a long interval between the issuing of a summons and its hearing and between setting down a case for trial and the actual date of the trial.

英国医疗诉讼非常昂贵，因此大多数原告都得到了法律援助的支持。在澳大利亚，除非预期会有大笔支出，否则通常情况并非如此。索赔书概述了索赔的性质，应由被告做出回应，承认或驳回指控。受法律援助的诉讼律师具有相当大的优势，因为法律援助基金可以承担所有费用，并且通常不会因未获得赔偿而罚款。

Medical litigation is expensive, and it is not therefore surprising that most plaintiffs in the UK are supported by Legal Aid. In Australia, this is often not the case unless a large payout is expected. The Statement of Claim outlines the nature of the claim, and it is up to the defendant to respond and either acknowledge or refute the allegations. The legally aided litigant has considerable advantages, as the Legal Aid fund meets all costs and there is usually no penalty for failure of a claim.

审判本身是一个对抗性过程，原告人有责任证明医务人员没有提供合理的临床服务，使患者遭受了不必要的伤害。

The trial itself is an adversarial process, and the onus is on the plaintiff to prove that the staff failed to provide a

✓ **经验**

英国和澳大利亚为了加速解决医疗诉讼，已通过《民事诉讼程序法规》引入了新的规定，新规定作为对专家证人的指导，从 2002 年 4 月开始实施。

法规规定专家主要需对法院负责，优先于其他人的指示或提供报酬者。

原告和被告双方提供标准化的报告后进行交换，一些法院会建议双方各将一份书面问题报告提交给专家。双方必须在报告送达后的 28 天内提出这些问题，并且必须在下一个 28 天内回应。

法院现在的惯例是命令专家开会讨论双方律师提出的共同议程，撰写一份联合报告，概述同意和不同意的部分。联合报告应概述任何不同意见的原因，并帮助案件在庭外解决，从而减少诉讼的费用。

To speed up the resolution of disputes in the UK and in Australia, new regulations have been introduced through the Civil Procedures Rules and were implemented as guidance to expert witnesses from April 2002.

The rules specify that the primary responsibility of an expert is to the Court and that this responsibility overrides any obligation to any other person from whom the expert has received instructions or payment.

After providing a report, the format of which has now been standardized, the reports of the plaintiff's and defendant's experts are exchanged, and some Courts advise the various parties to put one list of written questions to the experts. These questions must be put within 28 days of service of the report, and the questions must be answered within a further 28 days.

It is now common practice for the Court to order that the experts should also meet to discuss a common agenda submitted by the solicitors of both parties and to prepare a joint report outlining the extent of agreement and disagreement. The joint report should outline the reasons for any disagreements and should enable many cases to be resolved out of court, resulting in a substantial reduction in the legal costs involved.

reasonable level of care with the result that the patient suffered unnecessary injury.

在任何审判中，主要证据往往来自于病历记录。重要的是医务人员需记住病历记录会被仔细检查，并构成法律文件。因此，正确记录事实非常重要，病历记录应遵循以下准则。

During any trial, the major evidence tends to be drawn from the case records. As a resident medical officer, it is important to remember that case notes will be examined in detail and constitute a legal document. It is therefore important to record facts properly, and these guidelines should be followed:

- 病历记录的条目必须清晰、简明和真实，应详细说明当天的诊断、鉴别诊断、安排的检查和制订的管理计划。

- Entries into case notes must be clear, concise and factual and should detail the diagnosis, differential diagnoses, investigations arranged and plan of management to be instituted on that day.

- 第二天的病历记录应包括过去 24h 的进展、已行检查的结果、已安排的进一步检查（如果有），以及诊断或治疗的任何变化。

- The details written on the next day should include the progress over the previous 24 hours, the results of investigations that are to hand, further investigations arranged (if any) and any change in the diagnosis or treatment to be given.

- 术中并发症或问题应详细说明，最好由手术中年资最高的人撰写。

- All entries concerning intraoperative complications or problems should be detailed and preferably written by the most senior person in the operating theatre at the time.

- 记录应始终有签名和日期，并应及时完成。尽管缩写的签名可以识别作者的身份，但如果需要，最好在医疗文件上打印签名或盖章，其中包括其医疗注册号。在产房、重症监护病房和急诊室中，及时完成记录特别重要，在这些地方，紧急情况发生的可能性更大，需要评估急救的及时性。

- Entries should always be initialled and dated, and preferably timed. Although initialling should allow identification of the writer in the future, if required, it is better if the identification of the writer is printed or stamped in and the medical registration number included. Timing of the record writing is particularly important in the delivery suite, intensive care unit and emergency department where emergencies are more likely and the rapidity of care needs to be assessed.

- 未进行变更登记说明更改原因时，不得尝试更改病历记录中的内容。可以将有关不良事件的回顾性信息添加到病历中，并写明最新进展，需注明时间、签名并写明事实依据。

- No attempt should be made to alter entries in case records without countersigning the alteration and indicating why it has been made. Retrospective information concerning an adverse event can be added to the medical record, providing it is dated, appropriately signed and factual.

如果收到律师的来信，要求提供法律诉讼需要的信息，重要的是做到以下几点。

If a letter is received from a solicitor asking for information with a view to initiating legal action, it is important to:

- 通知医院法务人员。
- Notify one's medical defence organization
- 通知医院的投诉负责人员，他们会通知律师代表他们。
- Notify the complaints officer in the hospital concerned, who will usually then notify the solicitors who represent them
- 手术后或胎儿娩出后，若发生围产儿死亡或新生儿出现脑功能障碍或骨骼神经损伤（如臂丛神经损伤），患者常提起诉讼。
- Litigation commonly ensues when there are complications following a surgical procedure or where there is a perinatal death or the birth of a child who has brain dysfunction or skeletal or nerve injuries such as Erb's palsy.

✓ 经验

文献证据表明，少于 10% 的脑瘫或智力低下与分娩期发生的事件有关。但是，法官面临的困难在于，在平衡各种可能后，判断是否可以通过在分娩期提供更适当的管理来避免或减轻不良后果。如果法官决定支持原告，则将根据儿童残疾程度和预期寿命来裁决赔偿数额。这可能是几百万英镑或美元的赔偿。

All the evidence available in the literature suggests that fewer than 10% of cases of cerebral palsy or mental retardation are related to the events that occur during labour. However, the difficulty that judges have is deciding whether, on the balance of probabilities, the adverse outcome could have been avoided or reduced in severity by more appropriate care during labour. If the judge decides in favour of the plaintiff, the quantum of the award will be assessed on the level of disability and the life expectancy of the child. This may amount to an award of several million pounds or dollars.

肩难产导致臂丛神经损伤是产科诉讼的常见原因。在这种情况下提出的论点是，需要判断是否可以通过预测肩难产发生风险后行剖宫产或在较早孕周分娩来避免难产，或者是否可以通过避免过度牵引，或者将患者置于 McRobert 位以改善进入骨盆入口的角度并耻骨上加压以娩出前肩，或者进行适当内旋转来避免臂丛神经损伤。

Shoulder dystocia resulting in damage to the brachial plexus is a common cause for litigation in obstetrics. The arguments proffered in such cases are that either the dystocia could have been avoided by predicting the likelihood of shoulder dystocia and delivering the child by caesarean section or delivering vaginally but at an earlier gestation when the baby was smaller, or that the damage to the brachial plexus could have been avoided by not using excessive traction and by changing the angle of entry of the pelvic brim by placing the patient in McRobert's position and exerting directed suprapubic pressure to deliver the anterior shoulder or using appropriate internal manoeuvres.

针对产科医生的其他诉讼包括以下内容。

Other reasons for litigation against an obstetrician include:

- 孕期对胎儿异常的评估不到位，因为如果提前发现异常，患者会要求终止妊娠。
- Inadequate screening for a possible fetal abnormality during the antenatal period because the patient would have requested termination had the abnormality been defined.
- 未能识别胎儿生长受限，并说明原因。
- Failure to recognize a baby was growth restricted and defining why.
- 未能预料有胎死宫内的可能，并采取适当的预防措施。
- Failure to recognize a baby was going to die in utero and performing appropriate monitoring to prevent this.
- 未能在产程中评估异常胎心监护的重要性。
- Failure to adequately assess the significance of a fetal heart rate abnormality seen on the cardiotocographic record obtained during labour.
- 第二产程过长，导致产妇括约肌损伤，导致大便失禁。
- Allowing the second stage of labour to last too long, resulting in sphincter injury leading to bowel incontinence problems.
- 发生胎儿窘迫，决定剖宫产的时间到实际分娩时间间隔太长，导致新生儿不良结局。
- Too long a delay between the time a decision was made to perform a caesarean section on the grounds of fetal distress and the actual time the baby was delivered, resulting in adverse outcome to the newborn.
- 未充分控制产后出血，导致患者需要进行子宫切除术以控制出血。

- Not adequately treating a postpartum haemorrhage, resulting in the patient requiring a hysterectomy to control the life-threatening bleeding.

妇科诉讼通常与绝育术后避孕失败、妇科手术（尤其是腹腔镜手术）术中或术后并发症或漏诊或延迟诊断恶性肿瘤相关。

Litigations in gynaecology are often related to sterilization or contraception failure, complications occurring during or after gynaecological surgery (particularly when this has been performed laparoscopically) or failure or delay in diagnosing a malignancy in a patient.

大多数产科医生 / 妇科医生在其职业生涯中被诉讼，但可以通过以下方法将风险降至最低。

Most obstetricians/gynaecologists will be the subject of a litigious claim during their professional careers, but the risk can be minimized by:

- 不进行未经充分培训或未获得资质的手术操作。

- Careful adherence to the principle of not undertaking procedures for which one is inadequately trained or supervised.

- 在进行任何外科手术之前，应向患者仔细解释该手术本质和可能出现的并发症。

- Careful and considerate provision of information to the patient before any surgical procedure concerning the nature of the procedure and the possible complications.

- 检查结果异常应立刻采取干预措施，例如，分娩时对胎心率异常进行决策，决定继续观察并采集头皮血样用于 pH 测量，还是进行分娩。忽略胎心监护结果是不可接受的。检查结果和决策必须记录在病历中，这涉及未来进一步的治疗。

- Prompt action if there are abnormal findings in any tests that necessitate intervention; for example, an abnormal fetal heart rate during labour demands a decision. The decision may be to continue observation, to take a scalp blood sample for pH measurement or to deliver the baby. It is not acceptable to ignore the recording. The findings must be recorded in the notes as well as the decision concerning the further plan of care.

三、患者机密性（包括数据保护）[Patient confidentiality (including data protection)]

医生有对所有患者可能在诊治期间披露的人格

细节保密的道德义务；但是，此义务不是绝对的，在特殊情况下医生可能会违背保密原则。必须记住，未经患者同意而擅自披露信息虽不是刑事犯罪，但医师需要接受国家医事委员会或医务委员会的纪律调查。披露信息可能涉及公共利益，特别是在患者有暴力倾向，或者可能传播 HIV 病毒给公众或直系亲属时。

The doctor normally has an ethical obligation to keep secret all details of a personal nature that may be revealed during consultation and treatment. The duty is not, however, absolute, as confidentiality may be breached under special circumstances. It must be remembered that unauthorized disclosure of information without the patient's consent is not a criminal offence, but it does expose the doctor to disciplinary procedures by the medical board or medical council of the country concerned. Disclosure may involve matters of public interest, particularly where the patient may constitute a risk of violence or transmission of infections such as AIDS to the public or to the immediate relatives.

根据法规感染人类免疫缺陷病毒不是必须申报的，但在英国，通用医学委员会（GMC）建议医生"应尽一切努力说服艾滋病患者让其全科医生和性伴侣知情"。

Human immunodeficiency virus infection is not notifiable by statute, although in the UK, the General Medical Council (GMC) advises that doctors 'should make every effort to persuade a patient of the need for their General Practitioners and sexual partners to be informed of a positive diagnosis'.

根据法律规定，某些披露行为是必需的，但在不同国家 / 地区有所不同，其中包括以下情形。

Some acts of disclosure are compulsory by law, but do vary in different countries, and these include:

- 告知出生和死亡信息。

- Notification of births and deaths

- 告知体外受精治疗周期。

- Notification of a treatment cycle of in vitro fertilization

- 告知供精人工授精。

- Notification of artificial insemination by donor

在澳大利亚，HIV 病毒感染和与艾滋病相关的死亡是必须通报的情况。指定人员（医生和病理学家）必须通知其各自的州或辖区卫生部门，然后再将编码数据转发给国家艾滋病监测计划。通知者必须提供此人姓的前 2 个字母、名的前 2 个字母和邮政编码。不应提供被诊断人员的全名或地址。

In all Australian States and Territories, HIV infections and AIDS-related deaths are notifiable conditions. The designated persons (doctors and pathologists) must notify their respective State or Territory health authorities who then forward coded data to the National HIV Surveillance Program. The notifier must provide the first 2 letters of the person's family name, the first 2 letters of the person's given name and the postcode. The full name or the address of the person diagnosed should not be provided.

由于对医生或医院采取法律诉讼的时限规定，所有医疗记录必须保存至少 7 年，如果包括产科治疗，则必须保存 25 年，以防分娩的胎儿发生问题。

Because of the time scales of possible legal action being taken against a doctor or hospital, it is necessary for all medical records to be stored for at least 7 years, or 25 years if the record includes pregnancy care, in case a problem occurs in the baby produced by that pregnancy".

四、有关流产的规则（The rules regarding abortion）

英国的《流产法》（1967 年）从根本上改变了英国终止妊娠的惯例，使流产合法化和自由化。

The Abortion Act (1967) in the UK radically changed the availability of termination of pregnancy in the UK and had the effect of both legalizing and liberalizing abortion.

根据该法律，可以在以下四个条件下终止妊娠。

Under this law, termination of pregnancy can be performed under the following four conditions:

- 妊娠未超过第 24 周，与终止妊娠相比，持续妊娠将带来更大的风险，孕妇或家中任何现有子女的身体或精神健康会受到伤害。

- That the pregnancy has not exceeded its twenty-fourth week and that continuance of the pregnancy would involve greater risk, than if the pregnancy were terminated, of injury to the physical or mental health of the pregnant woman or any existing children of her family

- 为防止对孕妇的身体或精神健康造成严重永久性伤害而终止妊娠。

- That the termination is necessary to prevent grave permanent injury to the physical or mental health of the pregnant woman

- 与终止妊娠相比，继续妊娠会增加孕妇死亡风险。

- That the continuance of the pregnancy would involve

risk to the life of the pregnant woman greater than if the pregnancy were terminated

- 如果该孩子出生，发生严重的身体或精神异常，导致严重畸形的风险大。

- That there is a substantial risk that if the child were born it would suffer from physical or mental abnormalities to be seriously handicapped

根据现有法案，终止妊娠必须得到两名执业医师的同意，除非该执业医师"出于诚信善意的原则，认为终止妊娠是挽救生命或防止对孕妇的身体或精神健康造成严重永久性伤害所必需的"。

Under the conditions of the Act, the decision to terminate a pregnancy must be agreed by two practitioners unless the practitioner 'is of the opinion, formed in good faith, that the termination is immediately necessary to save life or to prevent grave permanent injury to the physical or mental health of the pregnant woman'.

终止妊娠必须在英国卫生大臣为履行其根据《国家卫生服务法案》（1977）规定的职能而授权的医院中进行。换言之，医院必须获得许可才能终止妊娠。此外，在妊娠 22 周后终止妊娠时，必须确保胎儿不会活着出生。通常需要行超声引导下胎儿心内注射氯化钾或其他物质，以使胎儿死亡。

Termination of pregnancy must be carried out in a hospital vested by the Secretary of State for the purposes of his or her functions under the National Health Services Act (1977). In other words, premises must be licensed for termination of pregnancy. In addition, the need to ensure the fetus will not be born alive is a requirement where the pregnancy is terminated after 22 weeks of gestation. This often necessitates the injection of potassium chloride or other substances into the fetal heart under ultrasonic guidance to result in fetal death.

法律规定对终止妊娠的目的、执行情况和术中或术后的任何并发症进行告知。告知十分重要，尽管法案本身非常自由，并没有把妊娠和绝育纳入其法律框架。

Notification is also a statutory requirement, first of the intention to perform an abortion and second of the performance of the termination and any complications during or after the event. This is perhaps why so much emphasis is still laid on notification when the Act itself is very liberal and in a legal framework that does not require notification of conception or sterilization.

在其他国家，有关终止妊娠的规定及其可行性差异很大。在某些国家 / 地区不允许流产，任何进行流产的医生或患者都可能被判重罪并受到惩罚。在澳大利亚没有关于流产的统一规定，在大多数州但并非所有州都可以进行。那些允许流产的州，所遵循的规则与英国先前制定的规则相似。在维多利亚州，多年以来一直采用与英国一致的 Menhennitt 规定。目前，只有在澳大利亚首都地区和维多利亚州流产是合法的。

In other countries, the rules concerning pregnancy termination and the availability of it vary dramatically. In some countries, abortion is not allowed, and any doctor performing an abortion or patient having an abortion can be convicted of a felony and punished appropriately. In Australia, there is no universal rule concerning abortion, although it is readily available in most, but not all, of the states. Those states that allow it do so under similar rules to those defined earlier in the UK. In Victoria, for many years, the Menhennitt ruling was applied, with this ruling being like the rules in the UK. Currently only the Australian Capital Territory and Victoria have decriminalized abortion.

尽管存在防摧残儿童法案，因满足合法流产的必要条件，在澳大利亚的某些州还是可以进行晚孕期引产。执行此操作的公立医院会评估引产是否合理，并在得到专门医学和法律委员会的批准后行流产术。

Third trimester abortions are performed in some states in Australia, despite the existence of child destruction laws, presumably because they have satisfied the conditions necessary for legal abortion. In public hospitals performing such procedures, the appropriateness of such an abortion is usually assessed and the procedure approved by a special medical and legal committee before it can be performed.

五、辅助生殖技术在不孕症中的应用
（The use of assisted reproduction in infertility care）

《人类受精和胚胎法案》（1990 年）（在英国适用）规定了与辅助生殖技术有关的事项。该法案冗长且复杂，应由参与手术的所有人员阅读。该法案由人类受精和胚胎管理局执行，其人员组成如下。

The Human Fertilisation and Embryology Act (1990) (which applies in the UK) provides the statutory authority that regulates all matters relating to assisted reproduction. The Act is long and complex and should be read by all personnel involved in these procedures. The Act is administered by the Human Fertilisation and Embryology Authority, which consists of:

- 主席和副主席。

- A chairman and deputy chairman

- 卫生大臣任命的其他成员。

- Such numbers of other members as the Secretary of State appoints

人类受精和胚胎管理局有以下职责。

The Human Fertilisation and Embryology Authority has the following duties:

- 常规审查胚胎及胚胎后续发育的信息，以及法案所管理的医疗服务和活动，并在需要的情况下向卫生大臣汇报。

- To keep under review information about embryos and any subsequent development of embryos and about the treatment services and activities governed by this Act and to advise the Secretary of State, if asked to do so, about these matters

- 向公众宣传人类受精和胚胎委员会可提供的服务或按许可证规定可提供的服务。

- To publicize the services provided to the public by the Human Fertilisation and Embryology Authority or provided in pursuance of licenses

- 在适当的程度内，为有执照许可的人员、正在接受治疗患者、提供配子或胚胎以用于法案规定活动的人或希望这样做的人提供建议和信息。

- To provide, to such extent as it considers appropriate, advice and information for persons to whom licenses apply or who are receiving treatment services or providing gametes or embryos for use for the purpose of activities governed by this Act or may wish to do so

- 执行法规中明确的其他功能。

- To perform such other functions as may be specified in the regulations

总体而言，人类受精和胚胎管理局有权利发放执照，或监督提供辅助生殖技术中心，并决定哪些符合法案条目的手术是可进行的。它在临床法中也有广泛的权力，其中包括有正当理由时，拥有"必要时使用合理的力量"进入医疗中心的权利，以获得违反法律的证据，并采取必要的措施来保存此类证据。

Overall, the Human Fertilisation and Embryology Authority has the power to license and supervise centres providing assisted reproduction and to decide which procedures are acceptable within the terms of reference of the Act. It also has wide-ranging powers under the clinical law, including, under warrant, the rights to enter premises 'using such force as is reasonably necessary' to take possession of whatever may be required as evidence of breach of the law and to take the necessary steps to preserve such evidence.

在其他国家，存在类似的机构和法律，不仅管理将辅助生殖技术用于合适的"夫妻"，还包括对转移胚胎数量的建议，以减少多胎妊娠的可能性，以及植入前遗传学诊断地点，并确保所有接受这种治疗的患者（无论是否需要供体配子及受孕者）均已适当注册，以便随后对子代进行评估。任何通过辅助生殖技术出生的儿童均有权知道他或她的受孕方式，以及涉及谁的配子。

In other countries, similar bodies and legislation exist and control not only the availability of this treatment to appropriate 'couples' but also may include recommendations as to the number of embryos to be transferred to reduce the likelihood of multiple pregnancies and the place for pre-implantation genetic diagnosis and ensure that all patients having such treatment, whether donor gametes are required or not and who conceive, are appropriately registered for subsequent assessment by any child so produced. Any such child has a right to know how he or she was conceived and whose gametes were involved.

六、胎儿、孕妇、儿童和青春期女孩的相关法律地位（The relevant legal status of the fetus, the pregnant woman, the child and the pubertal girl）

尽管在某些国家／地区，一旦受孕，胎儿便拥有合法权利，但在大多数情况下，胎儿在妊娠的各个时期没有合法权利，而活产后就获得了合法权利。因此，熟悉所在国家／地区的法律，以了解妊娠后对胎儿的责任十分重要。

Although in some countries the fetus has legal rights as soon as conception occurs, in most the fetus has no legal rights in any trimester of the pregnancy but gets these as soon as it is born alive. It is therefore imperative that you are familiar with the law in the country in which you are working to understand what your responsibility is to the fetus when a woman is pregnant.

最近几年在美国，一些法院被要求裁定是否在胎儿出现问题或有其他剖宫产指征时，强迫拒绝剖宫产的孕妇行剖宫产手术。在另一些国家，孕妇的权利被认为凌驾于胎儿的权利之上，可以继续妊娠。在许多国家，孕妇的权利明显凌驾于胎儿的权利之上，没有人代表胎儿权益向法院提出申请。

During the last few years in the United States, some

Courts have been asked to decide whether a woman can be forced to allow a caesarean section to be performed on the grounds of an identified problem within the fetus but where she has refused such treatment, and in some instances caesarean section has been ordered. In others, the rights of the mother have been deemed to override those of the fetus and the pregnancy has been allowed to continue. In many other countries, the rights of the pregnant woman have clearly overridden those of the fetus, and Court applications allegedly on behalf of the fetus have not been made.

一旦孩子出生，尽管母亲拒绝，但法院通常会支持对孩子进行抢救或为减少严重并发症而进行的治疗（如输血或交叉配血）。

Once the child has been born, a Court will usually approve treatment of the child which has been refused by the mother, where that treatment may be lifesaving (such as blood transfusion for blood group immunization) or would reduce the likelihood of significant morbidity.

在儿童期，通常由父母代表儿童同意接受治疗，这适用于大多数医疗管理，其中包括严重疾病的治疗、急诊处理和必要的手术操作，但不包括绝育手术。如果孩子存在精神障碍，大多数治疗需要父母同意才能进行；但是，绝育、流产和使用某些避孕措施（如宫内节育器或 Depo-Provera 避孕药）通常需要政府机构，如负责处理残疾儿童或成人权利的监护委员会的批准。

During childhood consent for treatment is usually given by the parents, with this generally accepted as being appropriate for most medical care, including serious illnesses, emergency care and for necessary operative procedures but *not* for sterilization. If the child is mentally disabled, again parental consent is appropriate for most treatment required. However, sterilization, abortion and the use of some forms of contraception such as an intrauterine device or Depo-Provera would usually require the approval of a Government Body, such as a Guardianship Board, which deals with the rights of a disabled child or adult.

尽管在大多数国家，儿童要到 18 岁才成年并可行使成年人的权利，其中包括同意接受治疗或手术，但 18 岁以下的儿童也被认为已经足够成熟可以在某些情况下做出决定。这些情况定义了 Gillick 胜任能力或 Fraser 指南，该指南指的是 1982 年在英国发生的一起案件，一名女性向法院提起诉讼，阻止未经父母同意向未满 16 岁的儿童提供避孕建议或治疗。最终，此案通过以下方式在上议院解决：孩子能否行知情同意，将取决于孩子的成熟度和理解力以及所需同意的具体事项。若儿童能够对所提议的治疗方法的优缺点进行合理的评估，则可以恰当公平地描述为真正的同意。为了满足 Fraser 指南，以下情况必须满足。

Although by definition a child does not become an adult and achieve full adult's rights until the age of 18 years in most countries, thereby obtaining the ability to consent to treatment or the performance of operative procedures, a child younger than 18 years has been deemed mature enough to make such decisions under certain circumstances. These circumstances define Gillick competency or satisfaction of the Fraser Guidelines, which refer to a case in the UK in 1982 where a woman took a case to Court to prevent contraceptive advice or treatment being given to a child under the age of 16 years without parental consent. Ultimately, this case was settled in the House of Lords as follows: 'whether or not a child is capable of giving the necessary consent will depend on the child's maturity and understanding and the nature of the consent required. The child must be capable of making a reasonable assessment of the advantages and disadvantages of the treatment proposed, so the consent, if given, can be properly and fairly described as true consent.' In order to satisfy the Fraser guidelines, the doctor concerned must be satisfied that:

- 年轻人能够理解专业人士的建议。

- The young person will understand the professional's advice

- 无法说服年轻人通知其父母。

- The young person cannot be persuaded to inform their parents

- 年轻人可能在接受或未接受避孕药的情况下开始或继续进行性交。

- The young person is likely to begin, or to continue having, sexual intercourse with or without contraceptive treatment

- 除非年轻人接受避孕药治疗，否则他们的身心健康或两者都有可能受到伤害。

- Unless the young person receives contraceptive treatment, their physical or mental health, or both, are likely to suffer

- 为保障年轻人的最大利益，在有或没有父母同意的情况下他们都需要接受避孕建议或治疗。

- The young person's best interests require them to receive contraceptive advice or treatment, with or without parental consent

对于有关避孕的分歧，因为如果孩子有 "Gillick 能力"，可以阻止父母查看他或她的病历。

The ramifications of this decision extend beyond that of the provision of contraception, because if the child is 'Gillick competent', he or she can prevent the parents from viewing his or her medical record.

许多国家 / 地区接受了英国关于 Gillick 能力的规定，该规定现在适用于大多数发达国家 / 地区。

Many countries have accepted the UK decision on Gillick competence, and this rule now applies in most developed countries.

七、医生在儿童保护中的作用（The role of the doctor in child protection）

儿童可能被虐待或忽视时，所有医生都应在儿童保护中发挥作用。这种虐待可能是身体虐待、性虐待，或者被拒绝进行恰当必要的治疗。医师需要与相关机构的工作人员，其中包括上级医师和社工共享信息，即使孩子或其父母不同意、不可能或不适合征求他们的同意。医生应就是否需要将儿童移交给其他机构做出决定，并且有必要了解有关机构的职责、政策和做法。

All doctors have a role in child protection when the possibility of child abuse or neglect is defined. This abuse can be physical abuse, sexual abuse or the denial of appropriate and necessary therapy. Relevant information needs to be shared with other staff members of the institution concerned, including senior medical personnel and medical social workers, even where the child or their parent does not consent, or it is not possible or it is inappropriate to ask for such consent. A decision should then be made concerning the need for referral to external agencies, and an understanding of the roles, policies and practices of such agencies in the country concerned would be necessary.

附录 D 客观结构化临床考试站点：问题与答案
OSCE stations: Questions and Answers

Paul Duggan　著　　杨慧霞　译　　石玉华　校

一、客观结构化临床考试站点的形式
（Format of and approach to OSCE stations）

OSCE 是客观结构化临床考试的缩写。OSCE 站点的设计符合"2 + 8"形式，即每站包括 2min 的阅读时间和 8min 的表现时间。

OSCE is the abbreviation used for objective structured clinical examination. The OSCE stations are written to comply with the '2 + 8' format. This involves 2 minutes' reading time and 8 minutes' performance per station.

OSCE 用于评估临床技能，其良好表现包括获取相关的临床信息 [病史和（或）检查]、安排和解释检查，以及制订和解释管理计划等部分。不同站点对这些部分的重视程度不相同，并非所有部分都必须包含在特定站点中。在表现期间，学员可能还需要回答患者 / 演员提出的问题。

OSCEs are used for assessment of clinical skills. Typically, a sound performance includes acquiring pertinent clinical information (history and/or examination), requesting and interpreting investigations and formulating and explaining your plan of management. The degree of emphasis on these components varies, and not all will necessarily be included in any particular station. You might during the performance also be required to answer questions posed by the patient/actor.

如何评估学员的 OSCE 表现？不同单位使用不同的评分表，但都有一个共同点，学员的表现情况与课程的学习成果相关。一些评分系统按不同领域进行分类，如专业、知识、推理和临床实践。

How is an OSCE performance assessed? Different organizations use different tools, but they all have in common that the performance criteria are linked to the learning outcomes for your course. Some marking systems categorize performance by domains, such as Professionalism, Knowledge, Reasoning and Clinical Practice.

学员应该如何为 OSCE 做准备？要了解考点，多与患者、朋友和同事练习技能。下面请阅读并回答问题！

How should you prepare for an OSCE? Know the subject; practise your skills as appropriate with patients, friends and colleagues; and read and answer the question!

二、OSCE 站点：问题（OSCE stations: Questions）

第 6 章（Chapter 6）

环境：普通产科门诊。

Setting: Outpatient clinic, general maternity unit

角色：低年资医生（实习生）。

Role: Junior doctor (intern)

场景：玛丽·麦克斯韦（Mary Maxwell）是一名 35 岁的女性，目前第 3 次怀孕，正在当地的医院妇产科进行常规产检。麦克斯韦女士是一名全职教师，与丈夫和他们 4 岁的孩子住在一起。这次是计划妊娠。她目前每天服用阿替洛尔 50mg 和叶酸 5mg，并且没有过敏史。

麦克斯韦女士已称重，测量了血压（BP）并进行了尿液分析。

检查结果如下。

- 身高 160cm，体重 88kg，体重指数（BMI）34.4kg/m²。血压 140/90mmHg（用大号袖带测量）。

- 尿液分析：葡萄糖阳性，蛋白质、酮体、白细胞和亚硝酸盐阴性。

Scenario: Mary Maxwell is a 35-year-old woman in her third pregnancy attending her local maternity unit for a routine booking visit. Ms Maxwell works full time as a teacher and lives with her husband and their 4-year old child. This pregnancy is planned. Her current medications are atenolol 50 mg daily and folic acid 5 mg daily. She has no allergies.

Ms Maxwell has been weighed, her blood pressure (BP) has been recorded and urinalysis performed.

The results are:

Height, weight, body mass index (BMI): 160 cm, 88 kg, 34.4 kg/m²

Blood pressure: 140/90 mmHg (large cuff)

Urinalysis: positive for glucose; negative for protein, ketones, white blood cells and nitrites

任务（Tasks）

- 从麦克斯韦女士那里采集产科史和病史（6min）。

- 告知她，您将为她安排的后续产检内容（1min）。

- 回答她可能有的任何问题（1min）。

Take an obstetric and medical history from Ms Maxwell. (6 minutes)

Advise Ms Maxwell of the next steps that you will arrange in relation to her ongoing care in this pregnancy. (1 minute)

Answer any questions she might have. (1 minute)

注意：演员可能没有上述身体特征。

Note: The actor might not have the stated physical characteristics.

第 7 章（Chapter 7）

环境：普通产科门诊。

Setting: Outpatient clinic, general maternity unit

角色：低年资医生（实习生）。

Role: Junior doctor (intern)

场景：希尔达·汉弗莱斯（Hilda Humphries）是一名 27 岁的女性，第一次怀孕，现妊娠 7 周。她是一名全职厨师，与 32 岁的老公约翰·杰米森住在一起，后者是一名长途卡车司机。

希尔达有不孕症和多囊卵巢综合征病史。她通过节食和定期锻炼减轻 10kg 后自然受孕。她目前的体重是 82kg（BMI 29.8kg/m²）。

她想和你讨论妊娠期是否需要对饮食和锻炼进行调整，以及如何调整。

Scenario: Hilda Humphries is a 27-year-old woman at 7 weeks' gestation in her first pregnancy. She works full time as a cook and lives with her 32-year-old partner John Jamieson, who is a long-distance truck driver.

Hilda has a history of subfertility and polycystic ovarian syndrome. She conceived spontaneously after losing 10 kg in weight by dieting and with regular exercise. Her current weight is 82 kg (BMI 29.8 kg/m²).

She wants to discuss with you the adjustments, if any, she should make to her diet and in her exercise routine at the gym during her pregnancy.

任务（Tasks）

- 采集汉弗莱斯女士的病史（5min）。

- 建议她注意有关饮食和锻炼，以及其他有利于健康和妊娠结局的事项（2min）。

- 回答她可能有的任何问题（1min）。

Take a directed history from Ms Humphries. (5 minutes)

Advise Ms Humphries regarding diet and exercise and any other matters you uncover that are relevant to optimizing her health and the outcome of her pregnancy. (2 minutes)

Answer any questions she might have. (1 minute)

注意：演员可能没有上述身体特征。假定日期是确定的。

Notes: The actor might not have the described physical characteristics. Assume the dates are certain.

第 8 章（Chapter 8）

设置：普通产科观察室。

Setting: Assessment unit, general maternity unit

角色：低年资医生（实习生）。

Role: Junior doctor (intern)

情景：弗里达·费舍尔（Freda Fisher）是一名 33 岁的女性，第二次怀孕，因阴道出血到当地医院妇产科急诊观察室就诊。

费舍尔女士目前怀孕 34 周。

检查结果如下。

- 脉搏 72 次 / 分；血压 130/70mmHg。

- 腹部触诊为腹软，胎儿臀位。

- 宫底高度 34cm；胎心率（手持多普勒仪）140 次 / 分。

- 尿液分析：红细胞阳性，白细胞、硝酸盐、蛋白质和酮体阴性。

Scenario: Freda Fisher is a 33-year-old woman in her second pregnancy who has presented to the acute assessment unit at her local maternity unit with vaginal bleeding.

Ms Fisher is currently at 34 weeks' gestation.

The assessment unit midwife has recorded the following observations:

Pulse: 72 beats/min

Blood pressure: 130/70 mmHg

Abdominal palpation: soft abdomen, breech presentation

Symphysial fundal height: 34 cm

Fetal heart rate (hand-held Doppler device): 140 bpm

Urinalysis: positive for blood; negative for leukocytes, nitrites, protein, ketones

任务（Tasks）

- 从费舍尔女士那里采集相关病史（6min）。

- 向她解释您将为她安排的后续产检内容（1min）。

- 回答她可能有的任何问题（1min）。

Take a relevant history from Ms Fisher. (6 minutes)

Explain to Ms Fisher the next steps that you will arrange in the assessment unit. (1 minute)

Answer any questions she might have. (1 minute)

注意：演员可能没有上述身体特征。

Note: The actor might not have the stated physical characteristics.

第 9 章（Chapter 9）

环境：普通产科产前咨询诊室。

Setting: Prenatal counselling clinic, general maternity unit

角色：低年资医生（实习生）。

Role: Junior doctor (intern)

情景：玛丽·莫里斯（Mary Morris）是一名 33 岁的女性，既往 G_3P_1，家庭医生将她转诊到您的诊所进行产前咨询。

莫里斯女士与她的伴侣和他们 4 岁的女儿住在一起。她是凝血因子 V Leiden 基因突变的纯合子，多年来每天服用华法林。

她和她的伴侣想再要一个孩子。

患者目前的 BMI 为 28kg/m²，血压为 120/70mmHg。

Scenario: Mary Morris is a 33-year-old G_3P_1 woman referred to your clinic by her local doctor for prenatal counselling.

Ms Morris lives with her partner and their 4-year-old daughter. She is homozygous for the factor V Leiden gene mutation and has been taking warfarin on a daily basis for several years.

She and her partner want to have another child.

The patient's current BMI is 28 kg/m² and her blood pressure is 120/70 mmHg.

任务（Tasks）

- 向莫里斯女士采集相关病史（6min）。

- 向她解释您将为她安排的后续产检内容（1min）。

- 回答她可能有的任何问题（1min）。

Take a relevant history from Ms Morris. (6 minutes)

Explain to Ms Morris the next steps that you will arrange in relation to her prenatal care. (1 minute)

Answer any questions she might have. (1 minute)

注意：演员可能没有上述身体特征。

Note: The actor might not have the stated physical characteristics.

第 10 章（Chapter 10）

环境：普通产科门诊。

Setting: Outpatient clinic, general maternity unit

角色：低年资医生（实习生）。

Role: Junior doctor (intern)

场景：艾莉森·奥尔布赖特（Alison Albright）是一名 39 岁的女性，第四次怀孕，正在当地医院妇产科进行产前检查。

奥尔布赖特女士目前妊娠 34 周（孕 8 周时已超声核对孕周）。她没有规律产检，一直在照顾生病的母亲，并独自操持着有 3 个学龄儿童的忙碌家庭。她的丈夫已被派往海外服兵役 5 个月，还要再过一个月才能回国。

在上次就诊时（妊娠 30 周），常规检查发现血压 110/80mmHg，胎儿为臀位，宫底高度为 28cm。

当日检查结果：血压 110/80mmHg；宫底高度 28cm；胎儿臀位。尿液分析正常。

Scenario: Alison Albright is a 39-year-old woman in her fourth pregnancy attending her local maternity unit for an antenatal visit.

Ms Albright is currently at 34 weeks' gestation (based on a dating scan at 8 weeks' gestation). She has not attended several routine clinic appointments. She has been caring for her ill mother and has been managing by herself a busy household comprising her three school-aged children. Her husband has been posted overseas on military service for 5 months now and is not due to return home for another month.

At the previous visit (30 weeks' gestation), routine observations included blood pressure 110/80 mmHg, breech presentation and symphysial-fundal height 28 cm.

At today's visit:

Blood pressure: 110/80 mmHg

Symphysial-fundal height: 28 cm

Breech presentation

Urinalysis: normal

任务（Tasks）

• 向奥尔布赖特女士了解简要病史（3min）。

• 告知她，今天您将为她安排的产检内容（1min）。

• 然后你会得到一些检查结果，阅读结果（1min）。

• 向奥尔布赖特女士解释结果，并告知您为她安排的后续产检计划（2min）。

• 回答她可能有的任何问题（1min）。

Take a brief directed history from Ms Albright. (3 minutes)

Advise Ms Albright of the investigations that you will arrange today. (1 minute)

You will then be provided with some results. Read the results. (1 minute)

Explain the results to Ms Albright and advise her of your

plan of management. (2 minutes)

Answer any questions she might have. (1 minute)

注意：演员可能没有上述身体特征。

Note: The actor might not have the stated physical characteristics.

第 11 章（Chapter 11）

环境：普通产科病房分娩室。

Setting: Delivery suite seminar room, general maternity unit

角色：低年资医生（实习生）。

Role: Junior doctor (intern)

场景：您正在与一名护理专业的一年级学生共同参加该单元简短的"实习"课程。

您的学生是芭芭拉·贝恩（Barbara Bain），她从未进入过妇产科。贝恩女士请您向她解释在产房中如何使用产程图和胎心监护仪。您将使用本单元教学产程图和 20 min 的产时心电图（CTG）完成此任务。

Scenario: You are undertaking a 'teaching on the run' session with a first-year nursing student on a brief attachment to the unit.

Your student is Barbara Bain, who has not set foot in a maternity unit before. Ms Bain has asked you to explain to her the use of a partogram and cardiotography machine in the delivery suite. You will do this using one of the unit's teaching partograms and a supporting 20-minute section of a cardiotograph (CTG) trace taken in labour.

临床病例简介

• G_1P_0，正常足月妊娠。

• 12h 前在家中出现宫缩，并胎膜破裂。

• 10h 前出现规律宫缩，进入产房（开始绘制产程图）。

在阅读期间，仅可使用复制的产程图。

The clinical case synopsis:
G_1P_0, normal-term pregnancy.

Spontaneous onset of contractions with rupture of the membranes occurring at home 12 hours ago.

Admission to delivery suite with regular painful contractions 10 hours ago (partogram commenced).

Copy ONLY of the partogram is available during the reading time.

房间内的设备：产程图的副本；20min 的产时胎

心监护图。

Equipment in room:

Copy of the partogram.

Reproduced image of 20-minute section of a deidentified CTG trace in labour.

任务：根据提供的产程图和胎心监护图向贝恩女士解释以下内容。

- 两种检查使用指征。

- 产程图上的正常和异常部分。

- 胎心监护上的正常和异常部分。

- 您对两种检查结果的解释，以及您认为需要采取的干预。

回答贝恩女士可能提出的任何问题（1min）。

Tasks:

Explain to Ms Bain, using the partogram and CTG trace provided:

- The indications for use of both items
- The normal and abnormal features shown on the partogram
- The normal and abnormal features shown on the CTG
- Your interpretation of the situation, including any intervention you believe is indicated

Answer any questions Ms Bain might have. (1 minute)

第 12 章（Chapter 12）

设置：医学院的教室。

Setting: Medical school tutorial room

角色：低年资医生（实习生）。

Role: Junior doctor (intern)

场景：您在替一名同事为正在产科轮转的医学生进行"快速"补习。

您的学生是弗雷德·法洛斯（Fred Fallows），教学主题是人工助产。

Scenario: You are filling in at short notice for a colleague who had agreed to undertake a 'catch-up' tutorial for a medical student on an obstetrics rotation.

Your student is Fred Fallows, and the tutorial topic is assisted vaginal delivery.

临床病例简介

- G_1P_0 正常足月妊娠。

- 昨晚 23 时自然临产，8h 前行硬膜外无痛分娩。

- 8h 前开始静脉注射催产素。

- 7h 前插入尿管，排出大量清澈的尿液。

- 4h 前宫口开全。

- 2h 前开始用力，进展缓慢。

- 胎心率正在出现深大变异减速和胎儿心动过速，基线为 170 次 / 分。

- 硬膜外镇痛效果达到峰值，镇痛效果良好。

- 腹部检查：先露未触及。

- 阴道检查：宫口开全，胎头 S+2，左枕前位，胎头塑形阳性。

The clinical case synopsis:

G_1P_0 normal-term pregnancy

Spontaneous onset of labour 23:00 last night Epidural inserted 8 hours ago

IV oxytocin infusion commenced 8 hours ago

Indwelling urinary catheter inserted 7 hours ago-draining copious clear urine

Fully dilated 4 hours ago

Pushing commenced 2 hours ago with slow progress

Fetal heart rate now showing deep variable decelerations and baseline tachycardia 170 bpm

Epidural now topped and fully functional

Abdominal examination: presenting part not palpable

Vaginal examination: full dilatation, station +2, position left occipitoanterior, caput and moulding positive

房间内设备

- 符合当地医院使用标准的胎吸装置：吸杯、橡皮管和吸引器。

- 出口产钳。

- 足月胎儿全真模型。

Equipment in room:

Vacuum extractor cup, tubing and pump model and type per local norms

Outlet forceps

Full-size model of term fetus

任务：向法洛斯先生解释下列事项。

- 您做如下决定的理由。

- 建议人工助产。

- 工具选择（1min）。

向法洛斯先生演示（请他根据需要提供协助）以下内容。

- 将您选择的工具置于胎头。

- 牵引的方向。

- 注意事项、使用说明和限制条件（共 5min）。

回答法洛斯先生可能提出的任何问题（1min）。

Tasks:

Explain to Mr Fallows:

- Your reason(s) for:
- Advising assisted delivery now
- The choice of instrument (1 minute)

Demonstrate to Mr Fallows (ask him to assist as required):

- The application of your preferred instrument to the fetal head.
- The direction of pull.
- Precautions, caveats and restrictions. (5 minutes total)

Answer any questions Mr Fallows might have. (1 minute)

第 13 章（Chapter 13）

环境：产后病房。

Setting: Postnatal ward of a maternity unit

角色：低年资医生（实习生）。

Role: Junior doctor (intern)

情景：您被产后病房助产士呼叫，为 31 岁的旺达·沃灵顿（Wanda Warrington）（G_1P_1）提供避孕建议。

沃灵顿女士和她出生 1 天的儿子威廉（William）准备一起出院。

威廉在孕 40 周时自然分娩。他的出生体重为 3800g，Apgar 评分是 1 分钟 8 分和 5 分钟 10 分。

威廉已被新生儿科批准出院。

沃灵顿女士的出院前检查均正常。

Scenario: You have been paged by the postnatal ward mid- wife to provide advice on contraception for Wanda Warrington (G_1P_1), aged 31 years.

Ms Warrington is ready for discharge together with her

1-day-old son William.

William was born vaginally after spontaneous labour at 40 weeks' gestation. His birth weight was 3800 g and Apgar scores were 8 and 10 at 1 and 5 minutes, respectively.

William has been cleared for discharge by the neonatology team.

The pre-discharge midwifery check for Ms Warrington is normal.

任务（Tasks）

- 采集沃灵顿女士的病史（5min）。

- 向她提供避孕建议（2min）。

- 回答她可能提出的任何问题（1min）。

Take a relevant history from Ms Warrington. (5 minutes)

Advise Ms Warrington regarding her options for contraception. (2 minutes)

Answer any questions Ms Warrington might have. (1 minute)

第 14 章（Chapter 14）

环境：产后病房。

Setting: Postnatal ward of a maternity unit

角色：低年资医生（实习生）。

Role: Junior doctor (intern)

情景：您被产后病房助产士呼叫，对 31 岁的安东涅塔·艾灵顿（Antonietta Allington）（G_3P_2）进行检查。

助产士担心艾灵顿女士的心理健康状况，她在过去 24h 内显得孤僻和"淡漠"。

艾灵顿女士在 3 天前通过紧急剖腹产分娩，此前她已怀孕 30 周并伴有产前出血。产前胎心监护中出现深大变异减速，来不及使用糖皮质激素即分娩。安德鲁（Andrew）从出生起就需要机械通气，今天早上被诊断为 II 级脑室内出血。

艾灵顿女士既往有产后抑郁史。她有一个 3 岁的女儿艾梅（Aimee），目前由其祖母照顾。艾灵顿女士今年早些时候与她的伴侣安东尼（Anthony）分居。安东尼是这两个孩子的父亲。

Scenario: You have been paged by the postnatal ward mid-wife to review Antonietta Allington (G3P2), aged 31 years.

The midwife is concerned about the mental health state of

Ms Allington, who has in the last 24 hours appeared withdrawn and 'flat'.

Ms Allington delivered by emergency caesarean section 3 days ago following a presentation at 30 weeks' gestation with antepartum haemorrhage. Deep variable decelerations were observed on cardiotocography, and there was no time for antenatal corticosteroids. Andrew has required ventilation since birth and this morning has been diagnosed with a grade II intraventricular haemorrhage.

Ms Allington has a prior history of postnatal depression. She has a 3-year-old daughter, Aimee, who is currently being cared for by her grandmother. Ms Allington separated from her partner Anthony earlier this year. Anthony is the father of both children.

任务（Tasks）

- 向艾灵顿女士采集相关病史（6min）。

- 向艾灵顿女士提供后续治疗建议（2min）。

Take a relevant history from Ms Allington. (6 minutes)
Advise Ms Allington regarding her continuing management. (2 minutes)

注意：不要对她进行正式的精神病学评估。

Note: DO NOT perform a formal psychiatric evaluation.

第 15 章（Chapter 15）

设置：医学院的模拟器具。

Setting: Medical school simulation suite

角色：仿真器具演示。

Role: Simulation suite demonstrator

场景：您被安排一对一教授一组二年级医学生如何采集宫颈样本进行衣原体和淋病聚合酶链反应（PCR）检测。

你的学生是帕特里克·普莱斯（Patrick Price）。

Scenario: You are rostered to teach 1:1 a group of second-year medical students how to take a cervical sample for polymerase chain reaction (PCR) testing for Chlamydia and gonorrhoea.

Your student is Patrick Price.

任务（Tasks）

- 向普莱斯先生解释在进行此项检查之前您会如何与患者沟通。（2min）

- 演示如何使用模型和仪器进行此项检测，以及包括回答普莱斯先生在此期间提出的任何问题。（6min）

Explain to Mr Price what you would tell a patient prior to undertaking this test. (2 minutes)

Demonstrate using the model and equipment provided the procedure for this test, including answering any questions Mr Price might pose whilst you do so. (6 minutes)

第 16 章（Chapter 16）

设置：全科（家庭）医生。

Setting: General (family) practice

角色：轮转全科医生（GP）的第一年医学院毕业生。

Role: First-year medical graduate on general practitioner (GP) rotation

场景：您将为 42 岁的女性伊莱扎·埃瑟里奇（Eliza Etheridge）做咨询，已向其告知。

埃瑟里奇女士被转诊到当地医院妇科治疗顽固性月经量过多。3 个月前她进行了宫腔镜检查并置入了左炔诺孕酮宫内节育器。

现按照妇科要求进行后续随访。

她的病史概要如下。

伊莱扎·埃瑟里奇，单身，独居，是大律师事务所首席合伙人的全职私人助理。

药物：左炔诺孕酮宫内节育器

手术：宫腔镜检查，结果正常（活检结果：增生期子宫内膜）。

产科：未妊娠。

妇科：月经量大，缺铁性贫血。炔诺酮、甲芬那酸和氨甲环酸治疗无效。

宫颈癌筛查：最新检查示正常。

实习护士刚刚完成了常规检查（体重和血压正常）。在此期间，埃瑟里奇女士向护士透露，她对迄今为止的治疗结果并不满意，正在考虑进行子宫切除术。

Scenario: You are about to undertake a consultation for Eliza Etheridge, a 42-year-old woman who is known to the practice.

Ms Etheridge had been referred to the local hospital gynaecology unit for management of refractory heavy menstrual bleeding. They undertook hysteroscopy and insertion of a levonorgestrel intrauterine system 3 months ago.

This is the planned follow-up visit as requested by the gynaecology unit.

The synopsis of her medical record is:

Eliza Etheridge

Single, lives alone, works full time as personal assistant to chief partner of large legal firm.

Medications: levonorgestrel intrauterine device Surgical: hysteroscopy-normal findings (biopsy result: disordered proliferative phase endometrium)

Obstetric: never pregnant

Gynaecological: heavy menstrual bleeding and Fe-deficiency anaemia. Unresponsive to courses of norethisterone, mefenamic acid and tranexamic acid.

Cervical screening test: normal and up to date

The practice nurse has just completed taking routine observations (normal weight and blood pressure). During this Ms Etheridge confided to the nurse that she has not been happy with the results of her management to date and was thinking about having a hysterectomy.

任务（Tasks）

• 向埃瑟里奇女士了解病史（4min）。

• 与她讨论进一步的治疗方案（3min）。

• 回答她可能提出的任何问题（1min）。

Take a directed history from Ms Etheridge. (4 minutes)

Discuss further management with Ms Etheridge. (3 minutes)

Answer any questions Ms Etheridge may have. (1 minute)

第 17 章（Chapter 17）

设置：全科（家庭）医师。

Setting: General (family) practice

角色：正在全科医生轮转的第一年医学院毕业生。

Role: First-year medical graduate on GP rotation

场景：您正在与您的培训主管进行"平行咨询"。您将要为 2 周前到临时全科医生那看病的一对夫妇进行随访。

这是临时全科医生为这对夫妇咨询的概要：

Scenario: You are 'parallel consulting' with your training supervisor. You are about to undertake a follow-up consultation for a couple who were seen by a locum practitioner 2 weeks ago.

This is the synopsis of the locum GP's consultations for this couple:

简·约翰逊，年龄 32 岁。

不孕：试孕 18 个月，未孕。

病史：无。

与罗伯特·罗伯逊 [（Robert Robertson），35 岁] 同居 4 年。

药物：补充叶酸。

手术：无。

要求检查：盆腔超声。

Jane Johnson age 32 years

Unable to get pregnant-trying for 18 months. Has never been pregnant.

Well, no medical history.

De facto (Robert Robertson, age 35)-have lived together last 4 years.

Medications: folic acid supplement

Surgical: nil

Investigation requested: pelvic ultrasound

罗伯特·罗伯逊，年龄 35 岁。

病史：无。

与（简·约翰逊，32 岁）同居 4 年。

药物：无。

手术：无。

要求检查：精液分析。

Robert Robertson age 35 years

Well, no medical history.

De facto (Jane Johnson, age 32)-have lived together last 4 years

Medications: nil

Surgical: nil

Investigation requested: semen analysis

结果（Results summary）

• 盆腔超声：正常。

• 精液分析：精子浓度 10M/ml（正常≥ 15M/ml），正常形态 3%（正常≥ 4%），其他功能正常。

这对夫妇急于了解他们的检查结果并寻求帮助

以解决不孕症。

- Pelvic ultrasound: normal

- Semen analysis: sperm concentration 10 M/mL (normal≥15 M/mL), normal morphology 3% (normal ≥4%), all other features normal.

The couple are anxious to learn the results of their tests and for assistance with their infertility.

任务（Tasks）

- 向这对夫妇解释检查结果（1min）。

- 从这对夫妇那里采集更多的病史（5min）。

- 将您的治疗计划告知他们，并回答他们可能提出的任何问题（2min）。

Explain the test results to this couple. (1 minute)

Take additional history from the couple. (5 minutes)

Advise them of your plan of management and answer any questions they may have. (2 minutes)

第 18 章（Chapter 18）

地点：综合医院急诊室。

Setting: General hospital emergency department

角色：第一年医学院毕业生。

Role: First-year medical graduate

情景：埃尔维拉·埃文顿（Elvira Evington），女，24 岁，已被列入您的急诊名单中，这是您毕业后的第一位患者。

分诊护士的记录如下。

Scenario: Elvira Evington, a 24-year-old woman, has been triaged to your list in the emergency department-your very first patient since graduation.

The record made by the triage nurse is:

埃尔维拉·埃文顿，年龄 24。

自主步入诊室。

从昨晚开始出现下腹痛，早晨 4 时开始阴道出血，最初有大量血凝块（+++），现在流血减少。

已妊娠，上周超声显示 6 周。

检查结果：患者看起来无不适，脉搏 72 次 / 分，血压 130/80mmHg，氧饱和度 99%，床旁血红蛋白（Hb）110g/L。

尿 **hCG**：阳性。

尿液分析：正常。

Elvira Evington age 24 years

Self-referred walk-in

Lower abdominal pain since last night, onset 04:00 vaginal bleeding-initially heavy with clots +++, now settled to very light bleeding

Pregnant, scan last week = 6 weeks

Observations: looks comfortable, pulse 72 bpm, BP 130/80 mmHg, O$_2$ sat 99%, point-of-care haemoglobin (Hb) 110 g/L

Urinary hCG: positive

Urinalysis: normal

计划：让实习生对病情进行回顾。

Plan: intern review

任务（Tasks）

- 采集埃文顿女士的病史。（5min）

- 解释您要进行的检查。（1min）

- 然后，您将获得一些检查结果，阅读提供的信息（1min）。

- 告知埃文顿女士您的目前诊断和治疗计划（1min）。

Take a history from Ms Evington. (5 minutes)

Explain the examination you propose to undertake. (1 minute)

You will then be provided with some examination findings.

Read the information provided. (1 minute)

Inform Ms Evington of your provisional diagnosis and plan of management. (1 minute)

第 19 章（Chapter 19）

设置：全科医生。

Setting: General practice

角色：轮转的第一年医学院毕业生。

Role: First-year medical graduate on rotation

情景：费莉希蒂·法林顿（Felicity Farrington），女，32 岁，今天被列入您的咨询名单中。您的上级医生要求您处理她的避孕需求。

法林顿女士多年来一直是该医院的患者。病历记录如下。

Scenario: Felicity Farrington, a 32-year-old woman, has been allocated to your consultation list today. Your supervisor has asked you to manage her request for contraception.

Ms Farrington has been a patient of this practice for several years. The practice record includes:

费莉希蒂·法林顿，年龄 32 岁。

职业：当地小学助理教师。

婚姻状况：已婚，丈夫是莫德雷德·麦卡勒姆（Mordred McCallum）。

其他家属：一个孩子，马丁·麦卡勒姆（Martin McCallum），现 3 岁，健康。

手术：剖宫产。

产科史：G_1P_1（计划外——避孕套避孕失败）；因胎儿窘迫行急症子宫下段剖宫产。

药物：无。

上次就诊时间：6 个月前例行健康检查。

Felicity Farrington age 32 years

Occupation: Teachers' aide at local primary school

Marital status: Married (Mordred McCallum)

Dependents: One child (Martin McCallum-current age 3 years; healthy)

Surgery: Caesarean section

Obstetric: G_1P_1 (unplanned condom failure); emergency lower segment caesarean section (LSCS) at term for fetal distress

Medical: nil

Last visit to the practice: 6 months ago for routine health check

任务（Tasks）

- 从法林顿女士那里采集相关病史（5min）。

- 与法林顿女士讨论可选择的避孕方式并回答她的问题（3min）。

Take a relevant history from Ms Farrington. (5 minutes)

Discuss with Ms Farrington her options for contraception and answer her questions. (3 minutes)

第 20 章（Chapter 20）

环境：普通门诊。

Setting: General practice

角色：轮转的第一年医学院毕业生。

Role: First-year medical graduate on rotation

场景：吉安娜·吉安诺普洛斯（Giana Giannopoulos）是一位 35 岁的女性，今天被列入您的咨询名单中。

吉安诺普洛斯女士预约了这次咨询，目的是讨论她是否应该同意让其 11 岁的女儿海莉（Haley）在学校接种人乳头瘤病毒（HPV）疫苗。海莉非常健康，是吉安诺普洛斯女士唯一的孩子。

此外，自 12 年前就诊于该诊所以来，吉安诺普洛斯女士的记录中有一个"危险"提示，提示她未进行常规宫颈癌筛查。

Scenario: Giana Giannopoulos, a 35-year-old woman, has been allocated to your consultation list today.

Ms Giannopoulos booked the appointment to discuss whether she should give consent for her 11-year-old daughter Haley to be vaccinated at school against human papilloma virus (HPV). Haley is completely healthy and is the only child of Ms Giannopoulos.

In addition, there is a 'red flag' alert in Ms Giannopoulos's records related to her non-attendance for routine cervical screening tests since she joined the practice 12 years ago.

任务（Tasks）

- 解决吉安诺普洛斯女士对 Haley 接种疫苗的担忧。（4min）

- 与她讨论她进行宫颈癌筛查的问题。（4min）

Address Ms Giannopoulos' concerns regarding Haley's vaccinations. (4 minutes)

Discuss with Ms Giannopoulos her own participation in the cervical screening programme. (4 minutes)

第 21 章（Chapter 21）

环境：普通妇科门诊。

Setting: A general gynaecology outpatient clinic

角色：低年资医生（实习生）。

Role: Junior doctor (intern)

场景：您即将看到一位由当地全科医生转诊来的新患者。

以下内容为推荐信的正文。

Scenario: You are about to see a new patient referred by her local general practitioner.

This is the text of the referral letter:

亲爱的医生

Re：奥利维亚·奥利芬特（Olivia Oliphant），

56 岁。

感谢您接诊奥利芬特女士，她有长期的尿失禁和阴道脱垂问题。盆底锻炼没有效果。是否适合手术治疗？当前药物：无。

您真诚的，

当地的 B 医生。

以下是患者的详情。

年龄：56 岁。

婚姻状况：单身。

身高：160cm。

体重：90 公斤。

体重指数：31.1kg/m^2。

产次：0 次。

过敏：膏药和外科胶带。

Dear Doctor

Re: Olivia Oliphant, age 56 years

Thank you for seeing Ms Oliphant regarding long-standing urinary incontinence and vaginal prolapse. There has been no response to pelvic floor exercises. Is surgery appropriate?

Current medications: nil Yours sincerely,

Dr B Local

These are the patient's booking details:

Age: 56 years

Marital status: single Height: 160 cm

Weight: 90 kg

BMI: 31.1 kg/m^2

Parity: 0

Allergies: sticking plasters and surgical tape

任务（Tasks）

- 向奥利芬特女士采集病史（4min）。

- 向她解释您要进行的检查（1min）。

- 阅读检查结果（1min）。

- 解释你的治疗方案（1min）。

Take a directed history from Ms Oliphant. (4 minutes)

Explain to Ms Oliphant the examination and investigations you require. (1 minute)

Read the available examination findings and investigation results. (1 minute)

Explain your proposed management. (1 minute)

注意：演员可能没有上述身体特征。

Note: The actor might not have the stated physical characteristics.

附录 A（Appendix A）

环境：大医院的普通妇科病房。

Setting: A general gynaecology ward in a metropolitan hospital

角色：低年资医生（实习生）。

Role: Junior doctor (intern)

场景：上午 8 时您正在进行例行术后查房。您将要查房的患者是玛德琳·麦格拉斯（Madeline McGrath）女士，42 岁。

麦格拉斯女士昨天入院并接受了腹腔镜辅助阴式子宫切除术和阴道前壁修补术（阴道缝合术），以治疗月经量大和 POP-Q$_2$ 期前盆腔脱垂。该手术是在 23h 前进行的。您查房后患者将出院。

麦格拉斯女士躺在病床上（或手术推车上），穿着病号服。

以下是手术记录的全文。

Scenario: You are undertaking a scheduled (routine) postoperative ward round at 08:00. The patient you are about to see is Ms Madeline McGrath, aged 42 years.

Ms McGrath had been admitted yesterday for laparoscopically assisted vaginal hysterectomy and anterior vaginal wall repair (anterior colporrhaphy) for heavy menstrual bleeding and POPQ stage 2 anterior compartment prolapse. The procedure was undertaken 23 hours ago. The patient is scheduled for discharge home following your review.

Ms McGrath will be lying propped up in a hospital bed (or barouche) and wearing hospital clothing.

This is the text of the operation note:

玛德琳·麦格拉斯，42 岁。

手术名称：腹腔镜辅助阴式全子宫切除术、右侧输卵管卵巢切除术、左侧输卵管切除术、阴道前壁修补术。

术中所见：2 期前盆腔脱垂、多发性子宫肌瘤、子宫增大至 14 周大小、右卵巢子宫内膜异位囊肿直径 4cm，故行右卵巢切除术。

术后指导：夜里 12 时拔除尿管。术后 23h 后实习生检查后，出院回家。

以下是她术后情况的概要。

夜里有中等程度不适，需要羟考酮 10mg，每 6 小时一次。

夜里 12 时拔掉尿管；到早晨 6 时为止还没有排尿。

脉搏：84 次 / 分。

血压：120/80mmHg。

体温：37.4℃。

Madeline McGrath, age 42 years

Procedure summary: laparoscopically assisted vaginal hysterectomy, right salpingo-oophorectomy, left salpingectomy, anterior vaginal repair.

Findings: stage 2 anterior compartment prolapse, multiple uterine fibroids, uterus enlarged to 14 w size, 4 cm endometrioma right ovary-elected also to perform right oophorectomy.

Postoperative instructions: remove urinary catheter midnight.Discharge home per 23-hour policy following intern review.

The following is the synopsis of her postoperative observations:

Moderately uncomfortable night, requiring oxycodone 10 mg 6-hourly

Urinary catheter removed midnight; has not passed urine as of 06:00

Pulse: 84 bpm

BP: 120/80 mmHg

Temperature: 37.4°C

任务（Tasks）

• 向麦格拉斯女士采集简要病史（3min）。

• 对她进行腹部检查（1min）。

• 解释您的后续方案（3min）。

• 回答她的问题（1min）。

Take a directed history from Ms McGrath. (3 minutes)

Perform an abdominal examination. (1 minute)

Explain your proposed management. (3 minutes)

Answer Ms McGrath's questions. (1 minute)

附录 C（Appendix C）

地点：大医院的普通妇科门诊。

Setting: A general gynaecology outpatient clinic in a metropolitan hospital

角色：低年资医生（实习生）。

Role: Junior doctor (intern)

场景：您在门诊进行咨询。您将要见到的是佐伊·色诺芬（Zoe Xenophon）女士，现年 52 岁。

当地妇科医生将色诺芬女士转诊到您的门诊，以治疗绝经后出血。

以下是推荐信的正文。

Scenario: You are consulting in an outpatient clinic. The woman you are about to see is Ms Zoe Xenophon, aged 52 years.

Ms Xenophon has been referred by her local gynaecologist for management of postmenopausal bleeding.

This is the text of the referral note:

亲爱的医生

Re：色诺芬，52 岁。

感谢您将要对色诺芬女士的治疗。她 3 年前绝经。在过去的 3 个月里她出现阴道不规则的流血，量同月经量。

盆腔超声提示子宫内膜厚度为 1.5cm。

宫颈癌筛查和液基细胞学结果正常。

当前药物：无。

过敏：无。

诊断：超重，2 型糖尿病（饮食控制）。

社会方面：已婚，做全职清洁工。

手术史：32 岁因 CIN2 行 LLETZ 手术。

产科史：1 个孩子，现年 24 岁。

我在我的诊室里尝试行宫腔镜检查。由于患者不适（宫颈狭窄），放弃操作，无法获取子宫内膜样本。

请您进行治疗。

Dear Doctor

re: Zoe Xenophon, age 52 years

Thank you for on-going management of Ms Xenophon. Her menopause was 3 years ago. For the past 3 months she has noticed irregular, period-like vaginal bleeding.

Pelvic ultrasound identified endometrial thickness of 1.5 cm.

Cervical screening test and liquid-based cytology results are normal.

Current medications: nil

Allergies: nil

Medical: overweight, type 2 diabetes diet controlled

Social: married, works full time as cleaner

Surgical: LLETZ procedure age 32 for CIN2

Obstetric: 1 child now aged 24 years

I attempted hysteroscopy in my rooms. The attempt was abandoned due to patient discomfort (cervical stenosis). Unable to obtain endometrial sample.

Please see and treat.

任务（Tasks）

• 采集色诺芬女士的简要病史（2min）。

• 向色诺芬女士解释评估她的疾病需要进行的操作，其中包括风险、获益和替代方案（如果有的话）（4min）。

• 回答她可能有的任何问题（2min）。

Take a brief, directed history from Ms Xenophon. (2 minutes)

Explain to Ms Xenophon the procedure that is required to evaluate her problem, including risks, benefits and alternatives (if any). (4 minutes)

Answer any questions she might have. (2 minutes)

三、OSCE 站点：答案（OSCE stations: Answers）

第 6 章（Chapter 6）

在这个情景中，一位不明孕周的孕妇正在就诊。该患者肥胖，正在接受高血压治疗，并且正在服用大剂量的叶酸。她和丈夫住在一起，没有提到孩子。她的糖尿呈阳性，这是一个干扰项。

In this scenario, a pregnant woman of unstated gestational age is presenting for a booking visit. The woman is obese, is on treatment for hypertension and is taking high-dose folic acid. She is living with her husband with no mention of children. She is positive for glycosuria, which is a distractor.

您应该从病史中确定孕周、她过去两次妊娠的详细信息、家族史、遗传病史、既往病史、手术史和目前妊娠的情况。以及患者可能有的顾虑和提出的开放性问题。

You should establish from the history the gestational age, the details of her two past pregnancies, history of familial or inheritable disorders, general medical and surgical history and progress to date in the current pregnancy. Include open questions regarding any concerns the patient might have.

在这种情况下，治疗高血压是关键。确定该患者服用阿替洛尔的时间、高血压的潜在病因（如果知道的话），以及她最近的血液检查结果。询问未控制满意的高血压的症状，如果孕周为 20 周或以上，考虑诊断子痫前期。

Treated hypertension is a key feature in this case. Establish how long the woman has been taking atenolol, the underlying cause of hypertension, if known, and what her recent blood measurements have been. Enquire regarding symptoms of poorly controlled hypertension, and consider pre-eclampsia if the gestational age is 20 weeks or more.

第二个关键点是该患者正在服用大剂量叶酸。问她为什么要服用这么高的剂量。这可能与之前怀孕出现过神经管缺陷有关，或者可能表明患者有血栓形成倾向。

The second key feature is that the woman is taking highdose folic acid. Ask her why she is taking this high dose. It might be related to neural tube defect in a previous pregnancy. Or it could indicate a thrombophilia.

第三个关键点是该患者肥胖。这增加了她患妊娠合并症的风险，其中包括妊娠期糖尿病。尿糖是一个干扰项。尽管如此，请考虑为筛查妊娠期糖尿病和其他妊娠合并症（子痫前期、胎儿异常、胎儿生长受限）要进行的检查。

The third key feature is that the woman is obese. This increases her risk of pregnancy complications, including gestational diabetes. Glycosuria is a distractor. Nevertheless, consider what screening or diagnostic tests for gestational diabetes and other pregnancy complications (pre-eclampsia, fetal anomalies, perturbation in fetal growth) are appropriate.

综合您获得的信息并向患者解释您的诊断和治疗计划。除了您的筛查和（或）诊断性检查外，这个病例的风险较高，还需要根据当地临床常规由专家进行保健。

Synthesize the data you have acquired and explain to the actor your working diagnosis/diagnoses and plans for management. In addition to screening and/or diagnostic tests, this case is high risk and requires specialist management per local protocols.

最后，准备好回答演员的简单问题。可能是询问诊断和管理方案，妊娠期阿替洛尔的安全性，或有关的其他社会问题，例如，她继续承担压力较大的全职工作是否合适。

Finally, be prepared for simple questions from the actor. These could be for clarification of diagnosis and management, safety of atenolol in pregnancy or related to a social issue such as appropriateness of her continuing to work full time in a stressful occupation.

第 7 章（Chapter 7）

在这个情景中，一位女士正在询问在妊娠期她应该如何调整饮食和锻炼。该患者超重，患有多囊卵巢综合征，并通过改变饮食和锻炼成功减轻了体重。

In this scenario, a woman is enquiring about adjustments during her pregnancy that she should make to her diet and exercise routine. The woman is overweight, has polycystic ovarian syndrome and has successfully lost weight through changes to her diet and with exercise.

她的核心要求是建立妊娠期饮食和运动习惯。应回答该患者担心的任何问题。

The key requirements are to establish what her current diet and exercise habits are. This should include open questions regarding any concerns the woman has.

关于妊娠期间的合理饮食的证据是有限的，部分原因是大多数研究是回顾性的，并且人们饮食类型广泛。然而，一些一般性原则可能适用于您所在的医院，其中包括建议孕前常规补充叶酸，以及产前常规补充口服铁剂。食用垃圾食品和软饮料会增加子痫前期和妊娠期糖尿病的风险，其他饮食因素包括钙和碘摄入不足（如不吃乳制品和碘盐）。一些素食者在没有膳食补充剂的情况下可能出现维生素 B_{12} 摄入量不足。这个患者的职业容易暴饮暴食，应该评估她每日热量摄入量。

Evidence regarding what constitutes an adequate diet in pregnancy is limited in part due to the retrospective nature of most studies and the wide range of diets people have. However, some generalizations are likely to apply to your locale, including recommendations for routine prepregnancy supplementation with folic acid and routine antenatal supplementation with oral Fe regimens. A diet that consists largely of junk food and soft drinks increases the risk of pre-eclampsia and gestational diabetes. Other dietary factors include inadequate calcium and iodine intake (e.g. by avoidance of dairy foods and iodized salt). Some vegetarians might, without dietary supplementation, have inadequate vitamin

B_{12} intake. The woman's occupation creates opportunities for overeating. Estimation of daily calorie intake should be covered in the enquiry.

此外，询问相关非食物物质的摄入量，其中包括酒精和香烟，并考虑她是否有足够的阳光照射以产生足够的维生素 D。

In addition, enquire about intake of relevant non-food substances, including alcohol and cigarettes, and consider whether she has adequate sun exposure for sufficient vitamin D production.

怀孕期间的运动可以限制体重过度增加，且有氧运动可以保持或改善健康状况。运动与饮食相结合可以降低妊娠期糖尿病和剖宫产的风险。然而，没有足够的证据去据此调整个人的饮食和运动习惯。但是，也有实际的考虑，如患者是否存在腰痛或关节痛等可能在妊娠期加剧并影响其锻炼的问题？如果有，您将如何推荐她的热量摄入量？

Exercise in pregnancy appears to limit excessive weight gain, and aerobic exercise maintains or improves fitness. Exercise in combination with diet appears to reduce the risk of gestational diabetes and caesarean delivery. Unfortunately, there is insufficient evidence to tailor this general information to an individual's diet and exercise habits. However, there are pragmatic considerations, for example, does the woman have an existing condition such as low back pain or joint pain that might be exacerbated during pregnancy and impact her ability to exercise? If so, how would you address that in relation to her recommended calorie intake?

准备好回答诸如"我应该吃双人餐吗？""继续我的日常健身计划会伤害胎儿或导致早产吗？"和"我在妊娠后期可以做哪些运动？"等问题。

Be prepared to answer questions such as 'Should I eat for two?' 'Will continuing with my daily gym circuit harm the baby or bring labour on early?' and 'What exercises can I do later in pregnancy?'

第 8 章（Chapter 8）

在这个情景中，一名第二次妊娠的患者在孕晚期出现了产前出血。这名患者已由一名助产士接管。她临床情况稳定，胎心率正常，腹部柔软，宫底高度与孕周一致，胎儿是臀位。血尿可能是由样本污染导致。

In this scenario, a woman in her second pregnancy presents with a third-trimester antepartum haemorrhage. The woman has been triaged by a midwife. She is clinically stable, the fetal heart rate is normal, abdomen soft and symphysial-fundal height is consistent with dates and with a breech presentation. The haematuria is likely explained by contamination of the sample.

首先通过"床边"观察形成对患者身体和精神状态的印象。虽然这不是一个真正的场景，但要注意演员的暗示，这些暗示表明情况比观察到的更为严重。

Begin by forming an impression of the patient's state both physically and mentally by 'end of the bed' observations. Although this is not a real encounter, be alert to cues from the actor that might suggest the situation is more acute than indicated by the observations provided.

根据病史，确定出血的情况和原因，相关或诱发因素，以及这是首次发作还是复发。产前出血通常分为疼痛性 [提示胎盘早剥和（或）早产] 或无痛性（提示前置胎盘或局部出血）。确认出血时间很关键，询问之前的检查如既往超声提示的胎盘位置、血型和血型抗体很重要。必须建立产科档案。如果患者曾有子宫下段剖宫产术史，则考虑前置胎盘植入的可能。

From your history, establish the onset and nature of the bleeding, associated or precipitating factors and whether this is the first or a recurrent episode. Antepartum haemorrhage is conventionally categorized as painful (suggesting placental abruption and/or pre-term labour) or painless (suggesting placenta praevia or a local cause of bleeding). Confirming dates is critical, as is enquiring about prior investigations such as previous placental location by ultrasound, and blood group and antibody status. The obstetric history must also be established. If the patient has had a prior lower segment caesarean delivery, consider placenta praevia accreta.

接下来的检查包括再次腹部检查、用窥器行阴道检查，以及安排心电图（CTG）和相关的血液检查。为谨慎起见，可行尿液显微镜检查和培养。大多数急诊室配备便携式超声机，这将用于检查胎盘位置。所有这一切都应该以明确条目形式向演员进行解释。在您的解释中应包括进行额外检查的原因，说明您要诊断或排除的疾病。当地临床常规可能包括向该患者提供倍他米松，并且可能会要求她在评估室或医院接受短时间观察。但是对于高风险患者，您应该告知该患者，同时由高年资医师进行评估。

The next steps include repeating the abdominal examination, performing a speculum examination and arranging in the unit a cardiotograph (CTG) and relevant blood tests. It would be prudent also to request a formal urine microscopy and culture. Most acute assessment units will have a portable ultrasound, and this would be used to check the presentation and placental localization. All of this should be explained to the actor in clear lay terms. Include in your explanation the reasons for performing the additional examination and tests, i.e. say what you are looking to find or exclude. Local protocol might include that this patient be offered betamethasone and likely will require her to be observed for a minimum period either in the assessment unit or admitted to the ward. However, as this is a high-risk situation, you should indicate that the patient will also be reviewed by a senior member of the medical staff.

最后，患者会担心出血，如果她家里有孩子，还会担心在她在院观察期间如何照顾孩子的问题。关于胎儿安全，可适当谨慎地保证，同时认识到这是一种不可预测的情况，可能会出现足月前手术分娩。目前该患者出院并不安全，需要考虑安排托儿服务。

Finally, the patient will be anxious about the bleeding and, if she has a child at home, about arrangements for that child's care whilst she remains under observation. In relation to fetal safety, cautious reassurance is appropriate whilst recognizing this is an unpredictable situation that might yet result in pre-term operative delivery. It is not safe at present for the woman to leave hospital, so child care arrangements will need to be made with that in mind.

第 9 章（Chapter 9）

在这个情景中，一名有一个孩子和两次妊娠流产的患者正在进行孕前咨询。她患有易栓症（凝血因子 V Leiden 基因纯合突变），"近几年"服用华法林，血压正常。她可能反复出现血栓栓塞。

In this scenario, a woman with one child and two pregnancy losses is attending for prenatal counselling. She has thrombophilia (homozygous factor V Leiden), has been taking warfarin 'for several years' and is normotensive. She might have had recurrent thromboembolism.

由于这是孕前咨询，因此需要明确该患者的计划。她想什么时候妊娠？这对夫妇可能正在使用工具避孕或左炔诺孕酮宫内节育器。是否有生育力低下问题需要解决？是否有其他需要考虑的病史或家族史？她最近有接种疫苗吗？

As this is a prenatal presentation, establish what the woman's plans are. When does she want to become pregnant? The couple are probably using either barrier contraception or a levonorgestrel intrauterine system. Are there subfertility problems that need to be addressed? Are there any other health problems in the woman or in the family history that also must be considered? Are her vaccinations up to date?

华法林具有致畸作用，需要在受孕前更换为更安全的抗凝药物，如依诺肝素。该患者应了解她的易栓症及治疗方案，她上次怀孕时可能使用过依诺肝素。使用开放式问题，例如，"您为什么服用华法林？"和"您上次怀孕时是如何治疗这个疾病的？"详细了解产科病史，注意用药与早孕流产和宫内生长受限的关系。在最近一次妊娠中是否有需要提前分娩的并发症？新生儿出生体重是多少？孩子健康吗？

Warfarin is teratogenic and will need to be replaced with a safer anticoagulant, such as enoxaparin, prior to conception. The woman should be well informed about her thrombophilia and its management and might have used enoxaparin in her last pregnancy. Use open questions such as 'Why you are taking warfarin?' and 'How was this problem managed in your last pregnancy?' Establish in detail the obstetric history, being mindful of the association with early pregnancy loss and intrauterine growth restriction in such cases. Were there complications in the last pregnancy requiring early delivery? What was the birth weight? Is the child healthy?

由于这是一个较难的情景，下一步需要根据当地临床常规请产科医生或多学科团队进行处理。但是，您应说明您计划的管理方案，其中包括抗凝方案的变化，以及产科保健常规，例如，必要时重新接种疫苗和服用营养补充剂以尽量减少神经管缺陷的风险。

As this is an advanced topic, the next step in management requires engagement of an obstetrician or a multidisciplinary team per local protocols. However, you should also indicate what you expect will be done, including a managed change in the anticoagulation regimen, plus routine preventive health care, such as updated vaccinations where required and supplements to minimize risk of neural tube defect.

如果需要，患者可能只要求您解释您提出的治疗方案。

The actor is likely to ask only for clarification of your proposed management if that is required.

第 10 章（Chapter 10）

在这个情景中，一名妊娠 34 周（日期确定）没有规律产检的患者，到诊所接受常规产前检查。胎位为臀位，4 周内宫底高度没有变化，提示宫内生长受限（IUGR）。孕周是准确的，IUGR 需鉴别子痫前期，但似乎不能诊断。

In this scenario, a woman at 34 weeks' gestation (sure dates) and with limited antenatal care presents for a routine antenatal clinic review. There is a breech presentation and no change in the symphysial-fundal height in 4 weeks, suggesting intrauterine growth restriction (IUGR). The dates are accurate,

and pre-eclampsia, although on the differential diagnosis of IUGR, appears unlikely in this case.

采集病史时应询问患者是否注意到任何胎儿异常，询问胎动情况和 IUGR 的危险因素，包括母亲吸烟、母体慢性疾病、是否服用有潜在有害的药物、胎儿结构的筛查结果、经胎盘感染情况、既往妊娠是否出现产前出血和 IUGR 等。由于时间很短，演员将被安排对大多数或所有这些问题持否定回答。

The history should be directed at establishing whether the woman has noticed anything wrong, enquiring about fetal movements and about risk factors for IUGR, including maternal smoking, chronic maternal disease, potentially harmful medications, results of screening for fetal anomalies, transplacental infection, antepartum haemorrhage and IUGR in previous pregnancies. Because time is short, the actor will be scripted to answer in the negative for most or all of these problems.

需要立即进行检查以评估胎儿的健康状况并确诊或排除一些诊断。应行胎心监护和正式的超声评估，以评估胎儿生长参数、羊水量和血流速度 [根据当地临床常规，胎儿脐动脉和（或）胎儿大脑中动脉的血流速度]。其他检查通常可以推迟，先等待这些结果。用通俗的语言解释这些检查的内容和目的。

Prompt investigations are required to assess fetal wellbeing and rule in or rule out the provisional diagnosis. A CTG should be requested, as should formal ultrasound evaluation for assessment of fetal growth parameters, amniotic fluid volume and Doppler flow velocity (fetal umbilical artery plus or minus fetal middle cerebral artery per local protocol). Other investigations usually can be delayed pending these results. Explain the investigations-what they are and their purpose-using plain language.

检查结果会以报告形式提供给您（有些学校可能希望您解释未出报告的 CTG）。向患者解释这些检查。最后解释您的后续治疗计划，包括确认胎位是臀位的意义。由于这是一个复杂的案例，需要产科医生的介入。

You will then be provided with results in report form (some schools might expect you to interpret an unreported CTG). Explain your interpretation of these data to the actor. Conclude with an explanation of your management, including factoring in the significance of the breech presentation if confirmed. As this is a complicated case, input of an obstetrician is required.

患者可能只要求您解释后续治疗方案。

The actor is likely to ask only for clarification of your proposed management.

第 11 章（Chapter 11）

在这个情景中，会给您一份"教学用产程图"，该图是基于对足月自然分娩的初产妇超过 10h 的观察。妊娠并不复杂。产程图将展示一个常见的产科问题，很可能是与胎儿持续正枕后位（OP）或横位有关的产程进展缓慢，检测到羊水粪染，随后用胎儿头皮电极直接监测胎心率。CTG 可能是正常的，也可能有明显的异常，如反复出现的深大变异减速和基线心动过速。

In this scenario, you are provided in the reading time with a 'teaching partogram' based on observations over 10 hours of a primigravid woman presenting with spontaneous labour at term. The pregnancy is uncomplicated. The partogram will indicate a common obstetric problem, most likely poor progress of labour associated with a persisting, deflexed occiput posterior (OP) position or a deep transverse arrest, with meconium liquor detected and subsequent application of a fetal scalp electrode for direct monitoring of the fetal heart rate. The CTG could be normal, or it might have an obvious abnormality such as recurrent deep variable decelerations with a baseline tachycardia.

你的任务是用新手护士能听懂的语言（其中应包括专业术语和外行语言）识别和解释如何完成检查记录及其含义。

Your task is to recognize and explain in terms suitable for a novice student nurse (which should include technical terms with their explanation in lay language) how the recordings are done and what they mean.

演员可能会要求您解释后续治疗计划，或者您是否认为可以更好地管理产程；如果是，该如何管理。根据本医院临床常规处理不理想的时候才会问到最后一个问题，例如，与静脉内（IV）使用催产素或镇痛药物有关的问题。

The actor might ask for clarification of your proposed management or if you thought the labour could have been better managed and, if so, how. The latter question would only be asked if management was suboptimal in accordance with local protocol, e.g. in relation to use of intravenous (IV) oxytocin or use of analgesia.

第 12 章（Chapter 12）

在这个情景中，您正在向演员或真正的医学生描述在第二产程延长且胎心率异常的情况下如何阴道助产（出口产钳）。

In this scenario, you are describing to an actor, or perhaps a real medical student, assisted vaginal (outlet) delivery in a case of prolonged second stage and with an abnormal fetal

heart rate pattern.

简要解释为什么需要立即分娩，为什么腹部和阴道检查结果表明人工助产是安全的，以及为什么现在是最佳分娩时机（无痛，排空膀胱）。

Explain briefly why delivery is indicated, the abdominal and vaginal examination findings that indicate assisted vaginal delivery is safe and why the timing is now optimal (optimal analgesia, bladder empty).

助产器械的选择要根据当地临床常规。由于胎头吸引术肛门括约肌损伤的风险较低，通常作为首选。但是胎头吸引杯容易脱落。操作者的技能也是一个重要因素。考虑到这些因素，解释您为何选择该器械。

The choice of instrument might be determined by local protocol. If so, usually vacuum extraction is preferred due to the lower risk of anal sphincter trauma. However, the vacuum cup is more likely to pull off. Individual operator skill is an important factor. Explain your choice of instrument with these factors in mind.

然后，在胎儿模型上演示，并在学生 / 演员的帮助下，将您选择的器械置于胎头，并在这样做时解释使用该器械的注意事项、使用说明和限制条件。

Then, demonstrate on the model of the fetus and with the aid of the student/actor the application to the fetal head of the instrument you prefer, and explain as you do so the precautions, caveats and restrictions in the use of this device.

学生 / 演员可能会要求您解释您提出的治疗方案，如采用会阴切开术，如果分娩情况没有达到您的预期，您会怎么做，或者您会使用什么形式的胎儿监护。

The student/actor might ask for clarification of your proposed management, e.g. use of an episiotomy, what you would do if delivery was not achieved as you had anticipated or what form of fetal monitoring you would use.

第 13 章（Chapter 13）

在这个情景中，您需要提供产后避孕建议。要有效地做到这一点，请确定患者产前避孕方式的选择和偏好、社会和财务状况，其中包括她当前是否处于异性恋关系中、相关的病史和家族史、母乳喂养计划及未来生育计划。

In this scenario, you are required to provide advice on contraception in the postnatal period. To do so effectively, establish antecedent use and preference, social and financial circumstances including whether she is in a current heterosexual relationship, relevant medical and family history, plans for breast-feeding and plans for future children.

潜在的因素包括先前对某些避孕方法的负面经验，个人选择和偏好，根据病史或家族史不适合的避孕方法（如凝血因子 V Leiden 因子纯合突变），不打算母乳喂养，在妊娠期间与伴侣分开或不打算继续妊娠。

Potential permutations include prior negative experience of certain methods, personal choice and preference, medical or family history that render some methods unsuitable (e.g. homozygous factor V Leiden), intention not to breast-feed, a split from her partner during the pregnancy or intention not to have more children.

演员可能会要求您解释推荐的避孕方法，以及她何时可以恢复性行为，或她应该采取哪些措施来预防性传播感染。

The actor might ask for clarification of a recommendation, about when she can resume having sex or what she should do to prevent sexually transmitted infection.

第 14 章（Chapter 14）

在这个情景中，你需要评估一位已知有抑郁症风险因素的女性，她的行为在过去 24h 内发生了变化，并引起了关注。

In this scenario, you are asked to assess a woman with known risk factors for depression and whose behaviour in the past 24 hours has changed and given cause for concern.

你的首要任务是与演员建立融洽的关系，演员被指示回答你的问题，但很少有表情或情绪，并避免与你眼神接触。

Your first task is to develop rapport with the actor, who has been instructed to answer your questions but with little expression or emotion and to avoid eye contact.

自我介绍后，询问这位女士和她的孩子的病情进展。说明会面的目的。了解以下内容。

After introducing yourself, enquire about the woman's progress and that of her baby. Explain the purpose of the interview. Establish the following:

- 病史，精神病学、家庭和社会史。

- 产科和性病史，其中包括有无来自前伴侣的暴力和虐待的风险。

- 她伤害自己和孩子的风险。

- Medical, psychiatric, family and social history

- Obstetric and sexual history, including risk of violence and abuse from her ex-partner

- Risk of harm to self and her children

尽管这似乎是一个对女性及其子女进行心理健康评估和风险评估的案例，但也要考虑可能存在疾病（如甲状腺功能减退症）的可能性。您必须表明您会汇报给上级医师（包括产科医生和新生儿团队），表明您将咨询值班的精神科医生或心理健康团队的意见。如果艾灵顿女士和孩子们面临来自她前伴侣的暴力的风险，请说明您将联系一位社工为他们安排安全的住宿和紧急财务支持。如果您担心艾灵顿女士本人可能会给她的孩子带来风险，您需要根据法律要求亲自通知当地儿童福利机构。这需要公开信息，但在方式和措辞上要小心谨慎。

Although this appears to be a case involving evaluation of mental health and risk assessment for the woman and her children, consider also the possibility that there might be contributing medical conditions (e.g. hypothyroidism). You must indicate that you will involve senior medical staff, including the consultant obstetrician and neonatology team. Indicate that you will request an opinion from the on-call psychiatrist or mental health team. If Ms Allington and the children are at risk of violence from her ex-partner, indicate that you will involve a social services worker who will be able to arrange safe housing and emergency financial support. If you are concerned that Ms Allington might herself pose a risk to her children, you might be legally required to personally notify the local child welfare authorities. Open disclosure is required, but be careful and sensitive in manner and choice of words.

第 15 章（Chapter 15）

在这个情景中，您正在教授一名低年资医学生（或演员）如何进行检查前的咨询，并使用骨盆模型教授宫颈取样，以进行衣原体和淋病聚合酶链反应（PCR）检测。

In this scenario, you are teaching a junior medical student (or actor) pre-examination counselling and, using a model of a pelvis, the technique of taking a cervical sample for polymerase chain reaction (PCR) testing for Chlamydia and gonorrhoea.

您将获得阴道窥器和其他相关设备。虽然没有真实的病人，但应使模拟体验尽可能真实，咨询应以患者为中心（使用通俗的语言）。

You will be provided with a vaginal speculum and other relevant equipment. Although there is no live patient, to keep the simulation experience as authentic as possible, the recommended counselling should be patient focussed (use lay language).

第 16 章（Chapter 16）

在这个情景中，一名 42 岁的女性在植入左炔诺孕酮宫内节育器 3 个月后就诊，表示她希望行子宫切除术，因为她对口服非甾体抗炎药、抗纤溶药物、孕激素制剂和宫内节育器的效果均不满意。

In this scenario, a 42-year-old woman, presenting 3 months after insertion of a levonorgestrel intrauterine system, has indicated that she is seeking hysterectomy, as she is unhappy with the outcomes of oral non-steroidal antiinflammatory, anti-fibrinolytic and progestogen regimens and the intrauterine system.

明确她为什么对左炔诺孕酮宫内节育器不满意，以及她将子宫切除术作为下一步方案的原因。出血的原因是什么？是否有子宫内膜异位症的相关症状？尽管根据子宫内膜活检的结果，慢性盆腔感染似乎不太可能，但仍需与她确认是否有异常阴道分泌物，以及她是否接受过性传播疾病（STI）筛查。检查她对先前方案的依从性和使用时间。考虑治疗失败的其他原因，特别是凝血障碍——她容易瘀青吗？是否有出血倾向的家族史？她是否正在服用任何可能导致异常子宫出血的非处方药？确定她的性交史，包括她是否担心干预后永久丧失生育能力。她是否考虑过子宫切除术的替代方案，包括等待更长时间来确定当前治疗的疗效、使用口服避孕药中的药物活性片剂或子宫内膜消融术？

Establish why she is unhappy with the levonorgestrel system and her reasons for considering hysterectomy as the next step. What is the nature of the bleeding problem? Are there associated symptoms that might indicate endometriosis? Although chronic pelvic infection seems unlikely given the endometrial biopsy result, check if she has abnormal vaginal discharge and if she has been screened for sexually transmitted infection (STI). Check her compliance with and duration of use of the prior regimens. Consider other reasons for treatment failure, in particular, clotting disorders-Does she bruise easily? Is there a family history of bleeding tendencies? Is she taking any over-the-counter substances that might contribute to abnormal uterine bleeding? Establish her sexual history, including whether she has any concerns about permanent loss of fertility from an intervention. Has she considered alternatives to hysterectomy, including waiting longer to establish the efficacy of the current treatment, continuous active tablets from an oral contraceptive pill regimen or endometrial ablation?

演员可能会要求您解释您的建议，例如，在手术后能否返回工作岗位。

The actor might ask for clarification of a recommendation, for example, return to work after a surgical procedure.

第 17 章（Chapter 17）

在这个情景中，一对患有原发性不孕症的夫妇正在参加随访，以了解盆腔超声和精液分析的结果。精液分析结果显示轻度异常。但是，双方都没有足够的历史记录，您必须在推荐治疗方案之前补充这些记录。

In this scenario, a couple with primary infertility are attending a follow-up visit to learn the results of a pelvic ultrasound and semen analysis. The semen analysis result is mildly abnormal. However, neither partner has had an adequate history documented, which you are to rectify prior to recommending management.

确定月经史和性交史，询问雄激素过多症相关症状（痤疮、多毛症）、性行为的频率和时间、是否有勃起或射精问题、酒精和药物使用情况、性传播感染的危险因素，并考虑其他生活方式问题（如肥胖）。

Establish the menstrual and sexual history, enquire regarding hyperandrogenism (acne, hirsutism), frequency and timing of sex, problems with erection or ejaculation, alcohol and drug use, risk factors for STI and consider other lifestyle issues (e.g. obesity).

您的管理应旨在排除输卵管因素不孕和性传播疾病，如果存在生活方式问题，则应加以解决，应在禁欲至少 3 天后重复精液分析，并应转诊至专科医生。

Your management should aim to exclude tubal factor infertility and STI, lifestyle issues if present should be addressed, the semen analysis should be repeated after at least 3 days of abstinence and referral for specialist review should be discussed.

演员可能会要求您解释您的建议或对某些治疗方案的看法，例如行腹腔镜检查术或体外受精胚胎移植术。

The actors might ask for clarification of a recommendation or for your views on a specific aspect of management such as laparoscopy or in vitro fertilization.

第 18 章（Chapter 18）

在这个情景中，您需要评估一位在妊娠早期（孕 7 周）出现腹痛和阴道流血的患者。先前已确认宫内妊娠，所提供的信息表明该女性目前并无失血性休

633

克的风险。

In this scenario, you are asked to assess a woman who has presented in early pregnancy (≈7 weeks) with abdominal pain and vaginal bleeding. An intrauterine pregnancy has previously been confirmed, and the information provided indicates the woman is not currently on the verge of haemorrhagic shock.

询问疼痛和出血情况，以确认患者临床情况稳定或正在好转。然而，无论对身体上有何影响，以及是否计划妊娠，早孕流产都会带来情绪上的痛苦。承认这一点，并询问该患者是否需要联系家人以获得支持。委婉地询问是否是计划怀孕。如果这是避孕失败的结果，不要认为患者不想妊娠。还需要询问简要的病史，在这个年龄段通常无特殊病史。

Enquire regarding pain and bleeding to confirm the impression that the woman is clinically stable or improving. However, early pregnancy loss is emotionally distressing, regardless of physical impact, whether the pregnancy was planned or not. Acknowledge this and ask if the woman needs a support person to be contacted. Tactfully enquire if the pregnancy was planned. If this was the result of failure of contraception, do not assume that the pregnancy is not wanted. A brief medical history is also required, which in this age group is usually normal.

需要进行腹部和盆腔检查。这位女士之前可能没有接受过任何检查，因此请确认一下，并解释检查如何进行以及为何需要检查。然后将向您提供结果，这些结果将指导您进行诊断和下一步检查。一个典型的情景是宫颈口可容一指（即宫颈扩张），这表明完全流产。在大多数医院，这种诊断将通过超声波确认，并安排常规血液检查，其中包括全血细胞计数、血型和抗体筛查。如果妊娠物在阴道内，安排病理学检查并说明原因。必要时向患者解释当地的抗 D 免疫球蛋白给药方案。

Abdominal and pelvic examination is required. The woman might not have had either type of examination before, so check this and explain how the examination is done and why it is indicated. You will then be provided with the results, which will guide you regarding the provisional diagnosis and to the next step: investigations. A typical scenario is that the cervical os admits a finger (i.e. is widely dilated), suggesting complete miscarriage. In most units this provisional diagnosis will be confirmed by ultrasound, and routine blood tests, including a full blood count, blood group and antibody screen, arranged. If products of conception are in the vagina, indicate that histopathological examination will be arranged and why. Be prepared to explain the local protocol for administration of anti-D immunoglobulin if relevant.

第 19 章（Chapter 19）

在这个情景中，您需要处理一位 32 岁女性提出的避孕需求。

In this scenario, you are asked to manage a request for contraception made by a 32-year-old woman.

首先确定患者此次就诊的目的。她想要暂时或永久的避孕吗？如果她有生育计划，她有什么打算？如果她已经完成了生育计划，这对夫妇对输精管结扎术 / 输卵管结扎术有什么看法？是否有任何其他因素需要考虑，如月经、性或新的医学问题？

First establish what the patient's goals are from this visit. Does she want reversible or permanent contraception? If she wants more children, what are her plans? If she has completed her family, what are the couple's views regarding vasectomy/tubal ligation? Are there any co-existing factors to be considered, e.g. menstrual, sexual or new medical problems?

一旦您知道患者想要什么，向其解释合适的避孕选择，其中包括可靠性、成本、其他措施（非避孕）的好处和主要风险。

Once you have an idea of what the woman wants, explain suitable options, including reliability, cost, other (non-contraceptive) benefits and key risks.

演员可能会要求解释您的建议或您对特定问题（如预防性传播感染）的看法。

The actor might ask for clarification of a recommendation or for your views on a specific aspect of management such as prevention of STI.

第 20 章（Chapter 20）

在这个情景中，一名女性要求您提供信息，以帮助她决定她 11 岁的女儿是否应该参加学校提供的人乳头瘤病毒（HPV）疫苗接种计划。此外，该女性未及时接受宫颈癌筛查。

In this scenario, a woman is requesting information to help her decide whether her 11-year-old daughter should participate in a human papilloma virus (HPV) vaccination programme offered at school. In addition, the woman is not up to date with recommended cervical screening tests.

首先了解该女性对 HPV 和 HPV 疫苗接种计划的认识，以及她对女儿的担忧。吉安诺普洛斯女士会担心疫苗接种的安全性和有效性，也许还会认为这会鼓励更早性经历。如果在所在地区的学校疫苗计划中尚无 HPV 疫苗，则是否选用替代的自费疫苗也是一个问题。

Start by establishing what the woman already knows about HPV, the HPV vaccination programme and what her concerns for her daughter are. You can anticipate that Ms Giannopoulos will be concerned about vaccination safety and effectiveness and, perhaps, perceived encouragement of precocious sexual experience. A more technical nuance could be a question regarding the alternative of selffunding a nonovalent vaccine if that is not yet available in the school-based programme in your region.

自然而然地进入第二个问题。确定该女士对宫颈癌筛查计划的了解以及她不按诊所要求参加筛查的原因。你可以预料到她已经单身好几年了，没有性生活，所以觉得没有必要做检查，而且她最后一次检查又痛又尴尬，所以她不想再做一次阴道检查。如果是这样，准备讨论替代方案，即患者自行取样。

This part should segue naturally into the second task. Establish what the woman already knows about the cervical screening programme and her reasons for not responding to requests from the practice to participate in this programme. You can anticipate that she has been single and not sexually active for several years so felt there was no need to be tested and that her last test was painful and embarrassing, so she would prefer not to have another speculum examination. If so, be prepared to discuss patient self-collection as an alternative.

第 21 章（Chapter 21）

在这个情景中，一名 56 岁的未育女性因阴道脱垂和尿失禁而对盆底锻炼无效。转诊医生考虑是否需要手术治疗。

In this scenario, a 56-year-old nulliparous woman presents with vaginal prolapse and urinary incontinence unresponsive to pelvic floor exercises. The referring doctor has questioned whether surgery is indicated.

确定症状的详细信息，其中包括严重程度、危险因素（注意未育和肥胖）、性功能、心理健康情况、病史和手术史、尝试过的治疗方法和液体摄入量。具体询问是否有慢性咳嗽，如果有的话，询问可能的原因；是否有糖尿病、使用利尿药物、烦渴行为、抑郁、社会孤立、先前行过骨盆手术或放疗和职业问题（如需要提重物的工作）。她是如何学习盆底锻炼的，做多久了？

Establish the details of the presenting symptoms, including severity, risk factors (noting nulliparity and obesity), sexual function, psychological health, medical and surgical history, treatments tried and fluid intake. Specifically enquire regarding chronic cough and, if present, the possible causes; diabetes, diuretic medications, behavioural polydipsia, depression, social isolation, prior pelvic surgery or radiotherapy

and occupational issues (e.g. a job requiring heavy lifting). How did she learn and for how long has she been doing pelvic floor exercises?

这种情景很可能是混合性尿失禁患者，没有其他下尿路症状，肠道功能正常，最近在淋浴时发现阴道壁隆起。她可能近期没有性生活，理疗师教她进行盆底锻炼，并且完全依从了 6 个月，但没有任何效果。

The scenario is likely to be mixed urinary incontinence with no other lower urinary tract symptoms, normal bowel function and recent detection of a vaginal bulge whilst showering. She will not be in a sexual relationship and will have been taught the pelvic floor exercises by a physiotherapist and been fully compliant for 6 months, without benefit.

用通俗易懂的语言向演员解释你打算进行的检查。短时间内仅限于腹部和阴道（双合诊和窥器）检查以及尿液分析。解释您想要询问的内容，例如，是否有子宫和阴道壁的下移以及"下压"时尿漏。然后，演员将向您提供可用的检查结果。常见的情景是做 Valsalva 动作时和盆腔器官脱垂量化系统（POP-Q）2 期阴道前壁脱垂时可见漏尿。

Explain in plain language to the actor the examination you propose to undertake. In a short station it is reasonable this be restricted to abdominal and vaginal (bimanual and speculum) examination, plus urinalysis. Explain what you will be looking for, e.g. descent of the uterus and vaginal walls and urinary leakage with 'bearing down'. The actor will then provide you with the available examination findings. A common scenario is visible loss of urine with Valsalva and a pelvic organ prolapse quantification system (POPQ) stage 2 anterior vaginal compartment prolapse.

使用通俗易懂的语言，解释当前诊断和病因（如果已知），并建议下一步的治疗方案。请记住，盆底锻炼没有效果，而且患者从转诊信中看起来已经准备好考虑手术。对于所描述的检查结果，手术是一种合理的方法。但是，没有时间详细介绍。如果您认为有必要，需要转诊给专科医生以进一步考虑手术方法。

Using plain language, explain the provisional diagnosis and the underlying cause(s) of the condition(s), if known, and advise the next stage in management. Bear in mind there has been no response to pelvic floor exercises and that the patient appears from the referral letter to have been primed to consider a surgical solution. For the examination findings described, surgery is a reasonable approach. However, there is no time to go into details. Indicate that referral to a specialist is required to consider further a surgical approach if you believe that is indicated.

附录 A（Appendix A）

在这个情景中，您将确定患者在大型妇科手术后 23h 后是否适合根据术前的计划出院。然而，由于发现了右侧卵巢子宫内膜异位囊肿而切除了卵巢，所行的手术与预期不同。此外，该女性在数小时前拔掉导尿管后一直没有排尿，而且大剂量羟考酮不能很好地控制她的疼痛。

In this scenario, you are to establish if a woman 23 hours following major gynaecological surgery is fit to be discharged home per preoperative planning. However, the performed procedure is different from the booked procedure due to the discovery of a right endometrioma managed by oophorectomy. Furthermore, the woman has not passed urine since removal of the urinary catheter several hours ago, and her pain is not well controlled with oxycodone at high dose.

当你问她感觉如何时，从床旁观察这个患者。演员看起来很痛苦，并回应说她感觉不舒服，而且手术比她预期的更为疼痛。确定疼痛的性质和部位、加重和缓解因素，以及她是否能够起床排尿或使用便盆。

Observe the woman from the end of the bed as you ask her how she is feeling. The actor will be instructed to look distressed and respond that she is not feeling well and that the procedure was more painful than she had anticipated. Establish the nature and location of pain, exacerbating and relieving factors and whether she has been able to get up to pass urine or to use a bedpan.

以通俗易懂的语言向演员解释您打算进行的腹部检查，寻求检查的许可，并确保手卫生。由于答题时间有限，所以情景将发展为单一的术后并发症，可能是尿潴留或意外的手术损伤，如与右卵巢解剖相关的输尿管损伤或与术后出血或肠道损伤相关的腹膜炎症状（可能性较小，因为心动过速难以模仿）。演员也将被指示模仿适当的体征。

Explain in plain language to the actor the abdominal examination you propose to undertake and seek permission to perform it, ensuring appropriate hand hygiene technique. Time is short, so the scenario will develop as a single postoperative complication, which could be urinary retention or an unexpected surgical injury, e.g. ureteric injury related to the dissection of the right ovary or peritonism related to postoperative bleeding or bowel injury (less likely, as tachycardia is difficult to emulate). The actor will also be instructed to mimic appropriate signs.

用通俗易懂的语言解释您目前的诊断和治疗计划，其中应包括由经验丰富的医生进行检查。患者

没有计划切除右侧卵巢。这可能是您发现的唯一"阳性"特征，需要包含在您的解释中。如果患者对方案表示不满，请表示遗憾，并保证您会立即将此事告知外科医生。

Explain in plain language your provisional diagnosis and plan of management, which should include review by an experienced doctor. The patient was not scheduled to have her right ovary removed. This might be the only 'positive' feature that you uncover and will need to be included in your explanation. If the woman expresses discontent with that aspect of her management, express regret that she is unhappy with the management and reassure that you will promptly draw this to the attention of the surgeon.

附录 C（Appendix C）

在这个情景中，一名 52 岁女性出现绝经后出血和子宫内膜厚度明显增加，需要排除子宫内膜癌，她的妇科医生诊断宫颈狭窄后转诊，这可能继发于宫颈上皮内瘤变（CIN）的宫颈手术。现在需要安排在日间手术室进行宫腔镜检查和分段诊刮术。

In this scenario, the diagnosis of exclusion is endometrial cancer in a 52-year-old woman presenting with postmenopausal bleeding and significantly increased endometrial thickness. Her referring gynaecologist has diagnosed cervical stenosis, probably secondary to cervical surgery for cervical intraepithelial neoplasia (CIN). Hysteroscopy and dilatation and curettage in a day-case operating theatre are now indicated.

确定是否存在子宫内膜癌的主要危险因素（错配修复基因，如果下一次宫腔镜检查也不令人满意，既往诊断为非典型子宫内膜增生的病史会影响决策），并确认既往妇科手术情况和次数。患者是否有麻醉后或术前使用米索前列醇扩张宫颈后不适的病史？患者有什么特别的顾虑吗？她需要支持人员在场吗？

Establish if there are any other major risk factors for endometrial cancer (mismatch repair gene, prior diagnosis of atypical endometrial hyperplasia would impact decisionmaking if the next hysteroscopy was also unsatisfactory) and confirm the nature and number of prior gynaecological procedures. Does the patient have a medical history that raises concern for anaesthesia or for preoperative cervical priming with misoprostol? Does the patient have any particular concerns? Does she need a support person present?

用简单的语言解释当前诊断，承认这是临时的，癌症并没有确诊，但必须排除。用通俗的语言解释手术，并详细说明当地医院的知情同意书。这应该包括这是一个诊断性的而非治疗性的手术，并且需

要及时随访以给出结果并计划进一步的方案。该手术的风险不应被夸大，手术风险包括子宫穿孔，造成假通道导致无法令人满意地完成手术，出现米索前列醇的肠道不良反应（如果用于宫颈术前扩张）及麻醉相关并发症。你可以预料到，演员会问为什么不能简单进行子宫切除术来"彻底解决问题"。回答应包括病情可能是良性的，不需要子宫切除术，并且某些恶性肿瘤需要进行比简单的子宫切除术更复杂的分期手术。一定要表明在这种情况下需要高年资医师的参与。

Explain in simple language the provisional diagnosis, acknowledging that this is provisional and that cancer is not a certainty but that it must be excluded. Explain the procedure in lay language and in sufficient detail for local requirements for informed consent. This should include that this is a diagnostic, not curative, procedure and that prompt follow-up will be required to give the results and plan further management. Risks of the procedure should not be exaggerated, but they include uterine perforation, creation of a false passage resulting in failure to complete the procedure satisfactorily, gut side effects from misoprostol if used for preoperative priming of the cervix and complications related to anaesthesia. You can anticipate that the actor will ask why she can't simply have a hysterectomy 'to get it all over and done with'. The response should include that the condition could be benign and not require hysterectomy and that some malignancies require surgical staging procedures that are more complex than a simple hysterectomy. Be sure to indicate that involvement of a senior doctor is required in such cases.

附录 E　自我评估：问题与答案
Self-assessment: Questions & Answers

Kevin Hayes　著　　杨慧霞　译　　石玉华　校

一、问题（Questions）

第 1 章（Chapter1）

1. 对骨盆动脉血供最恰当的描述是什么？

A. 髂外动脉起源于腰骶关节水平，后沿骨盆边缘进入盆腔

B. 髂内动脉前支供应膀胱上、中、下动脉，为膀胱供应血液

C. 子宫动脉最初在阔韧带上缘腹膜下的脂肪中向下走行

D. 子宫动脉在阴道侧穹窿旁 0.5cm 处跨过输尿管

E. 卵巢动脉在相应的闭孔内肌表面的腹膜后下降，直到骨盆边缘

1. What is the most appropriate description of the arterial supply of the pelvis?

A. The external iliac artery arises at the level of the lumbosacral articulation and passes over the pelvic brim

B. The anterior division provides the superior, middle and inferior vesical arteries that provide the blood supply for the bladder

C. The uterine artery initially runs downward in the subperitoneal fat under the superior attachment of the broad ligament

D. The uterine artery crosses the ureter approximately 0.5 cm from the lateral fornix of the vagina

E. The ovarian arteries descend behind the peritoneum on the surface of the corresponding obturator internus muscle until they reach the brim of the pelvis

2. 阴道的特征包括下列哪项？

A. 前方是膀胱三角区和尿道，与之紧密相连

B. 直肠是其后侧唯一相连的结构

C. 由横纹肌构成

D. 性成熟未妊娠女性阴道的 pH 为 2.0～3.0

E. 阴道内壁为腺上皮

2. The vagina:

A. Is closely related anteriorly to the trigone of the bladder and the urethra

B. Has the rectum as its only direct relation posteriorly

C. Is composed of striated muscle

D. Has a pH in the sexually mature non-pregnant female of 2.0–3.0

E. Is lined by glandular epithelium

3. 关于子宫及其支撑结构，下列说法正确的是？

A. 子宫后方的宫骶韧带及其表面覆盖的腹膜构成道格拉斯窝的外侧边界

B. 阔韧带是子宫两侧的重要支撑结构

C. 在大约 50% 的女性中，子宫在道格拉斯窝内位于后倾位

D. 分娩时，子宫峡部（子宫下段）对娩出胎儿有重要作用

E. 前韧带和子宫膀胱腹膜反折对于维持子宫前倾起着重要作用

3. In regard to the uterus and its supporting structures, which of the following statements is true?

A. Posteriorly, the uterosacral ligaments and their peritoneal covering form the lateral boundaries of the rectouterine pouch (of Douglas)

B. Laterally, the broad ligaments form an important supporting structure for the uterus

C. In about 50% of women, the uterus lies in a position of retroversion in the pouch of Douglas

D. In labour, the isthmus (lower segment) of the uterus plays a significant role in expulsion of the fetus

E. The anterior ligaments and uterovesical folds play an important role in maintaining anteversion of the uterus.

4. 卵巢的特征包括下列哪项？

A. 与髂内血管关系密切

B. 血液供应来自卵巢动脉，卵巢动脉起源于髂内动脉

C. 表面为纤毛柱状上皮

D. 侧面由悬韧带支撑，悬韧带与输尿管关系密切

E. 含格雷夫卵泡，仅出现在中央髓质

4. The ovary:

A. Lies in close relation to the internal iliac vessels

B. Derives its blood supply from the ovarian artery, which arises from the internal iliac artery

C. Is covered by ciliated columnar epithelium

D. Is supported laterally by the suspensory ligament, which lies in close relation to the ureter

E. Contains Graafian follicles, which are found only in the central medulla of the organ

5. 关于子宫，以下哪一项是正确的？

A. 子宫下半部分的淋巴引流到浅表腹股沟淋巴结和邻近股骨淋巴结

B. 子宫痛觉是通过 $T_{11}\sim T_{12}$ 和 $L_1\sim L_2$ 的交感传入神经介导的

C. 子宫动脉在输尿管进入膀胱处位于输尿管下方

D. 子宫的血液供应完全来自子宫动脉

E. 部分子宫峡部（子宫下段）受阴部神经支配

5. With regard to the uterus, which one of the following is correct?

A. Lymphatic drainage from the lower part of the uterus passes to the superficial inguinal and adjacent superficial femoral nodes

B. Uterine pain is mediated through sympathetic afferent nerves passing up to T_{11}–T_{12} and L_1–L_2

C. The uterine artery lies beneath the ureter at the point where the ureter enters the bladder

D. The blood supply of the uterus is derived entirely from the uterine artery

E. The isthmus (lower segment) of the uterus is partly innervated by the pudendal nerve

第 2 章（Chapter 2）

1. 关于精子最恰当的说法是什么？

A. 尾部包含螺旋状的线粒体，为精子活动提供"动力"

B. 在通过输卵管时，精子经历了成熟的最后阶段（获能），这使得精子能有效地通过最后一段输卵管

C. 精子细胞质中含有高浓度的半乳糖，它是精子能量的主要来源

D. 精子头部与卵母细胞膜融合，精子头部和中段通过吞噬作用被吞入卵母细胞

E. 精子运动的速度为 6mm/min，几乎都靠精子活力

1. What is the most appropriate statement relating to spermatozoa?

A. The tail contains a coiled helix of mitochondria that provides the 'powerhouse' for sperm motility

B. During their passage through the Fallopian tubes, the sperm undergo the final stage in maturation (capacitation), which enables a more efficient transport along the last section of tube

C. Seminal plasma has a high concentration of galactose, which is the major source of energy for the spermatozoa

D. The sperm head fuses with the oocyte plasma membrane, and the sperm head and midpiece are ngulfed into the oocyte by phagocytosis

E. Sperm migration is at a rate of 6 mm/min, nearly all due to sperm motility

2. 以下哪一项最能描述 25 岁女性的正常卵泡生长？

A. 每个月经周期约有 100 个卵泡明显生长

B. 在大多数女性中，在该周期的第 5～6 天，一个卵泡成为优势卵泡

C. 在周期的第 6～14 天，优势卵泡每天增长约 1cm

D. 卵泡直径达到 4cm 左右时破裂

E. 另一个邻近的卵泡成为黄体

2. Which one of the following best describes normal follicular growth occurring in a 25-year-old woman?

A. About 100 ovarian follicles show obvious follicular growth in each menstrual cycle

B. In most women one follicle is selected to become the dominant follicle on about day 5–6 of that cycle

C. The dominant follicle grows by about 1 cm per day from

days 6 to 14 of the cycle

D. The follicle ruptures when it reaches about 4 cm in diameter

E. A separate but adjacent follicle becomes the corpus luteum

3. 下列关于减数分裂的说法中哪项是正确的?

A. 胎儿 6 个月时，卵巢内减数分裂产生了 700 万个生殖细胞

B. 第一次减数分裂在婴儿出生前完成

C. 第二次减数分裂在精子附着到卵母细胞时开始

D. 染色体内基因重排发生在精子染色体进入细胞核与卵子染色体结合后

E. 第一次减数分裂结束和第二次减数分裂开始之间的间隔是 37 岁以上女性受孕后染色体异常率增加的原因

3. Which one of the following statements about meiosis is correct?

A. Meiosis is the mechanism of production of the 7 million germ cells found in the ovary at 6 months of fetal life

B. The first meiotic division is completed prior to birth of the baby

C. The second meiotic division commences at the time of attachment of the sperm to the oocyte

D. Rearrangements of the genes within the chromosomes occur after the male zygote chromosomes have entered the nucleus and combine with those of the female zygote

E. The delay between the end of the first meiotic division and the commencement of the second meiotic division is the cause of the increased chromosome abnormality rate seen in women who conceive after the age of 37 years

4. 下列关于女性受精过程的叙述，哪一项是正确的?

A. 它通常发生在输卵管的末端

B. 雌配子决定了所产生胎儿的性别

C. 双胎妊娠是由于正常的抑制过程失败，在第一个精子附着到透明带后，未能阻止更多的精子进入卵母细胞

D. 受精可以发生在排卵后第 6 天

E. 精子获能发生在睾丸的生精上皮内

4. Which one of the following statements about the process of fertilization in the human female is correct?

A. It usually occurs within the outer end of the Fallopian tube

B. The female gamete determines the sex of a resulting fetus

C. A twin pregnancy is due to failure of the normal inhibitory process, where further sperm are prevented from entering the oocyte following attachment of the first sperm to the

zona pellucida

D. Fertilization can occur up to 6 days after ovulation

E. Sperm capacitation occurs within the seminiferous epithelium of the testis

5. 下列哪项关于着床的叙述是正确的?

A. 着床通常发生在受精后 2 天左右

B. 着床时胚胎通常处于八细胞阶段

C. 着床后不久由胚胎产生人绒毛膜促性腺激素(hCG)

D. 如果着床时的子宫内膜为增生期，则会发生自然流产

E. 着床后月经会延迟，预计在月经来潮后的 2～3 天尿妊娠试验将呈阳性

5. Which one of the following facts about implantation is correct?

A. Implantation usually occurs about 2 days after fertilization

B. At the time of implantation the embryo is usually at the eight-cell stage

C. Human chorionic gonadotropin (hCG) is produced by the implanting embryo soon after implantation has commenced

D. If the endometrial appearance at the time of implantation is proliferative, the pregnancy is lost as a spontaneous miscarriage

E. If implantation occurs, the period is always delayed, and a urinary pregnancy test performed 2–3 days after the day the period was expected will be positive

第 3 章（Chapter 3）

1. 关于妊娠期免疫的最恰当的表述是?

A. 绒毛滋养层不表达人类白细胞抗原（HLA）I 类或 II 类分子

B. 绒毛外滋养层不表达 HLA I 类或 II 类分子

C. 蜕膜淋巴细胞的主要类型是子宫浆细胞

D. 妊娠期细胞因子 Th1 比 Th2 比例中 Th1 增多

E. 胸腺在妊娠期间表现出一些可逆的退化，是由雌激素驱动的淋巴细胞从胸腺皮质外流引起的

1. What is the most appropriate statement regarding immunology in pregnancy?

A. The villous trophoblast never expresses human leucocyte antigen (HLA) class I or class II molecules

B. The extra-villous trophoblast never expresses HLA class I or class II molecules

C. The main type of decidual lymphocytes are the uterine plasma cells

D. The Th1:Th2 cytokine ratio shifts towards Th1 in pregnancy

E. The thymus shows some reversible involution during pregnancy, apparently caused by the oestrogen-driven exodus of lymphocytes from the thymic cortex

2. 关于心输出量增加，下列哪一项是正确的？

A. 发生在妊娠晚期

B. 它完全是由每搏输出量的增加导致的

C. 它与后负荷的增加有关

D. 它会导致患有心脏病的女性心力衰竭

E. 导致肺动脉压升高

2. Regarding the rise in cardiac output, which one of the following is correct?

A. It occurs in late pregnancy

B. It is entirely driven by a rise in stroke volume

C. It is associated with a rise in afterload

D. It can precipitate heart failure in women with heart disease

E. It causes an increase in pulmonary arterial pressure

3. 关于孕期呼吸功能，下列哪一项是正确的？

A. 孕酮使肾上腺髓质对 CO_2 敏感

B. 母体 PaO_2 上升约 15%

C. 母体 2,3–DPG 没有增加

D. 母体携氧能力提高约 18%

E. 每分钟通气量增加 80%

3. Considering respiratory function in pregnancy, which one of the following statements is correct?

A. Progesterone sensitizes the adrenal medulla to CO_2

B. Maternal PaO_2 rises by ≈15%

C. There is no increase in maternal 2,3-DPG

D. Maternal oxygen-carrying capacity rises by ≈18%

E. There is an 80% increase in minute ventilation

4. 关于妊娠期肾功能，下列哪一项是正确的？

A. 肾脏体积的增大多发生在妊娠晚期

B. 输尿管松软且没有张力

C. 肾小球滤过率（GFR）的升高激活了肾素–血管紧张素系统

D. 妊娠期间潴留了大约 1800 mmol 钠

E. 泌尿道感染在妊娠期间不太常见

4. Considering renal function in pregnancy, which one of the following statements is correct?

A. Most increase in renal size occurs in late pregnancy

B. The ureters are floppy and toneless

C. The rise in glomerular filtration rate (GFR) activates the renin-angiotensin system

D. About 1800 mmol sodium is retained during pregnancy

E. Urinary tract infections are less common in pregnancy

5. 关于孕期内分泌功能，下列哪一项是正确的？

A. 产生胰岛素抵抗

B. 糖尿不常见

C. 甲状腺异常

D. 肠道吸收更多的钙，但在尿液中丢失的更少

E. 皮肤色素沉着增加是由促甲状腺激素引起的

5. In relation to endocrine function in pregnancy, which one of the following statements is correct?

A. Insulin resistance develops

B. Glycosuria is not common

C. The thyroid involutes

D. The gut absorbs more calcium but less is lost in the urine

E. The increased skin pigmentation is caused by thyroid-stimulating hormone

第 4 章（Chapter 4）

1. 在早期胎盘发育中，以下哪一项是正确的？

A. 外层细胞滋养层侵入子宫内膜细胞和子宫肌层

B. 蜕膜细胞不支持侵入的滋养层

C. 随着胎盘的侵入，形成大的腔隙并充满胎儿血液

D. 叶状绒毛膜形成胎盘

E. 绒毛膜形成胎盘

1. In early placental development, which one of the following is correct?

A. The outer cytotrophoblast invades the endometrial cells and the myometrium

B. Decidual cells do not support the invading trophoblasts

C. With the placental invasion, large lacunae are formed and are filled with fetal blood

D. Chorion frondosum forms the placenta

E. Chorion laevae forms the placenta

2. 下列关于脐带的说法正确的是？

A. 它有两条静脉和一条动脉

B. 动脉血含氧量多

C. 一条动脉和一条静脉与胎儿生长和活婴相匹配

D. 脐动脉收缩压为 120mmHg

E. 血管被称为华通化胶的疏水性黏多糖包围

2. Which one of the following is correct regarding the umbilical cord?

A. It has two veins and one artery

B. The arterial blood has more oxygen

C. One artery and one vein are compatible with fetal growth and a live baby

D. Cord artery has a systolic pressure of 120 mmHg

E. The vessels are surrounded by a hydrophobic mucopolysaccharide called Wharton's jelly

3. 关于胎盘气体转运，下列哪一项是正确的?

A. 胎盘气体的转运是通过简单扩散

B. 葡萄糖的转移是通过简单扩散

C. 在主动转运中，胎儿血液中转运的物质浓度低于母体血液

D. 低分子量物质通过胞饮作用转运

E. 氨基酸通过易化扩散转运

3. Which one of the following is correct regarding placental transfer?

A. Transfer of placental gases is by simple diffusion

B. Transfer of glucose is by simple diffusion

C. In active transport the concentration of the substrate transported in fetal blood is lower than on the maternal blood

D. Low-molecular-weight substrates are transported by pinocytosis

E. Amino acids are transferred by facilitated diffusion

4. 胎盘功能不包括下列哪项?

A. 气体交换

B. 胎儿营养

C. 运走代谢废物

D. 内分泌功能

E. 感染屏障

4. Placental function includes all of the following except:

A. Gaseous exchange

B. Fetal nutrition

C. Removal of waste products

D. Endocrine function

E. A barrier for infections

5. 关于羊水，下列哪一项是正确的?

A. 羊水过多与胎儿异常有关

B. 孕 38 周的平均羊水量为 500～600ml

C. 长期严重羊水过少的唯一并发症是姿势畸形

D. 大多数宫内生长受限病例的羊水量正常

E. 胎心监护中观察到变异减速时，标准处理是羊膜腔灌注

5. Regarding amniotic fluid, which one of the following is correct?

A. Polyhydramnios is associated with fetal anomaly

B. On average amniotic fluid volume at 38 weeks' gestation is 500–600 mL

C. The only complication of long-standing severe oligohydramnios is postural deformities

D. Most cases of intrauterine growth restriction have normal liquor volume

E. Amnio-infusion is a standard procedure for variable decelerations observed on the cardiotocography

第 5 章（Chapter 5）

1. 以下哪一项关于围产儿死亡率的陈述是正确的?

A. 围产儿死亡率是国家财力的标志

B. 围产儿死亡率是指每 10 万次分娩中胎儿死亡和早期新生儿死亡数

C. 是孕产妇健康和母婴保健水平的重要标志

D. 世界卫生组织为每个国家设定了围产儿死亡率目标

E. 世界银行向围产儿死亡率最低的国家提供财政奖励

1. Which one of the following statements is true of perinatal mortality?

A. Perinatal mortality is an indication of the wealth of the nation

B. Perinatal mortality rate describes the number of stillbirths and early neonatal deaths per 105 total births

C. It is an important indication of maternal health and the standard of maternal and neonatal care

D. The World Health Organization has set targets of perinatal mortality for each country

E. The World Bank gives financial incentives to countries that have the best perinatal mortality rates

2. 下列关于胎儿死亡的说法中哪一项是正确的?

A. 胎儿死亡是每 10 万次分娩中胎儿死亡的数量

B. 使用 Wigglesworth 分类，大约 30% 胎儿死亡原因未知

C. 最常见的胎儿死亡原因是产时胎儿死亡

D. 世界上胎儿死亡率最高的地区是加勒比地区

E. 使用现代分类法，胎儿死亡最常见原因是胎儿生长受限

2. Which one of the following statements is true of stillbirth?

A. Stillbirths are the number of stillbirths per 105 total births.

B. Using the Wigglesworth Classification, around 30% are classified as of unknown antecedent

C. The most common cause of stillbirth is intrapartum stillbirth

D. The region with the highest stillbirth rate in the world is in the Caribbean

E. Using modern classifications, the most common cause of stillbirth is fetal growth restriction

3. 下列关于新生儿死亡的说法中哪一项是正确的？

A. 低出生体重是众所周知的直接原因

B. 在资源匮乏的国家，破伤风仍然是新生儿死亡的最重要原因之一

C. 发展中国家与早产相关的新生儿死亡率显著下降

D. 在英国（CMACE），极早早产儿占新生儿死亡人数的近一半

E. 改善新生儿死亡率的最佳办法是建造更多新生儿重症监护病房

3. Which one of the following statements is true of neonatal deaths?

A. Low birth weight is a well-known direct cause

B. In low-resource countries, tetanus remains one of the most important causes of neonatal deaths

C. The neonatal death rates related to prematurity in developing countries have shown a significant fall

D. In the UK (CMACE) extreme prematurity accounts for nearly half of the neonatal deaths

E. The best investment to improve the neonatal death rates is to build more neonatal intensive care units

4. 以下哪一项最准确地描述了孕产妇死亡？

A. 孕产妇死亡的直接原因是产前、产时或产后期间发生的妊娠特有的合并症或其处理

B. 两个或两个以上的原因导致母亲死亡是巧合

C. 英国的孕产妇死亡率定义为每 10 万活产中直接和间接死亡人数

D. 孕产妇死亡率反映了一个国家的产前保健状况

E. 可以通过增加医生和助产士的数量来降低孕产妇死亡率

4. Which one of the following statements most accurately describes maternal deaths?

A. Direct maternal deaths arise from complications or their management, which are unique to pregnancy, occurring during the antenatal, intrapartum or postpartum periods

B. Coincidental causes occur when two or more causes are noted to cause a mother's death

C. The maternal mortality rate in the UK is defined as the number of direct and indirect deaths per 100,000 live births

D. Maternal mortality rates reflect the state of antenatal care of a country

E. They can be reduced by increasing the number of doctors and midwives

5. 这些关于孕产妇死亡率的陈述中哪一项是正确的？

A. B 组链球菌是孕产妇死亡的主要原因

B. 心脏病是英国孕产妇直接死亡的主要原因

C. A 组链球菌脓毒症易于识别和治疗

D. A 组链球菌脓毒症是 2006—2008 年英国孕产妇死亡的主要原因

E. 静脉血栓栓塞现在是一种罕见的死亡原因

5. Which one of these statements is true of maternal mortality?

A. Group B streptococcus is a major cause of maternal mortality

B. Cardiac disease is the leading cause of direct deaths in the UK

C. Group A streptococcus sepsis is easily recognized and treated

D. Group A streptococcus sepsis was the leading cause of maternal deaths in the UK between 2006 and 2008

E. Venous thromboembolism is now a rare cause of death

第 6 章（Chapter 6）

1. 对妊娠期的生理变化最恰当的描述是什么？

A. 乳房肿块是妊娠期的一种生理性变化

B. 脸颊上出现红褐色色素沉着时应检查是否患狼疮［系统性红斑狼疮（SLE）］

C. 血红蛋白浓度降低主要是由于红细胞生成减少

D. 受孕期激素变化的影响，骨盆形状变得更加女性化

E. 骨盆入口后界为骶岬，前界为耻骨上支和耻骨联合上缘

1. What is the most appropriate description of recognized physiological changes in pregnancy?

A. Breast lumps are a physiological variant in pregnancy

B. A reddish-brownish pigmentation over the cheeks should prompt the investigation of possible concomitant lupus (systemic lupus erythematosus [SLE])

C. A reduction in Hb concentration is principally due to reduced red cell production

D. The pelvic shape becomes more gynaecoid under the influence of hormonal change in pregnancy

E. The pelvic inlet is bounded posteriorly by the sacral promontory and anteriorly by the superior pubic rami and upper margin of the pubic symphysis

2. 在询问产科病史时，以下哪项是正确的？

A. 以前的产科病史相对不重要，决策是根据当前妊娠的进展情况做出的

B. 末次月经（LMP）的第一天是计算预产期（EDD）

的可靠指标

C. 排卵前相对稳定，而排卵后的时期在一个典型的月经周期中表现出很大的变化

D. 孕晚期通过超声扫描可准确判断胎龄

E. 激素避孕药可能导致停药后第一个周期排卵延迟

2. In eliciting an obstetric history, which of the following is correct?

A. Previous obstetric history is relatively unimportant, as management decisions are made on how the current pregnancy has progressed

B. The first date of the last menstrual period (LMP) is a reliable indicator of the expected date of delivery (EDD)

C. The pre-ovulatory period is fairly constant, whereas the post-ovulatory period shows a wide variation in a typical menstrual cycle

D. Ultrasound scan in the third trimester accurately determines the gestational age

E. Hormonal contraception may be associated with a delay in ovulation in the first cycle after discontinuation

3. 关于妊娠的症状，以下哪一项正确？

A. 恶心和呕吐通常在月经延迟后的 10 周内发生

B. 妊娠剧吐的特点是晚孕期呕吐过度

C. 在妊娠的前 12 周，随着子宫上升到耻骨联合水平，尿频发生率增加

D. 血浆渗透压随着妊娠的进展逐渐增加

E. 女性坐直时，水负荷后的利尿反应增加

3. Regarding symptoms of pregnancy, which one of following statements is most appropriate?

A. Nausea and vomiting commonly occur 10 weeks after missing the first period

B. Hyperemesis gravidarum is characterized by excessive vomiting in the third trimester

C. Increased frequency of micturition tends to worsen after the first 12 weeks of pregnancy as the uterus rises above the symphysis pubis

D. Plasma osmolality gradually increases with advancing gestation

E. There is an increased diuretic response after water loading when the woman is sitting in the upright position

4. 妊娠期间，下列说法正确的是？

A. 患者平躺时记录血压，以获得最准确的读数

B. 每次产前检查时应在不同体位记录血压，交替使用不同手臂测血压

C. 如果长时间未发现下腔静脉受压，可能发生子宫胎盘循环减少而导致胎儿死亡

D. 舒张压应根据第四柯氏音（即声音衰减）确定

E. 低血容量循环引起的良性"血流杂音"很常见，没有意义

4. During pregnancy, which of the following statements is correct?

A. Blood pressure is recorded with the patient lying flat on her back to get the most accurate reading

B. Blood pressure should be recorded on different positions during each antenatal visit, alternating the blood pressure cuff on different arms

C. If inferior vena cava compression is not recognized for a prolonged period, fetal compromise may occur secondary to a reduction in uteroplacental circulation

D. Diastolic pressure should be taken with the fourth Korotkoff's sound (i.e. fading of the sound)

E. Benign 'flow murmurs' due to the hypodynamic circulation are common and are of no significance

5. 孕期盆腔检查，下列哪项是正确的？

A. 即使在免费提供超声波检查的情况下，也应进行常规盆腔检查以确认妊娠和孕周

B. 妊娠晚期产前出血的情况下禁行阴道检查，直到除外前置胎盘

C. 常规产前骨盆测量已被证明在预测初产妇分娩结果方面具有价值

D. 在正常女性或女型骨盆中，由于骶骨均匀弯曲，在骨盆出口处为胎头提供了最大的空间

E. 骨盆入口的直径通常前后（AP）径长于横径

5. In pelvic examination during pregnancy, which of the following is correct?

A. Routine pelvic examination to confirm pregnancy and gestation at booking should be performed, even in settings where an ultrasound scan is freely available

B. Digital vaginal examination is contraindicated in later pregnancy in cases of antepartum haemorrhage until placenta praevia can be excluded

C. Routine antenatal radiological pelvimetry has been shown to be of value in predicting outcome of labour in primigravid women

D. In a normal female or gynaecoid pelvis, because the sacrum is evenly curved, maximum space for the fetal head is provided at the pelvic outlet

E. The diameter of the pelvic inlet is usually longer in the anteroposterior (AP) diameter than the transverse diameter

第 7 章（Chapter 7）

1. 产前感染筛查旨在改善母亲和胎儿/新生儿的结局，

不建议将以下哪一项检查作为常规产前检查的一部分？

A. 乙型肝炎病毒

B. 巨细胞病毒

C. 梅毒

D. 风疹

E. 艾滋病病毒

1. Antenatal screening for infection is designed to provide the best outcome for the mother and the fetus/newborn. Which one of the following investigations is not recommended as part of routine antenatal care?

A. Hepatitis B

B. Cytomegalovirus

C. Syphilis

D. Rubella

E. HIV

2. 关于 B 族链球菌最恰当的说法是什么？

A. 它是一种革兰阴性菌

B. 它不是共生微生物

C. 它与早产风险增加有关

D. 所有国家产前都常规对其进行筛查

E. 如果尿培养发现 B 族链球菌，无须临产后治疗

2. What is the most appropriate statement regarding group B streptococcus?

A. It is a Gram-negative bacteria

B. It is not a commensal organism

C. It is associated with an increased risk of pre-term birth

D. Screening is routine in the antenatal period in all countries

E. If group B streptococcus is found in urine culture, there is no need to treat subsequently in labour

3. 以下所有情况都会增加妊娠糖尿病的风险，除外下列哪项？

A. 曾分娩体重＞ 4.5kg 的巨大儿

B. 母体体重指数（BMI）＞ 35

C. 一级亲属患糖尿病

D. 既往妊娠患妊娠期糖尿病

E. 产妇年龄＜ 20 岁

3. There is an increased risk of gestational diabetes in all of the following except:

A. Previous macrosomic baby weighing >4.5 kg

B. Maternal body mass index (BMI) >35

C. First-degree relatives with diabetes mellitus

D. Gestational diabetes in previous pregnancy

E. Maternal age <20

4. 以下所有情况均建议额外补充叶酸，但除外以下哪项情况？

A. 先前分娩过患有神经管缺陷的孩子

B. 服用抗癫痫药物的女性

C. 患有糖尿病的女性

D. 孕产妇体重指数（BMI）＞ 35

E. 生育过唐氏综合征婴儿

4. Extra folic acid supplementation is recommended in all of the following except:

A. Previous child with neural tube defects

B. Women on anti-epileptic medication

C. Women with diabetes mellitus

D. Maternal obesity with a body mass index (BMI) >35

E. Mothers who had a previous Down's syndrome baby

5. 以下哪一项是妊娠后最适合的建议？

A. 鼓励母亲减少运动、规律休息

B. 妊娠 8 周完全自然流产后常规使用抗 D 免疫球蛋白

C. 妊娠期适量饮酒是合理的、无害的

D. 吸烟对胎儿有害，应及时戒烟

E. 扑热息痛妊娠期使用是安全的

5. Which one of the following is the most appropriate advice in pregnancy?

A. Mothers are encouraged to reduce exercise and rest routinely

B. Anti-D Ig is routinely administered after complete spontaneous miscarriage at 8 weeks' gestation

C. Moderate alcohol consumption is not harmful in pregnancy and is reasonable

D. Smoking is harmful to the fetus and should be stopped promptly

E. Paracetamol is proven to be a safe drug in pregnancy

第 8 章（Chapter 8）

1. 对于 36 周的产前出血，最常见的原因是什么？

A. 前置胎盘

B. 胎盘早剥

C. 特发性

D. 宫颈病变

E. 前置血管

1. With regard to an antepartum haemorrhage at 36 weeks, what is considered the commonest cause?

645

A. Placenta previa

B. Placental abruption

C. Idiopathic

D. A cervical gynaecological lesion

E. Vasa previa

2. 关于妊娠期高血压，哪种说法最合适？

A. 孕早期开始血压升高是正常生理变化

B. 舒张压＞ 90mmHg 比收缩压＞ 150mmHg 的读数更严重

C. 子痫前期的定义为 20 周后出现高血压

D. 孕期母体血压最重要的调节因素是外周阻力下降

E. HELLP 综合征是子痫前期的轻度变异

2. With regard to hypertension in pregnancy, which statement is most appropriate?

A. Normal physiological change is for an increase in blood pressure from the first trimester onwards

B. A diastolic reading of >90 mmHg is more significant than a systolic reading of >150 mmHg

C. Pre-eclampsia is defined as the development of hypertension after 20 weeks

D. The most important regulatory factor of maternal blood pressure in pregnancy is a fall in peripheral resistance

E. The HELLP syndrome is a mild variant of pre-eclampsia

3. 在双胎妊娠中，最恰当的说法是什么？

A. 同卵（单卵）双胞胎的发生率因国家而异

B. 双峰征最常见于异卵双胎的孕早期超声检查中

C. 流产发生率较单胎妊娠低

D. 早产风险比单胎妊娠增加 2 倍

E. 双胎输血综合征仅在妊娠 24 周后出现

3. In twin pregnancy, what is the most appropriate statement?

A. The prevalence of identical (monozygotic) twins varies from country to country

B. The twin peak sign is most commonly seen on a first-trimester ultrasound in dizygotic twins

C. Miscarriage is less common than in singleton pregnancies

D. Pre-term delivery is increased by a factor of two with respect to a singleton pregnancy

E. The feto-fetal (twin-twin) transfusion syndrome presents only after 24 weeks' gestation

4. 以下哪个不是胎位不稳定的原因？

A. 前置胎盘

B. 羊水过多

C. 子宫纵隔

D. 初产

E. 双胎妊娠

4. The causes of an unstable lie include all of the following except:

A. Placenta previa

B. Polyhydramnios

C. Subseptate uterus

D. Primiparity

E. Twin pregnancy

5. 关于过期妊娠，以下哪一项是正确的？

A. "过期妊娠" 是指妊娠超过 294 天

B. "过期妊娠" 的特点是羊水过多

C. 过期妊娠与羊水粪染发生率增加有关

D. 与围产期并发症增加有关，不影响死亡率

E. 可以通过妊娠 40 周时引产进行管理

5. In prolonged pregnancy, which one of the following statements is correct?

A. 'Postmaturity syndrome' refers to pregnancy beyond 294 days

B. 'Postmaturity syndrome' is characterized by polyhydramnios

C. Postmaturity is associated with an increased incidence of meconium in the amniotic fluid

D. Is only associated with an increase in perinatal morbidity, not mortality

E. It is managed by induction of labour at 40 weeks' gestation

第 9 章（Chapter 9）

1. 妊娠期贫血最常见的原因是什么？

A. 镰状细胞病

B. 叶酸缺乏

C. 维生素 B_{12} 缺乏

D. 地中海贫血

E. 缺铁

1. Anaemia in pregnancy is most frequently caused by:

A. Sickle cell disease

B. Folate deficiency

C. B_{12} deficiency

D. Thalassaemia

E. Iron deficiency

2. 以下哪一个激素被认为不会增加妊娠期糖尿病风险？

A. 皮质醇

B. 胰高血糖素

C. 人胎盘催乳素

D. 雌激素

E. 孕酮

2. Which of the following is not considered a causative hormone that can increase the risk of gestational diabetes?

A. Cortisol

B. Glucagon

C. Human placental lactogen

D. Oestrogen

E. Progesterone

3. 在妊娠期急性静脉血栓栓塞中，下列哪一项是正确的？

A. 与左腿相比，右腿更容易发生

B. 可以通过检测 D- 二聚体来诊断

C. 是非孕期发生率的 2 倍

D. 是发达国家孕产妇死亡的主要原因

E. 首选华法林治疗

3. In acute venous thromboembolism in pregnancy, which one of the following statements is true?

A. Is more likely to occur in the right leg compared to the left

B. Can be diagnosed by the use of d-dimer measurements

C. Is two times more likely than in the non-pregnant state

D. Is a leading cause of maternal mortality in the developed world

E. Is treated by warfarin in the first instance

4. 关于妊娠期寨卡病毒感染，下列哪项是正确的？

A. 大约 80% 的女性会出现症状

B. 孕妇比非孕妇更容易感染

C. 建议对高危地区的无症状女性进行常规产前检查

D. 最常见的传播方式是性传播

E. 妊娠期主要的临床问题是先天性异常

F. 超声筛查的有效性相似

4. Which of the following infections is true regarding Zika virus in pregnancy?

A. Approximately 80% of women will be symptomatic

B. Pregnant women are more susceptible to infection than non-pregnant women

C. Routine antenatal testing of asymptomatic women in high-risk areas is recommended

D. The commonest method of transmission is sexual

E. The principal clinical concern in pregnancy is congenital abnormality

F. Similar efficacy of ultrasound screening

5. 关于癫痫和妊娠，以下哪项陈述是正确的？

A. 大多数女性在妊娠期间癫痫发生率增加

B. 患有癫痫的女性有 25% 的概率生出患有癫痫的孩子

C. 母亲使用抗癫痫药物最常见的胎儿异常是神经管缺陷和心脏异常

D. 应在孕前和整个早孕期每日服用 400 μg 叶酸

E. 应避免母乳喂养

5. Concerning epilepsy and pregnancy, which of the following statements is true?

A. The majority of women will have an increase in seizure frequency in pregnancy

B. Women with epilepsy have a 25% chance of having a child who develops epilepsy

C. Neural tube defects and cardiac abnormalities are the commonest abnormalities seen with anti-epileptic medication

D. 400 μg of folic acid should be taken pre-conceptually and throughout the first trimester

E. Breast-feeding should be avoided

第 10 章（Chapter 10）

1. 孕 20 周时胎儿解剖结构超声检查未检测到以下哪个器官系统的大部分异常？

A. 心脏

B. 中枢神经系统

C. 骨骼

D. 胃肠道

E. 泌尿生殖系统

1. Ultrasound of fetal anatomy at 20 weeks does not detect the majority of abnormalities in which of the following organ systems?

A. Cardiac

B. Central nervous system

C. Skeletal

D. Gastrointestinal

E. Urogenital

2. 一名 20 岁的女性（分娩唐氏综合征患儿的背景风险为 1：1500）进行了妊娠早期唐氏综合征筛查，报告风险为 1：150。关于这一点，以下哪些说法是正确的？

A. 筛查的阳性预测值高

B. 筛查的阴性预测值低

C. 她生下唐氏综合征婴儿的概率大约是同龄人的预期值的 1350 倍（1500–150=1350）

D. 她的孩子患唐氏综合征的概率不到 1%

E. 如果她行绒毛膜绒毛取样（CVS），她将有大约 1/50 的概率术后流产

2. A woman aged 20 years (with a background risk of delivering a baby with Down's syndrome of 1:1500) has a first-trimester screening test for Down's syndrome which reports a risk of 1:150. Which of the following statements is true regarding this?

A. The positive predictive value of the screening test is high

B. The negative predictive value of the screening test is low

C. Her chances of having a baby with Down's syndrome are approximately 1350 times (1500–150=1350) greater than we would expect in someone of her age

D. There is less than 1% chance her baby has Down's syndrome

E. If she has a chorionic villus sampling (CVS), she will have about a 1 in 50 chance of miscarrying from the procedure

3. 下列关于妊娠期胎儿生长评估的叙述中，哪一项是不正确的？

A. 超声测胎儿腹围是记录胎儿生长最好的单一参数

B. 超声测量的胎头和腹围的相对大小在临床实践中是一种有用的测量方法

C. 妊娠期连续测量耻骨联合 – 宫底高度将检测到 80% 以上的小于胎龄儿

D. 超声发现小于胎龄儿后，需要确认胎儿解剖结构正常

E. 超声发现小于胎龄儿后，需要多普勒超声评估脐动脉血流

3. Which one of the following statements about assessment of fetal growth in pregnancy is not correct?

A. Ultrasound measurement of fetal abdominal circumference is the best single parameter to record fetal growth

B. The relative size of fetal head and abdominal circumferences measured by ultrasound is a useful measure in clinical practice

C. Serial symphysio-fundal height measurements during pregnancy will detect over 80% of small-fordates fetuses

D. Identification of a small-for-dates fetus on ultrasound is an indication to confirm that fetal anatomy is normal

E. Identification of a small-for-dates fetus on ultrasound is an indication to assess blood flow in the umbilical artery with Doppler ultrasound

4. 下列哪项用于管理高危女性妊娠的检测已被随机对照试验证明可以改善胎儿结局？

A. 胎儿胎心监护

B. 多普勒超声记录的脐动脉血流

C. 孕妇计数胎动

D. 胎儿生物物理评分

E. 超声测量羊水量

4. Which of the following tests used in the management of women with high-risk pregnancies have been shown to improve fetal outcome in randomized controlled trials?

A. Fetal cardiotocography

B. Umbilical artery blood flow recorded with Doppler ultrasound

C. Maternal fetal movement counting

D. Fetal biophysical profile testing

E. Ultrasound measurement of amniotic fluid volume

5. 以下哪种染色体异常在筛查中最常见？

A. 45XO（特纳综合征）

B. 21 三体综合征（唐氏综合征）

C. 47 XXY（克氏综合征）

D. 18 三体（爱德华综合征）

E. 13 三体（帕陶综合征）

5. Which of the following chromosomal abnormalities is most commonly found on screening?

A. 45XO (Turner's)

B. Trisomy 21 (Down's)

C. 47 XXY (Klinefelter's)

D. Trisomy 18 (Edwards)

E. Trisomy 13 (Patau)

第 11 章（Chapter 11）

1. 以下哪一项可以诊断临产？

A. 发现"见红"

B. 胎膜破裂

C. 自述宫缩时疼痛

D. 规律有痛性宫缩伴宫颈改变

E. 背痛和腹痛

1. Which one of the following is diagnostic of labour?

A. The appearance of 'show'

B. Rupture of membranes

C. Self-reported painful uterine contractions

D. Regular painful uterine contractions with cervical change

E. Backache and abdominal pain

2. 第一产程进展缓慢最有可能是以下哪一种情况？

A. 胎儿体重＞4kg

B. 子宫收缩不协调

C. 胎头位置不正

D. 女型骨盆

E. 初产

2. Slow labour progress in the first stage of labour is most likely to be due to which one of the following:

A. Fetal weight of >4 kg

B. Incoordinate uterine contractions

C. Malposition of the fetal head

D. Gynaecoid pelvis

E. Primigravidity

3. 正常足月临产可能是由于以下哪项引起的？

A. 系统性用黄体酮的停药

B. 前列腺素分泌减少

C. 胎儿炎症反应下调

D. 胎盘产生促肾上腺皮质激素释放激素（CRH）

E. 羊膜腔感染

3. Normal-term labour appears to be initiated by which of the following mechanisms?

A. Systemic progesterone withdrawal

B. Reduced prostaglandin secretion

C. Downregulation of fetal inflammatory response

D. Placental production of the corticotrophin-releasing hormone (CRH)

E. Infection of the amniotic membranes

4. 硬膜外镇痛的并发症不包括以下哪项？

A. 穿刺部位出血

B. 意外的硬膜损伤

C. 高血压

D. 全脊髓阻滞

E. 意外神经损伤

4. The complications of epidural analgesia include all of the following except:

A. Blood-stained tap

B. Accidental dural tap

C. Hypertension

D. Total spinal blockade

E. Accidental nerve injury

5. 正常胎心监护的特点包括下列哪项？

A. 有胎心加速

B. 没有胎心加速

C. 存在变异减速

D. 没有基线变异

E. 有晚期减速

5. Electronic fetal monitoring features that are reassuring for the fetal state are:

A. Accelerations of the fetal heart rate

B. Absence of accelerations

C. Presence of variable decelerations

D. Absent baseline variability

E. Presence of late decelerations

6. 在早产管理中，以下哪项已经证明有临床获益？

A. 特布他林

B. 阿托西班

C. 糖皮质激素

D. 抗生素

E. 硝酸甘油（GTN）

6. In the management of pre-term labour, which of the following is associated with a proven clinical benefit?

A. Terbutaline

B. Atosiban

C. Corticosteroids

D. Antibiotics

E. Glyceryl trinitrate (GTN)

7. 以下哪一项不是公认的引产指征？

A. 过期妊娠

B. 妊娠期糖尿病

C. 巨大儿

D. 宫内生长受限

E. 足月子痫前期

7. Which one of the following is not an accepted indication for induction of labour?

A. Prolonged pregnancy

B. Diabetes in pregnancy

C. Macrosomic baby

D. Intrauterine growth restriction

E. Pre-eclampsia at term

8. 引产并发症不包括下列哪项？

A. 早产

B. 脐带脱垂

C. 胎儿窘迫

D. 子宫破裂

E. 减轻分娩疼痛

8. The following are all known complications of induction of labour except:

A. Prematurity

B. Cord prolapse

C. Fetal distress

D. Uterine rupture

E. Less painful labour

第 12 章（Chapter 12）

1. 在正常分娩中，以下哪一项是正确的？

A. 接受硬膜外镇痛的初产妇第二产程的正常持续时间通常被认为可长达 2h

B. 当先露最低点下降到坐骨棘的水平时，认为胎头衔接

C. 当子宫颈完全扩张时，母亲有一种要用力的感觉

D. 在整个宫缩期间持续用力是产妇分娩的首选方法

E. 胎头应保持屈曲姿势，直至通过阴道口

1. In normal delivery, which one of the following statements is correct?

A. The normal duration of the second stage of labour in a nulliparous woman who has received epidural analgesia is commonly regarded as lasting up to 2 hours

B. The fetal head is said to be engaged when the bony part of the vertex has descended to the level of the ischial spines

C. The mother experiences a sensation to bear down when the cervix becomes fully dilated

D. Continuous pushing throughout the duration of a contraction is the preferred method for maternal expulsion

E. The fetal head should be maintained in an attitude of flexion until it has passed through the introitus

2. 在会阴损伤和会阴切开术中，下列哪一项是正确的？

A. 与中线会阴切开术相比，中外侧会阴切开术与更多的会阴三度和四度损伤相关

B. 肛门外括约肌完全撕裂时诊断为三度会阴撕裂

C. 肛门内外括约肌均断裂时发生四度裂伤

D. 器械助产和持续性枕后位（OP）是严重会阴裂伤的危险因素

E. 未能修复肛门括约肌的损伤可能会导致短期而非长期的排气和排便失禁

2. In perineal injury and episiotomy, which one of the following statements is correct?

A. Mediolateral episiotomy compared to midline episiotomy is associated with more third- and fourthdegree perineal injuries

B. A third-degree perineal tear is diagnosed when the external anal sphincter is completely torn

C. A fourth-degree laceration has occurred when both the external and internal anal sphincters are disrupted

D. Instrumental delivery and persistent occipitoposterior (OP) position are risk factors for severe perineal tears

E. Failure to repair injury to the anal sphincter may result in short-term, but not long-term, incontinence of flatus and faeces

3. 关于剖宫产，以下哪一项是正确的？

A. 近年来剖宫产率上升导致器械助产率相应下降

B. 曾行子宫下段剖宫产（LSCS）的女性不应在随后的妊娠中尝试阴道分娩

C. 先前的 LSCS 比经典剖宫产具有更大的瘢痕裂开风险，因为下段更薄

D. 胎儿在第二产程中持续的枕后（OP）位是产钳或胎吸助产的禁忌证

E. 几乎所有临产时面先露的婴儿都是剖宫产分娩

3. Regarding caesarean section, which one of the following statements is correct?

A. The rising caesarean section rate witnessed over recent years has resulted in a corresponding decrease in the instrumental delivery rate

B. Women who have had one previous lower segment caesarean section (LSCS) should not attempt vaginal delivery in a subsequent pregnancy

C. A previous LSCS carries a greater risk of scar dehiscence than a classical caesarean section because the lower segment is thinner

D. A persistent occiput posterior (OP) position of the fetus in the second stage of labour is a contraindication for forceps or vacuum-assisted delivery

E. Almost all babies with a face presentation in labour are delivered by caesarean section

4. 关于手术阴道助产，以下哪一项是正确的？

A. 仅使用 McRobert 的手法在大约 50% 的肩难产病例中是成功的

B. 对所有巨大儿（＞4500g）行选择性剖宫产将避免大多数肩难产发生

C. 胎吸与产钳助产成功率一样

D. 与胎吸相比，产钳助产与更多会阴三度和四度裂

伤有关

E. 当宫颈未完全扩张且胎头位置不确定时，可以尝试胎吸，但不能使用产钳

4. Regarding operative vaginal delivery, which one of the following statements is correct?

A. McRobert's manoeuvre alone is successful in about 50% of cases of shoulder dystocia

B. Elective caesarean delivery of all macrosomic infants (>4500 g) will eliminate the majority of cases of shoulder dystocia

C. The vacuum extractor is just as successful as the obstetric forceps for assisted vaginal delivery

D. Forceps delivery compared with vacuum extraction is associated with more third- and fourth-degree perineal lacerations

E. Vacuum extraction, but not forceps delivery, may be attempted when the cervix is not completely dilated and the fetal head position is not certain

5. 关于产后出血（PPH），以下哪一项是正确的？

A. 至少 75% 的早期 PPH 是由子宫收缩乏力引起的

B. 积极管理第三产程并不能降低产后出血的风险

C. PPH 后 3h 内使用氨甲环酸可使死亡率降低 80%

D. 尽管产后出血在持续，麦角新碱也不应静脉给药，因为存在促进血管收缩的风险

E. 宫腔填塞可能通过阻止子宫肌肉的有效收缩来增加产后出血

5. Regarding postpartum haemorrhage (PPH), which one of the following statements is correct?

A. Uterine atony is responsible for at least 75% of primary PPH obstetric cases

B. Active management of the third stage of labour does not reduce the risk of postpartum bleeding

C. Tranexamic acid within 3 hours of PPH will reduce mortality by 80%

D. Ergometrine should not be administered intravenously despite continuing PPH because of the risk of vasoconstriction

E. Intrauterine tamponade may increase postpartum bleeding by preventing effective contraction and retraction of the uterine muscle

第 13 章（Chapter 13）

1. 产褥期的生理变化包括下列哪项？

A. 血清雌激素和孕激素水平升高

B. 凝血因子增加

C. 母乳喂养女性的催乳素水平降低

D. 血小板计数下降

E. 心输出量迅速减少

1. Physiological changes in the puerperium include:

A. Increase in serum levels of oestrogen and progesterone

B. Increase in clotting factors

C. Decrease in prolactin levels in women who breastfeed

D. Drop in platelet count

E. Sudden decrease in cardiac output

2. 肛门括约肌损伤的危险因素包括下列哪项？

A. 枕前位

B. 第二产程持续 1h

C. 硬膜外镇痛

D. 胎儿体重＜ 4kg

E. 多次分娩史

2. Risk factors for anal sphincter injury include:

A. Occipitoanterior position

B. Second stage of an hour

C. Epidural analgesia

D. A baby weight less than 4 kg

E. Multiparous pregnancy

3. 在英国，2016 年导致孕产妇死亡最常见的直接原因是什么？

A. 血栓栓塞

B. 心脏病

C. 出血

D. 脓毒症

E. 羊水栓塞

3. In the UK, the most common overall direct cause of maternal death in 2016 was:

A. Thromboembolism

B. Cardiac disease

C. Haemorrhage

D. Sepsis

E. Amniotic fluid embolism

4. 关于肺栓塞（PE）的产后抗凝治疗，以下哪一项是正确的？

A. 哺乳期禁用肝素

B. 哺乳期禁用华法林

C. 产后不能立即开始使用华法林

D. 抗凝治疗应持续至少 3 个月

E. 妊娠期间发生静脉血栓栓塞（VTE）的女性的产

后检查应由全科医生（GP）进行

4. With regard to postnatal anticoagulation for pulmonary embolism (PE), which one of the following statements is correct?

A. Heparin is contraindicated in breast-feeding

B. Warfarin is contraindicated in breast-feeding

C. Warfarin cannot be commenced immediately postpartum

D. Anticoagulant therapy should be continued for a total of at least 3 months

E. Postnatal review for women who develop venous thromboembolism (VTE) during pregnancy should be with the general practitioner (GP)

5. 在新生儿检查中，下列哪一项是正确的？

A. 绝大部分是正常的

B. 最理想的检查时间是 7 日龄

C. 第一个 24h 出现黄疸是正常的

D. 脐疝有死亡的风险，需要转诊给外科医生

E. 哭声尖锐是正常的

5. In examination of the newborn, which one of the following statements is correct?

A. Most commonly involves assuring normality

B. The ideal time for this is at 7 days of age

C. Jaundice in the first 24 hours is normal

D. Umbilical hernias carry a risk of strangulation and need referral to the surgeon

E. A high-pitch cry is normal

第 14 章（Chapter 14）

1. 关于妊娠期和分娩的精神障碍，下列哪一项陈述是正确的？

A. 它们影响不到 5% 的妊娠女性

B. 应在孕早期停用精神科药物

C. 与其他重大生活事件相比，妊娠和分娩不太可能诱发精神障碍

D. 它是孕产妇直接死亡的主要原因

E. 严重情绪障碍的发病率升高与自杀风险增加有关

1. Regarding psychiatric disorders of pregnancy and childbirth, which one of the following statements is true?

A. They affect less than 5% of women in pregnancy

B. Psychiatric medication should be stopped in the first trimester

C. Pregnancy and childbirth are less likely to precipitate psychiatric disorders than other major life events

D. It is a leading cause of direct maternal death

E. Elevated incidence of severe mood disorders is associated with increased risk of suicide

2. 关于妊娠期抑郁症，下列哪项陈述是错误的？

A. 停药会导致 50% 的母亲复发

B. 焦虑是一个突出的特征

C. 对于轻度至中度抑郁和焦虑，咨询和认知行为疗法比药物治疗更有效

D. 常用的抗抑郁药是选择性血清素再摄取抑制剂（SSRI）

E. 大多数女性在妊娠期间可以停止抗抑郁治疗

2. Regarding depressive illness in pregnancy, all of the following statements are true except:

A. Stopping medication will cause relapse in 50% of mothers

B. Anxiety is a prominent feature

C. Counselling and cognitive behavioural therapy are more effective than medication for mild to moderate depression and anxiety

D. Commonly used antidepressants are selective serotonin reuptake inhibitors (SSRIs)

E. Most women will be able to discontinue antidepressant therapy during pregnancy

3. 在产后精神病中，以下哪项陈述是正确的？

A. 总体发病率在产后 6～12 周最高

B. 抑郁症是最常见的先天精神疾病

C. 双相情感障碍稳定时，通常可以由产科进行管理

D. 疾病的症状和体征通常很微妙

E. 曾患过产后精神病的女性复发概率为 50%

3. In postpartum psychosis, which of the following statements is true?

A. The overall incidence is greatest between 6 and 12 weeks postnatal

B. Depression is the commonest antecedent psychiatric condition

C. Bipolar affective disorder, when stable, can usually be managed by the obstetric services

D. Symptoms and signs of the disease are commonly subtle

E. The chances of recurrence in a woman with previous postpartum psychosis is 50%

4. 选择性 5- 羟色胺再摄取抑制剂（SSRI）与以下哪项无关？

A. 胎儿先天畸形未增加

B. 流产率增加

C. 宫内生长受限

D. 新生儿肺动脉高压

E. 新生儿低血糖

4. Selective serotonin reuptake inhibitors (SSRIs) are associated with all of the following except:

A. No increase in congenital malformation in the fetus

B. Increased pregnancy loss

C. Intrauterine growth restriction

D. Pulmonary hypertension in the newborn

E. Neonatal hypoglycaemia

5. 关于孕期和产褥期的进食障碍，下列哪项是正确的？

A. 据报道，低出生体重和厌食症之间存在一定的关联

B. 据报道早产和厌食症之间存在一定的关联

C. 母婴关系更困难

D. 进食障碍在产前和产后的严重程度往往相同

E. 大多数患有进食障碍的孕妇都会透露自己的病情

5. Regarding eating disorders in pregnancy and the puerperium, which of the following is correct?

A. A consistent association between low birth weight and anorexia has been reported

B. A consistent association between prematurity and anorexia has been reported

C. Mother-baby relationships are recognized to be more difficult

D. Eating disorders tend to be of the same severity in the antenatal and postnatal periods

E. Most pregnant women with eating disorders disclose their illness

第 15 章（Chapter 15）

1. 在下列哪种情况下，阴道检查时没有陪护人员在场是合理的？

A. 如果患者认识检查的医生

B. 如果医生是女性

C. 如果检查是在诊所进行的，有护士在房间外

D. 患者表示不希望第三者在场的情况

E. 如果患者是老年人

1. In which of the following circumstances is it reasonable for a chaperone not to be present during vaginal examination?

A. If the doctor performing the examination is known to the patient

B. If the doctor is female

C. If the examination is performed in the clinic with a nurse outside the room

D. Where the patient has indicated that they do not wish a third person to be present

E. If the patient is elderly

2. 您正在对一名出现异常出血的 26 岁女性进行盆腔检查。解释了手术并获得口头知情同意后，您进行了阴道检查。但是当您插入窥器时，患者感到痛苦并要求您停止。除了肯定她的痛苦并为她的不适道歉外，以下哪项是最合适的？

A. 取出窥器并进行双合诊检查

B. 换较小的窥器再试

C. 说明如果不做检查，您将无法做出诊断并几分钟后再次检查

D. 停止检查，让患者穿好衣服并讨论替代方案

E. 说明检查只需要几秒钟，然后完成检查

2. You are performing a pelvic examination on a 26-yearold woman who has presented with abnormal bleeding. Having explained the procedure and obtained verbal consent, you perform the examination, but as you insert the speculum the patient becomes distressed and asks you to stop. In addition to acknowledging her distress and apologizing for the discomfort which of the following would be the most appropriate response?

A. Withdraw the speculum and proceed with bimanual pelvic examination

B. Change to smaller speculum and try again

C. Explain that without being to do the examination you will be unable to make a diagnosis and retry the examination again after a few minutes

D. Stop the examination, allow the patient to get dressed and discuss alternatives

E. Explain that the examination will only take a few more seconds and complete the examination

3. 对服用避孕药的 30 岁经产女性阴道内置入窥器行常规子宫颈抹片检查时，您注意到宫颈外口周围的上皮区域比其余部分的粉红色上皮看起来颜色更深，无异常分泌物、溃疡或接触性出血。巴氏涂片结果正常。两周后你会见她讨论结果。以下哪一项是最合适的处理？

A. 转诊进行阴道镜检查

B. 要求她在正常间隔时间后返回复查宫颈抹片检查

C. 从该区域取活检

D. 取尿样行衣原体聚合酶链反应（PCR）

E. 对受影响区域进行冷冻治疗

3. On performing a speculum examination for a routine Pap smear for a 30-year-old multiparous woman on the contraceptive pill, you notice an area of epithelium surrounding the cervical os that appears darker red than the pink epithelium covering the rest of the cervix. There is no abnormal discharge, ulceration or contact bleeding. The Pap smear result is normal. You see her 2 weeks later to discuss the results. Which of the following would be the most appropriate action to take?

A. Refer for colposcopic examination

B. Ask her to return for a further Pap smear at the normal screening interval

C. Take a punch biopsy from the area

D. Request a first-pass urine sample for Chlamydia polymerase chain reaction (PCR)

E. Organize for cryotherapy to the affected area

4. 双合诊盆腔检查的以下哪些结果可以被认为是正常的?

A. 摇摆宫颈时不适

B. 右侧附件区可触及 7cm 肿块

C. 可移动的后位子宫

D. 后穹窿结节

E. 非妊娠患者的子宫大小相当于孕 12 周

4. Which of the following findings on bimanual pelvic examination can be considered normal?

A. Increased discomfort on movement of the cervix

B. A 7-cm palpable mass in the right adnexal region

C. A mobile retroverted uterus

D. Nodularity in the posterior formix

E. A uterus equivalent in size to a 12-week pregnancy in a non-pregnant patient

5. 在以下哪一项门诊阴道检查中使用 Sims 窥器?

A. 进行宫颈涂片

B. 取阴道拭子

C. 评估阴道前壁脱垂

D. 盆底张力的评估

E. 置入宫内节育器

5. For which of the following is a Sims' speculum normally used in outpatient vaginal examinations?

A. Taking a cervical smear

B. Taking vaginal swabs

C. Assessment of anterior vaginal wall prolapse

D. Assessment of pelvic floor tone

E. Insertion of an intrauterine device

第 16 章（Chapter 16）

1. 一名 50 岁的绝经前期女性在超声检查后被转诊到妇科诊所，超声显示子宫后壁存在 7cm 的孤立性平滑肌瘤。她没有症状。以下哪一项是最合适的处理?

A. 让她放心，除非她出现症状，否则不需要治疗

B. 子宫动脉栓塞术（UAE）

C. 腹腔镜子宫肌瘤剔除术

D. 使用 6 个月的促性腺激素释放激素（GnRH）类似物

E. 子宫切除术

1. A 50-year-old premenopausal woman is referred to the gynaecology clinic following an ultrasound which indicates the presence of a 7-cm solitary leiomyoma in the posterior uterine wall. She is asymptomatic. Which one of the following would be the most appropriate management?

A. Reassure her that no treatment is necessary unless she develops symptoms

B. Uterine artery embolization (UAE)

C. Laparoscopic myomectomy

D. A 6-month course of gonadotrophin-releasing hormone (GnRH) analogues

E. Hysterectomy

2. 一位 45 岁的经产妇，月经规律，但月经量大。盆腔检查和近期巴氏涂片是正常的。她性行为活跃，但已生育并且正在使用避孕套进行避孕。全血细胞计数显示她贫血，血红蛋白为 104g/L，并且缺铁。她每天抽 10 支烟，但身体健康，没有明显的既往病史或家族史。以下哪一项是最适合她症状的治疗?

A. 月经期间，氨甲环酸 1g，每天 1 次

B. 每个周期的第 12~26 天每天 5mg 炔诺酮

C. 曼月乐（Mirena）宫内节育器（IUD）的置入

D. 子宫内膜切除术

E. 腹腔镜辅助阴式子宫切除术

2. A 45-year-old multiparous woman presents with regular heavy periods. Pelvic examination and recent Pap smear are normal. She is sexually active but has completed her family and is using condoms for contraception. A full blood count shows that she is anaemic with a haemoglobin of 104 g/L and an iron-deficient picture. She smokes 10 cigarettes a day but is otherwise in good health with no significant past medical or family history. Which of the following would be the most appropriate management for her symptoms?

A. Tranexamic acid 1 g qds during her periods

B. Norethisterone 5 mg bd day 12–26 of each cycle

C. Insertion of Mirena intrauterine device (IUD)

D. Endometrial resection

E. Laparoscopically assisted vaginal hysterectomy

3. 一名 22 岁女性，有 2 年月经稀发史，妊娠试验阴性。除了她的体重指数（BMI）为 30 外，其他检查均正常。盆腔超声检查正常。第 21 天的血清孕酮水平显示无排卵。除了催乳素水平略有升高和游离雄激素水平升高外，其他初步血液检查结果均正常。以下哪一项最有可能导致她的症状？

A. 垂体腺瘤

B. 卵巢早衰

C. 特纳综合征

D. 多囊卵巢综合征

E. 功能性下丘脑性闭经

3. A 22-year-old woman presents with a 2-year history of oligo-amenorrhoea and a negative pregnancy test. Examination is normal except that she has a body mass index (BMI) of 30. Pelvic ultrasound is normal. A day-21 serum progesterone level is consistent with anovulation. Results of other initial blood investigations are normal except for a marginally raised prolactin level and an increased free-androgen index. Which one of the following would be the most likely cause for her symptoms?

A. Pituitary adenoma

B. Premature ovarian failure

C. Turner's syndrome

D. Polycystic ovarian syndrome

E. Functional hypothalamic amenorrhea

4. 一名 8 岁女孩在第一次月经后被带到她的全科医生（GP）处。经检查，她的身高在第 95 百分位，乳房发育第二期，腋毛和阴毛发育。以下哪项是最可能的诊断？

A. 特发性

B. 中枢神经系统（CNS）肿瘤

C. 先天性肾上腺增生（非经典）

D. 卵巢颗粒细胞瘤

E. 卵巢滤泡囊肿

4. An 8-year-old girl is brought to her general practitioner (GP) after having had her first period. On examination she is on the 95th centile for her age in height, has stage 2 breast development and has some axillary and pubic hair development. Which of the following would be the most

likely diagnosis?

A. Idiopathic

B. Central nervous system (CNS) tumour

C. Congenital adrenal hyperplasia (non-classical)

D. Granulosa cell tumour of the ovary

E. Follicular cysts of the ovary

5. 一名 49 岁女性，除了 2 年前因月经过多而行子宫切除术外，没有明显的既往病史，因潮热而要求激素替代疗法（HRT）。如果她服用 HRT，她患以下哪些疾病的风险会增加？

A. 缺血性心脏病

B. 结肠癌

C. 骨质疏松症

D. 子宫内膜癌

E. 深静脉血栓形成

5. A 49-year-old woman with no significant past medical history except for a hysterectomy for heavy menstrual bleeding 2 years ago is requesting hormone replacement therapy (HRT) for hot flushes. Which of the following conditions would she be at increased risk of developing if she takes HRT?

A. Ischaemic heart disease

B. Colonic carcinoma

C. Osteoporosis

D. Endometrial cancer

E. Deep venous thrombosis

第 17 章（Chapter 17）

1. 一对夫妇接受了检查，发现该女性患有卵巢早衰，哪个化验结果支持这一点？

A. 促卵泡激素（FSH）升高、黄体生成素（LH）升高、雌二醇降低

B. FSH 升高、LH 下降、雌二醇下降

C. FSH 正常、LH 升高、雌二醇正常

D. FSH 下降、LH 下降、雌二醇正常

E. FSH 正常、LH 正常、雌二醇下降

1. A couple are investigated, and the woman is found to have premature ovarian failure. Which biochemical pattern would support this?

A. Elevated follicle-stimulating hormone (FSH), elevated luteinizing hormone (LH), suppressed oestradiol

B. Suppressed FSH, suppressed LH, suppressed oestradiol

C. Normal FSH, elevated LH, normal oestradiol

D. Suppressed FSH, suppressed LH, normal oestradiol

E. Normal FSH, normal LH, suppressed oestradiol

2. 以下哪个不是少精症原因？

A. 柳氮磺吡啶

B. 美沙拉嗪

C. 环磷酰胺

D. 诺龙

E. 大麻

2. Which of the following is not a recognized cause of oligospermia?

A. Sulfasalazine

B. Mesalazine

C. Cyclophosphamide

D. Nandrolone

E. Cannabis

3. 关于体外受精，以下哪一项是正确的？

A. 给予天然黄体生成素（LH）使达到峰值用于诱导卵母细胞最终成熟

B. 40 岁时单周期治疗后活产的概率约为 30%

C. 促性腺激素药物从月经期的黄体期开始使用

D. 胚胎在受精后 2 天到达囊胚阶段

E. 胚胎移植当天的子宫内膜厚度应超过 5mm 以提供良好的着床机会

3. Regarding in vitro fertilization, which one of the following statements is correct?

A. The natural luteinizing hormone (LH) surge is used to induce final oocyte maturation

B. The chance of a live birth after a single cycle of treatment at age 40 years is approximately 30%

C. Gonadotropin medications are given from the start of the luteal phase of the cycle

D. Embryos reach the blastocyst stage 2 days after fertilization

E. Endometrial thickness on the day of embryo transfer should exceed 5 mm in order to give a good chance of implantation

4. 以下哪一项不是体外受精（IVF）卵巢过度刺激综合征（OHSS）的特征？

A. 毛细血管通透性降低

B. 血清雌二醇升高

C. 胸腔积液

D. 心包积液

E. 腹水

4. Which of the following is not a feature of in vitro fertilization (IVF) ovarian hyperstimulation syndrome (OHSS)?

A. Decreased capillary permeability

B. Elevated serum oestradiol

C. Pleural effusion

D. Pericardial effusion

E. Ascites

5. 以下哪一项最适合植入前基因筛查（PGS）？

A. PGS 的目的是寻找已知携带者的单基因缺陷

B. 使用 PGS 的目的是选择最好的胚胎进行移植

C. 所有体外受精（IVF）病例均应使用 PGS 进行非整倍体筛查

D. PGS 已被证明可以提高试管婴儿周期的成功率

E. PGS 对年龄＜ 35 岁的孕妇最有用

5. Which of the following is most appropriate regarding pre-implantation genetic screening (PGS)?

A. The purpose of PGS is to look for single gene defects in known carriers

B. The aim is to use PGS to select the best embryo for transfer.

C. PGS should be used for aneuploidy screening in all cases of in vitro fertilization (IVF)

D. PGS has been shown to increase the success of IVF cycles

E. PGS has most utility with maternal age <35

第 18 章（Chapter 18）

1. 一名 45 岁的女性在第一次妊娠时孕 11 周时流产。她没有其他家族史或病史。以下哪一项最有可能导致她流产？

A. 同种免疫

B. 抗磷脂抗体综合征

C. 宫颈功能不全

D. 双角子宫

E. 胎儿染色体异常

1. A 45-year-old woman has a miscarriage in her first pregnancy at 11 weeks' gestation. She has no other family or medical history of note. Which one of the following would be the most likely cause for the loss of her pregnancy?

A. Isoimmunization

B. Antiphospholipid antibody syndrome

C. Cervical incompetence

D. Bicornuate uterus

E. Fetal chromosomal abnormality

2. 当染色体异常导致流产时，最可能的异常核型是什么？

A. 45–XO

B. 47–21 三体

C. 46XY/45XO 嵌合

D. 69– 三倍体

E. 不平衡罗伯逊易位

2. When chromosomal abnormality is responsible for a sporadic miscarriage, what is the most likely karyotypic abnormality?

A. 45-XO

B. 47-trisomy 21

C. 46XY/45XO mosaic

D. 69-triploidy

E. Unbalanced robertsonian translocation

3. 一名 26 岁的女性因下腹痛 12h 和阴道流血被送往当地一家小型医院的急诊科。她的最后一次月经是在 8 周前，她的尿妊娠试验呈阳性。检查时，她面色苍白、出汗，血压为 70/40mmHg，脉搏为 50 次 / 分。触诊时腹部柔软，没有肌紧张和反跳痛的迹象。在开放静脉通路开始抢救后，以下哪项是最合适的下一步治疗？

A. 安排超声检查宫内妊娠物

B. 带她去手术室进行腹腔镜检查以排除异位妊娠

C. 进行阴道窥器检查以检查妊娠物

D. 给予米索前列醇并安排 2 天的超声

E. 转运到最近的有妇科的医院

3. A 26-year-old is admitted to the emergency department of a small local hospital with a 12-hour history of lower abdominal pain and vaginal bleeding. Her last period was 8 weeks ago, and she has a positive urinary pregnancy test. On examination she is pale and sweaty with a blood pressure of 70/40 and a pulse of 50. Her abdomen is soft on palpation with no evidence of guarding or rebound. After obtaining intravenous access and starting resuscitation, which of the following would be the most appropriate next step in treatment?

A. Arrange an ultrasound scan to check for an intrauterine pregnancy

B. Take her to theatre for laparoscopy to exclude ectopic pregnancy

C. Perform a speculum examination to check for products of conception

D. Prescribe misoprostol and arrange ultrasound scan for 2 days' time

E. Arrange for transfer to the nearest hospital with a gynaecology department

4. 关于子宫异常和流产，以下哪一种子宫异常与流产的关联性最高？

A. 弓形

B. 双角

C. 纵隔

D. 单角

E. 狄德尔福斯子宫

4. Regarding uterine abnormalities and miscarriage, which one of the following uterine variations has the highest association with miscarriage?

A. Arcuate

B. Bicornuate

C. Subseptate

D. Unicornuate

E. Didelphus

5. 一名有明显疼痛的女性被诊断为异位妊娠后，关于治疗的最恰当说法是什么？

A. 甲氨蝶呤紧急给药是合理的方案

B. 如果对侧输卵管正常，则首选输卵管切开术

C. 与输卵管切除术相比，输卵管切开术后复发异位妊娠更常见

D. 输卵管切除术后持续性滋养细胞疾病更常见

E. 与输卵管切开术相比，输卵管切除术后的后续妊娠率较低

5. After diagnosis of an ectopic pregnancy in a woman with significant pain, what is the most appropriate statement regarding treatment?

A. Urgent methotrexate administration is a reasonable management plan

B. Salpingotomy is the preferred option if the contralateral tube is normal

C. Recurrent ectopic pregnancy is more common after salpingotomy compared to salpingectomy

D. Persistent trophoblastic disease is more common following salpingectomy

E. Subsequent pregnancy rates are lower following salpingectomy compared to salpingotomy

6. 下列哪种情况应予抗 D 免疫球蛋白预防？

A. 先兆流产

B. 完全流产

C. 不完全流产保守治疗

D. 腹腔镜输卵管切除术治疗异位妊娠

E. 未知部位妊娠（PUL）的保守治疗

6. Which of the following situations should be prescribed anti-D immunoglobulin prophylaxis?

A. Threatened miscarriage

B. Complete miscarriage

C. Incomplete miscarriage with conservative management

D. Ectopic pregnancy with laparoscopic salpingectomy

E. Pregnancy of unknown location (PUL) with conservative management

第 19 章（Chapter 19）

1. 一名 19 岁的女孩在性健康诊所就诊，因为她担心在最近的无保护性交后可能感染了性传播疾病（STI）。性伴侣告诉她，他有衣原体感染。她没有症状，检查完全正常。检查衣原体最合适的检查？

A. 阴道下段拭子培养

B. 阴道上段拭子培养

C. IgM 抗体检测

D. IgG 抗体检测

E. 聚合酶链反应（PCR）

1. A 19-year-old attends a sexual health clinic because she is concerned she may have contracted a sexually transmitted infection (STI) following recent unprotected sexual intercourse. That partner has informed her he has chlamydia. She is asymptomatic, and examination is completely normal. What would be the most appropriate investigation to test for chlamydia?

A. Low vaginal swab for culture

B. High vaginal swab for culture

C. IgM antibody testing

D. IgG antibody testing

E. Polymerase chain reaction (PCR)

2. 一位 25 岁的女性来咨询各种避孕方法的有效性，因为她有了新的性伴侣，她没有使用各种避孕措施的禁忌证。以下哪一项被认为在预防意外妊娠方面最有效？

A. 复合雌激素 / 孕激素口服避孕药

B. Nuva 阴道避孕环

C. 仅含去氧孕酮黄体酮的药丸

D. 3 个月注射一次 Depo-Provera

E. 植埋避孕

2. A 25-year-old woman comes for advice about the effectiveness of various contraceptive methods, as she has a new partner. There are no contraindications to any method.

Which one of the following would be considered to have the best efficacy in preventing an unwanted pregnancy?

A. The combined oestrogen/progestogen oral contraceptive pill

B. The Nuva vaginal contraceptive ring

C. A desogestrel progesterone-only pill

D. Three monthly injections of Depo-Provera

E. The Implanon contraceptive rod

3. 一位 26 岁女性，一直月经不调，前来咨询避孕事宜。她的体重指数（BMI）为 32，血压为 120/80mmHg，除了多毛症，临床检查正常。最适合开以下哪一种口服避孕药（OCP）？

A. 含有 20μg 乙炔雌二醇和左炔诺孕酮的 OCP

B. 含有 30μg 乙炔雌二醇和左炔诺孕酮的 OCP

C. 含有 50μg 乙炔雌二醇和左炔诺孕酮的 OCP

D. 含有乙炔雌二醇和醋酸环丙孕酮的 OCP

E. 仅含低剂量左炔诺孕酮的 OCP

3. A 26-year-old woman, who has always had irregular periods, presents for contraceptive advice. Her body mass index (BMI) is 32, blood pressure is 120/80 mmHg and clinical examination is normal apart from some hirsutism. Which one of the following oral contraceptive pills (OCP) would be most appropriate to prescribe?

A. An OCP containing 20 μg of ethinyl oestradiol and levonorgestrel

B. An OCP containing 30 μg of ethinyl oestradiol and levonorgestrel

C. An OCP containing 50 μg of ethinyl oestradiol and levonorgestrel

D. An OCP containing ethinyl oestradiol and cyproterone acetate

E. An OCP containing low-dose levonorgestrel only

4. 置入铜制宫内节育器（IUCD）后，第一次检查时看不到尾丝。以下哪个 IUCD 并发症不是未见尾丝的可能原因？

A. 妊娠

B. 子宫内膜感染

C. 宫内节育器排出

D. 宫内节育器倒置

E. 穿孔

4. Following insertion of a copper intrauterine contraceptive device (IUCD), the strings are not visible on first string check. Which of the following IUCD complications is not a possible cause of missing strings?

A. Pregnancy

B. Endometrial infection

C. Expulsion

D. Device inversion

E. Perforation

5. 对于深静脉血栓形成和复方口服避孕药（COCP）的使用，以下哪项最合适？

A. COCP 的血栓风险与妊娠相同

B. 相对风险是一般人群风险的 3 倍

C. 无论孕激素含量如何，风险都是相同的

D. 每年女性患血栓的相对风险约为 15/10 万

E. COCP 使用者越年轻，风险越高

5. Which of the following is most appropriate regarding deep venous thrombosis and combined oral contraceptive pill (COCP) use?

A. The risk with the COCP is equivalent to that in pregnancy

B. The relative risk is three times the general population risk

C. The risk is equivalent, regardless of progestogen content

D. The relative risk is around 15/100,000 women per year

E. The risk is higher in COCP users who are younger

第 20 章（Chapter 20）

1. 外阴癌患者常见以下哪项？

A. 外阴上皮内瘤变（VIN）

B. 分化 VIN

C. 佩吉特病

D. 尖锐湿疣

E. 单纯疱疹感染

1. Which of the following is commonly found with vulval cancer?

A. Vulval intraepithelial neoplasia (VIN)

B. Differentiated VIN

C. Paget's disease

D. Condyloma

E. Herpes simplex infection

2. 关于宫颈癌的一级预防，哪个说法最贴切？

A. 细胞学筛查已被证明是一种有效的一级预防措施

B. 双价疫苗针对两种高危亚型：HPV6 和 HPV11

C. 四价疫苗针对 4 种高危亚型

D. 人乳头瘤病毒（HPV）疫苗接种计划显示至少减少了 70% 高危 HPV

E. 初次性交后打 HPV 疫苗无效

2. Regarding primary prevention of cervical cancer, which is

the most appropriate statement?

A. Cytological screening has been shown to be an effective primary prevention measure

B. The bivalent vaccine targets the two high-risk subtypes: HPV 6 and 11

C. The quadrivalent vaccine targets four high-risk subtypes

D. Human papilloma virus (HPV) vaccination programmes have shown at least a 70% reduction in high-risk HPV

E. HPV vaccines are of no efficacy after sexual debut

3. 以下哪项是子宫内膜癌的诱发因素？

A. 口服避孕药

B. 多胎

C. 肥胖

D. 人乳头瘤病毒感染

E. BRCA 载体

3. Which of the following is a predisposing factor for endometrial cancer?

A. Oral contraceptive pills

B. Multiparity

C. Obesity

D. Human papillomavirus infection

E. BRCA carrier

第 21 章（Chapter 21）

1. 子宫骶韧带为哪个位置提供支持？

A. 膀胱

B. 直肠

C. 阴道上部分和宫颈

D. 尿道

E. 肛门外括约肌

1. The uterosacral ligaments provide support to:

A. The urinary bladder

B. Rectum

C. Upper vagina and cervix

D. Urethra

E. The external anal sphincter

2. 患有膀胱膨出的 58 岁患者通常表现为下列哪种情况？

A. 绝经后出血

B. 深度性交痛

C. 膀胱排空不全

D. 便秘

E. 尿急

2. A 58-year-old patient with a cystocele may commonly present with symptoms of:

A. Postmenopausal bleeding

B. Deep dyspareunia

C. Incomplete bladder emptying

D. Constipation

E. Urinary urgency

3. 一名 22 岁的分娩过 1 个孩子的患者有压力性尿失禁的症状。以下哪一项是治疗的第一步？

A. 盆底理疗

B. 建议使用尿道中段吊带

C. 安排膀胱压力检查

D. 奥昔布宁

E. 阴道前壁缝合术

3. A 22-year-old para 1 has symptoms of stress urinary incontinence. Which of the following would be the first step in management?

A. Pelvic floor physiotherapy

B. Advise a mid-urethral sling

C. Arrange bladder pressure studies

D. Oxybutynin

E. Anterior colporrhaphy

4. 一名 29 岁的 G1P1 女性出现子宫脱垂。她计划再妊娠。以下哪一项是最合适的管理？

A. 阴道子宫托

B. 曼彻斯特修补术

C. 阴道筋膜修复

D. 阴道网片修复

E. 安排盆底理疗，建议她推迟手术，直到她完成生育计划

4. A 29-year-old G_1P_1 presents with uterovaginal prolapse. She is planning to have further pregnancies. Which of the following would be the most appropriate management?

A. Vaginal pessaries

B. Manchester repair

C. Fascial repairs of the vagina

D. Graft (mesh) repairs of the vagina

E. Arrange pelvic floor physiotherapy and advise her to delay surgery until her family is completed

5. 以下哪一项最不可能成为女性急性尿潴留的原因？

A. 分娩时阴道裂伤

B. 后位妊娠子宫挤压

C. 外阴炎性病变

D. 阴道脱垂修复

E. 宫颈癌放疗

5. Which of the following is least likely to be a cause of acute retention of urine in women?

A. Vaginal tears during childbirth

B. Impacted retroverted gravid uterus

C. Inflammatory lesions of the vulva

D. Vaginal repair of prolapse

E. Radiotherapy for cervical cancer

附录 A（Appendix A）

1. 以下哪一项不是常规的术前检查？

A. 其他方面健康的患者的全血细胞计数

B. 育龄女性的妊娠试验

C. 其他方面健康患者的凝血功能筛查

D. 高龄患者的心电图

E. 使用袢利尿药的女性体内的尿素和电解质

1. Which of the following is not a routine preoperative investigation?

A. Full blood count in an otherwise healthy patient

B. Pregnancy test in a reproductive-age woman

C. Coagulation screen in an otherwise healthy patient

D. Electrocardiogram in patients of advanced age

E. Urea and electrolytes in a woman on loop diuretics

2. 关于世界卫生组织（WHO）的围术期检查，以下哪项最合适？

A. "签到"是任何手术的最后一个 WHO 阶段

B. 术前"讨论"应该包括管理人员，以减少错误识别患者的风险

C. "暂停"是任何手术的第一个 WHO 阶段

D. "签退"应包括计数纱布和器械

E. 世卫组织核查表虽然合理，但尚未证明可以降低发病率和死亡率

2. Regarding World Health Organization (WHO) perioperative checks, which of the following is most appropriate?

A. 'Sign in' is the final WHO stage of any procedure

B. The preoperative 'huddle' should include administrative staff to reduce the risk of wrong patient identification

C. 'Time out' is the first WHO stage of any procedure

D. 'Sign out' should include swab and instrument count

recording

E. WHO checklists, whilst sensible, have not yet been shown to reduce morbidity and mortality

3. 大手术前应避免使用下列哪些药物以降低血栓栓塞的风险？

A. 单纯黄体酮

B. 激素替代疗法（HRT）

C. 复方口服避孕药（OCP）

D. 用于异常子宫出血的促性腺激素释放激素（GnRH）激动剂

E. 手术开始前的抗生素预防

3. Which of the following medications should be avoided before major surgery to reduce the risk of thromboembolism?

A. Progesterone-only pill

B. Hormone replacement therapy (HRT)

C. Combined oral contraceptive pill (OCP)

D. Gonadotropin-releasing hormone (GnRH) agonists for abnormal uterine bleeding

E. Antibiotic prophylaxis before the start of the procedure

4. 截石位不合适会引起以下哪些并发症？

A. 气体栓塞

B. 皮肤坏死

C. 股疝

D. 脚踝疼痛

E. 急性骨筋膜室综合征

4. Which of the following complications could be caused by an inappropriate lithotomy position?

A. Gas embolization

B. Skin necrosis

C. Femoral hernia

D. Ankle pain

E. Acute compartment syndrome

5. 以下哪些因素不会增加尿路损伤的风险？

A. 子宫内膜异位症

B. 膀胱过度膨胀

C. 高龄

D. 耻骨上 Trocar 穿刺

E. 尿路感染

5. Which of the following factors do not increase the risk of urinary tract injuries?

A. Endometriosis

B. Bladder overdistension

C. Advanced age

D. Suprapubic trocar insertion

E. Urinary infection

6. 以下哪项不是术后低血压的常见原因？

A. 脱水

B. 出血

C. 肾功能衰竭

D. 心力衰竭

E. 硬膜外镇痛

6. Which of the following is not a common cause of postoperative hypotension?

A. Dehydration

B. Bleeding

C. Renal failure

D. Heart failure

E. Epidural analgesia

7. 下列说法中哪一项是正确的？

A. 克雷伯菌是手术部位损伤的常见微生物

B. 术后盆腔脓肿常由需氧菌群引起

C. 糖尿病是手术部位感染的危险因素，而吸烟有保护作用

D. 剃毛脱毛是一种保护因素

E. 放置引流管是手术部位感染的危险因素

7. Which one of the following statements is correct?

A. Klebsiella is a common microorganism in surgical site injuries

B. Postoperative pelvic abscesses are frequently caused by aerobic flora

C. Diabetes is a risk factor for surgical site infections, while smoking is protective

D. Hair removal by shaving is a protective factor

E. Surgical drains are a risk factor for surgical site infections

8. 关于择期手术的加速恢复计划，以下哪一项是正确的？

A. 加速恢复路径里下床活动增加，会导致初期疼痛增加

B. 加速恢复路径需要更多护理时间

C. 加速恢复途径的主要目的是减少术中损伤的影响

D. 加速恢复途径是通用的

E. 在麻醉前禁水 2h，以避免脱水

8. Concerning enhanced recovery programmes for elective surgery, which one of the following statements is correct?

A. Enhanced recovery pathways are associated with more initial pain due to increased mobilization

B. Enhanced recovery pathways require more nursing time

C. Enhanced recovery pathways are principally aimed at reducing the effects of intraoperative insult

D. Enhanced recovery pathways are generic

E. The period of starvation is reduced to 2 hours for clear fluids prior to anaesthetic to avoid dehydration

附录 B（Appendix B）

1. 以下哪一项被认为是在医疗环境中使用社交媒体的潜在缺点？

A. 患者访问健康信息

B. 专业的网络

C. 社交网络

D. 维护保密性

E. 轻松与许多人沟通

1. Which of the following is considered a potential disadvantage of using social media in a medical context?

A. Patients accessing health information

B. Professional networking

C. Social networking

D. Maintaining confidentiality

E. Communicating with large numbers easily

2. 关于通用数据保护条例（GDPR）数据保护，以下哪些说法是正确的？

A. GDPR 于 2016 年推出

B. GDPR 是欧盟数据保护法

C. GDPR 在英国以外没有职权范围

D. GDPR 中的关键术语涉及企业数据

E. GDPR 为人们提供了完全开放访问公司 / 组织持有的关于他们的信息的权利

2. Regarding General Data Protection Regulation (GDPR) data protection, which of the following statements is correct?

A. GDPR was introduced in 2016

B. GDPR is an EU data protection law

C. GDPR has no remit outside the UK

D. The key term in GDPR involves corporate data

E. GDPR offers rights for people to have completely open access to the information companies/organizations hold about them

3. 关于研究和临床审计，以下哪些说法是正确的？

A. 临床审计和临床研究解决类似问题以改善患者保健

B. 临床审计旨在根据商定的标准提高患者保健质量

C. 临床研究批判性地评估临床常规，以确定与实际服务中差距

D. 只有在有国家指南的情况下才进行临床审计

E. 临床研究通常由制药公司资助以测试他们的药物

3. Regarding research and a clinical audit, which of the following statements is correct?

A. A clinical audit and clinical research address similar questions in order to improve patient care

B. A clinical audit seeks to improve the quality of patient care against agreed standards

C. Clinical research critically appraises routine clinical practice to identify gaps in service provision

D. A clinical audit should only be done if there is a national guideline

E. Clinical research is usually funded by the pharma ceutical companies to test their drugs

4. 关于临床指南，下列哪项正确？

A. 临床指南是基于证据的陈述，可帮助临床医生做出适当的临床决策以改善患者护理

B. 一旦发布临床指南所有医院就必须落实

C. 指南通常由在医院工作的临床医生制订

D. 制订临床指南的不同组织定期协商并遵循相似的方法学

E. 临床指订南建议基于成本效益数据

4. Regarding clinical guidelines, which of the following statements is correct?

A. Clinical guidelines are evidence-based statements to assist clinicians to make appropriate clinical decisions in order to improve patient care

B. It is mandatory for all organizations to implement all clinical guidelines once they are published

C. Guidelines are usually developed by clinicians working in the hospitals

D. Different organizations developing clinical guidelines regularly consult each other and follow similar methodology

E. The clinical guidelines recommendations are based on cost-effectiveness data

5. 在研究中，下列哪一项是正确的？

A. 描述性研究提供有关人群疾病流行的信息

B. 病例对照和队列研究比较了患病者和未患病者

C. 随机临床试验涉及根据临床医生的善意分配不同的治疗（干预）

D. 临床医生通常知道他们的患者正在接受活性药物还是安慰剂治疗

E. 新药的临床试验必须排除孕妇和在研究期间希望怀孕的人

5. In research, which one of the following statements is correct?

A. Descriptive studies provide information on disease prevalence in a population

B. Case control and cohort studies compare people with the disease and those without it

C. Randomized clinical trials involve allocation of different treatments (interventions) on good faith of the clinicians

D. Clinicians are usually aware of whether their patients are being treated with an active or a dummy preparation

E. Clinical trials of new drugs must exclude pregnant women and those who wish to become pregnant during the study

6. 关于循证医疗临床实践，以下哪项陈述是正确的？

A. 循证医学临床实践应确保风险管理策略到位，以降低所有患者的风险

B. 临床风险管理策略应仅关注孕产妇和新生儿死亡病例

C. 临床事件报告涉及针对所有参与管理特定患者的人员设立调查小组

D. 应鼓励患者投诉工作人员，因为这有助于改善护理

E. 组织内几乎死亡事件的调查应私下进行，以降低组织的风险

6. Regarding evidence-based health care, which of the following statements is correct?

A. Evidence-based health care should ensure that risk management strategies are in place to reduce risk to all patients

B. Clinical risk management strategies should only focus on cases of maternal and neonatal mortality

C. Clinical incident reporting involves setting up investigation panels against all those involved in the care of a specific patient

D. Patients should be encouraged to complain against staff, as it helps to improve care

E. The investigations of near-misses within an organization should be privately conducted to reduce risk to the organization

附录 C（Appendix C）

1. 一名 49 岁女性因行开腹子宫切除术和双侧输卵管

卵巢切除术入院。她作为医院的门诊患者接受了全面检查，并被诊断出患有功能失调性子宫出血（DUB）导致的严重贫血。已经进行了输血。您是将进行手术的外科登记员，但您之前从未见过该患者。您有一份关于此类手术风险的书面文件；这是由该国家的妇产科学院制作的。下列关于获得知情同意的说法中哪一项是正确的？

A. 同意书必须经过手术科室的主治医生的讨论和见证

B. 因为她已经在门诊接受过评估，所以不需要进一步讨论护理事宜

C. 您无须讨论任何风险低于 1% 的潜在并发症

D. 您必须讨论可能的替代方案、手术过程中可能发生的并发症、发生此类并发症时所需的护理，以及术后并发症和护理

E. 您必须提供关于向患者提议的手术可能出现的并发症的书面声明

1. A 49-year-old woman is admitted to hospital for the performance of a total abdominal hysterectomy and bilateral salpingo-oophorectomy. She has been fully investigated as an outpatient of the hospital and diagnosed with severe anaemia due to dysfunctional uterine bleeding (DUB). A blood transfusion has been given. You are the surgical registrar who will be performing the surgery, but you have not seen this patient previously. You have available a written document concerning the risks of such surgery; this has been produced by the College of Obstetrics and Gynaecology of the country concerned. Which one of the following statements regarding the obtaining of informed consent is correct?

A. The consent form must have been discussed and witnessed by the consultant of the surgical unit

B. Because she has been evaluated in the outpatient clinic, there is no need to discuss the care further

C. There is no need for you to discuss any potential complications where the risk of these is under 1%

D. You must discuss the possible alternatives to the proposed surgery, the complications which might occur during the surgery, the care required if such a complication occurred and the postoperative complications and care

E. You must provide the written college statement concerning the possible complications of the surgery proposed to the patient

2. 46 岁女性，10 天前因子宫肌瘤行全腹子宫切除术。手术本身显然并不复杂。然而，术后期间发生了深静脉血栓形成。她目前正在接受华法林治疗，计划至少持续 6 个月。应该遵循关于保留女性医疗记录的哪些规则？

A. 保留 5 年

B. 保留 7 年

C. 保留 10 年

D. 保留 15 年

E. 保留 25 年

2. A 46-year-old woman had a total abdominal hysterectomy for uterine fibroids 10 days ago. The operation itself was apparently uncomplicated; however, a deep vein thrombosis occurred during the postoperative period. She is currently on treatment with warfarin, and this is planned to continue for at least 6 months. Which of the following rules regarding retention of the medical records of the woman should apply?

A. Retention for 5 years

B. Retention for 7 years

C. Retention for 10 years

D. Retention for 15 years

E. Retention for 25 years

3. 下列哪一种方法评估治疗特定病症的特定方法是最好的？

A. 来自该领域专家的专家意见

B. 偶发病例报告

C. 多个病例报告

D. 回顾性病例 / 对照研究

E. 随机对照临床试验

3. Which one of the following methods of evaluating the adequacy of a particular method of treatment of a specific condition is best?

A. Expert opinion from a specialist in the field

B. Occasional case reports

C. Multiple case reports

D. Retrospective case/control studies

E. Randomized controlled clinical trials

4. 一位 34 岁的女性刚刚分娩了一个 4500g 的婴儿。头部已分娩，由助产士接生，但当确定肩难产时，您被要求完成接生。不幸的是，分娩的婴儿患有 Erb 麻痹症。您在分娩后立即填写的医疗记录中必须包含以下哪一项信息，以防 Erb 麻痹无法消失并且患者对您或医院提起诉讼？

A. 胎头娩出的时间和接生者

B. 您和其他人用于娩出胎儿肩部及其余部分的技术的详细信息，并由您签名

C. 胎儿完全娩出的确切时间

D. 胎儿出生时的 Apgar 评分

E. 以上所有

4. A 34-year-old woman has just been delivered of a 4500-g baby. The head was delivered by a midwife, but when shoulder dystocia was defined, you were requested to complete the delivery and did so. Unfortunately, the baby has Erb's palsy. Which one of the following pieces of information must be included in the medical record you are completing immediately after the delivery in case the Erb's palsy does not resolve and litigation occurs against you or the hospital?

A. The exact date and time the baby's head was delivered and by whom

B. Detailed information of all of the techniques you and others used to effect delivery of the shoulders and the remainder of the baby and signed by you

C. The exact time the remainder of the baby was delivered

D. The Apgar score of the baby at the time of birth

E. All of the above

5. 一个 15 岁的女孩进入您的诊室，因为她希望获得口服避孕药（OCP）的处方，以便她可以开始与一个"了不起的人"过性生活。她以前没有性生活。他向她表明他不准备使用安全套。她表示不希望告知她的父母，因为他们不允许这种性行为。以下哪一项是最适合给她的建议？

A. 鉴于她的年龄，给她吃避孕药是违法的

B. 要给她吃药，她需要同意让她的父母知道

C. 要给她吃药，她需要同意相关的卫生部门被告知

D. 为了给她服用避孕药，需要获得有关男性的更多信息

E. 她应该让她的伴侣使用避孕套

5. A 15-year-old girl attends your surgery because she wishes a prescription for the oral contraceptive pill (OCP) so that she can commence a sexual relationship with a 'wonderful man'. She has not been sexually active previously. He has indicated to her that he is not prepared to use condoms. She indicates that she does not wish her parents to be informed, as they would not allow such sexual activity. Which one of the following would be the most appropriate advice to give her?

A. It is illegal to give her the contraceptive pill because of her age

B. To give her the pill, she would need to give consent for her parents to be informed

C. To give her the pill she would need to give consent for the appropriate health department to be informed

D. To give her the pill more information about the male involved would need to be obtained

E. She should just get her partner to use condoms

二、答案（Answers）

第 1 章（Chapter 1）

1. 对骨盆动脉血供最恰当的描述

B 是正确的。髂内动脉起源于腰骶关节水平并越过骨盆边缘，继续向下到达真骨盆腔的后侧壁。前支供应膀胱上、中、下动脉，并为膀胱提供血液供应。子宫动脉初段沿阔韧带下缘附着下行，穿行于腹膜下脂肪。在该结构进入膀胱前，子宫动脉在距离阴道穹窿外侧 1.5～2cm 处，横跨输尿管。卵巢动脉在腹膜后沿腰大肌表面下行，直至骨盆边缘。

1. What is the most appropriate description of the arterial supply of the pelvis?

B is correct. The internal iliac artery arises at the level of the lumbosacral articulation and passes over the pelvic brim, continuing downward on the posterolateral wall of the cavity of the true pelvis. The anterior division provides the superior, middle and inferior vesical arteries that provide the blood supply for the bladder. The uterine artery initially runs downward in the subperitoneal fat under the inferior attachment of the broad ligament. The uterine artery crosses over the ureter shortly before that structure enters the bladder approximately 1.5–2 cm from the lateral fornix of the vagina. The ovarian arteries descend behind the peritoneum on the surface of the corresponding psoas muscle until they reach the brim of the pelvis

2. 阴道

A 是正确的。阴道是表面衬有无角化鳞状上皮的平滑肌管状结构。阴道前部紧邻膀胱和尿道的三角区。阴道后部下 1/3 与肛管被会阴体隔开，中间 1/3 紧邻直肠，上 1/3 靠近道格拉斯窝。性成熟未妊娠女性的阴道 pH 为 4.0～5.0，对降低盆腔感染的风险提供了重要的抗菌作用。

2. The vagina:

A is correct. The vagina is a tube of smooth muscle lined by non-cornified squamous epithelium. Anteriorly, it is intimately related to the trigone of the urinary bladder and the urethra. Posteriorly, the lower third is separated from the anal canal by the perineal body, the middle third is related to the rectum and the upper third to the rectouterine pouch (pouch of Douglas). The pH of the vagina in the sexually mature nonpregnant female is between 4.0 and 5.0, which has an important antibacterial function in reducing the risk of pelvic infection.

3. 子宫及其支撑结构

A 是正确的。子宫前部韧带是筋膜圆索状结构，与邻近的膀胱子宫反折腹膜一起自宫颈前方跨越膀胱表面延伸到前腹壁腹膜，有较弱的支撑作用。同样的，阔韧带的支撑作用也比较弱。后方的宫骶韧带对于支撑子宫和阴道穹窿起着重要作用，这些韧带和表面被覆腹膜构成了直肠子宫陷凹（道格拉斯窝）的侧缘。妊娠期间，子宫峡部扩大形成子宫下段，在分娩时成为产道的一部分，但对胎儿娩出的作用不大（子宫后倾的发生率约为 10%）。

3. Uterus and its supporting structures:

A is correct. The anterior ligament is a fascial condensation which, with the adjacent peritoneal uterovesical fold, extends from the anterior aspect of the cervix across the superior surface of the bladder to the peritoneal peritoneum of the anterior abdominal wall. It has a weak supporting role. Likewise, the broad ligament plays only a minor supportive role. Posteriorly, the uterosacral ligaments play a major role in supporting the uterus and the vaginal vault, and these ligaments and their peritoneal covering form the lateral boundaries of the rectouterine pouch (of Douglas). In pregnancy, the isthmus of the uterus enlarges to form the lower segment of the uterus, which in labour becomes a part of the birth canal but does not contribute greatly to the expulsion of the fetus. (The incidence of uterine retroversion is about 10%.)

4. 卵巢

D 是正确的。卵巢位于阔韧带的后表面上，靠近髂外血管和骨盆侧壁上的输尿管。它通过卵巢的悬韧带附着在骨盆边缘。卵巢表面被覆立方上皮或低层柱状生发上皮。血液供应来自卵巢动脉，卵巢动脉直接来自腹主动脉。卵泡位于卵巢的皮质和髓质中。

4. The ovary:

D is correct. The ovary lies on the posterior surface of the broad ligament in close proximity to the external iliac vessels and the ureter on the lateral pelvic wall. It is attached to the pelvic brim by the suspensory ligament of the ovary. The surface of the ovary is covered by a cuboidal or low columnar type of germinal epithelium. The blood supply is derived from the ovarian artery, which arises directly from the aorta. The follicles are found in both the cortex and medulla of the organ.

5. 子宫

B 是正确的。子宫的血液供应主要来自子宫动脉，其分支在阔韧带上方与卵巢血管分支吻合，即使在髂内动脉结扎后也能确保子宫有足够的侧支供应。淋巴引流沿着血管。子宫痛觉通过交感传入神经传达至 $T_{11}\sim T_{12}$ 和 $L_1\sim L_2$。阴部神经（躯体神经）供应外阴和盆底。

5. Uterus:

B is correct. The blood supply to the uterus comes largely from the uterine artery, but branches of this anastomose with branches of the ovarian vessels in the upper part of the broad ligament, assuring adequate collateral supply to the uterus even following internal iliac ligation. Lymphatic drainage follows the blood vessels. Uterine pain is mediated through sympathetic afferent nerves passing up to T11-T12 and L1-L2. The pudendal nerve (somatic nerve) supplies the vulva and pelvic floor.

第 2 章（Chapter 2）

1. 关于精子最恰当的说法

D 是正确的。精子头部与卵母细胞膜融合，精子头部和中段通过吞噬作用被吞入卵母细胞。精子体部包含一个屈曲螺旋状的线粒体为精子活动提供"动力"。尾部中央轴由 2 根纵向微管和周围 9 对双联微管组成，这些纤维终止于不同的点，最末端止于一根卵圆形的微丝。这些具有收缩功能的纤维推动精子运动。在精子通过输卵管的过程中，精子经历了成熟的最后阶段（获能），使得它能够穿透透明带。精浆中含有高浓度的果糖，果糖是精子的主要能量。在最适情况下，精子以 6mm/min 的速度迁移，这比单靠精子自身移动的速度快得多，宫腔的积极支持作用有助于精子运动。

2. What is the most appropriate statement relating to spermatozoa?

D is correct. The sperm head fuses with the oocyte plasma membrane, and the sperm head and midpiece are indeed engulfed into the oocyte by phagocytosis. The body contains a coiled helix of mitochondria that provides the 'powerhouse' for sperm motility. The tail consists of a central core of two longitudinal fibres surrounded by nine pairs of fibres that terminate at various points until a single ovoid filament remains. These contractile fibres propel the spermatozoa. During their passage through the Fallopian tubes, the sperm undergo the final stage in maturation (capacitation), which enables penetration of the zona pellucida. Seminal plasma has a high concentration of fructose, which is the major source of energy for the spermatozoa. Under favourable circumstances, sperm migrate at a rate of 6 mm/min. This is much faster than could be explained by the motility of the sperm and must therefore also be dependent on active support within the uterine cavity.

2. 正常的卵泡生长

B 是正确的。在正常排卵的月经周期中，周期的第 5~6 天会有一个卵泡被选择成为优势卵泡（因此 B 是正确的）；另有多达 10 个卵泡生长，但速度明显比优势卵泡慢（因此 A 是不正确的）。此后优势卵泡每天增长 2mm（C 因此不正确）并在直径约 2cm 时破裂（因此 D 不正确），破裂的卵泡在卵母细胞释放后成为黄体（因此 E 不正确）。

2. Normal follicular growth:

B is correct. In a normal ovulatory menstrual cycle, one follicle is selected to become the dominant follicle on day 5–6 of the cycle (B is therefore correct); however, up to 10 show obvious but lesser growth than the dominant follicle (A is therefore incorrect). The dominant follicle grows by 2 mm per day thereafter (C is therefore incorrect) and ruptures at about 2 cm in diameter (D is therefore incorrect), and this ruptured follicle becomes the corpus luteum after release of the oocyte (E is therefore incorrect).

3. 减数分裂

C 是正确的。胎儿期产生的 700 万个生殖细胞是由有丝分裂产生的，而不是减数分裂产生的（因此 A 是不正确的）。第一次减数分裂发生在宫内胎儿期，但停止于减数分 Ⅰ 期。直到在某次月经周期黄体生成素激增后继续分裂，第一次减数分裂在精子与卵母细胞受精之前完成（因此 B 是不正确的）。精卵相遇导致第二次减数分裂开始（因此 C 是正确的）。同源染色体配对过程发生在第一次减数分裂前期，而不是第一次减数分裂完成后（因此 D 是不正确的）。胎儿体内第一次减数分裂停止后，距离该周期重新开始的长时间间隔（可能是 40~45 年后）是高龄产妇染色体异常发生率增加的原因（E 是因此不正确）。

3. Meiosis:

C is correct. The 7 million germ cells produced during fetal life are produced by mitosis, not meiosis (A is therefore incorrect). The first meiotic division commences in utero in the fetus but ceases in prophase. It does not recommence its division until the luteinizing hormone surge occurs in the particular menstrual cycle, and this first meiotic division is completed just prior to fertilization of the oocyte by the sperm (B is therefore incorrect). The attachment of the sperm results in the commencement of the second meiotic division (C is therefore correct). The crossover process between adjacent copies of the same chromosome occurs during prophase of meiosis I, not after meiosis I has been completed (D is therefore incorrect). The long delay between the cessation of prophase I in fetal life and the time when it recommences in the cycle concerned (which can be 40–45 years later) is the reason for the increased incidence of chromosomal abnormalities associated with advanced maternal age (E is therefore incorrect).

4. 关于女性的受精过程

A 是正确的。雌性配子只含有一条 X 染色体，因此不能决定所产生胎儿的性别，这是由雄配子决定的，雄配子含有 X 或 Y 染色体（B 因此是不正确的）。双胎是由胚胎分裂成双胎（单绒毛膜双胎妊娠）或两个独立的卵母细胞被两个独立的精子受精（双绒毛膜双胎妊娠，因此 C 是不正确的）而产生。排卵后卵母细胞可以受精的确切时间尚不确定，但认为如果间隔时间超过 36h 通常不会受精（因此 D 不正确）。精子获能通常发生在女性的生殖道内（因此 E 是不正确的）。

4. Regarding the process of fertilization in the human female:

A is correct. The female gametes only contain an X chromosome and therefore cannot determine the sex of the resulting fetus. This is determined by the male gamete, which will contain either an X or Y chromosome (B is therefore incorrect). Twin pregnancies occur due to division of the embryo (identical or monochorionic twin pregnancy) or if two separate oocytes are fertilized by two separate sperm (a dichorionic twin pregnancy; therefore C is incorrect). The exact time during which the oocyte can be fertilized after ovulation is uncertain, but it is believed fertilization does not occur if this time interval is in excess of 36 hours (D is therefore incorrect). Sperm capacitation to facilitate fertilization generally occurs within the genital tract of the woman (E is therefore incorrect).

5. 着床

C 是正确的。着床通常发生在排卵和受精后 5～6 天（因此 A 不正确），此时胚胎处于囊胚阶段（B 因此是不正确的）。人绒毛膜促性腺激素（hCG）在着床后很快产生（因此 C 是正确的），如果妊娠进展正常，则血浆 hCG 水平每 48 小时增加 1 倍。子宫内膜必须是分泌型才能着床（因此 D 不正确），然后子宫内膜转化为蜕膜。如果子宫内膜是增生型的，则不会发生着床，因此不会妊娠。即使在胚胎高度异常的情况下，也可能发生着床和产生 hCG，在这种情况下，月经会在预期的时间到来，而这时患者永远不会知道她在那个周期中确实妊娠了（因此 E 不正确）。月经开始 2～3 天后进行的尿妊娠试验将呈阴性。

5. Implantation:

C is correct. Implantation generally occurs 5–6 days

after ovulation and fertilization (A is therefore incorrect), at which time the embryo is at the blastocyst stage (B is therefore incorrect). Human chorionic gonadotropin (hCG) is produced soon after the implantation process commences (C is therefore correct), and then the plasma levels double every 48 hours if the pregnancy is progressing normally. The endometrium must be secretory in type to allow implantation (D is therefore incorrect) and is then converted to the appearance of decidua. Implantation will not occur if the endometrium is proliferative in type so a pregnancy will not result. Implantation and hCG production can occur even where the embryo is very abnormal, under which circumstances the period occurs at the expected time and the woman concerned never knows she was actually pregnant in that cycle (E is therefore incorrect). A urinary pregnancy test performed 2–3 days after the period commenced will be negative.

第 3 章（Chapter 3）

1. 关于妊娠期免疫最恰当的表述

A 是正确的。只有两种类型的胎儿胎盘组织，即绒毛和绒毛外滋养层（EVT）与母体组织直接接触，实际上母体免疫系统没有 T 细胞或 B 细胞对人类滋养层细胞免疫攻击。被母体血液浸泡的绒毛滋养层不表达人类白细胞抗原（HLA）Ⅰ 类或 Ⅱ 类分子。EVT 与子宫内膜 / 蜕膜组织直接接触，不表达主要的 T 细胞配体如 HLA-A 或 HLA-B，但表达 HLA Ⅰ 类滋养层特异性 HLA-G，具有强烈的免疫抑制作用，并与 HLA-C 和 HLA-E 一同表达。蜕膜淋巴细胞的主要类型是子宫自然杀伤（NK）细胞。胸腺在妊娠期间表现出一些可逆的退化，显然是由孕激素驱动的淋巴细胞从胸腺皮质外流引起的。Th1 ∶ Th2 细胞因子比率向 Th2 占优势的状态转变。

1. What is the most appropriate statement regarding immunology in pregnancy?

A is correct. Only two types of feto-placental tissue come into direct contact with maternal tissues: the villous and extra-villous trophoblast (EVT), and there are effectively no systemic maternal T- or B-cell responses to trophoblast cells in humans. The villous trophoblast, which is bathed by maternal blood, never expresses human leucocyte antigen (HLA) class I or class II molecules. EVT, which is directly in contact with endometrial/decidual tissues, does not express the major T-cell ligands, HLA-A or HLA-B, but does express the HLA class I trophoblast-specific HLA-G, which is strongly immunosuppressive, along with HLA-C and HLA-E. The main type of decidual lymphocytes is the uterine natural killer (NK) cells. The thymus shows some reversible involution during pregnancy, apparently caused by the progesterone-driven exodus of lymphocytes from the thymic cortex, and the Th1:Th2 cytokine ratio shifts towards Th2.

2. 关于心输出量增加

D 是正确的。从妊娠早期心输出量开始增加。心输出量的增加是由每搏输出量增加和心率加快共同引起的。这与后负荷下降有关。由于需要泵出额外 40% 的血容量，心脏已经不堪重负，而对于那些患有心脏病的女性来说，它可能会破坏平衡并导致心力衰竭，尤其是在他们贫血或感染的情况下。正常母亲的心肺系统能够适应增加的血流量而不会引起肺动脉高压。

2. Regarding the rise in cardiac output:

D is correct. The rise in cardiac output is seen from early pregnancy. The increase in cardiac output is brought about by increase in the stroke volume and the heart rate. It is associated with a fall in the afterload. The heart is already strained due to the need to pump an extra 40% of blood volume, and in those with heart disease it can tip the balance and cause heart failure, especially if they are anaemic or if they contract an infection. The pulmonary vasculature in a mother is able to accommodate the increased blood flow without causing pulmonary hypertension.

3. 孕期呼吸功能

D 是正确的。孕酮使延髓而非肾上腺髓质对 CO_2 的敏感度增加。这会导致一定程度的过度通气，从而降低母体二氧化碳水平，使胎儿能够将二氧化碳转移到母体。母体的 PaO_2 未增加，但血液的携氧能力增加了 18%。母体 2,3-DPG 的增加使母体氧解离曲线向右移动，从而促进母体向胎儿侧输送氧气。每分钟通气量增加了 40%，使得潮气量从 500ml 增加到 700ml。

3. Considering respiratory function in pregnancy:

D is correct. Progesterone sensitizes the medulla oblongata and not the adrenal medulla to CO_2. This causes some over-breathing, which reduces the CO_2 level that allows the fetus to offload its CO_2 to the maternal side. Not the maternal PaO_2 but the oxygen-carrying capacity of blood increases by 18%. There is an increase in maternal 2,3-DPG that shifts the maternal oxygen dissociation curve to the right, thus facilitating the downloading of oxygen to the fetus. There is a 40% increase in minute ventilation due to increase in tidal volume from 500 to mL.

4. 关于孕期肾功能

C 是正确的。除了肾盂肾盏系统和输尿管增粗外，肾实质体积增加导致肾体积增加高达 70%，从

妊娠早期就开始出现这种变化。由于孕酮的影响和尿量增加，输尿管变粗，但张力良好，并不松弛。由于血容量增加，肾小球滤过率（GFR）增加 50%，继而激活肾素 – 血管紧张素系统。妊娠期间有大约 900mmol 而非 1800mmol 钠潴留。由于输尿管进入膀胱处的括约肌肌力不足，导致输尿管扩张和尿液反流，尿潴留的发生率较高，因此妊娠期尿路感染的发生率较高。

4. Considering renal function in pregnancy:

C is correct. There is an increase in renal size of up to 70% due to an increase in size of the parenchyma in addition to the enlargement of the pelvicalyceal system and the ureter, but the increase is seen from early pregnancy. The ureters increase in size due to the influence of progesterone and increased urinary output, but they are not floppy and have good tone. Because of an increase in blood volume there is a 50% increase in glomerular filtration rate (GFR) that activates the renin-angiotensin system. About 900 and not 1800 mmol of sodium are retained during pregnancy. Because of ureteric dilatation and reflux of urine due to lack of sphincteric action at the point entry of the ureter into the bladder and higher incidence of urinary stasis, there is higher incidence of urinary tract infection in pregnancy.

5. 关于孕期内分泌功能

A 是正确的。由于激素环境的变化，胰岛素抵抗随着妊娠的发展而发展。孕 28 周后人胎盘催乳素显著增加，因此一些女性会患妊娠期糖尿病。由于肾小球滤过率增加，更多的葡萄糖进入肾脏，在一些母亲体内，摄入的葡萄糖量超过了肾小管最大吸收能力，因此出现血糖水平不高的"肾性"糖尿。由于新陈代谢增加，甲状腺体积增大。肠道虽然吸收更多的钙，但尿液会丢失更多的钙，加之部分地区饮食中钙缺乏，因此需要补充钙。孕妇皮肤色素沉着是由促黑素细胞激素分泌增加导致的。

5. In relation to endocrine function in pregnancy:

A is correct. Insulin resistance develops with progress of pregnancy due to the change in the hormonal milieu. There is a significant increase in human placental lactogen after 28 weeks as a result of which some women develop gestational diabetes. Due to increased glomerular filtration rate, more glucose is presented to the kidneys, and in some mothers the quantity of glucose exposed for absorption exceeds the tubular maximal absorption capacity and hence presents as 'renal' glycosuria without a high blood glucose level. Because of increased metabolism, the thyroid increases in size. The gut absorbs more calcium but more is also lost in the urine and in areas of dietary deficiency, so calcium supplementation becomes necessary. Skin pigmentation is caused by an increase in melanocyte-secreting hormone.

第 4 章（Chapter 4）

1. 早期胎盘发育

D 是正确的。绒毛包括内部细胞滋养层和外部合体滋养层，它们侵入子宫内膜和子宫肌层。蜕膜细胞为入侵的滋养层提供初始营养。螺旋小动脉被滋养细胞侵入，形成充满母体血液的大腔隙，三级绒毛浸润在这些腔隙中，完成呼吸、营养和排泄功能。叶状绒毛膜形成胎盘。绒毛膜位于胎盘表面，与子宫腔融合。

1. In early placental development:

D is correct. The villi have an inner cytotrophoblast and an outer syncytiotrophoblast that invade the endometrium and myometrial layers. Decidual cells provide the initial nutrition for the invading trophoblasts. The spiral arterioles are invaded by the trophoblasts making large lacunae that are full of maternal blood, and the tertiary villi bathe in these lacunae to accomplish the respiratory, nutrition and excretory functions. Chorion frondosum forms the placenta. Chorion laevae is the layer surrounding the membranes, and it fuses with the uterine cavity.

2. 关于脐带

C 是正确的。脐带有两条动脉和一条静脉。胎儿将血液通过两条动脉输送到胎盘以获得更多的氧气并排出二氧化碳，因此与静脉相比，动脉血的氧气较少。每 200 个胎儿中就有 1 个胎儿只有一根动脉和一根静脉，但它们会正常生长，最终获得活产。脐动脉压在 60～70mmHg。这些血管被一种称为华通化胶的亲水性黏多糖包裹。

2. Regarding the umbilical cord:

C is correct. The umbilical cord has two arteries and one vein. The fetus pumps the blood through these arteries to the placenta to get more oxygen and excrete the carbon dioxide, and hence arterial blood has less oxygen compared with the vein. One in 200 babies has only one artery and one vein, and they grow normally and live birth is achieved. Cord arterial pressure is between 60 and 70 mmHg. The vessels are surrounded by a hydrophilic mucopolysaccharide known as *Wharton's jelly.*

3. 胎盘转运

A 是正确的。简单扩散是根据浓度梯度进行的，这有助于氧气和二氧化碳向正确方向的转运。葡萄糖根据浓度梯度转运，但需要能量，即易化扩散。主动运输需要能量驱动物质逆梯度转运，因此在某些情况下，胎儿血液中该物质的浓度可能已经更高，这个过程发生在氨基酸和水溶性维生素上。更高分子量的物质通过胞饮作用转运。

3. Placental transfer:

A is correct. Simple diffusion is according to the concentration gradients, and this facilitates transfer of oxygen and carbon dioxide in the right direction for the fetus. Glucose is transferred according to the gradient, but it needs energy, i.e. facilitated diffusion. Active transport needs energy for transport and to drive the substances against the gradient, and hence there could be cases where the concentration may be already higher in the fetal blood. This process occurs with amino acids and water-soluble vitamins. Higher-molecular-weight substrates are transferred by pinocytosis.

4. 胎盘功能

E 是正确的。胎盘有多种功能。它有助于气体交换，是将营养传递给胎儿和排泄胎儿废物的重要器官。它产生多种激素——最初是人绒毛膜促性腺激素，后来是雌激素和孕激素，这些都是维持妊娠所必需的。但它对感染的屏障作用很差。因此，胎儿会受到疟疾、梅毒、艾滋病病毒、巨细胞病毒（CMV）和弓形虫病的影响。

4. Placental function:

E is correct. The placenta has multiple functions. It helps with gas exchange and is an important organ for transferring nutrition to the fetus and excreting waste products from the fetus. It produces a number of hormones-initially human chorionic gonadotrophin and later oestrogens and progesterones, which are all essential for maintenance of pregnancy. But it is a poor barrier against infections; thus the fetus is affected by malaria, syphilis, HIV, cytomegalovirus (CMV) and toxoplasmosis.

5. 羊水

A 是正确的。羊水过多可能提示胎儿异常，如神经管缺陷、无脑畸形、肠道闭锁和其他几种已知的病理情况。羊水量随着胎儿的生长和胎龄增大而迅速增加，在 38 周时达到最大，约 1000ml。肢体挤压变形是长期严重羊水过少的并发症之一。这种情况导致的一个主要问题是肺发育不全。胎儿需要足够的羊水来推动肺泡和细支气管的扩张，否则会导致肺发育不全。大多数宫内生长受限病例与羊水减少有关，因为肾灌注减少会导致尿量减少。羊膜腔灌注可能会使变异减速消失，但试验表明术后临床结果没有改善，因此它不是标准手术操作。

5. Amniotic fluid:

A is correct. Polyhydramnios may suggest fetal anomaly such as neural tube defects, anencephaly, gut atresia and several other known pathologies. The amniotic fluid volume increases rapidly in parallel with fetal growth and gestational age up to a maximum volume of around 1000 mL at 38 weeks. Postural deformities are one of the complications of long-standing severe oligohydramnios. A major problem with this situation is pulmonary hypoplasia. Adequate fluid is needed to push the alveoli and bronchioles to expand; if not, it results in lung hypoplasia. Most cases of intrauterine growth restriction would be associated with reduced amniotic fluid due to less urine production caused by less renal perfusion. Amnio-infusion may abolish the variable decelerations, but trials have shown no improvement in clinical outcome, and hence it is not a standard procedure.

第 5 章（Chapter 5）

1. 围产期死亡率

C 是正确的。围产期死亡率是指每 1000 次分娩（包括活产和死产）中胎儿死亡和早期新生儿死亡的数量。这代表了孕产妇健康情况和母儿保健的标准。通过改善社会经济条件、产科管理质量、新生儿保健，以及积极筛查常见先天性异常，可以显著改善围产期死亡率。世界卫生组织有两个目标来评估改善孕产妇健康方面的进展 [千禧年发展目标（MDG）5]。这些措施在 1990—2015 年期间将孕产妇死亡率降低了 75%，并在 2015 年实现普遍的生育健康。

1. Perinatal mortality:

C is correct. Perinatal mortality rate describes the number of stillbirths and early neonatal deaths per 1000 total births (live births and stillbirths). This gives a picture of maternal health and the standard of care provided to mothers and their newborn babies. By improving socio-economic conditions, the quality of obstetric and neonatal care and an active screening programme for common congenital abnormalities, perinatal mortality rates can be significantly improved. The World Health Organization has two targets for assessing progress in improving maternal health (Millennium Development Goal [MDG] 5). These are reducing the maternal mortality ratio by 75% between 1990 and 2015 and achieving universal access to reproductive health by 2015.

2. 关于胎儿死亡

E 是正确的。胎儿死亡是指每 1000 次分娩中胎儿死亡的数量。直到 2011 年，英国母婴咨询中心已经发布了每年的围产期报告。报告显示，胎死率和新生儿早期死亡均显著降低。胎死率体现了产前保健和筛查计划的质量，并且是决定围产期死亡率的最大因素。大多数胎儿死亡发生在产前。传统系统，如 Wigglesworth 和 Aberdeen（产科）分类一致报告系统，多达 2/3 的胎儿死亡原因不明。ReCoDe（死亡相关条件）系统是英国开发的系统，对胎儿死亡时的相关条件进行分类。通过使用该系统发现，胎儿死亡的最常见原因是胎儿生长受限（43%），只有 15.2% 的死亡原因不明。中非撒哈拉以南地区的胎儿死亡率最高。

2. Regarding stillbirths:

E is correct. Stillbirths are the number of stillbirths per 1000 total births. Until 2011, the Centre for Maternal and Child Enquiries has published annual perinatal reports for the UK. The report showed a significant reduction in both stillbirth rates and early neonatal deaths. Stillbirth rates indicate the quality of antenatal care and screening programmes and are the largest contributors to perinatal mortality. Most stillbirths occur antenatally. The traditionally used systems such as the Wigglesworth and the Aberdeen (Obstetric) classifications consistently reported up to two-thirds of stillbirths as being from unexplained causes. The ReCoDe (Relevant Condition at Death) system, which classifies the relevant condition present at the time of death, was developed in the UK. By using this system, the most common cause of stillbirth was fetal growth restriction (43%), and only 15.2% remained unexplained. The sub-Saharan regions of central Africa have the highest stillbirth rates.

3. 关于新生儿死亡

B 是正确的。出生体重无疑是孕产妇健康和营养的指标。低出生体重虽然不是新生儿死亡的直接原因，但却是一个重要的相关因素。许多孕产妇没有接种破伤风疫苗，新生儿破伤风仍然是分娩时污染和脐带护理不足环境中新生儿死亡的常见原因。早产仍然是发展中国家围产儿死亡率的一个重要决定因素，与提供更多新生儿重症监护病房相比，改善孕产妇健康和产科保健是改善结局的更重要的措施。在英国，孕产妇死亡保密调查（CMACE）使用的新生儿分类着眼于新生儿死亡的主要原因和相关因素。过去，近一半的新生儿死亡是早产造成的，但新分类将极早早产限制在妊娠 22 周以下的病例中，发现其仅导致 9.3% 的新生儿死亡。

3. Regarding neonatal deaths:

B is correct. Birth weight is no doubt an indication of maternal health and nutrition. Low birth weight, although not a direct cause of neonatal death, is an important association. Neonatal tetanus remains a common cause of neonatal death in settings where lack of hygiene and inadequate cord care are prevalent, as many women are not immunized against tetanus. Prematurity remains a significant contributor to perinatal mortality rates in developing countries, and improving maternal health and obstetric care is a more important step to improving the outcome than providing more neonatal intensive care units. In the UK, the neonatal classification used by the Confidential Enquiry into Maternal Deaths (CMACE) looked at the primary cause and associated factors for neonatal deaths. In the past, nearly half of the neonatal deaths were due to immaturity, but the new classification restricted extreme prematurity to only cases below 22 weeks' gestation, resulting in only 9.3% of neonatal deaths.

4. 关于孕产妇死亡的描述

A 是正确的。产妇直接死亡的定义是，在产前、产时或产后期间，由于妊娠特有的条件或并发症或其管理而造成的死亡。非直接相关死亡是由发生在妊娠或产褥期的于妊娠无关的原因引起的。孕产妇死亡的定义可能因地区和国家而异。由于英国拥有准确的分母数据（包括活产和死胎）的优势，因此将其孕产妇死亡率定义为每 10 万产次中直接或间接因素死亡的人数，作为更准确的分母，以表明处于危险中的女性人数。产次被定义为任何孕周活产或法律要求告知的在妊娠 24 周或之后发生的胎死宫内的妊娠次数。提高女性的社会经济地位，加上改善孕产妇健康和产前保健，是降低孕产妇死亡率的关键。

4. Regarding the description of maternal deaths:

A is correct. Direct maternal deaths are defined as those resulting from conditions or complications or their management that are unique to pregnancy, occurring during the antenatal, intrapartum or postpartum periods. Coincidental (fortuitous) deaths occur from unrelated causes which happen to occur in pregnancy or the puerperium. Definitions of maternal death can vary across the regions and between countries. As the UK has the advantage of accurate denominator data, including both live births and stillbirths, it has defined its maternal mortality rate as the number of direct and indirect deaths per 100,000 maternities as a more accurate denominator to indicate the number of women at risk. Maternities are defined as the number of pregnancies that result in a live birth at any gestation or stillbirths occurring at or after 24 completed weeks of gestation and are required to be notified by law. Improving the socio-economic status of women, coupled with improved maternal health and antenatal care, is key to the improvement of maternal mortality rates.

5. 孕产妇死亡率

D 是正确的。在 2006—2008 年英国孕产妇死亡保密调查报告中，直接死亡的主要原因是脓毒症，尤其是 A 组链球菌引起的脓毒症。这种感染可以在产前至产后期间的任何时间发生，并且起病可能是隐匿的和非特异性的。心脏病仍然是间接死亡的主要原因。静脉血栓栓塞死亡人数的减少主要是由于英国所有产科病房采用了最新的筛查和血栓预防指南；然而，它仍然是一个重要且可避免的死亡原因。

5. Maternal mortality:

D is correct. In the 2006–2008 UK Confidential Enquiry into Maternal Deaths Report, the leading cause of direct deaths was sepsis, particularly from group A streptococcus. This infection can occur at any time during the antenatal or postpartum period, and the onset can be insidious and non-specific. Cardiac diseases remained the leading cause of indirect deaths. The reduction in the number of deaths from venous thromboembolism is due mainly to improved screening and thromboprophylaxis guidelines adopted by all maternity units in the UK. However, it remains an important and avoidable cause of death.

第 6 章（Chapter 6）

1. 孕期生理变化

E 是正确的。据报道，妊娠期间的乳腺癌与进展快速和预后不良有关。因此，任何乳房"肿块"都提示应进行详细的乳房检查。许多女性在脸颊上会出现一种称为黄褐斑的红褐色色素沉着，这是正常现象，在没有任何其他症状或体征的情况下无须检查。由于相对血液稀释（血浆增加大于红细胞增加），血红蛋白浓度会出现生理性降低。骨盆形状自出生开始就保持不变。骨盆入口平面以骶骨岬为后界，外侧为髂耻线，前侧为耻骨上支和耻骨联合上缘。

1. Physiological changes in pregnancy:

E is correct. Breast cancer during pregnancy is reportedly associated with rapid progression and poor prognosis. Hence, any complaint of a 'lump' in the breast should prompt a detailed breast examination. Many women develop a reddish-brownish pigmentation called chloasma over the cheeks, which is normal and needs no investigation in the absence of any other symptoms or signs. There is a physiological reduction in Hb concentration due to a relative haemodilution (plasma expansion is greater than red cell expansion). The pelvic shape remains unchanged in itself-it is what is from birth. The plane of the pelvic inlet or pelvic brim is bounded posteriorly by the sacral promontory, laterally by the iliopectineal lines and anteriorly by the superior pubic rami and upper margin of the pubic symphysis.

2. 在询问产科病史时

E 是正确的。过去的产科病史对于管理当前妊娠至关重要，例如，糖尿病、高血压或精神疾病的既往史将有助于更好地管理此次妊娠。许多女性无法准确记住末次月经（LMP），如果设备允许，会在早孕期通过超声评估妊娠情况，并根据孕早期超声计算预产期（EDD）。月经周期中排卵后的时间相对稳定，大约是 14 天，无论周期是长还是短。如果基于妊娠晚期超声核对孕周，大约 ±3 周，如果基于妊娠早期扫描，大约 ±1 周。激素避孕可将下一个排卵期推迟到用药结束。

2. In eliciting an obstetric history:

E is correct. Past obstetric history is pivotal to managing the index pregnancy, e.g. past history of diabetes, hypertensive or psychiatric illness would help us to plan management better. Many women do not remember the last menstrual period (LMP) accurately, and when facilities permit, the gestation is assessed by ultrasound in the first trimester and estimated date of delivery (EDD) is calculated based on the early scan. The postovulatory period is fairly constant and is about 14 days whether the cycle is long or short. Ultrasound for dating can be + or -3 weeks if it is based on thirdtrimester scans, while it is + or -1 week if it is based on a first-trimester scan. Hormonal contraception may delay the first ovulatory cycle after discontinuation of the method.

3. 关于妊娠的症状

E 是正确的。恶心和呕吐可在经期推迟的 2 周内开始，这被认为是由于人绒毛膜促性腺激素（hCG）升高导致，至少是部分原因。严重且持续地呕吐导致产妇脱水、尿酮和电解质失衡，被称为妊娠剧吐，主要出现在早孕期。排尿频率增加是由于尿量增加，以及除了妊娠子宫对膀胱的压力外，血容量增加 40% 后肾小球滤过率增加所致。孕 12 周后子宫进入腹腔后，这种压力会减轻，此后尿频减轻。由于血管内容量增加和血浆蛋白减少，血浆渗透压随着妊娠的进行而降低。当女性坐直时，由于灌注增加，导致水负荷后利尿作用增加。

3. Regarding symptoms of pregnancy:

E is correct. Nausea and vomiting can start within 2 weeks of the missed period, and it is believed to be secondary to the rise, at least partly, of human chorionic gonadotrophin (hCG). Severe and persistent vomiting leading to maternal dehydration, ketonuria and electrolyte imbalance is termed hyperemesis gravidarum and is typical in the first trimester only. The frequency of micturition is due to the increased urine production, which is due to an increased glomerular filtration

rate following 40% expansion of the blood volume in addition to the pressure on the bladder by the gravid uterus. This pressure is relieved after 12 weeks when the uterus becomes an intra-abdominal organ-hence the frequency lessens. Plasma osmolality reduces with advancing gestation due to increased intravascular volume and reduced plasma proteins. There is increased diuresis after water loading when the woman is sitting in an upright position, perhaps due to increased perfusion.

4. 妊娠期间

C 是正确的。血压（BP）是在患者坐起或以 45° 斜躺时记录的，而不是在她仰卧时记录，因为静脉回流可能会减少，从而影响心输出量和血压读数。每次就诊时应使用合适尺寸的袖带在同一位置记录血压——肥胖女性需要更大的袖带。如果下腔静脉受压时间过长，很可能会影响母亲的心输出量和子宫胎盘循环，可能会危及胎儿。目前的建议是考虑柯氏第五音，如果无法确定声音消失的点，则使用柯氏第四音。血流杂音是由超动力循环引起的，除非有症状或其他令人担忧的相关临床特征，否则通常没有意义；在这种情况下，它们应与心脏病引起的杂音区分开来。

4. During pregnancy:

C is correct. Blood pressure (BP) is recorded when the patient is sitting up or lying at a 45-degree incline and not whilst she is lying on her back because the venous return may be reduced, affecting the cardiac output and the reading. BP should be recorded in the same position during each visit using an appropriate size cuff-obese women would need a larger cuff. If inferior venocaval compression is prolonged, it is likely to affect the cardiac output of the mother and hence the uterine circulation, which could compromise the baby. Current recommendation is to consider the Korotkoff's fifth sound, and if the point at which the sound disappears cannot be identified, then use the Korotkoff's fourth sound. The flow murmurs are due to the hyper-dynamic circulation and are generally of no significance unless associated with symptoms or other worrying clinical features, where they should be differentiated from any murmur due to cardiac pathology.

5. 孕期盆腔检查

B 是正确的。有了早孕期超声，就没有必要进行常规盆腔检查。当晚孕期出现无痛性出血时，应排除前置胎盘。前置胎盘时行阴道检查可能导致大出血，需要紧急剖宫产；因此，阴道检查是禁忌的。骨盆的放射检查在预测分娩结果方面价值不大，因为分娩是一个动态过程，随着婴儿头部俯曲、形态改变和骨盆"弹性"而变化。女性型骨盆在骨盆的所有水平上都是"宽敞的"，允许头部下降。骨盆入口的直径通常在横向直径上大于前后（AP）直径。

5. In pelvic examination during pregnancy:

B is correct. With the availability of first-trimester scanning, it is not essential to perform a routine pelvic examination. When there is painless bleeding in late pregnancy, placenta praevia should be excluded. Digital vaginal examination in cases of placenta praevia may cause torrential haemorrhage and require an emergency caesarean section; hence, it is contraindicated. Radiological examination of the pelvis is of little value in predicting labour outcome, as labour is a dynamic process with changes in dimensions occurring with flexion of the baby's head, moulding and pelvic 'give'. The gynaecoid pelvis is 'roomy' at all levels of the pelvis to allow cephalic descent. The diameter of the pelvic inlet is usually longer in the transverse diameter than the anteroposterior (AP) diameter.

第 7 章（Chapter 7）

1. 关于感染的产前筛查

B 是正确的。乙型肝炎病毒筛查是常规进行的。乙型肝炎很容易通过产道传播给胎儿和新生儿。如果母亲有乙肝抗原，需要进一步检测表面（s）抗原或核心（e）抗原是否呈阳性。核心抗原阳性者被认为病毒复制活跃，对胎儿有高达 85% 的传播率。在大多数国家，如果 e 抗原呈阳性，则给予丙种球蛋白和活性疫苗；如果 s 抗原阳性，则仅接种疫苗。如果感染传播，发生肝硬化及继发肝细胞癌的可能较高；因此，需要对新生儿进行积极的免疫接种。不需要常规筛查巨细胞病毒（CMV），因为重复感染并不少见，并且无法根据检测采取预防措施。应给出一般建议，若儿童出现咳嗽、感冒和流感，并可能导致易于传播的 CMV 感染，避免儿童去托儿所。梅毒并不常见，但如果被发现，则可以很好地治疗，以避免感染胎儿及其后遗症。

检查丈夫 / 伴侣和接触者追踪很重要。如果母亲早孕期感染风疹，25%～50% 的胎儿会有严重的先天性畸形。如果母亲没有被免疫，则应该在产后接种疫苗。HIV/AIDS 筛查并不普遍，但建议将其作为常规筛查。如果发现阳性，抗逆转录病毒治疗、选择性剖宫产和避免母乳喂养将垂直传播的发生率从 45% 降低到不到 2%。

1. Regarding antenatal screening for infection:

B is correct. Screening for hepatitis B is routinely carried out. Hepatitis B is easily transmitted to the fetus and then the newborn whilst it traverses the birth canal. If the mother has hepatitis B antigens, further testing is required to confirm if they are positive for surface (s) antigens or core (e) antigens. Those who are positive for core antigens are considered to have active viruses and may have a high transmission rate of up to 85% to the fetus. In most countries newborns are given gamma globulins and the active vaccine if e positive and only the vaccine if they are s positive. If the infection is transmitted, there is a high possibility of liver cirrhosis followed by hepatocellular cancer, hence the need to actively immunize the newborn. No routine screening is done for cytomegalovirus (CMV), as re-infection is not uncommon and no preventive action can be taken based on the test. General advice should be given to avoid child nurseries where children have coughs, colds and influenza and may harbour CMV infection that is easily transmitted. Syphilis is uncommon, but if detected it is eminently treatable to avoid infection of the fetus and its sequelae. Checking the husband/partner and contact tracing are important. Rubella infection causes major congenital malformations in 25–50% if the mother is infected in the first trimester of pregnancy. If the mother is not immune, she should be immunized postpartum. HIV/AIDS screening is not universal, but it is advisable to make it a routine screening. If found positive, antiretroviral therapy, elective caesarean delivery and avoidance of breast-feeding have reduced the incidence of vertical transmission from 45% to less than 2%.

2. B 组链球菌

C 是正确的。B 组链球菌是一种革兰阳性菌，是一种存在于鼻、口咽、鼻咽、肛管和阴道中的共生菌。泌尿生殖道 B 组链球菌的定植与较高的早产和胎膜破裂的发生率有关。并非在所有国家都例行筛查。在英国通常不进行筛查，但如果有高危病史，应采取适当的预防措施，特别是如果母亲在阴道或直肠拭子中有链球菌定植或尿培养中有 GBS 生长，则产时应采取青霉素治疗。

2. Group B streptococcus:

C is correct. Group B streptococcus is a gram-positive bacterium and is a commensal organism found in the nose, oropharynx, nasopharynx, anal canal and vagina. Group B streptococcal colonization of the genitourinary tract is associated with higher incidence of pre-term labour and pre-labour rupture of membranes. Screening is not routine in all countries. In the UK screening is not performed, but should there be a high-risk history, suitable precautions are taken, especially intrapartum penicillin therapy if the mother had streptococcal colonization in the vaginal or rectal swab or growth in urine culture.

3. 妊娠期糖尿病

E 是正确的。妊娠期糖尿病患者易孕育巨大儿，而那些在前一次妊娠胎儿出生体重较高的女性更容易患妊娠期糖尿病。巨大儿诊断（即＞4kg 或 4.5kg）的界值因研究人群而异。孕妇体重指数（BMI）＞35 与妊娠期糖尿病相关。有妊娠期糖尿病史的女性很可能患早发性 2 型糖尿病，在随后的妊娠中患妊娠期糖尿病的概率更高。年龄＞35 岁的高龄母亲较年轻母亲更容易患妊娠期糖尿病。

3. Gestational diabetes:

E is correct. Gestational diabetes predisposes to macrosomic babies, and those who had higher-birthweight babies in the previous pregnancy are more prone to gestational diabetes. The cut-off value of when to consider the baby to be macrosomic, i.e. >4 or 4.5 kg, varies with the population studied. Maternal body mass index (BMI) >35 has a known association with gestational diabetes mellitus in pregnancy. Gestational diabetes in previous pregnancy identifies those who are likely to develop early-onset type 2 diabetes in their life, and they also indicate a higher chance of getting gestational diabetes in subsequent pregnancies. Older mothers >35 years of age are more prone to gestational diabetes and not younger mothers.

4. 额外补充叶酸

E 是正确的。众所周知，叶酸可降低先天性畸形的总体发病率。叶酸促进细胞分裂，是任何生长或修复过程中的重要维生素。额外的叶酸补充剂（每天 5mg）可减少神经管缺陷，因此对于分娩过神经管缺陷孩子的母亲来说，在妊娠前和妊娠早期服用叶酸非常重要。患有癫痫病的母亲，尤其是服用抗癫痫药物的母亲，生出神经管缺陷孩子的概率更高，应该建议她们补充更高剂量的叶酸。这也适用于患有糖尿病的母亲和具有高体重指数（BMI）的母亲。唐氏综合征是一种染色体问题，通常是 21 三体，不能通过服用额外的叶酸来降低发病率。

4. Extra folic acid supplementation:

E is correct. Folic acid is well known to reduce the overall incidence of congenital malformations. Folic acid facilitates cell division and is an important vitamin in any growth or reparative process. Extra folic acid supplementation (5 mg per day) reduces neural tube defects, and hence it is important to take prior to and in early pregnancy in mothers who had a previous child with neural tube defects. Mothers who have epilepsy, especially those who are on antiepileptic medication, have a higher chance of having children with neural tube defects, and they should be advised on higher-dose folic acid supplementation. This also applies to mothers with diabetes and those with a high body mass index (BMI), e.g. >35. Down's syndrome is a chromosomal problem, commonly trisomy 21, and the incidence cannot be reduced by taking extra folic acid.

5. 关于孕期建议

D 是正确的。适度的运动如游泳，是无害的，值得鼓励。剧烈运动和活动量大的竞争性运动是禁忌的。在未进行手术清宫的情况下，在孕 12 周以下完全自然流产后，不常规使用抗 D 免疫球蛋白。关于最低限度饮酒量及其对胎儿的影响存在争议。适度饮酒可能对胎儿有害，而大量饮酒与胎儿酒精综合征有关，后者与小头畸形和智力低下有关。吸烟对妊娠有害，众所周知吸烟与宫内生长受限有关。扑热息痛妊娠期使用是安全的，但没有任何药物被证明绝对安全。在晚孕期大量服用非甾体抗炎药可能导致羊水过少和动脉导管早闭。

5. Regarding advice in pregnancy:

D is correct. Moderate exercise for recreation, including swimming, is harmless and is encouraged. Strenuous exercise and competitive sports with active movements are contraindicated. Anti-D Ig is not routinely administered after complete spontaneous miscarriage under 12 weeks' gestation in the absence of surgical evacuation. There is controversy about minimal alcohol consumption and its effects on the fetus. Moderate alcohol consumption may be harmful to the fetus, and severe alcohol consumption is associated with fetal alcohol syndrome, which is associated with microcephaly and mental retardation. Smoking is harmful to the pregnancy and is well known to be associated with intrauterine growth restriction. Paracetamol appears to be safe in pregnancy, though no drug is proven to be completely safe. Non-steroidal anti-inflammatory drugs taken in significant amounts in the third trimester may cause oligohydramnios and premature closure of the ductus arteriosus.

第 8 章（Chapter 8）

1. 36 周产前出血

C 是正确的。尽管胎盘早剥（正常位置的胎盘剥离）和前置胎盘（低置胎盘）是孕产妇和围产儿发病并发症发射率和死亡率的主要原因，但每种情况的发生率都低于 1%。特发性最常见。全身和腹部的临床检查、阴道窥器检查（排除宫颈或阴道病变，并观察血液是否通过宫颈口流出）和超声检查（检查胎盘位置、胎位、胎先露和羊水量）对于确定病因，排除"特发性"诊断至关重要。

1. Antepartum haemorrhage at 36 weeks:

C is correct. Although placental abruption (separation

of normally situated placenta) and placenta praevia (low-lying placenta) are major causes of maternal and perinatal morbidity and mortality, the incidence of each of these conditions is less than 1%. The commonest reason is idiopathic. Clinical examination, both general and abdominal, and a speculum examination (to exclude cervical or vaginal lesion and to visualize whether blood is emerging via the cervical os) and an ultrasound examination (to check the placental position and to visualize the fetal lie and presentation and liquor volume) are vital to identify the other causes and to come to the diagnosis by exclusion of 'idiopathic'.

2. 妊娠期高血压

D 是正确的。正常的生理变化是从妊娠早期开始血压（BP）下降，随后在妊娠晚期缓慢上升至孕前水平。现在更多地强调收缩压读数，尤其是＞160mmHg，因为脑出血的倾向更大，强烈建议立即治疗并使收缩压＜150mmHg，最好＜140mmHg。在没有蛋白尿的情况下，妊娠 20 周后的高血压诊断为妊娠期高血压，如果额外存在明显的蛋白尿，则诊断为子痫前期。有几个因素可能导致血压升高，但重要的因素是血管舒张激素（包括雌激素和孕激素）会导致外周阻力下降。子痫前期中，血小板和血管内皮细胞释放的血管收缩剂血栓素和血管扩张剂前列环素起主要作用。HELLP 综合征包括溶血、肝酶升高和血小板减少，它表示严重的子痫前期已经影响了几个系统。HELLP 的预后很差，建议谨慎管理和尽早分娩。

2. Hypertension in pregnancy:

D is correct. Normal physiological change is for a decrease in blood pressure (BP) from the first trimester onwards with a later gentle rise to pre-pregnancy levels in the third trimester. More emphasis is now paid to the systolic reading, especially >160 mmHg, as there is a greater tendency for cerebral haemorrhage, and there is a strong recommendation to immediately treat and bring the systolic BP <150 mmHg and preferably <140 mmHg. Hypertension after 20 weeks is gestational in the absence of proteinuria, and the diagnosis would be pre-eclampsia in theadditional presence of significant proteinuria. Several factors may contribute to a rise in BP, although it is known that there is a fall in peripheral resistance due to vasodilatory hormones, including oestrogen and progesterone. In pre-eclampsia the vasoconstrictor thromboxane and vasodilatory prostacyclin, mainly liberated by the platelets and endothelial cells of blood vessels, play a major role. HELLP syndrome stands for haemolysis, elevated liver enzymes and low platelets, and it signifies a serious form of the pre-eclamptic process which has affected several systems. It has a poor prognosis, and careful management and early delivery are advised.

3. 在双胞妊娠中，最恰当的说法

B 是正确的。在许多国家，同卵双胎的发生率似乎都相似。胎膜子宫附着处的双峰征或 lambda 征表示羊膜之间的额外绒毛膜层，用于诊断双胎性质。妊娠的所有并发症在双胎中发生率都增加，流产也不例外。双胎早产是单胎妊娠的 2 倍，胎儿平均分娩胎龄远小于单胎。双胎输血综合征最早可在 18 周出现，许多中心会在这个阶段进行超声检查并决定下一次超声的日期。通过激光横断吻合血管进行早期诊断和治疗，将获得更好的结局。

3. In twin pregnancy, what is the most appropriate statement?

B is correct. The prevalence of identical twins appears to be uniformly similar in many countries. Twin peak sign or lambda sign at the attachment of the membranes to the uterus signifies additional chorionic layers in between the amniotic membranes and the diagnosis of dizygotic twins. All complications of pregnancy are increased in twins, and miscarriage is not an exception. Pre-term delivery in twins is twice that of singleton pregnancy, and the average gestational age of delivery of the fetuses are much less than singletons. Twin-totwin transfusion can appear as early as 18 weeks, and many centres would scan at this stage and decide on the date of the next scan. Earlier diagnosis and treatment by laser transection of anastomotic vessels are associated with better outcome.

4. 以下哪个不是胎位不稳定的原因

D 是正确的。前置胎盘占据子宫下段并妨碍胎儿头部或臀位下降到骨盆中。羊水过多使得胎儿"漂浮"在其中，而不能通过子宫肌张力和正常羊水量将胎儿固定在纵产式。纵隔子宫限制了宫腔的空间，一些胎儿可能会出现横位或斜位。初产时常有正常子宫和腹部肌张力，应该有利于稳定的纵产式。在双胎妊娠中，第一个胎儿通常是纵产式，但第二个胎儿可能处于异常胎位，如果羊水过多，则发生率更高。

4. The causes of an unstable lie include all of the following except:

D is correct. Placenta praevia occupies the lower segment and prevents the head or breech from settling down in the pelvis. Polyhydramnios allows the fetus to 'float' around instead of binding the fetus to a longitudinal lie by the uterine muscular tone and normal amount of amniotic fluid volume. Subseptate uterus limits the space of the uterine cavity, and some fetuses may present with transverse or oblique lie. Primiparity is generally associated with good uterine and abdominal muscle tone and should favour a stable longitudinal lie. In twin pregnancy the first twin usually presents in the longitudinal lie, but the second twin can be in an abnormal lie, and the incidence is made greater if it is associated with polyhydramnios.

5. 关于过期妊娠，以下哪一项是正确的

C 是正确的。术语"过度成熟综合征"指的是婴儿的状况和具有特征性的特点。这是宫内营养不良的表现，因此如果存在胎盘功能障碍，则可能发生在妊娠的任何阶段。胎儿过熟综合征是通常与羊水过少、羊水粪染的发生率增加及胎儿宫内吸入粪染羊水的风险增加有关。2% 的孕 41 周妊娠和高达 5% 的孕 42 周妊娠发生胎儿过熟综合征。过期妊娠与围产儿发病率和死亡率增加有关。大多数公认的专业机构的指南建议根据随机对照研究的证据在 41 周零 3 天前进行引产，以降低并发症率和死亡率。

5. In prolonged pregnancy, which one of the following statements is correct?

C is correct. The term *postmaturity syndrome* refers to the condition of the infant and has characteristic features. These are all indicators of intrauterine malnutrition and may therefore occur at any stage of the pregnancy if there is placental dysfunction. Postmaturity is often associated with oligohydramnios, an increased incidence of meconium in the amniotic fluid and an increased risk of intrauterine aspiration of meconiumstained fluid into the fetal lungs. It is found in 2% of pregnancies at 41 weeks and up to 5% of pregnancies at 42 weeks. Prolonged pregnancy is associated with increased perinatal morbidity and mortality. The guidelines from most recognized professional bodies suggest induction by 41 weeks and 3 days to avoid morbidity and mortality based on the evidence from randomized controlled studies.

第 9 章（Chapter 9）

1. 孕期贫血

E 是正确的。妊娠会导致血浆体积和红细胞量增加。需要增加铁和叶酸的摄入，而母亲的饮食并不能满足。此外，胎儿对这两种营养素都有需求。对铁的需求增加大于对叶酸的需求。虽然镰状细胞贫血和地中海贫血可导致妊娠期贫血，但与缺铁相比，这两种情况要少得多。

1. Anaemia in pregnancy:

E is correct. Pregnancy causes an increase in both plasma volume and red cell mass. This requires an increase in iron and folate, which is not always met by maternal diet. In addition there are fetal requirements for both these nutrients. The increased requirement for iron isgreater than that for folate.

Whilst sickle cell disease and thalassaemia can cause anaemia in pregnancy, this is much less common than iron deficiency.

2. 妊娠期糖尿病的原因

E 是正确的。妊娠会诱发糖尿病状态。这主要是因为胎盘产生的抗胰岛素的激素（雌激素、人胎盘催乳素、胰高血糖素和皮质醇）对胰岛素的抵抗作用增加，妊娠期间母体糖皮质激素和甲状腺激素的产生增加也促进了这一点。作为回应，母体胰腺必须增加胰岛素的分泌来对抗这种情况。在一些女性中，这没有实现，结果患妊娠期糖尿病。孕酮是列出的唯一一种没有胰岛素抵抗作用的物质。

2. Causes of gestational diabetes:

E is correct. Pregnancy induces a diabetogenic state. This is predominantly because of increased resistance to the actions of insulin due to the placental production of the anti-insulin hormones (oestrogen, human placental lactogen, glucagon and cortisol), though the increased production of maternal glucocorticoids and thyroid hormones during pregnancy also contribute to this. In response, the maternal pancreas must increase its production of insulin to combat this. In some women this is not achieved, and gestational diabetes is the result. Progesterone is the only one listed that does not oppose insulin action.

3. 妊娠期急性静脉血栓栓塞

D 是正确的。静脉血栓栓塞是发达国家孕产妇死亡的主要原因。与未妊娠女性相比，妊娠期间发生这种情况的可能性要高 10 倍。由于左髂总静脉受压，深静脉血栓更常发生在左腿。D- 二聚体测量在妊娠期间的用途有限，因为假阳性结果很常见。肝素是一线治疗药物；妊娠期间使用华法林与胚胎病和胎儿出血问题有关。

3. Acute venous thromboembolism in pregnancy:

D is correct. Venous thromboembolism is a leading cause of maternal mortality in the developed world. It is 10 times more likely to occur in pregnancy compared to when a woman is not pregnant. Deep vein thrombosis occurs more frequently in the left leg due to compression of the left common iliac vein. d-Dimer measurements are of limited use in pregnancy, as falsepositive results are common. Heparin is the first-line treatment; warfarin use in pregnancy is associated with an embryopathy and with fetal bleeding problems.

4. 妊娠期寨卡病毒

E 是正确的。大多数感染寨卡病毒的人（80%）没有任何症状。孕妇并不比非孕妇更容易受到感染。大多数寨卡病毒病例是通过受感染的蚊虫叮咬获得

的。然而，也报道了一些性传播病例和通过输血传播的病例。不建议对无症状孕妇进行检测。在对截至 2016 年 5 月 30 日的文献进行系统综述后，世界卫生组织（WHO）得出结论，妊娠期间感染寨卡病毒是胎儿先天性大脑异常的原因之一。

4. Zika virus in pregnancy

E is correct. Most people (80%) infected with Zika virus have no symptoms. Pregnant women are no more susceptible to infection than non-pregnant women. The majority of cases of Zika virus are acquired from infected mosquito bites; however, a few cases of sexual transmission and some through blood transfusions have been reported. Testing of asymptomatic pregnant women is not recommended. Following a systematic review of the literature up to 30 May 2016, the World Health Organization (WHO) concluded that Zika virus infection during pregnancy is a cause of congenital brain abnormalities.

5. 癫痫和妊娠

C 是正确的。妊娠对癫痫的影响是有差异的。通常癫痫发作频率没有变化，但少数女性癫痫发作会增加。不同的抗癫痫药给胎儿带来不同的风险，丙戊酸钠的风险最大，育龄女性应避免使用。在患有癫痫的女性中，胎儿先天性异常的风险更高（3%，而一般人群为 1%～2%）；如果女性正在服用抗癫痫药物，这种风险会进一步增加（4%～9%）。主要异常是神经管缺陷和心脏异常。

由于神经管缺陷的风险增加，建议使用更高剂量（5mg）的叶酸。患有癫痫症女性的孩子有 4%～5% 的概率也会患上这种疾病；如果他们的父亲也受到影响，这一比例会增加到 20%。母乳喂养对大多数使用抗癫痫药物的女性来说是安全的。

5. Epilepsy and pregnancy:

C is correct. The effect of pregnancy on epilepsy is variable. Usually the seizure frequency is unchanged, but a minority of women will have increased seizures. Different anti-epileptics confer different risks to the fetus; however, sodium valproate has the greatest risks and should be avoided in women of reproductive age. In women with epilepsy there is a higher risk of congenital abnormalities (3% compared with 1–2% in the general population); this risk is increased further if a woman is taking anti-epileptic drugs (4–9%). The main abnormalities are neural tube defects and heart abnormalities.

As there is an increased risk of neural tube defects, a higher (5 mg) dose of folic acid is recommended. Children of women with epilepsy have a 4–5% chance of developing the condition themselves; this increases to up to 20% if their father is also affected. Breast-feeding is safe for women on most anti-epileptic medications.

第 10 章（Chapter 10）

1. 孕 20 周 B 超异常

A 正确。超声仅检测到 25% 的胎儿心脏异常。60%～90% 的中枢神经系统（CNS）畸形被发现。超过 90% 的骨骼畸形被发现。60%～90% 的特定胃肠道异常能被诊断出来。在大多数情况下，85% 的泌尿生殖系统异常能被发现。

1. Abnormalities detected by ultrasound at 20 weeks: A is correct. Only 25% of cardiac anomalies are detected. About 60–90% of the central nervous system (CNS) malformations are picked up. More than 90% of skeletal malformations are identified. Depending on the specific gastrointestinal anomaly, 60–90% are diagnosed. In most series about 85% of urogenital anomalies are detected.

2. 早孕期唐氏综合征筛查试验

D 正确。婴儿筛查阴性的可能性超过 99%（149/150）。因此筛查试验的阳性预测值低至 1/150。由于这种疾病的可能性很小，因此此类筛查试验的阴性预测值非常高。背景发生率为 1:1500，但测试已将概率设为 1:150（高 10 倍）。在妊娠的这个阶段，绒毛取样是该类女性的一种选择，但该手术有 0.5%～1% 的概率导致手术相关的流产。

2. First-trimester screening test for Down's syndrome: D is correct. There is an over 99% chance (149/150) that the baby does not have the diagnosis. As a result the positive predictive value of the screening test is low at 1/150. As the disease is very unlikely, the negative predictive value of this type of screening test is very high. The background incidence is 1:1500, but the test has placed the chance to be 1:150 (10 times higher). At this stage of pregnancy chorionic villus sampling is an option for this woman, but this procedure has a 0.5–1% chance of leading to a procedure-related miscarriage.

3. 孕期胎儿生长评估

C 是唯一不正确的答案。连续腹围测量提供了胎儿生长的最佳监测方法。如果胎儿（大或小）腹围和头围在同一百分位数，更有可能是原发性 / 遗传；如果它们是不同的（例如，小胎儿头部大于腹部，或者大胎儿头部小于腹部），则更可能存在病理性胎儿生长。连续的耻骨联合－宫底高度测量可检测到 20% 的小于或大于胎龄儿。胎儿异常与病理性生长有关，在 20 周的排畸超声中可能会遗漏这一点。因此，在宫内生长受限（IUGR）的情况下，排除胎儿异常很重要。在胎儿生长受限的情况下，脐动脉（UA）多普勒记录将显示其严重程度，并指导管理决策。

3. Assessment of fetal growth in pregnancy:

C is the only answer which is not correct. Progressive abdominal circumference measurement provides the best measure of fetal growth. If the abdominal and head circumferences are on the same centile in a fetus that is small or large, it is more likely that the extreme of size is constitutional/genetic; if they are divergent (e.g. with head larger than abdomen in a small fetus or head smaller than abdomen in a large fetus), then it is more likely that there is pathological fetal growth. Serial symphysial-fundal height measurements detect as few as 20% of small- or large-for-dates fetuses. Fetal abnormality is associated with growth pathology, and that can have been missed at the 20-week detailed scan; thus it is important to exclude fetal anomaly in cases of intrauterine growth restriction (IUGR). In cases where the fetus is growth restricted, the umbilical artery (UA) Doppler recording will indicate its severity and inform management decisions.

4. 可改善胎儿结局的高危妊娠试验

B 是正确的。唯一能改善胎儿结局的产前胎儿功能测试是脐动脉多普勒检查。

4. Tests in high-risk pregnancies which improve fetal outcome:

B is correct. The only antenatal fetal function test that has shown to improve fetal outcome is the umbilical artery Doppler measurements.

5. 最常见的染色体异常

B 是正确的。最常见的异常是与 21 三体或唐氏综合征相关的异常。在这种情况下，在至少 92% 的病例中，染色体异常是每个细胞具有 3 条而不是 2 条 21 号染色体（大约 8% 的病例是易位）。其次最常见的是性染色体异常 [Klinefelter 综合征，有一条额外的性染色体，为 2 条 X 染色体和 1 条 Y 染色体；Triple-X 综合征，有 1 条额外的性染色体，形式为 3 条 X 性染色体；Turner 综合征只有 1 条性染色体（一条 X 染色体）；然后是 13 三体和 18 三体（分别是 Patau 和 Edwards 综合征）]。

5. Most common chromosomal abnormalities:

B is correct. The commonest abnormality is that associated with trisomy 21 or Down's syndrome. In this condition, in at least 92% of cases the chromosomal abnormality is that each cell has three rather than two number 21 chromosomes (about 8% of cases are translocations). The next most common are abnormalities of the sex chromosomes (Klinefelter's syndrome with one extra sex chromosome in the form of two X chromosomes and one Y chromosome, Triple-X syndrome with an extra sex chromosome in the form of three X chromosomes and Turner's syndrome with only one sex chromosome [an X chromosome] followed by trisomies 13 and 18 [Patau and Edwards syndromes, respectively]).

第 11 章（Chapter 11）

1. 临产诊断

D 是正确的。带血的黏液栓的排出或胎膜破裂，可能与临产有关，但可以独立发生而不临产。一些母亲出现胎膜"突出"或破裂后，需要几天时间才能临产。行两次连续的阴道检查后若发现疼痛性宫缩与宫颈消失和宫口扩张或两者有关，可以诊断临产。宫缩疼痛可能会持续数小时而没有宫颈变化，而疼痛可能会在几天后重新开始。背痛和腹痛不是诊断临产的充分指标。

1. Diagnosis of labour:

D is correct. 'Show', which is the discharge of the bloodstained mucus plug or rupture of membranes, may be associated with the onset of labour but can take place independently without progressing to labour. Some mothers have 'show' or rupture of membranes and will take days before going into labour. The painful contractions should be associated with cervical effacement and dilatation or both on two consecutive vaginal examinations to diagnose labour. Painful contractions may persist for several hours without cervical changes, and the pain may subside only to restart in a few days' time. Backache and abdominal pain are not sufficient indicators to diagnose labour.

2. 第一产程进展缓慢

C 是正确的。4kg 甚至更重的胎儿与异常产程无关。不协调的子宫收缩只是对收缩模式的描述，即 2 个或 3 个宫缩一起出现，然后出现 1 个宫缩，然后以不同的间隔再次 2 个或 3 个宫缩。不协调的收缩并不意味着无效的收缩，因为进行性宫颈扩张可能伴随不协调的宫缩发生。胎头位置不正时进入骨盆的径线较大，并可能导致相对头盆不称并导致产程进展缓慢。女型骨盆是宽敞的，因此不应导致进展缓慢。与经产妇相比，初产妇的分娩速度较慢，但在大多数情况下不会过于缓慢。

2. Slow labour progress in first stages of labour:

C is correct. A fetal weight of 4 kg or even more may have no association with abnormal labour progress. Incoordinate uterine contractions are just the description of how the contraction patterns appear, i.e. two or three together and then one and again two or three together at varying intervals. Incoordinate contractions do not mean inefficient contractions, as progressive cervical dilatation can take place with incoordinate contractions. Malposition of the head presents a larger diameter to the pelvis and can cause relative disproportion and lead to slow progress of labour. A gynaecoid pelvis is roomy and so should not cause slow progress. The labour is slower in primigravid compared with multigravida but is not abnormally slow in most cases.

3. 临产

E 是正确的。临产涉及局部孕酮下降与雌激素和前列腺素作用的增加。调节这些变化的机制尚未查明，可能是胎盘产生的肽类激素促肾上腺皮质激素释放激素（CRH）导致的。整个妊娠期间的胎盘发育导致发生 CRH 基因转录的合体滋养层细胞的细胞核数量呈指数增长。这种成熟过程导致母体和胎儿血浆 CRH 水平呈指数增长。CRH 对胎盘有直接作用，可增加雌激素合成，减少孕激素合成。在胎儿中，CRH 直接刺激胎儿肾上腺的区产生脱氢表雄酮（DHEA），这是胎盘雌激素合成的前体。CRH 还通过细胞膜刺激前列腺素的合成。孕酮的下降以及雌激素和前列腺素的增加导致连接蛋白 43 的增加，从而促进子宫肌细胞之间的连接，并改变子宫肌细胞的电兴奋性，进而导致子宫整体宫缩。羊膜感染似乎是早产的重要病因。

胎头位置不正和头盆倾势不均会导致胎头进入骨盆时径线变大，可能会导致第二产程停滞。硬膜外镇痛消除了"弗格森反射"和由于宫颈和阴道上部扩张以及相关的子宫活动增加引起的催产素的反射释放，因此可能导致第二产程延长。产妇力竭可能是一个原因，应该通过防止早期鼓励母亲用力来避免这种情况。最好等到头部下降到会阴时再用力。胎儿窘迫不会导致第二产程延长；相反，延长的第二产程可能会导致胎儿窘迫。

3. Initiation of labour:

E is correct. The onset of labour involves local progesterone withdrawal and an increase in oestrogen and prostaglandin action. The mechanisms that regulate these changes are unresolved but are likely to involve placental production of the peptide hormone corticotrophin-releasing hormone (CRH). Placental development across gestation leads to an exponential increase in the number of syncytio-trophoblast nuclei in which transcription of the CRH gene occurs. This maturational process leads to an exponential increase in the levels of maternal and fetal plasma CRH. The

CRH has direct actions on the placenta to increase oestrogen synthesis and reduce progesterone synthesis. In the fetus the CRH directly stimulates the fetal zone of the adrenal gland to produce dehydroepiandrosterone (DHEA), the precursor of placental oestrogen synthesis. CRH also stimulates the synthesis of prostaglandins by the membranes. The fall in progesterone and increase in oestrogens and prostaglandins lead to increases in connexin 43 that promote connectivity of uterine myocytes and change uterine myocyte electrical excitability, which in turn leads to increases in generalized uterine contractions. Infection of the amniotic membranes seems to be an important pathological cause of pre-term labour.

Malposition and asynclitism of the fetal head present larger diameters to the pelvis and may cause delay in the second stage of labour. Epidural analgesia abolishes the 'Ferguson's reflex' and reflex release of oxytocin due to distension of the cervix and upper vagina and associated increased uterine activity and hence may cause a prolonged second stage. Maternal exhaustion can be a cause, and this should be avoided by preventing early encouragement for the mother to bear down-one should ideally wait until the head descends to the perineal phase. Fetal distress does not cause delay in the second stage; on the contrary, the delayed second stage may cause fetal distress.

4. 硬膜外镇痛的并发症

C 是正确的。并发症包括穿刺部位出血和意外的硬膜损伤，如果在没有意识到的情况下注射药物，可能会导致完全脊髓阻滞。极少数情况下，可能会发生神经损伤。它会因血管舒张引起低血压，而不是高血压。

4. Complications of epidural analgesia:

C is correct. Complications include blood-stained tap and accidental dural tap, and if the medication is injected without realizing, this may lead to total spinal blockade. Extremely rarely, nerve injury may take place. It causes hypotension due to vasodilatation and not hypertension.

5. 电子胎心监护

A 是正确的。胎心加速表明胎儿健康状况良好，不太可能出现酸中毒。没有加速可能是由于感染、胎儿睡眠、服用镇静药和镇痛药，以及罕见的颅内病变或既往损伤导致。变异减速提示脐带受压，晚期减速提示胎盘功能不全，需要关注并观察其他特征，如基线上升和基线变异性下降。胎心率变异消失可能表明胎儿已经缺氧或受到伤害。

5. Electronic fetal monitoring:

A is correct. Accelerations of the fetal heart rate indicate good fetal health, and the fetus is unlikely to be acidotic. Absence of accelerations may be due to infection, fetal sleep phase, administration of sedatives and analgesics and, rarely, intracranial pathology or previous injury. The presence of variable decelerations is suggestive of cord compression, and late decelerations are suggestive of placental insufficiency and are of concern and need to be observed for additional features of concern such as rising baseline rate and reduction in baseline variability. Absent fetal heart rate variability may suggest that the fetus is already hypoxic or has suffered injury.

6. 早产管理

C 是正确的。除了其他器官未成熟外，肺透明膜病和新生儿呼吸窘迫综合征是早产的主要问题。给予糖皮质激素（地塞米松或倍他米松 12mg，间隔 12h 或 24h）可降低透明膜疾病的严重程度。为了有时间使胎儿成熟，分娩必须在没有感染等禁忌证的情况下通过使用宫缩抑制药延长至少 48h。尚未证明宫缩抑制药（特布他林、阿托西班和 GTN）具有临床益处。仅在与胎膜早破相关的早产情况下，抗生素被证明是有价值的。

6. Management of pre-term labour:

C is correct. Hyaline membrane disease and respiratory distress syndrome are the major concerns with prematurity in addition to concern about other organ maturation. The severity of hyaline membrane disease is reduced by the administration of corticosteroids (dexamethasone or betamethasone 12 mg 12 or 24 hours apart). In order to have the time to bring about this maturity, the labour has to be delayed for at least 48 hours in the absence of contraindications such as infections, and this is achieved by the use of tocolytics. Tocolytic agents (terbutaline, atosiban and GTN) in themselves have not been proven to confer clinical benefit. Antibiotics are shown to be of value in cases of pre-term labour associated with pre-labour rupture of membranes only.

7. 可接受的引产指征

C 是正确的。与糖尿病、过期妊娠、子痫前期和宫内生长受限相关的高危妊娠的并发症率和死亡率增加。没有证据表明巨大儿的引产对母体、胎儿或新生儿有好处。

7. Accepted indication for induction of labour:

C is correct. There are increased morbidity and mortality in high-risk pregnancies associated with diabetes, prolonged pregnancy, pre-eclampsia and intrauterine growth restriction. There is no evidence to suggest that there is maternal, fetal or neonatal advantage by induction for macrosomia.

8. 引产并发症

E 是正确的。如果未正确核对孕周，早产是一种已知的引产并发症。在现代临床工作中，在早孕期用超声核对胎龄日益容易。脐带脱垂是一种可能性，相较于广泛使用前列腺素，人工破膜导致脐带脱垂更常见。然而，需要在破膜前排除脐带先露，并且在胎头较高时破膜应谨慎。使用催产素或前列腺素可能会过度刺激子宫并导致医源性胎儿窘迫。引产时子宫破裂是罕见的，但在有剖宫产史（CS）的女性和产次多的高龄患者中可能发生。引产通常比自然分娩的时间长，并且可能伴随更多的宫缩，自然会更痛苦。

8. Complications of induction of labour:

E is correct. Prematurity is a known complication of induction if the gestation is not checked correctly. In modern practice this is less of a problem with ultrasound estimation of gestational age in the first trimester. Cord prolapse is a possibility and is less due to wider use of prostaglandins instead of depending on artificial rupture of membranes. However, one needs to exclude cord presentation prior to rupture and should be cautious when rupture is carried out with a high head. The use of oxytocin or prostaglandin may hyperstimulate the uterus and cause iatrogenic fetal distress. Uterine rupture is rare with induction but is a possibility in women with previous caesarean section (CS) and in grand multiparous women. Induced labour is usually longer than spontaneous labour and may be associated with more contractions and naturally is likely to be more painful.

第 12 章（Chapter 12）

1. 正常分娩

B 是正确的。如果不存在不利的临床因素，在接受硬膜外镇痛的初产妇中，第二产程的正常可持续长达 3h。当胎头下降到或超过坐骨棘水平时，就认为已经发生了衔接。在第二产程的胎头下降阶段，母亲通常不会在头部到达盆底和会阴阶段之前体验到用力的感觉。产妇应向下用力结合呼吸让前进的头部处的阴道和会阴组织放松并延伸。作为正常分娩机制的一部分，当胎头"着冠"时，胎儿仰伸后分娩。

1. Normal delivery:

B is correct. Provided no adverse clinical factors are present, a normal duration of the second stage of labour is commonly regarded as lasting up to 3 hours in a nulliparous woman who has received epidural analgesia. Engagement is considered to have occurred when the fetal head has descended to or beyond the level of the ischial spines. During the descent phase of the second stage of labour, the mother does not normally experience the sensation of bearing down until the head has reached the pelvic floor and perineal phase. Maternal expulsive effort should combine short pushing spells with periods of panting to allow vaginal and perineal tissues to relax and stretch over the advancing head. As part of the mechanism of normal labour, the fetal head is delivered by extension when 'crowning' of the head occurs.

2. 会阴损伤及会阴切开术

D 是正确的。在进行会阴切开术时，推荐的术式是取中外侧切口，以减少延裂到肛门外括约肌的风险。会阴三度裂伤根据外括约肌损伤是否 < 50%（3a）、> 50%（3b）或完全裂伤（3c）分为三个等级。四度裂伤涉及肛门 / 直肠黏膜及肛门括约肌复合体。器械助产，尤其是产钳助产，以及胎头枕后（OP）位分娩可能会导致会阴过度扩张，导致会阴损伤。产科肛门括约肌损伤，特别是如果损伤未被识别和充分修复，可能导致长期排气和排便失禁。

2. Perineal injury and episiotomy:

D is correct. Where episiotomy is performed, the recommended technique is a mediolateral incision to reduce the risk of extension involving the external sphincter and anus. Third-degree injury to the perineum is classified into three subcategories according to whether the damage to the external sphincter is <50% (3a), >50% (3b) or complete (3c). A fourth-degree laceration involves the ano/rectal mucosa as well as the external and internal sphincter complex. Instrumental delivery, especially forceps delivery, and delivery of a deflexed fetal head in the occiput posterior (OP) position may result in over-distension of the perineum, resulting in perineal injury. Obstetric anal sphincter injuries may lead to long-term incontinence of flatus and faeces, especially if the injury was not recognized and adequately repaired.

3. 剖宫产

E 是正确的。尽管在大多数发达国家剖宫产的发生率为 25%～30% 或更高，但器械助产率几年来一直保持在 10% 左右。有过一次无并发症的子宫下段剖宫产的女性且此次妊娠无剖宫产指征者，可以尝试阴道分娩，前提是不存在其他不利的临床因素。先前进行过传统剖宫产手术患者的瘢痕裂开或破裂的风险要大得多，并且可能发生在临产前。如果操作者接受过足够的培训，大多数枕后位和横位的胎头都可以通过产钳或胎吸安全地进行分娩。尽管一些面先露的婴儿可能会经阴道分娩，但由于与这种异常胎位相关的风险，大多数产科医生会进行剖宫产。

3. Caesarean section:

E is correct. Despite incidences of 25–30% or greater for caesarean deliveries in most developed countries, the instrumental vaginal delivery rates have remained around 10% for several years. Women who have had one uncomplicated previous lower segment caesarean section for a non-recurrent indication may attempt a vaginal delivery in a subsequent labour, provided no other adverse clinical factors are present. The risk of scar dehiscence or rupture is much greater with a previous classical caesarean section and may occur before the onset of labour. Provided the operator has been adequately trained, most occipitoposterior and transverse positions of the fetal head can be managed safely by forceps or vacuum delivery. Although some babies with a mentoanterior face presentation may deliver vaginally, most obstetricians will perform a caesarean delivery because of the risks associated with this malpresentation.

4. 手术阴道分娩

D 是正确的。McRobert 的手法在大多数肩难产病例中是成功的。只有少数巨大儿出现肩难产，大多数发生在体重小于 4000g 婴儿的分娩中。在几乎所有比较产钳助产和胎吸助产的报道中，使用产钳成功分娩的婴儿比使用胎吸多。与胎吸助产相比，产钳分娩引起的会阴裂伤严重得多。胎吸的先决条件与产钳相同，即宫颈应充分扩张，胎头位置和先露已知。

4. Operative vaginal delivery:

D is correct. McRobert's manoeuvre is successful in the majority of cases of shoulder dystocia. Only a minority of macrosomic infants will experience shoulder dystocia, and the majority of cases will occur in normal labours with infants weighing less than 4000 g. In almost all reports comparing forceps and vacuum delivery, more infants are successfully delivered with forceps than the vacuum extractor. Significantly more severe perineal lacerations are associated with forceps delivery than vacuum extraction. The prerequisites for vacuum delivery are the same as for the forceps, namely, there should be full dilatation of the cervix and a known position and attitude of the fetal head.

5. 产后出血

A 是正确的。许多重要的产科因素导致子宫收缩乏力，使其成为产后出血（PPH）的最常见原因。尽管如此，正常分娩后也可能会出现子宫收缩乏力。毫无疑问，第三产程的积极管理可减少产后出血，应作为推荐。PPH 后 3h 内给予氨甲环酸可使 PPH 的死亡率降低 30%。如果已排出胎盘且静脉注射催产素，但出血仍在继续，且母亲没有高血压或心脏病，则应静脉注射麦角新碱。最近，宫腔球囊填塞已成为一种相对简单的方法，通常是治疗持续性 PPH 的有效方法。

5. Postpartum haemorrhage:

A is correct. A number of important obstetric factors predispose to atonic uterus, making it the most common cause of postpartum haemorrhage (PPH). Nevertheless, uterine hypotonia may occur following normal delivery. There is little doubt that active management of the third stage of labour reduces postpartum bleeding and should be recommended as preferred management of the third stage. Administration of tranexamic acid within 3 hours of PPH will reduce mortality from PPH by 30%. If the placenta has been expelled and the haemorrhage continues despite the administration of intravenous oxytocin, ergometrine should be administered intravenously, provided the mother does not have hypertension or a cardiac condition. Recently, uterine tamponade with balloon catheters has become a relatively simple method and is usually effective management for persisting PPH.

第 13 章（Chapter 13）

1. 产褥期生理变化

B 是正确的。随着胎儿和胎盘的娩出，产生激素的胎儿胎盘单位与母亲分离。这会导致这些激素减少并在 6 周内逐渐降低到非妊娠水平。在第三产程和产后短时间内凝血因子增加作为防止过度出血的防御机制，这可能会导致一些高危女性血栓栓塞。催乳素随着泌乳而增加。血小板计数稳定或尽在血小板消耗量增加时略有增加，除非消耗量增加。患者心输出量保持稳定，但随着尿液排出和血容量逐渐恢复正常而下降。

1. Physiological changes in the puerperium:

B is correct. With the delivery of the fetus and placenta, the hormone-producing fetoplacental unit is detached from the mother. This causes a reduction of these hormones that gradually reduce to non-pregnant levels by 6 weeks. There is an increase in clotting factors in the third stage of labour and immediate puerperium as a defence mechanism to prevent excessive bleeding, which in some women at risk may cause thromboembolism. Prolactin increases with lactation. Platelet counts are stable or increase slightly unless there is increased consumption. Cardiac output remains stable but gradually comes down with diuresis and return of the blood volume to normal.

2. 肛门括约肌损伤的危险因素

C 是正确的。正枕后位胎头径线最大，枕前位胎头的径线最小不容易出现三度裂伤。第二产程的正常持续时间是否会增加肛门括约肌损伤的发生率是未知的。

麻醉的使用与肛门括约肌损伤的轻微增加有关，可能是由于麻醉后器械助产率较高。体重超过 4.5kg 或不低于 4.0kg 的婴儿与会阴三度裂伤有关。多产不是肛门括约肌损伤的独立危险因素。

2. Risk factors for anal sphincter injury:

C is correct. Occipitoanterior position presents the smallest diameter and has less association with thirddegree tears compared with a direct occipitoposterior delivery when a larger diameter is presented. Normal duration of the second stage of labour is not known to increase the incidence of anal sphincter injury.

Use of an epidural is associated with a slight increase in anal sphincter injury, probably due to its higher rate of instrumental delivery. Babies that weigh more than 4.5 kg and not less than 4.0 kg are linked to third-degree tears. Multiparous pregnancies are not an independent risk factor for anal sphincter injury.

3. 英国最常见的孕产妇死亡总原因（2006—2008 年）

D 是正确的。根据《母亲和婴儿：通过全英国审计和秘密调查降低风险》（MBRRACE-UK）2016 年的报告，脓毒症是孕产妇发病和死亡的主要原因。尽管 2009—2014 年英国产妇脓毒症的直接死亡率从 0.67/10 万降至 0.29/10 万，它仍然是英国和伦敦孕妇总死亡（直接和间接因素）的第二大常见原因，它是 2016 年孕产妇直接死亡的主要原因。

3. The UK's most common overall cause of maternal death (2006–2008):

D is correct. Sepsis is a leading cause of maternal morbidity and mortality according to the *Mothers and Babies: Reducing Risk through Audits and Confidential Enquiries across the UK* (MBRRACE-UK) report in 2016. Despite the UK direct death rate from sepsis falling from 0.67 to 0.29 per 100,000 maternities between 2009 and 2014, it remains the second commonest cause of total (combined direct and indirect) deaths in the UK and in London. It was the leading cause of direct maternal deaths in 2016.

4. 关于产后抗凝

D 是正确的。肝素和华法林并非母乳喂养的禁忌证。由于"华法林胚胎病"而在产前阶段不鼓励使用华法林。由于华法林给药方便且效果更好，那些服用肝素的患者在 2～3 天后转换为华法林。对于因肺栓塞（PE）或近端血栓形成而发生血栓栓塞的患者，通常建议接受 3 个月的治疗，以使凝块完全消退，凝血功能障碍状态完全减轻。产后随访最好由血液科医生进行，其可以根据检测结果控制药物剂量，也可以对长期随访提出建议。

4. Regarding postnatal anticoagulation:

D is correct. Heparin and warfarin are not contraindicated with breast-feeding. Use of warfarin is discouraged in the antenatal period due to fear of 'warfarin embryopathy'. Those who were on heparin are converted to warfarin after an interval of 2–3 days due to ease of administration and better effectiveness. Generally 3 months of treatment is advised for those who had thromboembolism for pulmonary embolism (PE) or proximal thrombosis to allow for full resolution of the clots and for the coagulopathy status to have completely abated. Postnatal follow-up is best done by the haematologist, who will be able to control the dosage based on the test results and will also be able to give advice on the long-term follow-up.

5. 新生儿检查

A 是正确的。新生儿的检查是为了排除全身、心血管、呼吸、腹部和肌肉骨骼系统的任何异常体征后向父母告知新生儿正常。最佳的检查时间是在分娩后 24h 内，必须在母婴出院之前。黄疸并不是所有婴儿的正常特征，尤其是在最初的 24h 内——需要观察，并应排除感染和其他原因。新生儿的脐疝可能很小，大多会在 1～2 年后消退。需要儿科医生随访，无须立即转诊。如果有较大的缺陷，要手术修复。尖锐的哭声是不正常的——应该检查可能存在的脓毒症和脑膜刺激征，如果婴儿出现呕吐、发烧或痉挛的症状，可能需要额外的检查。

5. Examination of the newborn:

A is correct. Examination of the newborn is to assure normality to the parents by excluding any abnormal signs on general, cardiovascular, respiratory, abdominal and musculoskeletal systems. The best time is within 24 hours of delivery and certainly before the mother and baby are discharged from the hospital. Jaundice is not a normal feature of all babies, particularly in the first 24 hours-it needs to be observed, and infection and other causes should be ruled out. Umbilical hernia in a newborn may be small and should regress by the end of 1–2 years. Follow-up by the paediatrician is needed, and there is no need for immediate referral or surgical repair unless there is a large defect. Highpitched cry is not normal-possible sepsis and meningeal irritation should be checked for, and additional tests may be needed if the baby develops symptoms of vomiting, fever or fits.

第 14 章（Chapter 14）

1. 分娩时的精神障碍

E 是正确的。精神疾病在妊娠期间很常见，因为妊娠往往会引发这种情况，可能至少有 1/10 的妊娠受到一定程度的影响。如果母亲正在服用精神药物，则应分析其风险和益处；停药可能会导致精神疾病复发，但是某些药物的致畸性更高。精神疾病是孕产妇间接死亡的第三大常见原因。严重的情绪障碍（情感障碍）与自杀风险增加有关。

1. Psychiatric disorders of childbirth:

E is correct. Psychiatric disorders are common in pregnancy, as pregnancy often precipitates the condition-probably at least 1:10 pregnancies are affected in some way. If the mother is on psychiatric medication, the risks and benefits should be analyzed; stopping the drug may cause relapse of the psychiatric condition, and certain drugs can be more teratogenic. Psychiatric disorder is the third commonest single cause of indirect maternal deaths. Elevated severe mood disorders (affective) are linked to increased risk of suicide.

2. 孕期抑郁症

D 是正确的。停药后，50% 的母亲可能会复发抑郁症。焦虑是抑郁症的一个显著特征。与药物相比，咨询和认知行为疗法对与焦虑相关的轻度至中度抑郁症效果良好。选择性 5- 羟色胺再摄取抑制剂（SSRI）是最常见的抗抑郁药，在妊娠期间使用并继续使用的药物。大多数女性在妊娠期间需要继续抗抑郁治疗。

2. Depressive illness in pregnancy:

D is correct. Depressive illness is likely to recur in 50% of mothers when medication is stopped. Anxiety is a prominent feature in depression. Counselling and cognitive behavioural therapy work well for mild to moderate depression associated with anxiety compared with medication. Selective serotonin reuptake inhibitors (SSRIs) are the commonest antidepressant drug that is used and is continued in pregnancy. Most women will need to continue antidepressant therapy during pregnancy.

3. 产后精神病

E 是正确的。该病有以下特点：

- 在分娩后的最初几天突然发病，每天都在恶化。一半产妇会在产后第一周出现，大部分会在 2 周内出现，几乎全部会在分娩后 3 个月内出现。

- 精神病、妄想、恐惧和茫然、困惑和激动，有时还会出现幻觉。

- 大约 50% 曾患有双相情感障碍或产后精神病的女性会出现躁动和严重的情绪紊乱。

3. Postpartum psychosis in pregnancy:

E is correct. The illness is characterized by the following:

- Sudden onset in the early days following delivery, deteriorating on a daily basis.
- Half will present within the first postpartum week, the majority within 2 weeks and almost all within 3 months of delivery.
- Psychosis, delusions, fear and perplexity, confusion and agitation and sometimes hallucinations.
- Agitation and severe disturbance.

Approximately 50% of women with a previous bipolar illness or postpartum psychosis will become ill.

4. 选择性血清素再摄取抑制剂（SSRI）

A 是正确的。SSRI 与先天性畸形有关，尤其是室间隔缺损。流产和宫内生长受限的发生率增加。体温过低、低血糖和肺动脉高压的发生率也有所增加。

4. Selective serotonin reuptake inhibitors (SSRIs):

A is correct. SSRIs are associated with congenital malformation, especially ventricular septal defects. There is increased pregnancy loss and intrauterine growth restriction. There is also an increased incidence of hypothermia, hypoglycaemia and pulmonary hypertension.

5. 孕期及产褥期饮食失调

C 是正确的。已经发现厌食症和低出生体重或早产有关，但这些发现并未在所有研究中重现。母亲和她未出生的孩子之间的关系经常受到影响。对妊娠有矛盾或后悔情绪的母亲更有可能难以与宝宝建立温暖的关系。产后进食障碍很可能会进一步升级。患有活动性进食障碍的母亲可能会隐瞒病情的严重程度。

5. Eating disorders in pregnancy and the puerperium:

C is correct. Some association with anorexia and low birth weight or prematurity have been found, but these findings haven't been reproduced in all studies. The relationship between mother and her unborn is often affected. Mothers who have ambivalent or regretful emotions about being pregnant are more likely to have difficulty establishing a warm relationship with their baby. It is highly likely that postnatally the eating disorder behaviours will escalate further. It is probable that mothers with active eating disorders may be concealing the

extent of their illness.

第 15 章（Chapter 15）

1. 阴道检查期间的陪护

D 是正确的。即使医生是女性，也应始终有陪护人员在场。如果患者不想要陪护，您应该记录提议被提出并被拒绝。如果有陪护人在场，您应该记录该事实并记下陪护人的身份。如果出于正当的实际原因您不能提供陪护人，您应该向患者解释，并在可能的情况下推迟检查时间。

1. Chaperone during vaginal examination:

D is correct. A chaperone should always be present, even if the doctor is female. If the patient does not want a chaperone, you should record that the offer was made and declined. If a chaperone is present, you should record that fact and make a note of the chaperone's identity. If for justifiable practical reasons you cannot offer a chaperone, you should explain to the patient and, if possible, offer to delay the examination to a later date.

2. 盆腔检查

D 是正确的。如果患者在检查期间表示他们已不再同意检查，您必须立即停止检查。尽管可以讨论再尝试一次检查，如使用另一种工具，应该明确患者已同意；考虑到患者所处的情景，患者是否真正自由地表示同意可能存在问题。一个更好的选择是在那个时候放弃检查。替代方案可能包括安排另一次会面进行检查和（或）讨论替代方法。

2. Pelvic examination:

D is correct. If a patient indicates during an examination that they have withdrawn their consent you must cease the examination immediately. Although it may be possible to discuss a further attempt at examination, for example, with another instrument, it should be clear that the patient has consented to this and, given the position the patient is in, there could be some question over whether the patient is truly giving consent freely. A better alternative would be to abandon the examination at that time. Alternatives might include scheduling the examination for another appointment and/or discussing alternative methods.

3. 巴氏涂片

B 是正确的。外观是典型的宫颈外翻，即宫颈阴道部被覆柱状上皮，这是正常的，尤其是在服用避孕药的生育年龄的女性中。除非有接触史，否则没有指征对这个年龄的无症状女性进行性传播感染（STI）检测。尽管可以用冷冻疗法治疗外翻，但如果患者无症状，则没有治疗的指征。她应该在正常的筛查间隔（例如，在她这个年龄在英国每 3 年一次）来进行下一次涂片检查。

3. Pap smear:

B is correct. The appearance is typical of a cervical ectropion, which is the presence of columnar epithelium on the ectocervix, and is normal, especially in reproductive women on the contraceptive pill. There is no indication to offer sexually transmitted infection (STI) testing in a woman of this age who is asymptomatic unless there is a history of contact. Although ectropions can be treated with cryotherapy, this is not indicated if the patient is asymptomatic. She should come for her next smear at the normal screening interval (e.g. every 3 years at her age in the UK).

4. 双合诊

C 是正确的。10% 的女性中发现后位子宫，是正常解剖变异。它可能与道格拉斯窝中的病变有关，但如果子宫是可移动的，则这种可能性较小。道格拉斯窝内结节是典型的子宫内膜异位症。虽然在一个瘦弱的女性中，可以在附件区域触及卵巢，但它的大小通常应该小于 5cm（包括生理性囊肿）。宫颈摇摆疼痛（宫颈刺激）与血液或炎症引起的腹膜刺激有关。

4. Bimanual pelvic examination:

C is correct. Uterine retroversion is a normal anatomical variant found in 10% of women. It may be associated with pathology in the pouch of Douglas, but this is less likely if the uterus is mobile. Nodularity in the pouch of Douglas is typical of endometriosis. Although in a thin woman the ovary may be palpable in the adnexal region, this should normally be less than 5 cm in size (to include physiological cysts). Pain on cervical movement (cervical excitation) is associated with peritoneal irritations from blood or inflammation.

5. Sims 窥器

C 是正确的。大多数医生使用双瓣（如 Cuscoe）窥器进行子宫颈检查，插入宫内节育器和采集拭子。盆底肌张力通常用指检评估。只有使用沿着阴道后壁插入的 Sims 窥器才能看到阴道前壁的运动。双瓣窥器可以掩盖这一点，因为它妨碍了前壁和后壁的可视化。

5. Sims' speculum:

C is correct. Examination of the cervix, insertion of an intrauterine device and taking swabs are performed by most doctors using a bivalve (e.g. Cuscoe's) speculum. Pelvic floor tone is normally assessed by digital examination. Movement of the anterior vaginal wall can only be seen using the Sims' speculum inserted along the posterior vaginal wall. A bivalve speculum can mask this, as it gets in the way of visualizing the anterior and posterior walls.

第 16 章（Chapter 16）

1. 子宫后壁 7cm 孤立性平滑肌瘤的治疗

A 是正确的。大多数肌瘤是无症状的，不需要治疗。对于有症状的女性，选择的治疗可取决于患者对未来生育的愿望、子宫保留的重要性、症状严重程度和肿瘤特征等因素。虽然所有的治疗都有效，但没有一个会在没有症状的情况下被建议。恶变风险很小（约 1/1000），除非肌瘤开始迅速扩大或引起疼痛，否则无治疗指征。在正常情况下，肌瘤会在绝经后缩小。生育能力在这时不太可能成为问题，因此不建议进行子宫动脉栓塞术（UAE）。促性腺激素释放激素（GnRh）治疗因对骨密度的影响而应用减少。

1. Treatment of 7-cm solitary leiomyoma in the posterior uterine wall:

A is correct. Most fibroids are asymptomatic and do not require treatment. In symptomatic women the choice of approach may be dictated by factors such as the patient's desire for future fertility, the importance of uterine preservation, symptom severity and tumour characteristics. Although all the treatments are effective, none would be indicated in the absence of symptoms. There is a small risk of malignant change (approximately 1:1000), but this would not normally be considered an indication for treatment unless the fibroid began to enlarge rapidly or cause pain. In the normal course of events the fibroid will regress after menopause. Fertility is highly unlikely to be an issue here, so uterine artery embolization (UAE) would not be indicated. Gonadotropin-releasing hormone (GnRh) treatment would be limited by its effect on bone density.

2. 月经过多的处理

C 是正确的。当有规律的大量出血而没有潜在的结构性病变时，大量月经出血（HMB）通常是原发性子宫内膜疾病的结果，其调节局部子宫内膜 "止血" 机制受到干扰。释放左炔诺孕酮的宫内节育系统被广泛推荐为无使用禁忌证且不希望妊娠的女性 HMB 药物治疗的首选。

2. Treatment of regular heavy periods:

C is correct. When there is regular heavy bleeding with no underlying structural lesion, heavy menstrual bleeding (HMB) is usually the result of a primary endometrial disorder where the mechanisms regulating local endometrial 'haemostasis' are disturbed. The levonorgestrel-releasing intrauterine system is widely recommended as the first choice for medical therapy of HMB in those women who do not have contraindications to its use and do not desire pregnancy.

3. 月经稀发和妊娠试验阴性

D 是正确的。多囊卵巢综合征（PCOS）的诊断标准是以下三项满足任意两项足以确认诊断：

- 少排卵或无排卵。
- 雄激素过多症（化验结果或临床）。
- 超声检查中的多囊卵巢。

在 15% 的 PCOS 患者中催乳素水平升高（通常轻微）。

3. Oligo-amenorrhoea and a negative pregnancy test:

D is correct. The diagnostic criteria for polycystic ovarian syndrome (PCOS) are any two of the following; three are sufficient to confirm the diagnosis:

- Oligo-ovulation or anovulation
- Hyperandrogenism (biochemical or clinical)
- Polycystic ovaries on ultrasound examination

Prolactin levels are increased (usually mildly) in 15% of cases of PCOS also.

4. 性早熟

A 是正确的。在女孩中，性早熟被定义为在 8 岁之前出现青春期的体征，通常从乳房早熟进展到月经初潮，因为乳房组织对雌激素的反应比子宫内膜更快。只要维持正常的发育顺序（乳房发育、肾上腺素能初现、生长突增和初潮的顺序），大多数病例就没有病理问题。在 4 岁以上的女孩中，不太可能找到特定原因，大多数是特发性的（80%）。

4. Precocious puberty:

A is correct. In girls precocious puberty is defined as the development of the physical signs of puberty before the age of 8 years. It usually progresses from premature thelarche to menarche because breast tissue responds faster to oestrogen than the endometrium. The majority of cases do not have a pathological basis as long as normal consonance (sequence of thelarche, adrenarche, growth spurt and menarche) is maintained. In girls older than 4 years old specific causes are less likely to be found, with the majority being idiopathic (80%).

5. 激素替代疗法（HRT）

E 是正确的。由于她接受了子宫切除术，因此她只需要雌激素治疗，显然不会发展为子宫内膜癌。尽管对老年女性进行联合 HRT 的研究显示心血管疾病增加，但在年轻女性或仅使用雌激素治疗的女性中并未发现这种情况。HRT 与结肠癌和骨质疏松症的风险降低有关。仅雌激素治疗与乳腺癌（长期）、静脉血栓形成和胆石症的增加有关。

5. Hormone replacement therapy (HRT):

E is correct. As she has had a hysterectomy, she would require oestrogen-only treatment and obviously cannot develop endometrial cancer. Although studies in older women on combined HRT showed an increase in cardiovascular disease, this was not seen in younger women or with oestrogen-only treatment. HRT is associated with a reduced risk of carcinoma of the colon and osteoporosis. Oestrogen-only treatment is associated with an increase in breast cancer (long term), venous thrombosis and cholelithiasis.

第 17 章（Chapter17）

1. 卵巢早衰

A 是正确的。这些是排卵障碍的特征性临床和激素表现：由于卵巢功能衰竭，高促性腺激素性性腺功能减退；由垂体的脉冲式促性腺激素分泌失败引起的性腺功能减退症；正常促性腺激素无排卵，最常由多囊卵巢综合征引起；外源性雌二醇抑制促卵泡激素（FSH）和促黄体生成素（LH）。

1. Premature ovarian failure:

A is correct. These are the characteristic clinical and hormone profiles of disorders of ovulation: hypergonadotropic hypogonadism, due to ovarian failure; hypogonadal hypogonadism resulting from failure of pulsatile gonadotropin secretion from the pituitary; normogonadotropic anovulation, most commonly caused by polycystic ovary syndrome; and suppression of follicle-stimulating hormone (FSH) and luteinizing hormone (LH) by exogenous oestradiol in the pill.

2. 少精症的原因

B 是正确的。精子发生和精子功能可能会受到多种毒素和治疗剂的影响。各种毒素和药物可作用于生精小管和附睾，抑制精子发生。化学治疗剂，特别是烷化剂会抑制精子功能；常用于治疗克罗恩病的柳氮磺吡啶，可降低精子活力和密度；而用于健美的合成代谢类固醇可能会产生严重的精子生成不足。美沙拉秦与异常精子参数无关。

2. Causes of oligospermia:

B is correct. Spermatogenesis and sperm function may be affected by a wide range of toxins and therapeutic agents. Various toxins and drugs may act on the seminiferous tubules and the epididymis to inhibit spermatogenesis. Chemotherapeutic agents, particularly alkylating agents, depress sperm function; and sulfasalazine which is frequently used to treat Crohn's disease, reduces sperm motility and density; and anabolic steroids used for bodybuilding may produce profound hypospermatogenesis. Mesalazine is not associated with abnormal sperm parameters.

3. 体外受精

E 是正确的。在 40 岁时接受一个周期的治疗后，活产的概率约为 12%。胚胎在受精后 5 天达到囊胚阶段。体外受精（IVF）涉及使用重组或尿源性促性腺激素刺激多个卵泡发育，同时使用促性腺激素释放激素（GnRH）激动药或拮抗药，以防止在获得卵母细胞之前过早的黄体生成素（LH）激增导致排卵。

3. In vitro fertilization:

E is correct. The chance of a live birth after a single cycle of treatment at age 40 is approximately 12%. Embryos reach the blastocyst stage 5 days after fertilization. In vitro fertilization (IVF) involves stimulation of multiple ovarian follicle development using recombinant or urinary-derived gonadotropins, with concurrent use of a gonadotropin-releasing hormone (GnRH) agonist or antagonist to prevent a premature luteinizing hormone (LH) surge and ovulation before oocytes are harvested.

4. 体外受精（IVF）卵巢过度刺激综合征（OHSS）

A 是正确的。OHSS 导致明显的卵巢增大，液体从血管内腔转移到第三间隙，导致腹水、胸腔积液、钠潴留和少尿。患者可能出现低血容量和低血压，并可能出现肾功能衰竭、血栓栓塞和成人呼吸窘迫综合征。这种情况的病理生理学似乎与毛细血管通透性增加有关。

4. In vitro fertilization (IVF) ovarian hyperstimulation syndrome (OHSS):

A is correct. OHSS results in marked ovarian enlargement with fluid shift from the intravascular compartment into the third space, leading to ascites, pleural effusion, sodium retention and oliguria. Patients may become hypovolaemic and hypotensive and may develop renal failure as well as thromboembolic phenomena and adult respiratory distress syndrome. The pathophysiology of this condition appears to be associated with an increase in capillary vascular permeability.

5. 胚胎植入前基因筛查（PGS）

B 是正确的。PGS 的目的是筛查胚胎中的非整倍体，尽管父母双方都没有发现基因异常。PGS 已被用于反复流产、高龄产妇、反复 IVF 不成功或严重的男性因素不孕。目的是使用 PGS 选择最佳胚胎进行移植。一直提倡在所有 IVF 病例中使用 PGS 进行非整倍体筛查，但不加区别地使用时是否有助于改善成功率仍有待证明。

5. Pre-implantation genetic screening (PGS):

B is correct. The purpose of PGS is to screen for aneuploidy in embryos, although both parents have no identified genetic abnormality. PGS has been used in cases of recurrent pregnancy loss, advanced maternal age, repeated unsuccessful in vitro fertilization (IVF) cycles or severe male factor infertility. The aim is to use PGS to select the best embryo for transfer. The use of PGS for aneuploidy screening in all cases of IVF has been advocated, but the contribution to improve success rates when used indiscriminately remains to be proven.

第 18 章（Chapter 18）

1. 流产

E 是正确的。50% 的自然流产与染色体异常有关，尤其是在高龄时。这是她第一次妊娠，因此造成反复流产的原因不太适用。宫颈功能不全通常在妊娠后期表现为无痛性宫颈扩张。

1. Miscarriage:

E is correct. Fifty per cent of spontaneous miscarriages are associated with chromosome abnormality, particularly at her advanced maternal age. This was her first pregnancy, so the causes of recurrent miscarriage are less likely to apply. Cervical incompetence normally presents with painless cervical dilation later in pregnancy.

2. 染色体异常

B 是正确的。染色体异常是早期流产的常见原因。在任何形式的流产中，高达 57% 的妊娠物有异常核型。最常见的染色体缺陷是常染色体三体，占异常的一半，而多倍体和 X 单体分别占 20%。虽然染色体异常在散发性流产中很常见，但只有 2%～5% 的反复流产发现父方染色体异常，最常见的是平衡易位或罗伯逊（Robertsonian）易位或嵌合体。

2. Chromosomal abnormalities:

B is correct. Chromosomal abnormalities are a common

cause of early miscarriage. In any form of miscarriage up to 57% of products of conception will have an abnormal karyotype. The most common chromosomal defects are autosomal trisomies, which account for half the abnormalities, while polyploidy and monosomy X account for a further 20% each. Although chromosome abnormalities are common in sporadic miscarriage, parental chromosomal abnormalities are present in only 2–5% of partners presenting with recurrent pregnancy loss. These are most commonly balance reciprocal or robertsonian translocations or mosaicisms.

3. 早孕期出血

C 是正确的。与妊娠早期出血相关的失血性休克通常是由于异位妊娠破裂或不全流产导致。在这种情况下，脉率降低表明妊娠物使宫颈膨胀刺激了迷走神经，没有腹膜炎的表现可除外异位破裂。当务之急是寻找妊娠物并从子宫颈中取出组织。这将确认流产的诊断，延迟这样做将导致持续失血，因为即使使用麦角新碱，子宫也无法正常收缩。

3. Bleeding in early pregnancy:

C is correct. Haemodynamic shock associated with bleeding in early pregnancy is usually due either to ruptured ectopic pregnancy or incomplete miscarriage. In this case the low pulse rate suggests vagal stimulation from products of conception distending the cervix, and the absence of abdominal signs of peritonism is against ruptured ectopic. The immediate priority would be to look for products of conception and remove tissue from the cervix. This will confirm a diagnosis of miscarriage, and delay in doing this will cause ongoing blood loss, as the uterus will not be able to contract properly, even with the administration of ergometrine.

4. 子宫异常和流产

D 是正确的。宫腔先天畸形，如双角子宫或纵隔子宫，对流产的确切影响仍然存在争议。反复流产女性子宫异常率从不到 2% 到高达 38%。子宫异常的影响取决于异常的类型，妊娠中期流产女性的子宫异常的发病率更高。有子宫纵隔的胎儿存活率最高，而单角子宫的胎儿存活率最差。子宫内膜和子宫内壁受损后，表面可能会粘连，从而部分地闭塞子宫腔 [阿舍曼（Asherman）综合征]。这些粘连的存在可能导致反复流产。

4. Uterine abnormalities and miscarriage:

D is correct. The exact contribution that congenital abnormalities of the uterine cavity, such as a bicornuate uterus or subseptate uterus, make to miscarriage remains controversial. The reported incidence of uterine anomalies in women with recurrent miscarriage varies from less than 2% to up to 38%. The impact of the abnormality depends on the nature of the

anomaly, and the prevalence appears to be higher in women with second-trimester miscarriage. The fetal survival rate is best where the uterus is septate and worst where the uterus is unicornuate. Following damage to the endometrium and inner uterine walls, the surfaces may become adherent, thus partly obliterating the uterine cavity (Asherman's syndrome). The presence of these synechiae may lead to recurrent miscarriage.

5. 异位妊娠

B 是正确的。异位妊娠的药物和保守治疗不适用于有明显疼痛或血流动力学不稳定的人。一旦确诊，即采用如下治疗方案。

- 输卵管切除术：如果输卵管严重受损，或对侧输卵管看起来很健康，正确的治疗方法是移除患侧输卵管。

- 输卵管切开术：如果异位妊娠包含在管内，则可以移除妊娠物并输卵管成形。这在对侧输卵管已丢失的情况下尤为重要。缺点是在高达 6% 的病例中滋养细胞组织持续存在，需要进一步手术或药物治疗。

尽管输卵管切开术后异位妊娠复发的风险更大，但两种类型治疗后的宫内妊娠率相似。

5. Ectopic pregnancy:

B is correct. Medical and conservative management of ectopic pregnancy is not appropriate for someone with significant pain or haemodynamic instability. Once the diagnosis is confirmed, the options for treatment are:

- Salpingectomy-If the tube is badly damaged, or the contralateral tube appears healthy, the correct treatment is removal of the affected tube.
- Salpingotomy-Where the ectopic pregnancy is contained within the tube, it may be possible to conserve the tube by removing the pregnancy and reconstituting the tube. This is particularly important where the contralateral tube has been lost. The disadvantage is the persistence of trophoblastic tissue requiring further surgery or medical treatment in up to 6% of cases.

Subsequent intrauterine pregnancy rates are similar after both types of treatment, although the risk of recurrent ectopic pregnancy is greater after salpingotomy.

6. 抗 –D 免疫球蛋白

D 是正确的。未致敏 Rh 阴性的女性所有手术治疗的流产和异位妊娠应接受抗 D 免疫球蛋白治疗。对于只接受过药物或期待治疗的流产或异位妊娠、先兆流产或妊娠位置不明的女性不需要给予抗 D 免疫球蛋白。

6. Anti-D immunoglobulin administration:

D is correct. Non-sensitized rhesus (Rh)-negative women should receive anti-D immunoglobulin for all miscarriages and ectopic pregnancies managed surgically Anti-D immunoglobulin does not need to be given for women who have had only medical or expectant management for miscarriage or ectopic pregnancy, who have a threatened miscarriage or who have a pregnancy of unknown location.

第 19 章（Chapter 19）

1. 性传播感染（STI）检测

E 是正确的。发达国家最常见的 STI 微生物是沙眼衣原体。这最好通过尿液聚合酶链反应（PCR）检测来确定。最不可能在阴道下部或阴道上部拭子中发现。阴道拭子可用于筛查细菌性阴道病，如加德纳菌感染、念珠菌感染和 B 组链球菌（GBS）筛查。对于衣原体，抗体筛查不如 PCR 准确。

1. Testing for sexually transmitted infection (STI):

E is correct. The most common STI organism in the developed world is Chlamydia trachomatis. This is best defined by polymerase chain reaction (PCR) testing of urine. It is most unlikely to be found in low vaginal or upper vaginal swabs. Vaginal swabs are useful for screening for bacterial vaginosis such as Gardnerella infection, Candida infection and group B streptococcus (GBS) screening. Antibody screening is less accurate than PCR for Chlamydia.

2. 避孕有效性

E 是正确的。皮下埋植剂避孕棒的失败率最低，尽管在植入后 3～6 个月内的月经通常非常不规则且不可预测。在给定的其他方法中，A、B 和 D 的失败率相似，但 C 的失败率略高。

2. Contraceptive efficacy:

E is correct. The Implanon contraceptive rod has the lowest failure rate whether assessed overall or just with perfect use, although the periods in the 3–6 months after insertion are often very irregular and unpredictable. Of the other methods given A, B and D have similar failure rates, but the failure rate of C is slightly higher.

3. 选择合适的避孕药

D 是正确的。该女性很可能具有多囊卵巢综合征（PCOS）的临床特征，因此不应服用含有由睾酮衍生的孕激素的药物（A、B 和 C），而应服用含

有抗雄激素的药丸醋酸环丙孕酮。低剂量孕激素药丸的失败率太高，考虑到她的生育欲望，不予考虑，尤其是对于超重的女性。

3. Choice of the appropriate contraceptive to prescribe:

D is correct. This woman is likely to have the clinical features of polycystic ovarian syndrome (PCOS) and thus should not be given a pill containing a progestogen derived from testosterone (A, B and C) but should be given the one containing the anti-androgen cyproterone acetate. The failure rate of the low-dose progestogen pill is too high to be validly considered in view of her reproductive desires, particularly in women who are overweight.

4. 宫内节育器（IUCD）并发症

B 是正确的。如果女性或临床医生发现尾丝消失，则必须假设发生了以下情况之一：妊娠，节育器已被排出，节育器已在宫腔内转动并拉起尾丝，或节育器已穿出子宫并部分或完全位于腹膜腔内。宫内感染不是尾丝消失的原因。

4. Intrauterine contraceptive device (IUCD) complications:

B is correct. If the woman or clinician notices that the strings of the device are missing, it must be assumed that one of the following has occurred: pregnancy, the device has been expelled, the device has turned in the uterine cavity and drawn up the strings or the device has perforated the uterus and lies either partly or completely in the peritoneal cavity. Intrauterine infection is not a cause of missing strings.

5. 复方口服避孕药（COCP）的风险

B 正确。静脉血栓形成的风险从每年 5/10 万增加到 15/10 万（RR=3），并且在吸烟者和有静脉血栓形成史的女性中进一步增加。风险随着年龄的增长而增加。相比之下，每 10 万名女性中有 60 人在妊娠期和产褥期有静脉血栓形成的风险。几项研究表明，与含有其他孕激素的药物相比，含有去氧孕烯、孕二烯酮或屈螺酮的所谓第三代和第四代复方药物的静脉血栓形成风险要高 2 倍，尽管这些研究中静脉血栓形成的风险低于之前的报道。

5. Risks of the combined oral contraceptive pill (COCP):

B is correct. The risk of venous thrombosis is increased from 5/100,000 to 15/100,000 women per year (RR = 3) and is further increased in smokers and women with a previous history of venous thrombosis. Risk increases with age. This compares to a risk of venous thrombosis in pregnancy and the puerperium of 60/100,000 women. Several studies have suggested that so-called third- and fourth-generation combined pills containing desogestrel, gestodene or drospirenone are associated with a twofold greater risk of venous thrombosis than those containing other progestogens, although the risk of venous thrombosis was lower in these studies than had previously been reported.

第 20 章（Chapter 20）

1. 外阴癌

B 是正确的。外阴癌有两种不同的组织学表现，具有两种不同的危险因素。常见的基底细胞样 / 疣状型主要发生在年轻女性中，并且与常见的外阴上皮内瘤变（VIN）和人乳头瘤病毒（HPV）感染有关，这些感染的危险因素与宫颈癌相似。角化类型发生在老年女性，与硬化性苔藓有关。VIN 分为普通 VIN（经典 VIN 或鲍温病）和基于独特病理特征的分化 VIN。

1. Vulvar cancer:

B is correct. Vulvar cancer has two distinct histological patterns with two different risk factors. The more common basaloid/warty types occur mainly in younger women and are associated with usual vulvar intraepithelial neoplasia (VIN) and human papilloma virus (HPV) infection sharing similar risk factors as cervical cancer. The keratinizing types occur in older women and are associated with lichen sclerosis. VIN is categorized into usual VIN (classic VIN or Bowen's disease) and differentiated VIN based on the distinctive pathological features.

2. 宫颈癌的一级预防

D 是正确的。由于我们现在知道宫颈癌的主要原因是人乳头瘤病毒（HPV）感染，因此预防 HPV 感染将是最好的初级预防措施。已经开发出预防性 HPV 疫苗。二价和四价疫苗已上市约 10 年。二价疫苗针对两种高危亚型 HPV16 和 HPV18；而四价疫苗涵盖 HPV16 和 HPV18，以及两种低危亚型 HPV6 和 HPV11，它们会导致生殖器疣。预防 HPV16 和 HPV18 感染理论上可以预防超过 70% 的宫颈癌病例。事实上，澳大利亚在使用 10 年后的证据表明，18—24 岁女性的高危 HPV 血清型减少了 77%，并且高级别鳞状上皮内病变（HSIL）减少 30%～50%，生殖器疣减少 90%。这些疫苗在接触病毒之前接种最有效，即在首次性行为之前。一旦性活跃，它们可能仍然有一些功效。细胞学筛查已被证明是一种有效的二级预防措施。

2. Primary prevention of cervical cancer:

D is correct. Since we now know that the main cause for cervical cancer is human papilloma virus (HPV) infection, preventing HPV infections would be the best primary preventive measure. Prophylactic HPV vaccines have been developed. Bivalent and quadrivalent vaccines have been in the market for about a decade. The bivalent vaccine targets the two high-risk subtypes, HPV 16 and 18, while the quadrivalent vaccine covers HPV 16 and 18 as well as two low-risk subtypes, HPV 6 and 11, which cause genital warts. The prevention of HPV 16 and 18 infections could theoretically prevent more than 70% of cases of cervical cancer, and indeed evidence from Australia after a decade of use has shown a 77% reduction in high-risk HPV serotypes in women aged 18–24 and a 30–50% reaction in highgrade squamous intraepithelial lesion (HSIL) with a 90% reduction in genital warts. These vaccines are most effective when given before any exposure to the virus, i.e. before sexual debut. They may still have some efficacy once sexually active. Cytological screening has been shown to be an effective secondary prevention measure.

3. 子宫内膜癌的诱发因素

C 是正确的。特定因素与子宫体癌风险增加有关，如未生育、绝经晚、糖尿病和高血压，也可以遗传。患有遗传性非息肉病性结直肠癌（HNPCC）综合征的女性患子宫内膜癌、卵巢癌及结直肠癌的风险增加。以下为与高雌激素状态相关的最重要的风险因素。

- 肥胖。

- 外源性雌激素。

- 内源性雌激素。

- 产生雌激素的卵巢肿瘤。

- 他莫昔芬治疗乳腺癌。

- 子宫内膜增生。

3. Predisposing factor for endometrial cancer:

C is correct. Specific factors are associated with an increased risk of corpus carcinoma, such as nulliparity, late menopause, diabetes and hypertension. It can also be hereditary. Women with hereditary non-polyposis colorectal cancer (HNPCC) syndrome have increased risk of endometrial cancer and ovarian cancer, as well as colorectal cancer. However, the most important risk factors associated with a hyper-oestrogenic state are:

- Obesity
- Exogenous oestrogens
- Endogenous oestrogens
- Oestrogen-producing ovarian tumours
- Tamoxifen in breast cancer

- Endometrial hyperplasia

第 21 章（Chapter 21）

1. 宫骶韧带

C 是正确的。子宫骶韧带负责为阴道上部分、宫颈和子宫，提供一级支撑。

1. Uterosacral ligaments:

C is correct. The uterosacral ligaments are responsible for providing level 1 support to the upper vagina and the cervix and the uterus.

2. 膀胱膨出

C 是正确的。典型的描述是，患者会抱怨阴道里 "有东西掉下来"。有时可能有膀胱排空不完全，这将与二次排尿有关，即在排尿明显完成后立即有重复排尿的愿望。患者可能有过必须手动将脱出物还纳到阴道以排尿的病史。尿急是膀胱过度活动症的症状，膀胱膨出本身不应引起便秘、出血或深度性交痛。

2. Cystocele:

C is correct. Typically patients complain of 'something coming down' per vaginam. At times there may be incomplete emptying of the bladder, and this will be associated with double micturition, the desire to repeat micturition immediately after apparent completion of voiding. The patient may give a history of having to manually replace the prolapse into the vagina to void. Urgency is a symptom of overactive bladder, and a cystocele per se should not cause constipation, bleeding or deep dyspareunia.

3. 压力性尿失禁

A 是正确的。压力性尿失禁最初应通过盆底理疗进行管理。手术治疗适用于保守治疗无效的情况。

3. Stress urinary incontinence:

A is correct. Stress incontinence should be managed initially by pelvic floor physiotherapy. Surgical treatment is indicated where there is a failure to respond to conservative management.

4. 子宫阴道脱垂

E 是正确的。如果后续阴道分娩，则可能需要重复手术修复。

4. Uterovaginal prolapse:

E is correct. Surgical repair may have to be repeated if vaginal delivery occurs later.

5. 急性尿潴留

E 是正确的。放疗更常与尿频或因瘘管形成而引起的尿失禁有关。

5. Acute retention of urine:

E is correct. Radiotherapy is more often associated with urinary frequency or incontinence from fistula formation.

附录 A（Appendix A）

1. 常规术前检查

C 是正确的。术前血液检查包括全血细胞计数、尿素和电解质，以筛查高血压或糖尿病患者的肾脏疾病，以及使用利尿药以及酗酒或肝病的女性患者的肝功能检查；在有出血风险的手术前行血型检查并配血，如果怀疑大量出血或存在抗体，则交叉配血。除非患者有已知的出血性疾病或正在服用导致抗凝的药物，否则不需要常规筛查凝血功能。

1. Routine preoperative investigations:

C is correct. Preoperative blood investigations include full blood count, urea and electrolytes for screening for renal disease in patients with hypertension or diabetes and in women on diuretics and liver function test for patients with alcohol abuse or liver disease; group and save prior to procedures with risk of bleeding, and cross-match if heavy bleeding is suspected or antibodies are present. A routine coagulation screen is not necessary unless the patient has a known bleeding disorder or has been on medication that causes anticoagulation.

2. 世界卫生组织（WHO）手术核查表

D 是正确的。WHO 手术安全检查表提供了一套在手术的三个阶段（签到、暂停和签出）进行的核查。术后的常规流程是确认正确的纱布数和器械数。管理人员通常不参与术前讨论。制订世卫组织手术安全检查表是为了减少错误和不良事件，以及增加手术中的团队合作和沟通。该核查表的使用与发病率、死亡率及术后并发症的显著降低有关。

2. World Health Organization (WHO) surgical checklists:

D is correct. The WHO surgical safety checklist provides a set of checks to be done at three stages of a surgical procedure (sign in, time out and sign out). A routine part of the postoperative sign out is an acknowledgement of correct swab and instrument counts. Administrative staff are not usually involved in the preoperative huddle. The WHO Surgical Safety Checklist was developed to reduce errors and adverse events, as well as increase teamwork and communication in surgery. The use of this checklist has been associated with significant reductions in both morbidity and mortality, as well as postoperative complications.

3. 术前禁忌证

C 是正确的。应在大手术前 4~6 周停用复方口服避孕药将静脉血栓栓塞（VTE）的风险降至最低。其他选项都没有重大的围术期血栓栓塞风险。

3. Contraindications prior to surgery:

C is correct. The combined oral contraceptive pill should be stopped 4–6 weeks prior to major surgery to minimize the risk of venous thromboembolism (VTE). None of the others carry a major perioperative risk of thromboembolism.

4. 术中 / 术后并发症

E 是正确的。截石位可能会使骨筋膜室的肌肉压力增加，引起缺血再灌注，缺血组织毛细血管渗漏，进一步增加组织水肿，导致神经肌肉损伤和横纹肌溶解，发生腿部间室综合征。腿托、充气压力袜、高体重指数和延长手术时间是危险因素。股神经病变继发于过度的髋关节屈曲、外展和髋关节外旋，这会导致神经受压。

4. Intraoperative/postoperative complications:

E is correct. Compartment syndrome in the legs may occur due to the lithotomy position when the pressure in the muscle of an osteofascial compartment is increased, causing ischaemia followed by reperfusion, capillary leakage from the ischaemic tissue and further increase in tissue oedema resulting in neuromuscular compromise and rhabdomyolysis. Leg holders, pneumatic compression stockings, high body mass index and prolonged surgical time are risk factors. Femoral neuropathy occurs secondary to excessive hip flexion, abduction and external hip rotation, which contribute to nerve compression.

5. 尿路损伤的危险因素

C 是正确的。膀胱损伤的危险因素包括子宫内膜异位症、感染、膀胱过度膨胀和粘连。外侧而不是耻骨上 Trocar 置入将降低膀胱损伤的风险。

5. Risk factors for urinary tract injuries:

C is correct. Risk factors for bladder injury include endometriosis, infection, bladder overdistension and adhesions. Lateral rather than suprapubic trocar insertion will reduce the risk of bladder injury.

6. 术后护理

C 是正确的。硬膜外镇痛、脱水和出血是术后低血压的常见原因。

6. Postoperative care:

C is correct. Epidural analgesia, dehydration and bleeding are common causes of postoperative hypotension.

7. 术后并发症

E 是正确的。腹部切口手术部位感染（SSI）中的常见微生物是金黄色葡萄球菌、凝固酶阴性葡萄球菌、肠球菌属和大肠埃希菌。术后盆腔脓肿通常与厌氧菌有关。危险因素包括糖尿病、吸烟、全身性类固醇药物治疗、放疗、营养不良、肥胖、住院时间延长和输血。与 SSI 相关的手术因素包括手术时间延长、失血过多、体温过低、术前剃毛和手术引流。

7. Postoperative complications:

E is correct. Common organisms in surgical site infections (SSIs) of abdominal incisions are Staphylococcus aureus, coagulase-negative staphylococci, Enterococcus spp. and Escherichia coli. Postoperative pelvic abscesses are commonly associated with anaerobes. Risk factors include diabetes, smoking, systemic steroid medication, radiotherapy, poor nutrition, obesity, prolonged hospitalization and blood transfusion. Surgical factors associated with SSIs include prolonged operating time, excessive blood loss, hypothermia, hair removal by shaving and surgical drains.

8. 加速恢复途径

E 是正确的。加速康复路径与减轻疼痛和护理需求以及提高患者满意度和生活质量有关。加速康复侧重于优化患者教育和围术期期望，减少围术期禁食期，维持血流动力学稳定性和正常体温，增加下床活动，提供有效的疼痛缓解，预防恶心和呕吐，以及减少尿管和引流管的使用。这些途径应个体化。加速康复的术中要素涉及麻醉师和外科医生。在手术当天，为了避免脱水，在麻醉前禁水减少到 2h。

8. Enhanced recovery pathways:

E is correct. Enhanced recovery pathways have been associated with reduced pain and nursing requirements and improved patient satisfaction and quality of life. Enhanced recovery focuses on optimizing patient education and perioperative expectations, decreasing the perioperative fasting period, maintaining haemodynamic stability and normothermia, increasing mobilization, providing effective pain relief, nausea and vomiting prophylaxis and decreasing use of catheters and drains. These pathways should be individualized as indicated. Intraoperative elements of enhanced recovery involve both the anaesthetists and surgeons. On the day of the surgical procedure, the period of starvation is reduced to 2 hours for clear fluids prior to anaesthetic to avoid dehydration.

附录 B（Appendix B）

1. 使用社交媒体

D 是正确的。如果医生和医疗保健专业人员使用社交媒体，他们也可能会有风险。虽然建立专业和社交网络以及公众从专业人员处获取与健康有关的信息具有优势，但在保持机密性以及维护专业和个人界限方面存在挑战。因此，重要的是所有医生都了解并遵守通用医学委员会关于使用社交媒体的指导。

1. Using social media:

D is correct. There are potential benefits and risks for doctors and health care professionals if they are engaging with social media. Whilst there are advantages of networking professionally and socially and the public accessing health-related information from professionals, challenges exist in maintaining confidentiality and professional and personal boundaries. It is therefore important that all doctors be aware of and adhere to the General Medical Council's guidance on the use of social media.

2. 通用数据保护条例（GDPR）数据保护

B 是正确的。GDPR 于 2018 年 5 月 25 日推出，用于更新个人数据规则。它是欧盟法律中关于欧盟和欧洲经济区（EEA）内所有个人的数据保护和隐私的强制性规定。它还解决了向欧洲经济区和欧盟以外出口个人数据的问题。因此，即使是在欧洲经济区和欧盟以外注册的公司和组织，但在欧洲境内经营也必须遵守这一规定。GDPR 中的两个关键术语涉及个人数据和敏感数据。从本质上讲，GDPR 为人们提供了访问公司/组织所持有的信息的新权利，组织有义务更好地管理数据，否则将面临新的罚款制度。

2. General Data Protection Regulation (GDPR) data protection:

B is correct. GDPR was introduced on 25 May 2018 to update personal data rules. It is a mandatory regulation in EU law on data protection and privacy for all individuals within the European Union and European Economic Area (EEA). It also addresses the export of personal data outside the EEA and EU. Therefore even companies and organizations registered outside the EEA and EU but operating within Europe must comply with this regulation. The two key terms in GDPR involve personal and sensitive data. Essentially GDPR offers new rights for people to access the information companies/organizations hold about them, and there are obligations for organizations for better management of data or to risk a new regimen of fines.

3. 研究和临床审计

B 是正确的。一个完整的临床审计周期体现了患者管理的改进，包括用于诊断、治疗的流程、相关资源使用和患者结局，而研究的主要目的是推动新知识的推广。对于临床研究，需要向研究伦理委员会申请批准，而对于临床审计则不需要这样的批准。重要的是，临床审计的第一个周期之后是进一步的审计周期，以证明持续改进过程。可能需要几个周期的临床审计来证明患者预后的显著改善。围绕研究的资助有明确的原则。一些组织为研究提供资金。

3. Research and clinical audit:

B is correct. One complete cycle of a clinical audit demonstrates improvement in patient care and that includes procedures used for diagnosis, treatment, associated use of resources and resulting outcome for the patient, whereas the primary aim of research is to drive generalizable new knowledge. For clinical research, application is made for approval from a research ethics committee, whereas no such approval is required for a clinical audit. It is important that the first cycle of a clinical audit is followed by further audit cycles in order to demonstrate continuing improvement process. This may require several cycles of clinical audits to demonstrate significant improvement in patient outcomes. There are clearly laid out principles around research funding. Several organizations provide funding for research.

4. 临床指南

A 是正确的。临床指南由许多组织制订，如世界卫生组织（WHO）、国家卫生和临床卓越研究所（NICE）、苏格兰校际指南网络（SIGN）和皇家学院。尽管指南以证据为基础并源自一级证据，但并非所有组织都遵循类似的方法。指南制订者通常会参考其他组织先前发布的指南，但不一定遵循他们的方法论。指南制作是一个非常紧张、耗时的过程，需要18～24 个月。指南推荐基于临床有效性。NICE 发布的指南也考虑了建议的成本效益。

4. Clinical guidelines:

A is correct. Clinical guidelines are developed by a large number of organizations such as World Health Organization (WHO), National Institute for Health and Care Excellence (NICE), Scottish Intercollegiate Guidelines Network (SIGN) and royal colleges, to cite a few. Although guidelines are evidence based and derived from level 1 evidence, not all organizations follow a similar methodology. The guideline developers usually consult previously published guidelines from other organizations, but they do not necessarily follow their methodology. Guidelines production is a very intense, time-consuming process taking between 18 and 24 months. Guidelines recommendations are based on clinical effectiveness. Guidelines published by NICE take account of cost-effectiveness of the recommendation as well.

5. 研究

E 是正确的。描述性研究测试了一个病因学假设——例如，过度吸烟会增加患肺癌的风险。病例对照研究将患病者与未患病者进行比较，而队列研究则将暴露于疑似病原体的人和未暴露于该病原体的人进行比较。未经伦理委员会批准，将患者随机分组是不道德的。此外，患者在进入临床试验前应给予有效的知情同意。如果患者不希望被随机分配到临床试验中，他们应该接受针对该病症的标准治疗。临床医生不应该知道他们的患者是在使用活性药物还是安慰剂进行治疗，应该以类似的方式进行治疗。应准确报告所有不良反应。但是，如果任何患者出现不良反应，无论他或她在试验中的分配组别如何，他或她都应立即退出试验。此后，他或她应该按照最佳实践指南进行治疗。最后，孕妇或希望妊娠的女性不应接触新药物或新干预措施，因为可能无法获得这些药物对胚胎发育的安全性数据。

5. Research:

E is correct. Descriptive studies test an aetiological hypothesis-such as excessive smoking increases the risk of cancer of the lung. Case control studies compare people with disease and those without it, whereas cohort studies compare people exposed to the suspected causative agent and those not exposed to it. It is unethical for patients to be randomized without ethics committee approval. Furthermore, patients should give valid, informed consent before they can be entered into a clinical trial. If patients do not wish to be randomized to a clinical trial, they should be treated with standard treatment for that condition. Clinicians should not be aware of whether their patients are being treated with an active drug or a dummy preparation and should be treated in a similar way. All side effects should be reported accurately. However, if any patient experiences an undesirable side effect, he or she should be withdrawn from the trial immediately, irrespective of his or her allocation in the trial. Thereafter he or she should be treated following the best practice guidelines. Finally, pregnant women or those who desire to become pregnant should not be exposed to new drugs or new interventions, as data may not be available on the safety of these drugs on embryonic development.

6. 循证医疗

A 是正确的。每个组织都应制订风险管理策略，不仅改善对女性的护理，而且还尽量减少对患者和医院的风险。临床风险管理策略包括收集以下患者护理各方面的数据，包括过程、治疗和结局的要素；因此，重点不应只放在严重的后果上，如孕产妇和新生儿死亡率。通过降低女性及其婴儿的风险，可以改善护理。重点应该是最小化风险，并从错误中吸取教训。这只能通过从接近过失事件中学习并由实施者来完成指导方针的制订。定期临床审计始终支持指南的成功实施，以确保对指南的遵守程度在90% 以上。当临床事故报告后，应以积极和建设性的方式对护理团队的所有成员进行调查。应该吸取教训并实施行动计划，以减少未来类似事件再次发生的风险。当患者确实对工作人员提出投诉时，以公开和透明的方式调查他们的投诉很重要，以确保患者发现的问题得到充分调查。应该吸取教训，组织应对患者投诉中发现的问题做出回应。

6. Evidence-based health care:

A is correct. The risk management strategy should be in place in each organization in order to not only improve care of women but also to minimize risk to patients and to the organization. A clinical risk management strategy involves collection of data on all aspects of patient care and that involves elements of process, treatment and outcome. Therefore the focus should not only be on serious outcomes such as maternal and neonatal mortality. By reducing risk to women and to their babies, care can be improved. The focus should be to minimize risk and to learn from errors. This can only be done by learning from near-misses and by implementation of guidelines.

Successful implementation of guidelines is always supported by regular clinical audits to ensure that level of adherence to guidelines is above 90%. When clinical incidents are reported, they should be investigated in a positive and constructive way involving all members of a care team. Lessons should be learned and an action plan be implemented to reduce the risk of recurrence of similar incidences in the future. When patients do complain against staff, it is important to investigate their complaints in an open and transparent way to ensure that issues identified by the patient have been investigated fully. Lessons should be learned and organizations should respond to the issues identified in the patient's complaints.

附录 C（Appendix C）

1. 知情同意

D 是正确的。作为手术外科医生，您有责任获得知情同意。你永远无法确定其他人到底讨论了什么；因此，您必须讨论该患者可用的其他治疗方案，以及如果实施计划中的手术可能会出现的潜在并发症，以及随后可能需要的进一步治疗。当获得所有这些信息时，她很可能会决定不接受计划中的手术，特别是如果手术并发症（尽管大部分不太可能发生，甚至风险低于1%）会给她带来相当大痛苦的话。提供的关于手术风险的书面声明是不完整的信息，即使提供，也不会涵盖所有知情同意要求，除非有时间详细讨论这些问题。

1. Informed consent:

D is correct. As the operating surgeon, it is your responsibility to obtain informed consent. You can never be sure exactly what was discussed by other individuals; therefore you must discuss the other treatment options available to this patient and the potential complications which could occur if the planned surgery was performed and the further treatment which might then be necessary. She may well decide against the planned surgery when given all of this information, especially if complications of the surgery, although most unlikely and even at a risk of less than 1%, would distress her considerably. Provision of the college statement on the risks of surgery would be incomplete information and, even if provided, would not cover the requirements of informed consent unless time was given for these matters to be discussed in detail.

2. 关于保留病历的法律要求

B 是正确的。对于与妊娠无关的问题，医疗记录必须保留至少7年，然后才能销毁。对于与妊娠相关的记录，这些记录需要在孩子18岁达到"成年"后保留7年。因此，母亲和孩子的医疗记录都必须保留25年。由于本例不涉及妊娠，正确答案为B。

2. Legal requirements regarding retention of medical records:

B is correct. For a problem unrelated to pregnancy, medical records must be retained for at least 7 years and can then be destroyed. For a pregnancy-related record, these need to be retained for 7 years after the child has reached 'maturity' at the age of 18 years. Both the maternal medical record and that of the child must therefore be retained for 25 years. As this case does not involve a pregnancy, the correct response is B.

3. 证据等级

E 是正确的。迄今为止，随机对照临床试验提供了最好的证据。其余选项在定义所给证据的充分性和准确性方面价值较低，这些选项的有效性从D到

A 逐渐下降。

3. Levels of evidence:

E is correct. By far the best level of evidence is provided by randomized controlled clinical trials. The remaining options are less valuable in defining the adequacy and accuracy of the evidence given, with these progressively declining in efficacy from level D to level A.

4. 全面的病历要求

E 是正确的。所有这些事项都需要详细记录。只有根据所有这些信息才能评估护理的充分性，并确定婴儿出现任何长期问题的可能原因。

4. Requirements of an adequate medical record:

E is correct. All of these matters need to be documented in detail. The adequacy of care can only be assessed and the possible cause of any long-term problem in the baby defined with all of this information.

5. 对要求避孕的15岁女孩的适当护理

D 是正确的。如果他比她大不到3岁，并且不是亲戚、老师或其他负责人，那么性行为就是合法的。如果他年龄较大，是近亲、教师或青年领袖等，则任何性关系都是非法的；如果实际关系得到确认，可向警方举报。只要她了解其中的含义，给她服用避孕药并不违法。不需要告知父母或卫生部门给她服用避孕药。使用避孕套可以让医生摆脱这个问题，但由于她的伴侣表示他不准备使用这种方法，因此可提供的避孕方法不够全面。

5. Appropriate care of a 15-year-old girl requesting contraception:

D is correct. If he is less than 3 years older than her and is not a relative, a teacher or other responsible person, then sex would be legal. If he is older, is a close relative, a teacher or youth leader, etc., any sexual relationship would be illegal and is potentially reportable to the police if the actual relationship is confirmed. It is not illegal to give her the pill, provided she understands the implications. Advising the parents or department of health is not necessary to give her the pill. Use of condoms would remove the doctor from the problem, but less-than-adequate contraception would be provided since her partner has indicated he is not prepared to use such methods.

拓展阅读
Further reading

杨慧霞　译　　石玉华　校

标有 * 的文献表示原著编辑认为过去 40 年来妇产科发展中具有里程碑意义的研究。这些主要是影响当代临床实践的临床试验或 Meta 分析。他们也深受研究生考试中简答题出题者的喜爱。尽管被高度引用，但其中许多研究一直是许多争论的来源，并不一定代表循证实践中的"最终结论"。我们确信本书的读者会对其他应该包括（或实际上应该被排除在此列表之外）的研究提出自己的建议。

Papers marked * indicate those the editors consider landmark studies in the development of obstetrics and gynaecology over the last 40 years. These are mainly clinical trials or meta-analyses that have influenced contemporary practice. They are also beloved of the setters of short-answer questions in postgraduate examinations. Although highly cited, many of these studies have been the source of much debate and do not necessarily represent the 'final word' in evidence-based practice. We are sure that readers of this book will have suggestions of their own as to other studies that should be included (or indeed should be excluded from this list).

第 2 章（Chapter 2）

Johnson MH. *Essential Reproduction*. 6th ed. Chichester: John Wiley; 2008.

Moore K. *The Developing Human: Clinically Oriented Embryology*. London: WB Saunders; 1988.

Philipp EE, Setchell M, eds. *Scientific Foundations of Obstetrics and Gynaecology*. London: Heinemann; 1991.

第 3 章（Chapter 3）

Broughton Pipkin F. Maternal physiology. In: Chamberlain GV, Steer P, eds. *Turnbull's Obstetrics*. 3rd ed. Edinburgh: Churchill Livingstone; 2001.

Broughton Pipkin F. Maternal physiology. In: Edmonds DK, ed. *Dewhurst's Textbook of Obstetrics and Gynaecology*. 8th ed. Oxford: Blackwell; 2007.

Cartwright JE, Duncan WC, Critchley HO, et al. Remodelling at the maternal-fetal interface: relevance to human pregnancy disorders. *Reproduction*. 2010;140:803-813.

James D, Steer P, Weiner C, et al. *High Risk Pregnancy: Management Options*. London: Elsevier Saunders; 2011.

第 4 章（Chapter 4）

De Swiet M, Chamberlain GVP. *Basic Science in Obstetrics and Gynaecology*. Edinburgh: Churchill Livingstone; 1992.

Erikson PS, Secher NJ, Weis-Bentson M. Normal growth of the fetal biparietal diameter and the abdominal diameter in a longitudinal study. *Acta Obstet Gynaecol Scand*. 1985;64:65-70.

Gardosi J, Chang A, Kalyan B, et al. Customised antenatal growth charts. *Lancet*. 1992;339:283-287.

Thorburn GD, Harding R. *Textbook of Fetal Physiology*. Oxford: Oxford University Press; 1994.

第 5 章（Chapter 5）

Centre for Maternal and Child Enquiries (CMACE). *Perinatal Mortality 2008 United Kingdom*. London: CMACE; 2010. Available: http://www.publichealth.hscni.net/sites/default/files/Perinatal%20Mortality%202008.pdf.

Centre for Maternal and Child Enquiries (CMACE). Saving mothers' lives: reviewing maternal deaths to make motherhood safer: 2006-08. The eighth report on confidential enquiries into maternal deaths in the United Kingdom. *BJOG*. 2011;118(suppl 1):1-203.

Gardosi J, Kady SM, McGeown P, et al. Classification of stillbirth by relevant condition at death (ReCoDe): population based cohort study. *BMJ*. 2005;331:1113-1117.

World Health Organization. *Beyond the Numbers: Reviewing Maternal Deaths and Complications to Make Pregnancy Safer.* Geneva: WHO Press; 2004. Available: http://apps.who.int/iris/handle/ 10665/42984.

World Health Organization. *Neonatal and Perinatal Mortality: Country, Regional and Global Estimates.* Geneva: WHO Press; 2006. Available: http://apps.who.int/iris/handle/10665/43444.

World Health Organization. *Neonatal and Perinatal Mortality: Country, Regional and Global Estimates 2004 /Elisabeth Åhman and Jelka Zupan.* Geneva: WHO Press; 2007. Available: http://apps.who.int/iris/bitstream/handle/10665/43800/9789241596145_eng.pdf?sequence=1.

World Health Organization. *Trends in Maternal Mortality: 1990 to 2008. Estimates Developed by WHO, UNICEF, UNFPA and The World Bank. 2010.* Geneva: WHO Press; 2010. Available: https://www.who.int/reproductivehealth/publications/monitoring/ 9789241500265/en/

第 6 章（Chapter 6）

Chandraharan E, Arulkumaran S. Female pelvis and details of operative delivery; shoulder dystocia and episiotomy. In: Arulkumaran S, Penna LK, Rao Basker, eds. *Management of Labour.* India: Orient Longman; 2005.

第 7 章（Chapter 7）

Australian Institute of Health and Welfare, Australian Government, Canberra. Australian Red Cross Blood Service. *Transfusion.* Available: www.transfusion.com.au

Laws PJ, Li Z, Sullivan EA. *Australia's Mothers and Babies 2008. Perinatal Statistics Series No. 24. Cat. No. PER 50.* Canberra: AIHW. National Health and Medical Research Council Immunization Handbook; 2010. Available: http://www.health.gov.au/internet/ immunise/publishing.nsf/Content/Handbook-home.

National Organisation for Fetal Alcohol Syndrome and Related Disorders (NOFASARD). Available: http://www.nofasard.org.au/.

Antenatal Care for uncomplicated pregnancies National Institute for Health and Care Excellence (NICE) Clinical Guideline CG62 Updated Feb 2019. Availlable: https://www.nice.org.uk/ guidance/cg62.

Qureshi H, Massey E, Kirwan D, et al. BCSH guideline for the use of anti-D immunoglobulin for the prevention of haemolytic disease of the fetus and newborn. *Transfus Med.* 2014;24:8-20.

Royal Australian and New Zealand College of Obstetrics and Gynaecology. Statement C-Obs 6 Guidelines for the use of Rh (D) Immunoglobulin (anti-D) in Obstetrics in Australia.Available: https://www.ranzcog.edu.au/Statements-Guidelines/ Obstetrics/RhD-Immunoglobulin-(Anti-D)-in-Obstetrics-in. Austr.

第 8 章（Chapter 8）

*CLASP collaborative group. CLASP: a randomised trial of low-dose aspirin for the prevention and treatment of pre-eclampsia among 9364 pregnant women. *Lancet.* 1994;343:619-629.

*Hannah ME, Hannah WJ, Hellman J, et al. Induction of labour as compared with serial antenatal monitoring in post-term pregnancy. *N Engl J Med.* 1992;326:1587-1592.

*Hannah ME, Hannah WJ, Hewson SA, et al. Planned caesarean section versus planned vaginal birth for breech presentation at term: a randomised multicentre trial (Term Breech Trial). *Lancet.* 2000;356:1375-1383.

*Hilder L, Costeloe K, Thilaganathan B. Prolonged pregnancy: evaluating gestation-specific risks of fetal and infant mortality. *BJOG.* 1998;105:169-173.

*Magpie Trial Follow-Up Study Collaborative Group. The Magpie Trial: a randomised trial comparing magnesium sulphate with placebo for pre-eclampsia. Outcome for children at 18 months. *BJOG.* 2007;114:289-299.

National Institute for Health and Clinical Excellence. *The Management of Hypertensive Disorders in Pregnancy. July 2013*; 2010. Available: https://www.nice.org.uk/guidance/qs35/chapter/ quality-statement-3-antenatal-blood-pressure-targets.

Royal College of Obstetricians and Gynaecologists Green-top Guideline No. 63. *Antepartum Haemorrhage*; 2011. Available: https://www.rcog.org.uk/globalassets/documents/guidelines/ gtg_63.pdf.

Royal College of Obstetricians and Gynaecologists Green-top Guideline No. 20b. *The Management of Breech Presentation*; 2017. Available: https://obgyn.onlinelibrary.wiley.com/doi/epdf/10.1111/1471-0528.14465.

Royal College of Obstetricians and Gynaecologists Green-top Guideline No. 27. *Placenta Praevia, Placenta Accreta.*

Diagnosis and Management. 27 A; 2018. https://www.rcog. org. uk/en/guidelines-research-services/guidelines/gtg27a/

Royal College of Obstetricians and Gynaecologists Green-top Guidelines No. 51. *Management of Monochorionic Twin Pregnancy*; 2016. Available: https://obgyn.onlinelibrary. wiley.com/ doi/pdf/10.1111/14711-0528.14188.

Smith GC, Pell JP, Dobbie R. Birth order, gestational age, and risk of delivery related perinatal death in twins: retrospective cohort study. *BMJ.* 2002;325:1004.

第 9 章（Chapter 9）

*Crowther CA, Hiller JE, Moss RJ, et al. Effect of treatment of gestational diabetes mellitus on pregnancy outcomes (ACHOIS). *N Engl J Med.* 2005;352:2477-2486.

*HAPO Study Cooperative Research Group. Hyperglycaemia and adverse pregnancy outcomes. *N Engl J Med.* 2008;358:1991-2002.

Royal College of Obstetricians and Gynaecologists Green-top Guideline No. 37b. *The Acute Management of Thrombosis and Embolism During Pregnancy and the Puerperium*; 2007, reviewed 2010. Available: https://www.rcog.org.uk/ globalassets/documen ts-guidelines/gtg_37b.pdf.

Royal College of Obstetricians and Gynaecologists & BASH - Management of Genital Herpes in Pregnancy. 2014. Available: https://www.rcog.org.uk/globalassets/documents/ guidelines/ management-genital-herpes.pdf.

Royal College of Obstetricians and Gynaecologists Green-top Guideline No. 13. Chickenpox in Pregnancy; 2015. Available: https:// www.rcog.org.uk/en/guidelines-research-services/guidelines/ gtg13/.

Royal College of Obstetricians and Gynaecologists Green-top Guideline No. 72. *Care of Women With Obesity in Pregnancy*; 2018. Available at: https://obgyn.onlinelibrary.wiley.com/doi/ full/10.1111/1471-0528.15386.

第 10 章（Chapter 10）

Baschat AA. Pathophysiology of fetal growth restriction: implications for diagnosis and surveillance. *Obstet Gynecol Surv.*2004;59:617-627.

Bottomley C, Bourne T. Dating and growth in the first trimester. *Best Pract Res Clin Obstet Gynaecol.* 2009;23:439-452.

Cosmi E, Ambrosini G, D'Antona D, et al. Doppler, cardiotocography, and biophysical profile changes in growth-restricted fetuses. *Obstet Gynecol.* 2005;106:1240-1245.

Devoe LD. Antenatal fetal assessment: contraction stress test, non-stress test, vibroacoustic stimulation, amniotic fluid volume, biophysical profile, and modified biophysical profile-an overview. *Semin Perinatol.* 2008;32:247-252.

Johnstone FD. *Clinical Obstetrics and Gynaecology.* London: Baillière Tindall; 1992.

Langford KS. Infectious disease and pregnancy. *Curr Obstet Gynaecol.* 2002;12:125-130.

*Malone FD, Canick J, Ball R, et al. First-trimester or second- trimester screening, or both, for Down's syndrome (FASTER). *N Engl J Med.* 2003;353:2001-2011.

Inducing Labour National Institute for Health and Care Excellence Clinical Guideline CG70 July 2008. Available at https://www. nice.org.uk/guidance/cg70.

Reed GB, Claireaux AE, Bain AD. *Diseases of the Fetus and Newborn.*London: Chapman and Hall; 1989.

Royal College of Obstetricians and Gynaecologists Green-top Guidelines No. 31. *The Investigation and Management of the Small-for-Gestational-Age Fetus*; 2013. Available: https:// www.rcog.org.uk/globalassets/documents/guidelines/gtg_31. pdf.

Spencer K, Spencer CE, Power M, et al. Screening for chromosomal abnormalities in the first trimester using ultrasound and maternal serum biochemistry in a one-stop clinic: a review of three years prospective experience. *BJOG.* 2003;110: 281-286.

*The GRIT study group. A randomised trial of timed delivery for the compromised preterm fetus: short term outcomes and Bayesian interpretation. *BJOG.* 2003;110:27-32.

Timor-Tritsch IE, Fuchs KM, Monteagudo A, et al. Performing a fetal anatomy scan at the time of first-trimester screening. *Obstet Gynecol.* 2009;113:402-407.

*Van Bulck B, et al. Infant wellbeing at 2 years of age in the Growth Restriction Intervention Trial. *Lancet.* 2004;364:513-520.

第 11 章（Chapter 11）

Baskett TF, Arulkumaran S. *Intrapartum Care for the MRCOG and Beyond.* London: RCOG Press; 2001. https://www. cambridge. org/core/books/intrapartum-care-for-the-mrcog-and-beyond/ 1D5FBAAFF75E23DD10341DE35F0521EC.

*Doyle LW, Crowther CA, Middleton P, et al. Magnesium sulphate for women at risk of preterm birth for neuroprotection of the fetus. *Cochrane Database Syst Rev.* 2009;(Issue 1):Art No: CD004661.

Fonseca EB, Celik E, Parra M, et al. Progesterone and the risk of preterm birth among women with a short cervix. *N Engl J Med.* 2007;357:462-469.

*Kenyon SL, Taylor DJ, Tarnow-Mordi W; ORACLE Collaborative Group. Broad-spectrum antibiotics for preterm, prelabour rupture of fetal membranes: the ORACLE I randomised trial. *Lancet.* 2001;357:979-988.

*Kenyon SL, Taylor DJ, Tarnow-Mordi W, ORACLE Collaborative Group. Broad-spectrum antibiotics for spontaneous preterm labour: the ORACLE II randomised trial. *Lancet.* 2001;357:989-994.

*MacDonald D, Grant A, Sheridan-Pereira M, et al. The Dublin randomised controlled trial of intrapartum fetal heart rate monitoring. *Am J Obstet Gynecol*. 1985;152:524-539.

Mahmood T, Owen P, Arulkumaran S, Dhillon C, eds. *Models of Care in Maternity Services*. London: RCOG Press; 2010. Available: https://www.cambridge.org/core/books/models- of-care-in-maternity-services/C903136D3328C459994BC009 8F67363D.

Intrapartum care for healthy women and babies NICE Clinical Guideline CG190 Feb 2017. Available: https://www.nice.org. uk/guidance/cg190.

*O'Driscoll K, Stronge JM, Minogue M, et al. Active management of labour. *BMJ*. 1973;3:135-137.

Royal College of Obstetricians and Gynaecologists Green-top Guideline No.50. *Umbilical Cord Prolapse*; 2014. Available: https:// www.rcog.org.uk/en/guidelines-research-services/ guidelines/ gtg50/

Royal College of Obstetricians and Gynaecologists Green-top Guideline *No. 7. Antenatal Corticosteroids to Reduce Neonatal Morbidity. Cross referenced to NICE guidelines on Preterm labour and birth. ND 25) of Nov 2015*; 2010. Available: http://www. rcog.org.uk/files/rcog-corp/ GTG 7.pdf https://www.nice.org.uk/ guidance/ng25?unl id=9291036072016213201257.

Royal College of Obstetricians and Gynaecologists Green-top Guideline No. 1b. *Tocolysis for Women in Preterm Labour. Cross Referenced to NICE Guidelines on Preterm Labour and Birth. ND 25 of Nov 2015*; 2011. Available: https://www.rcog. org.uk/en/ guidelines-research-services/guidelines/gtg1b/

Royal College of Obstetricians and Gynaecologists Green-top Guideline No. 42. *Shoulder Dystocia*; 2012. Available: http:// www.rcog.org.uk/files/rcog-corp/GTG 42_Shoulder dystocia 2nd edition 2012.pdf https://www.rcog.org.uk/globalassets/ documents/guidelines/gtg_42.pdf.

第 12 章（Chapter 12）

*Landon MB, Hauth JC, Leveno KJ, et al. Maternal and perinatal outcomes associated with a trial of labour after prior caesarean delivery. *N Engl J Med*. 2004;351:2581-2589.

Robson S, Higgs P. Third- and fourth- degree injuries. *Aust N Z J Obstet Gynaecol*. 2011;13(2):20-22.

Royal College of Obstetricians and Gynaecologists Green-top Guideline No. 52. *Prevention and Management of Postpartum Haemorrhage*; 2016. Available: https://www.rcog.org.uk/en/ guidelines-research-services/guidelines/gtg52/

Royal College of Obstetricians and Gynaecologists Green-top Guidelines No. 26. *Operative vaginal delivery*; 2011. Available: https://www.rcog.org.uk/en/guidelines-research-services/guide- lines/gtg26/

第 13 章（Chapter 13）

Benn C. Milk of humankind: best. *Aust N Z J Obstet Gynaecol*.

2011;13(2):40-41.

Coker A, Oliver R. *Definitions and Classifications in a Textbook of Post-partum Hemorrhage*. Sapiens Publishing; London 2006:11-16.

Kumarasamy R. Infection in the peuperium. *Aust N Z J Obstet Gynaecol*. 2011;13(2):17.

Royal College of Obstetricians and Gynaecologists Green-top Guideline No. 37b. *Thromboembolic Disease in Pregnancy and the Puerperium: Acute Management*; 2015. Available: https://www. rcog.org.uk/en/guidelines-research-services/ guidelines/gtg37b/

Royal College of Obstetricians and Gynaecologists Green-top Guideline No. 29. *The Management of Third and Fourth Degree Perineal Tears*; 2015. Available: https://www.rcog. org.uk/global assets/documents/guidelines/gtg-29.pdf.

Royal College of Obstetricians and Gynaecologists Green-top Guideline No. 47. *Blood Transfusion in Obstetrics*; 2015. Available: https://www.rcog.org.uk/en/guidelines-research-services/ guidelines/gtg47/

Royal College of Obstetricians and Gynaecologists Green-top Guideline No. 56. *Maternal Collapse in Pregnancy and the Peurperium*; 2011. Available: https://www.rcog.org.uk/ globalassets/ documents/guidelines/gtg_56.pdf.

Thakkar. *Guidelines on neonatal examination. CGCHealth005-1*. Milton Keynes, UK: Milton Keynes NHS Trust; 2004.

第 14 章（Chapter 14）

Antenatal and Postnatal Mental Health - Quality standard. QS115. 2016. Available: https://www.nice.org.uk/guidance/qs115.

British Association of Psychopharmacology Consensus Guidance on Use of Psychotropic Medication in Perinatal Period 2017. Available: https://www.bap.org.uk/pdfs/BAP_ Guidelines- Perinatal.pdf.

Howard L, Piot P, Stein A. No health without perinatal mental health. Lancet 2014;15;384(9956):1723-4. Available: www.th elancet.com/journals/lancet/article/PIIS0140-6736(14)62040- 7/fulltext.

Maternal Mental Health-Womens Voices RCOG Publications. 2017. Available: https://www.rcog.org.uk/globalassets/docu-ments/patients/information/maternalmental-healthwomens-voices.pdf. MBRRACE-UK:Saving Libes, Improving Mothers Care (2-14-2016). Available at: https://www.npeu. ox.ac.uk/mb rrace-uk/reports.

Mental Health in Pregnancy and the Postnatal Period - Fingertips Tool PHE. 2017. Available: https://fingertips.phe. org.uk/profile- group/mental-health/profile/perinatal-mental-health.

第 15 章（Chapter 15）

Critchley HOD, Munro MG, Broder M, et al. A five-year

international review process concerning terminologies, definitions and related issues around abnormal uterine bleeding. *Semin Reprod Med.* 2011;29:377-382.

第 16 章（Chapter 16）

*Garry R, Fountain J, Mason S, et al. The eVALuate study: two parallel randomised trials, one comparing laparoscopic with abdominal hysterectomy, the other comparing laparoscopic with vaginal hysterectomy. *BMJ.* 2004;328:129.

*Hulley S, Grady D, Bush T, et al. Randomised trial of estrogen plus progestin for secondary prevention of coronary heart disease in postmenopausal women (HERS). *J Am Med Ass.* 1998;280:605-613.

Royal College of Obstetricians and Gynaecologists Green-top Guideline No. 48. *Management of Premenstrual Syndrome*; 2017. Available: https://obgyn.onlinelibrary.wiley.com/doi/epdf/10.1111/1471-0528.14260.

NICE Guideline No 23 Menopause: diagnosis and managment No 2015. Available: https://www.nice.org.uk/guidance/ng23.

Royal College of Obstetricians and Gynaecologists Green-top Guideline No. 41. *The Initial Management of Chronic Pelvic Pain*; 2012. Available: https://www.rcog.org.uk/globalassets/documents/guidelines/gtg_41.pdf.

RANZCOG College Statement C-Gyn 9. Management of the Menopause; 2011. Available: https://www.ranzcog.edu.au/RANZCOG_ SITE/media/RANZCOG-MEDIA/Women%27s%20Health/ Statement%20and%20guidelines/Clinical%20-%20Gynae- cology/Management-of-the-Menopause-(C-Gyn-9)-Review- November-2014_1.pdf?ext=.pdf.

Sampson JA. Perforating hemorrhagic (chocolate) cysts of the ovary.Their importance and especially their relation to pelvic adenomas of the endometrial type ('adenomyoma' of the uterus, rectovaginal septum, sigmoid, etc.). *Arch Surg.* 1921;3:245-323.

*The Women's Health Initiative steering committee. Effects of conjugated equine estrogen in postmenopausal women with hysterectomy: the WHI randomised controlled trial. *J Am Med Ass.* 2004;291:1701-1712.

*Writing group for the Women's Health Initiative (WHI) randomised controlled trial. Risks and benefits of estrogen plus progestin in healthy postmenopausal women: principle results the WHI randomised controlled trial. *J Am Med Ass.* 2002;288:321-333.

第 17 章（Chapter 17）

Bhattacharya S, Porter M, Amalraj E, et al. The epidemiology of infertility in the north east of scotland. *Hum Reprod.* 2009;24(12):3096-3107.

Brosens J, Gordon A. *Tubal Infertility*. Philadelphia: J B

Lippincott; 1990.

Insler V, Lunenfeld B. *Infertility, Male and Female*. Edinburgh: Churchill Livingstone; 1986.

Lashen H. Investigations for infertility. *Curr Obstet Gynaecol.* 2001;11:239-244.

Ledger WL. In vitro fertilization. *Curr Obstet Gynaecol.* 2002;12:269-275.

Fertility Problems: assessment and treatment NICE Clinical Guideline CG156 Sept 2017. Available: https://www.nice.org. uk/guidance/cg156.

Royal College of Obstetricians and Gynaecologists Green-top Guidelines No. 24. *The Investigation and Management of Endomtreiosis. Cross Referenced to Guideline on the Management of Women With Endometriosis by ESHRE. Sept 2013*; 2006. Available: https://www.eshre.eu/Guidelines-and-Legal/Guidelines/ Endometriosis-guideline.aspx.

Taylor A. The subfertile couple. *Curr Obstet Gynaecol.* 2001;11:115-125.

Wakley G. Sexual dysfunction. *Curr Obstet Gynaecol.* 2002;12:35-40.

第 18 章（Chapter 18）

Abortion Act. London: HMSO; 1967.

Ankum A. Diagnosing suspected ectopic pregnancy. *BMJ.*2000;321:1235-1236.

*Clark P, Walker ID, Langhorne P, et al. Scottish pregnancy intervention (SPIN) study: a multicentre, randomised controlled trial of low molecular weight heparin and low dose aspirin in women with recurrent miscarriage. *Blood.* 2010;115: 4162-4167.

Demetroulis C, Saridogan E, Kunde D, et al. A prospective RCT comparing medical and surgical treatment for early pregnancy failure. *Hum Reprod.* 2001;16:365-369.

Department of Health, Department for Education and Employment, Home Office. *The Removal, Retention and Use of Human Organs and Tissue Post-Mortem Examination. Advice from the Chief Medical Officer.* London: Stationery Office; 2001.

Eliakim R, Abulafia O, Sherer DM. Hyperemesis: a current review.*Am J Perinatol.* 2000;17(4):207-218.

Graziosi GC, Moi BW, Ankum WM, et al. Management of early pregnancy loss-a systematic review. *Int J Gynaecol Obstet.* 2001;86:337-346.

National Institute for Health and Clinical Excellence. *NICE Clinical Guideline 154 Ectopic Pregnancy and Miscarriage: Diagnosis and Initial Management*; 2012. guidance. Available: https://www.nice.org.uk/guidance/cg154.

Regan L, Rai R. Epidemiology and the medical causes of miscarriage. *Best Pract Res Clin Obstet Gynaecol.* 2000;14(5):839-854.

Royal College of Obstetricians and Gynaecologists Green-top

Guideline No. 38. *Management of Gestational Trophoblastic Disease*; 2010. Available: https://www.rcog.org.uk/en/ guidelines- research-services/guidelines/gtg38/

Royal College of Obstetricians and Gynaecologists Green-top Guideline No. 17. *The Investigation and Treatment of Couples with Recurrent First-trimester and Second-trimester Miscarriage*; 2011. Available: https://www.rcog.org.uk/ globalassets/docu- ments/guidelines/gtg_17.pdf.

Speroff L, Glass RH, Kase NG. Ectopic pregnancy. In: Speroff L, Glass RH, Kase NG, eds. *Clinical Gynecologic Endocrinology and Infertility*. 32. Baltimore: Williams and Wilkins; 1994:947-964.

*Trinder J, Brocklehurst P, Porter R, et al. Management of miscar- riage: expectant, medical or surgical? Results of randomised controlled trial (MIST). *BMJ*. 2006;332:1235-1240.

Zhang J, Gilles JM, Barnhart K, et al. A comparison of medical management with misoprostol and surgical management for early pregnancy failure. *N Engl J Med*. 2005;353:761-769.

第 19 章（Chapter 19）

Adaikan PG, Chong YS, Chew SSL, et al. Male sexual dysfunction.*Curr Obstet Gynaecol*. 2000;10:23-28.

Barton SE. Classification, general principles of vulval infections.*Curr Obstet Gynaecol*. 2000;10:2-6.

Berek JS. *Berek and Novak's Gynecology*. 14th ed. Philadelphia: Lippincott, Williams & Wilkins; 2007.

Breen KJ, Cordner SM, Thomson CJH, et al. *Good Medical Practice: Professionalism, Ethics and Law*. Melbourne: Cambridge University Press; 2010.

Bignell CJ. Chlamydial infections in obstetrics and gynaecology.*Curr Obstet Gynaecol*. 1997;7:104-109.

Denman M. Gynaecological aspects of female sexual dysfunction.*Curr Obstet Gynaecol*. 1999;9:88-92.

Department of Health. *Handbook of Contraceptive Practice*. London: HMSO; 1990.

Hampton N. Choice of contraception. *Curr Obstet Gynaecol*.2001;11:50-53.

Hamoda H, Bignell C. Pelvic infections. *Curr Obstet Gynaecol*.2002;12:185-190.

Johnstone FD. *Clinical Obstetrics and Gynaecology*. London: Baillière Tindall; 1992.

Ledger WJ, Witkin SS. *Vulvovaginal Infections*. London: Manson Publishing; 2007.

Loudon N. *Handbook of Family Planning*. 2nd ed. Edinburgh: Churchill Livingstone; 1991.

Masters T, Everett S. Intrauterine and barrier contraception. *Curr Obstet Gynaecol*. 2002;12:28-34.

Robinson C, Kubba AA. Medical problems and oral contraceptives. *Curr Obstet Gynaecol*. 1997;7:173-179.

Royal Australian and New Zealand College of Obstetrics and

Gynaecology College Statement C-Gyn 11. *Emergency Contraception*; 2012. Available: http://www.ranzcog.edu.au/ compone-nt/docman/doc_view/1001-c-gyn-11-emergency-contraception. html?Itemid=341.

Sterilisation Familiy Planning Association (accessed 14th July 2019). Available: https://www.sexwise.fpa.org.uk/contracep-tion/sterilisation.

Royal College of Obstetricians and Gynaecologists. *Evidence-Based Guideline 7: The Care of Women Requesting Induced Abortion*. London: RCOG Press; 2011. Available: https:// www.rcog.org.uk/globalassets/documents/guidelines/ abortion-guideline_web_1.pdf.

Spagne VA, Prior RB. *Sexually Transmitted Diseases*. New York: Marcel Dekker; 1985.

Stewart P, Fletcher J. Therapeutic termination of pregnancy. *Curr Obstet Gynaecol*. 2002;12:22-27.

Szarciwski A, Guillebaud J. *Contraception*. Oxford: Oxford Univer- sity Press; 1994.

Walters WAW. *Clinical Obstetrics and Gynaecology*. London: Baillière Tindall; 1991.

第 20 章（Chapter 20）

Australian Government Department of Health. *National Cervical Screening Program*. (2017). Available: http://www. cancerscreen- ing.gov.au/cervical.

Berek JS, Neville F, Hacker NF. *Berek and Hacker's Gynecologic Oncology*. 5th ed. Philadelphia: Lippincott, William & Wilkins; 2009.

Brown V, Sridhar T, Symonds RP. Principles of chemotherapy and radiotherapy. *Obstet Gynaecol Reprod Med*. 2011;21 (12):339-345.

*Buys SS, Partridge E, Black A, et al. Effect of screening on ovarian cancer mortality: the prostate, lung, colorectal and ovarian cancer screening randomised controlled trial. *J Am Med Ass*. 2011;305:2295-2303.

Freeman S, Hampson F, Addley H, et al. Imaging of the female pelvis. *Obstet Gynaecol Reprod Med*. 2009;19(10):271-281.

Hannemann MH, Alexander HM, Cope NJ, et al. Endometrial hyperplasia: a clinician's review. *Obstet Gynaecol Reprod Med*. 2010;20(4):116-120.

Holland C. Endometrial cancer. *Obstet Gynaecol Reprod Med*. 2010;20(12):347-352.

Iyengar S, Acheson N. Premalignant vulval conditions. *Obstet Gynaecol Reprod Med*. 2008;18(3):60-63.

Kyrgiou M, Shafi MI. Colposcopy and cervical intra-epithelial neoplasia. *Obstet Gynaecol Reprod Med*. 2010;20(5):38-46.

Kyrgiou M, Shafi MI. Invasive cancer of the cervix. *Obstet Gynaecol Reprod Med*. 2010;20(5):47-54.

Palmer J, Gillespie A. Palliative care in gynaecological oncology.*Obstet Gynaecol Reprod Med*. 2012;22(5):123-128.

Peevor R, Fiander AN. Human papillomavirus (including

vaccina- tion). *Obstet Gynaecol Reprod Med.* 2010; 20(10): 295-299.

Robinson Z, Edey K, Murdoch J. Invasive vulval cancer. *Obstet Gynaecol Reprod Med.* 2011;21(5):129-136.

Shafi MI, Earl H, Tan LT. *Gynaecological Oncology.* Cambridge: Cambridge University Press; 2010.

Symonds IM. Screening for gynaecological conditions. *Obstet Gynaecol Reprod Med.* 2012. Available: https://doi. org/10.1016/ j.ogrm.2012.11.005.

Taylor SE, Kirwan JM. Ovarian cancer: current management and future directions. *Obstet Gynaecol Reprod Med.* 2012;22(2):33-37.

第 21 章（Chapter 21）

*Altman D, Väyrynen T, Engh ME et al; Nordic Transvaginal Mesh Group. Anterior colporrhaphy versus transvaginal mesh for pelvic-organ prolapse. *N Engl J Med.* 2011;364:1826-1836.

DeLancey JO. Anatomic aspects of vaginal eversion after hysterec- tomy. *Am J Obstet Gynecol.* 1992;166:1717.

National Institutes for Health and Clinical Excellence. Clinical Guideline 40. *Urinary Incontinence. The Management of Urinary Incontinence in Women*; 2006. Available: http:// www.nice. org. uk/nicemedia/pdf/CG40NICEguideline.pdf.

*Ward K, Hilton P, United Kingdom and Ireland Tension-free Vaginal Tape Trial Group. Prospective multicentre randomised trial of tension-free vaginal tape and colposuspension as primary treatment for stress incontinence. *BMJ.* 2002; 325:67-70.

附录 A（Appendix A）

Croissant K, Shafi MI. Preoperative and postoperative care in gynaecology. *Obstet Gynaecol Reprod Med.* 2009;(3):68-74.

National Institute for Clinical Excellence (NICE). Clinical Guidline 46. *Venous Thromboembolism: Reducing the Risk of Venous Throm-boembolism (Deep Vein Thrombosis and Pulmonary Embolism) in Inpatients Undergoing Surgery*; 2010. Available: https://www.ncbi. nlm.nih.gov/pmc/articles/ PMC1871784/

Royal College of Obstetricians and Gynaecologists Clinical Governance Advice No. 6. *Obtaining Valid Consent*; 2008. Available: http://www.rcog.org.uk/files/rcog-corp/CGA6-15072010.pdf.

Scottish Intercollegiate Guidelines Network (SIGN). *Postoperative Management in Adults. A Practical Guide to Postoperative Care for Clinical Staff.* Edinburgh: SIGN; 2004.

Sharp HT. Prevention and management of complications from gynecologic surgery. *Obstet Gynecol Clin N Am.* 2010;37(3): 461-467.

附录 B（Appendix B）

General Medical Council. Confidentiality: Supplementary Guidance. Available: www.gmc-uk.org.

General Medical Council. Research: The Role and Responsibilities of Doctors. Available: www.gmc-uk.org.

McSherry R, Pearce P, eds. *Clinical Governance: A Guide to Implementation for Healthcare Professionals.* 2nd ed. Oxford: Blackwell; 2007.

Royal College of Obstetricians & Gynaecologists Clinical Governance Advice No. 5. *Understanding Audit*; 2003. Available: https://www.rcog.org.uk/en/guidelines-research-services/guide- lines/clinical-governance-advice-5/

Royal College of Obstetricians and Gynaecologists. *Guideline Compendium: A Compendium of College Guidelines Available.* London: RCOG Press; 2006.

Royal College of Obstetricians and Gynaecologists Clinical Governance Advice No. 2. *Improving Patient Safety: Risk Management for Maternity and Gynaecology*; 2009. Available: https://www.rcog.org.uk/globalassets/documents/ guidelines/clinical-governance- advice/cga2improvingpatien.

Scottish Intercollegiate Guidelines Network. SIGN 50. *A Guideline Developer's Handbook.* Scottish Intercollegiate Guidelines Network; 2011:23-27. Available: https://www. sign.ac.uk/assets/ sign50_2011.pdf.

附录 C（Appendix C）

Breen KJ, Cordner SM, Thomson CJH, et al. *Good Medical Practice: Professionalism, Ethics and Law.* Melbourne: Cambridge University Press; 2010.

Chamberlain GVP, ed. *How to Avoid Medico-legal Problems in Obstetrics and Gynaecology.* 2nd ed. London: RCOG; 1992.

Clements RV. *Safe Practice in Obstetrics and Gynaecology. A Medico-legal Handbook.* Edinburgh: Churchill Livingstone; 1994.

更多网站（Further websites）

自上一版出版以来，在线资源的可用性呈指数级增长。其中许多是开源的，问题不再是读者是否可以在线访问信息，而是哪些信息对于想要更详细地研究某个领域的读者来说足够可靠和详细，且足够简洁。

Since the publication of the last edition, the availability of online resources has expanded exponentially. Many of these are open source, and the issue is no longer whether there is information the reader can access online, but which information is reliable and detailed enough for the student who wants to study an area in greater detail yet concise enough not to overwhelm them.

我们在相关部分中包含了许多在线资源，但应该注意的是，英国皇家妇产科学院（RCOG）、澳大利亚和新西兰皇家妇产科学院（RANZCOG）和英国国家卫生与临床优化研究所（NICE）发布有关临床实践的声明和指南。这些不仅提供了每个国家／地区被认为是最佳实践的摘要，而且本身通常包含指向其他材料和参考原始证据的进一步链接。它们具有比大多数教科书更定期更新的额外优势。应该注意的是，随着文档的更新，URL 可能会发生变化。如果您无法使用章节中列出的网址访问相关网页，您可以将该网址复制到您的搜索引擎中，搜索此处给出的相关内容网页，并按名称搜索信息。

We have included a number of online resources within the relevant sections, but it should be noted that both the Royal College of Obstetrics and Gynaecology (RCOG) in the UK and the Royal Australian and New Zealand College of Obstetrics and Gynaecology (RANZCOG) and the National Institute for Health and Care Excellence publish statements and guidelines about clinical practice. These not only provide a summary of what is considered best practice in each country but often themselves contain further links to other material and reference original evidence. They have the added advantage of being more regularly updated than most textbooks. It should be noted that as documents are updated the URL may change. If you are unable to access the relevant webpage using the URLs listed in the chapters, you can copy the URL into your search engine for the relevant contents webpage given here and search by name for the information.

英国国家卫生与临床优化研究所指南

The National Institute for Clinical Excellence guidelines

http://www.nice.org.uk/guidance/index.jsp?action=byTopic &o=7252.

英国皇家妇产科学院（RCOG）

The Royal College of Obstetrics and Gynaecology (RCOG)

Green-top 指南

Green-top guidelines

http://www.rcog.org.uk/guidelines?filter0%5B%5D=10.

临床治理建议

Clinical governance advice

http://www.rcog.org.uk/guidelines?filter0%5B%5D=6.

联合指导方针

Joint guidelines

http://www.rcog.org.uk/guidelines?filter0%5B%5D=11.

国家循证指南

National evidence-based guidelines

http://www.rcog.org.uk/guidelines?filter0%5B%5D=12.

澳大利亚和新西兰皇家妇产科学院 (RANZCOG) 关于女性健康的声明

Royal Australian and New Zealand College of Obstetrics and Gynaecology (RANZCOG) statements on women's health

产科学

Obstetrics

https://www.ranzcog.edu.au/statements-Guidelines/Obstetrics.

妇科学

Gynaecology

https://www.ranzcog.edu.au/Statements-Guidelines/Gynaecology.

一般内容

General

https://www.ranzcog.edu.au/Statements-Guidelines/General.

英国国家健康电子图书馆有关于英国和美国的指导方针的链接

The National Electronic Library for Health has links to guidelines for both the UK and United States on: http://www.evidence.nhs.uk.

英国孕产妇死亡保密调查的最新版本

The most recent version of the Confidential Enquiry into Maternal Deaths in the United Kingdom: http://onlinelibrary.wiley.com/ doi/10.1111/bjo.2011.118.issue-s1/issuetoc.

澳大利亚卫生和福利研究所关于澳大利亚孕产妇死亡的最新报告

The most recent report on maternal deaths in Australia from the Australian Institute of Health and Welfare: http://www.aihw.gov.au/ WorkArea/DownloadAsset.aspx?id=10737421514.

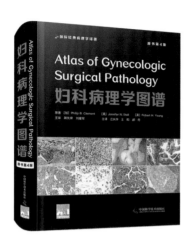

主译：江庆萍 王 昀 胡 丹
定价：458.00元

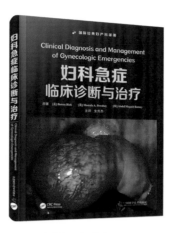

主译：生秀杰
定价：148.00元

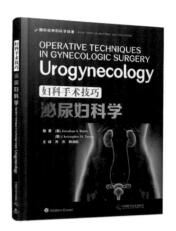

主译：乔 杰 韩劲松
定价：128.00元

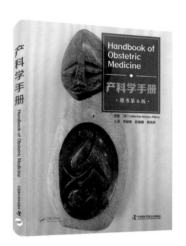

主译：李映桃 陈娟娟 韩凤珍
定价：180.00元

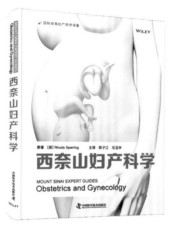

主译：陈子江 石玉华
定价：198.00元

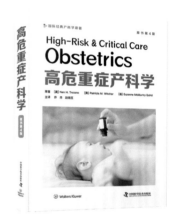

主译：乔 杰 赵扬玉
定价：198.00元

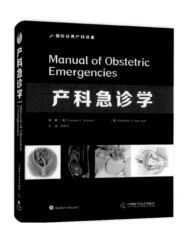

主译：赵扬玉
定价：268.00元

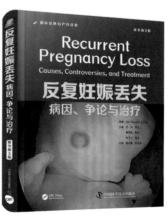

主译：曹云霞 向卉芬
定价：158.00元

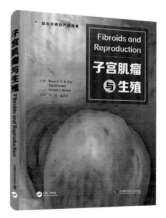

主译：李 萍 蒋清清
定价：108.00元